Comprehensive Review in *Toxicology* for Emergency Clinicians

---

Third Edition

Comprehensive Review in *Toxicology* for Emergency Clinicians

Third Edition

Peter D. Bryson, M.D.

Director, Denver Institute
of Clinical Toxicology
Denver, Colorado

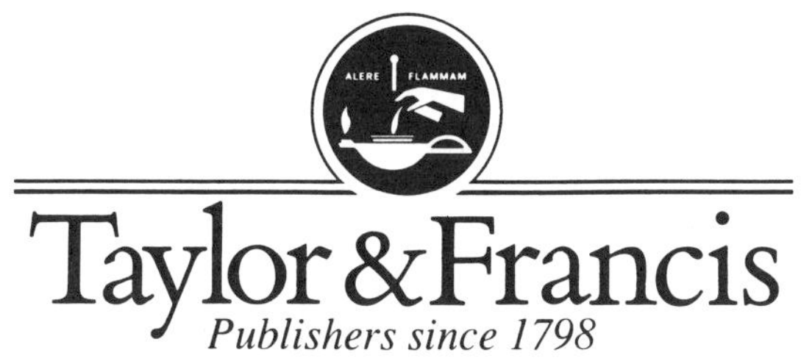

Taylor & Francis
Publishers since 1798

USA	Publishing Office:	Taylor & Francis 1101 Vermont Avenue, NW, Suite 200 Washington, DC 20005-3521 Tel: (202) 289-2174 Fax: (202) 289-3665
	Distribution Center:	Taylor & Francis 1900 Frost Road, Suite 101 Bristol, PA 19007-1598 Tel: (215) 785-5800 Fax: (215) 785-5515 E-mail: bkorders@tandfpa.com
UK		Taylor & Francis Ltd. 1 Gunpowder Square London EC4A 3DE Tel: 0171 583 0490 Fax: 0171 583 0581
World Wide Web		http://www.tandf.co.uk

Comprehensive Review in Toxicology for Emergency Clinicians, Third Edition

---

The author and editors have made every effort to ensure the accuracy of the information herein, particularly with regard to drug selection and dose. However, appropriate information sources should be consulted, especially for new or unfamiliar procedures. It is the responsibility of every practitioner to evaluate the appropriateness of a particular opinion in the context of actual clinical situations and with due considerations of new developments. The Author, editors, and the publisher cannot be held responsible for errors or for any consequences arising from the use of the information contained herein.

1 2 3 4 5 6 7 8 9 0 E B E B 9 8 7 6

Printing and binding by Edwards Brothers, Inc.

A CIP catalog record for this book is available from the British Library.
♾ The paper in this publication meets the requirements of the ANSI Standard Z39.48-1984 (Permanence of Paper)

Library of Congress Cataloging-in-Publication Data

Bryson, Peter D.
Comprehensive review in toxicology for emergency clinicians / Peter D. Bryson. —
3rd ed.
p. cm.
Includes bibliographical references and index.
1. Toxicological emergencies. 2. Toxicology. 3. Drugs of abuse—Toxicology. 4.
Drugs—Overdosage. I. Title.
[DNLM: 1. Poisoning. 2. Emergencies. 3. Poisons. 4. Substance Abuse. QV 600 B915c 1997]
RA 1224.5.B79 1997
615.9—dc20
DNLM/DCL
for Library of Congress 96-9209
CIP

ISBN 1-56032-612-3

Contents

X. Metals and Antagonists

XI. Miscellaneous Agents

XII. Botanical Agents

XIII. Toxins in Food

XIV. Venomous Creatures

XV. Environmental Agents

Comprehensive Review in *Toxicology* for Emergency Clinicians

---

Third Edition

PART I

GENERAL PRINCIPLES OF OVERDOSE MANAGEMENT

CHAPTER 1

General Management of the Overdosed Patient

Toxicology is that branch of pharmacology that deals with the undesirable effect of chemicals in biologic systems. In addition, toxicology involves the analysis, both qualitative and quantitative, of these agents in biologic materials as well as the development of procedures for the treatment of the poisoning (1). *Medical toxicology* is concerned with the clinical manifestations, differential diagnoses, and treatment regimen of the accidental or deliberate acute overdose or chronic poisoning. It also encompasses the acute and chronic exposure to toxins in the workplace, as well as exposure to environmental toxins.

Poisonings and drug overdoses, both accidental and intentional, continue to be a major medical problem. The field of medical toxicology is constantly expanding and changing, and in the last decade there have been many important advances that aid in both the diagnosis and the treatment of poisoned patients (2). It is vitally important for the practitioner to be aware of the most up-to-date treatment protocols so as to improve the chances of the patient's survival.

Any drug under certain circumstances can be toxic, and this toxicity can present itself as various signs and symptoms (3). The poisoned patient may represent a clinical challenge to the emergency department physician, who must be aware of the potential for multisystem involvement. Whenever a patient who appears to be ill presents with a history or symptom complex that is unusual or confusing, purposeful or accidental ingestion or exposure to a toxic chemical should be considered (4). This may be the critically ill patient who presents with an altered mental status, unexplained cardiotoxicity, unexplained metabolic acidosis, seizures, or head trauma for which there is no satisfactory explanation. Although the most common route for accidental exposure to poisons is the gastrointestinal tract, toxic effects may also be produced by accidental absorption of the toxin through the skin, inhalation through the lungs, or parenteral administration (5). This chapter is a general overview of the patient who has ingested or been exposed to a toxic material and who may or may not be manifesting toxic symptoms. It will look at toxins by the signs and symptoms that they may produce, so as to accurately and quickly compose a differential diagnosis, and treatment regimen.

There is often no difference between the mechanism of action of a drug and that of a poison, only an extension of effect. A drug may be administered in dosages that alter physiologic function to produce a desired therapeutic effect. When a drug is administered in greater than therapeutic quantities, toxic effects may be noted. It may be difficult to diagnose drug toxicity when the poisoning is of a chronic nature, especially when a relevant history is unavailable.

INITIAL EVALUATION

The initial evaluation of the patient should include obtaining as reliable a history as possible and performing a thorough but quick physical examination (6–9). In conjunction with appropriate laboratory analyses, these provide essential data for appropriate patient management (Table 1–1).

History

A history may not always be easy to obtain and may be inaccurate, especially if the patient is a toddler who cannot relate a good and accurate history or an adult intent on causing himself or herself harm who will purposely not give an accurate account (10). In addition, poisoning as a manifestation of child abuse has been reported and should be considered, especially in the very young or in children who repeatedly "overdose" (11,12). In the infant, poisoning is largely a result of therapeutic overdosing (11). In children 1 to 5 years old, ingestions are most often accidental. A child older than 6 or 7 years at the time of overdose must be evaluated for psychological dysfunction, because in this age group overdose is rarely an accident (13).

When eliciting the history, it is important to obtain information regarding the type of poison ingested, the amount taken, the time since ingestion, any antidotes that may have been given, and the presence of any allergies or underlying illnesses.

TABLE 1–1. *Items in the initial patient evaluation*

History
- Patient history
- Corroborative history
- Worst possible scenario

Physical examination
- Vital signs
  - Blood pressure
    - Hypertension (see Table 1–2)
    - Hypotension (see Table 1–3)
  - Pulse
    - Tachycardia
    - Bradycardia (see Table 1–4)
    - Dysrhythmia
  - Respiratory rate
    - Tachypnea (see Table 1–5)
      - Respiratory alkalosis
      - Metabolic acidosis
  - Temperature
    - Hyperthermia (see Table 1–6)
    - Hypothermia
- Skin and mucous membranes
  - Burns
  - Cyanosis
  - Bullous lesions (see Table 1–7)
  - Diaphoresis (see Table 1–8)
  - Jaundice (see Table 1–9)
- Odors (see Table 1–11)
- Neurologic examination (see Table 1–12)
- Emesis
  - ? Pill fragments
  - ? Amount
  - ? Hematemesis

There will be a period of time immediately after an ingestion of the toxin that evidence of poisoning will not be present. This can be referred to as the preclinical phase. During this phase, estimation of toxicity and management of the patient will need to be based on the best history of the maximum possible ingested dose coupled with the available knowledge of the drug's kinetics and toxicity. It is wise to consider the history as the worst possible scenario so as not to minimize the effect of the potential toxin (14).

Corroborative History

It is wise in all cases of overdose to obtain a separate history from a friend, a relative, or the person who brought the patient to the emergency department to corroborate the patient's history. The family, friends, or paramedical personnel should be asked about any known prescription or over-the-counter medications found in the house or known to be used by the patient (15). Conversations by telephone with the patient's family and friends may also yield information about previous overdose attempts, medications and chemicals available in the home.

The Size of a "Swallow"

Many times the physician may be given a history of the amount ingested in terms of a "swallow." Although there is no rigid amount, approximately 5 mL is the average swallow of a child from a relatively large orifice container containing a water-like, low-viscosity fluid. Orifice size can influence the swallow volume in that reducing the orifice size reduces the volume (16). The average swallow in the adult is 10–30 mL.

PHYSICAL EXAMINATION

A brief physical examination should be performed shortly after the patient arrives. The physical examination should include vital signs, a careful search for trauma, and a good neurologic examination. Reassessment should be done frequently. This will determine what immediate treatment may be necessary as well as provide clues to the practitioner as to what was ingested or the extent of toxicity when the ingested agent is known.

Vital Signs

A clue as to what was ingested may be discovered by a critical examination of the patient's vital signs. An accurate measurement of each parameter, including the respiratory rate and temperature, should be obtained.

Heart rate and blood pressure: tachycardia and hypertension. Persistent tachycardia and hypertension, if drug-induced, may be caused by a monoamine oxidase (MAO) inhibitor, phencyclidine or by acute withdrawal from a central nervous system (CNS) depressant, alcohol, clonidine, or β-adrenergic blocking agents (Table 1–2) (10,17). Tachycardia also suggests anticholinergic or sympathomimetic poisoning. Because these poisonings present with similar symptoms, they are difficult to differentiate, though the patient with sympathomimetic overdose may have prominent piloerection and sweating, which are absent in anticholinergic poisoning (10,17,18). Hypertension and tachycardia may also result from late ganglionic stimulation during organophosphate insecticide intoxication. Drugs that cause initial stimulation resulting in hypertension or tachycardia may be followed by generalized depression.

Hypertension, when caused primarily by intense α-receptor-mediated vasoconstriction, is frequently accompanied by reflex bradycardia. This may be noted with phenylephrine, phenylpropanolamine, and other α-stimulatory agents.

Heart rate and blood pressure: hypotension and tachycardia. Hypotension accompanied by tachycardia may be due to fluid loss, third spacing, or direct depression of cardiac contractility with peripheral vascular collapse

TABLE 1–2. *Substances causing hypertension and tachycardia*

Anticholinergics
Antidepressants
Antihistamines
Antipsychotics
Antiparkinsonian medicines
Mushrooms (*Amanita muscaria*)
Over-the-counter medicines
Plants (Jimson weed)
Sympathomimetics
Amphetamines
Amphetamine derivatives
Methylenedioxyamphetamine (MDA)
Methylenedioxymethamphetamine (MDMA)
Methylenedioxyethamphetamine (MDEA)
Caffeine
Cocaine
Lysergic acid diethylamide (LSD)
"Look-alikes" (phenylpropanolamine, caffeine, ephedrine)
Monoamine oxidase inhibitors
Theophylline
Phencyclidine
Substances associated with withdrawal syndromes
Alcohol
β-Blocking agents
Centrally acting α_2 agonists
Aldomet
Clonidine
Central nervous system depressants
Sedative-hypnotics
Nicotinic action
Nicotine
Organophosphates

(10). Hypotension may be due to α-receptor blockade or β-adrenergic stimulation and has been seen in overdoses with cyanide, iron, sedative-hypnotics, theophylline, and carbon monoxide (Table 1–3).

Heart rate and blood pressure: hypotension and bradycardia. Hypotension associated with bradycardia may be due to calcium channel blockers, central depression of sympathetic output, overdose with membrane depressant drugs or digitalis, or peripheral blockade of α-adrenergic receptors (Table 1–3) (17).

Bradycardia. Bradycardia may be caused by digitalis preparations, α-adrenergic blockers, calcium channel blockers, clonidine, and acetylcholinesterase inhibitors (parasympathomimetic agents). Bradycardia may also occur as a response to hypertension caused by α-adrenergic drugs (17). Additional agents are listed in Table 1–4.

Respiratory rate. The respiratory rate and depth may be increased by sympathomimetics such as amphetamine, cocaine, or caffeine. The respiratory rate and pattern may also be the first clue that the patient has an acid-base disorder (Table 1–5). As an example, tachypnea may represent a drug-induced primary respiratory alkalosis (from salicylates or dinitrophenol) or a compensation for an underlying and potentially dangerous metabolic acidosis (ethylene glycol, methanol, and others). Treatment of tachypnea should therefore never consist of paper bag rebreathing, even in the patient who may have primary hyperventilation syndrome (19). For the patient thought to be hyperventilating due to anxiety and whose oxygenation is not known, oxygen should be used along with other measures of reassurance that do not affect the con-

TABLE 1–3. *Substances associated with hypotension*

Hypotension and tachycardia
α-Adrenergic blockers
Carbon monoxide
Cyanide
Disulfiram
Iron
Narcotics
Nitrites
Phenothiazines
Sedative-hypnotics
Theophylline
Tricyclic antidepressants
Hypotension and bradycardia
α-Adrenergic blockers
β-Adrenergic blockers
Calcium channel blockers
Cholinergics
Centrally acting α_2 agents
Digoxin
Membrane-stabilizing drugs
Quinidine
Procainamide
Local anesthetics
Tricyclic antidepressants (TCAs)
Organophosphate insecticides

TABLE 1–4. *Substances associated with bradycardia*

α-Adrenergic blockers
β-Adrenergic blockers
Calcium channel blockers
Cardiac glycosides
Cholinergics
Clonidine
Hypertensives
Insecticides (organophosphates)
Local anesthetics
Mushrooms (cholinergic)
Nicotine
Tricyclic antidepressants (late)

TABLE 1–5. *Substances associated with tachypnea*

Drug-associated respiratory alkalosis
Dinitrophenol
Pentachlorophenol
Salicylates
Drug-associated metabolic acidosis
Drug-associated hepatic failure
Sympathomimetics

TABLE 1–6. *Substances associated with hyperthermia*

Anticholinergics
Antihistamines
Antidepressants
Antipsychotics
Mushrooms (*Amanita muscaria*)
Over-the-counter medications
Plants (Jimson weed)
Uncoupling of oxidative phosphorylation
Dinitrophenol
Pentachlorophenol
Salicylates
Sympathomimetics
Amphetamines
Cocaine
Thyroid
Phencyclidine
Drug withdrawal
Miscellaneous
Monoamine oxidase inhibitors
Metal fume fever

centration of inspired gases. It should be remembered that tachypnea may be a normal and universal response to even moderate stress (19).

Hypoventilation associated with respiratory depression may result from an overdose of any central nervous system depressant. It is usually due to depression of the reticular activating system and the respiratory drive center in the brain, and endotracheal intubation may be required to protect the patient.

Temperature. Hyperthermia secondary to drug overdose may be an immediate threat to life and must be quickly recognized and treated (Table 1–6). Hyperthermia caused by any drug can lead to extensive muscle breakdown and renal failure as well as direct brain injury. It may result from impaired thermoregulatory mechanisms, muscle hyperactivity, or increased metabolic rate (17). Hypothermia is a common problem seen with a substantial overdose. It is frequently caused by a central nervous system depressant and may be the result of exposure to a cool ambient temperature in a patient with inadequate physiologic responses to body cooling due to the ingested drug.

Skin and Mucous Membranes

The skin is an important organ for absorption of various compounds, therapeutic as well as environmental. Absorption of a compound is directly related to the degree of hydration of the skin and is inversely related to the thickness. The systemic availability for an identical percutaneous dose of a drug will be approximately three times greater in an infant than in an adult (20).

Not only may drugs penetrate the skin unchanged, but they also may be metabolized in the skin or interact with receptors present on or in epidermal cells. The enzyme system responsible for drug metabolism in the skin resembles that of the liver. Both oxidative and reductive reactions occur in the skin. The skin is therefore not the inert barrier it was traditionally thought to be.

In any patient presenting with an altered mental state, the skin should be examined for evidence of needle marks. Needle "tracks" should be especially looked for in the antecubital fossae, the neck, the supraclavicular areas, the groin, the dorsum of the feet, and under the tongue. Drugs have also been found hidden in the vagina or rectum.

Bullous lesions may be a clue to the examiner that a sedative-hypnotic was ingested, that the patient was exposed to carbon monoxide, that the patient was bitten by an insect or a snake, or that the patient may have come in contact with a chemical that, owing to its caustic nature, has caused a burn (Table 1–7) (17). Diaphoresis may be profuse and may be the clue to the agent ingested (Table 1–8). Jaundice is not an immediate effect of a toxin but may also be noted 48 to 72 hours after exposure to a hepatotoxin (Table 1–9).

TABLE 1–7. *Substances causing bullous lesions*

Caustic agents
Acids
Alkalis
Environmental hazards
Carbon monoxide
Snake bite
Insect bite
Sedative-hypnotic agents
Barbiturates
Diphenoxylate (Lomotil)
Glutethimide (Doriden)
Meprobamate (Equanil, Miltown, Equagesic)

TABLE 1–8. *Substances causing diaphoresis*

Acetaminophen
Acetylcholinesterase inhibitor insecticides
Drugs causing hypoglycemia
Mushrooms (cholinergic)
Nicotine
Salicylates
Withdrawal of substances of abuse
Sympathomimetics

TABLE 1–9. *Substances causing jaundice*

Acetaminophen
Amanita phalloides and related mushrooms
Arsenic
Carbon tetrachloride
Chloroform
Ethanol
Iron
Methotrexate
Phenacetin
Phenothiazines
Phosphorus
Toluene
Trichloroethane
Trichloroethylene

TABLE 1–10. *Drugs absorbed by transdermal patch*

Clonidine
Estradiol
Fentanyl
Nicotine
Nitroglycerin
Scopolamine
Testosterone

Transdermal Delivery Systems

Transdermal delivery systems deliver drugs to the systemic circulation by means of the skin (Table 1–10). One advantage of such a system is that the first-pass effect of the liver on drug metabolism is avoided, although some degree of analogous metabolism may take place in the skin.

Odors

Odors on the breath and body may help indicate the nature of the ingested toxin (21). For example, the odor of alcohol is frequently encountered in the emergency department and is well recognized. Alcohol, however, is associated with many drug ingestions and may only indicate that the patient is intoxicated with alcohol in addition to an overdose of another substance (22).

The odor of garlic may suggest the ingestion of arsenic (or arsine gas inhalation), organophosphate insecticide, or phosphorus rodenticide or the topical application of dimethyl sulfoxide (DMSO). Cyanide may have the odor of bitter almonds or macaroons, and the odor of rotten egg may indicate hydrogen sulfide gas. Other odors that may be helpful in diagnosing an unknown overdose are noted in Table 1–11. Although the presence of certain odors may aid the diagnosis, their absence is not a reliable means of excluding intoxication.

TABLE 1–11. *Substances causing characteristic odors*

Odor	Substance
Acetone	Ethyl Alcohol
	Isopropyl alcohol
	Lacquer
Bitter almond	Amygdalin
	Apricot pits
	Cyanide
Burned rope	Marijuana
Carrot	Cicutoxin
Garlic	Arsenic
	Arsine gas
	Dimethyl sulfoxide
	Organophosphates
	Phosphorus
	Selenium
	Thallium
Mothballs	Naphthalene
	Paradichlorobenzene
Peanuts	Rodenticides
Pear	Chloral hydrate
	Paraldehyde
Pungent aromatic	Ethchlorvynol
Rotten eggs	Hydrogen sulfide
	Mercaptans
	Sewer gas
Shoe polish	Nitrobenzene
Violets	Turpentine
Wintergreen	Methyl salicylate

Emesis

History of emesis should be ascertained and documented on the patient's chart. Emesis before arrival in the emergency department may explain why a patient remains asymptomatic after having ingested what appeared to be a toxic amount of substance. Further questioning concerning approximate amount of emesis and whether there was accompanying hematemesis should also be documented.

Neurologic Examination

A brief neurologic examination (Table 1–12) should include evaluating the patient's mental status which reflects the clinical state of cognitive and emotional functioning of an individual in his or her environment (23). The neurologic examination should also include looking for evidence of previous seizure activity (Table 1–13), evaluating the size and reactivity of the pupils (Table 1–14), observing for the presence of nystagmus (Table 1–15), and testing for the presence or absence of the gag reflex (24).

For simplicity, the formal mental status evaluation can be divided into six categories: appearance, behavior, and attitude; disorders of thought; disorders of perception; mood and affect; insight and judgment; and sensorium and intelligence (23). A routine history and physical examination will provide a general impression concern-

TABLE 1–12. *Items in the neurologic examination of the overdosed patient*

Focal signs
Gag reflex
Mental status
Affect
Behavior and appearance
General intellectual functioning
Perceptual disorders
Thought content
Thought process
Nystagmus (see Table 1–15)
Pupil size/reactivity (see Table 1–14)
Seizure activity (see Table 1–13)

TABLE 1–13. *Substances causing seizure activity (Acronym: WITH L.A. COPS)*

W	Withdrawal
I	Isoniazid
T	Theophylline
H	Hypoglycemic agents
	Hypoxia
L	Lead
	Lithium
	Local anesthetics
A	Anticholinergics
	Amphetamines
C	Camphor
	Carbon monoxide
	Carbamazepine (Tegretol)
	Chlorinated hydrocarbons (DDT, lindane)
	Cholinergics
	Cocaine
	Cyanide
O	Organophosphates (malathion, parathion)
P	Phencyclidine
	Phenothiazines
	Phenytoin (Dilantin)
	Propoxyphene (Darvon)
S	Salicylates
	Strychnine
	Sympathomimetics

TABLE 1–14. *Substances causing characteristic eye changes*

Mydriasis
Anticholinergics
Glutethimide (Doriden)
Meperidine (Demerol)
Mushrooms (anticholinergics)
Withdrawal of abused substances
Sympathomimetics
Miosis
α-Adrenergic blockers
Cholinergics
Clonidine (Catapres)
Insecticides (cholinergic)
Mushrooms (cholinergic)
Narcotics
Nicotine
Phenothiazines
Phencyclidine

ing five of six categories, but will not test cognitive function. For this, specific tests of higher cognitive function need to be included in a patient's evaluation (25).

Seizure activity. Seizure is a relatively common feature of poisoning by many drugs and toxins. The most common causes of toxin-induced seizures are cyclic antidepressants, theophylline, isoniazid, sympathomimetics, and withdrawal from alcohol or sedative-hypnotics (17). The acronym "WITH L.A. COPS" is presented for the drug causes of seizure (Table 1–13). Seizures may result in pulmonary aspiration, hypoxia, and lactic acidosis and may ultimately cause rhabdomyolysis and acute renal failure.

TABLE 1–15. *Toxins causing nystagmus (Acronym: SALEM TIP)*

S	Sedative-hypnotic
	Solvents
A	Alcohols
L	Lithium
E	Ethanol
	Ethylene glycol
M	Methanol
T	Thiamine depletion
	Tegretol (carbamazepine)
I	Isopropanol
P	Phencyclidine
	Phenytoin (Dilantin)

Eye changes. There are many classes of compounds that cause changes in the eyes, such as mydriasis, miosis (Table 1–14), or nystagmus (Table 1–15). Pupil size is controlled by the autonomic nervous system and is determined by the relative balance between the parasympathetic and sympathetic systems. Dilation is mediated by α_1-adrenoceptors, and constriction is mediated by muscarinic cholinergic receptors (26). Antimuscarinic drugs would therefore be expected to cause mydriasis. Although phenothiazines have some antimuscarinic side effects, they may cause miosis because of a predominant α-blocking action (17).

Sympatholytic agents, narcotics, and cholinergics usually cause miosis. Although phencyclidine is considered a sympathomimetic agent, its cholinergic properties predominate and miosis may be frequently noted. The acronym "SALEM TIP" is presented for drugs that cause nystagmus (Table 1–15).

Radiopacity of Substances

There are a number of pills with different chemical compositions that exhibit varying degrees of radiopacity (24). Although clinical experience has led to the development of the acronym "CHIPS" (24), an updated

TABLE 1–16. *Substances that may be radiopaque (Acronym:BET A CHIP)*

B	Barium
E	Enteric-coated tablets
T	Tricyclic antidepressants
A	Antihistamines
C	Chloral hydrate, cocaine packets, calcium
H	Heavy metals
I	Iodides
P	Potassium, phenothiazines

acronym, "BET A CHIP," is suggested to describe the more common radiopaque medications (Table 1–16). For a substance to be radiopaque, it should have stability in the gastric or intestinal contents, low water solubility, and the ability to decrease gastrointestinal motility.

Radiographs are of little use in most ingestions (24), yet for those pills that are consistently visible on a plain abdominal roentgenogram a radiographic diagnosis may be possible. A postemesis or lavage radiograph may also be used to assess the effectiveness of the gastric emptying procedure.

Compounds containing iron and other heavy metals are the most radiopaque class of medications. This is not necessarily true for vitamin tablets containing iron, which are not consistently radiopaque. Calcium carbonate is strongly radiopaque, but other calcium compounds may be radiolucent. Potassium preparations are also among the most radiopaque substances. The tricyclic antidepressants and the phenothiazines demonstrate a highly variable degree of radiopacity. Although enteric-coated tablets are part of the acronym, there is variability in the degree of radiopacity of the particular compounds (26). Antihistamines with and without enteric coating frequently demonstrate radiopacity. In addition, swallowed drug packets or condoms may sometimes be visible on plain radiographs.

CLASSIFICATION OF COMA

Although there are many systems to describe an altered mental status, there is not one description that is universally accepted (27). Rather than using terms such as *lethargy*, *semicoma*, and *coma*, which may not adequately communicate to another person what the examiner intended, it is more important to describe specific findings, such as response to pain and gag reflex, as well as circulatory or respiratory depression. One such system is divided into five stages as follows (28).

Stage 0: The patient is asleep but easily aroused and has normal response to pain and an intact gag reflex (this constitutes the majority of patients seen).

Stage 1: The patient is comatose, withdraws from painful stimuli, and has an intact gag reflex (gastric contents may be evacuated without prior nasotracheal intubation).

Stage 2: The patient is comatose and does not withdraw from pain, but the gag reflex is intact (gastric contents may be evacuated without prior nasotracheal intubation).

Stage 3: The patient is comatose, does not withdraw from pain, and has lost the gag reflex. There is no circulatory or respiratory depression (requires endotracheal intubation prior to gastric evacuation).

Stage 4: The patient is comatose, does not withdraw from pain, and has lost the gag reflex; cyanosis and circulatory and/or respiratory depression are present (requires the basics of emergency medicine followed if necessary by gastric lavage).

TABLE 1–17. *Suggested therapy for patients with altered mental status (Acronym: DONT)*

	Drug	Dosage
D	Dextrose	Adult: 50 mL of $D_{50}W$ (25 g) Child: 1 mL/kg of same solution diluted 1:1
O	Oxygen	As necessary
N	Naloxone	2 mg IV up to 10 mg
T	Thiamine	50 to 100 mg IV

THERAPEUTIC AGENTS

In the past, it has been considered standard of care that all adult patients presenting with an altered mental status should receive oxygen, an intravenous injection of 50 mL of 50% glucose, 50–100 mg thiamine, and 2 mg of naloxone (the DONT regimen) (Table 1–17) (26,29). During the last few years investigators have reported some potential adverse effects concerning the administration of glucose (30). Because of this, a brief discussion and recommendation of the potentially useful therapeutic agents will follow.

Naloxone

Since naloxone was introduced in 1967, it has greatly improved the treatment of patients with opiate overdose. It has been available since 1986 as a generic product, which has markedly reduced its cost.

Naloxone is a pure narcotic antagonist and in the absence of a narcotic it will not cause any further deterioration of the patient's condition. Most sources advocate that naloxone be administered to any patient with an altered mental status, although some would advocate that naloxone be administered to patients with an altered mental status and bradypnea (31).

The optimal dose of naloxone for endotracheal use remains unknown (32). Starting with the recommended intravenous dose and repeating the dose as needed to achieve the desired therapeutic endpoint is best until definitive guidelines become available (33).

There is some risk of opioid withdrawal seizures in neonates whose mothers have been maintained on methadone during pregnancy. Withdrawal seizures are not seen in adults or children after chronic opioid dependency or massive acute overdose (34).

Recommendation

In the patient with an altered mental state and respiratory depression, 2 mg of naloxone should be administered (31). This may be repeated to a total of 10 mg. If an intravenous route cannot be established, other acceptable routes of administration of naloxone are sublingual and endotracheal.

Although the pupils are generally constricted in narcotic overdose, meperidine poisoning may not produce miosis. In addition, as the narcotic poisoned patient's brainstem becomes hypoxic the pupils will dilate; one should therefore never use a lack of pupillary constriction as an excuse not to administer naloxone to lethargic or comatose patients (18).

Glucose

The empiric administration of intravenous glucose has become a standard of care in the emergency management of the comatose patient (35). It has been generally accepted that hypoglycemia is harmful and must be immediately identified and treated (31). In addition to the association of hypoglycemia and diabetes, several medications can cause hypoglycemia, including ethanol, insulin, β-blockers, salicylates, and sulfonylureas (18). In addition, certain drugs are known to alter glucose metabolism in patients undergoing therapy for diabetes (35).

Potential Detrimental Cerebral Effects of Glucose

Although it is known that D50W might worsen hyperglycemia and hyperosmolality, alter serum potassium, and cause skin necrosis if infiltrated subcutaneously, these complications are considered rare (36,37). Recent evidence suggests that under certain circumstances, such as cerebral ischemia, acute stroke, impending cardiac arrest, severe hypotension, or patients receiving cardiopulmonary resuscitation (CPR) (35), the administration of 50% dextrose intravenously may result in increased neurologic damage (35). It has therefore been suggested that administration of 50% dextrose be reserved for those patients in whom hypoglycemia is either highly suspected or confirmed, or where a quick venous sample cannot be obtained (29).

The detrimental effect of glucose on ischemic brain tissue is thought to be mediated by lactic acid that accumulates through anaerobic glycolysis (35). The amount of lactate that accumulates during complete ischemia appears to be determined by the preischemic tissue glucose stores. If hyperglycemia is as deleterious as has been suggested, then a policy of aggressive glucose control at the time of hospitalization may be warranted and efficacious (36). However, if hyperglycemia is merely a marker for severity of infarction, then a clinical policy of aggressive glucose control would have negligible benefit and, in fact, may be dangerous (38). Although consistent with the hypothesis that hyperglycemia itself leads to poor outcomes, the clinical evidence does not establish a causal link (18).

Although bedside fingerstick blood glucose estimations are relatively easy to perform, their accuracy in severely hypotensive patients has been seriously questioned; they should therefore not be relied upon in patients in shock. Fortunately, accurate, rapid and inexpensive methods of blood glucose determination have been recently developed and shown to be accurate in the prehospital and emergency department environment (29).

Visually read reagent strips for rapid determination of blood glucose concentration are commonly used to guide initiation of emergent treatment of hypoglycemia (31). Testing of venous blood using reagent strips correlates closely with results obtained by laboratory analysis (29). Four strips that are available in the United States are Chemstrip, Dextrostix, Glucostix, and Visidex II (6). Problems that might affect the accuracy of visually read strips in an emergency department (ED) setting include interobserver variability, improper storage, and extremes of hematocrit. The extent to which abnormal hematocrit levels will affect diagnoses using glucose reagent strips is unclear (6,31). Manufacturers of these products caution that improper storage with various degrees of exposure to heat, moisture, air, or light may markedly affect strip performance. Nevertheless, for reasons of convenience and economy, visually read strips have become widely used for emergent blood glucose monitoring (6).

Recommendation

In the adult patient with an altered mental status, glucose may be withheld if an accurate estimation of serum glucose can be obtained immediately. If this cannot be obtained, 50 mL of 50% glucose should be strongly considered (37,39).

The recommended dose of dextrose in a child is 0.5 to 1.0 g/kg, which usually is administered as 2 to 4 mL/kg of $D_{25}W$ for the child or 50 mL of $D_{50}W$ for the teenager (34).

Thiamine

Thiamine (vitamin B1) is an essential vitamin required for the proper functioning of many enzymes in several metabolic pathways. Many of these pathways involve glucose. Thiamine is also necessary in the synthesis of acetylcholine. Thiamine deficiency states commonly lead to medical problems, both overt and subclinical. Peripheral neuropathy, beriberi, Wernicke's encephalopathy, Korsakoff's psychosis, and subacute necrotizing encephalomyelopathy all represent either local or systemic deficiency of some active form of this vitamin (40). Because thiamine is necessary for the metabolism of glucose, when glucose is administered to a thiamine-depleted patient who is not yet showing clinical signs of thiamine depletion, the remaining thiamine stores may be

TABLE 1–18. *Conditions associated with Wernicke's encephalopathy*

Acquired immunodeficiency syndrome (AIDS)
Anorexia/bulimia
Cancer patients
Chronic alcoholism
Chronic renal failure
Gastric bypass surgery
Gastrointestinal obstruction syndromes
Hyperemesis gravidarum
Malabsorption syndromes
Nonalcoholic cirrhosis
Patients receiving total parenteral nutrition
Prolonged parenteral nutrition
Uncontrolled diabetes

used in the metabolism of the administered glucose, precipitating an acute Wernicke's encephalopathy (41).

Wernicke's Encephalopathy

Although Wernicke's encephalopathy has been associated with the alcoholic, this is not the only group of concern. Wernicke's encephalopathy has been associated with nonalcoholic cirrhosis, malabsorption syndromes, as well as many other medical conditions (Table 1–18) (42).

Because the clinical findings in Wernicke's encephalopathy may be subtle and one or more of the classic findings may be absent, thiamine should be administered whenever a malnourished or alcoholic patient is evaluated in the emergency department, especially if glucose is administered.

Toxicity of Thiamine

Cases of anaphylaxis from the parenteral administration of thiamine have been reported (40). Because there are several reports in the literature involving serious and sometimes fatal reactions to parenteral thiamine, some hospital personnel have refused to allow patients to receive IV thiamine (41).

Both an anaphylactoid reaction as well as an overdose response has occurred after the administration of thiamine. The anaphylactoid response typically occurs after many large doses are administered at relatively frequent intervals. The reactions are often preceded by allergic symptoms such as sneezing or transient local or generalized pruritus on prior injections (40). It is important to note that these reactions occur not only after IV doses but also after subcutaneous and intramuscular administration (41).

The second type of response, that of overdosage, occurs also after large doses, sometimes orally administered over a long period of time. Symptoms that develop may resemble those of hyperthyroidism, which may disappear after cessation of the drug.

It appears that any prejudice against IV thiamine dosing in favor of other parenteral routes is unwarranted because anaphylactoid reactions seem to occur with equal frequency in IV, IM, or subcutaneous injections (41). The intravenous route therefore appears to be as safe as deep intramuscular injections for patients. Intradermal test doses before the administration of thiamine have been advocated. Because severe reactions with IV thiamine are rare, testing is considered unwarranted except in patients with a history of an allergic response such as itching, sneezing, wheezing, or frank anaphylactic shock with a previous injection (40).

Recommendation

The detection of subclinical thiamine deficiency is difficult and biochemical defects precede clinical pathology. Because of this, thiamine should be administered intravenously to all patients at significant risk for thiamine deficiency. This is especially important in a patient who has been given intravenous glucose (Table 1–17) (41).

ESSENTIALS OF OVERDOSE MANAGEMENT

There are four essentials of overdose management that should be considered for every patient (26):

1. Supportive care (the mainstay of care)
2. Prevention of further absorption (see Chapter 2)
3. Enhancement of excretion (see Chapter 3)
4. Administration of an antidote if available

Supportive Care

One of the important aspects in the management of the poisoned patient is supportive care (43). For the most part, patients will detoxify as the ingested compound is metabolized by normal body processes. The highest priorities in the treatment of patients who have ingested toxins are assigned to the establishment of an airway, providing adequate ventilation, and maintenance of adequate vital signs. Support of the vital signs, in addition to good pulmonary hygiene, will enhance any of the other more specific methods (44). Because the cardiac status is unknown, the patient should be observed on a cardiac monitor until medically cleared. The need for more specific therapy should be based on the patient's clinical condition and the results of toxicologic screening.

A large group of acutely poisoned patients can be treated with supportive care, which includes the appropriate treatment of common complications that may occur during intoxication (hypotension, cardiac dysrhythmias, and seizures) (26). The drug will be progressively eliminated over the next 12 to 36 hours in most patients, and many times this is all the care that is necessary.

The poisoned patient may be in shock for a number of reasons. Pooling of blood in an expanded vascular bed caused by vasodilation may have occurred. Hypovolemia from lack of fluid intake during prolonged unconsciousness or from a direct myocardial depressant effect of the drug may also be involved. In some cases of poisoning, hypotension should be treated initially with the intravenous infusion of isotonic fluids. Fluid and electrolyte management may be complex (45). Monitoring body weight, central venous pressure, pulmonary capillary wedge pressure and arterial blood gases may be necessary to ensure adequate but not excessive administration of fluid.

In general, seizures should be treated initially with intravenous diazepam. A rectally administered benzodiazepine can be used for the initial control of seizures if intravenous access cannot be obtained (46).

Position of the Patient

The left lateral position has been found to be associated with the slowest rate of absorption of ingested medication. It is thought that, because of gravity, there is a layering out of gastric contents along the greater curvature of the stomach (45,47). In addition, oropharyngeal drainage is also improved, there is an easy access for suction as well as the prevention of aspiration of emesis in the patient with central nervous system depression (45). Other positions, such as the right lateral decubitus position and the sitting position increase the rate of absorption probably because they favor gravitational and peristaltic emptying into the small intestine (47).

Route of Administration of Fluids

Although supportive care should consist of the establishment of an IV line, this may not always be the case. There are times, in infants and young children especially where an IV line is not easy to establish. In this situation, other routes of fluid and drug therapy should be considered.

Endotracheal Administration

The potential utility of endotracheal delivery of medications has been recognized for more than 20 years. Due to the large surface area, many drugs are rapidly absorbed through the mucous membranes and pulmonary epithelium of the respiratory tract. Emergency drugs that can be safely delivered by the endotracheal route include epinephrine, atropine, and naloxone (Table 1–19). Saline should be used as the diluent for the endotracheal delivery of these drugs. Distilled water should be the diluent if lidocaine is to be administered. The volume of fluid should be in the range of 5 to 10 mL in the young child or with 10 to 20 mL in the older child or adult. Providing five positive pressure breaths immediately after instillation of the drug into the airway will force the drug distally and increase its absorption.

Bicarbonate, calcium, and glucose solutions produce serious lung damage when instilled in the airway and, therefore, cannot be administered endotracheally.

TABLE 1–19. *Drugs and endotracheal administration*

Can be administered	Cannot be administered
Epinephrine	Bicarbonate
Atropine	Calcium
Naloxone	Glucose

Intraosseous Administration

The use of intraosseous infusions in patients has undergone a relatively recent resurgence of popularity after a long period of quiescence since first introduced in the early part of this century (48,49). Any drug or solution that can be administered intravenously can be given by the intraosseous route, including crystalloid and colloid solutions for volume resuscitation (25). In actuality, intraosseous infusion is an infusion through blood vessels within the bone marrow, which are held open by a rigid, noncollapsible bony wall (25).

Intraosseous infusion is a practical and effective route for the administration of sodium bicarbonate, calcium, and glucose, none of which can be given by the endotracheal route (Table 1–20) (25). Many other drugs such as atropine, epinephrine, and diazepam may also be safely administered by the intraosseous route (49). This route is usually reserved for potentially life-threatening emergency situations.

PREVENTION OF ABSORPTION

Prevention of absorption of a toxin is another important facet to the care of the poisoned patient (50). This is due to the fact that once a toxin is absorbed there may be very little that can be done to enhance the excretion of the

TABLE 1–20. *Drugs and interosseous administration*

Can be administered
Atropine
Calcium
Diazepam
Epinephrine
Glucose
Sodium bicarbonate

particular compound. Methods for the prevention of absorption include decontamination of the skin, administration of syrup of ipecac, gastric lavage, administration of activated charcoal (51), and use of a cathartic. These methods are discussed in detail in Chapter 2.

ENHANCEMENT OF EXCRETION

Although there are various methods for enhancing the excretion of drugs and toxins, their use in toxicology is limited. Procedures intended to enhance the excretion of the ingested agent from the body include forced diuresis, alteration of urine pH, dialysis, hemoperfusion, interruption of the enterohepatic circulation, "intestinal dialysis," plasmapheresis, and exchange transfusion. The various methods available for enhancing excretion are listed in Table 1–21 and are discussed in Chapter 3.

TABLE 1–21. *Methods to enhance drug elimination*

Diuresis
Neutral diuresis
Alkaline diuresis
Acid diuresis
Dialysis
Hemodialysis
Peritoneal dialysis
Hemoperfusion
Multiple doses of activated charcoal
Interruption of enterohepatic recirculation
"Intestinal dialysis"
Plasmapheresis
Exchange transfusion

ADMINISTRATION OF AN ANTIDOTE

Certain patients present to the emergency department with toxic symptom complexes that may respond to the administration of an antidote. The antidote is rarely the essence of the management of a poisoned patient. Antidotal therapy may not be necessary, but to have the antidote available and to know when and how to use it may be lifesaving (52–54). Although there are a number of specific antidotes known for poisoning, their use should not take the place of good general supportive measures. A list of available antidotes is given in Table 1–22.

DRUGS TO AVOID

Analeptic Agents

Analeptics act on the central nervous system to stimulate respiration. In the past, analeptics were sometimes advocated for those patients who presented with central nervous system depression. The use of such agents is condemned because they may cause a seizure when the patient is not in control of his or her airway (55,56). Although analeptic agents may be of some benefit in the operating room, they have no place in emergency medicine and toxicology (Table 1–23).

Antidotes

Many "antidotes" that were used in the past are now considered obsolete, or more importantly, dangerous to the patient. Some examples include mineral oil cathartics which, when aspirated, may cause chemical pneumonitis; the "universal antidote," which contains tannic acid, which is now replaced by activated charcoal; and fluid extract of ipecac, which is 14 times more potent than syrup of ipecac and associated with fatalities. Apomorphine has been associated with fatalities secondary to central nervous system and respiratory depression and protracted vomiting. Levallorphan and nalorphine, used in the past, are more dangerous and less effective than naloxone, and copper sulfate and sodium chloride, have been replaced by syrup of ipecac. Finally, oral dilution with water can actually increase the absorption and toxicity of certain drugs and should only be used with caution in corrosive agent ingestion (57).

COMPLICATIONS OF OVERDOSE

There are a number of complications that can occur after an overdose (Table 1–24). These potential complications may arise from overly vigorous fluid replacement with ensuing fluid overload or as a direct result of the toxin, with seizures, hypothermia, rhabdomyolysis (58), aspiration, and acid-base disorders as consequences. The clinician should be prepared for these complications. Many lethal toxins depress the CNS, resulting in obtundation or coma. Comatose patients frequently lose their airway protection and their respiratory drive. Thus, they are likely to die as a result of airway obstruction by the flaccid tongue, aspiration of gastric contents into the tracheobronchial tree, or respiratory arrest.

Cardiovascular toxicity is also frequently encountered in poisoning. Hypotension, hypertension, dysrhythmias, hypoxemia, seizures, and acid-base disturbances all increase the likelihood of significant medical sequelae. A careful monitoring of these problems, many times with only symptomatic care given is all that is necessary. Management of poisoning requires thorough knowledge of how to treat hypoventilation, coma, shock, seizures, and psychosis.

THE GERIATRIC PATIENT

Profound physiologic changes occur as the human body ages and predispose the elderly to both adverse

TABLE 1–22. *Antidotes and their dosages*

Antidote	Use	Dosage	Chapter
N-Acetylcysteine	Acetaminophen	140 mg/kg orally (loading) 70 mg/kg every 4 hours, 17 doses (maintenance)	56
Activated charcoal	General adsorbent	10× by weight of ingested toxin	1,2,3
Atropine	Organophosphate and carbamate insecticides; symptomatic bradycardia	2 to 4 mg or more as needed	81
Botulism antitoxin	*Clostridium botulinum*	As necessary	72
Calcium gluconate	Calcium channel blockers; oxalates; ethylene glycol; fluorides; hydrofluoric acid	500 mg to 1 g	22,28,39
Deferoxamine	Iron	10 to 15 mg/kg/hr	64
Dextrose 50%	Hypoglycemia; altered mental state	Adult: 25 g	1
Digoxin Fab antibody fragment	Digoxin; Digitoxin; Oleander	As necessary	21
Dimercaprol (BAL)	Heavy metals	As necessary	60
Disodium EDTA	Heavy metals	As necessary	60
Epinephrine	Anaphylaxis	0.02–0.03 mg subcutaneously	9
Ethanol	Ethylene glycol; methanol	1 mL/kg of 95% solution, diluted (loading) 0.1 mL/kg/hour, diluted (maintenance)	39
Flumazenil	Benzodiazepines	0.2 mg IV repeated to 3 mg	48
Fuller's earth	Paraquat	As needed	82
Glucagon	β-Blockers; calcium channel blockers; hypoglycemia	1 to 5 mg IV	15,22
Magnesium sulfate	Cathartic	Adult: 15 to 30 g Child: 250 mg/kg	2
Methylene blue	Methemoglobinemia	1 to 2 mg/kg of 1% solution	35
Naloxone	Opioids	2 mg IV up to 10 mg	1,44,45
Oxygen	Carbon monoxide	100% nonrebreathing; HBO	32
Penicillamine	Heavy metals	As needed	60
Physostigmine	Antimuscarinics	Adult: 1 to 2 mg IV slowly Child: 0.5 mg or 0.02 mg/kg as needed	10
Pralidoxime	Organophosphate insecticides	1–2 g IV	81
Protamine sulfate	Heparin	As needed	
Pyridoxine	Isoniazid; *Gyromitra* mushroom	2–5 g IV slowly	68,70
Sodium bicarbonate	Tricyclics	1–3 Meq/kg	16
Sodium chloride	Bromide	As needed	1
Sodium nitrite	Cyanide	Adult: 300 mg Child: 10 mg/kg	33
Sodium thiosulfate	Cyanide	Adult: 12.5 g IV Child: 1.5 mL/kg	33
Snake antivenin	*Crotalidae* and *Elapidae*	As needed	74
Sorbitol	Cathartic	Adult: 100 to 150 mL of 70% solution Child: 1 to 2 mL/kg of 70% solution	1,2
Starch	Iodine	As needed	
Succimer	Lead	As needed	60,62
Thiamine	Thiamine deficiency; ethylene glycol	50–100 mg IV	38,40
Vitamin K1	Warfarin-like anticoagulants	As needed	79

drug reactions as well as a heightened sensitivity to drugs (Table 1–25). Contrary to the many myths regarding the aging process, physiologic changes with age can occur at dramatically different rates for different individuals (22). No easy and accurate way of assessing biologic age exists. For this reason, most studies on aging have arbitrarily defined elderly as an individual having a chronologic age of 65 years or over (46). This definition, although not perfect, is a practical choice (22). Although the aging human body becomes increasingly susceptible to illnesses and age-related changes, improved medical care has dramatically extended life expectancy (59).

The elderly exhibit a high incidence of reduced gastric acid secretion, which is associated with a delay in gastric emptying (59). Aging does not affect the absorption of most drugs, but once absorbed into the body, a drug may have very different kinetics in the elderly as compared with the younger adult (60).

The glomerular filtration rate decreases markedly with advancing age, resulting in decreased clearance of many medications. Renal function declines, on average, about

TABLE 1–23. *Contraindicated agents in toxicology*

Agent
Analeptic agents
Amphetamine
Bemegride
Caffeine
Nikethamide (Coramine)
Picrotoxin
Mineral oil cathartics
"Universal antidote"
Fluid extract of ipecac
Apomorphine
Nalorphine

TABLE 1–24. *Complications of overdose*

Complication
Respiratory
Airway occlusion
Aspiration
Hypoxemia
Pneumonia
Pulmonary edema
Respiratory depression
Cardiovascular
Dysrhythmias
Cardiovascular collapse
Hypotension
Neurologic
Cerebral edema
Central nervous system depression
Coma
Seizures
Renal
Myoglobinuria
Renal failure
Miscellaneous
Acid-base disorder
Decubitus ulcers
Hypothermia
Sepsis

TABLE 1–25. *Changes in the geriatric patient*

Change
Reduced gastric acid secretion
Delay in gastric emptying
Decreased glomerular filtration rate
Decreased renal function
Reduced hepatic metabolism
Decreased hepatic function
Increased incidence of multiple chronic illnesses

10% each decade after age 40 (46). This decreased clearance prolongs the half-lives of renally excreted drugs thereby increasing the toxicity.

Hepatic enzyme activity may decline, leading to reduced metabolism and longer plasma half-lives of many agents. Hepatic function also decreases due to reductions in both hepatic blood flow and activity of many enzymatic pathways including enzymatic oxidation, reduction, and hydrolysis (46).

The elderly are especially vulnerable to drug side effects and interactions for both physiologic and epidemiologic reasons. Also, geriatric patients frequently have multiple chronic diseases and therefore take many medications concurrently. Reduced homeostatic reserve generally renders them less tolerant of drug interactions than younger patients. It is imperative therefore to consider drug "overdose" in this group of patients presenting with an altered mental status and with no history of acute overdose. The altered pharmacokinetics of the elderly is further discussed in Chapter 6.

TABLE 1–26. *Partial listing of nontoxic substances*

Substance
Pharmaceuticals
Antacids
Antibiotics
Contraceptives
Corticosteroids
Laxatives
Mineral oil
Household products
Ballpoint pen inks
Bath oil
Bathtub floating toys
Candles
Crayons
Dehumidifying packets (silica gel)
Deodorants
Felt-tip pens
Magic markers
Matches
Pencils
Skin conditioners
Teething rings
Thermometers
Toothpaste
Soaps and detergents
Bar soap
Bath foam
Bubble bath soap
Fabric softeners
Hair conditioners
Cosmetics
Eye makeup
Hand lotion
Lipstick
Makeup
Perfume
Suntan preparations
Toilet water
Miscellaneous
Chalk
Clay
Lubricating oil
Motor oil
Paint (water-based)
Pistol caps
Play Doh
Starch
Sweetening agents

THE "NONTOXIC" INGESTION

Toxicity is a matter of degree, so that, in a sense, anything in excess may cause toxicity. The substances listed in Table 1–26 are those that are relatively nontoxic and for which no treatment may be indicated (33,61,62). Accidental ingestion of a substance known to be nontoxic may be dealt with by reassurance alone.

Simple antacids are generally nontoxic in a single acute ingestion. Antibiotics may, in general, cause diarrhea or an allergic reaction, but they do not typically cause any more serious medical problems.

Ballpoint pen inks of the black or blue variety contain tannic acid, gallic acid, and ferrous sulfate and are nontoxic (31). Purple, green, and red inks may contain aniline dyes, which are hazardous if taken in large amounts. Household bleach contains approximately 5% sodium hypochlorite and typically causes no more than erythema (62). Candles contain beeswax or paraffin, which are inert (61). Toy pistol caps and matches contain potassium chlorate, which in the amount that might be ingested is nontoxic (61). Chalk contains calcium carbonate (62). Corticosteroids do not cause toxicity from a single ingestion (63). Crayons of the AP and CP markings are nontoxic (62). Dehumidifying packets contain silica gel or charcoal.

Anionic and nonionic detergents are essentially nontoxic but are irritants and may cause vomiting and diarrhea (63). Dishwasher or laundry detergents may contain surfactants and builders, which may be very toxic. Soaps are mild irritants that may affect the skin, eyes, or gastrointestinal tract; nausea, vomiting, and diarrhea are common after their ingestion, but mucosal erosion or ulceration does not occur. Cationic detergents are the most toxic of the detergents.

Mineral oil may cause diarrhea. Oral contraceptives can be regarded as nontoxic, although withdrawal bleeding may occur. Water-based paints must be distinguished from oil-based paints, in which the hydrocarbon solvents may be dangerous.

Pencils contain no lead but do contain graphite and coloring agents. The ingredients in Play-Doh may be nontoxic, but the material may cause physical obstruction (62). Solvents and most perfumes contain alcohol, but the small amounts ingested are rarely enough to cause harm (63). Wet shampoos may cause nausea and vomiting, but dry shampoos may contain carbon tetrachloride, trichloroethylene, or other hydrocarbons that may result in systemic toxicity. Most shoe polishes contain no aniline dyes, but the ingestion of shoe polish may result in the development of methemoglobinemia. Teething rings and bathtub floating toys contain water and glycerin, which are not toxic; however, toxicity may develop from any pathogenic organisms that might be present. Toothpaste may contain stannous fluoride, which might cause nausea and vomiting.

PSYCHIATRIC EVALUATION

The depressed patient and the potentially suicidal patient are among the most common psychiatric conditions that face the emergency physician (64). Many times there is a negative attitude toward patients who have attempted suicide by overdose. This may be due to the physician's own natural feelings of frustration and hopelessness when confronted with a depressed, suicidal patient (23).

A patient who has attempted suicide may have a number of reasons for this behavior (65). Any patient in whom suicidal ideation or intent is suspected should be questioned directly in this area. Once a patient is assessed as being suicidal, he or she must not be left alone or sent home.

It is easy for emergency department personnel to become insensitive to the overdosed individual, who may be hard to handle and who may also be intoxicated with alcohol (66). Often it is forgotten that these individuals are in psychological distress. Although they may be difficult for emergency personnel to care for, these individuals need someone to talk with them and to try to calm them down (67). If the physician and nurse taking care of the patient can spend that extra time, it might make it easier for all concerned (23). Medical professionals should regard the event with empathy and as an overreaction to a short-lived crisis that usually resolves (68).

Demographics of Suicide

For every completed suicide, approximately eight people will attempt suicide (64). Although women attempt suicide more frequently than men, more men will be successful in their suicide attempt. Whereas men complete 80% of suicides, 60% to 70% of attempts are made by women (69). The elderly depressed patient represents a special challenge because they often have concurrent medical illnesses and are taking multiple medications. There has been a recent dramatic increase in the rate of suicide among teenagers and young adults, particularly in young men 15 to 24 years old (68).

For attempted suicide, overdosage of medication is by far the most common method employed, whereas for completed suicide, the use of firearms is most common (64).

Predictors of Suicide

Patients who are considered at high risk for suicide are those with a history of previous suicide attempts (Table 1–27). About 50% of the people who commit suicide have a history of previous attempts. Any history of a previous attempt, even if it is in the distant past, should be taken seriously, especially if potentially lethal means were employed (69).

TABLE 1–27. *Predictors and demographics of suicide*

Suicidal attempts
Women > men
Completed suicides
Men > women
Increased risk
Previous suicide attempt
History of depression
Divorced/widowed
Recent loss of spouse or employment
Social isolation

Although suicide is not always preceded by clinical depression, depression remains as one of the major risk factors for subsequent suicide. Marital status has a significant impact on suicide rates (70). Those who are divorced or widowed have the highest rates, followed by those who are single and finally those who are married (71). Recent significant loss of employment or a spouse, and social isolation are independent risk factors for suicide. Sleep is frequently disturbed. Insomnia with difficulty in falling asleep and early morning awakening are common although hypersomnia may also occur (72).

Leaving Against Medical Advice

If a potentially suicidal patient threatens to leave the ED before the evaluation is completed, all states have statutes permitting detention by physicians of individuals deemed dangerous to themselves or others (69). The patient should remain under close observation. In some cases physical or pharmacologic restraint may be needed. The legal justifications for the application of such restraint vary from state to state. The physician should become familiar with the commitment laws in that state, as well as any policies in place at the facility regarding restraining of patients. From a purely legal perspective, it is much easier to defend oneself against a charge of unwarranted hospitalization than it is if a patient is allowed to leave the hospital and later commits suicide (64).

Explaining that all states allow physicians to hospitalize patients who present a threat to themselves or others may encourage suicidal persons to opt for voluntary hospitalization (23). If necessary, the emergency physician can involuntarily admit a suicidal patient without fear of legal retribution.

In all cases, detailed documentation is necessary regarding the emergency intervention and treatment, and the rationale for selecting that particular intervention (70).

Evaluating the Suicidal Patient

The physical examination of the depressed or potentially suicidal patient should be directed toward uncovering possible organic causes for the depression (70). One should look for physical signs of substance abuse. A careful mental status examination should also be performed to detect an organic brain syndrome (23,64).

This examination should begin with a mental status examination with assessment of orientation to time, place, and person (73). Memory is also checked, including memory for recent events (74). Direct questioning of the patient concerning suicidal thoughts and ideation should be attempted. A patient who has attempted suicide may have a number of reasons for this behavior. It may represent a cry for help, the actual intent to die, an expression of anger, a means of conferring guilt on someone else, or an impulsive act of rage (69).

It is a lingering myth that the discussion of suicidal ideation with depressed patients will put the thought into their minds and contribute to the risk for subsequent suicide (64). Quite the opposite is in fact true; an open and honest discussion of suicide with an empathetic physician in the ED is often the first step toward treatment and recovery. Asking about suicide should be part of any review of systems, and will allow many covertly suicidal patients to voice their concerns. Most patients will not be insulted if such inquiry is made in a concerned and forthright manner (69). It is important to learn if the patient actually has the means to execute the plan, and to consider how lethal this method is likely to be. In general, the more detailed and lethal the plan, the greater the risk. Family and friends should also be interviewed, preferably in private and away from the patient.

Patient Disposition

Protecting patients until their crisis has passed is the central goal of emergency management (34). Suicidal episodes usually last only a few hours or days. Immediate treatment includes determining whether patients require hospitalization, obtaining psychiatric consultation, and laying the groundwork for long-term intervention (70). Protecting the patient from self-harm is the first priority. ED staff members never should leave suicidal patients unobserved. Someone must accompany these patients at all times, even if they need to use the rest room. All potentially harmful objects must be removed from the vicinity (70).

If a patient is to be discharged from the emergency department the first priority is that the patient is cleared from having any medical effects or complications of the overdose (64). The patient should then be cleared in a psychiatric perspective (Table 1–28). The above criteria may be useful, but in addition other criteria that must be fulfilled before considering discharge home from the ED include (a) the patient is not intoxicated, delirious, demented, or psychotic; (b) the patient no longer feels suicidal; (c) the acute precipitants to this crisis have been identified, addressed, and in some way resolved; (d) the

TABLE 1–28. *Psychiatric clearance*

Patient has normal mental status
Patient no longer feels suicidal
Identification of acute precipitants
Patient's agreement to return to emergency department
Removal of suicidal objects
Arrangement for early psychiatric follow-up
Evaluate patient's social support system
Physician believes that patient will comply

patient is able to promise to return to the ED before harming himself or herself if suicidal ideas recur; (e) any pills or firearms at home have been removed; (f) treatment for underlying psychiatric problems has been arranged; (g) the emergency physician believes the patient will follow through on the treatment plan (69).

The most important resource to evaluate is the patient's social supports. Meeting with family members and contacting collateral sources are key steps in deciding how reliable the patient may be and in corroborating the patient's account of his circumstances (64).

Because of the delayed response of many psychiatric disorders to treatment, psychiatric follow-up is especially important. An appointment should be available within 48 hours of discharge from the ED, with a clear plan for what the patient should do if the appointment falls through (69).

It would be best if the physician could follow up on the treatment plan to ensure it is carried out by or on behalf of the patient. If the patient is released with recommendations for further therapy, follow up with the patient to make sure that the therapy has been initiated. If not, consider the need for initiating commitment proceedings or taking other actions, such as warning others.

SUMMARY

The overdosed patient many times represents a diagnostic dilemma in that there may be no way to obtain an accurate history of the preceding events. It is therefore important to use the clues obtained from a thorough physical examination. The establishment of an intravenous line and continuous cardiac monitoring in the potentially overdosed patient is considered good prophylactic care should the patient deteriorate or have an underlying dysrhythmia secondary to the ingested compound (Table 1–29).

TABLE 1–29. *Summary of generalized treatment of the overdosed patient*

Peripheral intravenous line
Continuous cardiac monitoring
Vital sign monitoring
History, including route of administration
Physical examination
Appropriate laboratory studies (see Chapter 4)
Toxicology screen with selected blood levels
Complete blood count
Serum electrolytes
Blood urea nitrogen
Urinalysis
Administration of therapeutic agents
Glucose
Naloxone
Oxygen
Thiamine
Evacuation of stomach and intestine (see Chapter 2)
Administration of activated charcoal and cathartic (see Chapter 3)
Administration of an antidote if available
Psychiatric evaluation when medically cleared

REFERENCES

1. Spyker D, Minocha A: Toxicodynamic approach to management of the poisoned patient. *J Emerg Med* 1988;6:117–120.
2. Arena J: The clinical diagnosis of poisoning. *Pediatr Clin North Am* 1970;17:477–494.
3. Kaufman R, Levy S: Overdose treatment. *JAMA* 1974;227:411–416.
4. Ficarra H: Toxicologic states treated in an emergency department. *Clin Toxicol* 1980;17:1–43.
5. Sunshine I: Basic toxicology. *Pediatr Clin North Am* 1970;17:509–513.
6. Cheeley R, Joyce S: A clinical comparison of the performance of four blood glucose reagent strips. *Am J Emerg Med* 1990;8:11–15.
7. Oderda G, Klein-Schwartz W: General management of the poisoned patient. *Crit Care Q* 1982;4:1–18.
8. Saxena K, Kingston R: Acute poisoning—management protocol. *Postgrad Med* 1982;71:67–77.
9. Sullivan J, Rumack B, Peterson R: Management of the poisoned patient in the emergency department: poisonings and overdose. *Top Emerg Med* 1979;1:1–12.
10. Benowitz N, Rosenberg J, Becker C: Cardiopulmonary catastrophes in drug-overdosed patients. *Med Clin North Am* 1979;63:267–296.
11. Dine M, McGovern M: Intentional poisoning of children—an overlooked category or child abuse: report of seven cases and review of literature. *Pediatrics* 1982;70:32–35.
12. Gaudreault P, McCormick M, Lacouture P, et al: Poisoning exposures and use of ipecac in children less than 1 year old. *Ann Emerg Med* 1986;15:808–810.
13. Atwood S: The laboratory in the diagnosis and management of acetaminophen and salicylate intoxications. *Pediatr Clin North Am* 1980; 27:871–879.
14. Cashman T, Shirkey H: Emergency management of poisoning. *Pediatr Clin North Am* 1970;17:525–534.
15. Nicholson D: The immediate management of overdose. *Med Clin North Am* 1983;67:1279–1293.
16. Saylor J: Volume of a swallow: role of orifice size and viscosity. *Vet Hum Toxicol* 1987;29:79–82
17. Olson K, Pentel P, Kelley M: Physical assessment and differential diagnosis of the poisoned patient. *Med Toxicol* 1987;2:52–81.
18. Sieber F, Traystman R: Special issues: glucose and the brain. *Crit Care Med* 1992;20:104–111.
19. Callaham M: Hypoxic hazards of traditional paper bag rebreathing in hyperventilating patients. *Ann Emerg Med* 1989;18:622–628.
20. Reed M, Besunder J: Developmental pharmacology: ontogenic basis of drug disposition. *Pediatr Clin North Am* 1989;36:1053–1074.
21. Goldfrank L, Weisman R, Flomenbaumm N: Teaching the recognition of odors. *Ann Emerg Med* 1982;11:684–686.
22. Steinhart C, Pearson-Shaver A: Poisoning. *Crit Care Clin* 1988; 4:845–872
23. Zun L, Howes D: The mental status evaluation: application in the emergency department. *Am J Emerg Med* 1988;6:165–172.
24. Savitt D, Hawkins H, Roberts J: The radiopacity of ingested medications. *Ann Emerg Med* 1987;16:331–339.
25. Orlowski J, Julius C, Petras R, et al: The safety of intraosseous infu-

sions: risks of fat and bone marrow emboli to the lungs. *Ann Emerg Med* 1989;18:1062–1067
26. Goldberg M, Spector R, Park G, et al: An approach to the management of the poisoned patient. *Arch Intern Med* 1986;146q:1381–1385.
27. Stein L, Weiss S: Treatment of the drug-overdosed patient in the intensive care unit. *Anes Clin North Am* 1991;9:327–345.
28. Reed C, Driggs M, Foote C: Acute barbiturate intoxication: a study of 300 cases. *Ann Intern Med* 1952; 37:290–292.
29. Atkin S, Dasmahapatra A, Jaker M, et al: Fingerstick glucose determination in shock. *Ann Intern Med* 1991:114:1020–1024.
30. Shuster M, Chong J: Pharmacologic intervention in prehospital care: a critical appraisal. *Ann Emerg Med* 1989;18:192–196.
31. Hoffman J, Schriger D, Luo J: The empiric use of naloxone in patients with altered mental status: a reappraisal. *Ann Emerg Med* 1991;20:246–252.
32. Goldfrank L: Medical toxicology. *JAMA* 1992;268:375–376.
33. Mofenson H, Greensher J: The nontoxic ingestion. *Pediatr Clin North Am* 1970;17:583–590.
34. Fine J, Goldfrank L: Update in medical toxicology. *Pediatr Clin North Am* 1992;39:1031–1051.
35. Browning R, Olson D, Stueven H, et al: 50% dextrose: antidote or toxin? *Ann Emerg Med* 1990;19:683–687.
36. Pulsinelli W, Waldman S, Rawlinson D, et al: Moderate hyperglycemia augments ischemic brain damage: a neuropathologic study in the rat. *Neurology* 1982;32:1239–1246.
37. Longstreth W, Inui T: High blood glucose level on hospital admission and poor neurological recovery after cardiac arrest. *Ann Neurol* 1984;15:59–63.
38. Matchar D, Divine G, Heyman A, et al: The influence of hyperglycemia on outcome of cerebral infarction. *Ann Intern Med* 1992;117:449–456.
39. Candelise L, Landi G, Orazio E, et al: Prognostic significance of hyperglycemia in acute stroke. *Arch Neurol* 1985;42:661–663.
40. Stephen J, Grant R, Yeh C: Anaphylaxis from administration of intravenous thiamine. *Am J Emerg Med* 1992:10:61–63.
41. Wrenn K, Murphy F, Slovis C: A toxicity study of parenteral thiamine hydrochloride. *Ann Emerg Med* 1989;18:867–870.
42. Marx J: The varied faces of Wernicke's encephalopathy. *J Emerg Med* 1985;321:442–454.
43. Brett A, Rothschild N, Gray R, et al: Predicting the clinical course in intentional drug overdose. *Arch Intern Med* 1987;147:133–137.
44. Carlton F: Toxidromes for altered mental status. *Top Emerg Med* 1991;13:46–53.
45. Vance M, Selden B, Clark R: Optimal patient position for transport and initial management of toxic ingestions. *Ann Emerg Med* 1992;21:243–246
46. Nolan L, O'Malley K: Prescribing for the elderly: part II. *J Am Geriatr Soc* 1988;36:245–254.
47. Thomas H, Schwartz E, Petrilli R: Droperidol versus haloperidol for chemical restraint of agitated and combative patients. *Ann Emerg Med* 1992;21:407–413.
48. Brickman K, Krupp K, Rega P, et al: Typing and screening of blood from intraosseous access. *Ann Emerg Med* 1992;21:414–417.
49. Grisham J, Hastings C: Bone marrow aspirate as an accessible and reliable source for critical laboratory studies. *Ann Emerg Med* 1991; 20:1121–1124.
50. Woodard J, Shannon M, Lacouture P, et al: Serum magnesium concentrations after repetitive magnesium cathartic administration. *Am J Emerg Med* 1990;8:297–300.
51. Krenzelok E, Lush R: Container residue after the administration of aqueous activated charcoal products. *Am J Emerg Med* 1991: 9:144–146.
52. Conner C, Robertson N, Murphrey K, et al: Rational use of emergency antidotes: poisonings and overdose. *Top Emerg Med* 1979;1:27–41.
53. Meredith T, Caisley J, Volans G: Emergency drugs: agents used in the treatment of poisoning. *Br Med J* 1984;289:742–747.
54. Litovitz T: The anecdotal antidotes. *Emerg Med Clin North Am* 1984;2:145–158.
55. Matthew H: Acute poisoning: some myths and misconceptions. *Br Med J* 1971;1:519–522.
56. Wright N: Common errors in the management of poisoning. *J R Coll Physicians Lond* 1980;14:114–116.
57. Schlager D, Sanders A, Wiggins D, et al: Ultrasound for the detection of foreign bodies. *Ann Emerg Med* 1991;20:189–191.
58. Chaikin H: Rhabdomyolysis secondary to drug overdose and prolonged coma. *South Med J* 1980;73:990–994.
59. Greenblatt D, Harmatz J, Engelhardt N, et al: Sensitivity to triazolam in the elderly. *N Engl J Med* 1991;324:1691–1698.
60. Scott R, Mitchell M: Aging, alcohol, and the liver. *J Am Geriatr Soc* 1988;36:255–265.
61. Done A: Poisoning from common household products. *Pediatr Clin North Am* 1970;17:569–581.
62. Mofenson H, Greensher J, Caraccio T: Ingestions considered nontoxic. *Emerg Med Clin North Am* 1984; 2:159–174.
63. Henry J. Wiseman H: Non-poisons. *Br Med J* 1984;289:240–241.
64. Hofmann D, Dubovsky S: Depression and suicide assessment. *Emerg Med Clin North Am* 1991;9:107–121.
65. Dilsaver S: The mental status examination. *Am Fam Physician* 1990; 41:1489–1496
66. Jorden R: Initial evaluation of the patient with altered mental status. *Top Emerg Med* 1991;13:1–9.
67. Wagemaker H, Lippman S, Cade R: Acutely psychotic patients: a treatment approach. *South Med J* 1985;78:833–837.
68. McAlpine D: Suicide: recognition and management. *Mayo Clin Proc* 1987;62:778–781.
69. Buzan R, Weissberg M: Suicide: risk factors and therapeutic considerations in the emergency department. *J Emerg Med* 1992;10:335–343.
70. Dwyer B: Strategies for recognizing and managing suicidal patients. *Emerg Med Rep* 1993;14:91–98.
71. Pulsinelli W, Levy D, Sigsbee B, et al: Increased damage after ischemic stroke in patients with hyperglycemia with or without established diabetes mellitus. *Am J Med* 1983;74:540–544.
72. Hurlbut K: Drug-induced psychoses. *Emerg Med Clin North Am* 1991;9:107–121.
73. Cavanaugh S: Psychiatric emergencies. *Med Clin North Am* 1986; 70:1185–1202.
74. Tintinalli J, Peacock F, Wright M: Emergency medical evaluation of psychiatric patients. *Ann Emerg Med* 1994;23:859–871.

ADDITIONAL SELECTED REFERENCES

Barnes J: Toxic substances and the nervous system. *Sci Basis Med* 1969; 183–201.

Cereda J, Scott J, Quigley E: Endoscopic removal of pharmacobezoar of slow release theophylline. *Br Med J* 1986;293:1143.

Comstock E, Stewart E: Current literature on medical toxicology. *Clin Toxicol* 1979;15:91–95.

Done A: For particulars on poisons. *Emerg Med* 1982; 14:102–104.

Eriksson M, Catz C, Yaffe S: Drugs and pregnancy. *Clin Obstet Gynecol* 1973;16:199–224.

Fazen L, Lovejoy F, Crone R: Acute poisoning in a children's hospital: a 2-year experience. *Pediatrics* 1986;77:144–151.

Gilles C, Ford P, Lovejoy F, et al: Management of pediatric poisoning. *Pediatr Nurs* 1980;6:33–44.

Gossel T, Wuest J: The right first aid for poisoning. *RN* 1981;44:73–75.

Keller E: Poisoning in children. *Postgrad Med* 1979; 65:177–186.

Walton W: An evaluation of the Poison Prevention Packaging Act. *Pediatrics* 1982;69:363–370.

Weisman R, Price D, Wald P: Outpatient management of acute and chronic poisoning. *Primary Care* 1986;13:151–156.

White L, Driggers D, Wardinsky T: Poisoning in childhood and adolescence: a study of 111 cases admitted to a military hospital. *J Fam Pract* 1980;11:27–31.

Woolf A, Lewander W, Gilippone G, et al: Prevention of childhood poisoning: efficacy of an educational program carried out in an emergency clinic. *Pediatrics* 1987;80:359–363.

Yaffe S, Sjoeqvist F, Alvan F: Pharmacological principles in the management of accidental poisoning. *Pediatr Clin North Am* 1970;17:495–507.

CHAPTER 2

Methods of Preventing Absorption

Absorption into the blood is significantly influenced by the route of administration. In addition to the intravenous route, which bypasses the absorption process, the important routes of administration are oral, inhalational, topical, transdermal, subcutaneous, intramuscular, and buccal or sublingual (Table 2–1). Less commonly, the intra-arterial, intrathecal, and rectal routes may be used.

The attempt at preventing absorption of a drug or toxin is of utmost priority in lessening the likelihood that subsequent toxicity will ensue (1). This chapter discusses the various methods of preventing absorption of drugs and toxins. The major areas of discussion cover the role of skin decontamination, gastric emptying techniques, activated charcoal, cathartics, and activated charcoal as the sole agent of decontamination in treating the poisoned patient.

SKIN DECONTAMINATION

Systemic drug absorption through the skin is highly dependent on the site, and the condition of the skin. Important factors include skin thickness, vascularity, and whether the skin is intact, broken, or inflamed. There are a number of toxins that are absorbed through the skin or directly injure the skin. Skin decontamination in select cases should therefore not be overlooked because it may be the only method available to prevent further absorption of the toxin or physically remove it. Decontamination may not only be useful but in certain circumstances may be lifesaving. As an example, the organophosphates can be absorbed through the intact skin, and unless decontamination is performed continuous absorption will occur. Other toxins for which decontamination is both necessary and beneficial are listed in Table 2–2.

Skin decontamination may be carried out after attending to life-threatening problems. Decontamination may be performed with at least two soap-and-water washes. For most agents, protective clothing (gloves, gown, and mask) should be used to protect personnel from being contaminated.

GASTROINTESTINAL TRACT

The oral route is most commonly used because of its convenience and, for most, drugs, efficiency of absorption. However, the acid and enzymes secreted by the patient and the biochemical activity of the resident microbiologic flora also have the capacity to destroy some drugs before they are absorbed.

The primary site of absorption for most medications is the small intestine because of its large surface area, thin epithelium, and low electrical resistance. Even drugs that are highly water-soluble or readily cross cell membranes in an acid medium, such as ethanol and salicylate, have only limited absorption directly through the gastric mucosa because of its unique characteristics, particularly its much smaller absorptive surface area (2). Factors that would delay gastric emptying into the small intestine should, therefore, decrease the rate of systemic absorption and limit the onset of potential toxic effects of ingested drug.

Many factors influence the rate of gastric emptying and, consequently, may affect the rate of drug absorption in the poisoned patient. Many of these factors cannot be controlled (presence of food, alcohol, other drugs, preexisting illness, etc.).

Delayed Gastrointestinal Absorption

It is common with a drug overdose for delayed absorption to occur either because of the formation of a large,

TABLE 2–1. *Potential routes of drug administration*

Buccal
Inhalational
Intra-arterial
Intramuscular
Intrathecal
Intravenous
Oral
Rectal
Subcutaneous
Sublingual
Transdermal

TABLE 2–2. *Toxins for which skin decontamination is effective*

Aniline dyes
Caustic agents
Cyanide
Dimethyl sulfoxide (DMSO)
Hydrocarbons
Mace (CS, CN gas)
Methanol
Pesticides
Radiation

poorly soluble drug mass or a drug-induced decrease in gastric motility. As an example, the absorption of aspirin with normal dosing is completed within 1 hour; however, in an overdose situation, absorption may be delayed for more than 6 hours. In addition, sustained release preparations may substantially delay peak drug effects for as much as 36 hours after ingestion. Narcotic analgesics directly increase the tone of gastric smooth muscle, interfere with normal peristalsis, and delay gastric emptying. Drugs with antimuscarinic activity such as atropine and antidepressants reduce gastric motility and cause gastric relaxation.

GASTRIC EMPTYING

Gastric emptying was recommended as a therapeutic intervention for acute self-poisoning as early as the 1800s (3). In the case of an overdose by ingestion, the generally accepted standard of care for the patient continues to be an attempt at preventing further absorption of the toxin by gastric emptying with gastric lavage, followed by the administration of activated charcoal and a cathartic (4–6). Other methods of decreasing gastrointestinal absorption have been whole gut lavage and removal of material by surgical or endoscopic intervention (7). This has occasionally been reported for foreign body removal, bezoars, or gastric concretions (1,8,9). Gastrointestinal decontamination is currently one of the most controversial areas of medical toxicology (1,8–10).

In the last few years, many of the traditional methods of gastrointestinal decontamination have been challenged as being ineffective and possibly dangerous (3,5,6). Yet, because of inconsistent protocols and differences in lavage technique among the various studies, there is great confusion in the current medical literature (10).

EMETICS

Many methods have at one time been advocated to induce vomiting. Most have been discarded because evidence revealed that they were either potentially toxic or unreliable (11). Although syrup of ipecac is considered the only acceptable emetic, the relative usefulness of other emetics is also briefly discussed below.

Syrup of Ipecac

Syrup of ipecac is the emetic of choice in both children over the age of 6 months and in adults (4,11–13). Although ipecac has been known for many years as a potent emetic, its common use as an antidotal agent in the treatment of accidental ingestion of poisons began in the 1960s. Ipecac is the dried root of *Cephaelis ipecacuanha*, which is found in South and Central America (1). The principal alkaloids of ipecac are emetine and cephaline (14). Emetine, which constitutes more than one half of the total alkaloid, is cardiotoxic, while cephaline causes nausea and vomiting (14). During the last few years, ipecac syrup has been prepared from powdered ipecac, not from the fluid extract that had been reported as the source of toxicity. The concentration of the alkaloid in the syrup is one fourth that of the powdered ipecac. In the United States, ipecac is available without a prescription in 15- and 30-mL bottles. In two thirds of the countries in Europe, it is available only by prescription (15). Fluid extract of ipecac, 14 times more potent than ipecac syrup, is no longer available in the United States (16).

Mechanism of Action

Ipecac has a dual mechanism by which it causes an emesis; it acts both locally in the stomach and has a delayed effect on the chemoreceptor trigger zone located in the floor of the fourth ventricle (1,14). The chemoreceptor trigger zone then activates the vomiting center located in the reticular formation, resulting in an emesis (14,17). Early vomiting is due to the direct local irritant action of ipecac on the gastric mucosa, whereas late vomiting is a result of central stimulation of the vomiting center (18,19).

Dosage

The therapeutic dose of syrup of ipecac for an adult is 30 mL. The suggested dose for children 6 months of age and older is 10–15 mL. This dose may be repeated in 20 to 30 minutes if necessary. Recently, it has been shown that an initial dose of 30 mL in children produces an emesis significantly faster than the traditional dose. In addition, when 30 mL of syrup of ipecac is administered no repeat doses of the emetic may be necessary (12).

Adjunctive Methods

After the initial dose of syrup of ipecac is administered, ingestion of fluids should be encouraged to empty the stomach more adequately: 12 to 16 ounces is recommended for an adult and 4 to 8 ounces for a child (1,20). Children younger than one year should drink 15 mL/kg body weight of water (16). Larger volumes of fluids may be counterproductive because they may promote more rapid gastric emptying, placing the ingested toxin beyond retrieval. There also does not appear to be any benefit from walking compared with remaining stationary at bedrest (21). In addition, patient position after ipecac syrup administration does not affect results (16).

There is no difference in the speed at which emesis occurs if the fluid is administered before or after syrup of ipecac (1). Although almost any available nontoxic liquid may be administered, milk is not recommended because it has been shown to increase significantly the time before onset of vomiting (1,14,22,23). Carbonated beverages do not appear to have an adverse effect on the onset or amount of emesis (24).

Repeating Ipecac

If the patient has received ipecac but has not had an effective emesis in 15 to 20 minutes, it is advisable to attempt to stimulate the gag reflex with a tongue blade before administering a second dose (1). This stimulation may cause the desired emesis. In general, 60% of patients will have an emesis within the first 15 minutes and 90% will have an emesis within the first 30 minutes (1,25–27). Although not recommended, even ipecac that is expired produces an emesis in a comparable period and is not accompanied by more severe side effects (1,28).

Safety of Ipecac in Children

Syrup of ipecac is safe to use in children older than 6 months of age and, when used properly, should not exacerbate the patient's condition (12,15,17,25). The use of ipecac syrup in infants younger than 6 months of age is generally not advocated because of risk of aspiration, although there are no data to substantiate this concern (1,29,30).

Ipecac and Antiemetics

Many of the phenothiazine derivatives are effective antiemetics and are believed to act centrally by depression of the vomiting center in the medulla. Ipecac has been shown, however, to be effective for these antiemetics, probably as a result of its direct irritant action on the gastrointestinal tract (12,14,25,26). Thus, the same initial dose should be administered (1). If the patient has had a documented antiemetic overdose and there has been no effective emesis within a reasonable period of time, the ipecac and the ingested material should be retrieved by means of gastric lavage.

Ipecac and Activated Charcoal

Although it has been assumed that activated charcoal and syrup of ipecac should not be administered at the same time because of the adsorption of ipecac by the charcoal (1,31), it has been shown that a 10-minute interval between the administration of 60 mL of syrup of ipecac and activated charcoal prevents the inhibition of the emetic properties of ipecac and allows a successful emesis to occur (32,33). Nevertheless, more documentation as to whether conventional amounts of ipecac would also be effective is necessary before this method is advocated.

Disadvantages of Ipecac

The prolonged time to emesis is the major disadvantage of ipecac syrup because the delay results in continued absorption of the ingested toxin (1). In addition, it may delay the administration of activated charcoal. Because prolonged vomiting after administration of syrup of ipecac has been a frequent problem, attempts have been made to shorten the time of emesis. The intravenous use of prochlorperazine (Compazine) as an effective and safe treatment has been described (34), but because experience with this method is lacking, it can be neither advocated nor condemned. One potential disadvantage of this regimen might be the potential side effects associated with this antiemetic.

Ipecac should be avoided with specific toxins with rapid absorption that can lead to early central nervous system disturbance or cardiovascular dysfunction. These are best treated by immediate removal from the gastrointestinal tract by lavage. Examples of such toxins are strychnine, tricyclic antidepressants, cyanide, camphor, propoxyphene, the rapidly acting barbiturates, and toxic liquids (8).

Toxicity of Ipecac

Clinically significant toxicity from the use of syrup of ipecac is unusual, and there are few reports of serious toxicity directly attributable to the use of the emetic in recommended doses (12,14,20,35–37). Side effects, including diarrhea and mild drowsiness, are minimal with therapeutic doses (Table 2–3) (1,20,26,38–41). Rare reports of gastrointestinal side effects from the fluid extract include hemorrhage and ulceration of the small bowel, gastritis, and a Mallory-Weiss syndrome (42). Diarrhea due to increased peristalsis caused by emetine

TABLE 2–3. *Potential toxic effects of ipecac*

Acute administration
General
Emesis
Drowsiness (mild)
Gastrointestinal
Mallory-Weiss tears
Diarrhea
Vomiting
Chronic administration
Neuromuscular
Weakness
Muscle aches
Muscle tenderness
Tremor
Seizure
Cardiovascular
Electrocardiographic abnormalities
Atrial premature contractions
ST-T wave changes
QRS prolongation
Prolongation of PR interval
Cardiomyopathy

as well as to local irritation of the mucosa of the gastrointestinal tract has also been noted (1).

Recommendation

Ipecac Use in the Emergency Department

Available evidence suggests that ipecac-induced emesis in the emergency department setting does not provide any clinical advantage in the treatment of poisonings by ingestion (43). In fact, ipecac administration may prolong the emergency department stay, may result in an increased rate of complications, and may delay the administration of more effective therapy (16). There has therefore been a noticeable and consistent trend in emergency departments toward limiting use of syrup of ipecac as a first stop in gastric emptying (10).

Ipecac Use in the Home

In the home setting, where ipecac can be given immediately after ingestion, there is some limited evidence of possible efficacy of ipecac syrup because of its convenience and ready availability within minutes of the ingestion (16). Until further studies confirm or refute its usefulness, ipecac syrup will continue to be recommended for home administration. The benefit of keeping ipecac in the home appears to clearly outweigh the risks. Home administration of ipecac has been associated with decreased time from ingestion to therapy and fewer emergency room visits for ingestions. Giving ipecac without professional consultation seems to be uncommon (44).

Chronic Ipecac Toxicity

General Considerations

Ipecac alkaloid toxicity primarily involves the gastrointestinal tract and cardiovascular and neuromuscular systems (45). In very large doses, when fluid extract was mistakenly given in place of syrup of ipecac, or with chronic administration of the syrup, reports of central nervous system depression and of cardiovascular effects, including tachycardia, hypotension, and electrocardiographic abnormalities have been noted (17).

Syrup of ipecac may be chronically abused by patients with anorexia nervosa and bulimia nervosa (20,39). This has resulted in cumulative toxicity from the various alkaloids in ipecac. Syrup of ipecac has been implicated as the causal factor in the deaths of several women with bulimia and anorexia who used it on a long-term basis to induce vomiting after eating binges (46). This drug is chosen because it is a relatively inexpensive, nonprescription item that is effective in producing an emesis (20). Patients with these eating disorders may use the drug daily in doses that are higher than recommended and over a long period of time (47). Because the rate of excretion of emetine is slow, the ingestion of daily oral doses may produce an accumulation that approaches the single fatal parenteral dose (20).

Neuromuscular Manifestations of Chronic Toxicity

The neuromuscular manifestations of ingestion of emetine are weakness, aching, tenderness, and stiffness of the skeletal muscles, particularly those in the proximal extremities and the neck (17,39). Myopathy has developed in patients who chronically used excessive doses for weight reduction (47). This has been found to be reversible unless complicated by cardiovascular toxicity (22,46,48). Other signs of neuromuscular toxicity include skeletal muscular weakness, tremor, and generalized tonic-clonic seizures. The neuromuscular toxicities may be caused by a block of norepinephrine release by acetylcholine at adrenergic nerve terminals (Table 2–3) (49)

Cardiovascular Manifestations of Chronic Toxicity

Signs of cardiovascular toxicity from emetine include electrocardiographic abnormalities such as alterations in the QRS duration, ST and T wave alterations, prolongation of the PR interval, and atrial prematurity (39). This is due to decreased metabolic activity, which results in a decrease in contractile function in the myocardium (17,20,50). The delay in clinical signs is attributable to the time required for the inhibition of the biosynthesis of new contractile proteins.

TABLE 2–4. *Contraindicated methods to induce emesis*

Apomorphine
Copper sulfate
Detergents and soaps
Mechanical induction
Mustard water
Salt water

Pneumomediastinum and retropneumoperitoneum have also been reported (36,46). Both these events occur after prolonged vomiting. Syrup of ipecac, when used in appropriate doses, should not cause any of the above problems.

Methods Not Advocated

There are several methods of inducing emesis that are contraindicated (Table 2–4).

Mechanical Induction

An attempt at mechanical pharyngeal stimulation with a finger or other blunt object is a simple method that may produce an emesis, but the volume produced is small. This method has been ineffective for adequate retrieval of toxin and has the potential of causing physical harm; therefore its use is not recommended (12,50).

Salt Water

At one time salt water was recommended as an emetic, and although an effective emesis may occur, serious side effects have been found with its use (1). Electrolyte disorders, such as fatal hypernatremia, seizures, and intestinal damage, have occurred. Because of the nonuniformity of the product and the side effects, salt water is considered too dangerous and is therefore contraindicated.

Copper Sulfate

Copper sulfate is an irritant to the gastrointestinal tract and typically will cause an emesis. When absorbed, however, copper sulfate has the ability to produce severe renal and hepatic toxicity (1,51). Copper sulfate has led to elevated serum copper levels, raising the possibility of copper toxicity. Because of its local corrosive effect, which has caused mucosal erosions and a hemorrhagic gastroenteritis, and its potential for systemic toxicity, its use is also contraindicated (52).

Mustard Water

Mustard water is difficult to induce patients to drink. In addition it is unreliable as an emetic, and time should not be wasted with its administration.

Detergents and Soaps

The emetic response to soaps is thought to be the result of gastrointestinal irritation rather than stimulation of the chemoreceptor trigger zone. Although anionic detergents (soaps) may be useful in causing emesis and have a rather quick emetic response (1,19,53), confusion may arise as to what product should be used and the more corrosive detergents may be easily mistaken for anionic soaps. This confusion might lead to a more dangerous detergent being administered. For example, liquid soaps used for dishes (such as Palmolive) may only cause nausea and vomiting, whereas dishwasher soaps (such as Electrosol and Cascade) have corrosive properties due to the alkaline builders such as the sodium salts of phosphates, carbonates, metasilicates, and silicates. The general pH ranges of automatic dishwasher detergents is from 10.5 to 12.0 (54). Industrial strength detergents and the new liquid products may have pH values as high as 13.0. This confusion may be even more dangerous now that liquid dishwasher soaps are available. For this reason, the use of soaps as a routine measure for inducing emesis should be avoided.

Apomorphine

Apomorphine is a morphine congener prepared by reacting morphine with a strong mineral acid (1). It induces emesis in a relatively short period of time by stimulation of the chemoreceptor trigger zone in the medulla oblongata. It is inactive if administered orally (14).

The advantage of this drug is that it can be administered intramuscularly to an uncooperative patient who would refuse orally administered ipecac. The usual dose is 0.1 mg/kg to a maximum of 6 mg in adults or 0.07 mg/kg in children (1). It offers a high degree of success, with a latency period averaging 5 minutes, and promotes a forceful emesis with reflux of the proximal small bowel contents (14). There is also a high incidence of serious side effects relating to the drug's narcotic-like action, however, including central nervous system (CNS) depression, apnea, and hypotension in previously nondepressed individuals (14). In addition, these individuals may have a variable response to the narcotic antagonist naloxone.

Apomorphine is unstable in solution and must be prepared for injection by placing a tablet in a syringe, dissolving it in normal saline, and then sterilizing the solution before use. With so many potential dangers and disadvantages, its use is not recommended (55,56).

GASTRIC LAVAGE

Gastric lavage is another method for removing substances from the stomach that has been described in detail in the medical literature as early as 1819, but its utility has been debated vigorously ever since. Gastric lavage can be considered essentially equal to the use of syrup of ipecac in the amount of material retrieved (57), although this has long been an area of controversy, with many studies showing conflicting results (8,11,25,57–60). If gastric lavage is used, it should be accomplished with the largest tube that can be passed through the oropharynx. An orogastric tube 26 to 28F or larger for children and 32 to 40F for adults should be chosen (8,61,62). The Ewald tube, a soft rubber tube with a single distal aperture, is considered less effective than other tubes with additional lateral holes (8). The tube should therefore have a number of lateral holes (1). Large-bore oral tubes increase the return of pill fragments, decrease the likelihood of tube occlusion, and increase the rapidity with which gastric lavage is performed.

Technique of Lavage

The technique of lavage involves placing the patient in the Trendelenburg, left lateral decubitus position with knees flexed, which should give maximal abdominal wall relaxation and maximal gastric emptying.(1,8,59,63). In addition, this position has been suggested to reduce the risk of aspiration should vomiting occur (64).

The lavage tube should be advanced gently. The tube should be preferably placed through the mouth because large-bore tubes passed through the nose can damage the mucosa or turbinates, resulting in epistaxis (16). After it is inserted, it is essential to determine that it is correctly placed before initiating the lavage. Proper location of the tube in the stomach can be assessed by auscultating the stomach while injecting air into the tube (8). Coughing, cyanosis, or respiratory distress may indicate that the tube has entered the larynx. Aspiration of the stomach contents confirms its proper location (10). If the patient has demonstrated an intact gag reflex, lavage may be performed without prior endotracheal intubation. If the patient has lost the gag reflex, and this is associated with CNS depression, then adequate protection of the airway should be performed before lavage.

Typically, a passive lavage system can be used. The stomach should be completely aspirated until no return is obtained (8). The choice of lavage fluid is based on the patient's age. In an adult, tap water can be safely used

TABLE 2–5. *Substances causing concretions (acronym: BIG MESS)*

B	Barbiturates
I	Iron
G	Glutethimide
M	Meprobamate
E	Extended-release theophylline
SS	Salicylates

(17,65) because there are no resultant changes in serum electrolytes or serum osmolality (63). Children under 5 years require normal saline to avoid possible free water absorption and dilutional hyponatremia (16).

Lavage is then begun with 50 mL of warm tap water instilled into the stomach and retrieved. After repeating this procedure, 200-mL to 300-mL aliquots of warm saline or warm tap water are then flushed down the large-bore tube and retrieved either by suction or by lowering the tube to the floor and siphoning out the effluent (63). For pediatric patients, the amount of saline during each lavage is 10 mL/kg (1,8). For adults, larger aliquots (300 to 500 mL) are preferable to smaller aliquots (50 mL) in that the distension of the stomach can inhibit stomach contractions, and the larger aliquots tend to open up the rugae in the stomach so that pills, pill fragments, or other toxic substances in the rugal folds are exposed (1,63). Warm lavage solution is recommended because it can increase the rate of dissolution of pills while also decreasing gastric peristalsis, thereby decreasing the potential loss of medication through the pylorus. The patient is lavaged until there is a clear return, and for a greater margin of safety 1 or 2 L more lavage solution should then be instilled and retrieved. Generally, 5 to 20 L of fluid is required (1).

A left upper quadrant massage is recommended when there is the possibility of a drug that can cause concretions (Table 2–5) (65). The massage is an attempt to loosen existing or potential concretions. Although this method is empiric and anecdotal, there does not appear to be any harm associated with its use, and there is good possibility for benefit.

Complications of Lavage

Although rare, there is the possibility for significant complications from an attempt at lavage (61,66). Laryngospasm, cyanosis, aspiration of stomach contents, gastric erosion, and esophageal tears may be caused by the lavage tube (Table 2–6) (1,8,67). Epistaxis may occur after gastric lavage if the tube has been placed through the nose. Mediastinitis can be a potentially devastating complication (8). A case of legionnaire's disease caused by *Legionella pneumophila* was documented after an 18-year-old male patient aspirated postgastric lavage fluid when tap water was used (68).

TABLE 2–6. *Complications of lavage*

Aspiration
Cyanosis
Gastric erosion
Epistaxis
Esophageal tears
Laryngospasm
Mediastinitis

CONTRAINDICATIONS FOR IPECAC OR LAVAGE

In addition to the complications that are possible from the use of lavage or ipecac, there are also contraindications for their use (15). Neither should be used to retrieve any agent that might burn the gastrointestinal tract, because an additional burn may occur. In the absence of other neurologic signs and symptoms, an absent gag reflex should not be considered a contraindication to emesis because a demonstrable gag reflex is not present in a significant percentage of normal people (1). Ipecac should not be administered, however, to a patient who has lost the gag reflex, and the patient should only be lavaged after the airway has been protected with a cuffed endotracheal tube. In addition, hydrocarbons such as kerosene, gasoline, coal oil, fuel oil, paint thinner, cleaning fluid, and furniture polish should, for the most part, be left in the gastrointestinal tract (Table 2–7).

TABLE 2–7. *Substances for which ipecac or lavage are contraindicated*

Caustic agents
Acids
Alkalis
Ammonia
Automatic dishwasher detergent
Coffee pot cleaners
Drain cleaners
Hair bleaches
Lye
Metal cleaners
Mildew removers
Oven cleaners
Rust removers
Toilet bowl cleaners
Wart removers
Petroleum distillates
Furniture polish
Gasoline
Kerosene
Lighter fluid
Linseed oil
Mineral spirits
Naphtha
Oils
Paint and lacquer thinners
Petroleum solvents
Pine oil cleaners
Turpentine
Wood stains

WHOLE BOWEL IRRIGATION

A method of bowel preparation for barium enemas was developed in the mid 1970s (69). This technique consisted of perfusing the gastrointestinal tract with large volumes of electrolyte solution through a nasogastric tube (70), which induced a copious diarrhea and was found to be a quick, safe, and an effective means of cleansing the gut (71). Early on, solutions that contained saline, potassium chloride, and sodium bicarbonate were used. Because of the sodium load, and the fact that this solution was absorbed, electrolyte problems ensued (72).

Whole bowel irrigation (WBI), as it is now called, has been suggested as a gastrointestinal decontamination procedure (73–77). The lavage solutions currently in clinical use contain polyethylene glycol and sodium sulfate as the chief osmotic agents. This specific solution was formulated to prevent the net absorption or secretion of fluid or electrolytes across the gastrointestinal epithelium (77).

Whole bowel irrigation has been suggested for large ingestions of toxic substances, for patients presenting hours after ingestion when much of the drug is presumed to have passed the pylorus, for ingestions of delayed-release preparations, for tablet bezoars, and for drugs such as iron and lithium that are not adsorbed by activated charcoal (Table 2–8) (70). Whole bowel irrigation has also been successfully used in decontamination of patients attempting to conceal packets of controlled substances (10). Although the effects that large volumes of fluids may have on leaking or poorly wrapped condoms or drug packets are of concern, there is not data to document that WBI will accelerate dissolution or rupture (78).

TABLE 2–8. *Whole bowel irrigation*

Possible indications
Concretions (Bezoars)
Delayed presentation from ingestion
Delayed release preparations
Drugs not absorbed by activated charcoal
Iron
Lithium
Large ingestions of toxic substances
Packets of controlled substances
Patient on commode
Instill 1–2 L/hr polyethylene glycol
Adverse effects
Abdominal cramps
Diarrhea
Vomiting
Contraindications
Gastrointestinal hemorrhage
Ileus
Obstruction
Perforation

Technique of Whole Bowel Irrigation

Proponents of this method suggest seating the patient on a commode and instilling of 1 to 2 L of polyethylene glycol electrolyte (Golytely, Colyte) solution per hour, either orally or through a gastric tube (74). This has been recommended for adult patients and children older than 5 years. Administration rates of 150 to 500 mL/hr in children up to age 5 years have been used (16). The solution is administered until rectal discharge has the same appearance as the ingested fluid. This may take from 6 to 12 hours (16).

Adverse Effects

Adverse effects include profuse diarrhea, vomiting, and abdominal cramping. Hyperchloremia has also been reported (16). Additional drawbacks of WBI are that it is time-consuming and requires that patients be alert, cooperative, and able to sit on a bedside commode or toilet for up to several hours while having protracted diarrhea (16).

Contraindications to the use of WBI include ileus, obstruction, perforation, and significant gastrointestinal hemorrhage (72).

Recommendations

Whole bowel irrigation is not recommended as a routine procedure because of the lack of experience of most physicians in its use and because it appears to be awkward and cumbersome. At present, WBI is still considered an investigational procedure for GI decontamination of toxic substances. It should be considered for tablet bezoars, delayed release preparations, and for drugs not adsorbed by activated charcoal.

Bezoars (Concretions)

The term *bezoar* is derived from the Arabic word meaning "antidote". It was once believed that bezoars extracted from animals had healing powers and they were used to treat such ailments as plaque and snake bites (79). Three categories based on composition can be used to describe bezoars: (a) phytobezoars or undigested food material; b) trichobezoars or undigested hair; c) miscellaneous material, such as inanimate objects and medications. The bezoars noted in the area of toxicology involve the latter category (80).

Because bezoars or concretions may form from the ingestion of certain drugs, it may possibly explain why a patient may have continual absorption when it was thought that the gastrointestinal tract was adequately emptied. The possibility of concretions should always be considered when patients do not respond to adequate therapy or when blood concentrations of the toxin do not diminish as expected. Concretion may also explain why a patient may have a waxing and waning clinical status (80).

Concretions usually develop after the ingestion of a large number of pills or capsules in a short period of time (52,62,81). There appears to be little relationship between the drug's chemical nature and the fact that it can cause concretions (8,9). Drugs that can cause concretions are listed in Table 2–5. The method of massage of the left upper quadrant described above is an attempt to break up these concretions so that they are more easily solubilized and retrieved. That a drug may cause a concretion has no relation to its degree of radiopacity (72). Gastroscopy and even gastrotomy may be required to remove a toxic concretion (1,8,82).

ACTIVATED CHARCOAL

General Considerations

There is an incomplete return with the use of either ipecac or lavage. Although this incomplete return may represent material absorbed from the intestine, it also represents material still present in the gastrointestinal tract. Because of this it is important that additional methods be attempted to decrease the absorption of the material still remaining in the gastrointestinal tract. This is accomplished through the use of activated charcoal and a cathartic (83).

The capacity of charcoal to bind chemicals has been recognized for centuries and the first systematic studies of charcoal as an antidote were performed in the early 1800s (84). Activated charcoal is not absorbed from the gut and can adsorb a wide variety of ingested substances, holding them during gut passage and decreasing their systemic absorption (16). The use of activated charcoal in the management of most acute toxicologic emergencies has emerged from the role of adjunctive intervention to being recognized as the standard of care (85).

Activated charcoal or activated carbon is a residue from the distillation of various organic materials such as sawdust, wood, paper, and bone. Most carbon-based compounds can be converted to activated charcoal, which is "activated" by heating with steam, oxygen, and acids at temperatures in excess of 600°C in the absence of air (1,86–88). This activation process not only cleans the charcoal but expands each grain, producing a fine network of external and internal pores that increase the surface area of the material and thereby its adsorptive power. The size and number of pores that develop determine the surface area of the activated charcoal and its adsorptive capacity (86,88). Activated charcoal adsorbs toxic substances within the gastrointestinal tract, forming an activated charcoal–toxin complex and thus preventing absorption of the toxin (89,90). The adsorption of a toxin to charcoal is a reversible process, and with prolonged gastrointestinal transit time the process may shift toward desorption. However, if adequately high doses of activated charcoal are used the desorption is seldom significant in clinical situations (32,84).

Activated charcoal is an inert, fine, black, odorless, tasteless powder with a gritty consistency (91–93). It is available as a powder, can be supplied as an aqueous charcoal slurry, or can be mixed with water before administration to make an aqueous slurry (83). In addition, activated charcoal is marketed as a suspension of 20% activated charcoal in 70% sorbitol. This is also a bacteriostatic concentration of sorbitol (1,94–97). Activated charcoal can be instilled into the stomach through a lavage tube or a nasogastric tube. If the patient is conscious and cooperative it can be administered orally. Activated charcoal is most effective when administered early in treatment (30).

TABLE 2–10. *Substances with little or no adsorption by activated charcoal*

Acids
Boric acid
Mineral acids
Alcohols
Ethanol
Methanol
Alkalis
Potassium hydroxide
Sodium hydroxide
Sodium metasilicate
Cyanide
Insecticides
Carbamates
Chlorinated hydrocarbons (DDT)
Organophosphates
Metals
Iron
Lead
Lithium
Mercury

Indications for Use

Activated charcoal is a safe, effective, and inexpensive gastrointestinal adsorbent and is universally advocated for adsorbing a wide range of chemicals, including alkaloids, salicylates, barbiturates, phenothiazines, tricyclic antidepressants, sulfonamides, and selected inorganic compounds in nonionized form (Table 2–9) (5,86,98–102). In general, most drugs and household products are adsorbed well enough for the administration of activated charcoal to be clinically useful (103). The substance is ineffective for inorganic compounds in ionic form, such as mineral acids and bases, boric acid, cyanide, iron, lithium, and other small ionized molecules (Table 2–10) (1,8,86).

TABLE 2–9. *Substances adsorbed by activated charcoal*

Acetaminophen	Glutethimide	Phenolphthalein
Aconitine	Hexachlorophene	Phenothiazines
Alcohol	Imipramine	Phenylbutazone
Amphetamines	Iodine	Phenyl propanolamine
Antimony	Ipecac	Phenytoin
Antipyrine	Isoniazid	Phosphorus
Arsenic	Kerosene	Potassium
Atropine	Malathion	Primaquine
Barbiturates	Mefenamic acid	Probenecid
Camphor	Meprobamate	Propantheline
Cantharides	Mercuric chloride	Propoxyphene
Carbamazepine	Methotrexate	Quinacrine
Chlordane	Methyl salicylate	Quinidine
Chloroquine	Methylene blue	Quinine
Chlorpheniramine	Morphine	Salicylamide
Chlorpromazine	Muscarine	Salicylates
Cocaine	Narcotics	Selenium
Colchicine	Nicotine	Silver
Dapsone	Nortriptyline	Stramonium
2,4-Dichlorophen-oxyacetic acid	Opium	Strychnine
Digitalis	Oxalates	Sulfonamides
Digitoxin	Paracetamol	Theophylline
Diphenylhydantoin	Parathion	Tricyclic antidepressants
Ergotamine	Penicillin	
Ethchlorvynol	Phenobarbital	

Adapted with permission from *Clin Pediatr* 1985;24:678–684. Philadelphia: Lippincott.

Dosage

Activated charcoal is an excellent adsorbent and will adsorb not only the poison but also other substances (99,100). For this reason, activated charcoal should be administered after ipecac has induced vomiting (26), although a recent study suggests that there is no interference with the efficacy of ipecac when 60 mL of the emetic is administered initially (31). It does not appear to adsorb sorbitol or magnesium sulfate.

Completeness of adsorption depends greatly on the ratio of charcoal to poison, because according to the mass law there is an equilibrium between free and adsorbed poison (104). The higher the charcoal–poison ratio, the more complete is the adsorption (84). Gastrointestinal contents impair the adsorption of drugs to activated charcoal, however the slowing of the absorption of food allows charcoal more time to effectively adsorb drugs in the gastrointestinal tract (1,84,96).

A dose of activated charcoal that provides a charcoal-to-poison ratio of 10:1 ensures optimal binding. If this ratio cannot be achieved with a single dose, then serial dosing may be required (1,8,86,94,105,106). The usual adult doses of activated charcoal are 30 to 100 g mixed with water as a slurry (240 mL of water/20 g or 30 g of activated charcoal). For children up to 10 to 12 years of age, doses of 15 to 30 g are recommended (1,8,86,94,95,

TABLE 2–11. *Activated charcoal preparations by trade name*

Acta-Char
Actidose
Adsorba
Arm-a-char
Charcoaid
Insta-char
Norit-A
Nuchar
Superchar

105). In infants, the dose is 1 to 2 g activated charcoal/kg body weight (16).

The mixture of activated charcoal and water should be stirred constantly to ensure uniform distribution and delivery of the full dose to the patient (85).

Because activated charcoal sticks to the walls of a bottle during storage, the bottle should be rinsed. Sealed aqueous suspensions of activated charcoal can be stored for at least 1 year without measurable loss of activity (107).

Activated charcoal USP, Norit-A, Nuchar, and Actidose are among the many acceptable charcoal preparations (Table 2–11) (1,107). Tablets of activated charcoal are ineffective because once activated charcoal is compressed into a tablet its effective surface area is drastically lowered, the result being a much less effective adsorbent than an equal amount of granular activated charcoal (108). The adsorptive capacity of the pills is not restored by crushing or chewing the tablets (109).

Superactivated Charcoal

A superactivated charcoal preparation appears to have a greater adsorption capability in vitro than regular activated charcoal (86,110). This substance, previously available as Superchar, has an extremely large internal surface area, two to three times that of regular activated charcoal (87,111). This substance may reduce the quantities of activated charcoal required yet still provide the same adsorptive capacity as regular activated charcoal (87). Currently superactivated charcoal is not available commercially in the United States (16,111).

Factors Limiting Use

The factors limiting the use of activated charcoal are inconvenience of admixture and the repugnant and unpalatable physical characteristics of the substance (88). There may be problems with patient compliance because the black color of the slurry, its gritty texture, and its tendency to adhere to the throat all tend to limit its acceptability. The use of activated charcoal is strongly recommended, however, because it may adsorb much of the compound still remaining in the gastrointestinal tract. Besides acting as an adsorbent, activated charcoal can also serve as a fecal marker, providing evidence that the poison has passed through the gastrointestinal tract. Contrary to popular belief, activated charcoal taken orally does not appear to induce emesis unless syrup of ipecac has been administered earlier (112).

The time of administration of activated charcoal is influenced by whether ipecac-induced emesis or gastric lavage is used to empty the gastrointestinal tract of poison. In many patients, activated charcoal may not be tolerated for some time after ipecac-induced vomiting, which constitutes a serious drawback to the use of ipecac.

Attempts To Increase Palatability

Because patients dislike the black color and gritty consistency, placing the activated charcoal in a covered cup may remove some of the aversion (16). Thickening agents such as bentonite (2.5 g per 10 g of activated charcoal) and sodium carboxymethylcellulose have been suggested as additives to activated charcoal (1,113). These agents can provide a smooth yet tasteless consistency that may enhance patient compliance without interfering with the binding capacity of the activated charcoal (42).

Most attempts at flavoring charcoal or mixing it with ice cream have met with little success because most of these flavoring agents are well adsorbed by the charcoal and thereby decrease its available binding sites (88,113). There are some premixed charcoal preparations that contain sorbitol, either in cathartic doses, or in smaller doses as a flavoring agent to increase patient acceptance (85). The addition of sorbitol appears to improve palatability more than aqueous solutions and does not compromise the efficacy of the activated charcoal (83,97,114). Clinicians should know whether the available preparation contains sorbitol and at what concentration to avoid iatrogenic cathartic overdose (85).

Safety of Activated Charcoal

Activated charcoal has been investigated for inherent toxicity on skin contact, via inhalation, and during ingestion. No detectable harmful effects have been noted on prolonged skin contact (92), and inhalation has also produced no significant toxic effects (93). If charcoal were aspirated into the lungs, the particles would remain inert and would not produce an inflammatory reaction (10,100). Toxicity may occur though from coaspiration of stomach contents or sorbitol (103). Activated charcoal can therefore be considered a safe, inert, nontoxic material. The most common side effect of activated charcoal administration is vomiting, especially when charcoal is given after ipecac syrup (103). Other complications include constipation, black stools, and gastrointestinal obstruction (103).

Activated charcoal is contraindicated in ingestions of caustic substances. Charcoal does not adsorb significant amounts of these chemicals, obscures endoscopic visualization of esophageal and gastric injuries, and predisposes to vomiting and reexposure of the esophagus to caustic injury. In addition, there may be times when an interaction of the charcoal with therapeutic methods may be detrimental. There are, however, no absolute contraindications for its use in that activated charcoal has not of itself been associated with specific toxicity (84).

In some cases the binding of drugs and toxins to a single dose of activated charcoal is far from complete, although the charcoal has been given at an appropriate time (84). This may be due to inadequate administration of charcoal, to low affinity of the ingested poisons to charcoal, to the reversibility of adsorption of that particular substance, or to the saturation of the adsorbing capacity of charcoal by the drug or other gastrointestinal tract contents (85). In addition, the release rates of drugs from various pharmaceutical formulations and in various intoxications may vary considerably (10). This makes the adsorption to a single charcoal dose sometimes less complete than when multiple charcoal doses were given (84).

Recommendation

The efficacy of charcoal is expected to be good in poisonings where adsorption capacity will not be saturated, and its administration does not prevent gastric emptying being performed later. The immediate administration of activated charcoal before other time-consuming procedures should be considered in most intoxications (115). The early administration of charcoal neither prevents later gastric emptying nor does it cause serious adverse effects, as long as pulmonary aspiration in obtunded patients is prevented (84).

The absorption of drugs in life-threatening overdosages may be considerably prolonged. Therefore, there is no exact time at which charcoal should no longer be administered to prevent gastrointestinal absorption in intoxications (116).

Activated Charcoal As a Sole Agent for Decontamination

The use of activated charcoal as a sole means for preventing absorption of an ingested compound is a subject of much research (117). Some investigators have questioned the utility of gastric emptying procedures unless performed within 1 hour of ingestion in obtunded patients (5). In addition, a variety of reports have concluded that the sole use activated charcoal is superior to standard gastric emptying procedures and some have called for the abandonment of the traditional means of gastric decontamination (3). Although this should be kept in mind, further studies are needed to confirm this conclusion (117).

Because there are conflicting reports concerning the role of activated charcoal as the sole agent for preventing absorption of a toxin (118), until further work is performed it would not be prudent to limit treatment of the overdosed patient solely to activated charcoal. Until that time, when not contraindicated, lavage should be induced because the patient's history may be inaccurate, gastric motility may be reduced, or concretions of the drug may have been formed in the stomach. Some investigators believe that gastric emptying has value up to 24 hours after ingestion of certain long-acting compounds (1,86). In view of the efficacy and safety of activated charcoal, however, it is in the best interests of the patient to begin this treatment as quickly as possible after admission to the emergency department (117).

Although many toxicologists have begun to recommend administration of activated charcoal without prior gastric emptying for the management of minor ingestions, they continue to perform gastric emptying procedures for patients with potentially serious overdoses and for those who have ingested poisons not adsorbed by activated charcoal. Unfortunately, many of these studies include only a small number of patients with potentially lethal ingestions. For this reason, until further investigations involving large samples of patients with severe poisoning have been completed, gastric emptying techniques should not be abandoned (10). These findings do certainly provoke a number of questions about the gastric emptying techniques that have been considered standard of care. Yet, what may have been demonstrated is that the majority of overdose patients have mild intoxications and are likely to have a satisfactory clinical outcome regardless of the gastric emptying procedure.

Studies have not yet proven that patients with serious or massive ingestions can be safely treated without gastric emptying procedures. This research is just a beginning and does not yet constitute a justification to abandon the accepted gastric emptying techniques. Instead it provides compromise and provides guidance regarding situations when it may be appropriate to utilize activated charcoal as the sole intervention to prevent absorption of a toxin.

Multiple-Dose Activated Charcoal

In addition to the role of activated charcoal as an adsorbent for ingested material, there also appears to be a role for its use with toxins that undergo enterohepatic or enterogastric circulation (13,119). Drugs such as digitalis, tricyclic antidepressants, and phencyclidine undergo either enterohepatic circulation or secretion into the stom-

TABLE 2–12. *Drugs for which multiple-dose activated charcoal may be of benefit*

Carbamazepine (Tegretol)
Cyclic antidepressants
Dapsone
Digitoxin
Glutethimide (Doriden)
Meprobamate (Equanil, Miltown)
Nadolol (Corgard)
Phenobarbital
Phenylbutazone (Azolid, Butazolidin)
Theophylline

ach, and the activated charcoal remaining in the small intestine appears to expedite the removal of the toxic substance from the body by binding the drug within the lumen of the small intestine, thereby making it unavailable for reabsorption (86,120). Therefore, repeated doses of activated charcoal without a cathartic (119), also known as "pulse" charcoal or multiple-dose activated charcoal (MDAC), may further decrease drug absorption if the drug undergoes enterogastric or enterohepatic recirculation (Table 2–12) (13). Intestinal dialysis can also be used to increase the clearance of certain drugs through repeated doses of activated charcoal (86,88,96,119–123). This is discussed further in Chapter 3.

"Universal Antidote"

Activated charcoal should not be confused with the "universal antidote," for which there are two preparations: (a) the hospital preparation is a mixture of activated charcoal, magnesium oxide, and tannic acid; (b) the household preparation consists of burnt toast, tea, and Milk of Magnesia (124). In theory, the "universal antidote" has a three-way action, with (a) adsorption of the toxic substance by the activated charcoal or burnt toast, (b) a neutralization and precipitation of acidic poisons by the magnesium oxide or Milk of Magnesia, and (c) neutralization and precipitation of alkaline poisons by the tannic acid or tea. In actual practice the "universal antidote" is less effective in detoxifying drugs than is activated charcoal alone, and there is the potential for toxicity from the tannic acid. This combination is therefore useless and potentially dangerous and should not be used (124).

CATHARTICS

The rationale for cathartics is to decrease the toxin's intestinal transit time, thus minimizing the availability of nonabsorbed toxin for gut absorption. Theoretically, the quicker a poison passes through the gastrointestinal tract the less will be its desorption. Thus, many recommend the use of cathartics as an adjunct to charcoal to hasten the elimination of the charcoal–poison complex (84).

Types of Cathartics

Five classes of cathartics are currently available: bulk-forming agents, stimulants or irritants, softeners, saline and osmotic agents, and lubricants (125). The saline and osmotic agents are the most common cathartics and are the only agents advocated as adjunctive therapy for poisoning (126).

Oil-based cathartics, such as castor oil, are no longer used because they can produce serious lipoid pneumonitis if aspirated (16). The stimulant cathartics include cascara, castor oil, bisacodyl, senna, and phenolphthalein; they act by increasing peristalsis and also increase secretion of enteral fluid. The osmotic cathartics are of greater interest and use in toxicology. They are generally classified as saline or saccharide cathartics (126). Although controlled studies have demonstrated the effectiveness of activated charcoal in decreasing serum levels of many toxins, the use of a cathartic is based primarily on empiric and anecdotal evidence (84,119,125). Most toxicologists agree with the use of a cathartic as a method of decreasing gastrointestinal transit time of the toxin and thereby of decreasing the likelihood that the toxin will be absorbed (125,127).

Saline Cathartics

The saline cathartics include the magnesium and sodium cathartics such as magnesium sulfate, citrate, and hydroxide and sodium sulfate and phosphate (Table 2–13) (71). These agents produce catharsis on an osmotic basis by causing a large volume of fluid to be retained in the stomach, which leads to an increase of small bowel peristalsis, decreases toxin transit time, and causes defecation (83,90,125).

TABLE 2–13. *Saline and saccharide cathartics and their dosages*

Drug	Dosage
Sorbitol	Adult: 100 to 150 mL of 70% solution Child: 1 to 2 mL/kg of 70% solution
Magnesium sulfate (Epsom salts)	Adult: 15 to 30 g Child: 250 mg/kg
Magnesium citrate	Adult: 15 to 30 g Child: 250 mg/kg
Sodium sulfate (Glauber's solution)	Adult: 15 to 30 g Child: 250 mg/kg
Disodium phosphate (Fleet enema)	15 to 30 mL diluted 1:4

The intraluminal wall of the small intestine acts as a semipermeable membrane to magnesium and its salts, retaining most of these osmotic ions in the gut. The osmotic character of the saline cathartics draws fluids intraluminally. Theoretically, the extra fluid from the gastrointestinal blood supply creates a "bulk" or diarrheal state. This state activates peristalsis and propulsion (14). In actuality, the mechanisms may be more complex (90).

Sodium sulfate presents a large sodium dose and should be avoided in patients with congestive heart failure (16). In the past, magnesium sulfate (Epsom salts) has been the cathartic of choice. An adult can be given 15 to 30 g as a 10% solution along with the activated charcoal because there is no significant adsorption of the cathartic to the charcoal. The pediatric dose of magnesium sulfate is 250 mg/kg (1,119). Magnesium sulfate and citrate have caused significant hypermagnesemia in some patients, especially those with renal failure, and even have produced elevated magnesium levels in patients with normal renal function who received standard doses (128). Hypermagnesemia may also be a consequence of using multiple-dose magnesium cathartics in the patient with renal impairment as well as in the patient with normal renal function (119,128–130).

Signs and symptoms of hypermagnesemia (131) may include initial hypotension, nausea, vomiting, muscular paralysis, respiratory depression, electrocardiographic abnormalities, bradycardia, coma, and hypothermia, altered mental status, decreased deep tendon reflexes, decreased respiration, coma, and death from cardiac arrest (126,127,132–134).

Fleet Enema

Fleet enemas contain 16 g sodium biphosphate and 6 g sodium monophosphate (135). Acting as osmotic laxatives, Fleet enema can cause an increase in fluid volume in the colon, the colon is distended, peristalsis becomes more vigorous, and defecation occurs. It was once thought that phosphate was poorly absorbed from the colon and that phosphate enemas could be safely used as cathartics (131). Prolonged retention of these enemas in a dilated atonic colon, however, can result in a large "third" space within the colon causing dehydration, and hypernatremia (128,130). Life-threatening hyperphosphatemia and hypocalcemia and tetany can also occur secondary to the absorption of large amounts of phosphate from a distended colon with increased luminal permeability (131). Because significant morbidity has resulted from its use, phosphate solutions are therefore not recommended (127,133,135).

Saccharide Cathartics

The saccharide cathartics are sorbitol, mannitol, and lactulose (119). Recently, sorbitol has been shown to be more efficacious than some of the other available cathartics.

Sorbitol, a hexahydric alcohol that is 50% to 60% as sweet as sucrose, has been suggested as an additive to activated charcoal to make it more palatable (96). Although in the past saline cathartics were recommended, many toxicologists are now preferring sorbitol as the cathartic of choice because the combination of sorbitol and activated charcoal has been demonstrated to be more effective in producing a stool in a shorter period of time compared with saline cathartics (94,95,102,119, 129). After an orally administered dose, sorbitol is slowly absorbed and metabolized to fructose; that which remains in the gut acts osmotically to draw free water into the lumen and cause diarrhea (94–96,119).

The addition of sorbitol to activated charcoal imparts sweetness to the suspension, and its viscosity may mask the grittiness of the charcoal and maintains the particles in suspension for a prolonged period of time without reducing the adsorptive properties of the charcoal. Sorbitol has also been shown to enhance the antidotal activity of charcoal when the two are combined (81,86,94,95, 136).

The dose of sorbitol in adults is 1 to 2 g/kg of a 35% solution. This should not exceed 150 mg/dose. Pediatric doses of sorbitol are 1 to 1.5 g/kg of a 35% solution, not to exceed 50 g/dose (16,86,94,95). Because sorbitol has caused protracted diarrhea and severe fluid and electrolyte disturbances, including severe hypernatremia and hypokalemia in both children and adults, it should therefore be used cautiously in dehydrated individuals (16,96).

Contraindications

There are several documented reports of severe toxicity from the use of cathartics in the treatment of poisoning; therefore, a cathartic should be avoided with patients who have adynamic ileus because they may not respond (127), a patient who overdoses and has concomitant intestinal obstruction (a rare circumstance) should not be given a cathartic because it may worsen the patient's condition and cause a perforation of the intestine, and a patient with diarrhea does not require a cathartic.

In a patient with potential myoglobinuria and subsequent renal failure, a saline cathartic other than the magnesium salt should be selected. Sodium cathartics should be avoided in patients in whom restricted salt intake is indicated and in patients with a history of congestive heart failure (125). Oil-base cathartics such as castor oil or mineral oil, which are advocated by some (especially after an ingestion of glutethimide), are contraindicated because they may be hazardous if aspirated (1). Finally, a cathartic should be used cautiously in the very young and the very old.

Osmotic cathartics have the potential to cause hypernatremic dehydration. Because both the ileum and the colon have the ability to absorb sodium against a large concentration gradient, and because the normal passive transfer of water is retarded by the presence of the osmotically active substance, the sodium concentration in the stool may be considerably less than its concentration in the plasma (137).

SUMMARY

Attempts at preventing absorption of a compound may be the most important aspect of the early care of the poisoned patient. Yet, there is no one "correct" technique or combination of techniques for decreasing systemic absorption of ingested toxicants for all patients. All gastrointestinal decontamination procedures have potential adverse effects (138). Each patient with an ingestion poisoning must thus be considered individually in terms of ingestants, clinical presentation, and available resources to determine the optimal treatment regimen.

Preventing the absorption of an orally ingested material usually consists of lavage followed by activated charcoal and a cathartic. Because of the importance of using activated charcoal and the prolonged vomiting that occurs secondary to administration of ipecac, gastric lavage is advocated in significant overdoses if carried out in a timely fashion. Although magnesium sulfate had previously been the cathartic of choice, sorbitol now appears to be superior. Finally, there is an increasing importance being ascribed to the administration of activated charcoal both as single therapy and, in select cases, in a multiple-dose regimen.

REFERENCES

1. Rodgers G, Matyunas N: Gastrointestinal decontamination for acute poisoning. *Pediatr Clin North Am* 1986;33:261–285.
2. Thomas H, Schwartz E, Petrilli R: Droperidol versus haloperidol for chemical restraint of agitated and combative patients. *Ann Emerg Med* 1992;21:407–413.
3. Merigian K, Woodard M, Hedges J, et al: Prospective evaluation of gastric emptying in the self-poisoned patient. *Am J Emerg Med* 1990; 8:479–483.
4. Gaudreault P. McCormick M, Lacouture P, et al: Poisoning exposures and use of ipecac in children less than 1 year old. *Ann Emerg Med* 1986;15:808–810.
5. Kulig K, Bar-Or D, Cantrill S, et al: Management of acutely poisoned patients without gastric emptying. *Ann Emerg Med* 1985;14:562–567.
6. Tenenbein M, Cohen S, Sitar D: Efficacy of ipecac induced emesis, or gastric lavage, and activated charcoal for acute drug overdose. *Ann Emerg Med* 1987;16:838–841.
7. Fleisher G, Kearney T, Henretig F, et al: Gastric decontamination in the poisoned patient. *Pediatr Emerg Care* 1991;7:378–381.
8. Lanphear W: Gastric lavage. *J Emerg Med* 1986;4:43–47.
9. North D: Meprobamate and bezoar formation. *Ann Emerg Med* 1987;16:472–473.
10. Harris C, Filandrinos D: Accidental administration of activated charcoal into the lung: aspiration by proxy. *Ann Emerg Med* 1993;22: 1470–1473.
11. Corby D, Decker W, Moran M, et al: Clinical comparison of pharmacologic emetics in childhood. *Pediatrics* 1968:42:361–364.
12. Dean B, Krenzelok E: Syrup of ipecac: 15 mL versus 30 mL in pediatric poisonings. *Clin Toxicol* 1985;23:165–170.
13. Neuvonen P: Clinical pharmacokinetics of oral activated charcoal in acute intoxications. *Clin Pharmacokinet* 1982;7:465–489.
14. Wheeler-Usher D, Wanke L, Bayer M: Gastric emptying: risk versus benefit in the treatment of acute poisoning. *Med Toxicol* 1986; 1:142–153.
15. Chafee-Bahomon C, Lacouture P, Lovejoy F: Risk assessment of ipecac in the home. *Pediatrics* 1985;75:1105–1109.
16. Hall A, Krenzelok E: Gastrointestinal decontamination: sifting through supportive therapeutic options. *Emer Med Rep* 1991;12: 171–178.
17. Manno B, Manno J: Toxicology of ipecac: a review. *Clin Toxicol* 1977;10:221–242.
18. Moran D, Crouch D, Finkle B: Absorption of ipecac alkaloids in emergency patients. *Ann Emerg Med* 1984;13;1100–1102.
19. Weaver J, Griffith J: Induction of emesis by detergent ingredients and formulations. *Toxicol Appl Pharmacol* 1969;14:214–220.
20. King W: Syrup of ipecac: a review. *Clin Toxicol* 1980;17:353–356.
21. Eisenga B, Meester W: Evaluation of the effect of motility on syrup of ipecac-induced emesis. *Vet Hum Toxicol* 1978;20:462–465.
22. Palmer E, Guay A: Reversible myopathy secondary to abuse of ipecac in patients with major eating disorders. *N Engl J Med* 1985; 313:1457–1459.
23. Klein-Schwartz W, Litovitz T, Oderda G, et al: The effect of milk on ipecac-induced emesis. *J Toxicol Clin Toxicol* 1991;29:505–511.
24. Uden D, Davison G, Kohen D: Effect of carbonated beverages on ipecac-induced emesis. *Ann Emerg Med* 1981;10:79–81.
25. Easom J, Lovejoy F: Efficacy and safety of gastrointestinal decontamination in the treatment of oral poisoning. *Pediatr Clin North Am* 1979;26:827–836.
26. Manoguerra A, Krenzelok E: Rapid emesis from high-dose ipecac syrup in adults and children intoxicated with antiemetics or other drugs. *Am J Hosp Pharm* 1978;35:1360—1362.
27. Amitai Y, Mitchell A, McGuigan M, et al: Ipecac induced emesis and reduction of plasma concentrations of drugs following accidental overdose in children. *Pediatrics* 1987;80:364–367.
28. Grbcich P, Lacouture P, Kresel J, et al: Expired ipecac syrup efficacy. *Pediatrics* 1986;78:1085–1089.
29. Czajka P, Russell S: Nonemetic effects of ipecac syrup. *Pediatrics* 1985;75:1101–1104.
30. Krenzelok E, Dean B: Syrup of ipecac in children less than one year of age. *Clin Toxicol* 1985;23;171–176.
31. Cooney D: In vitro evidence for ipecac inactivation by activated charcoal. *J Pharm Sci* 1978;67:426–427.
32. Freedman G, Pasternak S, Krenzelok E: A clinical trial using syrup of ipecac and activated charcoal concurrently. *Ann Emerg Med* 1987;16:164–166.
33. Krenzelok E, Freedman G, Pasternak S: Preserving the emetic effect of syrup of ipecac with concurrent activated charcoal administration: a preliminary study. *Clin Toxicol* 1986;24:159–166.
34. Ordog G, Vann P, Owashi N, et al: Intravenous prochlorperazine for the rapid control of vomiting in the emergency department. *Ann Emerg Med* 1984;13:253–258.
35. McClung H, Murray R, Braden N, et al: Intentional ipecac poisoning in children. *Am J Dis Child* 1988;142:637–639.
36. Wolowodiuk O, McMicken D, O'Brien P: Pneumomediastinum and retropneumonoperitoneum: an unusual complication of syrup of ipecac-induced emesis. *Ann Emerg Med* 1984;13:1148–1151.
37. Smith R, Smith D: Acute ipecac poisoning—report of a fatal case and review of literature. *N Engl J Med* 1961;265:523–525.
38. Klein-Schwartz W, Gorman R, Oderda G, et al: Ipecac use in the elderly: the unanswered question. *Ann Emerg Med* 1984;13: 1152–1154.
39. Brushwood D, Tietze K: Regulatory controversy surrounding ipecac use and misuse. *Am J Hosp Pharm* 1986;43:157–161.
40. Rumack B: Ipecac use in the home. *Pediatrics* 1985;75:1148.
41. Rumack B, Rosen P: Emesis: safe and effective? *Ann Emerg Med* 1981;10:551.
42. Tandberg D, Liechty E, Fishbein D: Mallory-Weiss syndrome: an unusual complication of ipecac-induced emesis. *Ann Emerg Med* 1981;10:521–523.
43. Bond G, Requa R, Krenzelok E, et al: Influence of time until emesis on the efficacy of decontamination using acetaminophen as a marker in a pediatric population. *Ann Emerg Med* 1993;22:1403–1407.

44. Steinhart C, Pearson-Shaver A: Poisoning. *Crit Care Clin* 1899;4: 845–872.
45. Miser J, Robertson W: Ipecac poisoning. *West J Med* 1978;128: 440–443.
46. Adler A, Walinsky P, Krall R, et al: Death resulting from ipecac-syrup poisoning. *JAMA* 1980;243:1927–1928.
47. Wrenn K, Rodewald L, Dockstader L: Potential misuse of ipecac. *Ann Emerg Med* 1993;22:1408–1412.
48. Bennett H, Spiro A, Pollack M, et al: Ipecac-induced myopathy simulating dermatomyositis. *Neurology* 1982;32:91–94.
49. Brotman M, Forbath N, Garfinkel P, et al: Myopathy due to ipecac syrup poisoning in a patient with anorexia nervosa. *Can Med Assoc J* 1981;125:453–454.
50. MacLeod J: Ipecac intoxication—use of a cardiac pacemaker in management. *N Engl J Med* 1963;268:146–147.
51. Stein R, Jenkins D, Korns M: Death after use of cupric sulfate as emetic. *JAMA* 1976;235:801.
52. Schwartz E, Schmidt E: Refractory shock secondary to copper sulfate ingestion. *Ann Emerg Med* 1986;15:952–954.
53. Gieseker D, Troutman W: Emergency induction of emesis using fluid detergent products: a report of fifteen cases. *Clin Toxicol* 1981;18:277–282.
54. Krenzelok E: High-pH automatic dishwashing detergents. *Ann Emerg Med* 1987;16:470.
55. MacLean W: A comparison of ipecac syrup and apomorphine in the immediate treatment of ingestion of poisons. *J Pediatr* 1973;82: 121–124.
56. Schofferman J: A clinical comparison of syrup of ipecac and apomorphine use in adults. *JACEP* 1976;5:22–25.
57. Auerbach P, Osterloh J, Braun O, et al: Efficacy of gastric emptying: gastric lavage versus emesis induced with ipecac. *Ann Emerg Med* 1986;15:692–698.
58. Arnold F, Hodges J, Barta R, et al: Evaluation of the efficacy of lavage and induced emesis in the treatment of salicylate poisoning. *Pediatrics* 1959;23:286–301.
59. Burke M: Gastric lavage and emesis in the treatment of ingested poisons: a review and a clinical study of lavage in ten adults. *Resuscitation* 1972;1:91–105.
60. Young W, Bivins H: Evaluation of gastric emptying using radionuclides: gastric lavage versus ipecac-induced emesis. *Ann Emerg Med* 1993;22:1423–1427.
61. Matthew H: Gastric aspiration and lavage. *Clin Toxicol* 1970;3: 179–183.
62. McDougal C, MacLean M: Modifications in the technique of gastric lavage. *Ann Emerg Med* 1981;10:514–517.
63. Rudolph J: Automated gastric lavage and a comparison of 0.9% normal saline solution and tap water irrigant. *Ann Emerg Med* 1985;14: 1156–1159.
64. Torres A, Serra-Batlles J, Ros E, et al: Pulmonary aspiration of gastric contents in patients receiving mechanical ventilation: the effect of body position. *Ann Intern Med* 1992;116:540–543.
65. Bartecchi C: A modification of gastric lavage technique. *JACEP* 1974;3:304–305.
66. Blake D, Bramble M, Grimley-Evans J: Is there excessive use of gastric lavage in the treatment of self poisoning? *Lancet* 1978;2: 1362–1364.
67. Askenasi R, Abramowicz M, Jeanmart J, et al: Esophageal perforation: an unusual complication of gastric lavage. *Ann Emerg Med* 1984;13;146.
68. Doumon E, Bure A, Desplaces N, et al: Legionnaires' disease related to gastric lavage with tap water. *Lancet* 1982;1:797–798.
69. Kirshenbaum L, Sitar D, Tenenbein M: Interaction between whole-bowel irrigation solution and activated charcoal: implications for the treatment of toxic ingestions. *Ann Emerg Med* 1990;19:1129–1132.
70. Rosenberg P, Livingstone D, McLellan B: Effect of whole bowel irrigation on the antidotal efficacy of oral activated charcoal. *Ann Emerg Med* 1988;17:681–683.
71. Porter R, Baker E: Drug clearance by diarrhea induction. *Am J Emerg Med* 1985;3:182–186.
72. Burkhart K, Kulig K, Rumack B: Whole bowel irrigation as treatment for zinc sulfate overdose. *Ann Emerg Med* 1990;19:1167–1170.
73. Boba A: Rapid whole-gut evacuation. *IMJ* 1979;155:156–157.
74. Davis G, Santa Ana C, Morawski S, et al: Development of a lavage solution associated with minimal water and electrolyte absorption or secretion. *Gastroenterology* 1980;78:991–995.
75. Porter R, Baker E: Drug clearance by diarrhea induction. *Am J Emerg Med* 1985;3:182–186.
76. Tenenbein M: Whole bowel irrigation for toxic ingestions. *Clin Toxicol* 1985;23:177–184.
77. Tenenbein M: Inefficacy of gastric emptying procedures. *J Emerg Med* 1985:3:133–136.
78. Hoffman R, Smilkstein M, Goldfrank L: Whole bowel irrigation and the cocaine body packer. *Am J Emerg Med* 1990;8:523–527.
79. Bellomo R, Kearly Y, Parkin G, et al: Treatment of life-threatening lithium toxicity with continuous arteriovenous hemodiafiltration. *Crit Care Med* 1991;19:836–839.
80. Carrougher J, Barrilleaux C: Esophageal bezoars: the sucralith. *Crit Care Med* 1991;19:837–839.
81. Cereda J, Scott J, Quigley E: Endoscopic removal of pharmacobezoar of slow-release theophylline. *Br Med* 1986;293:1143.
82. Marstellar H, Gigler R: Endoscopic management of toxic masses in the stomach. *N Engl J Med* 1977;296:1003–1004
83. Czajka P, Konrad J: Saline cathartics and the adsorptive capacity of activated charcoal for aspirin. *Ann Emerg Med* 1986;15:548–551.
84. Neuvonen P, Olkkola K: Oral activated charcoal in the treatment of intoxications. Role of single and repeated doses. *Med Toxicol* 1988;3:33–58.
85. Krenzelok E, Lush R: Container residue after the administration of aqueous activated charcoal products. *Am J Emerg Med* 1991;9: 144–146.
86. Mofenson H, Caraccio T, Greensher J, et al: Gastrointestinal dialysis with activated charcoal and cathartic in the treatment of adolescent intoxications. *Clin Pediatr* 1985;24:678–684.
87. Curd-Sneed C, Parks K, Bordelon J, et al: In vitro adsorption of sodium pentobarbital by Superchar, USP and Darco G-60 activated charcoals. *Clin Toxicol* 1987;25:1–11.
88. Katona B, Siegel E, Cluxton R: The new black magic: activated charcoal and new therapeutic uses. *J Emerg Med* 1987;5:9–18.
89. Neuvonen P, Vartiainen M, Tokola O: Comparison of activated charcoal and ipecac syrup in prevention of drug absorption. *Eur J Clin Pharmacol* 1983;24:557–562.
90. Harvey R, Read A: Mode of action of the saline purgatives. *Am Heart J* 1975;89:810–813.
91. Comstock E, Boisaubin E, Comstock B, et al: Assessment of the efficacy of activated charcoal following gastric lavage in acute drug emergencies. *J Toxicol Clin Toxicol* 1982;19:149–165.
92. Nau C, Neal J, Stembridge V: A study of the physiological effects of carbon black: II: skin contact. *Arch Ind Health* 1958:18:511–520.
93. Nau C, Neal J, Stembridge V, et al: Physiological effects of carbon black: inhalation. *Arch Environ Health* 1962:4:415–420.
94. Minocha A, Herold D, Bruns D, et al: Effect of activated charcoal in 70% sorbitol in healthy individuals. *J Toxicol Clin Toxicol* 1985;22: 529–534.
95. Minocha A, Krenzelok E, Spyker D: Dosage recommendations for activated charcoal-sorbitol treatment. *Clin Toxicol* 1985;23:579–587.
96. Farley T: Severe hypernatremic dehydration after use of an activated charcoal-sorbitol suspension. *J Pediatr* 1986;109:719–722.
97. Mayersohn M, Perrier D, Picchioni A: Evaluation of a charcoal-sorbitol mixture as an antidote for oral aspirin overdose. *Clin Toxicol* 1977;11:561–567.
98. Neuvonen P, Elonen E: Effect of activated charcoal on absorption and elimination of phenobarbitone, carbamazepine, and phenylbutazone in man. *Eur J Clin Pharmacol* 1980;17:51–55.
99. Holt L, Holz P: The black bottle. *J Pediatr* 1970;63:306–314.
100. Hayden J, Comstock E: Use of activated charcoal in acute poisoning. *Clin Toxicol* 1975;8:515–533.
101. Kulig K: Interpreting gastric emptying studies. *J Emerg Med* 1984;1:447–448.
102. Krenzelok E, Keller R, Stewart R: Gastrointestinal transit times of cathartics combined with charcoal. *Ann Emerg Med* 1985;14: 1152–1155
103. Elliott C, Colby T, Kelly T, et al: Charcoal lung. Bronchiolitis obliterans after aspiration of activated charcoal. *Chest* 1989;96: 672–674.
104. McKinney P, Gillilan R, Watson W: The preadministration of activated charcoal and aspirin absorption. *J Toxicol Clin Toxicol* 1992; 30:549–556.
105. Olkkola K, Neuvonen P: Do gastric contents modify antidotal efficacy of oral activated charcoal? *Br J Clin Pharmacol* 1984;18: 663–669.

106. Browning R, Olson D, Stueven H, et al: 50% dextrose: antidote or toxin? *Ann Emerg Med* 1990;19:683–687.
107. Picchioni A, Chin L, Laird H: Activated charcoal preparations—relative antidotal efficacy. *Clin Toxicol* 1974;7:97–108.
108. Keller R, Schwab R, Krenzelok E: Contribution of sorbitol combined with activated charcoal in prevention of salicylate absorption. *Ann Emerg Med* 1990;19:654–656
109. Tsuchiya T, Levy G: Drug adsorption efficacy of commercial activated charcoal tablets in vitro and in man. *J Pharm Sci* 1972;61: 624–625.
110. Chung D, Murphy J, Taylor T: In-vivo comparison of the adsorption capacity of "superactive charcoal" and fructose with activated charcoal and fructose. *J Toxicol Clin Toxicol* 1982;19:219–224.
111. Katona B, Siegel E, Roberts J, et al: The effect of "superactive" charcoal and magnesium citrate solution on blood ethanol concentrations and area under the curve in humans. *J Toxicol Clin Toxicol* 1989;27: 129–137.
112. Curtis R, Barone J, Biacona W: Efficacy of ipecac and activated charcoal/cathartic: prevention of salicylate absorption in a simulated overdose. *Arch Intern Med* 1984;144:48–52.
113. Gwilt P, Perrier D: Influence of thickening agents on the antidotal efficacy of activated charcoal. *Clin Toxicol* 1976;9:89–92.
114. Levy G, Soda D, Lampman T: Inhibition by ice cream of the efficacy of activated charcoal. *Am J Hosp Pharm* 1975:32:289–291.
115. McNamara R, Aaron C, Genborys M, et al: Efficacy of charcoal cathartic versus ipecac in reducing serum acetaminophen in a simulated overdose. *Ann Emerg Med* 1989;18:934–938.
116. Goulbourne K, Cisek J: Small-bowel obstruction secondary to activated charcoal and adhesions. *Ann Emerg Med* 1994;24:108–114.
117. Kronberg A, Dolgin J: Pediatric ingestions: charcoal alone versus ipecac and charcoal. *Ann Emerg Med* 1991;20:648–651.
118. Burton B, Bayer M, Barron L, et al: Comparison of activated charcoal and gastric lavage in the prevention of aspirin absorption. *J Emerg Med* 1984;1:411–416.
119. Jones J, Heiselman D, Dougherty J, et al: Cathartic induced magnesium toxicity during overdose management. *Ann Emerg Med* 1986;15:1214–1218.
120. Amitai Y, Degani Y: Treatment of phenobarbital poisoning with multiple dose activated charcoal in an infant. *J Emerg Med* 1990;8: 449–450.
121. Berlinger W, Spector R, Goldberg G, et al: Enhancement of theophylline clearance by oral activated charcoal. *Clin Pharmacol Ther* 1983;33:351–356.
122. True R, Berman J, Mahutte C: Treatment of theophylline toxicity with oral activated charcoal. *Crit Care Med* 1984;12:113–119.
123. Rowden A, Spoor J, Bertino J: The effect of activated charcoal on phenytoin pharmacokinetics. *Ann Emerg Med* 1990;19:1144–1147
124. Picchioni A, Chin L, Verhulst H, et al: Activated charcoal vs "universal antidote" as an antidote for poisons. *Toxicol Appl Pharmacol* 1966;8:447–454.
125. Shannon M, Fish S, Lovejoy F: Cathartics and laxatives: do they still have a place in the management of the poisoned patient? *Med Toxicol* 1986;1:247–252.
126. Gerard S, Hernandez C, Khayam-Bashi H: Extreme hypermagnesemia caused by an overdose of magnesium-containing cathartics. *Ann Emerg Med* 1988;17:728–731.
127. Riegel J, Becker C: Use of cathartics in toxic ingestions. *Ann Emerg Med* 1981;10:79–81.
128. Weber C, Santiago R: Hypermagnesemia. A potential complication during treatment of theophylline intoxication with oral activated charcoal and magnesium-containing cathartics. *Chest* 1989;95: 56–59.
129. Krenzelok E: Sorbitol—a safe and effective cathartic. *Ann Emerg Med* 1987;16:729–730.
130. Smilkstein M, Smolinske S, Kulig K, et al: Severe hypermagnesemia due to multiple-dose cathartic therapy. *West J Med* 1988;148: 208–211.
131. Wason S, Tiler T, Cunha C: Severe hyperphosphatemia, hypocalcemia, acidosis, and shock in a 5-month old child following the administration of an adult Fleet enema. *Ann Emerg Med* 1989; 18:696–700.
132. Cheeley R, Joyce S: A clinical comparison of the performance of four blood glucose reagent strips. *Am J Emerg Med* 1990;8:11–15.
133. Martin R, Lisehora G, Braxton M, et al: Fatal poisoning from sodium phosphate enema. *JAMA* 1987;257:2190–2192.
134. Gren J, Woolf A: Hypermagnesemia associated with catharsis in a salicylate-intoxicated patient with anorexia nervosa. *Ann Emerg Med* 1989;18:200–203.
135. Korzets A, Dicker D, Chain C, et al: Life-threatening hyperphosphatemia and hypocalcemic tetany following the use of Fleet enemas. *J Am Geriatr Soc* 1992;40:620–621.
136. Harchelroad F, Cottington E, Krenzelok E: Gastrointestinal transit times of a charcoal/sorbitol slurry in overdose patients. *J Toxicol Clin Toxicol* 1989;27:91–99.
137. Lis R, Lief P: Extracorporeal methods in the intensive care unit. *Anes Clin North Am* 1991;9:245–263.
138. Albertson T, Derlet R, Foulke G, et al: Superiority of activated charcoal alone compared with ipecac and activated charcoal in the treatment of acute toxic ingestions. *Ann Emerg Med* 1989;18:56–59.

ADDITIONAL SELECTED REFERENCES

Goulding R, Volans G: Emergency treatment of common poisonings: emptying the stomach. *Proc Royal Soc Med* 1977;70:766–770.

Morris M, Levy G: Absorption of sulfate from orally administered magnesium sulfate in man. *J Toxicol Clin Toxicol* 1983;20:107–114.

Pollack M, Dunbar B, Holbrook P, et al: Aspiration of activated charcoal and gastric contents. *Ann Emerg Med* 1981;10:528–529.

Schwartz H: Acute meprobamate poisoning with gastrostomy and removal of a drug-containing mass. *N Engl J Med* 1976;295:1177–1178.

Stewart J: Effects of emetic and cathartic agents on the gastrointestinal tract and the treatment of toxic ingestion. *J Toxicol Clin Toxicol* 1983;20: 199–253.

Thoman M: The use of emetics in poison ingestion. *Clin Toxicol* 1970;3: 185–188.

Vale J, Rees A, Widdop B, et al: Use of charcoal haemoperfusion in the management of severely poisoned patients. *Br Med J* 1975;1:5–9.

Varipapa R, Oderda G: Effect of milk on ipecac induced emesis. *N Engl J Med* 1977;296:112–113.

CHAPTER 3

Methods of Enhancing Drug Excretion

The elimination of certain drugs from the body may be aided by methods that make use of pharmacokinetic parameters that affect drug excretion (1). These include forced diuresis with or without ion-trapping methods; the use of multiple-dose activated charcoal; dialysis; hemoperfusion; hemofiltration; and plasmapheresis (Table 3–1) (2–8). Except for the use of activated charcoal, these methods have one feature in common: the vasculature must deliver the drug to the site of removal, whether this be the chamber of an extracorporeal machine, the peritoneal space, or the kidney (9).

FORCED DIURESIS

The processes involved in the urinary excretion of drugs include glomerular filtration, active tubular secretion, and tubular reabsorption. Only the last process can be influenced so that drug elimination is significantly enhanced. If tubular reabsorption is inhibited, less drug is allowed back into the body and more is excreted by the kidney. Decreasing the concentration gradient between the urine and the blood by diluting the urine by diuresis may decrease tubular reabsorption. This process shortens the time of a drug's exposure to the reabsorptive sites in the distal tubules (10).

Factors Involved in Diuresis

A major factor accounting for the renal elimination of a drug or metabolite is the chemical molecule's polarity. Most lipid drugs, which are nonpolar, are not readily excreted unchanged by the kidney because of their ability to be readily reabsorbed through the membrane of the kidney tubules. If the liver adds more polar groups to the molecule, the drug becomes more soluble in water and renal excretion can occur. Addition of polar groups is achieved by acetylation, conjugation (with acetate, glycine, sulfate, or glucuronic acid), reduction, oxidation, or hydroxylation. In most cases, however, an attempt to increase urine flow and output will not result in an increase in renal clearance unless a reasonable fraction of the drug is eliminated through the kidneys in comparison with other routes of elimination, such as metabolism or fecal excretion. In general, for many drugs, elimination by renal excretion is independent of urine flow rates. Therefore, the enhancement of excretion of only a few drugs is increased solely by forced diuresis. In general, drugs with a large volume of distribution or a high degree of plasma protein binding will not be removed by forced diuresis. The few drugs whose excretion can be enhanced by a neutral diuresis with sodium chloride are isoniazid (controversial), and bromides (Table 3–2). It is more likely that the excretion of isoniazid is enhanced by an alkaline diuresis. Bromide intoxication is rarely seen due to the discontinuance of most bromide-containing compounds. Because of the very few compounds whose excretion could be enhanced, diuresis with normal saline is usually not necessary for the overdosed patient.

TABLE 3–1. *Methods to enhance drug elimination*

Diuresis with or without ion trapping
Normal saline diuresis
Alkaline diuresis
Acid diuresis
Dialysis
Hemodialysis
Peritoneal dialysis
Hemoperfusion
Hemofiltration
Plasmapheresis
Multiple-dose activated charcoal
Interruption of enterohepatic circulation
"Intestinal dialysis"

TABLE 3–2. *Drugs whose excretion can be enhanced by diuresis or ion trapping*

Neutral diuresis
Bromides
Lithium (controversial)
Isoniazid (controversial)
Alkaline diuresis
Phenobarbital
Primidone
Mephobarbital
Salicylates
Isoniazid (controversial)
Lithium (controversial)
Acid diuresis
Phencyclidine (not advised)
Amphetamines (not advised)

Ion-Trapping Methods

Ion-trapping methods essentially cause a solution to become more alkaline or acidic, depending on the pKa of the substance, so that the substance is trapped in the kidney and excretion is enhanced. Low degrees of ionization and high lipid solubility favor rapid movement across membranes. Weak acids are more ionized in an alkaline medium, and weak bases are more ionized in an acidic medium. If there is a pH difference across a membrane, ion trapping will occur, and drug will accumulate in the compartment where ionization is greater because the nonionized form crosses the lipid–cell membrane much more readily than the ionized form.

Ion trapping can be helpful in increasing the elimination of some drugs (Table 3–2). Most drugs are weak acids or bases that exist in the nonionized or ionized form. Nonionized molecules, in contrast to ionized molecules, are lipid-soluble and cross cell membranes by nonionic diffusion. Tubular transport is bidirectional and a concentration gradient is created for reabsorption of the lipid-soluble drug back into blood. Increasing intraluminal pH increases the degree of ionization of weak acids and reduces tubular reabsorption, whereas the reverse applies to weak bases. Dissociation is determined by both the drug dissociation constant pKa and pH gradient across the tubular epithelium. Drugs that have a dissociable group, either acidic or basic, carry a charge at a pH value that is distant from their pKa value (at a pH equal to the pKa, a drug is half dissociated and half undissociated).

Renal elimination of weak acids is increased in alkaline urine if the drug pKa lies between 3.0 and 7.5, and for weak bases if the drug pKa is 7.5 to 10.5. For forced diuresis to be effective, the drug must be predominantly eliminated in the unchanged form via the kidney; be a weak electrolyte, with a pKa in the appropriate acidic or basic pKa range; and be distributed, with minimal protein binding, in the extracellular fluid compartment (11).

Alkaline Diuresis

Both salicylate and phenobarbital are weak acids. By promoting an alkaline urine these drugs will become more ionized in the distal tubular lumen, which will slow tubular reabsorption and allow a larger fraction of drug to be excreted without being reabsorbed back into the body. This mechanism makes use of more effective renal excretion rather than saturation of the liver. This concept of ion trapping also allows phenobarbital and salicylate to move from the central nervous system into the blood compartment and then to be trapped in the tubular lumen of the kidney and excreted in the urine.

Drugs whose excretion can be enhanced by an alkaline diuresis are therefore the long-acting barbiturates, such as phenobarbital and drugs converted to phenobarbital in the body (mephobarbital and primidone), as well as salicylates, and possibly isoniazid (12) (Table 3–2). It has been shown that alkali alone may achieve similar quantities of salicylate removal obtained with "forced diuresis" in patients with moderate salicylate poisoning, avoiding the inherent dangers of high-volume fluid administration (11). Because short-acting barbiturates such as secobarbital and pentobarbital have a pKa greater than 8.0, renal clearance cannot be enhanced greatly by alkalinization of urine in the physiologic range (13). In addition, the short- and intermediate-acting barbiturates must be metabolized before being excreted by the kidney (14).

How to Set Up Alkaline Diuresis

An alkaline diuresis is achieved by administering one or two ampules of sodium bicarbonate dissolved in a liter of one-half normal saline. It is necessary to check the pH of the urine both before and after an effective urine flow is obtained. Potassium depletion should be carefully monitored, and the addition of potassium chloride may be necessary to ensure the adequate alkalinization of the urine. Sodium bicarbonate can increase urinary pH by 2 or 3 units, which will have a pronounced effect on the renal clearance of weakly acidic drugs.

Acetazolamide (Diamox) is a carbonic anhydrase inhibitor that will cause an alkaline urine through bicarbonate loss. It will also cause a hyperchloremic metabolic acidosis (non-anion-gap metabolic acidosis), however, and should not be used for urinary alkalinization.

Acid Diuresis

Drugs whose excretion can be enhanced by an acid diuresis include amphetamines and phencyclidine. Although acidifying the urine to enhance the excretion of these two drugs has been suggested and may be effective, many physicians do not recommend its use owing to the possibility of developing acute tubular necrosis secondary to rhabdomyolysis. In other words, although there is the potential for enhancing the renal excretion of these compounds, there is also the likelihood that these compounds will cause rhabdomyolysis with subsequent myoglobinemia and myoglobinuria (15). Because the excretion of myoglobin is decreased in an acid urine, there is a greater likelihood of causing an acute tubular necrosis. It is therefore held that the risks of the procedure outweigh the potential benefit (15).

How to Set Up Acid Diuresis

It has been suggested that 500 mg to 1 g of ascorbic acid should be added to each liter of normal saline to acidify the urine. There have been some questions raised regarding the efficacy of intravenous and oral preparations of ascorbic acid in producing an acid urine (1,15,16). Ammonium chloride, 75 mg/kg intravenously or orally per day, has also been suggested, but caution is advised for patients with kidney or liver disease.

Complications of Diuresis

Because forced diuresis involves the administration of large fluid quantities which might be either acidic or alkaline, the procedure may require careful observation of urine pH, plasma pH, and electrolytes. Complications of forced diuresis include pulmonary edema, hypokalemia, hyperkalemia, acidemia, and alkalemia, urinary infection from bladder catheter, and complications from Swan-Ganz lines used to assess fluid balance (Table 3–3) (11). Because of these potential complications, forced diuresis should be reserved for an overdose with a positive history of ingestion of one of the above substances.

TABLE 3–3. *Complications of forced diuresis*

Fluid overload
Pulmonary edema
Cerebral edema
Electrolyte disorders
Hypokalemia
Hyperkalemia
Acid-base disturbances
Infection
Indwelling catheter infection
Swan-Ganz line infection

THE ROLE OF EXTRACORPOREAL MEANS FOR DRUG REMOVAL

Hemodialysis, hemoperfusion, hemofiltration, and plasmapheresis are considered the state of the art in invasive detoxification. There are certain similarities among these procedures (17). They all require an extracorporeal chamber through which blood is passed, either a membrane dialyzer (dialysis) or a bed of charcoal or other sorbent (hemoperfusion and plasmapheresis). They make use of blood anticoagulation treatments, pumps, and safety devices to detect or prevent air embolism. The major processes of extracorporeally facilitated drug removal, diffusion (dialysis), adsorption (hemoperfusion), and convection (hemofiltration) also differ markedly in their ability to remove drugs (18).

Pharmacokinetic principles indicate the reasons dialysis or hemoperfusion would be infrequently useful in treating drug overdose (19). An underlying assumption, that is incorrect, is that the toxic effect of any drug is in some way related directly to the plasma concentration of the toxin; hence, attempts have been made to control the plasma concentration. Yet adequate extracorporeally facilitated drug removal refers to the relief of the total body's drug burden, not just that in the vascular compartment. The larger the volume of distribution, the less likelihood that there will be substantial delivery of the drug to the extracorporeal drug removal device as drug removal will be insignificant relative to the total body drug burden.

"Rebound" Effect

Most substances are distributed at varying rates to extravascular tissues and are not confined to the vascular compartment. If the rate of distribution of the agent from extravascular tissues is slower than the overall elimination rate, the agent will be removed from the blood more rapidly than it can be replaced from tissue stores (20). This occurrence results in a rebound in blood concentration of the agent on cessation of extracorporeal removal. This effect is seen more when the volume of distribution is large (>1 L/kg). Unfortunately, most reported studies have not considered these principles. Thus, reported declines of blood concentrations following the use of extracorporeal devices are useless for evaluating a significant reduction in total body stores of an agent unless the amount of drug removed in the effluent is measured (19).

Change in Kinetics

It is possible that first-order kinetics of an agent may become concentration-dependent and approach zero-order kinetics in an overdose situation (Chapter 5). This change in kinetics may be a consequence of decreased metabolic clearance at high plasma concentration. Since many drugs may be subject to concentration-dependent kinetics, and only limited pharmacokinetic data are available for toxic doses of many drugs, it is incorrect to extrapolate kinetics during overdose from data derived during therapeutic dosage studies. Therefore, whenever possible, determination of the elimination half-life of a drug should be made in intoxicated patients to indicate the benefit derived from dialysis or hemoperfusion therapy (19).

Dialysis

Concept of Dialysis

In practice, hemodialysis is performed by withdrawing blood continuously from the circulation and pumping it through plastic tubes that serve as a semipermeable membrane. A dialysate solution bathes the other side of the membrane. Continuously pumping the blood and dialysate at specific flow rates permits maintenance of concentration gradients for appropriate diffusion. Adjustment of resistance to flow permits the creation of hydrostatic and pressure gradients (21).

The solute composition of the blood is altered by exposing the blood to a modified salt solution, which is the dialysate, separated by a semipermeable membrane. In hemodialysis, this membrane is artificial, whereas with peritoneal dialysis, the peritoneum acts as the dialysis membrane (19). Solutes and water pass across the semipermeable membrane through the processes of diffusion and ultrafiltration. The movement of solutes is directly proportional to the magnitude of existing concentration gradients. The concentration gradient can be manipulated by the measured addition of substances to the dialysate concentration. A typical blood flow rate with standard equipment is between 200 and 300 mL/min.

The dialysate has direct access across the semipermeable membrane to the patient's bloodstream and with each dialysis session, the patient is exposed to approximately 120 L of dialysate. For this reason, maintaining a quality water supply is a major focus in hemodialysis. Several contaminants of water can directly affect the patient's health (14).

Exposure of blood to dialysis membranes initiates the clotting cascade, and anticoagulation is used routinely to prevent occlusion of the dialyzer (22). Heparin is widely used as an initial bolus followed by a constant infusion. Coagulation is monitored using either the whole blood partial thromboplastin time, the activated clotting time, or the Lee-White clotting time, in which a 50% increase in clotting time is sufficient. Bleeding is a frequent complication of systemic heparin use and is particularly common in patients with bleeding disorders or liver disease.

Patients may be dialyzed without any heparin or citrate. Anticoagulant free dialysis is particularly useful in patients with prolonged bleeding times; however, steps must be taken to decrease the incidence of clotting in the dialyzer (17).

Peritoneal Dialysis

The principles that govern peritoneal dialysis are similar to those for hemodialysis. Peritoneal dialysis is limited by the rate of mesenteric blood flow, which cannot be adjusted as in hemodialysis. Because the clearance of toxins depends on both the blood flow rate and the dialysate flow rate, hemodialysis is a more rapid and efficient means of dialyzing the poisoned patient (11). Peritoneal dialysis clearances rarely exceed 10 mL/min (23). This technique is, therefore, rarely useful for treating poisonings unless conducted over prolonged intervals (14,19).

Criteria for Dialysis

No single criterion determines the dialyzability of any drug; often there may be a complex relationship that determines this factor. Essentially, to be dialyzed a substance should (a) be of small molecular weight, (b) have limited protein and lipid binding, (c) have a small volume of distribution, and (d) diffuse readily across a dialysis membrane (Table 3–4). Therefore, agents that are highly protein-bound, have low aqueous solubility, or are poorly distributed in plasma water are poorly dialyzable.

Molecular weight. Drugs with a low molecular weight cross the dialysis membrane more readily than compounds with high molecular weight because the membrane's pores allow the smaller compounds to pass. Removal by dialysis of an agent from either peritoneal fluid or blood decreases as the molecular weight of the agent increases: a small solute such as lithium (74 daltons) is dialyzable, but a larger drug such as vancomycin (1,800 daltons) is not, despite its low protein binding (10%). Small molecules (<500 daltons) exhibit high membrane permeability with a rapid decline in blood to dialysate gradient; the limiting determinants of clearance are blood and dialysate flow rates. In contrast, large molecules exhibit low membrane permeability, maintain a gradient across the membrane,

TABLE 3–4. *Pharmacokinetic properties important to extracorporeal therapy*

A.	Will passive diffusion through a membrane be possible?	Most drugs are eliminated by passive diffusion; therefore, the existence of a concentration gradient and molecular size are important.
B.	Is the drug lipid-soluble?	Lipid-soluble drugs accumulate in lipid-rich tissues and are not accessible for elimination.
C.	Does the drug ionize at physiologic pH?	Ionization inhibits drug transport across body membranes. This can aid in elimination by trapping the ionized form of the drug on one side of the membrane. Drugs that ionize remain in the serum and are more available for elimination.
D.	Is the drug highly protein-bound?	Only the unbound form of the drug participates in the diffusion equilibrium.
E.	What is the drug's volume of distribution?	A high volume of distribution is consistent with high tissue concentrations; therefore, less drug is accessible for extracorporeal removal.
F.	Is there a high degree of variability in equilibrium for various tissues?	If there is, changes in one compartment may not accurately reflect changes in other compartments. Serum levels may fall quickly, but if tissue levels lag behind, the clinical effect of the intoxication will continue.

From Steinhart C and Pearson-Shaver A, *Crit Care Clin* 1988; 4:850, with permission.

and their clearance is dependent on membrane surface area rather than the rate of blood or dialysate flow. Therefore, a low cardiac output in the intoxicated patient may preclude the effectiveness of either peritoneal or hemodialysis by reducing blood flow rates and compromising the effective membrane surface area (19).

Water solubility. Drugs that are poorly solubilized in water are poorly diffused in the aqueous dialysate solution because they do not diffuse from the blood into the aqueous dialysate medium. For example, despite a low molecular weight of 252 daltons, phenytoin is insoluble in water at a pH of 7.4, highly protein-bound, and therefore is not dialyzed (19).

Volume of distribution. If the apparent volume of distribution is large, only a small amount of the drug will be available for elimination by dialysis because only a small amount of the drug is in the vascular compartment.

Protein binding. Albumin is not well filtered by the kidneys, so that drugs bound to proteins in the plasma are also not diffusible through the dialysis membrane. Therefore, only the free drug is available for removal.

Active metabolites. All these criteria apply as well to active metabolites of the parent compound (Table 3–5).

Indications for Dialysis

Immediate dialysis. Immediate dialysis is indicated for only two drugs, ethylene glycol and methanol, which cause toxicity because of their breakdown products. If a patient presents with a history of ingestion of either of these compounds and is acidotic or has visual symptoms, then dialysis should be instituted immediately.

TABLE 3–5. *Pharmacologically active metabolites of drugs*

Drug	Metabolite
Acetylsalicylic acid	Salicylic acid
Amitriptyline	Nortriptyline
Chloral hydrate	Trichloroethanol
Chlordiazepoxide	Desmethylchlordiazepoxide
Codeine	Morphine
Diazepam	Desmethyldiazepam
Digitoxin	Digoxin
Flurazepam	Desmethylflurazepam
Glutethimide	4-Hydroxyglutethimide
Imipramine	Desipramine
Lidocaine	Desethyllidocaine
Meperidine	Normeperidine
Methamphetamine	Amphetamine
Phenacetin	Acetaminophen
Phenylbutazone	Oxyphenbutazone
Prednisone	Prednisolone
Primidone	Phenobarbital
Procainamide	N-Acetylprocainamide
Propranolol	4-Hydroxypropranolol

Adapted from Rowland M, Tozer T. *Clinical pharmacokinetics: concepts and application.* Philadelphia: Lea & Febiger;1980:125, with permission.

TABLE 3–6. *Drugs for which dialysis is indicated on the basis of patient condition*

Alcohols	Phenobarbitol
Amphetamines	Potassium
Bromides	Quinidine
Chloral hydrate	Salicylate
Ethylene glycol	Strychnine
Isoniazid	Theophylline
Isopropanol	Thiocyanate
Lithium	
Methanol	

Dialysis on the basis of patient condition. Although dialysis may be effective in the removal of certain other drugs (Table 3–6), it is usually not necessary unless certain conditions exist (Table 3–7). Even then, dialysis is usually reserved for salicylates, theophylline, long-acting barbiturates, and lithium.

Dialysis has been shown to not be effective for many of the drugs previously thought to yield an effective return from dialysis (Table 3–8).

Substances Removed by Hemodialysis (Table 3–6)

Alcohols

Ethanol is the most common intoxicant in this class of drugs. Ethanol causes severe chronic consequences as well as life-threatening acute toxic syndrome; however, because this drug is rapidly metabolized and does not cause the accumulation of toxic metabolites, hemodialy-

TABLE 3–7. *Conditions for which dialysis is required*

A.	Progressive deterioration despite intensive supportive therapy
B.	Severe intoxication with hypoventilation, hypothermia, or hypotension
C.	Impairment of normal excretory function due to hepatic, cardiac, or renal insufficiency
D.	Development of coma or other complications during therapy (i.e., pneumonia or sepsis) or the existence of conditions predisposing to such complications (i.e., obstructive airway disease)
E.	Potentially lethal ingestion and probable absorption of the intoxicant
F.	Toxin metabolized to more toxic substances (methanol, ethylene glycol)
G.	Poisoning by agents with delayed toxicity

From Steinhart C and Pearson-Shaver A, *Crit Care Clin* 1988; 4:851, with permission.

TABLE 3–8. *Drugs for which dialysis is contraindicated*

Antidepressants	Glutethimide
Antihistamines	Methaqualone
Benzodiazepines	Methyprylon
Digitalis	Opiates
Ethchlorvynol	Phenothiazines

sis has almost no place in the treatment of acute ethanol intoxication (24).

Hemodialysis removes both isopropanol and acetone efficiently, thus shortening the duration of coma and potentially reversing the hemodynamic consequences of the intoxication. The rate of removal of these two compounds is 40 to 50 times faster through dialysis than via renal excretion. Hemodialysis is indicated for isopropanol ingestion with refractory hypotension, evidence of myocardial depression or tachyarrhythmias, or renal failure (14).

In conjunction with the ethanol-induced blockade of the action of alcohol dehydrogenase, hemodialysis is effective in reducing the mortality rate and the permanent optic sequelae of methanol poisoning. Dialysis not only accelerates the elimination of the parent compound but also its toxic metabolites and corrects the metabolic acidosis.

In ethylene glycol intoxication, one should aggressively attempt to correct the metabolic acidosis with sodium bicarbonate, the achievement and maintenance of an adequate ethanol level, and the institution of hemodialysis using a bicarbonate bath. With this combination, even severe acidosis can be reversed and the metabolism of ethylene glycol is retarded while both the parent compound and its toxic metabolites are effectively cleared by dialysis (11).

Lithium

Hemodialysis is highly effective in the removal of lithium. During dialysis, the extraction ratio of lithium is 90%, and serum levels decrease dramatically. However because of the relatively slow equilibration of intracellular and extracellular lithium, a "rebound" of serum levels occurs following cessation of dialysis. This rebound can be obviated by extending the duration of dialysis to 8 or even 10 hours, or by repeating the dialysis, depending upon the severity of the intoxication (25).

Salicylate

The volume of distribution V_d of salicylates is small and removal of substantial quantities by extracorporeal devices is excellent. Both hemoperfusion and hemodialysis clear salicylate from the blood; however, hemodialysis is the superior method because of the frequent association of salicylate poisoning with acid-base, electrolyte, and extracellular fluid volume disturbances (26).

Long-Acting Barbiturates

Long-acting compounds like phenobarbital, and drugs that are converted to phenobarbital have a low pKa value, increased water solubility, decreased protein binding, and effective removal by hemodialysis. The short and intermediate barbiturates are not effectively removed by dialysis.

Theophylline

Although hemodialysis removes theophylline, hemoperfusion is more efficient. There are two major reasons why hemoperfusion is superior to hemodialysis for theophylline intoxication. First, theophylline is present in plasma and in red blood cells in almost equal concentrations. Charcoal hemoperfusion is capable of extricating theophylline as efficiently from plasma as from red blood cells; thus, the total amount of drug removed depends on blood flow rather than on plasma flow. Second, cardiac arrhythmias have hemodynamic instability as major problems in patients with severe theophylline toxicity, and they are more likely to be aggravated by hemodialysis than by hemoperfusion, which appears to be less prone to cause hypotension and hemodynamic instability (14).

Dialysis in Perspective

Although dialysis can be a useful means of removing endogenous wastes in the event of poor renal function, it has a limited application in toxicology (17). The use of hemodialysis in the treatment of drug overdose has waned in recent years because of the good results obtained with conservative management and the poor clearance of many drugs with standard dialysis procedures (19). The overwhelming majority of overdosed patients can be treated conservatively, and procedures such as peritoneal dialysis and hemodialysis are seldom indicated in the modern treatment of drug intoxication. In many instances, claims of efficacy have been based on uncontrolled observations. With very few exceptions, dialysis should be considered only a part of the supportive care of a poisoned patient and not the primary form of treatment.

Hemoperfusion

Hemoperfusion, first described approximately 40 years ago (27), is a procedure in which blood is passed through various adsorbent materials, such as activated charcoal or amberlite (a polymeric resin that has an affinity for lipid-soluble organic molecules) (27,28). These adsorbent materials contain granules of either activated charcoal or resins coated with a semipermeable membrane through which blood may pass. The cartridges are disposable, and conventional hemodialysis tubing, pumps, and monitoring devices are used. Hemoperfusion is essentially dialysis against an adsorbent. Hemoperfusion removes substances from the blood by direct contact within adsorbent material. Any material that has greater affinity than blood for a given substance removes both native and foreign substances (27,29–31).

Early column use was plagued with complications including febrile reactions, destruction of blood cells, embolization of charcoal particles, electrolyte disturbances, and thrombosis. The development in the early 1970s of coated charcoal, fixed-bed charcoal, and the discovery of newer polymer resins overcame these technical problems (19). Resin cartridges are no longer available, presumably because they offer only marginal advantages over charcoal in the extraction of lipid-soluble poisons and have a more limited range of applicability.

Advantages and Disadvantages of Hemoperfusion

The advantage of hemoperfusion is that it circumvents some of the physical drug characteristics, such as molecular weight, water solubility, and protein binding, that limit dialysis (Table 3–9) (32). Agents that are highly protein-bound, have a low aqueous solubility, or are poorly distributed in plasma water are poorly dialyzable. With these agents, the technique of hemoperfusion may be appropriate. In general, drugs are removed from the blood at a more rapid rate by hemoperfusion than by dialysis. For example, a 2-or 3-hour hemoperfusion may remove as much drug as an 8-hour hemodialysis (9). The adsorptive capacity of most charcoal columns is large, but the nonspecificity allows many blood-borne substances to adhere to the charcoal, which quickly reduces its capacity to adsorb desired toxins. Consequently, removal rate declines progressively with prolonged use, necessitating column replacement (19).

Limitations of Hemoperfusion

Pharmacokinetic parameters such as volume of distribution limit the applicability of hemoperfusion. In addition, the affinity of the drug for the adsorbent material and the binding capacity of the adsorbent material must be considered as well as the hazards involved in the procedure (29).

TABLE 3–9. *Charcoal hemoperfusion*

Advantages over hemodialysis
Circumvents molecular weight
water solubility
protein binding
More rapid removal than hemodialysis
Complications of hemoperfusion
Bacteremia
Bleeding to heparinization
Damage to blood-forming elements
Destruction of platelets
Destruction of red and white blood cells
Embolization of adsorbent particles
Hypocalcemia
Hypoglycemia
Hypotension
Hypothermia
Infection at blood access site
Removal of normal body fluids
Indications for hemoperfusion
Long-acting barbiturates
Salicylates
Theophylline

Complications of Hemoperfusion

Because direct contact of blood with activated charcoal results in significant damage to blood-forming elements, embolization of adsorbent particles, destruction of red and white blood cells, and, more commonly, destruction of platelets and the removal of certain normal body fluids such as plasma proteins and solutes are frequent consequences of the procedure (33). Complications from hemoperfusion include a drop in platelet count that averages about 30% which rarely causes bleeding, hypoglycemia, and some decrease in the white blood cell count. Other complications are common to all methods that require extracorporeal blood circulation and include bleeding due to heparinization, the possibility of infection at the blood access site, bacteremia, and hypotension due to hemodynamic changes (11).

Since the 1960s most clinical investigators have used encapsulated filters (34), which embed the charcoal on a column (21,35), but complications such as platelet destruction, hypotension, hypothermia, hypocalcemia, and the risks associated with heparinization still exist (10,36). Another important aspect of hemoperfusion is that it does not correct any acid-base or electrolyte disorders that may be secondary to the ingestion of the drug (37).

Indications for Hemoperfusion

Hemoperfusion is indicated for a massive intoxication when the extracellular distribution of the drug is significant and when the plasma level of the drug is at its maximum (22,27,32,34,38,39). Typically, hemoperfusion is successful with the same compounds that can be dialyzed (barbiturates, salicylates, and theophylline) and has been found to be ineffective for drugs with weak extracellular distribution (digoxin, tricyclic antidepressants, heavy metals, and glutethimide) (38–41). Some investigators seriously question the efficacy of hemoperfusion in comparison to supportive and conservative care (42). Others hold that hemoperfusion should never be employed for drug overdose, especially in view of its drawbacks (41,42).

Hemodialysis vs. Hemoperfusion

Hemodialysis is less effective than is hemoperfusion for the majority of poisons because the necessity of preventing the leakage of blood components into the large fluid volume of the dialysate (while withstanding a substantial hydrostatic pressure gradient) dictates that dialysis membranes must have a relatively low porosity and great thickness. Furthermore, the total surface of the dialyzing membrane has an upper limit of just a few square meters. By contrast, hemoperfusion cartridges are characterized by ultrathin membranes of high porosity and extensive surface area (14).

The absolute clearances obtained by hemoperfusion cannot be matched by any other existing extracorporeally facilitated drug removal process (36). For highly protein-bound poisons, hemoperfusion offers the best opportunity for rapid removal. For dialysable poisons with a small V_d, acute hemodialysis seems the most reasonable approach. However, both hemoperfusion and acute hemodialysis are short-lived procedures and the possibility of post-therapy "rebound" in blood concentration exists. The contribution of dialysis or hemoperfusion to the overall clearance of a drug must be determined by first considering the intrinsic plasma clearance of the drug without extracorporeal removal.

Hemofiltration

Continuous arteriovenous hemofiltration (CAVH) is an extracorporeal method of removing plasma water and solutes via hemofiltration. CAVH is a bedside modality, generally used in the intensive care unit. It does not require specialty-trained personnel such as dialysis nurses or technicians (20).

The principle of CAVH depends on the diffusion of substances along a concentration gradient (18). The hydraulic pressure of CAVH causes blood solutes to be removed by convective transport through semipermeable artificial membranes over a continuous period. This differs from that of hemoperfusion, in that perfusion removes via sorbent-binding (20). Anticoagulation, usually with heparin, is necessary to prevent blood from clotting and occluding the filter.

Because only the unbound drug in plasma water is filterable, the extent of filtration is limited by the amount of binding to plasma proteins (43). Hemofiltration is also dependent upon the volume of distribution of a particular drug. Drugs that are highly tissue bound will not be filtered significantly because not enough of the drug will reach the hemofilter.

In the appropriate clinical setting, CAVH is suggested to offer certain specific advantages. When compared with hemodialysis, CAVH allows for less hemodynamic instability, gradual changes in osmolality, no complement activation or leukopenia, and a decreased need for specialized personnel (20).

There are no reported absolute contraindications to CAVH. A relative contraindication to CAVH is active bleeding or the presence of a coagulopathy. Filter rupture, with blood leakage into the environment or from a communication between the blood and ultrafiltrate space is the major reported problem intrinsic to the filter. Despite these apparent advantages, it has been demonstrated that more complications occur with CAVH per liter of urea cleared than with intermittent hemodialysis (20).

Plasmapheresis

Plasmapheresis uses the technique of phlebotomy and modifies it so that the cellular components of the blood are returned to the patient (44). The plasma and plasma proteins are then replaced with fresh plasma or a suitable colloid (45). Although modifications of this procedure were used for centuries, it was successfully utilized for clinical manifestations of hyperviscosity in the 1960s (45). Since that time it has been suggested for many disorders but only in anecdotal reports, not in controlled studies.

Plasmapheresis can be considered a modification of exchange transfusion (9). Many of the same requirements for hemodialysis or hemoperfusion also apply to plasmapheresis, especially that the drug have a small volume of distribution so that it will be present in sufficient quantity in the plasma for there to be an effective extraction. If the drug has a large volume of distribution, even an efficient system of plasmapheresis will remove only a small amount. In addition, both hemoperfusion and hemodialysis are generally able to clear much larger volumes of plasma than plasmapheresis. Plasmapheresis is most useful with drugs that are strongly protein- bound, have a long half-life, and are not well dialyzed or hemoperfused (44).

Plasmapheresis can be run using either a veno-venous or arteriovenous circuit (44). A pump is necessary to run veno-venous plasmapheresis, but arteriovenous plasmapheresis can be either driven by a pump or by the patient's own blood pressure. Provided the patient has a stable circulation with a mean arterial pressure > 60 mm Hg, blood pressure driven arteriovenous plasmapheresis is a useful alternative if a pump is not available. It is less efficient than hemoperfusion and hemodialysis but works with highly protein-bound drugs that have small volumes of distribution (13).

Many of the side effects associated with other extracorporeal methods are noted with plasmapheresis, including bleeding from anticoagulation, extracorporeal blood clotting, thrombotic complications, hypocalcemia, fluid overload, citrate toxicity, infection, and problems associated with vascular access. In addition, plasmapheresis can be a very expensive procedure.

MULTIPLE-DOSE ACTIVATED CHARCOAL

In the past, the applicability of charcoal was thought to be limited to its ability to bind whatever drug remained in the gastrointestinal tract after emesis or gastric lavage was performed. It is now widely accepted that the clearance of some drugs and poisons is increased when activated charcoal is administered in multiple oral doses; for this reason, activated charcoal has recently emerged as a valuable new modality to increase the elimination of certain agents (46,47). This intervention is now frequently used in the management of many overdosed patients, in large part because this therapy is innately attractive to clinicians (24). It is reasonable to expect that an increased clearance of a toxin from the body should result in a decreased duration of toxicity. It is, however, a controversial area in toxicology (24).

There are three ways in which activated charcoal can be effective. One involves prevention of absorption of a toxin, and the other two involve enhancing excretion of the toxin (48). The first makes use of a single dose of activated charcoal, which is effective because it prevents primary absorption of the toxin. Multiple-dose activated charcoal may aid excretion of drugs by two different mechanisms: interruption of enterohepatic recirculation of certain drugs, and adsorption of drug secreted across intestinal membranes into the bowel lumen (intestinal dialysis) (25,49,50).

Preventing Primary Absorption of a Drug

Activated charcoal may adsorb any remaining drug in the gastrointestinal tract. There is ample documentation that this is clinically important (see Chapter 2).

Enhancing Elimination of a Drug

Interruption of Enterohepatic Circulation

The activity of some drugs, particularly the high molecular weight polar compounds, can be decreased if their natural cycle of enterohepatic recirculation is interrupted. Because of enterohepatic circulation, these drugs are reabsorbed into the stomach or intestine through the biliary system. Interruption of this pathway facilitates fecal elimination of the toxin (48).

Agents that interfere with enterohepatic recirculation include anionic exchange resins such as cholestyramine or colestipol (Table 3–10). Activated charcoal is another agent that appears to have a useful role in binding drugs in the gastrointestinal tract that are recycled enterohepatically. At this time, such methods are promising but still in the experimental stage because no definite advantage has been shown in controlled studies.

TABLE 3–10. *Drugs that undergo enterohepatic recirculation or secretion into the stomach*

Carbamazepine
Digitoxin
Glutethimide
Meprobamate
Nadolol
Phencyclidine
Phenylbutazone
Tricyclic antidepressants

"Intestinal Dialysis"

Most nonionized drugs and poisons dissolved in the blood can diffuse across gastrointestinal membranes. Furthermore, many drugs can be concentrated in gastrointestinal fluids by ion trapping as predicted by the pH partition gradient (25). Therefore, there exists a persistent concentration gradient favoring the passive diffusion of poison into the gastrointestinal lumen. Intestinal dialysis is an attempt at using the mesenteric capillaries and intestinal epithelium as a dialysis membrane. Drugs or poisons that can easily diffuse across gastrointestinal membranes and also have small volumes of distribution (less than 1 L/kg) are effectively removed by multiple-dose activated charcoal. Drugs with large volumes of distribution are not effectively removed by orally administered activated charcoal (26). Overall, the principles that govern the ability of oral activated charcoal to increase the clearance of drugs and poisons from the body are analogous to the principles that govern the effectiveness of hemodialysis and hemoperfusion for removing drugs and poisons (43). It has been postulated that gastrointestinal dialysis is comparable in effect to peritoneal dialysis. It is believed that a large amount of unbound charcoal in the intestine creates a large drug concentration gradient between the blood and intestinal contents, favoring diffusion of the drug from the circulation into the intestinal lumen and onto the charcoal. This increases the clearance of some compounds from the body. For example, substantial decreases in serum half-life have been reported for theophylline, phenobarbital, and dapsone (51). In theory, multiple-dose activated charcoal may also be effective for enhancing the elimination of salicylates. In addition, multiple-dose activated charcoal may prevent desorption of drug from the charcoal as it passes down the gastrointestinal tract. For this reason, many toxicologists advocate the use of multiple-dose activated charcoal as a safe alternative to extracorporeal methods of drug removal in mild to moderate poisonings with these drugs (26).

Considerations in the Use of Multiple-Dose Activated Charcoal

As can be seen, not many compounds undergo enhanced elimination by multiple-dose activated charcoal, and the pharmacokinetic characteristics of the compound should be considered before patients are treated in this way (51). A drug whose excretion may be enhanced by multiple-dose activated charcoal must have a small volume of distribution, not be extensively bound to plasma proteins or other blood compartments, must be lipophilic (uncharged), or it must undergo enterohepatic or enteroenteric circulation (26). Most compounds have some degree of protein binding, so that the upper limit of hepatic blood flow will only apply to the clearance of unbound drug. The administration of activated charcoal should not replace supportive care, nor should it be relied on as the sole treatment of an intoxication (24).

Method of Administration

The optimal dose and frequency of administration of activated charcoal (AC) are not well defined. The dosage usually recommended for adults is 20 to 100 g every 2 to 8 hours until objective evidence and clinical observations indicate that serum drug concentrations have declined to a subtoxic range. A dosage of 5 to 10 g every 4 to 8 hours is recommended for children. It should be noted that both the dosage of AC and the dosing interval have been arbitrarily established. It appears that the more frequent use of smaller doses of AC is equally as efficacious as the 4-hour administration regimen (51). When using this method, it is important to keep the gut continuously full of charcoal, at least as far as is practical, and it may not be necessary to administer sorbitol or other cathartics more than once (25). There is also the potential for fluid and electrolyte depletion if sorbitol or other cathartics are used with each dose of activated charcoal in a multiple-dose regimen. Aspiration is an even more serious complication. Although charcoal is relatively unreactive and the acidic gastric contents are known to be the cause of the aspiration syndrome, the repeated administration of charcoal risks triggering vomiting episodes (52).

Multiple-Dose Cathartic

Treatment with multiple-dose cathartic has been associated with many reports of adverse reactions (52–54). Osmotic cathartics have the potential to cause hypernatremic dehydration. Because both the ileum and the colon have the ability to absorb sodium against a large concentration gradient, and because the normal passive transfer of water is retarded by the presence of the osmotically active substance, the sodium concentration in the stool may be considerably less than its concentration in plasma (48). This minimal electrolyte content coupled with the large stool volumes induced by sorbitol may lead to water depletion and hypernatremia unless vigorous water replacement is provided. In addition to water losses in the stools, repetitive doses of sorbitol could cause excessive losses of potassium and bicarbonate, resulting in hypokalemia and normal anion-gap metabolic acidosis (54).

Multiple doses of saline cathartics, such as magnesium sulfate, should not be administered because this regimen has resulted in hypermagnesemia with acute neuromuscular deterioration that required dialysis (53). Furthermore, gastrointestinal obstruction has been reported after repeated doses of activated charcoal along with a cathartic (55). Repeated doses of activated charcoal may also adsorb orally and parenterally administered drugs necessary for the management of the overdosed patient. These medications may therefore have to be administered more frequently.

SUMMARY

Although there are methods to enhance excretion of various compounds, they are effective for very few compounds. Forced diuresis, dialysis, and hemoperfusion are all limited in the number of compounds for which they are effective. Many of the advantages and disadvantages of extracorporeal means of drug removal are not likely to change markedly as a result of improved technology because it is the chemical characteristics of toxic substances that limit the role of these procedures. Multiple-dose activated charcoal appears to offer the advantage of not having dangerous side effects but still being an effective means for removing certain compounds.

REFERENCES

1. Arena J: The clinical diagnosis of poisoning. *Pediatr Clin North Am* 1970;17:477–494.
2. Cashman T, Shirkey H: Emergency management of poisoning. *Pediatr Clin North Am* 1970;17:525–534.
3. Gilles C, Ford P, Lovejoy F, et al: Management of pediatric poisoning. *Pediatr Nurs* 1980;6:33–44.
4. Gossel T, Wuest J: The right first aid for poisoning. *RN* 1981;44:73–75.
5. Kaufman R, Levy S: Overdose treatment. *JAMA* 1974;227:411–416.
6. Keller L: Poisoning in children. *Postgrad Med* 1979;65:177–186.
7. Sullivan J, Rumack B, Peterson R: Management of the poisoned patient in the emergency department: poisonings and overdose. *Top Emerg Med* 1979;1:1–12.
8. Sunshine J: Basic toxicology. *Pediatr Clin North Am* 1970;17:509–513.
9. Peterson R, Peterson L: Cleansing the blood: hemodialysis, peritoneal dialysis, exchange transfusion, charcoal hemoperfusion, forced diuresis. *Pediatr Clin North Am* 1986;33:675–689.
10. Watanabe A, Rumack B, Peterson R: Enhancement of elimination in poisonings. *Top Emerg Med* 1979;1:19–26.
11. Winchester J: Poisoning: is the role of the nephrologist diminishing? *Am J Kid Dis* 1989;13:171–183.
12. Matthew H: Acute poisoning: some myths and misconceptions. *Br Med J* 1971;1:519–522.
13. Schlager D, Sanders, A, Wiggins D, et al: Ultrasound for the detection of foreign bodies. *Ann Emerg Med* 1991;20:189–191.
14. Garella S: Extracorporeal techniques in the treatment of exogenous intoxications. *Kidney Int* 1988;33:735–754.
15. Barton C, Sterling M, Thomas R, et al: Ineffectiveness of intravenous ascorbic acid as an acidifying agent in man. *Arch Intern Med* 1981;141:211–212.
16. Nahata M, Shimp L, Lampman T, et al: Effect of ascorbic acid on urine pH in man. *Am J Hosp Pharm* 1977;34:1231–1237.

17. Jameson M, Wiegmann T: Principles, uses, and complications of hemodialysis. *Med Clin North Am* 1990;74:945–960.
18. Golper T, Bennett W: Drug removal by continuous arteriovenous haemofiltration. A review of the evidence in poisoned patients. *Med Toxicol* 1988;3:341–349.
19. Cutler R, Forland S, Hammond P, et al: Extracorporeal removal of drugs and poisons by hemodialysis and hemoperfusion. *Ann Rev Pharmacol Toxicol* 1987;27:169–191.
20. Nahman N, Middendorf D: Continuous arteriovenous hemofiltration. *Med Clin North Am* 1990;74:975–984.
21. Lis R, Lief P: Extracorporeal methods in the intensive care unit. *Anes Clin North Am* 1991;9:245–263.
22. Vale J, Rees A, Widdop B, et al: Use of charcoal hemoperfusion in the management of severely poisoned patients. *Br Med J* 1975;1:5–9.
23. Steinhart C, Pearson-Shaver A: Poisoning. *Crit Care Clin* 1988;4:845–872.
24. Tenenbein M: Multiple doses of activated charcoal: time for reappraisal? *Ann Emerg Med* 1991;20:529–531.
25. Campbell J, Chyka P: Physiochemical characteristics of drugs and response to repeat-dose activated charcoal. *Am J Emerg Med* 1992;10:208–210.
26. Dolgin J, Nix D, Sanchez J, et al: Pharmacokinetic simulation of the effect of multiple-dose activated charcoal in phenytoin poisoning—report of two pediatric cases. *DICP Ann Pharmacother* 1991;25:646–649.
27. Rosenbaum J, Kramer M, Raja R: Resin hemoperfusion for acute drug intoxication. *Arch Intern Med* 1976;136:263–265.
28. Rosenbaum J, Kramer M, Raja R, et al: Current status of hemoperfusion in toxicology. *Clin Toxicol* 1980;17:493–500.
29. Lorch J, Garella S: Hemoperfusion to treat intoxications. *Ann Intern Med* 1979;91:301–304.
30. Muirhead E, Reid A: A resin artificial kidney. *J Lab Clin Med* 1948;33:841–844.
31. Okonek S: Hemoperfusion in toxicology: basic considerations of its effectiveness. *Clin Toxicol* 1981;18:1185–1198.
32. Bismuth C, Fournier P, Galliot M: Biological evaluation of hemoperfusion in acute poisoning. *Clin Toxicol* 1981;18:1213–1223.
33. Mamdani B, Dunea C: Long-term hemoperfusion with coated activated charcoal. *Clin Toxicol* 1980;17:543–546.
34. Trafford A, Horn C, Sharpstone P, et al: Hemoperfusion in acute drug toxicity. *Clin Toxicol* 1980;17:547–556.
35. Chang T: Clinical experience with ACAC-coated charcoal hemoperfusion in acute intoxication. *Clin Toxicol* 1980;17:529–542.
36. De Groot G, Maes R, Van Heijst A: A toxicological evaluation of different adsorbents in hemoperfusion. *Clin Toxicol* 1981;18:1199–1211.
37. Koffler A, Bernstein M, LaSette A, et al: Fixed-bed charcoal hemoperfusion. *Arch Intern Med* 1978;138:1691–1694.
38. Gelfand M, Winchester J: Hemoperfusion in drug overdosage: conservative management is not sufficient. *Clin Toxicol* 1980;17:583–602.
39. Gelfand M: Hemoperfusion in drug overdose. *JAMA* 1978;240:2761–2762.
40. Gibson T: Hemoperfusion of digoxin intoxication. *Clin Toxicol* 1980;17:501–513.
41. Garella S, Lorch J: Hemoperfusion for acute intoxications. *Clin Toxicol* 1980;17:515–527.
42. Dumont C, Rangno R: Argument against hemoperfusion in drug overdose. *JAMA* 1979;242:1611.
43. Bellomo R, Kearly Y, Parkin G, et al: Treatment of life-threatening lithium toxicity with continuous arterio-venous hemodiafiltration. *Crit Care Med* 1991;19:836–839.
44. Laussen P, Shann F, Butt W, et al: Use of plasmapheresis in acute theophylline toxicity. *Crit Care Med* 1991;19:288–290.
45. Jones J, Dougherty J: Current status of plasmapheresis in toxicology. *Ann Emerg Med* 1986;15:474–482.
46. Levy G: Gastrointestinal clearance of drugs with activated charcoal. *N Engl J Med* 1982;307:676–678.
47. Pond S: Role of repeated oral doses of activated charcoal in clinical toxicology. *Med Toxicol* 1986;1:3–11.
48. Ros S, Black L: Multiple-dose activated charcoal in management of phenytoin overdose. *Pediatr Emerg Care* 1989;5:169–170.
49. Park G, Spector R, Goldberg M, et al: Expanded role of charcoal therapy in the poisoned and overdosed patient. *Arch Intern Med* 1986;146:969–973.
50. Katona B, Siegel E, Cluxton R: The new black magic: activated charcoal and new therapeutic uses. *J Emerg Med* 1987;5:9–18.
51. Ilkhanipour K, Yealy K, Krenzrelok E: The comparative efficacy of various multiple-dose activated charcoal regimens. *Am J Emerg Med* 1992;10:298–300.
52. Wax P, Wang R, Hoffman R, et al: Prevalence of sorbitol in multiple-dose activated charcoal regimens in the emergency departments. *Ann Emerg Med* 1993;22:1807–1812.
53. Jones J, Herselman D, Dougherty J, et al: Cathartic induced magnesium toxicity during overdose management. *Ann Emerg Med* 1986;15:1214–1218.
54. Allerton J, Strom J: Hypernatremia due to repeated doses of charcoal-sorbitol. *Am J Kid Dis* 1991;17:581–584.
55. Watson W, Cremer K, Chapman J: Gastrointestinal obstruction associated with multiple-dose activated charcoal. *J Emerg Med* 1986;4:401–407.

ADDITIONAL SELECTED REFERENCES

Krenzelok E, Keller R, Stewart R: Gastrointestinal transit times of cathartics combined with charcoal. *Ann Emerg Med* 1985;14:1152–1155.

Mofenson H, Caraccio T, Greensher J, et al: Gastrointestinal dialysis with activated charcoal and cathartic in the treatment of adolescent intoxications. *Clin Pediatr* 1985;24:678–684.

Oderda G, Klein-Schwanz W: General management of the poisoned patient. *Crit Care Q* 1982;4:1–18.

Ordog G, Vann P, Owashi N, et al: Intravenous prochlorperazine for the rapid control of vomiting in the emergency department. *Ann Emerg Med* 1984;13:253–258.

Watanabe A: Pharmacokinetic aspects of the dialysis of drugs. *Drug Intell Clin Pharm* 1977;1:407–416.

CHAPTER 4

The Role of the Laboratory

The laboratory can provide a great deal of information to the emergency department physician and can aid in the diagnosis and care given to the overdosed patient (1). Some physicians, however, have unrealistic expectations of how the laboratory can be of help. In the toxicologic setting, the laboratory can aid the physician diagnostically in a qualitative manner through a toxicologic screen for the presence of one or more suspected toxins, or prognostically through a quantitative analysis of a particular toxin. The laboratory can also aid in the therapeutic monitoring of drugs and in testing for drugs of abuse (2). However, the majority of toxicologic diagnoses and therapeutic decisions are made on a clinical basis, even though technology has provided the ability to measure almost any toxin (3).

Certain specific intoxicants require specific antidotal therapies; in these cases expedient laboratory investigation is warranted. For example, the presence of acetaminophen, ethylene glycol, lithium, methanol, iron, salicylates and others should be confirmed as soon as possible so that aggressive therapeutic procedures may be undertaken (4). For most other substances, little change in supportive therapy may be needed, and, if the patient is stable and properly monitored, laboratory work may not be urgently required (5).

Because relatively few classes of drugs are responsible for the great majority of drug intoxications, most laboratories can routinely identify prototypical members of these drug classes (6). Yet, screens do not identify all toxins, and the limited scope of such a test must be understood by the practitioner (5,7).

Methods such as spectrophotometry and spectrophotofluorometry can measure serum drug concentrations of milligrams per liter, which is the typical concentration when drugs are given in doses of several hundred milligrams (8). Some of the new techniques such as gas chromatography, mass spectrometry, and the immunoassays can determine fractions of nanograms or less. This is an important advance in toxicology as well as in the area of therapeutic monitoring of drugs. Many hospitals have the increased capability of performing limited emergency toxicology testing using commercially available reagents compatible with clinical instrumentation (9–11). Supplementing these are the reference laboratories which provide expanded toxicology services with broadened, more sophisticated analytical techniques. Unfortunately, toxicology results, especially in a rural area, do not usually return from outside laboratories in timely fashion.

Appropriate use of the laboratory entails knowing which specific tests to order, whether the presence of a substance (qualitative results) or the concentration of the substance in the blood (quantitative results) is most important, what the "turnaround time" for the results will be, and the type of specimen that should be obtained (e.g., urine or blood) (12). The clinician should communicate to the laboratory as much information as possible about the patient's status to facilitate the selection of screening priorities (13). The patient's signs and symptoms, possibly associated with clinical patterns of drug intoxication, can be used to suspect the presence or absence or narcotics, sedative-hypnotics, stimulants, hallucinogens, and/or antipsychotics (4). (For therapeutic and toxic laboratory values, see Appendix A.)

QUALITATIVE TESTING

The "Tox Screen"

Although it may be important to know whether a patient's altered mental status is caused by ingestion or exposure to a drug or toxin, often it is not mandatory to know the concentration of the toxin to initiate treatment (5). For instance, it is useful to know from a toxicologic screen whether a barbiturate is causing the picture of central nervous system (CNS) depression in a particular patient, but knowing the exact concentration is not as important as following the patient clinically and determining the necessary treatment (14).

Qualitative drug screening continues to be a prevalent practice despite its limitations. A toxicologic screen may be referred to as an "overdose panel," "comprehensive screen," "tox screen," "coma panel," or "drug screen" (15). The name given might imply that a toxicologic screen is truly comprehensive, but a negative screen is not conclusive evidence that no drug that can account for a patient's symptoms has been ingested because most laboratories observe an abridged procedure limited to a few sequential analyses (16). A screen is performed for only certain classes of compounds, and each laboratory uses a different type of screen (17). Because there is no one accepted screen that is uniformly performed and because the protocol for a toxicologic screen is typically determined by the historic needs of the institution, it is of the utmost importance to know exactly what is not included in a toxicologic screen for a particular laboratory (6,7). It is extremely important to have good ongoing communication between emergency department personnel and laboratory technicians so that the most efficient job can be performed by both parties (6,18).

A toxicology screen, therefore, is a combination of many procedures aimed at identifying most of the common drugs in emergency toxicology (19). Screens may include as many procedures as necessary for identification of target drugs or can be focused or abbreviated to give rapid turnaround for a few common critical or difficult-to-recognize drugs (3).

Many methods are employed to detect toxins. Each method differs in cost, complexity, speed, and accuracy (20). The practitioner should become acquainted with the particular methods used, their specificity for each drug group, the substances detected by a particular laboratory's screening, and the length of time it takes to obtain results (21). Justification for the use of toxicologic screening includes the following:

To confirm a diagnosis, when necessary.
As a guide to therapy
For medicolegal evidence.
For allocation of resources.

URINE COMPARED WITH BLOOD SCREENING

Though blood samples are submitted most frequently for the analysis of drugs, urine is the specimen of choice for preliminary studies. Gastric contents are useful only if a recent ingestion is suspected in an overdose (22).

Generally, quantitative analysis is performed on blood or plasma samples, whereas urine is required to perform the qualitative drug screen. The importance of a urine sample in facilitating the toxicology analyses cannot be understated because, as a general rule, urine has a much higher drug concentration than blood. In fact, urine is the best sample for finding the greatest number of drugs in easily detectable quantities (23). Urine produces the highest rate of positive findings when compared with serum or gastric aspirates (24). Adding a blood sample to a urine specimen produces a slightly greater overall yield of positives. The belief lingers, however, that blood is the preferred sample for a general evaluation (18).

TYPES OF TESTING

There are many different methods for drug analysis, and the laboratory must decide on the appropriate degree of sophistication. Laboratories can choose spot tests; thin-layer, gas, liquid, or high-performance liquid chromatography; spectrophotometry; immunoassays, including radioimmunoassay and enzyme-modified immunoassay; gas chromatography with mass spectroscopy; and, recently, nuclear magnetic resonance spectroscopy (18). Whichever method or methods are used in the screening process, it is important to remember that a confirmation of the presumptive presence of drugs be made by an alternative methodology (20).

Methods that are normally used in measuring serum drug concentrations usually do not differentiate between drugs bound to serum proteins (which are therefore inactive) and those that are free. In most situations, however, free drug concentration is a fairly constant percentage of the total, which makes total serum drug levels indicative of the active drug concentration (25).

Typically, laboratory methodology is an area of relative ignorance for the emergency department physician. The following discussion is not meant to be an in-depth analysis of each laboratory test but is an attempt to familiarize the physician with the various laboratory procedures available (Table 4–1). There are a variety of instruments, analytic techniques, and reagent systems currently available to screen for drugs in urine and blood. Each methodology has certain advantages and disadvantages. However, in consideration of the methods used in the screening processes, one must have a basic understanding

TABLE 4–1. *Toxicologic laboratory analyses*

Spot tests
Chromatography
Thin-layer chromatography (TLC)
Gas chromatography (GC)
Liquid chromatography (LC)
Gas-liquid chromatography (GLC)
High-performance (pressure) liquid chromatography (HPLC)
Electrophoresis
Immunoassay
Radioimmunoassay (RIA)
Enzyme-modified immunoassay (EMIT)
Fluorescence polarization immunoassay
Latex particle immunoassay
Enzymatic methods
Spectroscopy
Visible
Ultraviolet
Infrared
Fluorometry
Nuclear magnetic resonance (NMR)
Mass spectroscopy
Gas chromatography with mass spectroscopy (GC-MS)

of the various tests and the results obtained with each methodology.

Comprehensive screening using spot tests, immunoassays, thin-layer chromatography (TLC), and gas chromatography (GC) procedures may require 3 to 4 hours of intense labor. During the application of multiple procedures, many drugs may be confirmed by any two of the procedures. Presently, most laboratories will not report a drug identification unless it is present on two procedures or unless the single method is known to be highly specific for a highly prevalent intoxicant. Initial identification of a drug would be considered only presumptive.

Spot Tests

Spot tests are simple colorimetric tests that rely on a change in the sample color after addition of certain reagents (6). Spot tests are among the simplest and quickest initial screening processes. Although this method is inexpensive, it is characterized by both poor sensitivity and specificity and also requires subjective interpretation (Table 4–2). Drugs such as salicylates, phenothiazines, acetaminophen, phencyclidine, methadone, chloral hydrate, and the tricyclics rely on the chemical reactivity of the drug with specific reagents. These are not usually applied in settings in which a high degree of sensitivity or specificity is required but have found excellent utility when applied to urine in emergency settings because of high drug concentrations present, ease of application, and quick turnaround (26).

Electrophoresis

Electrophoresis is a separation technique based on the movement of charged particles under the influence of an external electric field. Different molecules can be separated in an electric field if they carry different charges. The electric field is applied to a solution through oppositely charged electrodes placed in the solution and a particular ion then travels through the solution toward the electrode of opposite charge. Electrophoresis is not used very often in toxicology (25).

TABLE 4–2. *Spot tests and their sensitivity and specificity*

Drug	Sensitivity	Specificity
Acetaminophen	+	+
Carbamates	+	–
Carbon monoxide	–	–
Ethanol	+	–
Ethchlorvynol	+	+
Iron	–	–
Imipramine	–	–
Phenothiazines	–	–
Salicylate	+	+

Chromatography

Chromatography refers to a group of separation processes of closely related compounds by adsorption from a solution to an adsorbent medium. These methods are classified according to the physical state of the solute or mobile phase. Three types of chromatography are currently employed by clinical laboratories. These are thin-layer chromatography, gas chromatography, and liquid-solid chromatography, commonly referred to as high-performance liquid chromatography (HPLC) (20). Thin-layer, gas, and high-performance liquid chromatography are all based on the flow of a liquid or gas over a solid or liquid stationary phase that contains the unknown compound. Characteristic patterns of drug distribution between the stationary and mobile phases occur.

Chromatographic assays are widely used in emergency toxicology because a large number of drugs may be detected in a single chromatogram. Sensitivity is adequate for many common pharmaceuticals at concentrations seen in overdose. For most chromatographic procedures, drugs must first be extracted from serum, gastric material, or urine. In many cases, further chemical derivatization is necessary in order to make the drug compatible with the chromatographic phase or detection system.

Thin-Layer Chromatography

The earliest technical approaches to drug screening were primarily based on thin-layer chromatography. TLC is one of the most widely used screening procedures; it is inexpensive and requires no automation. It is an excellent method for screening or for the confirmation of drugs (27,28). The results from TLC are qualitative in nature, and positive results cannot be quantified (27).

In TLC, a liquid solvent containing the sample diffuses through a solid adsorbent, which may be glass plates coated with silica (Fig. 4–1) (27). Different compounds migrate by capillary action across this uniform thin layer at different rates, resulting in a separation of the sample constituents. When the solvent reaches the top of the plate some drugs may simultaneously reach the top of the plate, whereas others may not have moved at all (20). The compounds of interest will be located on the plate somewhere between these two extremes. Drugs are detected by spraying chemical reactants on the plate and comparing their location with the co-migrated reference drugs. The fractional distance that each constituent travels is called the migration distance, or Rf value. Visualization of the spots on the thin layer can be achieved through illumination with ultraviolet or fluorescent light. An experienced technician is of utmost importance because of the subjectivity of data interpretation (6).

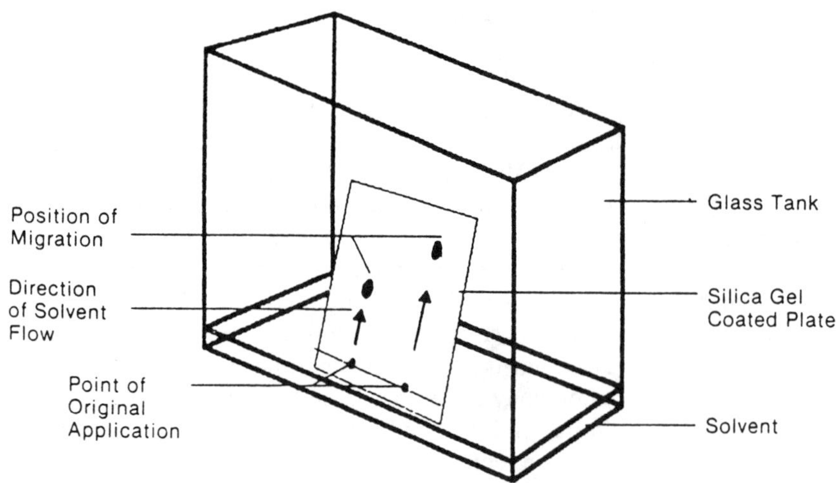

FIG. 4–1. Diagram of thin-layer chromatography. (From Osterloh J, *Emerg Med Clin North Am* 1990;8: 703, with permission.)

Advantages of TLC

TLC, for a number of years, has been the workhorse of analytic methodologies used in the broad-spectrum screening of drugs in urine. It is rather simple to use and the results can be available within approximately 1 hour. TLC for drug detection in emergency situations has become standardized with the use of commercially prepared TLC systems (5,28).

Disadvantages of TLC

Thin-layer chromatography is one of the least sensitive screening methods; a negative result from TLC may be positive from some other, more sensitive method. With TLC, most drugs are detected only when their concentration in urine is 1,000 to 2,000 ng/mL (27). Although this is usually adequate for drug overdoses, there is a lack of specificity associated with TLC, so that its results must always be compared with those of a confirmatory test. The confirmatory test should always be based on a different principle of analysis and should be more specific than the screening test. Another disadvantage of TLC is the relatively long turnaround time required.

Recently, better performance has been obtained through the use of small-particle size derivatized silica, and it is possible to obtain useful separation of many therapeutic drugs. This technique is known as high-performance thin-layer chromatography. The advent of high-performance or high-efficiency TLC has greatly reduced its disadvantages, and many modern techniques are highly specific. In some cases the specificity is beyond that of gas chromatography.

Gas Chromatography

Gas chromatography (GC), or gas-liquid chromatography (GLC) is a rigorous and complicated technique that allows a multitude of compounds within a single sample to be separated and measured simultaneously (29). In GC, molecules in a vaporized sample are separated by means of a glass or metal tube that is packed with material of a particular polarity (27). The stationary phase may be either liquid or solid; the gas is the mobile phase.

When a mixture of substances is injected at the inlet of the column and vaporized, each component is swept through the column and toward a detector. If the substance in question has no affinity for the solvent, then it is deposited on the solid packing material of the column. The column therefore permits graded retardation of the components of the mixture to establish a relatively clean separation among groups of similar molecules. GC requires that the extracted drug be volatile at temperatures inside the GC column (80 to 300°C). To be analyzed by GC, if a drug is not volatile, it may derivatize to form a more volatile form of the substance. Drugs eluting (leaving) from the column can be detected by thermal conductivity, combustivity, ability to donate electrons, capture beta particle beams (electron capture), and ionization.

Once these groups are separated, they leave the column and enter the detection system. When a particular molecule reaches the detector, a signal is produced. The most direct interpretation of this signal may be obtained from a tracing on a flat-bed recorder. The height of each peak is measured and converted to concentration units after comparison with a standard. The time between injection of the sample and appearance of the signal is referred to as the retention time and is characteristic of each substance.

Separation of drugs by GC, then, is based on the characteristic vapor pressures that different compounds establish above the liquid phase of a stationary separation medium. Theoretically, any compound that can be vaporized or converted to a volatile derivative can be analyzed by GC. The technique is usually limited to organic molecules because inorganic compounds lack sufficient volatility. For screening purposes, samples can be chromatographed on a single column or injected into various compound-selective columns to enhance specificity and sensitivity.

Although GC is an excellent tool for analysis, it requires several steps to prepare the samples for analysis. Relatively large volumes of blood or urine are required for the extraction process, although recent advances have made microsampling possible on a more routine basis. One of the major disadvantages of GC is the complexity of instrumentation, which necessitates a highly trained and skilled analyst. As a result of the introduction of capillary columns, narrow-bore open tubular columns with the stationary phase coated on the inner surface, GC has gained popularity as the preferred method to screen for a large number of drugs in a single analysis. Moreover, by equipping the capillary GC with two columns of differing polarities and with two detectors, one is able to screen for drugs and "confirm" in the same analysis (4).

High-Performance Liquid Chromatography

High-performance (pressure) liquid chromatography (HPLC) is similar to GC except that liquid pressurization rather than evaporation is used to force the sample through the adsorbent. HPLC can analyze complex mixtures from microsamples and is rapid and specific, but it is also expensive. The advantage of HPLC is the high resolution of similar compounds, which is made possible by the separating power of the system. HPLC is therefore most useful in situations where more than one substance is being measured. The power of HPLC also lies in its ability to separate structurally similar drugs, such as tricyclics and benzodiazepines.

Most commonly, theophylline and related compounds, antiepileptic drugs, tricyclics, procainamide, disopyramide, the aminoglycosides, and a host of other drugs can be measured by HPLC systems. HPLC and other chromatographic methods are similar in many respects, so that HPLC complements rather than supplants these other methods. The greatest limitation of HPLC is the success of competing immunoassay systems. Although it is quite selective and sensitive, HPLC is too expensive, cumbersome, and time-consuming to be used in general screening, yet HPLC is the method of choice for many drugs not routinely monitored in most clinical labs or for which there are no commercial immunoassays (20).

Immunoassays

Immunoassays are widely employed in drug assays because they provide a high degree of sensitivity and specificity (30). Immunoassays measure substances by exploiting the immunochemical reaction between antigen and antibody. Antigens are substances that induce an immune response. The most potent antigens are macromolecules with molecular sizes greater than 100,000 daltons. Drugs usually have molecular sizes that are too small for them to act as antigens, so that it is necessary to couple the drug to a larger molecule, which is usually a protein. The most commonly used protein is albumin, which is taken from a species other than that in which the antibody is to be raised.

The general theory concerning the immunoassay is that a labeled drug is competitively displaced from an antibody complex by an unlabeled drug in a sample. The amount of labeled drug that is displaced from the antibody is proportional to the amount of unlabeled drug in the sample. Immunoassays for toxic substances use radioisotopic labels, fluorescent labels, latex particles, red cells, and enzymes (30). These techniques differ according to how the drug is labeled and in the method of detection of the displaced labeled drug. Because clinical laboratories frequently have sensitive spectrophotometers and technologists who are experienced in the handling of enzyme-based systems, emphasis has recently shifted to the use of enzyme markers.

Quantitation in serum can also be performed using modified immunoassays for selected drugs. There are a number of commercially available assays that are supplied as a kit. This is only available for a limited number of drugs. All of the available assays have analytic sensitivity in excess of that needed to detect overdose concentrations. These tests are rapid, easy to perform, and have been used as presumptive tests within the emergency department (ED). The immunoassays, then, are often used as initial screens and then confirmed by a second method. The most common type in use is the enzyme immunoassay (EIA) (6) or the enzyme-modified immunoassay (EMIT), but fluorescent polarization inhibition (32,33) and radioimmunoassays (34) are also used in many laboratories.

Radioimmunoassay

In radioimmunoassay (RIA), known quantities of drug-specific antibody and known amounts of isotopically labeled drug are mixed with a sample. The mixture is then scanned for the emission of gamma radiation after the displacement of the labeled antigen by the drug in the sample (6,35). Labeled and unlabeled drug molecules compete for a limited number of binding sites on a specific drug antibody. The amount of displaced label correlates directly with the concentration of drug in the added sample. The sensitivity of this procedure can be at the picogram or nanogram level (35).

The sensitivity of RIA results primarily from the binding affinity between antigen and antibody. The specificity of RIA is a reflection of the uniqueness of fit between an antigen and its corresponding antibody. The affinity of the unknown drug for the antibody is plotted as a curve, which is compared with standard curves so that the unknown drug can be identified (35). Because there is no difference between the bound and free labeled drug, it is necessary to separate the two before measurement; therefore, these assays are referred to as heterogeneous immunoassays. The major advantages of RIA are its microcapability, accuracy, relative rapidity, and ease of operation. The disadvantages are that it is limited to those drugs for which antibodies are available and that its specificity is limited to classes of compounds rather than to individual drugs (36). The most popular RIA method of screening for drugs in urine is available commercially as a kit (4).

Fluorescence Polarization Immunoassay

Fluorescence polarization immunoassay makes use of competitive binding principles and directly measures the binding of labeled drug without the need for a separation process (Fig. 4–2). With fluorescence polarization immunoassay the unknown sample and a known labeled substance compete for a limited and known number of antibody sites specific for the drug. The more drug present, the lower the measured fluorescence polarization of the labeled drug (Fig. 4–3).

As with other immunoassays, standard curves are prepared from calibrated drug concentrations, and the unknown is determined from the standard curve (33,37). Although this procedure has great potential, it has seen little clinical utility primarily because of a lack of a simple, low-cost, high-performance instrumentation.

Enzyme-Modified Immunoassay

Assays in which the antibody or hapten is bound to an enzyme are called enzyme-modified (or multiplied) immunoassays (38). Enzyme-multiplied immunoassay technique (EMIT) has been found to be accurate, specific, and easier to use than RIA. This technique generally requires only the addition of one, two, or three reagents in an orderly, timed sequence. The sample size rarely exceeds 100 μL. In addition, EMIT is applicable to

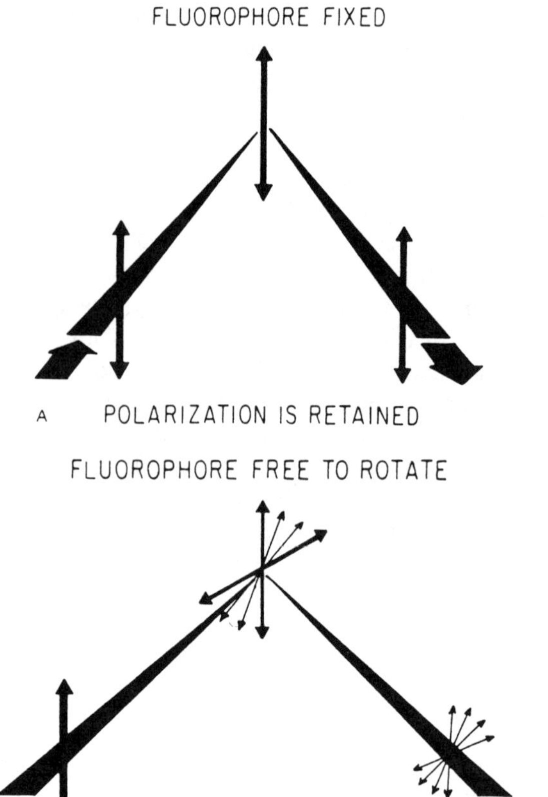

FIG. 4–2. Fluorescence polarization. **A:** The plane of emitted light is the same as that of exciting light when a molecule is in a fixed position. **B:** As molecules rotate between the time of excitation and the time of emission, the polarization of emitted light is diminished. (From Gerson B. *Essentials of therapeutic drug monitoring.* New York: Igaku-Shoin; 1983, with permission.)

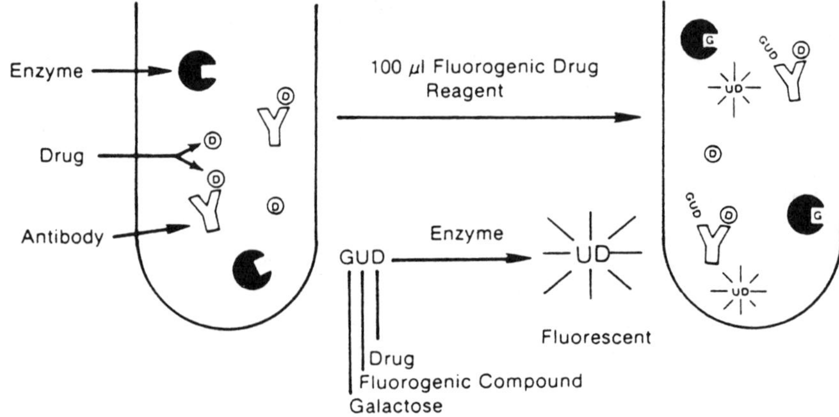

FIG. 4–3. Performance of substrate-labeled fluorescence immunoassay. First, drug, enzyme, and antibody are incubated. The fluorogenic drug reagent (the complex) is added, initiating the competition for binding sites. (From Gerson B. *Essentials of therapeutic drug monitoring.* New York: Igaku-Shoin; 1983, with permission.)

TABLE 4–3. *Drugs that can be assayed by EMIT*

Urine	Serum	Therapeutic monitoring
Amphetamines	Acetaminophen	Amikacin
Barbiturates	Barbiturates	Disopyramide
Benzodiazepines	Benzodiazepines	Ethosuximide
Cannabinoids	Ethyl alcohol	Gentamicin
Cocaine metabolites	Phencyclidine	Lidocaine
Ethyl alcohol	Tricyclic antidepressants	Methotrexate
Methadone	Carbamazepine	Netilmicin
Methaqualone	Digoxin	Phenobarbital
Opiates	Phenytoin	Primidone
Propoxyphene		Theophylline
		Tobramycin
		Valproic acid

Adapted with permission from *Emerg Med Clin North Am* 1986;4:367–376. WB Saunders Company.

many classes of compounds (39). This system makes use of a nonisotopic label and is usually less sensitive than RIA; nevertheless, it has become the prevailing means of toxicologic analysis in hospital laboratories during the past few years because it can be performed directly and expeditiously on a given sample (40).

In EMIT, the inhibition of an enzyme-substrate reaction is proportional to the amount of drug in the sample (Fig. 4–4). A labeled hapten is added to an unlabeled sample to be assayed; that is, the drug is labeled by chemical attachment to an enzyme, which is then allowed to equilibrate with a specific antibody. When the enzyme-labeled drug becomes bound to an antibody to the drug, the activity of the enzyme is reduced. The remaining enzyme activity is then measured by adding a known amount of substrate; the amount of added substrate needed to neutralize the remaining enzyme equals the concentration of the hapten being measured.

Because there is a difference between the free and bound labeled drug, no separation step is necessary (41,42). These immunoassays are therefore referred to as homogeneous immunoassays. A wide variety of homogeneous immunoassays are available as commercial kits that identify many common poisons (Table 4–3). In contrast to RIA, the shelf-life of EMIT reagents is usually long (41). This system is adaptable to many automated and semiautomated instruments, so that with enzyme immunoassay technology hundreds of specimens can be run per day with a turnaround time of approximately 20 minutes. The use of automation has significantly reduced reagent costs because a small volume of material can be used.

Enzyme-modified immunoassay is designed to achieve accurate measurement in the therapeutic range of the drug being assayed. Biochemically accurate measurement of higher concentrations requires dilution of sam-

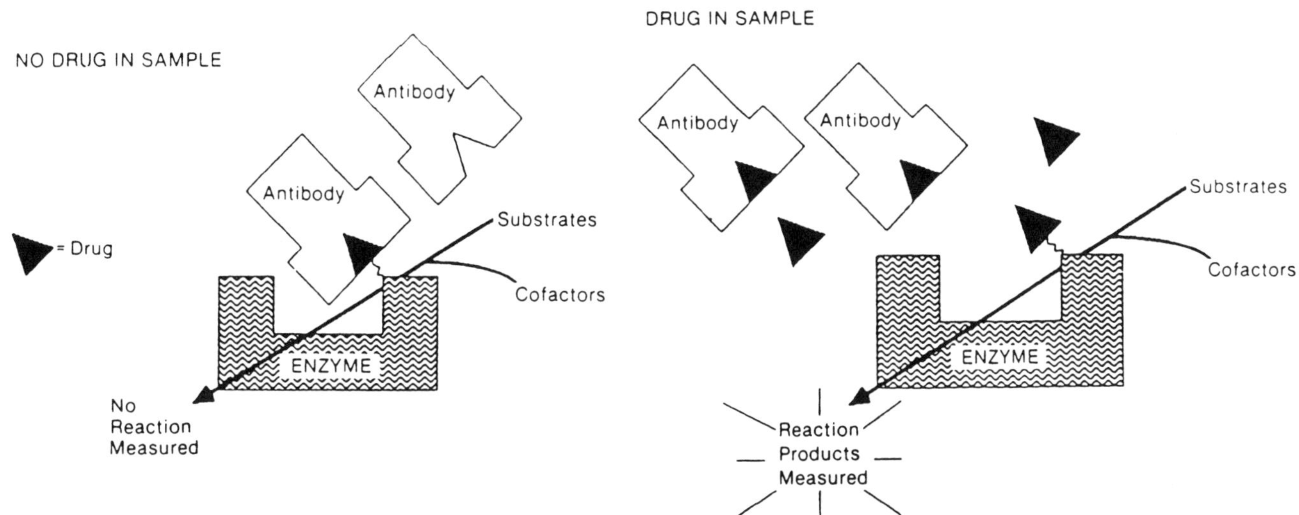

FIG. 4–4. Principle of enzyme immunoassay. A drug-specific antibody that inhibits an enzyme reaction due to drug label on enzyme. The greater the free drug is from the sample, the less the inhibition is by the antibody and the faster the reaction of the enzyme system. (From Osterloh J, *Emerg Med Clin North Am* 1990; 8:702, with permission.)

ples with drug-free serum. Concentrations below the therapeutic range are also less accurately measured.

Enzyme-modified immunoassay measures total drug concentration and does not separate free from protein-bound drug. To this effect, it does not give an estimate of the pharmacologically active drug but only of the total, potentially available drug circulating in the serum. In addition, it does not measure metabolic products in a single system that may or may not contribute to pharmacologic action or toxicity.

Although this procedure gives the highest percentage of positive results, by itself it does not provide the necessary comprehensive result. Therefore, confirmation of a presumptive positive finding carried out by a second analytically distinct method is prudent because it ensures the quality of the data reported.

Spectrophotometry

Spectrophotometry was the chief, and at one time the only, technique for drug detection. The development of the more sensitive and specific methods described previously has supplanted most but not all assays using visible or ultraviolet absorption as an endpoint.

Spectroscopy

Spectroscopy measures the ability of a substance to absorb electromagnetic radiation. The wavelengths of maximum absorbance and the shape and pattern of the spectrum identify the compound. There are many types of spectrophotometry, although many have drawbacks for practical use in an emergency setting. The three types of spectrophotometry most often used in toxicology are ultraviolet spectroscopy, fluorescence spectroscopy, and nuclear magnetic resonance spectroscopy. Mass spectroscopy, a very specific and sensitive testing procedure, requires highly skilled personnel. Reference laboratories may be equipped with mass spectroscopy, and many times this is combined with gas chromatography.

Ultraviolet Spectroscopy

Ultraviolet spectroscopy identifies a substance by measuring its pattern of peak absorbance of light of monochromatic wavelength. Ultraviolet spectroscopy has a relatively poor specificity unless the unknown drug is isolated by other procedures. This is because many compounds have overlapping or similar ultraviolet spectra. This method is useful as a confirming test or in conjunction with immunoassay techniques (6).

Fluorescence Spectroscopy

Fluorescence spectroscopy is one of the most widely used luminescence techniques primarily because of its intrinsic sensitivity and selectivity. This technique measures the intensity of emitted energy of a compound after it is exposed to an exciting light source. Some drugs have natural fluorescence, such as quinine and imipramine, and some have derivatives that fluoresce.

Nuclear Magnetic Resonance Spectroscopy

Nuclear magnetic resonance (NMR) spectroscopy measures a molecule's absorption of energy in an externally applied magnetic field. As the frequency of incident radio waves changes, the molecules undergo characteristic atomic resonances that are recorded as a spectrum, which identify the chemical structure of the drug. Although NMR spectroscopy is used in many institutions to detect disease states and can be adapted for use in toxicology, it is rarely used for this purpose at present, primarily because of its high cost.

Mass Spectrometry

Mass spectrometry (MS) is the only instrument technique to yield a positive identification of a drug or metabolite. Mass spectrometers operate on the principle that charged particles moving through a magnetic or an electric field can be separated from other charged particles according to their mass-to-charge ratios (43). A record of the ions is formed and the relative abundance of each issued as a fingerprint to determine the identity of the original samples. The reconstructed molecular spectra are compared with those in a library and a closeness of match is made with a certain confidence level. Contemporary mass spectrometers incorporate a computer system for control of the instrument and for the acquisition, display, manipulation, and interpretation of data. However, because of its cost and the complexity of analysis, MS is not generally used as a broad-spectrum screening tool (4). Recently, several benchtop MS units have been introduced. GC/MS is generally accepted as a rigorous confirmation technique for all drugs, because it provides the best level of confidence in the result (43).

Gas Chromatography with Mass Spectrometry

Although gas-liquid chromatography is one of the most versatile instrumental techniques for performing separation of complex mixtures and has become a widely accepted separation technique primarily because of its sensitivity, speed in analysis, and versatility, the rapid development of new GC instrumentation and separation phases has extended analytical capabilities far beyond those imagined by its originators (43). Recent developments in capillary columns have enabled chromatographers to separate hundreds of compounds in a single analysis routinely. No other instrumental technique approaches this kind of separation of complex mixtures.

Computer-assisted gas chromatography with mass spectroscopy is a sophisticated but not readily available method of testing. It has long been recognized as the most definitive technique for positive identification of compounds. The drug must generally be extracted from the sample before GC can be performed, and the drug must either be volatile or derivatized to make it volatile.

GC-MS can be used both qualitatively and quantitatively and has a sensitivity of nanograms to picograms. It is applicable to a wide range of samples, there being more than 30,000 known standards (44). These standards are listed in computer libraries by the mass of the parent compound and its characteristic fragments. Not surprisingly, GC-MS requires a high level of sophistication to operate the equipment and is therefore usually reserved for certain reference laboratories (27).

Two widespread misconceptions about mass spectrometry are that GC/MS is a specific "method," and that GC/MS is 100% accurate. In fact, GC/MS is a technique with many variations and a diverse variety of instrumental configurational possibilities. There are countless methodologies based on GC/MS techniques, each with its own set of advantages and disadvantages.

Miscellaneous Testing

Breath

Breath alcohol analyzers, similar to those used by law enforcement agencies, have been used to obtain rapid blood ethanol in the ED. If this device is used with a cooperative patient, a high degree of correlation with laboratory-obtained blood alcohol is obtained. In uncooperative patients, however, due in part to their difficulty in controlling exhalation, the correlation is less strong. There are many variables that can affect the reliability of breath alcohol analyzers (Table 4–4), including the fact that breath analysis determinations require the use of a conversion factor and may be inaccurately high and not truly reflective of blood alcohol content (BAC); the ingestion of mouthwash or other substances that contain alcohol; whether vomiting or regurgitation has occurred; the skill of the examiner; the necessity for frequent machine recalibrations; time of collection; eructation of gastric contents; and subject-to-subject variability of breath alcohol ratios (45).

TABLE 4–4. *Use of alcohol breath analyzers*

Requires use of conversion factor
Coingestion of other alcohol products may confound results
Vomiting, eructation, or regurgitation may confound results
Skill of examiner is important
Machine requires frequent calibrations
Intersubject variability of breath alcohol ratios

Saliva

Drug concentration in saliva has been suggested as an approximation of the free drug concentration in the systemic circulation. Although rapid tests to detect drugs such as alcohol in saliva have been developed, they have many of the same limitations of alcohol breath analysis determinations (46). This is because saliva is generated from three pairs of glands and the saliva from these have different pH values. Quantification from the saliva of each would be expected to give different free drug concentrations. In addition, the relative proportions of saliva derived from each upon stimulation are not constant. Because of this, there is no reliable relation between saliva drug concentration and serum free drug level, and the use of saliva should be discouraged (45).

Gastric

There has been poor sensitivity of gastric contents as a drug screen, and gastric drug screens may actually fail to detect many of the drugs found in either the urine or blood. Many drugs are readily absorbed or quickly pass into the lower gastrointestinal tract and therefore may not be detected. In addition, other drugs and nonpharmacologic substances may be present in gastric fluid. Finally, dilution of the drug with gastric juice or lavage fluid commonly occurs, rendering drug identification more difficult (8). Unless the estimated time since ingestion is short, screens of gastric fluid generally add little to urine test results (8).

TABLE 4–5. *Substances and parameters that may require stat quantitative analysis*

Serum iron
Methanol
Ethylene glycol
Acetaminophen
Salicylates
Carbon monoxide (carboxyhemoglobin)
Ethanol
Digoxin
Lithium
Methemoglobin
Serum osmolality
Theophylline

Summary

In considering the comprehensive approach to drug screens, one must utilize as many screening methodologies as practical. For example, EMIT chemistries and spot tests can be used rather efficiently to quickly screen for and detect or rule out the presence of several drugs and classes of drugs that may be involved in an overdose. These initial screens may be best followed by TLC screens of urine for acidic, basic, and neutral drugs as possible confirmations. These previous findings may then be supplemented by a GC analysis of a urine extract. Additional confirmatory testing can be performed by GC/MS, if necessary.

DRUG TESTING IN THE EMERGENCY SETTING

Qualitative Compared with Quantitative Testing

When attempting to rule out a drug as a cause of coma, qualitative drug screening is often adequate (5,16,47). Nevertheless, for certain drugs or toxins the early clinical symptoms correlate poorly with the patient's eventual outcome (48). A quantitative screening for these drugs may be important in determining treatment. Also, some toxins must be identified quickly so that proper treatment can be promptly administered (49). A laboratory should therefore be prepared to perform the tests listed in Table 4–5 on an immediate (stat) basis, or it should have easy access to a reference laboratory that can perform these analyses. Methods of quantitation for various laboratory tests are listed in Table 4–6.

Drugs such as benzodiazepines, cocaine, narcotics, phenothiazines, sedative-hypnotics, and tricyclic antidepressants, if involved in a poisoning, need not be identified on an emergency basis because the basic supportive care of the patient can be accomplished with or without knowing the exact drug involved in the intoxication.

When "Stat" Quantitation Is Desirable

There may be substances whose levels it might be helpful to know, but in actuality such information would not change the treatment offered to the patient and so would just be obtained for scientific interest. These levels could be obtained, but it is not necessary to have them available on a stat basis.

Drug quantitations in overdose are used to diagnose whether toxicity is occurring but not yet clinically apparent, or whether toxicity will occur after a delay, and to monitor the course of the patient. In the emergency setting there are relatively few drugs that need to be quantitated. Two criteria need to be satisfied for quantitation to be useful. First, there should be an absence of good clinical indicators that would otherwise reveal the status or condition of the patient. For many drugs, the clinical indicators of toxicity are better than drug concentration. For example, the clinical manifestations of a tricyclic overdose indicate the course and severity of the ingestion better than drug concentrations. Most overdoses may be monitored by clinical signs. The second criterion for the use of drug concentrations is the existence of a concentration–effect relationship.

The following levels should be available on a stat basis because they will change or determine the treatment provided. These quantitations include acetaminophen, salicylates, theophylline, ethanol, methanol, ethylene glycol, iron, carbon monoxide, digoxin, methemoglobin, serum osmolality, lithium, and circumstances in which hazardous therapy may be used or evaluation of therapeutic efficacy is required. Conversions from SI units are noted in Table 4–7 and in Appendix.

TABLE 4–6. *Methods of quantitation of various toxins*

Acetaminophen	HPLC, immunoassay
Ethanol	GLC, enzyme assay
Ethylene glycol	GLC
Methanol	GLC
Phenytoin	HPLC, GLC, immunoassay
Salicylates	Spectrophotometry, HPLC
Theophylline	HPLC, GLC, immunoassay

Iron and Total Iron Binding Capacity

Although iron is a relatively specialized test and is typically not available on a stat basis, its usefulness in toxicol-

TABLE 4–7. *Common conversions using SI units*

Compound	SI unit	Conversion factor	Converted unit
Acetaminophen	μmol/L	0.15	μg/mL
Cyanide	μmol/L	0.002	mg/dL
Diazepam	nmol/L	0.00028	mg/L
Digoxin	nmol/L	0.78	ng/mL
Ethanol	mmol/L	4.6	mg/dL
Ethylene glycol	mmol/L	6.2	mg/dL
Iron	μmol/L	5.58	μg/dL
Lead	μmol/L	20.7	μg/dL
Mercury	nmol/L	0.02	μg/dL
Methanol	mmol/L	3.2	mg/dL
Phenobarbital	μmol/L	0.023	mg/dL
Phenytoin	μmol/L	0.252	μg/mL
Salicylate	mmol/L	13.81	mg/dL
Theophylline	μmol/L	0.18	μg/mL

Example:

A) To convert acetaminophen from SI units to μg/mL.

If acetaminophen level were 1,000 μmol/L, what would the APAP level be in μg/mL?

1,000 multiplied by 0.15 equals 150 μg/mL

B) A phenytoin level of 40 umol/L would be what as μg/mL?

40 multiplied by 0.252 equals 10.08 μg/mL

ogy cannot be overstated in a suspected case of iron overdose. If the iron is high, then specific chelation therapy is immediately required. The results of iron overload tests are unreliable, and such tests should not be attempted.

Methanol and Ethylene Glycol

The metabolites of methanol and ethylene glycol are extremely toxic, and immediate laboratory confirmation is necessary so that specific therapy can be instituted rapidly. Methanol concentration is relatively simple to measure. Most laboratories, however, are not able to measure ethylene glycol concentrations; for this reason, the diagnosis of ethylene glycol toxicity may be based on other findings, such as history, anion gap, metabolic acidosis, osmolar gap, and crystalluria.

Acetaminophen

Plotting the acetaminophen concentration on the acetaminophen nomogram is absolutely necessary because without this measurement there may be no accurate way to foresee which patient may go on to have hepatic necrosis and which patient may be discharged from the emergency department. Since acetaminophen concentrations exceeding the toxic range on the nomogram suggest the potential for hepatic necrosis, treatment with *N*-acetylcysteine would be indicated, and would be based on the number obtained by quantitation.

Salicylates

As with acetaminophen, it is important to measure the salicylate concentration and to plot it on the salicylate nomogram so as to have a prognostic indicator that will determine the extent of treatment necessary.

Carbon Monoxide

Carbon monoxide (carboxyhemoglobin) concentrations are important to know because the history may be spurious, and the diagnosis may be missed without an immediate test.

Ethanol

Ethanol concentrations are measured for comparison with the patient's condition. For example, a low ethanol concentration in the face of an advanced stage of coma would alert the physician that the coma is due to another cause. A high concentration, on the other hand, may not be the sole cause of coma. The patient's condition should continue to be monitored and will improve as the ethanol is metabolized.

Digoxin

A serum digoxin concentration may be diagnostic in the chronically overdosed patient, but it should not determine treatment. The condition of the patient determines the course of treatment because a serum digoxin concentration may not adequately reflect the clinical course in the acute overdose.

Lithium

Blood lithium concentrations should be measured because a toxic level may require dialysis. Early in an acute intoxication, however, blood lithium concentration may not adequately reflect the future clinical outcome. For lithium toxicity, multiple serum concentrations may assist in defining whether the drug is rapidly distributing. Elevated, but rapidly falling concentrations suggest an acute overdose which often results in only minor toxicity. Elevated or slowly rising concentrations of $>$ 4 mEq/L are indicative of a serious chronic overdose.

Methemoglobin

Because methemoglobinemia is a potentially fatal condition that can be treated with an antidote, tests for the measurement of methemoglobin should be readily available. A co-oximeter can measure both carboxyhemoglobin and methemoglobin concentrations in the same sample (50).

Serum Osmolality

A serum osmolality test by freezing point depression should be available to detect some of the more toxic alcohols such as methanol and ethylene glycol. This measurement is compared with the calculated serum osmolality for evidence of an osmolal gap.

Osmolality, as measured by vapor pressure instruments that use a vacuum, will cause a loss of volatile alcohols (methanol, ethanol, acetone), but not ethylene glycol. Low-molecular-weight anions, such as formate, lactate, and glycolate, tend not to be measured in the gap owing to low quantities and because doubling the counter ion (2×Na) accounts for these anions in the calculation. Renal failure also increases the osmolar gap. Sample tubes containing citrate, EDTA, or oxalate will falsely elevate the measured osmolality.

Theophylline

Measurement of the serum theophylline concentration may be helpful as an adjunct in deciding whether a patient requires extracorporeal means of drug removal (51,52).

Additional Laboratory Values (Table 4–8)

Arterial Blood Gas

Other areas of concern in the intoxicated individual are the arterial blood gases. Arterial blood gases aid in evaluating respiratory status due to depressant drugs; from pulmonary edema due to narcotic, salicylate, and iron overdoses; and from pneumonitis after aspiration of gastric contents or low-viscosity solvents. In addition, arterial blood gases are used in the evaluation of metabolic acidosis due to poisoning.

Serum Electrolytes

Electrolytes may also be useful as an indication of the acid-base status, as well as the actual electrolytes themselves. Low serum potassium concentrations are useful in assessing the severity of alkalosis and adrenergic stimulation, as both drive potassium into cells. Hypokalemia may occur with chronic diuretic use and also occurs in theophylline overdose. Hyperkalemia may result from increased muscle activity occurring with stimulant drugs, nonsteroidal anti-inflammatory drugs, seizures, and acute overdose from cardiac glycosides.

The anion gap is useful in assessing the presence of acids or drugs that produce acids that have neutralized bicarbonate.

Electrocardiogram

The EKG can be used to assess the toxicologic effects of several drugs. Owing to the slowing of the inward fast Na conductance of the action potential in the heart, widening of the QRS > 0.1 sec helps confirm the suspicion of a significant tricyclic overdose.

QT prolongation and QRS widening may occur in overdoses due to phenothiazines, quinidine, procainamide, and the tricyclics.

Enzymes

Certain enzyme assays are useful in evaluating acute liver and muscle damage. Liver toxins such as acetaminophen, amanitin, chlorinated hydrocarbons, nitrosamines, phosphorus, isoniazid, and iron can produce release of the hepatic enzymes aspartate aminotransferase (AST) and alaninine aminotransferase (ALT). Muscle damage may result from compression ischemia after coma due to narcotics and barbiturates, and from increased muscular activity, rigidity, or seizures due to stimulants such as cocaine, amphetamines, or phencyclidine. Such damage is indicated by increased creatine phosphokinase (CPK) activity and potassium concentrations in the serum (Table 4–9).

Radiography

Flat plate x-ray of the abdomen is also useful for recognizing certain formulated pharmaceuticals in tablet form while still in the gastrointestinal tract. A perforated viscus may be diagnosed by an upright chest x-ray that may indicate free-air under the diaphragm, or mediastinal air that may indicate an esophageal rupture.

TABLE 4–8. *Additional laboratory helpful in toxicology work-up*

Serum electrolytes
Arterial blood gases
Electrocardiogram
Liver and muscle enzymes
Chest or abdominal radiographs

TABLE 4–9. *Clinical chemistry parameters associated with organ and organ systems*

Heart
Creatine kinase and isoenzymes
Lactate dehydrogenase and isoenzymes
Liver
Alanine aminotransferase
Albumin
Alkaline phosphatase
Aspartate aminotransferase
Bilirubin
Gamma-glutamyltransferase
Lactate dehydrogenase and isoenzymes
Sorbitol dehydrogenase
Total protein
Kidney
Albumin
Chloride
Creatinine (urine and serum)
Glucose
Potassium
Protein (urine and serum)
Sodium
Urea nitrogen
Pancreas
Amylase
Glucose
Lipase
Calcium
Bone
Alkaline phosphatase and isoenzymes
Calcium
Phosphorus
Uric acid
Miscellaneous
Cholesterol (diet and liver)
Triglycerides (diet and liver)
High-density lipoprotein cholesterol
Lipoproteins
Glucose
Cholinesterase

APPENDIX

Conversion of SI and conventional units

Substance	Units		Conversion		Units	Substance	Units		Conversion		Units
Alcohols						**Sedative-Hypnotics**					
Ethanol	mg/dL	×	0.22	=	mmol/L	Chlordiazepoxide	μg/mL	×	3.3	=	μmol/L
	mmol/L	×	4.6	=	mg/dL		μmol/L	×	0.30	=	μg/mL
Ethylene glycol	mg/dL	×	0.16	=	mmol/L	Diazepam	μg/mL	×	3.515	=	nmol/L
	mmol/L	×	8.2	=	mg/dL		nmol/L	×	0.00003	=	μg/mL
Isopropanol	mg/dL	×	0.17	=	mmol/L	Ethchlorvynol	μg/mL	×	6.9	=	μmol/L
	mmol/L	×	6.0	=	mg/dL		μmol/L	×	0.145	=	μg/mL
Methanol	mg/dL	×	0.3	=	mmol/L	Glutethimide	μg/mL	×	4.6	=	μmol/L
	mmol/L	×	3.2	=	mg/dL		μmol/L	×	0.22	=	μg/mL
Analgesics						Meprobamate	μg/mL	×	4.6	=	μmol/L
Acetaminophen	μg/dL	×	6.62	=	μmol/L		μmol/L	×	0.22	=	μg/mL
	μmol/L	×	0.151	=	μg/dL	Methaqualone	μg/mL	×	4.0	=	μmol/L
Propoxyphene	μg/mL	×	2.946	=	μmol/L		μmol/L	×	0.25	=	μg/mL
	μmol/L	×	0.34	=	μg/mL	Methyprylon	μg/mL	×	5.46	=	μmol/L
Salicylates	mg/dL	×	0.072	=	mmol/L		μmol/L	×	0.025	=	μg/mL
	mmol/L	×	13.81	=	mmol/L	Pentobarbital	mg/dL	×	4.4	=	μmol/L
Antidepressants							μmol/L	×	0.18	=	mg/dL
Amitriptyline	ng/mL	×	3.6	=	nmol/L	Phenobarbital	mg/dL	×	43.1	=	μmol/L
	nmol/L	×	0.28	=	ng/mL		μmol/L	×	0.02	=	mg/dL
Desipramine	ng/mL	×	3.75	=	nmol/L	**Cardiac medication**					
	nmol/L	×	0.267	=	ng/mL	Digoxin	ng/mL	×	1.28	=	nmol/L
Doxepin	ng/mL	×	0.22	=	nmol/L		nmol/L	×	0.78	=	ng/mL
	nmol/L	×	0.28	=	ng/mL	Lidocaine	μg/mL	×	4.3	=	μmol/L
Imipramine	ng/mL	×	3.57	=	nmol/L		μmol/L	×	0.23	=	μg/mL
	nmol/L	×	0.28	=	ng/mL	Procainamide	μg/mL	×	4.2	=	μmol/L
Maprotiline	ng/mL	×	3.6	=	nmol/L		μmol/L	×	0.24	=	μg/mL
	nmol/L	×	0.28	=	ng/mL	Propanolol	ng/mL	×	3.85	=	nmol/L
Nortriptyline	ng/mL	×	3.8	=	nmol/L		nmol/L	×	0.26	=	ng/mL
	nmol/L	×	0.26	=	ng/mL						
Anti-seizure medication						**Miscellaneous**					
Carbamazepine	μg/mL	×	4.2	=	μmol/L	Iron	μg/dL	×	0.18	=	μmol/L
	μmol/L	×	0.24	=	μg/mL		μmol/L	×	5.6	=	μg/dL
Ethosuximide	μg/mL	×	7.0	=	μmol/L	Isoniazid	μg/mL	×	7.3	=	μmol/L
	μmol/L	×	0.14	=	μg/mL		μmol/L	×	0.14	=	μg/mL
Phenytoin	μg/mL	×	3.9	=	μmol/L	Lithium	mg/dL	×	1.4	=	mmol/L
	μmol/L	×	0.25	=	μg/mL		mmol/L	×	0.70	=	mg/dL
Primidone	μg/mL	×	4.6	=	μmol/L	Theophylline	μg/mL	×	5.5	=	μmol/L
	μmol/L	×	0.21	=	μg/mL		μmol/L	×	0.18	=	μg/mL
Valproic Acid	μg/mL	×	6.9	=	μmol/L	Warfarin	μg/mL	×	3.2	=	μmol/L
	μmol/L	×	0.14	=	μg/mL		μmol/L	×	0.3	=	μg/mL

REFERENCES

1. Arena J: The clinical diagnosis of poisoning.*Pediatr Clin North Am* 1970;17:477–494.
2. Hansen H, Caudill S, Boone J: Crisis in drug testing: results of CDC blind study. *JAMA* 1985;253:2382–2387.
3. Osterloh J: Utility and reliability of emergency toxicologic testing. *Emerg Clin North Am* 1990;8:693–723.
4. Batch R: Drug screening in hospital clinical laboratories. *Clin Lab Med* 1987;7:371–388.
5. Kellermann A, Fihn S, LoGergo J, et al: Impact of drug screening in suspected overdose. *Ann Emerg Med* 1987;16:1206–1216.
6. Epstein F, Hassan M: Therapeutic drug levels and toxicology screen. *Emerg Med Clin North Am* 1986;4:367–376.
7. Kulig K: Utilization of emergency toxicology screens [Editorial]. *Am J Emerg Med* 1985;6:573–574.
8. Kellerman A, Fihn S, LoGerfo J, et al: Utilization and yield of drug screening in the emergency department. *Am J Emerg Med* 1988;6:14–20.
9. Baselt R, Wright J, Cravey R: Therapeutic and toxic concentrations of more than one hundred toxicologically significant drugs in blood, plasma, or serum: a tabulation. *Clin Chem* 1975;21:44–62.
10. Jellett L: Plasma concentrations in the control of drug therapy. *Drugs* 1976;11:412–422.
11. Koch-Weser J: Serum drug concentrations as therapeutic guides. *N Engl J Med* 1972;287:227–231.
12. Kulig K: Initial management of ingestions of toxic substances. *N Engl J Med* 1992;326:1677–1681.
13. Wiley J: Difficult diagnoses in toxicology. Poisons not detected by the comprehensive drug screen. 1991;38:725–737.
14. Herr R, Swanson T: Pseudometabolic acidosis caused by underfill of vacutainer tubes. *Ann Emerg Med* 1992;21:177–180.
15. Schwartz J, Zollars P, Okorodudu A, et al: Accuracy of common drug screen tests. *Am J Emerg Med* 1991;9:166–170.
16. Bailey D: The role of the laboratory in treatment of the poisoned patient: laboratory perspective. *J Anal Toxicol* 1983;7:136–141.
17. Brett A: Implications of discordance between clinical impression and toxicology analysis in drug overdose. *Arch Intern Med* 1988;148:437–441.

18. Helper B, Sutheimer C, Sunshine I: Role of the toxicology laboratory in suspected ingestions. *Pediatr Clin North Am* 1986;33:245–260.
19. Mahoney J, Gross P, Stern T, et al: Qualitative serum toxic screening in the management of suspected drug overdose. *Am J Emerg Med* 1990;8:16–22.
20. Binder S: Chromatographic techniques for therapeutic drug monitoring. *Clin Lab Med* 1987;7:335–356.
21. Schlager D, Sanders A, Wiggins D, et al: Ultrasound for the detection of foreign bodies. *Ann Emerg Med* 1991;20:189–191.
22. Cannon D: Instrumentation and techniques for therapeutic drug monitoring. *Clin Lab Med* 1987;7:325–334.
23. Chan S, Gerson B: Free drug monitoring. *Clin Lab Med* 1987;7:279–287.
24. Schwartz R: Urine testing in the detection of drugs of abuse. *Arch Intern Med* 1988;148:2407–2412.
25. Nice A, Leikin J, Maturen A, et al: Toxidrome recognition to improve efficiency of emergency urine drug screens. *Ann Emerg Med* 1988;17:676–680.
26. Sangalli B: A new look at qualitative toxicology. Spot tests in the emergency department. *Vet Hum Toxicol* 1989;31:445–448.
27. Gold M, Dackis C: Role of the laboratory in the evaluation of suspected drug abuse. *J Clin Psychiatry* 1986;47:17–23.
28. Martel P, Lones D, Rousseau R: Application of ToxiLab: a broad spectrum drug detection system in emergency toxicology. *Am Assoc Clin Chem* 1983;2:1–4.
29. Finke B: A GLC-based system for the detection of poisons, drugs and human metabolites encountered in forensic toxicology. *J Chromatogr Sci* 1971;9:393–396.
30. Blecka L, Jackson G: Immunoassays in therapeutic drug monitoring. *Clin Lab Med* 1987;7:357–370.
31. Brattin W, Sunshine I: Immunological assays for drugs in biological samples. *Am J Med Tech* 1973;39:223–230.
32. Bakerman S: Substrate-labeled fluorescence immunoassay. *Lab Manage* 1983;21:13–16.
33. Jolley M, Stroupe S, Schwenzer K, et al: Fluorescence polarization immunoassay: part III: an automated system for therapeutic drug determination. *Clin Chem* 1981;27:1575–1579.
34. Skelley D, Brown L, Besch P: Radioimmunoassay. *Clin Chem* 1973;19:146–186.
35. Castro A, Mittleman R: Determination of drugs of abuse in body fluids by radioimmunoassay. *Clin Biochem* 1978;11:103–105.
36. Spector S: Application of radioimmunoassay to pharmacology. *Clin Pharmacol Ther* 1974;16:149–154.
37. Lu-Steffes M, Pittluck G, Jolley M, et al: Fluorescence polarization immunoassay: part IV: determination of phenytoin and phenobarbital in human serum and plasma. *Clin Chem* 1982;28:2278–2281.
38. Rubenstein K, Schneider R, Ullman E: Homogenous enzyme immunoassay: a new immunochemical technique. *Biochem Biophys Res Commun* 1972;47:846–854.
39. Drost R: EMIT-st drug detection system for screening of barbiturates and benzodiazepines in serum. *J Toxicol Clin Toxicol* 1982;19:303–312.
40. Shannon M, Saladino R, McCarty D, et al: Clinical evaluation of an acetaminophen meter for the rapid diagnosis of acetaminophen intoxication. *Ann Emerg Med* 1990;19:1133–1136.
41. Helper B, Sutheimer C, Sunshine I: The role of the toxicology laboratory in emergency medicine. *J Toxicol Clin Toxicol* 1982;19:-353–365.
42. Helper B, Sutheimer C, Sunshine I: The role of the toxicology laboratory in the treatment of acute poisoning. *Med Toxicol* 1986;1:61–75.
43. Lehrer M: Application of gas chromatography/mass spectrometry instrument techniques to forensic urine drug testing. *Clin Lab Med* 1990;10:271–288.
44. Ullucci P: A comprehensive GC/MS drug screening procedure. *J Anal Toxicol* 1978;2:33–38.
45. Wax P, Hoffman R, Goldfrank L: Rapid quantitative determination of blood alcohol concentration in the emergency department using an electrochemical method. *Ann Emerg Med* 1992;21:254–259.
46. Christopher T, Zeccardi J: Evaluation of the Q.E.D. saliva alcohol test: a new, rapid, accurate device for measuring ethanol in saliva. *Ann Emerg Med* 1992;21:1135–1137.
47. Baker S, Davey D: The predictive value for man of toxicological tests of drugs in laboratory animals. *Br Med Bull* 1976;26:208–211.
48. Green V: Use of the toxicology laboratory. *Crit Care Q* 1982;19–23.
49. Weisman R, Howland M: The toxicology laboratory. *Top Emerg Med* 1983;5:9–15.
50. Oles K: Therapeutic drug monitoring analysis systems for the physician office laboratory: a review of the literature. *DICP Ann Pharmacother* 1990;24:1070–1077.
51. Cook J, Platoff G, Koch T, et al: Accuracy and precision of methods for theophylline measurement in physicians' office. *Clin Chem* 1990;36:780–783.
52. Jones L, Bonzalez E, Venitz J, et al: Evaluation of the vision theophylline assays in the emergency department setting. *Ann Emerg Med* 1992;21:777–781.

ADDITIONAL SELECTED REFERENCES

Opheim K, Raisys V: Therapeutic drug monitoring in pediatric acute drug intoxications. *Ther Drug Monit* 1985;7:148–158.

Pippenger C: Rationale and clinical application of therapeutic drug monitoring. *Pediatr Clin North Am* 1980;27:891–925.

Teitelbaum D, Morgan J, Gray G: Nonconcordance between clinical impression and laboratory findings in clinical toxicology. *Clin Toxicol* 1977;10:417–422.

Vere D: The significance of blood levels of drugs. *Sci Basis Med* 1972;363–384.

CHAPTER 5

Pharmacokinetics and Toxicokinetics

Pharmacokinetics and toxicokinetics are relatively new areas of pharmacology and toxicology, respectively. An understanding of pharmacokinetics can greatly aid in the treatment of medical conditions and in therapy for substance overdose.

Pharmacokinetics is the study of the changes in a drug or its metabolites in the body from the time it enters the body until it is fully eliminated (1,2). It encompasses many factors, such as absorption, distribution, extent of body storage, amount of protein binding, metabolites of the parent compound and the toxicity associated with those metabolites, as well as the method and mode of excretion of the compound and metabolites (3,4). Pharmacologic principles are also important in predicting whether the various methods of enhancing elimination will be effective (these methods are discussed in Chapter 3).

Toxicokinetics has been coined to denote the absorption, distribution, excretion, and metabolism of toxins, toxic doses of therapeutic agents, and their metabolites. It is a mathematical conceptualization of clinical pharmacology in an overdosed patient. By using toxicokinetic principles, numbers (such as the volume of distribution) and rates are assigned to the biologic processes. An understanding of toxicokinetics is important in predicting how a drug acts in the body and why it acts in that manner. It may also explain why compounds are more easily removed from the body by extracorporeal methods or with multiple doses of activated charcoal. This chapter presents some of the terminology and concepts in pharmacokinetics and toxicokinetics.

Whereas *pharmacokinetics* refers to what the body does to the drug, *pharmacodynamics* refers to what the drug does to the system, and is the study of the effect of drugs on a target site (5). It describes drug effects over time and relates drug concentrations at sites of action to pharmacologic effects.

Overdosage of a drug can alter the usual pharmacokinetic processes. For example, dissolution of tablets or gastric emptying time may be altered so that peak effects of the toxin are delayed. Drugs may injure the gastrointestinal tract (GIT) and thereby alter absorption. If the capacity of the liver to metabolize a drug is exceeded, then more drug will be delivered to the circulation.

GENERAL CONSIDERATIONS

For a drug to exert the desired biologic effect, it must reach and interact with the site regulating that specific effect. The site of action of a drug is the location at which a given drug acts; this is also called the receptor site.

Receptors

The mechanism of action of a drug is the means by which, at a specific site, the drug initiates its biologic effect. The mechanism of action of most drugs depends on this chemical interaction with a functionally viable component of the physiologic system, the receptor. A receptor is a functional macromolecule found in the cell or on the cell surface. Drug–receptor interaction, or binding, requires a high degree of structural specificity; that is, the drug must fit its receptor exactly with regard to three-dimensional structure, areas of charge density, and lipophilicity (6).

After a drug is administered, the pharmacologic effect achieved is a direct consequence of the reversible formation of bonds between the drug and tissue receptors controlling a particular response (7). For most drugs, the intensity of a pharmacologic effect tends to be proportional to the drug concentration in extracellular fluid (8). For a drug to be therapeutically effective, it must reach the site of its intended pharmacologic activity within the body at a sufficient rate and in sufficient amount to yield an effective concentration. Factors important in determining the serum drug concentrations attained and eventually reflected at receptor sites include disease, drug pharmacokinetics, bioavailability, physiologic factors, patient compliance, and drug interactions.

Although the intensity of a drug effect is related to the concentration of the drug at its receptor or site of action, in most clinical situations, it is not possible to measure the concentration of a drug at its receptor. Instead, the steady-state plasma concentration of a drug is measured and used as an indirect indicator of drug concentration at the receptor site.

Agonists, Antagonists, and Partial Agonists

An *agonist* is a drug that binds to a receptor and elicits a maximal response. Drugs that bind to a receptor and inhibit the action of an agonist are called receptor *antagonists*. In the presence of an agonist, the antagonist and agonist may compete for receptor binding. The outcome will depend on the concentrations of the two drugs and their affinities for the receptor. A *partial agonist* is a drug that produces a less than maximal response even when it occupies 100% of the available receptors. Therefore, a partial agonist has an efficacy that is less than a full agonist but greater than an antagonist.

Drug–receptor binding is saturable, which means that there are a limited number of receptors, and when they are all occupied, a maximal therapeutic response is elicited. Once the receptors are saturated, not only will increasing the drug concentration not produce a greater therapeutic effect, but the risk of adverse drug effects is likely to increase.

ABSORPTION

Drugs must undergo absorption in order to exert a systemic effect. The small intestine is the principal site of oral drug absorption. Ideally, for absorption to occur, a drug must be in solution, lipophilic, and in a nonionized state (Table 5–1). In general, drugs are not well absorbed when ionized, as they cannot pass the lipid barrier of the gastrointestinal (GI) epithelium. At all levels of the GIT, therefore, the slowest rates of absorption are found with completely ionized drugs, such as the quaternary ammonium compounds. Absorption is also influenced by factors such as route of administration, product formulation, physical and chemical characteristics of the drug, and host characteristics.

The stomach is a significant site of absorption for many acidic and neutral compounds but not for basic compounds. For example, acidic drugs like salicylates and barbiturates, which exist as nonionized lipid-soluble molecules in the acid gastric contents, are readily absorbed, whereas basic drugs like the plant alkaloids, which exist largely as ions, are hardly absorbed at all.

In other portions of the alimentary tract where the intraluminal pH is closer to neutrality, many weak acids and bases are, to a considerable extent, nonionized and are absorbed at rates related to their lipid-to-water partition ratios.

The two most relevant clinical aspects of drug absorption are the rate and extent of drug absorption. Generally the rate of absorption depends on the rate of drug dissolution and the rate of gastric emptying. These factors help to define the onset of peak drug effect. For most drugs, food will decrease the rate of absorption without affecting the extent of absorption. The rate of absorption also would appear important in anticipating the onset of toxicologic symptoms in cases of drug overdoses.

With a drug overdose, it is common for delayed absorption to occur either because of the formation of a large, poorly soluble drug mass or a drug-induced decrease in gastric motility. For example, with normal dosing, the absorption of aspirin is completed within 1 hour; however, in an overdose situation, absorption may be delayed for more than 6 hours. In addition, with salicylates, bezoars or concretions may form, further limiting absorption. Sustained release preparations may substantially delay peak drug effects for as much as 36 hours after ingestion (9).

Drugs with anticholinergic activity such as atropine and antidepressants reduce gastric motility and cause gastric relaxation. Narcotic analgesics directly increase the tone of gastric smooth muscle, interfere with normal peristalsis, and delay gastric emptying. Alcohol can also delay gastric emptying. Interestingly, because weak acids are more likely to be absorbed in the stomach, slow gastric emptying will increase their absorption.

TABLE 5–1. *Pharmacokinetic parameters and factors affecting them*

Absorption
Drug must be in solution
Drug should be lipophilic
Drug should be nonionized
Route of administration
Product formulation
Physical and chemical characteristics
Host characteristics
Rate of absorption depends on rate of drug dissolution
Food decreases rate but not extent of absorption
Absorption may be delayed due to
concretions
decreased gastrointestinal motility (anticholinergics, narcotics, alcohol)

"Compartment" Models

The most commonly employed approach to the pharmacokinetic characterization of a drug is to represent the body as a system of compartments, even though these compartments usually have no physiologic or anatomic reality. One-compartment and two-compartment models are the most common although three- and four-compartment models have been described but are rarely used. It is important to realize that these "compartments" have no real physiologic meaning; they vary in extent depending on the particular drug under consideration.

One-Compartment Model

The one-compartment model, the simplest one, depicts the body as a single, kinetically homogeneous unit (10).

This model is particularly useful for drugs that distribute relatively rapidly throughout the body. This does not necessarily mean that the concentration of drug in plasma and other tissues is equal, rather, that the entire system is at equilibrium and changes in plasma drug concentrations quantitatively reflect changes in plasma drug concentrations occurring in other fluids and tissues.

Many drugs equilibrate between plasma and other tissues very rapidly. Furthermore, at the usual plasma sampling times, the one-compartment pharmacokinetic model adequately describes the data of time–plasma drug concentration curves. Therefore, this model, although the most elementary, is often the most appropriate pharmacokinetic model for many drugs.

Drugs that follow one-compartment kinetics exhibit log linear plasma concentrations as a function of time. This concept can be more easily understood using the concept of a "sink" or bathtub. In the sink model, a known quantity or amount of dye is added to a sink of known volume. A large sink will yield a smaller concentration than a smaller sink if the same quantity of dye is placed in each one (Fig. 5–1).

Two-Compartment Model

Most drugs cannot be described by a simple one-compartment model because they do not exhibit log linear plasma concentration versus time plots (11). Models having two or more compartments are necessary to describe such behavior. These models feature a rapidly perfused compartment, usually composed of the blood volume and those tissues or organs receiving high blood flow, termed the *central compartment*. In addition, one or more compartments, termed *peripheral* or *tissue compartments* are needed to describe the movement of drug into less well-perfused tissues or spaces. For example, tissues with high blood flow, like the adrenals, kidneys, heart, brain, and blood vessels, may compose the central compartment and receive drugs rapidly. All other tissues with lower blood flow constitute the peripheral compartment and, therefore, exchange drugs at a slower rate.

The two-compartment model, therefore, considers the fact that drugs distribute to different tissues at rates related to the blood flow in each tissue, and therefore, divides tissues primarily upon vascularization (9).

Distribution Phase

The distribution phase is the time required to distribute to these tissue compartments. Usually this is longer than distribution to the central compartment. Initially there may be higher concentrations because the drug is only in the central compartment. As distribution to the tissue compartments occurs, drug concentration decreases because the same quantity of drug is now in a larger volume (10).

Most drugs display a relationship between serum concentration and pharmacologic effect and it is possible to develop hypothetical models based on drugs moving between compartments (representing the body) that are

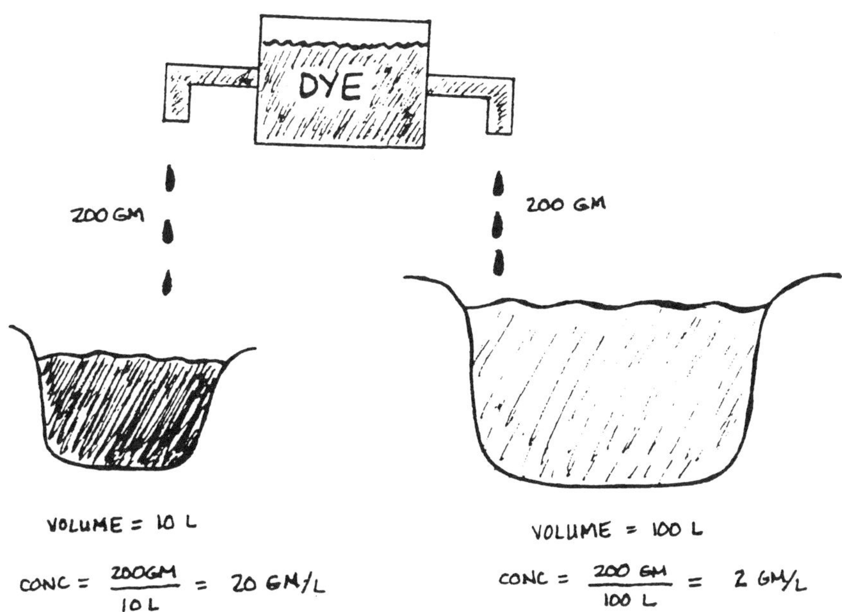

FIG. 5–1. The concentration of dye in two "sinks", one with a volume of 10 L and the other 100 L. This can be described by the equation: concentration = amount of dye/volume of the sink. If 200 g of dye are placed in each sink, the concentration of dye in the 100-L sink (2 g/L) will be lower than in the 10-L sink (20 g/L)

consistent with these empirically obtained mathematical equations.

For some drugs, such as quinidine and lidocaine, the pharmacologic "receptor site" appears to be located in the central compartment, therefore the rate of drug administration is important. Because serum levels will exceed "therapeutic" concentrations during the initial distribution phase before the drug has equilibrated with peripheral compartments, toxicity may occur. For many other drugs, the receptor site for pharmacologic activity appears to lie in the tissue compartment. Thus, initially high serum concentrations resulting from rapid administration of drug are not related to pharmacologic effect or toxicity.

The clinical implication is important: for drugs whose pharmacologic effect is related to tissue compartment concentrations, distribution phase drug samples are of limited value in predicting either pharmacologic effect or toxicity. Distribution to the peripheral compartment must be complete before drawing serum samples. Digoxin and lithium are two such examples.

BIOAVAILABILITY

Bioavailability, in simple terms, is the percentage or fraction of the administered dose which reaches the systemic circulation of the patient (12). By definition, a drug is 100% bioavailable after intravenous administration (13). The bioavailability of a drug after oral administration is thus a product of the fraction appearing in the portal circulation and the fraction remaining after any first-pass elimination (11–13).

Examples of factors that can alter bioavailability include the inherent dissolution and absorption characteristics of the administered drug, the dosage form (tablet, capsule), the route of administration, the stability of the active ingredient in the gastrointestinal tract, and the extent of drug metabolism prior to reaching the systemic circulation (Table 5–2). In addition, drugs can be metabolized by GI bacteria and by the GI mucosa before reaching the systemic circulation.

TABLE 5–2. *Pharmacokinetic parameters and factors affecting them*

Bioavailability
Inherent dissolution and absorption of drug
Dosage form (tablet, capsule)
Route of administration
Stability of the active ingredient in gastrointestinal tract
Extent of drug metabolism
Metabolism by GI bacteria or GI mucosa
Area under the plasma concentration curve (AUC) (Fig. 5–5)

"Area under the Plasma Concentration Curve"

An important concept that describes bioavailability is the area under the plasma concentration curve (AUC). This term is frequently used in discussing pharmacokinetics and is an indicator of total drug absorption. Because it reflects bioavailability, the AUC is more appropriate than peak serum level, which is dependent on the rate of drug absorption. The AUC, then, is the most important measurement of bioavailability and is based on serum concentration plotted against time (Fig. 5–2). The AUC represents the amount of drug that enters the systemic circulation during the distribution phase, early after administration. The distribution phase, or alpha phase, lasts approximately 30 minutes to 2 hours for most drugs. During this phase concentrations in the plasma decrease more rapidly than during the second phase, or elimination phase (beta phase) (9).

Effect of Drug Overdose

Bioavailability controls the amount of drug that reaches the systemic circulation. In overdose cases, the extent of absorption may be increased because of saturation of presystemic metabolism. This is especially true for drugs that normally exhibit this significant "first-pass" metabolism. Examples include narcotic analgesics, tricyclic antidepressants, and β-adrenergic antagonists.

DISTRIBUTION

After a drug is absorbed, it is distributed from the intravascular space to extravascular fluid and tissue. Both the degree and rate of this distribution are influenced by

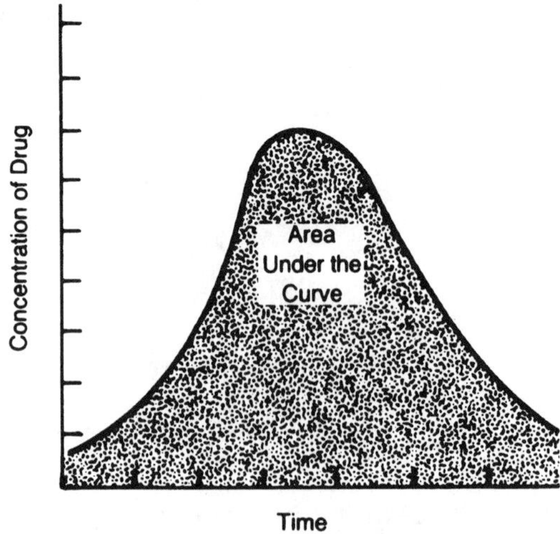

FIG. 5–2. Serum concentration plotted against time for hypothetical drug.

factors such as route of administration, protein binding, blood flow, blood pH, diffusion rates, and degree of partitioning to tissues (Table 5–3).

APPARENT VOLUME OF DISTRIBUTION

The apparent volume of distribution is a useful pharmacokinetic parameter that relates the plasma or serum concentration of a drug to the total amount of drug in the body (1,2). The measure of the compartment into which the drug distributes is termed the *apparent volume of distribution* (Table 5–4). The volume of distribution is defined as that volume of fluid into which a drug appears to distribute to a concentration equal to that in plasma. It is calculated from the dose of a drug administered and the resulting plasma concentration. A drug concentration in body fluids other than plasma may be used, but different values for the volume of distribution are obtained for each fluid. It is therefore important to note which fluid is being used. In this text, the volumes of distribution are based on plasma concentrations.

The volume of distribution for a drug does not necessarily refer to any identifiable compartment in the body (14). It is simply the site of a compartment necessary to account for the total amount of drug in the body if it were present throughout the body at the same concentration found in the plasma. The concept of volume of distribution is relatively simplistic because it assumes that the body acts as a single compartment with respect to the drug. In reality, this volume is a hypothetical value that does not refer to any actual physiologic space in the body (14).

Total body water can be divided into extracellular and intracellular compartments. The extracellular compartment can be divided further into the interstitial fluid and intravascular compartments (or plasma volume). In a 70 kg lean individual the volume of total body water is about 42 L. The volume in the vascular compartment is about 4 L, and the entire extracellular volume is approximately 14 L. Dividing the total amount of drug in the body in milligrams by the concentration of drug in the plasma or vascular compartment in milligrams per liter will give an apparent volume of distribution, in liters, in which the drug is dissolved. If a drug has an apparent volume of distribution of about 4 L, it would suggest that the drug was not distributing beyond the vascular compartment. A volume of distribution of approximately 42 L would indicate the drug has distributed throughout the total body water. Most drugs, however, are significantly bound in either the vascular or extravascular space (or both) (15).

TABLE 5–3. *Pharmacokinetic parameters and factors affecting them*

Distribution
Route of administration
Degree of protein binding
Blood flow
Blood pH
Diffusion rates
Degree of partitioning to tissues

TABLE 5–4. *Apparent volume of distribution*

"That volume of fluid into which a drug *appears* to distribute to a concentration equal to that in plasma." —States where a drug *goes* in the body—whether it is in vascular space or in the tissues of the body.

- Small volume of distribution—Vascular space
- Large volume of distribution—Tissues in body

- Basic drugs—Large volume of distribution
- Acidic drugs—Small volume of distribution

Factors affecting the volume of distribution
- Surface area
- Degree of obesity
- Sex
- Physical stress
- Thyroid condition
- Renal function
- Age
- Cardiac output
- Protein binding

Volume of distribution may aid in
- Calculating the amount of substance in the body
- Verifying history of quantity ingested
- Calculating drug amount to be administered in therapeutic situation
- Determining the amount of antidote needed
- Deciding how much drug to administer
- Deciding whether methods to enhance elimination are appropriate
- Calculating the approximate plasma level after overdose

The term *volume of distribution* gives some idea of the extent to which a drug is taken up by tissues in the body or whether a drug is found to a greater extent in the plasma. When the volume of distribution is large, the tissue concentration is large and plasma concentration is small (6). When the volume of distribution is small, most of the drug remains in the plasma (15).

Individual differences in the apparent volume of distribution of a drug will affect steady-state plasma concentrations and thus affect therapeutic response. For example, with increasing age, lean body mass is reduced, cardiac output drops, the percentage of total body fat increases and total body water volume decreases (16).

Such compartments of the body, since they constitute actual physical entities, may be considered real volumes of potential distribution. However, many drugs are not simply dissolved in these volumes but bind to cell surfaces and intercellular macromolecules. If the volume in which a drug is dissolved is computed by dividing the total amount of drug present in the body by the measured plasma concentration, the apparent volume of distribution is obtained. Because some drugs are almost 100% bound by tissue structures, leaving only a small amount in solution, the apparent volume of distribution may be extremely large, much larger than the total volume of the body. Although the apparent volume of distribution is obviously an abstract rather than a real entity, it is nevertheless more useful than the real volume of distribution for purposes of pharmacologic calculation.

The volume of distribution, then, is a measure of the compartment into which a drug distributes. The equation for the volume of distribution defines the relation between the amount of drug in the body and the amount of drug in the bloodstream. If a drug is highly concentrated in tissues, its apparent volume of distribution may be many times the total body water. Because the volume of distribution does not represent a real body space, it may be as small as the plasma volume or as large as several hundred liters. Often the volume of distribution is characteristic of a drug and constant over a wide dose range (16). The formula for the apparent volume of distribution is

$$V_d = A/(C_p)(M)$$

where V_d is the volume of distribution (in liters per kilogram), A is the amount of drug in the body (in milligrams), C_p is the concentration of drug in plasma (in milligrams per liter or micrograms per milliliter), and M is body weight (in kilograms).

The volume of distribution may also be affected by a number of different factors. These include the amount of body fat (because certain drugs distribute to fat to a greater or lesser extent), renal function, age (because both the very young and the elderly metabolize drugs differently and have different volumes of distribution), cardiac output (because all drugs are distributed by the bloodstream throughout the body), and the degree of protein binding for a drug. Drugs that are highly bound to albumin and other proteins, although they may have a small volume of distribution and are found to a great extent in the plasma, are inactive and therefore do not account for any drug activity (17–19). Binding to serum albumin thus decreases the maximum intensity of action of most drugs because it lowers the peak drug concentration achieved at the sites of action (1,20,21).

Basic drugs are quickly taken up by tissues and fat and thus have a large volume of distribution (greater than 1 L/kg). The volume of distribution then exceeds the volume of total body fluids. Acidic drugs are not taken up by fat and thus have a small volume of distribution (less than 1 L/kg). Selected drugs and their volumes of distribution are listed in Table 5–5. A more comprehensive list appears in Appendix B. In terms of body compartments, a drug with a volume of distribution of 4 L in a person weighing 70 kg can be thought of as being contained in the plasma volume. A volume of distribution of approximately 14 L in the same person is contained in the extravascular interstitial fluid and plasma. A drug such as alcohol has a volume of distribution of approximately 40 L and is thought of as being contained in total body water.

TABLE 5–5. *Volumes of distribution of selected drugs*

Drug	V_d (L/kg)
Acetaminophen	0.75–1.0
Acetylsalicylic acid	0.1–0.3
Amitriptyline	66.0
Benzodiazepines	3.0–10.0
Digoxin	5.0
Ethanol	0.6
Lithium	0.7–2.0
Narcotics	3.0–5.0
Phenobarbital	0.60–0.75
Phenytoin	0.75
Theophylline	0.46

In toxicology, the volume of distribution can be useful (a) in calculating the amount of substance in the body to help verify the history of the quantity ingested, (b) in determining the amount of antidote needed if the serum level of the ingested substance is known, (c) in deciding whether to attempt to enhance elimination of the toxic substance, (d) in deciding how much more drug to administer, or (e) in calculating the approximate plasma level of a drug. Knowledge of the volume of distribution may also provide a reasonable basis for the design of typical dosage regimens and may indicate whether dosage adjustments will be necessary in the event of renal impairment (21,22).

To Verify the History of an Ingested Substance

To verify the history of the quantity of an ingested substance after the plasma concentration is determined, the equation given above for the apparent volume of distribution is rearranged as

$$A = V_d \times C_p \times M.$$

For example, a patient weighing 70 kg states that he/she ingested approximately thirty 100-mg phenobarbital tablets (phenobarbital has a volume of distribution of 0.75 L/kg). Blood is drawn and sent to the laboratory, and the peak plasma concentration is determined to be 60 mg/L. The history is verified as follows.

$$A = V_d \times C_p \times M$$
$$A = 0.75 \text{ L/kg} \times 60 \text{ mg/L} \times 70 \text{ kg}$$
$$A = 3{,}150 \text{ mg}$$

The amount calculated from the equation is essentially equal to that from the patient's history, and the history is therefore verified.

Therapeutic Dosing

As another example, involving therapeutic dosing in an emergency situation, a 110-pound patient with a history of taking xanthine bronchodilators enters the emergency department with bronchoconstriction. If the plasma theophylline concentration is 5 μg/mL (therapeutic concentration, 10 to 20 μg/mL), the amount of aminophylline it would take to raise the patient's level to the midtherapeutic range (15 μg/mL) is calculated as follows. The necessary change in plasma concentration is 10 μg/mL. The change in the dose is then the volume of distribution (0.46 L/kg) multiplied by the patient's weight and the change in concentration.

$$A = V_d \times (\text{change in } C_p) \times M$$
$$A = 0.46 \text{ L/kg} \times 10\ \mu\text{g/mL} \times 50 \text{ kg}$$
$$A = 230 \text{ mg}$$

The dose required is 230 mg and can be given as a loading dosage over a 20-minute period (in actuality, this may be an underestimate because aminophylline is only 80% to 85% theophylline).

Calculating the Plasma Level

If the equation is rearranged, then the plasma concentration after a given quantity of drug has been ingested can also be estimated. For example, if a 60-kg patient ingests approximately 20 tablets of phenytoin (100 mg each; volume of distribution, 0.75 L/kg), the peak plasma concentration is calculated as follows:

$$C_p = A/(V_d)(M)$$
$$C_p = 2{,}000 \text{ mg}/0.75 \text{ L/kg} \times 60 \text{ kg} = 44.4\ \mu\text{g/mL}.$$

Knowing this level before receiving the laboratory report may aid in determining the extent of toxicity and treatment required.

As another example, an 8-month-old child weighing 10 kg is given 2 tablespoons of 80-proof bourbon to soothe teething pain. The peak plasma concentration of ethanol is calculated as follows. Two tablespoons (30 mL) of 80-proof whiskey (40% ethanol) is approximately 9.5 g of ethanol (40% of 30 mL, or 12 mL, times the density of ethanol, 0.79 g/mL). This is then divided by the volume of distribution (0.60 L/kg) times the child's weight to yield more than 150 mg/dL. This value means that the infant requires immediate attention, and appropriate measures must be taken to prevent complications (e.g., seizures, hypoglycemia, hypothermia, apnea, and hypotension). If a person weighing 70 kg ingests the same 2 tablespoons of bourbon, the plasma concentration is only about 23 mg/dL because this person has a markedly larger space into which the ethanol is distributed (70 kg ×0.6 L/kg), making the peak plasma level only 23 mg/dL.

$$12{,}500 \text{ mg}/42 \text{ L} \times 0.79 = 22.7 \text{ mg/dL}.$$

These examples show that the volume of distribution is not simply a concept but a number that can aid in certain predictions of outcome and the extent of toxicity in various therapeutic and overdose situations.

Drugs with a relatively small volume of distribution (less than 1 L/kg) are present in substantial amounts in the circulation at any given time and may be removed with some success by extracorporeal methods. This is by no means always true because there are many other variables that determine whether the excretion of a substance may be enhanced by extracorporeal means. The degree of protein binding and the volume of distribution of the compound are only two factors. Substances with a large volume of distribution (greater than 1 L/kg) are not present in the blood in high concentrations, and generally a significant fraction of the total drug in the body is not recovered by extracorporeal means.

Effect of Drug Overdose Situation

Changes that may occur in drug overdose can affect drug distribution. Cardiovascular alterations, such as hypotension, decreased cardiac output, and decreased vascular resistance can decrease the apparent volume of distribution and drug clearance. In an overdosed patient one might expect higher, more prolonged serum drug concentrations. Acid-base disturbances may alter the distribution of the drug into organs and tissues. For example, a decrease in blood pH can enhance salicylate distribution into the brain and augment toxicity.

PROTEIN BINDING

Often, drugs are transported in the blood in two forms: attached to carrier proteins, or unbound in solution. Interaction between binding proteins in the serum and drugs is a reversible event. The plasma protein binding of drugs is usually expressed as the percentage of total drug that is bound (9).

Most drugs are bound to plasma albumin, although α_1-acid glycoprotein and lipoproteins are other carrier proteins for many therapeutic agents. Basic drugs bind to albumin, α_1-acid glycoprotein, and lipoprotein, whereas acidic and neutral compounds bind primarily to albumin.

The drug concentration in extracellular fluid is in equilibrium with the drug concentration in plasma water (18,19,23,24). The latter, known as the *free drug concentration*, is an indirect measure of drug concentration at the site of action (25). On entering the systemic circulation, any drug that is characteristically protein-bound binds to the plasma proteins. Bound drug is unable to cross cell membranes and consequently exerts no biologic effect. This is because the drug–protein complex is usually a large molecule that cannot leave the blood to reach the cell membranes. Only the unbound or free drug is able to cross the various lipoprotein membranes and is dissolved in plasma water. It is then transported across cell membranes and interacts with specific receptors to elicit a desired pharmacologic response. A drug that is highly protein-bound has a small volume of distribution.

Each drug has its own characteristic protein binding pattern that is dependent on the physical and chemical properties of that drug. Drugs are either tightly or loosely bound, depending on their affinity for the plasma proteins.

Competition for Protein Binding

Because albumin and other plasma proteins possess a limited number of binding sites and these sites are rather nonselective with respect to the drugs that will bind, two drugs with an affinity for the same site will compete with one another for binding. Multiple drugs that are highly bound to plasma proteins may compete for binding sites. A drug that binds with a higher affinity can displace another drug (6). This would result in an increase in the intensity of pharmacologic action of the displaced drug, or possibly, an increase in the risk of adverse drug effect. Those drugs that are tightly bound are not displaced rapidly. Heredity, sex, age, disease, and other physiologic conditions may also affect the extent of drug binding to proteins (11). Displacement of a drug from its plasma protein binding site can, under certain circumstances, elevate free drug concentrations at the tissue receptor sites with resultant clinical toxicity, even though the total plasma drug concentration remains unchanged (Fig. 5-3).

As plasma protein-binding sites become saturated in overdose the unbound fraction of the drug increases, resulting in an increased volume of distribution for the drug. Increases in the amount of free drug may then lead to a greater clinical or toxic effect than would be expected from the drug's total concentration because free concentrations generally correlate more closely with clinical effect.

Clinical laboratory reports of drug concentration in plasma represent drug that is bound to plasma protein plus drug that is unbound or free. It is the free or unbound drug which is in equilibrium with the receptor site and is, therefore, the pharmacologically active moiety. Thus, the reported plasma drug concentration indirectly reflects the concentration of free or active drug.

Any factors such as competition for protein-binding sites by other drugs or a decrease in protein concentration will alter the percentage of unbound drug and can markedly affect pharmacologic response. Fortunately, this is of little consequence for drugs with less than approximately 90% protein binding, which constitutes the majority of available drugs. When bound drug is displaced from plasma proteins, the resulting increase in unbound drug concentration is rapidly equilibrated with tissue compartments. As an example, a patient with a low serum albumin and an apparently low plasma phenytoin concentration may still have a therapeutically acceptable plasma drug concentration when it is adjusted for the low serum albumin.

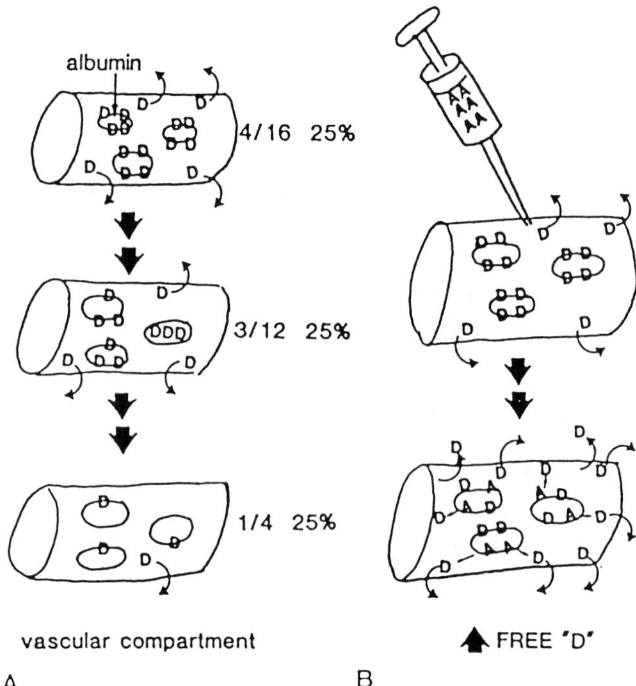

FIG. 5–3. A: Plasma protein binding. Binding to plasma proteins decreases the intensity and prolongs the action of drugs. The ratio of bound to free drug remains constant regardless of the total amount of drug in the plasma. The ratio in the figure represents free drug/total drug. *D* = drug. **B:** Drug displacement. Drugs with high plasma protein binding affinity (*A*) can displace other drugs (*D*) from plasma proteins. (From Schwertz D, *Nurs Clin North Am* 1991;26:249, with permission.)

Effect in Drug Overdose

In drug overdose, alterations in drug distribution may occur. Saturation of plasma protein binding sites can result in an increase in the free (or pharmacologically active) fraction of drug, which can manifest enhanced toxic effects. Saturation of tissue binding sites also may occur (9).

ROUTES OF EXCRETION AND ELIMINATION

Clearance

The elimination of drugs from the body can also be described quantitatively by the term *clearance*. Clearance is a measure of the amount of drug that is eliminated per unit time. It is important to emphasize that clearance is not an indicator of how much drug is being removed; it only represents the theoretical volume of blood or plasma which is completely cleared of drug in a given period of time. The amount of drug removed depends on the plasma concentration of drug as well as the clearance. This elimination may be accomplished through major routes, such as excretion by the kidneys or metabolism by the liver as well as through minor routes, such as the lungs, sweat, and feces. Clearance is generally assumed to be additive. How a drug is cleared and by what mechanism is important in deciding on a method for detoxification. For most drugs, clearance by glomerular filtration by the kidney and metabolism by the liver is directly proportional to the amount of free drug in the serum. Consequently, an increase in free drug concentration makes more drug available for elimination.

The clearance or elimination rate does not necessarily refer to the actual elimination of the drug from the body because drug metabolism converts drugs from pharmacologically active to inactive compounds. Thus, the pharmacologically active portion of the drug may be eliminated even though the metabolite is still present in the body. This type of elimination is dependent only on plasma concentration.

The liver transforms a drug into one or more metabolites, and the kidneys excrete variable amounts of a drug and its metabolites. That is why the liver is the most important organ to remove drugs by metabolism and the kidneys are the second in importance.

The body has intrinsic mechanisms for clearing drugs, and the total clearance is the sum of clearances by excretion by the kidneys, metabolism by the liver, and elimination by sweat, feces, and expired air.

TABLE 5–6. *Biotransformation reactions*

Phase I reactions—Drugs may still be active
Oxidation
Cytochrome P-450-dependent monooxygenase
Xanthine oxidase
Peroxidases
Amine oxidase
Monoamine oxidase
Dioxygenases
Reduction
Cytochrome P-450-dependent reductases
Ketoreductase
Glutathione peroxidases
Hydrolysis
Epoxide hydrolase
Ester hydrolysis
Carboxylesterases
Amidases
Alcohol dehydrogenases
Aldehyde dehydrogenases
Superoxide dismutase
Phase II reactions—Drugs usually rendered inert
Conjugation with:
Sulfotransferase
Glucuronosyltransferase
Glutathione *S*-transferase
Glucosyltransferase
Thioltransferase
Amide synthesis
Methylation
O-Methyltransferases
N-Methyltransferases
S-Methyltransferases
Acetylation
N-Acetyltransferase
Acyltransferases
Thiosulfate sulfurtransferase (rhodanese)

Biotransformation

Lipid-soluble drugs introduced into the body are usually not excreted until they undergo chemical changes that result in an increase in polarity. Because many drugs are lipophilic, biotransformation increases their water solubility. This solubility change restricts further penetration of the drug through cellular membranes, reduces systemic destruction, and promotes elimination through excretory systems such as the kidney.

Biotransformation or metabolism can take place in most cells and in the plasma, but the primary organ for drug metabolism is the liver, though the kidney, intestine, lung, adrenal, and skin are also capable of biotransforming certain compounds.

The four major biotransformation reactions that occur within the body are oxidation, reduction, hydrolysis, (Phase I reaction) and conjugation (Phase II reaction) (Table 5–6).

Phase I and Phase II Reactions

There are two stages of drug biotransformation within the hepatocyte. In the first stage, the mixed-function oxidase enzyme system that is associated with the smooth endoplasmic reticulum of liver cells catalyzes hydroxylation, oxidation, or hydrolysis of drugs. This cytochrome P-450 is now known to be a group of closely related proteins which catalyze a diverse number of oxidative reactions involved in metabolism of drugs (Table 5–7). This is referred to as Phase I reactions (5,6). In the second stage of biotransformation, a chemical moiety, such as glucuronic acid, glutathione, or glycine, is combined with a drug or a drug product from the first stage of biotransformation. This is referred to as Phase II reactions, also called conjugation reactions. Phase II reactions almost always result in drug inactivation and an increased rate of excretion.

Phase I reactions usually precede Phase II reactions, but in some cases Phase II reactions occur before those of Phase I. Alternately, a given drug may undergo only Phase II reactions. In other words, in general, conjugation reactions follow oxidation, reduction, or hydrolytic reactions. A conjugated drug is generally more polar and therefore more water-soluble; this greatly enhances renal

TABLE 5–7. *Oxidative reactions catalyzed by cytochrome P-450-dependent monooxygenase system*

Aliphatic hydroxylation
Aromatic hydroxylation
Epoxidation
N-Dealkylation
O-Dealkylation
S-Dealkylation
Deamination
Sulfoxidation
N-Oxidation
Oxidative dehalogenation
Desulfuration

excretion of the compound (26). Although most reactions yield compounds with less activity than the parent compound, some chemicals are metabolized to more toxic substances (Table 5–8).

First-Pass Effect

Drugs that are administered intravenously enter the systemic circulation as soon as they are injected. They then may be redistributed into various tissues or remain in the blood compartment. Drugs that are ingested orally first traverse the hepatic portal system before reaching the systemic circulation. Metabolism may inactivate or activate a fraction of the absorbed drug or have no effect. Usually, the drug is inactivated, which reduces the bioavailability of the drug. Thus, if a drug is extensively cleared by the liver, only a small fraction of it will reach the systemic circulation. This is called the *first-pass effect* and occurs with a number of therapeutic agents. It is also called the *extraction ratio*, the proportion of a drug that enters the liver and is then eliminated from the plasma in a single passage. Drugs with significant first-pass effect may not be effective orally because the liver may extract the drug before it reaches the systemic circulation.

TABLE 5–8. *Selected drugs that are metabolized to more toxic substances*

Acetaminophen
Acetanilid
Aniline
Benzene
Carbon tetrachloride
Chloral hydrate
Codeine
Ethylene glycol
Imipramine
Malathion
Methanol
Parathion

Drugs that have a significant first-pass effect can be administered as sublingual tablets or by rectal suppositories, which avoids the first pass through the portal circulation. For example, naloxone is absorbed by almost all routes with significant serum concentrations being achieved. This is not true for the oral route because of the significant first-pass effect; by this route, the drug is 2% as potent as when it is parenterally administered. Other drugs that have a significant first-pass effect are listed in Table 5–9. In the elderly, who have reduced liver blood flow, the first-pass effect is lessened so that more drug can reach systemic circulation.

Some orally administered drugs such as chlorpromazine are more extensively metabolized in the intestine than the liver. Thus, intestinal metabolism may contribute to the overall first-pass effect.

First-Order, Zero-Order, and Michaelis-Menten Elimination

Drugs are eliminated in one of three ways: first-order elimination, zero-order elimination, or a combination of the two (Table 5–10). Drugs that are charged or highly polar are either not metabolized or, what is more likely, the metabolism is rapid enough that the highly polar metabolites are excreted directly by the kidneys. This is referred to as *first-order elimination*. Drugs that are highly lipid-soluble are first metabolized by the liver to introduce a charge or highly polar group and are then excreted by the kidneys. When elimination depends in this way on metabolism and when the enzymes responsible for the breakdown of the compound are saturated, it is referred to as *zero-order elimination*. A combination of the two types of elimination in which a drug changes its elimination pattern from first order to zero order, is called *Michaelis-Menten elimination*.

TABLE 5–9. *Drugs that exhibit significant first-pass effect*

N-Acetylcysteine (Mucomyst)
Alprenolol
Chlorpromazine (Thorazine)
Hydralazine (Apresoline)
Isoproterenol (Isuprel)
Labetalol (Normodyne, Trandate)
Lidocaine (Xylocaine)
Meperidine (Demerol)
Metoprolol (Lopressor)
Morphine
Naloxone (Narcan)
Naltrexone (Trexan)
Nitroglycerin
Pentazocine (Talwin)
Propoxyphene (Darvon)
Propranolol (Inderal)
Salicylamide (Codalan, Korigesic)
Verapamil (Calan, Isoptin)

TABLE 5–10. *Types of elimination*

First order—A constant *fraction* of drug is eliminated per unit time.
- Considered renal elimination, but implies hepatic metabolism.
- The higher the plasma concentration, the more drug eliminated.
- Half-life can be useful parameter.
- Linear relationship between drug concentration and amount of drug in body.
- Clearance and volume of distribution remain constant.

Zero order—A constant *amount* of drug is eliminated per unit time.
- Implies hepatic metabolism with enzymes that are easily saturable.
- Constant amount of drug is eliminated per unit time.
- Greater degree of accumulation will occur.

Michaelis-Menten—Changing elimination from first-order to zero-order in *therapeutic* situation.

First-Order Elimination

The rate of elimination is proportional to the drug concentration; therefore, the amount of drug removed per unit of time will vary proportionately with drug concentration. The fraction or percentage of the total amount of drug present in the body that is removed at any instant in time, however, will remain constant and independent of dose. First-order elimination (renal elimination) means that the higher the plasma concentration of a drug, the greater the amount of drug excreted in a given time interval. This also means that, regardless of how much drug is in the body, one-half the total amount will be excreted in one drug half-life. Doubling the plasma concentration will thus result in a doubling of the rate at which the drug is eliminated. In other words, the rate of clearance is directly proportional to the concentration of the drug in the system. Because of this, there is a linear relation between plasma concentration of the drug and the total amount of drug. Renal elimination therefore is linear when plotted on semilogarithmic graph paper and is called first-order because a constant fraction of the drug is eliminated per unit of time (Fig. 5–4). Another important characteristic of first-order elimination is that both clearance and volume of distribution remain constant and do not vary with dose or concentration.

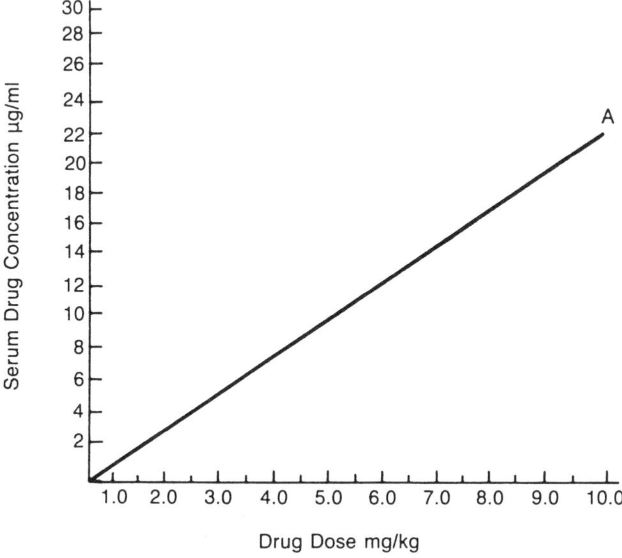

FIG. 5–4. Graph showing linear relation between plasma concentration of the drug and the total amount of drug. Adapted with permission from *Syva Monitor.* Palo Alto, CA: Syva Company; 1979:3.

The "Half-Life"

The half-life for first-order elimination is a constant. It can be a useful kinetic parameter as long as renal function is normal. In other words, the half-life can be used to determine how long it will take to effectively eliminate all of the drug from the body once a drug has been discontinued. It will take one half-life to eliminate 50%, two half-lives to eliminate 75%, three half-lives to eliminate 87.5%, and four half-lives to eliminate 93.75% of the total amount of drug in the body (Table 5–11). In most clinical situations it can be assumed that drug activity has been effectively eliminated after three to four half-lives. In a drug excreted by first-order elimination, a plasma concentration of 200 µg/mL will fall to 100 µg/mL after one half-life, to 50 µg/mL after two half-lives, and so on. It is important to note that half-life is a theoretical, population-based concept, and the real value may differ from patient to patient and from day to day in the same patient.

The half-life of a drug has practical implications. Drugs with short half-lives accumulate in the body minimally and with multiple doses reach steady-state concentrations shortly after initiation of therapy. They also leave the body rapidly once therapy has been discontinued. For

TABLE 5–11. *Percentage of steady-state plasma concentrations achieved at each half-life interval*

Number of half-lives	Percentage of steady-state concentration
1	50
2	75
3	88
4	94
5	97
6	98
7	99

Reprinted with permission from *Pediatr Clin North Am* 1980;27:906. WB Saunders Company.

drugs with long half-lives the converse is true; that is, they accumulate extensively in the body with multiple doses, reach steady-state concentration slowly, and leave the body slowly on termination of therapy.

Zero-Order Elimination

Zero-order elimination (hepatic metabolism) occurs with compounds that require degradation in the liver before excretion. This type of elimination involves enzymes that are easily saturable, and the rate at which a drug is metabolized can only be increased to a certain point, which is the maximal rate at which the particular enzyme can act. Since the enzyme system generally has a slow rate of metabolism, the rate of elimination is fixed and depends on the activity of the saturated enzymes irrespective of the drug concentration. Therefore, unlike the first-order in which the greater the plasma level the larger the amount of drug excreted, zero-order metabolism has an upper limit for metabolism that cannot go higher regardless of the plasma level. Once the hepatic enzymes are saturated, the plasma level increases abruptly (Fig. 5–5). This rate of elimination can be predicted by simply plotting it on linear graph paper, with concentration on the y-axis and time on the x-axis. An example of a drug that undergoes this type of elimination is ethanol, which is broken down at 15 to 25 mg%/hour regardless of the concentration.

At a certain concentration point, drug absorption, excretion, and biotransformation become independent of concentration. It is thought that all drugs convert from first-order to zero-order kinetics because a point is reached at which enzyme or transport mechanisms become saturated.

Most drugs never achieve concentrations in the body that approach the transition point from first-order to zero-order kinetics. In most cases, the serum concentrations of a drug achieved at therapeutic doses are low relative to the drug concentration necessary to saturate the particular system involved, and therefore most drugs follow first-order elimination. For most drugs, then, first-order kinetics is usually observed throughout the therapeutic range. When the drug elimination system is saturated, linear kinetics then switches to zero order, in which a constant amount of the drug that is present is eliminated per unit of time. This is typically seen when patients ingest toxic amounts of a drug.

Following drug overdose, alterations in the metabolic process occur owing to saturation of enzymes, inhibition of enzyme activity, reduction in enzyme affinity, depletion of cofactors, and partial enzyme inactivation. These changes may result in a change to a zero-order drug elimination process with a constant rate of elimination, regardless of serum drug concentration.

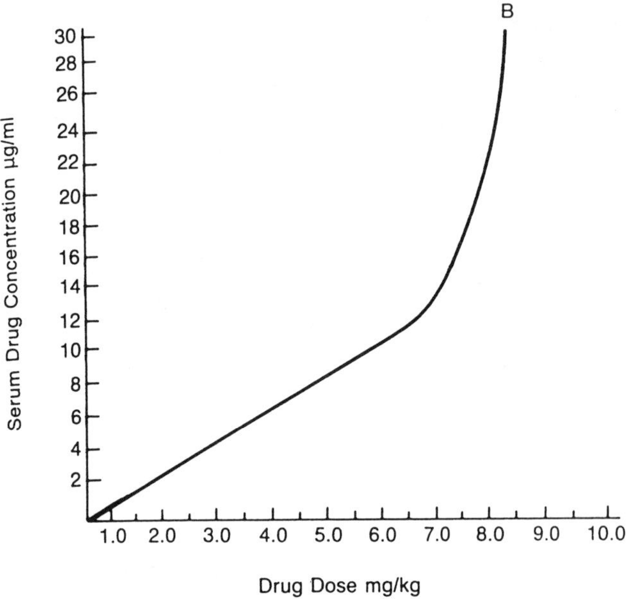

FIG. 5–5. Graph showing abrupt increase in plasma level irrespective of drug concentration. Adapted with permission from *Syva Monitor.* Palo Alto, CA: Syva Company; 1979:3.

Michaelis-Menten Elimination

There are some drugs, however, that, due to saturation of enzymes switch their kinetics in therapeutic amounts. This has important clinical ramifications. Salicylates, phenytoin, theophylline, and ethyl alcohol are examples of drugs that undergo dose-dependent or Michaelis-Menten elimination in the therapeutic range (Table 5–12). As concentration increases, the half-life of the drug increases as well because there is an early saturation of the various enzymes in the liver. Further administration of these drugs may result in accumulation of the drug, and a small change in dose may, over several days, result in anywhere from a modest to large change in plasma concentration. In other words, once the plasma level approaches the saturation concentration a very small change in dose will, over several days, result in a very large change in plasma concentration (1,2).

In this situation the proportion of drug elimination falls as the drug concentration rises, resulting in a longer elim-

TABLE 5–12. *Drugs that undergo Michaelis-Menten elimination at therapeutic concentrations*

Dicumarol
Ethanol
Phenylbutazone
Phenytoin
Probenecid
Salicylates
Theophylline

TABLE 5–13. *Drugs eliminated primarily by the kidneys*

Amantadine
Aminoglycosides
Atenolol
Captopril
Chlorpropamide
Clonidine
Digoxin
Disopyramide
Diuretics
Enalapril
Famotidine
Guanfacine
Lithium
Nadolol
Nizatidine
NSAIDs
Procainamide
Ranitidine
Tocainide

ination half-life. As an example, an overdose of phenytoin may change the drug's elimination half-life from 22 hours to 4 days because first-order elimination is changed to zero-order when the enzyme system is saturated. A 50% increase in the maintenance dose of aspirin has resulted in a 300% increase in steady-state salicylate concentrations in the plasma. Therefore, the half-life for drugs such as phenytoin and salicylates may not be constant, even in therapeutic doses, but can change as a result of the amount of drug in the body.

Renal Excretion

Urinary excretion is the major pathway for the elimination of drugs and drug metabolites, although most of these drugs have been metabolized by the liver. Only a small number of drugs are eliminated primarily by the kidneys (Table 5–13). Any change in renal function will alter plasma concentrations of drugs that are not metabolized extensively. If renal function is impaired, plasma drug concentrations may be elevated. Impaired renal excretion can be caused by preexisting or age-related renal dysfunction, direct toxic effect of the drug, saturation of active tubular secretion, reduced cardiac output, rhabdomyolysis, myoglobinuria, acute renal failure, or hemolysis (9)

Summary of Elimination

The difference between first-order and zero-order elimination is a matter of degree. Although first-order elimination is "equivalent" to renal elimination, almost all drugs require some degree of metabolism before excretion. That is why the liver is the most important organ for removing drugs by metabolism and the kidneys are the second in importance. When the metabolic processes are not saturated, then the drug does not accumulate and is said to be excreted by first-order elimination. When the metabolic processes are saturated early, then zero-order kinetics prevails. In most nonoverdose situations, first-order kinetics prevails. In certain nonpurposeful overdose situations, kinetics switches from first-order to zero-order as a result of enzyme saturation (Michaelis-Menten kinetics). In most large overdoses, in which hepatic metabolism of the substance is required, the enzymes are overwhelmed and zero-order kinetics prevails.

Therapeutic Index

When the difference between toxic and minimal therapeutic drug levels is small, the drug is said to have a narrow therapeutic window and a high inherent risk of adverse effect. Examples of drugs with a narrow therapeutic window include digoxin, lithium, and gentamicin (6).

Limitations of Use of Pharmacokinetic Data

The variability in pharmacokinetic parameters for most drugs may be as much or more than 10-fold, even if the population is quite homogeneous and the dose is corrected for body weight (27). These differences originate from variability in absorption and from differences in the metabolizing capacity of the liver caused by genetic or environmental factors (10). For most drugs, pharmacokinetic variables such as volume of distribution, clearance, and half-life are well described in the literature, but they are often based on population data from normal volunteer studies. Naturally, such general information is important for the common characterization of the drug in question but cannot be used to predict, with exactness, the precise plasma concentrations in individual patients (9).

Unlike the use of clinical pharmacokinetics in routine therapeutic drug monitoring, the application of individualized pharmacokinetics in drug overdose in based on limited data that are often anecdotal, incomplete, or unreliable. For example, an accurate clinical history that includes the identity, dose, and time of all drugs ingested is rarely obtainable; the presence of other disease states or chronically administered drugs and their effects on overdose pharmacokinetics are usually unknown at the time of ingestion; and serum drug sampling results are difficult to interpret because absorption and elimination phases may overlap. Nevertheless, a basic knowledge of pharmacokinetic processes and the effect of drug overdose on them, as well as an understanding of overdose interventions and the limitations of drug serum monitoring, can be useful in the management of overdose victims.

SUMMARY

The principles of pharmacokinetics and toxicokinetics can be used by emergency department personnel in many different ways. Knowledge of the volume of distribution of a substance can help in determining approximate plasma concentrations or aid in deciding whether elimination will be facilitated by diuresis, dialysis, or hemoperfusion. Drugs with a large volume of distribution are concentrated in the tissues and fat of the body and so are not found to a great extent in the serum. For that reason, diuresis, dialysis, and hemoperfusion are not effective. In addition, although many drugs undergo first-order kinetics in therapeutic situations, they may change their kinetics in the overdose situation and thereby accumulate and change their half-life.

REFERENCES

1. Gibaldi M, Levy G: Pharmacokinetics in clinical practice: concepts. *JAMA* 1976;235:1864–1867.
2. Gibaldi M, Levy G: Pharmacokinetics in clinical practice: applications. *JAMA* 1976;235:1987–1992.
3. Greenblatt D, Koch-Weser J: Clinical pharmacokinetics. *N Engl J Med* 1975;293:702–708.
4. Watanabe A: Pharmacokinetic aspects of the dialysis of drugs. *Drug Intell Clin Pharmacol* 1977;11:407–416.
5. Cheeley R, Joyce S: A clinical comparison of the performance of four blood glucose reagent strips. *Am J Emerg Med* 1990;8:11–15.
6. Schwertz D: Basic principles of pharmacologic action. *Nurs Clin North Am* 1991;26:245–262.
7. Gilette J: The importance of tissue distribution in pharmacokinetics. *J Pharmacokinet Biopharmacol* 1973;1:497–520.
8. Ariens E: Drug levels in the target tissue and effect. *Clin Pharmacol Ther* 1974 16:155–175.
9. Platt D: Pharmacokinetics of drug overdose. *Clin Lab Med* 1990;10:261–269.
10. Nightingale C, Carver P: Basic principles of pharmacokinetics. *Clin Lab Med* 1987;7:267–278.
11. Theodore W: Basic principles of clinical pharmacology. *Neurol Clin* 1990;8:1–13.
12. Greenblatt D, Sellers E, Shader R: Drug disposition in old age. *N Engl J Med* 1982;306:1081–1088.
13. Levy G: Pharmacokinetic control and clinical interpretation of steady-state blood levels of drugs. *Clin Pharmacol Ther* 1975;16:120–134.
14. Chiou W, Peng G, Nation R: Rapid estimation of volume of distribution after a short intravenous infusion and its application to dosing adjustments. *J Clin Pharmacol* 1978;18:266–271.
15. Pagliaro L, Benet L: Pharmacokinetic data: clinical compilation of terminal half-lives, percent excreted unchanged, and changes of half-life in renal and hepatic dysfunction for studies in humans with references. *J Pharmacokinet Biopharmacol* 1975 3:333–383.
16. Kowarski C, Kowarski A: Simplified method for estimating volume of distribution at steady state.*J Pharm Sci* 1980;69:1222–1223.
17. Wagner J: A modern view of pharmacokinetics. *J Pharmacokinet Biopharmacol* 1973;1:363–401.
18. Koch-Weser J, Sellers E: Binding of drugs to serum albumin, part I. *N Engl J Med* 1976;294:311–316.
19. Koch-Weser J, Sellers E: Binding of drugs to serum albumin, part 2. *N Engl J Med* 1976;294:526–531.
20. Gilman AG, Goodman L, Gilman A: *Pharmacological basis of therapeutics.* 6th ed. New York: Macmillan; 1980.
21. Klotz U: Pathophysiological and disease-induced changes in drug distribution volume: pharmacokinetic implications. *Clin Pharmacokinet* 1976;1:204–218.
22. Graham G, Chinwah P, Kennedy M, et al: Monitoring plasma concentrations of drugs. *Med J Aust* 1980;2:124–130.
23. Koch-Weser J: Bioavailability of drugs. *N Engl J Med* 1974;291: 233–237.
24. Vesell E: Factors causing interindividual variations of drug concentrations in blood. *Clin Pharmacol Ther* 1974;16:135–148.
25. Reed M, Besunder J: Developmental pharmacology: ontogenic basis of drug disposition. *Pediatr Clin North Am* 1989;36:1053–1074.
26. Yuen G: Altered pharmacokinetics in the elderly. *Clin Geriatr Med* 1990;6:257–267.
27. Hvidberg E: Why do we need pharmacokinetic studies? *Am J Obstet Gynecol* 1990;163:316–318.

CHAPTER 6

Pharmacokinetics and Age Extremes

Much of the important work in the last decade in the area of pharmacokinetics has been performed with young adults (1). Because of this, estimates of drug disposition in infants, children, and the elderly have been made with the use of pharmacokinetic parameters derived from the study of young adults (2). Patients in the extremes of age groups present special pharmacokinetic problems that must be considered in overdose situations (3). Neonates and the elderly, however, generally have a lower metabolic capacity compared with subjects between these extremes of age (2). There are many other reasons why these parameters may be incorrect, owing to the continuous and rapid physiologic changes associated with the basic stages of human development. Even in healthy elderly, the normal aging process creates important changes in many of the phenomena included under the heading of pharmacokinetics: absorption, distribution, metabolism, and excretion.

PLACENTAL TRANSFER OF DRUGS

At one time it was theorized that the placenta served as a means of protection to the fetus. With the belief that it was a barrier, it was assumed that harmful substances could not enter the fetal circulation. It is now known that one of the main functions of the placenta is to transport substances present in the maternal circulation to the fetus. Instead of a barrier, the placenta tends to serve as a sieve (4).

As is true also of other biologic membranes, drug passage across the placenta is dependent on the lipid solubility and degree of drug ionization (Table 6–1). Lipophilic drugs tend to diffuse readily across the placenta and enter the fetal circulation. The molecular weight of the drug influences the rate and amount of drug transferred across the placenta. Drugs with molecular weights of 250–500 can cross the placenta easily, depending upon their lipid solubility and degree of ionization; those with molecular weights of 500–1,000 cross the placenta with more difficulty; and those with molecular weights greater than 1,000 cross very poorly (5).

TABLE 6–1. *Placental transfer of drugs*

Placental transfer of drugs should have
Low molecular weight (250–500)
Low degree water solubility
Lipophilic properties

Impermeability of the placenta to polar compounds is relative rather than absolute. If high enough maternal–fetal concentration gradients are achieved, polar compounds can cross the placenta. Salicylate, which is almost completely ionized at physiologic pH, crosses the placenta readily. This occurs because the small amount of salicylate that is not ionized is highly lipid-soluble.

Two mechanisms help to protect the fetus from drugs in the maternal circulation. The placenta itself plays a role both as a semipermeable barrier and as a site of metabolism of some drugs passing through it. In addition, drugs that have crossed the placenta enter the fetal circulation via the umbilical vein. About 40–60% of umbilical venous blood flow enters the fetal liver; the remainder bypasses the liver and enters the general fetal circulation. After the first trimester of development, medications are not usually capable of producing structural changes, but they are able to alter the normal growth or functional development of the fetus (5).

MEDICATIONS POSSIBLY ASSOCIATED WITH FETAL ABNORMALITIES

Chronic consumption of ethanol during pregnancy, particularly during the first and second trimesters, results in the fetal alcohol syndrome. In this syndrome, the central nervous system (CNS), growth, and facial development are all affected.

The administration of warfarin during pregnancy may lead to the "fetal warfarin syndrome." If taken during the sixth to ninth week of gestation, bone marrow involvement, extremity hypoplasia, and nasal cartilage hypoplasia may occur. If warfarin is taken during the second and third trimesters, then CNS effects, vaginal bleeding, abruptio placentae, and stillbirth have been noted. Phenytoin taken during pregnancy may cause "fetal hydantoin syndrome" with abnormal genitalia, cleft palate and lip, hypoplasia of the distal phalanges, diaphragmatic hernia, and congenital heart and eye defects. Other medications possibly associated with fetal abnormalities are listed in Table 6–2.

PHARMACOKINETICS IN THE NEONATE AND CHILD (TABLE 6–3)

In the first 2 weeks of life, the microsomal enzymes responsible for metabolism are immature and not fully active. Furthermore, very young children do not have the necessary plasma-binding proteins. Shortly after 2 weeks until approximately 10 years of age the activity of these systems increases, and drug elimination usually occurs at a significantly higher rate than in adults because maturing organ function contributes to a greater drug effect per unit body weight than in the adult (6). At puberty (10 to 14 years of age), the child's physiologic pattern for metabolizing drugs rapidly approaches that of an adult. Children older than 15 years of age typically exhibit adult patterns of drug utilization. These changes are directly associated with the initial onset of puberty and are observed earlier in females than in males.

The major cause of age-related changes in drug disposition is the maturational increase in liver and kidney function. Age-dependent variations in plasma protein binding, tissue distribution, gastrointestinal absorption, and other physiologic parameters also contribute to the rapid changes.

Protein Binding

The premature infant has much less protein-binding ability than the neonate. Adult values for plasma protein may not be attained until the infant is over 1 year of age

TABLE 6–2. *Medications possibly associated with fetal abnormalities*

Antibiotics
- Chloroquine (Aralen)
- Tetracycline (Vibramycin, Terramycin)
- Aminoglycosides (Gentamicin, Kanamycin)
- Metronidazole (Flagyl)
- Nitrofurantoin (Furadantin, Macrodantin)
- Sulfonamides (Bactrim, Septra)
- Isoniazid
- Rifampin

Anticoagulants
- Dicumarol (Dicoumarin)
- Warfarin (Coumadin)

Anticonvulsants
- Phenytoin (Dilantin)
- Paramethadione (Paradione)
- Trimethadione (Tridione)
- Benzodiazepines (Valium, etc.)
- Phenobarbital

Antidiabetics
- Chlorpropamide (Diabinese)
- Tolbutamide (Orinase)

Antiemetics
- Meclizine (Antivert)
- Prochlorperazine (Compazine)
- Promethazine (Phenergan)
- Trimethobenzamide (Tigan)
- Doxylamine (Bendectin)

Anti-inflammatory agents
- Meclofenamate (Meclomen)
- Phenylbutazone (Butazolidin)
- Indomethacin (Indocin)
- Naproxen (Naprosyn)
- Salicylates (Aspirin)

Asthma medications
- Ephedrine
- Epinephrine
- Theophylline

Cardiovascular drugs
- Diazoxide (Hyperstat)
- Propranolol (Inderal)
- Digoxin

Central nervous system drugs
- Alprazolam (Xanax)
- Amphetamines
- Barbiturates
- Chlordiazepoxide (Librium)
- Haloperidol (Haldol)
- Hydroxyzine (Vistaril)
- Lithium
- Methaqualone (Quaalude)
- Tricyclic antidepressants

Diuretics
- Acetazolamide (Diamox)
- Furosemide (Lasix)
- Chlorothiazide (Diuril)
- Ethacrynic acid (Edecrin)

Miscellaneous agents
- Ethanol
- LSD
- Radiation
- Marijuana
- Tobacco
- Vaccinations

Narcotics
- Heroin
- Methadone (Dolophine)
- Pentazocine (Talwin)
- Propoxyphene (Darvon)

Synthetic hormones
- Clomiphene (Clomid)
- Diethylstilbestrol
- Estrogen (Premarin, Gynogen)
- Medroxyprogesterone (Provera)
- Progesterone (Progestin, Progestasert)
- Corticosteroids

TABLE 6–3. *Pharmacokinetics in the very young*

Protein binding
Less protein binding than adult
Increased amount of free drug
Possibly greater toxicity with "normal" plasma levels
Volume of distribution
Usually larger in neonate and premature infant
Higher percentage of body weight as water
Gastrointestinal factors
Alkaline gastric pH at birth
Adult levels of gastric acid reached age 5–12 years
Prolonged gastric emptying time in very young
Lower degree of gastrointestinal enzymes
Renal factors
Low glomerular filtration rate at birth—until 5 months of age
Low tubular secretion rate
Decreased clearance on renally eliminated drugs
Hepatic factors
Immature microsomal enzyme system until 2 weeks
Increased drug elimination until 10 years of age
Adult pattern—approximately age 15

(7). Albumin is the plasma protein with the greatest binding capacity. In general, protein binding of drugs is reduced in the neonate. This has been seen with local anesthetic drugs, diazepam, phenytoin, ampicillin, and phenobarbital. Therefore, the concentration of free drug in plasma is increased. This can result in greater drug effect or toxicity despite a normal or even low plasma concentration of total drug (8).

Volume of Distribution

As body composition changes with development, the relative volume into which a drug is distributed also changes. The neonate has a higher percentage of its body weight in the form of water than does the adult. The neonate and premature infant generally have a larger volume of distribution because of an increase in the extracellular fluid and the decreased ability of fetal plasma proteins to bind drugs.

Gastrointestinal Factors

Significant biochemical and physiologic changes occur in the neonatal gastrointestinal tract shortly after birth. In full-term infants, gastric acid secretion begins soon after birth and increases gradually over several hours. In premature infants, the secretion of gastric acid occurs more slowly, with the highest concentration appearing on the fourth day of life.

The gastric pH of a neonate is 6 to 8, but reaches adult values by 1 year of age. The fetal gastrointestinal tract is rapidly colonized by bacteria after birth, and the level of gastrointestinal microorganism flora is related to bile acid deconjugation activity and β-glucuronidase activity, both of which are significantly higher in neonates than in adults.

Gastric emptying time is prolonged in the first day or two of life. Therefore, drugs that are absorbed primarily in the stomach may be absorbed more completely than anticipated. However, in the case of drugs absorbed in the small intestine, absorption, and therefore therapeutic effect, are delayed. Because the neonate has irregular peristalsis and prolonged gastric emptying, absorption of drugs from the gastrointestinal tract (GIT) may be altered.

Gastrointestinal enzyme activities are lower in the newborn than in the adult. Activities of amylase and other pancreatic enzymes in the duodenum are low in infants up to 4 months of age. Neonates also have low concentrations of bile acids and lipase, which may decrease the absorption of lipid-soluble drugs.

Renal Factors

The glomerular filtration rate is much lower in newborns than in older infants, children, or adults, and this limitation persists during the first few days of life. It reaches adult levels at approximately 5 months of age. Drugs that depend on renal function for elimination are therefore cleared from the body very slowly in the first weeks of life. The tubular secretion rate reaches adult levels somewhat later than the glomerular filtration rate so that the premature infant has difficulty handling some drugs even though glomerular filtration is possible.

Hepatic Factors

The metabolism of most drugs occurs in the liver. The drug-metabolizing activities of the cytochrome P-450–dependent, mixed-function oxidases and the conjugating enzymes are substantially lower in early neonatal life than later. The point in development at which enzymatic activity is maximal depends upon the specific enzyme system in question. As an example, glucuronide formation reaches adult values between the third and fourth years of life. Although hepatic microsomal enzyme systems may be immature in neonates and young children, a higher proportion of drug may be excreted unchanged in the urine, and clearance remains comparable to adult values in many cases.

Clinical Application

Salicylate elimination in the infant is slower than in the adult, and consequently some infants have platelet dysfunction with hemorrhage. For this reason, salicylate use should be only occasional during pregnancy. It is of clinical importance that acetaminophen seems to be less poisonous in children than in adults. This may be explained, in part, by the compensatory routes of metabolism, although other mechanisms also may be operating. Theophylline is subject to extensive age-dependent changes in its metabolism. In premature infants, theophylline is eliminated virtually only by direct excretion, which is nonexistent in the adult.

There has been a recent identification of an endogenous digoxin-like immunoreactive substance (EDLIS) in the serum of neonates. The presence of this EDLIS falsely elevates the serum digoxin concentration by cross-reacting with laboratory reagents commonly used to measure digoxin in serum. Thus, until a routine laboratory assay becomes available that consistently discriminates between exogenously administered digoxin and EDLIS, available pharmacokinetic data must be interpreted cautiously.

Drugs and Lactation

Secretion of toxic compounds into the milk is not a major excretory route but it is extremely important because toxic material may be passed in the milk from the mother to the nursing child. Most drugs administered to lactating women are detectable in breast milk (9). Fortunately, the concentration of drug achieved in breast milk is usually low. Therefore, the total amount the infant would receive in a day is likely to be less than what would be considered a therapeutic dose. Toxic agents are excreted into the milk by simple diffusion; and because milk is more acidic than plasma, basic compounds may be concentrated in milk whereas acidic compounds attain a lower concentration in milk than in plasma water. To be transferred to milk, a compound must cross a number of cell membranes. Such a path will deter substances with high molecular weight, those that are ionized at milk pH, which is less than plasma pH of 7.40, and those that possess high water solubility (10).

Most antibiotics taken by nursing mothers can be detected in breast milk. Sulfonamides should not be taken in the early neonatal period, because they compete with bilirubin for binding to plasma albumin and increase the risk of kernicterus (10). Tetracycline concentrations in breast milk are approximately 70% of maternal serum concentrations and present a risk of permanent tooth staining in the infant. Chloramphenicol concentrations in breast milk are not sufficient to cause gray baby syndrome, but there is a remote possibility of causing bone marrow suppression, and chloramphenicol should be avoided during lactation (9).

TABLE 6–4. *Drugs that can be administered during lactation*

Digoxin
Diuretics (most)
Calcium channel blockers
β-Adrenergic blockers
Antibiotics (except metronidazole)
Warfarin
Heparin

TABLE 6–5. *Drugs that have moderate or significant excretion in milk*

	Moderate	Significant
Chloral hydrate		+
Chloramphenicol		+
Diazepam		+
Ethanol	+	
Heroin		+
Lithium		+
Methadone		+
Phenobarbital	+	
Phenytoin	+	
Propylthiouracil		+
Tetracycline	+	
Theophylline	+	

Most sedative-hypnotics achieve concentrations in breast milk sufficient to produce a pharmacologic effect in the infant.

Digoxin is not detected in the plasma of nursing infants whose mothers are receiving digoxin chronically (Table 6–4) (11). Most diuretics, calcium channel blockers, and β-blockers are considered safe. Most antibiotics, one exception being metronidazole, are safe. This includes antiviral and antifungal agents. Maternal warfarin is safe to the nursing infant because it is 99% bound to maternal plasma protein and hence unavailable for transport to milk. Heparin, being a protein, does not cross in any detectable amount. Thyroid preparations are safe. Propylthiouracil is safe; should concern be expressed over the infant's thyroid function, the appropriate thyroid assays should be done on the infant.

For short-term therapy of less than 10 days, all nonsteroidal anti-inflammatory drugs (NSAIDs) are safe except for aspirin in the very young infant of less than 2 months of age.

Short-term narcotic use such as codeine, morphine, and meperidine is not harmful to the baby. Caffeinated beverages are safe. One cup of coffee containing about 100 mg of caffeine will provide an accumulated dosage of 1 mg or less to the nursing infant over the ensuing 24 hours. A nursing mother can probably drink up to 6 cups of coffee per day without effect on the infant. Caffeinated soft drinks have too little caffeine to be detected in the mother's milk; most soft drinks have between 40 and 50 mg caffeine per 12 oz (9).

On the other hand, an infant's plasma level of lithium can be one-third to one-half that of the mother taking therapeutic doses of a lithium salt (Table 6–5). Ethanol is a nonionized, small molecular weight compound with lipid solubility. It is transported quickly to milk.

PHARMACOKINETICS IN THE ELDERLY

General Statement

There has been relatively little research in the area of geriatric clinical pharmacology. Fortunately, the situation is now changing with an increasing number of studies in the elderly involving a combined kinetic and dynamic approach (12). The elderly use more prescription and nonprescription drugs than younger persons and as a consequence of increased drug use and physiologic changes of aging, therapeutics in the elderly are more complex and are more commonly associated with adverse drug effects or iatrogenic problems. Understanding the pharmacologic consequences of the physiologic changes associated with aging is critical to safe and effective therapeutics (13). The recognition and treatment of toxicity is critical, and the clinician who is familiar with these physiologic and pharmacologic differences in the elderly will be prepared to individualize treatment and critically evaluate the response to drugs in this population (14).

Profound physiologic changes occur as the human body ages and predispose the elderly to both adverse drug reactions as well as a heightened sensitivity to drugs. Contrary to the many myths regarding the aging process, physiologic changes with age can occur at dramatically different rates for different individuals. No easy and accurate way of assessing biologic age exists. For this reason, most studies on aging having arbitrarily defined *elderly* as an individual having a chronologic age of 65 years or over. The elderly as a group actually represent a highly diverse group of individuals with changing physiology and, thus, variable kinetics and dynamics in the handling of drugs.

Drug therapy in this age group acquires a greater importance because of several factors. Persons over 65 consume nearly a third of all prescription medications, although they comprise only 12% of the population. Most elderly who are taking medicines frequently are taking more than one and they may often get them from multiple sources (15). The medications are costly and are often changed, and patients may or may not take them as prescribed.

The elderly are especially vulnerable to drug side effects and interactions for both physiologic and epidemiologic reasons. Reduced homeostatic reserve generally renders them less tolerant of drug interactions than younger patients. It is imperative therefore to consider drug "overdose" in this group of patients presenting with an altered mental status and with no history of acute overdose (16).

Factors Affecting the Elderly (Table 6–6)

The elderly exhibit a high incidence of reduced gastric acid secretion, which is associated with a delay in gastric emptying (2). Aging does not affect the absorption of most drugs, but once absorbed into the body, a drug may have very different kinetics in the elderly as compared with the younger adult (17). Although the aging human body becomes increasingly susceptible to illnesses and age-related changes, improved medical care has dramatically extended life expectancy (18).

Drug Absorption

There appears to be no difference in the rate or extent of absorption of most drugs in the elderly. However, propranolol and lidocaine appear to have increased systemic bioavailability after an oral dose in the elderly. This appears to be due to a decreased first-pass effect (19).

Body Mass

There is a loss of skeletal muscle mass with advancing age, combined with an increase in fatty tissue. Thus, the percentage of total body weight that is lean body mass declines as the proportion of total body weight occupied by fat rises. Fat content increases from 15% of body weight to 30% of body weight, tissue decreases from

TABLE 6–6. *Factors affecting the elderly*

Gastrointestinal
Reduced gastric acid secretion
Delayed gastric emptying
Body mass
Loss of skeletal muscle mass
Increased fatty tissue
Result is decreased lean body mass
Volume of distribution
Lipophilic drugs—larger volume of distribution
Longer elimination half-life of benzodiazepines
Polar drugs—lower volume of distribution
Higher initial plasma levels of
ethanol
digoxin
cimetidine
Changes in serum proteins
Reduced serum albumin
Increased amount of free drug
Results in larger volume of distribution
Renal changes
Decreased glomerular filtration rate
Decreased tubular secretion rate
Decreased creatinine clearance
Decreased renal mass and functioning nephrons
Results in reduction in renal elimination of drugs
Hepatic changes
Decreased liver size
Decreased hepatic blood flow
Decreased Phase I metabolism (oxidation, hydroxylation)
Higher serum levels for drugs with significant first-pass effect (Table 5–9)

17% to 12%, and intracellular water decreases from 42% to 33% in the average 25-year-old compared with the average 75-year-old, respectively (19).

Volume of Distribution

Because of the above noted changes in body mass, lipophilic drugs would be expected to have a slightly larger volume of distribution per body weight in the elderly than in younger individuals. The volume of distribution of water-soluble drugs is smaller in the elderly, with increased initial concentrations in the central compartment (higher plasma levels). Consequently, water-soluble drugs or polar drugs such as ethanol, digoxin, and cimetidine have higher initial plasma concentrations because of decreased volumes of distribution, and lipid-soluble drugs such as diazepam have larger volumes of distribution in the elderly with longer elimination half-lives. Conversely, lipid-soluble drugs tend to have a larger distribution in older persons because of their increased body fat (20).

Protein Binding

Because the unbound or free drug is considered to be the amount of drug available to bind to pharmacologic receptors, decreases in protein binding with aging may enhance the pharmacologic or toxicologic actions of the drug observed in the patient for a given total concentration. Albumin concentration has been shown to be significantly reduced in the elderly and may drop as much as 20% with increasing age. In addition, reduced albumin levels in the aged may also occur from poor nutrition and concomitant illness. Therefore, drugs that are highly bound to albumin would be expected to have an increased amount of unbound (free) drug as less drug is bound to albumin. This would result in a larger volume of distribution as more drug is free to distribute to the rest of the body (21). This is usually modest and does not result in drug-binding changes of major clinical importance. However, important aberrations in drug effect can be seen with pathologically low levels of serum albumin, sometimes seen in malnourished or chronically ill elderly patients (22).

There is usually a decrease in serum albumin, which binds many drugs, especially weak acids. There may be a concurrent increase in α-acid glycoprotein, which binds many basic drugs. Thus, the ratio of bound to free drug may be significantly altered.

Renal Changes

The most predictable alteration in pharmacokinetics with advanced age is the reduction in the rate of renal elimination of drugs. This is due to a decline in both the glomerular filtration rate (GFR) and the tubular secretion rate, which accounts for the decreased creatinine clearance that occurs with aging. The decline of renal tubular secretion and absorption is at a rate of approximately 7% per decade. Decreased renal plasma flow as well as structural changes in the kidney, including fewer or more sclerotic glomeruli and thickened vessel walls, impair clearance of drugs dependent on renal excretion. Renal mass is decreased by approximately 30%, and there is a significant loss of functional nephrons. This reduction in renal function appears to reduce both GFR and tubular secretion of substances.

Although the number of functioning nephrons decreases with increasing age, because of the large reserve, this does not in itself pose a major problem. In addition, a decrease in renal blood flow of approximately 50% to 60% by the age of 70 years occurs primarily because of a decrease in or redistribution of cardiac output. Together, these changes lead to a 20% to 50% decrease in GFR. This decrease in glomerular filtration may not be mirrored adequately by the serum creatinine concentration, because creatinine production also decreases with age and can result in a seemingly “normal” serum creatinine concentration. The seemingly normal creatinine and blood urea nitrogen are due to both a decreased lean body mass and a decreased production of creatinine.

Hepatic Changes

For many medications, metabolism in the liver is the main route of drug deactivation. Important changes have been found in the capacity of the liver to metabolize medications in old age. Changes in liver anatomy and function appear to occur late in the aging process. A decrease in liver size may be noted after the age of 70 years, yet the functional reserve capacity of the liver as an excretory organ does not appear to be severely compromised in the elderly. A decrease in hepatic blood flow, thought to be caused by an age-related reduction and/or redistribution of cardiac output, may affect the hepatic elimination of certain drugs (18).

Phase I metabolism appears to be the most impaired with advancing age. Phase I includes processes such as oxidation, hydroxylation, and phosphorylation. By contrast, there appears to be relative sparing of the Phase II metabolic processes, such as conjugation. This distinction is important in choosing among various available medications within a class, because those that require only conjugation will be metabolized and thus cleared more readily than those that require more complex forms of Phase I metabolism by the aging liver (13).

The aging process is also associated with a diminution in liver size and hepatic blood flow. As a result, those medications that have first-pass metabolism as an important component of their clearance will have higher serum levels in older than in younger patients. The bioavailability of drugs is generally unchanged in the elderly except in the case of drugs that are extracted at a high rate by the liver (23).

Clinical laboratory tests for liver function do not appear to change with aging in the absence of concurrent disease states. Despite this fact, there are age-related alterations in hepatic microsomal metabolism.

Miscellaneous Factors

It has been shown that for some receptors, with aging, there is an increased sensitivity to drugs. This increased receptor sensitivity will create an enhanced drug effect in target organs and nontarget organs alike. For example, receptors in the central nervous system (CNS) are more sensitive to a number of agents in the elderly, even drugs whose "target" organs are not in the CNS (24). Thus, increased adverse effects as well as increased efficacy or toxicity in the target organs themselves can be expected in the aged because of these pharmacodynamic changes (11).

Conversely, for some medications there appears to be a decrease in receptor sensitivity with advancing age. These medications include the β-adrenergic agents, both agonist and antagonist. Evidence indicates that higher doses are needed in older patients to produce an acceleration or deceleration of the heart. It is not known why some receptors appear to lose sensitivity with aging while other receptors appear to gain in sensitivity (23).

Physiologic changes, such as reduced peripheral venous tone, altered baroreceptor response, or depletion of cellular receptors or neurotransmitters such as dopamine and acetylcholine, can all alter responses to, for example, antihypertensive and neuroleptic drugs.

In addition to normal physiologic changes, the elderly tend to have more acute and chronic diseases, which can produce further alterations in renal excretion, hepatic metabolism, and protein binding of drugs.

SPECIFIC DRUGS

Sedative-Hypnotics

Lipid-soluble, or nonpolar drugs such as diazepam tend to have a larger distribution in older persons because of older persons' increased body fat (25). When the volume of distribution of drug is increased, the result may be a prolonged action because of a longer elimination half-life. Elderly persons appear to be sensitive to the short-term effects of benzodiazepines on the CNS (24).

The half-lives of many benzodiazepines and barbiturates increase 50–150% between ages 30 and 70. The age-related decline in renal function and the presence of liver disease both contribute to the reduction in elimination of these compounds (26).

Calcium Channel Blockers

As a group, the calcium antagonist drugs in use undergo extensive first-pass hepatic extraction after oral administration and are considered high-clearance drugs. Elderly patients have decreased clearance of these drugs in relationship to younger patients (27). Based on the pharmacokinetic changes of aging, one might predict greater antihypertensive effect in the elderly and, in the case of verapamil and diltiazem, a greater prolongation of atrioventricular conduction.

Opioids

The opioids show variable changes in pharmacokinetics with age. The elderly are often markedly more sensitive to the respiratory effects of these agents because of age-related changes in respiratory function (21).

Major Tranquilizers

When major tranquilizers are administered, the initial doses should be small because the elderly are particularly vulnerable to the side effects of these drugs (15). Antidepressant agents are likely to cause postural hypotension, urinary retention, and sedation. Doses should be reduced or given at bedtime. Nonsteroidal anti-inflammatory drugs have an increased risk of causing hyperkalemia or renal failure and death from gastrointestinal hemorrhage. With diuretic therapy, the elderly are more susceptible to fluid and electrolyte disorders, including volume depletion, hypokalemia, hyponatremia, and hypomagnesemia (22).

In general, the highly anticholinergic, low potency agents are less useful in the elderly than are higher potency agents, such as haloperidol or fluphenazine. Water-soluble, or polar drugs, such as ethanol, cimetidine, and digoxin, will have a reduced volume of distri-

TABLE 6–7. *Drugs that have increased toxicity in elderly*

Antihypertensives
Barbiturates
Benzodiazepines
Calcium channel blockers
Digitalis products
Diuretics
Methyldopa
Nonsteroidal anti-inflammatory agents
Salicylates
Sympathomimetics
Theophylline

TABLE 6–8. *Examples of age-related alterations in drug sensitivity*[a]

Cardiovascular
Propranolol ↓
Verapamil ↑ ↓
Furosemide ↓
Theophylline ↑
Central nervous system
Benzodiazepines ↑
Halothane ↑
Narcotic analgesics ↑
Metoclopramide ↑
Endocrine
Insulin sensitivity ↓
Cortisol suppression ↓
Immune/Antihistamine
Antibody response to vaccination ↓
Hydroxyzine ↑
Respiratory
Theophylline ↓
Anticoagulants
Warfarin ↑

[a]↓ Decreased, ↑ increased, ↑↓ both, depending on organ or function studied.

bution in the elderly, with increased initial concentrations in the central compartment and resultant higher plasma concentrations.

β Blockers

The pharmacokinetics of β-adrenergic blocking agents change in a predictable manner in elderly individuals. Decreased drug clearance associated with increased steady-state plasma drug concentration has been documented for propranolol, metoprolol, atenolol, sotalol, and practolol. The pharmacodynamic effects of agonists and antagonists acting on β_1-adrenergic receptors are blunted in the elderly, with an increased drug concentration required to achieve a similar pharmacodynamic effect when compared with younger individuals. To block β_1-adrenergic responses in the elderly requires increased drug dose and concentration. In contrast, β_2-adrenergic responses may be less affected by the aging process.

Summary

Drugs most commonly implicated in adverse drug reactions in the elderly include digoxin, sympathomimetics, nonsteroidal anti-inflammatory agents, benzodiazepines, calcium channel blockers, diuretics, theophylline, and methyldopa (Table 6–7). Other examples of age-related alterations in drug sensitivity are noted in Table 6–8 (16).

REFERENCES

1. Gibaldi M, Levy G: Pharmacokinetics in clinical practice: concepts. *JAMA* 1976;235:1864–1867.
2. Greenblatt D, Sellers E, Shader R: Drug disposition in old age. *N Engl J Med* 1982;306:1081–1088.
3. Kelso T: Laboratory values in the elderly. Are they different? *Emerg Med Clin North Am* 1990;8:241–254.
4. Ariens E: Drug levels in the target tissue and effect. *Clin Pharmacol Ther* 1974;16:155–175.
5. Halpern J, Davis J: Use of drugs during pregnancy. *J Emerg Nurs* 1983;9:160–168.
6. Pippenger C: Rationale and clinical application of therapeutic drug monitoring. *Pediatr Clin North Am* 1980;27:891–925.
7. Koch-Weser J, Sellers E: Binding of drugs to serum albumin, part I. *N Engl J Med* 1976;294:311–316.
8. Koch-Weser J, Sellers E: Binding of drugs to serum albumin, part 2. *N Engl J Med* 1976;294:526–531.
9. Berlin C: Drugs and chemicals: exposure of the nursing mother. *Pediatr Clin North Am* 1989;36:1089–1097.
10. Reed M, Besunder J: Developmental pharmacology: ontogenic basis of drug disposition. *Pediatr Clin North Am* 1989;36:1053–1074.
11. Abernethy R: Altered pharmacodynamics of cardiovascular drugs and their relation to altered pharmacokinetics in elderly patients. *Clin Geriatr Med* 1990;6:285–292.
12. Montamat S, Cusack B, Vestal R: Management of drug therapy in the elderly. *N Engl J Med* 1989;321:303–309.
13. Wall R: Use of analgesics in the elderly. *Clin Geriatr Med* 1990;6:345–364.
14. Vesell E: Factors causing interindividual variations of drug concentrations in blood. *Clin Pharmacol Ther* 1974;16:135–148.
15. LeSage J: Polypharmacy in geriatric patients. *Nurs Clin North Am* 1991;26:273–289.
16. Feely J, Coakley D: Altered pharmacodynamics in the elderly. *Clin Geriatr Med* 1990;6:269–283.
17. Messerli F, Losem C: Antihypertensive therapy in the elderly. *Clin Geriatr Med* 1990;6:335–344.
18. Rocci M, Vlasses P, Abrams W: Geriatric clinical pharmacology. *Cardiol Clin* 1986;4:213–336.
19. Yuen G: Altered pharmacokinetics in the elderly. *Clin Geriatr Med* 1990;6:257–267.
20. O'Malley K: Geriatric clinical pharmacology. *Clin Geriatr Med* 1990;6:229–234.
21. Hughey J: Pain medication and the elderly. *Top Emerg Med* 1989;11:61–71.
22. Fox F, Auested A: Geriatric emergency clinical pharmacology. *Emerg Clin North Am* 1990;8:221–239.
23. Williams L, Lowenthal D: Drug therapy in the elderly. *South Med J* 1992;85:127–131.
24. Prinz P, Vitiello M, Raskind M, et al: Geriatrics: sleep disorders and aging. *N Engl J Med* 1990;323:520–525.
25. Shorr R, Bauwens S, Landefeld C: Failure to limit quantities of benzodiazepine hypnotic drugs for outpatients: placing the elderly at risk. *Am J Med* 1990;89:725–732.
26. Greenblatt D, Harmatz J, Shapiro L, et al: Sensitivity to triazolam in the elderly. *N Engl J Med* 1991;324:1691–1698.
27. Nolan L, O Malley K: Prescribing for the elderly. Part I: Sensitivity of the elderly to adverse drug reactions. *J Am Geriatr Soc* 1988;245–253.

CHAPTER 7

Drug Interactions

The increase in the potency and number of new drugs has contributed immeasurably to modern drug therapy, but like all progress it has also created new problems. A problem of increasing concern is the greater incidence of adverse effects when two or more drugs are given concurrently. Interactions between drugs are predictable and avoidable, or at least manipulable. Physicians should know about potential drug interactions and take precautions to avoid adverse clinical outcomes whenever they prescribe or administer medications (1) (Table 7–1).

It is clear that either the therapeutic or toxic effects of a drug can be greatly modified by interactions with other drugs, foods, environmental substances (e.g., aromatic hydrocarbons and insecticides), or endogenous substances (e.g., hormones, neurohumeral transmitters, and vitamins). Deaths or serious hypertensive crises have been reported when monoamine oxidase inhibitors (MAOIs) were administered with some prescription drugs such as amphetamines and tricyclic antidepressants, over-the-counter drugs such as phenylpropanolamine in cold preparations, and some foods containing tyramine (2).

There are several mechanisms by which drugs may interact, but most can be categorized as pharmacokinetic (absorption, distribution, metabolism, excretion), pharmacodynamic, or combined toxicity (3). Knowledge of the mechanism by which a given drug interaction occurs is often clinically useful because the mechanism may influence both the time course and the methods of circumventing the interaction (4). Some important drug interactions occur as a result of two or more mechanisms (5).

Drug interactions can lead to any one of three undesirable outcomes (1). One drug can increase the level or effectiveness of another drug, leading to toxicity. For example, a person on theophylline for asthma started on cimetidine for peptic ulcer disease can develop theophylline toxicity, because cimetidine inhibits the first drug's hepatic metabolism (2). One drug can decrease the level or effectiveness of another drug, leading to therapeutic failure. For instance, a person taking quinidine to suppress atrial fibrillation given phenobarbital for new-onset seizures will have increased hepatic metabolism of quinidine; without proper dosage adjustment, the patient may experience uncontrolled atrial fibrillation from inadequate levels of quinidine (3). Drug combinations can produce toxic reactions that do not occur when any one drug is used independently. As an example, serious complications or even death may occur in a patient taking a MAOI for depression who then receives meperidine for pain. The drug interaction can cause excitation, rigidity, hypertensive crisis, or hypotension and coma within minutes of absorption (5).

When drugs with similar pharmacologic effects are administered concurrently, an additive or synergistic response is usually seen. The two drugs may or may not act on the same receptor to produce such effects (5). Conversely, drugs with opposing pharmacologic effects may reduce the response to one or both drugs. Pharmacodynamic drug interactions are relatively common in clinical practice, but adverse effects can be minimized if the interactions are anticipated and appropriate countermeasures are taken (6).

COMBINED TOXICITY

The combined use of two or more drugs, each of which has toxic effects on the same organ, can greatly increase the likelihood of organ damage (7). For example, concurrent administration of two nephrotoxic drugs can produce kidney damage even though the dose of either drug alone may have been insufficient to produce toxicity. Furthermore, some drugs can enhance the organ toxicity of another drug even though the enhancing drug has no intrinsic toxic effect on that organ (8).

Certain Chemical Properties of Drugs

Drug interactions may occur for a number of reasons. Some drugs interact directly because of specific properties. For example, acidic compounds, such as heparin, may be inactivated by basic drugs, such as protamine (9).

TABLE 7–1. *Significant Drug Interactions of Selective Agents*

Drug name	Interacts with	Clinical effect
A		
ACE inhibitors	Furosemide	Inc. antihypertensive action
ACE inhibitors	K-sparing diuretics	Hyperkalemia
ACE inhibitors	NSAIDs	Dec. antihypertensive action
ACE inhibitors	Thiazide diuretics	Inc. antihypertensive action
Acetaminophen	Barbiturates	Dec. acetaminophen effect
Acetaminophen	Ethanol	Inc. acetaminophen toxicity
Acetaminophen	Metoclopramide	Inc. acetaminophen absorption
Acetazolamide	Lithium	Dec. lithium levels
Acetazolamide	Thiazide diuretics	Severe hypokalemia
Adenosine	Carbamazepine	Dec. adenosine effect
Adenosine	Dipyridamole	Inc. adenosine effect
Adenosine	Methylxanthines	Dec. adenosine effect
Adrenergic agents	MAOIs	Adrenergic crisis
Alcohol	Benzodiazepines	Inc. CNS depression
Alcohol	Chloral hydrate	Inc. CNS depression
Alcohol	Chlorpropamide	Antabuse-type reaction
Alcohol	Metronidazole	Antabuse-type reaction
Alcohol	Oral hypoglycemics	Inc. hypoglycemia
Alcohol	Quinacrine	Antabuse-like reaction
Alcohol	Sulfonylureas	Inc. hypoglycemic effect
Allopurinol	Azathioprine	Inc. azathioprine toxicity
Allopurinol	Oral hypoglycemics	Inc. hypoglycemic effect
Allopurinol	Phenytoin	Inc. phenytoin level
Allopurinol	Theophylline	Inc. theophylline effect
Allopurinol	Warfarin	Inc. warfarin effect
α-Adrenergics	β Blockers	Inc. incidence of hypertension
α Blockers	Epinephrine	Hypotension
α Blockers	Nicotinic acid	Hypotension
Aluminum antacids	Ursodiol	Dec. ursodiol absorption
Amantadine	Anticholinergics	Inc. anticholinergic toxicity
Amantadine	MAOIs	Adrenergic crisis
Amiloride	Digoxin	Inc. digoxin levels
Amiloride	Indomethacin	Hyperkalemia
Aminoglycosides	Ethacrynic acid	Inc. ototoxicity
Aminoglycosides	Furosemide	Inc. ototoxicity
Aminoglycosides	Neuromuscular blocker agents	Inc. respiratory depression
Aminophylline	Dobutamine	Physical incompatibility
Aminophylline	Dopamine	Physical incompatibility
Aminophylline	Epinephrine	Physical incompatibility

TABLE 7–1. *Continued*

Drug name	Interacts with	Clinical effect
Aminophylline	Isoproterenol	Physical incompatibility
Amiodarone	Digoxin	Inc. digoxin level
Amiodarone	Phenytoin	Inc. phenytoin levels
Amiodarone	Procainamide	Inc. procainamide effect
Amiodarone	Quinidine	Inc. quinidine effect
Amiodarone	Warfarin	Inc. prothrombin time
Amphotericin B	Digoxin	Inc. digoxin toxicity
Antacids	Digoxin	Dec. digoxin absorption
Antacids	Iron	Dec. iron absorption
Antacids	Isoniazid	Dec. isoniazid absorption
Antacids	Ketoconazole	Dec. ketoconazole absorption
Antacids	Oral tetracyclines	Dec. tetracycline absorption
Antacids	Phenothiazines	Dec. phenothiazine absorption
Antacids	Phenytoin	Dec. phenytoin level
Antacids	Prednisolone	Dec. prednisolone absorption
Antacids	Quinolones	Dec. quinolone absorption
Antacids	Ranitidine	Dec. ranitidine absorption
Antacids	Tetracycline	Dec. tetracycline absorption
Anticholinergics	Amantadine	Inc. anticholinergic toxicity
Anticholinergics	Antispasmodics	Inc. anticholinergic effect
Anticholinergics	Digoxin	Inc. digoxin effect
Anticholinergics	Disopyramide	Inc. anticholinergic effect
Anticholinergics	Metoclopramide	Dec. metoclopramide efficacy
Anticholinergics	TCAs	Inc. anticholinergic effect
Anticoagulants	Ethanol	Inc. hypoprothrombinemic effect
Antidiabetic agents	β Blockers	Altered response to hypoglycemia
Antidiabetic agents	Ethanol	Alcohol-antabuse reaction
Antidiarrheal agents	Digoxin	Dec. digoxin absorption
Antimuscarinics	Levodopa	Dec. levodopa levels
Antiparkinsonian agents	Bromocriptine	Inc. incidence of dyskinesias/ neuropsychiatric effect
Antispasmodics	Anticholinergics	Inc. anticholinergic effect
Antithyroid drugs	Warfarin	Dec. response to anticoagulants
Aspirin	Heparin	Prolonged bleeding time
Astemizole	Clarithromycin	Life-threatening arrhythmias
Astemizole	Erythromycin	Life-threatening arrhythmias

TABLE 7–1. *Continued*

Drug name	Interacts with	Clinical effect
Astemizole	Itraconazole	Life-threatening arrhythmias
Astemizole	Ketoconazole	Life-threatening arrhythmias
Astemizole	Troleandomycin	Life-threatening arrhythmias
Atropine	Sodium bicarbonate	Physical incompatibility
Azathioprine	Allopurinol	Inc. azathioprine toxicity
B		
Barbiturates	Acetaminophen	Dec. acetaminophen effect
Barbiturates	β Blockers	Dec. effect of β blockers
Barbiturates	CCBs	Inc. CCB metabolism
Barbiturates	CNS depressants	Inc. CNS depression
Barbiturates	Corticosteroids	Inc. steroid metabolism
Barbiturates	Digitoxin	Dec. digitoxin effect
Barbiturates	Estrogen	Inc. estrogen metabolism
Barbiturates	Metronidazole	Dec. metronidazole effect
Barbiturates	Oral contraceptives	Inc. barbiturate effect
Barbiturates	Oral hypoglycemics	Dec. hypoglycemic effect
Barbiturates	Phenothiazines	Inc. phenothiazine metabolism
Barbiturates	Quinidine	Dec. quinidine levels
Barbiturates	TCAs	Dec. TCA effect
Barbiturates	Theophylline	Dec. theophylline levels
Barbiturates	Valproic acid	Dec. phenobarbital metabolism
Barbiturates	Vitamin D	Possible vitamin D deficiency
Barbiturates	Warfarin	Dec. warfarin effect
Benzodiazepines	Alcohol	Inc. CNS depression
Benzodiazepines	β Blockers	Inc. CNS depression
Benzodiazepines	Cimetidine	Inc. benzodiazepine effect
Benzodiazepines	Ranitidine	Inc. benzodiazepine effect
Benzodiazepines	Rifampin	Dec. benzodiazepine effect
β Blockers	Alpha adrenergic stimulants	Inc. incidence of hypertension
β Blockers	Antidiabetic agents	Dec. response to hypoglycemia
β Blockers	Barbiturates	Dec. β blocker effect
β Blockers	Benzodiazepines	Inc. CNS depression
β Blockers	CCBs	Inc. bradycardia incidence
β Blockers	Chlorpromazine	Dec. metabolism of propranolol
β Blockers	Cimetidine	Inc. β blocker effect
β Blockers	Clonidine	Paradoxical hypertension

TABLE 7–1. *Continued*

Drug name	Interacts with	Clinical effect
β Blockers	Digoxin	Inc. bradycardia incidence
β Blockers	Diltiazem	Inc. bradycardia incidence
β Blockers	Epinephrine	Inc. pressor response
β Blockers	Methyldopa	Paradoxical hypertension
β Blockers	Metoclopramide	Inc. β blocker absorption
β Blockers	Morphine	Inc. β blocker effect
β Blockers	Oral hypoglycemics	Inc. hypoglycemic effect
β Blockers	Oral hypoglycemics	Dec. hypoglycemic response
β Blockers	Phenytoin	Inc. β blocker metabolism
β Blockers	Ranitidine	Inc. β blocker effect
β Blockers	Rifampin	Inc. β blocker metabolism
β Blockers	Verapamil	Bradyarrhythmias
Bile acid resins	Cephalexin	Dec. cephalexin effect
Bile acid resins	Digoxin	Dec. digoxin levels
Bile acid resins	L-thyroxine	Dec. L-thyroxine effect
Bile acid resins	Methotrexate	Dec. methotrexate effect
Bile acid resins	Naproxen	Dec. naproxen effect
Bile acid resins	Penicillin	Dec. penicillin effect
Bile acid resins	Phenylbutazone	Dec. phenylbutazone effect
Bile acid resins	Picroxicam	Dec. picroxicam effect
Bile acid resins	Propranolol	Dec. propranolol effect
Bile acid resins	Tetracycline	Dec. tetracycline effect
Bile acid resins	Thiazide diuretics	Dec. thiazide effect
Bile acid resins	Vitamins A, D, E, K	Dec. vitamin effect
Bile acid resins	Vitamin B_{12}	Dec. B_{12} effect
Bile acid resins	Warfarin	Dec. warfarin effect
Bromocriptine	Antiparkinsonian agents	Inc. incidence of dyskinesias/ neuropsychiatric effect
Buspirone	Digoxin	Inc. digoxin levels
C		
Calcium	Corticosteroids	Dec. calcium absorption
Calcium	Digoxin	Inc. digoxin toxicity
Calcium	Iron	Dec. iron absorption
Calcium	Phenytoin	Dec. phenytoin absorption
Calcium	Sodium bicarbonate	Physical incompatibility
Calcium	Tetracycline	Dec. tetracycline absorption
Captopril	Potassium chloride	Poss. hyperkalemia
Carbamazepine	Adenosine	Dec. adenosine effect

TABLE 7–1. *Continued*

Drug name	Interacts with	Clinical effect
Carbamazepine	Cimetidine	Inc. carbamazepine effect
Carbamazepine	Diltiazem	Dec. carbamazepine metabolism
Carbamazepine	Erythromycin	Inc. carbamazepine levels
Carbamazepine	Fluoxetine	Dec. carbamazepine metabolism
Carbamazepine	Haloperidol	Inc. haloperidol metabolism
Carbamazepine	Isoniazid	Inc. carbamazepine levels
Carbamazepine	Propoxyphene	Dec. carbamazepine metabolism
Carbamazepine	Ranitidine	Inc. carbamazepine effect
Carbamazepine	TCAs	Inc. TCA metabolism
Carbamazepine	TCAs	Inc. TCA toxicity
Carbamazepine	Theophylline	Dec. carbamazepine effect
Carbamazepine	Verapamil	Dec. carbamazepine metabolism
Carbamazepine	Warfarin	Dec. warfarin effect
Catecholamines	Oral hypoglycemics	Dec. hypoglycemia
CCBs	Barbiturates	Inc. CCB metabolism
CCBs	β Blockers	Inc. bradycardia incidence
CCBs	Cimetidine	Inc. CCB effect
CCBs	Ranitidine	Inc. CCB effect
CCBs	Rifampin	Dec. CCB metabolism
Cephalexin	Bile acid resins	Dec. cephalexin effect
Cephalosporins	Probenecid	Inc. cephalosporin effect
Chloral hydrate	Alcohol	Inc. CNS depression
Chloramphenicol	Oral hypoglycemics	Inc. hypoglycemic effect
Chloramphenicol	Phenytoin	Inc. phenytoin levels
Chloramphenicol	Warfarin	Inc. warfarin effect
Chlorpromazine	β Blockers	Dec. propranolol metabolism
Chlorpromazine	Prazosin	Inc. hypotensive effect
Chlorpropamide	Alcohol	Antabuse-type reaction
Chlorpropamide	Probenecid	Inc. chlorpropamide effect
Cholesterol-lowering drugs	Digoxin	Dec. digoxin absorption
Cholestyramine	Ursodiol	Dec. ursodiol absorption
Chronic alcohol intake	Lovastatin	Inc. hepatotoxicity incidence
Cigarette smoking	Theophylline	Dec. theophylline levels
Cimetidine	Benzodiazepines	Inc. benzodiazepine effect
Cimetidine	β Blockers	Dec. β blocker metabolism
Cimetidine	β Blockers	Inc. β blocker effect
Cimetidine	Carbamazepine	Inc. carbamazepine effect

TABLE 7–1. *Continued*

Drug name	Interacts with	Clinical effect
Cimetidine	CCBs	Inc. CCB effect
Cimetidine	Corticosteroids	Inc. steroid toxicity
Cimetidine	Digitoxin	Inc. digitoxin effect
Cimetidine	Encainide	Inc. encainide effect
Cimetidine	Flecainide	Inc. flecainide effect
Cimetidine	Ketoconazole	Inc. ketoconazole absorption
Cimetidine	Lidocaine	Inc. lidocaine effect
Cimetidine	Metronidazole	Inc. metronidazole effect
Cimetidine	Oral hypoglycemics	Inc. effect of oral hypoglycemics
Cimetidine	Phenytoin	Inc. phenytoin effect
Cimetidine	Procainamide	Inc. procainamide effect
Cimetidine	Quinidine	Inc. quinidine effect
Cimetidine	Salicylates	Inc. salicylates effect
Cimetidine	TCAs	Inc. TCA effect
Cimetidine	Theophylline	Inc. theophylline effect
Cimetidine	Valproic acid	Inc. valproic acid effect
Cimetidine	Warfarin	Dec. anticoagulant metabolism
Ciprofloxacin	Theophylline	Inc. theophylline levels
Ciprofloxacin	Warfarin	Inc. warfarin effect
Clarithromycin	Astemizole	Life-threatening arrhythmias
Clarithromycin	Terfenadine	Life-threatening arrhythmias
Clofibrate	Lovastatin	Severe myositis
Clofibrate	Warfarin	Inc. anticoagulant effect
Clonidine	β Blockers	Paradoxical hypertension
Clonidine	Digoxin	Inc. bradydysrhythmias
Clonidine	TCAs	Dec. clonidine effect
CNS depressants	Barbiturates	Inc. CNS depression
CNS depressants	Ethanol	Inc. CNS depression
CNS depressants	Metoclopramide	Inc. CNS depression
Colchicine	Food	Dec. absorption of vitamin B_{12}
Colestipol	Ursodiol	Dec. ursodiol absorption
Corticosteroids	Barbiturates	Inc. steroid metabolism
Corticosteroids	Calcium	Dec. calcium absorption
Corticosteroids	Cimetidine	Inc. steroid toxicity
Corticosteroids	Erythromycin	Inc. corticosteroid levels
Corticosteroids	NSAIDs	Inc. peptic ulcer disease
Corticosteroids	Oral hypoglycemics	Dec. hypoglycemic effect
Corticosteroids	Phenytoin	Dec. corticosteroids effect
Corticosteroids	Rifampin	Dec. corticosteroids effect

TABLE 7–1. *Continued*

Drug name	Interacts with	Clinical effect
Cyclosporine	Lovastatin	Inc. lovastatin toxicity
D		
Dexamethasone	Phenytoin	Dec. phenytoin levels
Diazepam	Oral contraceptives	Inc. diazepam effect
Digitalis glycosides	Amphotericin B	Inc. digitalis levels
Digitoxin	Barbiturates	Dec. digitoxin levels
Digitoxin	Cimetidine	Inc. digitoxin levels
Digitoxin	Phenylbutazone	Dec. digitoxin levels
Digitoxin	Phenytoin	Dec. digitoxin effect
Digitoxin	Ranitidine	Inc. digitoxin levels
Digitoxin	Rifampin	Dec. digitoxin levels
Digitoxin	Tamoxifen	Inc. digitoxin levels
Digoxin	Amiloride	Inc. digoxin levels
Digoxin	Amiodarone	Inc. digoxin levels
Digoxin	Antacids	Dec. absorption of digoxin
Digoxin	Anticholinergics	Inc. digoxin levels
Digoxin	Antidiarrheal agents	Dec. digoxin absorption
Digoxin	β Blockers	Inc. incidence of bradycardia
Digoxin	Bile acid resins	Dec. digoxin levels
Digoxin	Buspirone	Inc. digoxin levels
Digoxin	Cholesterol-lowering drugs	Dec. digoxin absorption
Digoxin	Clonidine	Inc. bradydysrhythmias
Digoxin	Diltiazem	Inc. digoxin levels
Digoxin	K-depleting diuretics	Inc. digoxin toxicity
Digoxin	Methyldopa	Inc. bradydysrhythmias
Digoxin	Metoclopramide	Dec. digoxin absorption
Digoxin	Quinidine	Inc. digoxin levels
Digoxin	Spironolactone	Inc. digoxin levels
Digoxin	Thiazide diuretics	Inc. digoxin levels
Digoxin	Triamterene	Inc. digoxin levels
Digoxin	Verapamil	Inc. digoxin levels
Diltiazem	β Blockers	Inc. bradycardia incidence
Diltiazem	Carbamazepine	Dec. carbamazepine metabolism
Diltiazem	Digoxin	Inc. digoxin levels
Dipyridamole	Adenosine	Dec. adenosine effect
Disopyramide	Anticholinergics	Inc. anticholinergic effect
Disopyramide	Oral hypoglycemics	Inc. hypoglycemia
Disopyramide	Phenytoin	Dec. disopyramide effect
Disopyramide	Procainamide	Inc. procainamide effect
Disopyramide	Propranolol	Inc. propranolol effect
Disopyramide	Quinidine	Inc. quinidine effect
Disopyramide	Rifampin	Dec. disopyramide effect
Disopyramide	Sulfonylureas	Inc. hypoglycemic effect
Disopyramide	Verapamil	Inc. incidence of congestive heart failure
Disulfiram	Ethanol	Alcohol intolerance

TABLE 7–1. *Continued*

Drug name	Interacts with	Clinical effect
Disulfiram	Phenytoin	Inc. phenytoin level
Disulfiram	Warfarin	Dec. anticoagulant metabolism
Diuretics	Theophylline	Inc. diuretic effect
Dobutamine	Aminophylline	Physical incompatibility
Dobutamine	Phenytoin	Physical incompatibility
Dobutamine	Sodium bicarbonate	Physical incompatibility
Dopamine	Aminophylline	Physical incompatibility
Dopamine	Phenytoin	Physical incompatibility
Dopamine	Sodium bicarbonate	Physical incompatibility
Doxycycline	Phenytoin	Dec. doxycyline effect
E		
Encainide	Cimetidine	Inc. encainide effect
Encainide	Ranitidine	Inc. encainide effect
Enteral nutrition	Phenytoin	Dec. phenytoin level
Epinephrine	α Blockers	Hypotension
Epinephrine	Aminophylline	Physical incompatibility
Epinephrine	β Blockers	Inc. pressor response
Epinephrine	Calcium salts	Physical incompatibility
Epinephrine	Sodium bicarbonate	Physical incompatibility
Epinephrine	TCAs	Inc. pressor response
Erythromycin	Astemizole	Life-threatening arrhythmias
Erythromycin	Theophylline	Inc. theophylline levels
Erythromycin	Carbamazepine	Inc. carbamazepine levels
Erythromycin	Corticosteroids	Inc. corticosteroid levels
Erythromycin	Phenytoin	Inc. phenytoin levels
Erythromycin	Terfenadine	Life-threatening arrhythmias
Erythromycin	Theophylline	Inc. theophylline levels
Erythromycin	Warfarin	Inc. warfarin levels
Estrogen	Barbiturates	Inc. estrogen metabolism
Estrogen	Oral hypoglycemics	Dec. hypoglycemic effect
Estrogens	Ursodiol	Inc. ursodiol absorption
Estrogens	Warfarin	Dec. warfarin action
Ethacrynic acid	Aminoglycosides	Inc. ototoxicity
Ethanol	Acetaminophen	Inc. APAP toxicity
Ethanol	Anticoagulants	Inc. hypoprothrom-binemic effect
Ethanol	Antidiabetic agents	Alcohol-antabuse reaction
Ethanol	CNS depressants	Inc. CNS depression
Ethanol	Disulfiram	Alcohol intolerance
Ethanol	Sedative-hypnotics	Inc. CNS depression
F		
Flecainide	Cimetidine	Inc. flecainide effect
Flecainide	Ranitidine	Inc. flecainide effect
Fluoxetine	Carbamazepine	Dec. carbamezepine metabolism
Fluoxetine	Phenytoin	Inc. phenytoin level
Folic acid	Phenytoin	Dec. phenytoin level
Food	Colchicine	Dec. absorption of vitamin B_{12}
Furosemide	ACE inhibitors	Inc. antihypertensive action

TABLE 7–1. *Continued*

Drug name	Interacts with	Clinical effect
Furosemide	Aminoglycosides	Inc. ototoxic effect
Furosemide	NSAIDs	Dec. diuretic effect
G		
Gemfibrozil	Lovastatin	Inc. lovastatin toxicity
Gemfibrozil	Oral hypoglycemics	Dec. hypoglycemic effect
Glutethimide	Warfarin	Inc. anticoagulant metabolism
Guanethidine	Neuroleptics	Dec. antihypertensive effect
Guanethidine	Oral hypoglycemics	Inc. hypoglycemia
Guanethidine	TCAs	Dec. guanethidine effect
H		
Haloperidol	Carbamazepine	Inc. haloperidol metabolism
Haloperidol	Methyldopa	Confusion
Haloperidol	Phenytoin	Dec. haloperidol effect
Heparin	Aspirin	Prolong bleeding time
Heparin	Platelet inhibitors	Prolong bleeding time
Heparin	Protamine	Dec. heparin effect
High-protein diet	Theophylline	Dec. theophylline levels
Hydralazine	NSAIDs	Dec. antihypertensive effect
I		
Immunosuppressives	Live vaccines	Inc. likelihood infection
Indomethacin	Amiloride	Hyperkalemia
Indomethacin	Lithium	Inc. lithium toxicity
Iron	Antacids	Dec. iron absorption
Iron	Calcium	Dec. iron absorption
Isoniazid	Antacids	Dec. isoniazid absorption
Isoniazid	Carbamazepine	Inc. carbamazepine levels
Isoniazid	Phenytoin	Inc. phenytoin level
Isoniazid	Warfarin	Inc. warfarin effect
Itraconazole	Astemizole	Life-threatening arrhythmias
Itraconazole	Terfenadine	Life-threatening arrhythmias
K		
Ketoconazole	Astemizole	Life-threatening arrhythmias
Ketoconazole	Antacids	Dec. ketoconazole absorption
Ketoconazole	Anticholinergics	Dec. ketoconazole absorption
Ketoconazole	H2 Blockers	Dec. ketoconazole absorption
Ketoconazole	Cimetidine	Inc. ketoconazole absorption
Ketoconazole	Terfenadine	Life-threatening arrhythmias
L		
L-thyroxine	Bile acid resins	Dec. L-thyroxine effect
Levodopa	Antimuscarinics	Dec. levodopa levels
Levodopa	MAOIs	Adrenergic crisis

TABLE 7–1. *Continued*

Drug name	Interacts with	Clinical effect
Levodopa	Metoclopramide	Inc. levodopa absorption
Levodopa	Neuroleptics	Dec. levodopa effect
Levodopa	TCAs	Hypertension
Lidocaine	Cimetidine	Inc. lidocaine effect
Lidocaine	Ranitidine	Inc. lidocaine effect
Lithium	Acetazolamide	Dec. lithium levels
Lithium	Indomethacin	Inc. lithium toxicity
Lithium	Metoclopramide	Inc. lithium absorption
Lithium	NSAIDs	Inc. lithium toxicity
Lithium	TCAs	Inc. mania and tremor
Lithium	Theophylline	Dec. lithium levels
Lithium	Thiazide diuretics	Inc. lithium toxicity
Live vaccines	Immunosuppressives	Inc. likelihood infection
Lovastatin	Chronic alcohol intake	Inc. incidence of hepatotoxicity
Lovastatin	Clofibrate	Severe myositis
Lovastatin	Cyclosporine	Inc. lovastatin toxicity
Lovastatin	Gemfibrozil	Inc. lovastatin toxicity
M		
MAOIs	Adrenergic agents	Adrenergic crisis
MAOIs	Amantadine	Adrenergic crisis
MAOIs	Levodopa	Adrenergic crisis
MAOIs	Meperidine	Excitation, hypertension
MAOIs	Metoclopramide	Adrenergic crisis
MAOIs	Oral hypoglycemics	Inc. hypoglycemic effect
MAOIs	Phenylephrine	Hypertension
MAOIs	Pseudoephedrine	Hypertension
MAOIs	Sympathomimetics	Adrenergic crisis
MAOIs	TCAs	Adrenergic crisis
MAOIs	Tyramine	Adrenergic crisis, hypertension
Meperidine	MAOIs	Excitation, hypertension
Meperidine	Oral contraceptives	Inc. meperidine effect
Meperidine	Phenytoin	Dec. meperidine effect
Methadone	Phenytoin	Dec. methadone levels
Methotrexate	Bile acid resins	Dec. methotrexate effect
Methotrexate	Probenecid	Dec. methotrexate concentration
Methyldopa	β Blockers	Paradoxical hypertension
Methyldopa	Digoxin	Bradycardia
Methyldopa	Haloperidol	Confusion
Methyldopa	Oral contraceptives	Inc. methyldopa effect
Methyldopa	TCAs	Dec. antihypertensive effect
Methylxanthines	Adenosine	Dec. adenosine effect
Metoclopramide	Acetaminophen	Inc. acetaminophen absorption
Metoclopramide	Anticholinergics	Dec. metoclopramide efficacy
Metoclopramide	β Blockers	Inc. β blocker absorption
Metoclopramide	CNS depressants	Inc. CNS depression

TABLE 7–1. *Continued*

Drug name	Interacts with	Clinical effect
Metoclopramide	Digoxin	Dec. digoxin absorption
Metoclopramide	Levodopa	Inc. levodopa absorption
Metoclopramide	Lithium	Inc. lithium absorption
Metoclopramide	MAOIs	Adrenergic crisis
Metoclopramide	Salicylates	Inc. salicylates absorption
Metronidazole	Alcohol	Alcohol-antabuse reaction
Metronidazole	Barbiturates	Dec. metronidazole effect
Metronidazole	Cimetidine	Inc. metronidazole effect
Metronidazole	Ranitidine	Inc. metronidazole effect
Metronidazole	Warfarin	Inc. response to anticoagulant
Mexiletine	Phenytoin	Dec. mexiletine levels
Milk/dairy products	Oral tetracyclines	Dec. concentration of tetracycline
Moricizine	Cimetidine	Inc. moricizine level
Moricizine	Digoxin	Inc. digoxin effect
Moricizine	Propranolol	Inc. propranolol effect
Moricizine	Theophylline	Inc. theophylline effect
N		
Naproxen	Bile acid resins	Dec. naproxen effect
Narcotics	Sedative-hypnotics	Inc. CNS depression
Neuroleptics	Guanethidine	Dec. antihypertensive effect
Neuroleptics	Levodopa	Dec. neuroleptic activity
Neuroleptics	Levodopa	Dec. levodopa effect
Neuromuscular blockers	Aminoglycosides	Inc. resp.depression
Nicotinic acid	α Blockers	Hypotension
Norepinephrine	TCAs	Inc. pressor response
Nortriptyline	Phenytoin	Dec. nortriptyline effect
NSAIDs	ACE inhibitors	Dec. antihypertensive action
NSAIDs	Corticosteroids	Inc. peptic ulcer disease
NSAIDs	Furosemide	Dec. diuretic effect
NSAIDs	Hydralazine	Dec. antihypertensive effect
NSAIDs	Lithium	Inc. lithium toxicity
NSAIDs	Prazosin	Dec. antihypertensive effect
NSAIDs	Triamterene	Inc. renal insufficiency
O		
Oral contraceptives	Barbiturates	Inc. barbiturate effect
Oral contraceptives	Diazepam	Inc. diazepam effect
Oral contraceptives	Meperidine	Inc. meperidine effect
Oral contraceptives	Methyldopa	Inc. methyldopa effect
Oral contraceptives	TCAs	Inc. TCA effect
Oral hypoglycemics	Alcohol	Inc. hypoglycemia

TABLE 7–1. *Continued*

Drug name	Interacts with	Clinical effect
Oral hypoglycemics	Allopurinol	Inc. hypoglycemic effect
Oral hypoglycemics	Barbiturates	Dec. hypoglycemic effect
Oral hypoglycemics	β Blockers	Inc. hypoglycemic effect
Oral hypoglycemics	Catecholamines	Dec. hypoglycemia
Oral hypoglycemics	Chloramphenicol	Inc. hypoglycemic effect
Oral hypoglycemics	Cimetidine	Inc. hypoglycemic effect
Oral hypoglycemics	Corticosteroids	Dec. hypoglycemic effect
Oral hypoglycemics	Disopyramide	Inc. hypoglycemia
Oral hypoglycemics	Estrogen	Dec. hypoglycemic effect
Oral hypoglycemics	Gemfibrozil	Dec. hypoglycemic effect
Oral hypoglycemics	Guanethidine	Inc. hypoglycemia
Oral hypoglycemics	MAOIs	Inc. hypoglycemic effect
Oral hypoglycemics	Phenylbutazone	Inc. hypoglycemic effect
Oral hypoglycemics	Phenytoin	Dec. hypoglycemic effect
Oral hypoglycemics	Probenecid	Inc. hypoglycemic effect
Oral hypoglycemics	Ranitidine	Inc. oral hypoglycemic effect
Oral hypoglycemics	Rifampin	Dec. oral hypoglycemic effect
Oral hypoglycemics	Salicylates	Inc. hypoglycemia
Oral hypoglycemics	Sulfonamides	Inc. hypoglycemic effect
Oral hypoglycemics	Thyroid hormone	Dec. hypoglycemia
Oral hypoglycemics	Thiazide diuretics	Dec. hypoglycemic effect
Oral tetracyclines	Antacids	Dec. conc. tetracycline
Oral tetracyclines	Milk/dairy prod.	Dec. conc. tetracycline
Oxazepam	Phenytoin	Dec. oxazepam effect
P		
Penicillin	Bile acid resins	Dec. penicillin effect
Penicillin	Probenecid	Inc. penicillin effect
Phenothiazines	Antacids	Dec. absorption of phenothiazines
Phenothiazines	Barbiturates	Inc. phenothiazine metabolism
Phenylbutazone	Bile acid resins	Dec. phenylbutazone effect
Phenylbutazone	Digitoxin	Dec. digitoxin levels
Phenylbutazone	Oral hypoglycemics	Inc. hypoglycemic effect
Phenylbutazone	Warfarin	Inc. response to anticoagulant
Phenylephrine	MAOIs	Hypertension
Phenytoin	Allopurinol	Inc. phenytoin levels

TABLE 7–1. *Continued*

Drug name	Interacts with	Clinical effect
Phenytoin	Amiodarone	Inc. phenytoin levels
Phenytoin	Antacids	Dec. phenytoin levels
Phenytoin	β Blockers	Inc. β blocker metabolism
Phenytoin	Calcium	Dec. phenytoin absorption
Phenytoin	Chloramphenicol	Inc. phenytoin levels
Phenytoin	Cimetidine	Inc. phenytoin levels
Phenytoin	Corticosteroids	Dec. effect of steroids
Phenytoin	Dexamethasone	Dec. phenytoin levels
Phenytoin	Digitoxin	Dec. digitoxin levels
Phenytoin	Disopyramide	Dec. disopyramide effect
Phenytoin	Disulfiram	Inc. phenytoin levels
Phenytoin	Doxycycline	Dec. doxycycline effect
Phenytoin	Enteral nutrition	Dec. phenytoin levels
Phenytoin	Erythromycin	Inc. phenytoin levels
Phenytoin	Fluoxetine	Inc. phenytoin levels
Phenytoin	Folic acid	Dec. phenytoin levels
Phenytoin	Haloperidol	Dec. haloperidol effect
Phenytoin	Isoniazid	Inc. phenytoin levels
Phenytoin	Meperidine	Dec. meperidine effect
Phenytoin	Methadone	Dec. methadone levels
Phenytoin	Mexiletine	Dec. mexiletine levels
Phenytoin	Nortriptyline	Dec. nortriptyline effect
Phenytoin	Oral hypoglycemics	Dec. hypoglycemic effect
Phenytoin	Oxazepam	Dec. oxazepam effect
Phenytoin	Quinidine	Dec. quinidine levels
Phenytoin	Ranitidine	Inc. effect of phenytoin
Phenytoin	Rifampin	Dec. phenytoin effect
Phenytoin	Sucralfate	Dec. phenytoin levels
Phenytoin	Theophylline	Dec. theophylline levels
Phenytoin	Theophylline	Dec. phenytoin levels
Phenytoin	Verapamil	Dec. verapamil levels
Phenytoin	Warfarin	Dec. warfarin effect
Picroxicam	Bile acid resins	Dec. picroxicam effect
Platelet inhibitors	Heparin	Prolong bleeding time
K-sparing diuretics	ACE inhibitors	Hyperkalemia
K-depleting diuretics	Digoxin	Inc. digoxin toxicity
K-sparing diuretics	Potassium chloride	Poss. hyperkalemia
Potassium chloride	Captopril	Poss. hyperkalemia
Potassium chloride	Potassium-sparing diuretics	Poss. hyperkalemia
Prazosin	Chlorpromazine	Inc. hypotensive effect
Prazosin	NSAIDs	Dec. antihypertensive effect
Prazosin	Quinidine	Inc. syncope incidence
Prazosin	Thioridazine	Inc. hypotensive effect
Prednisolone	Antacids	Dec. prednisolone absorption
Primaquine	Quinacrine	Inc. primaquine toxicity
Primidone	Warfarin	Inc. anticoagulant metabolism
Probenecid	Cephalosporins	Inc. cephalosporin effect

TABLE 7–1. *Continued*

Drug name	Interacts with	Clinical effect
Probenecid	Chlorpropamide	Inc. chlorpropamide effect
Probenecid	Methotrexate	Dec. methotrexate conc.
Probenecid	Oral hypoglycemics	Inc. hypoglycemic effect
Probenecid	Penicillins	Inc. penicillin effect
Probenecid	Salicylates	Dec. probenecid effect
Probenecid	Thiazide diuretics	Inc. diuretic effect
Procainamide	Amiodarone	Inc. procainamide effect
Procainamide	Cimetidine	Inc. procainamide effect
Procainamide	Disopyramide	Inc. procainamide effect
Procainamide	Ranitidine	Inc. procainamide effect
Propafenone	β Blockers	Inc. β blocker level
Propafenone	Cimetidine	Inc. propafenone level
Propafenone	Digoxin	Inc. digoxin level
Propafenone	Quinidine	Inc. propafenone level
Propafenone	Warfarin	Inc. warfarin effect
Propoxyphene	Carbamazepine	Dec. carbamazepine metabolism
Propranolol	Bile acid resins	Dec. propranolol effect
Propranolol	Disopyramide	Inc. propranolol effect
Propranolol	Theophylline	Inc. theophylline levels
Protamine	Heparin	Dec. heparin effect
Pseudoephedrine	MAOIs	Hypertension
Q		
Quinacrine	Alcohol	Antabuse-like reaction
Quinacrine	Primaquine	Inc. primaquine toxicity
Quinidine	Amiodarone	Inc. quinidine effect
Quinidine	Barbiturates	Dec. quinidine effect
Quinidine	Cimetidine	Inc. quinidine levels
Quinidine	Digoxin	Inc. digoxin level
Quinidine	Disopyramide	Inc. quinidine effect
Quinidine	Phenytoin	Dec. quinidine levels
Quinidine	Prazosin	Inc. syncope incidence
Quinidine	Ranitidine	Inc. quinidine effect
Quinidine	Rifampin	Dec. quinidine levels
Quinidine	TCAs	Inc. cardiotoxicity incidence
Quinidine	Verapamil	Inc. quinidine levels
Quinolones	Antacids	Dec. quinolone absorption
Quinolones	Sucralfate	Dec. quinolone absorption
R		
Ranitidine	Antacids	Dec. ranitidine absorption
Ranitidine	Benzodiazepines	Inc. benzodiazepine effect
Ranitidine	β Blockers	Inc. β blocker effect
Ranitidine	Carbamazepine	Inc. carbamazepine effect
Ranitidine	CCBs	Inc. CCB effect
Ranitidine	Digitoxin	Inc. digitoxin effect
Ranitidine	Encainide	Inc. encainide effect

TABLE 7–1. *Continued*

Drug name	Interacts with	Clinical effect
Ranitidine	Flecainide	Inc. flecainide effect
Ranitidine	Lidocaine	Inc. lidocaine effect
Ranitidine	Metronidazole	Inc. metronidazole effect
Ranitidine	Oral hypoglycemics	Inc. effect of oral hypoglycemics
Ranitidine	Phenytoin	Inc. phenytoin effect
Ranitidine	Procainamide	Inc. procainamide effect
Ranitidine	Quinidine	Inc. quinidine effect
Ranitidine	Salicylates	Inc. salicylates effect
Ranitidine	TCAs	Inc. TCA effect
Ranitidine	Theophylline	Inc. theophylline effect
Ranitidine	Valproic acid	Inc. valproic acid effect
Rifampin	Benzodiazepines	Dec. benzodiazepine effect
Rifampin	β Blockers	Inc. β blocker metabolism
Rifampin	CCBs	Dec. CCB metabolism
Rifampin	Corticosteroids	Dec. corticosteroid effect
Rifampin	Digitoxin	Dec. digitoxin effect
Rifampin	Disopyramide	Dec. disopyramide effect
Rifampin	Oral hypoglycemics	Dec. hypoglycemic effect
Rifampin	Phenytoin	Dec. phenytoin effect
Rifampin	Quinidine	Dec. quinidine levels
Rifampin	Theophylline	Dec. theophylline levels
Rifampin	Verapamil	Dec. verapamil effect
Rifampin	Warfarin	Dec. warfarin effect
S		
Salicylates	Cimetidine	Inc. salicylate effect
Salicylates	Metoclopramide	Inc. salicylate absorption
Salicylates	Oral hypoglycemics	Inc. hypoglycemia
Salicylates	Probenecid	Dec. probenecid effect
Salicylates	Ranitidine	Inc. salicylate effect
Salicylates	Sulfonylureas	Inc. hypoglycemic effect
Salicylates	Warfarin	Increased bleeding risk
Sedative-hypnotics	Ethanol	Inc. CNS depression
Sedative-hypnotics	Narcotics	Inc. CNS depression
Sodium bicarbonate	Atropine	Physical incompatibility
Sodium bicarbonate	Dobutamine	Physical incompatibility
Sodium bicarbonate	Dopamine	Physical incompatibility
Sodium bicarbonate	Isoproterenol	Physical incompatibility
Spirololactone	Digoxin	Inc. digoxin toxicity
Sucralfate	Phenytoin	Dec. phenytoin levels
Sucralfate	Quinolones	Dec. quinolone absorption

TABLE 7–1. *Continued*

Drug name	Interacts with	Clinical effect
Sulfinpyrazone	Warfarin	Inc. response to anticoagulant
Sulfonamides	Oral hypoglycemics	Inc. hypoglycemic effect
Sulfonamides	Warfarin	Inc. response to anticoagulant
Sulfonylureas	Alcohol	Inc. hypoglycemic effect
Sulfonylureas	Disopyramide	Inc. hypoglycemic effect
Sulfonylureas	Salicylates	Inc. hypoglycemic effect
Sympathomimetics	MAOIs	Adrenergic crisis
Sympathomimetics	TCAs	Inc. pressor response
Sympathomimetics	Theophylline	Inc. adrenergic stimulation
T		
Tamoxifen	Digitoxin	Inc. digitoxin levels
Tamoxifen	Warfarin	Inc. bleeding incidence
TCAs	Anticholinergics	Inc. anticholinergic effect
TCAs	Barbiturates	Dec. TCA effect
TCAs	Carbamazepine	Inc. TCA toxicity
TCAs	Cimetidine	Inc. TCA effect
TCAs	Clonidine	Dec. clonidine effect
TCAs	Epinephrine	Inc. pressor response
TCAs	Guanethidine	Dec. guanethidine effect
TCAs	Levodopa	Hypertension
TCAs	Lithium	Inc. mania and tremor
TCAs	MAOIs	Adrenergic crisis
TCAs	Methyldopa	Dec. antihypertensive effect
TCAs	Norepinephrine	Inc. pressor response
TCAs	Oral contraceptives	Inc. TCA effect
TCAs	Quinidine	Inc. cardiotoxicity incidence
TCAs	Ranitidine	Inc. TCA effect
TCAs	Sympathomimetics	Inc. sympathomimetic effects
Terfenadine	Ketoconazole	Life-threatening arrhythmias
Tetracycline	Antacids	Dec. tetracycline absorption
Tetracycline	Bile acid resins	Dec. tetracycline effect
Tetracycline	Calcium	Dec. tetracycline absorption
Theophylline	Allopurinol	Inc. theophylline effect
Theophylline	Barbiturates	Dec. theophylline levels
Theophylline	Carbamazepine	Dec. carbamazepine effect
Theophylline	Cigarette smoke	Dec. theophylline conc.
Theophylline	Cigarette smoking	Dec. theophylline levels
Theophylline	Cimetidine	Inc. theophylline levels
Theophylline	Ciprofloxacin	Inc. theophylline levels

TABLE 7–1. *Continued*

Drug name	Interacts with	Clinical effect
Theophylline	Diuretics	Inc. diuretic effect
Theophylline	Erythromycin	Inc. theophylline levels
Theophylline	High-protein diet	Dec. theophylline levels
Theophylline	Lithium	Dec. lithium levels
Theophylline	Phenytoin	Dec. theophylline levels
Theophylline	Phenytoin	Dec. phenytoin levels
Theophylline	Propranolol	Inc. theophylline levels
Theophylline	Ranitidine	Inc. theophylline effect
Theophylline	Rifampin	Dec. theophylline levels
Theophylline	Smoking	Dec. theophylline levels
Theophylline	Sympathomimetics	Inc. adrenergic stimulation
Theophylline	Troleandomycin	Inc. theophylline levels
Theophylline	Tube feeding	Dec. theophylline absorption
Theophylline	Verapamil	Inc. theophylline levels
Thiazide diuretics	ACE inhibitors	Inc. antihypertensive action
Thiazide diuretics	Acetazolamide	Severe hypokalemia
Thiazide diuretics	Bile acid resins	Dec. thiazide effect
Thiazide diuretics	Digoxin	Inc. digoxin toxicity
Thiazide diuretics	Lithium	Inc. lithium levels
Thiazide diuretics	Oral hypoglycemics	Dec. hypoglycemic effect
Thiazide diuretics	Probenecid	Inc. diuretic effect
Thioridazine	Prazosin	Inc. hypotensive effect
Triamterene	Digoxin	Inc. digoxin levels
Triamterene	NSAIDs	Inc. incidence of renal insufficiency
Thyroid hormone	Oral hypoglycemics	Dec. hypoglycemia
Troleandomycin	Astemizole	Life-threatening arrhythmias
Troleandomycin	Terfenadine	Life-threatening arrhythmias
Troleandomycin	Theophylline	Inc. theophylline levels
Tube feeding	Theophylline	Dec. theophylline absorption
Tyramine in foods	MAOIs	Adrenergic crisis
U		
Ursodiol	Aluminum antacids	Dec. ursodiol absorption
Ursodiol	Cholestyramine	Dec. ursodiol absorption
Ursodiol	Colestipol	Dec. ursodiol absorption
Ursodiol	Estrogens	Inc. ursodiol absorption
V		
Valproic acid	Barbiturates	Dec. phenobarbital metabolism
Valproic acid	Cimetidine	Inc. valproic acid effect
Valproic acid	Ranitidine	Inc. valproic acid effect
Verapamil	β Blockers	Bradyarrhythmias
Verapamil	Carbamazepine	Dec. carbamazepine metabolism
Verapamil	Digoxin	Inc. digoxin levels
Verapamil	Disopyramide	Inc. incidence of congestive heart failure
Verapamil	Phenytoin	Dec. verapamil levels
Verapamil	Quinidine	Inc. quinidine levels
Verapamil	Rifampin	Dec. verapamil effect
Verapamil	Theophylline	Inc. theophylline levels
Vitamins A, D, E, K	Bile acid resins	Dec. vitamin effect
Vitamin B_{12}	Bile acid resins	Dec. B_{12} effect
Vitamin D	Barbiturates	Possible vitamin D deficiency
Vitamin K	Warfarin	Dec. warfarin effect
W		
Warfarin	Allopurinol	Inc. warfarin effect
Warfarin	Amiodarone	Inc. protime
Warfarin	Antithyroid drugs	Dec. response to anticoagulants
Warfarin	Barbiturates	Dec. warfarin effect
Warfarin	Bile acid resins	Dec. warfarin effect
Warfarin	Carbamazepine	Dec. warfarin effect
Warfarin	Chloramphenicol	Inc. warfarin effect
Warfarin	Cimetidine	Dec. anticoagulant metabolism
Warfarin	Ciprofloxacin	Inc. warfarin effect
Warfarin	Clofibrate	Inc. anticoagulant effect
Warfarin	Disulfiram	Dec. anticoagulant metabolism
Warfarin	Erythromycin	Inc. warfarin levels
Warfarin	Estrogens	Dec. warfarin action
Warfarin	Glutethimide	Inc. anticoagulant metabolism
Warfarin	Isoniazid	Inc. warfarin effect
Warfarin	Metronidazole	Inc. anticoagulant effect
Warfarin	Phenylbutazone	Inc. response to anticoagulant
Warfarin	Phenytoin	Dec. warfarin effect
Warfarin	Primidone	Inc. anticoagulant metabolism
Warfarin	Rifampin	Dec. warfarin effect
Warfarin	Salicylates	Increased bleeding risk
Warfarin	Sulfinpyrazone	Inc. response to anticoagulant
Warfarin	Sulfonamides	Inc. response to anticoagulant
Warfarin	Tamoxifen	Inc. bleeding incidence
Warfarin	Vitamin K	Dec. warfarin action

ACE, angiotensin-converting enzyme; CCBs, calcium channel blockers; Dec., decreased; Inc., increased; MAOIs, monoamine oxidase inhibitors; NSAIDs, nonsteroidal anti-inflammatory drugs; TCAs, tricyclic antidepressants.

Changes in Gastrointestinal Absorption

The gastrointestinal (GI) absorption of drugs may be affected by concurrent use of other agents that (a) have a large surface area upon which the drug can be absorbed, (b) bind or chelate, or (c) alter GI motility. One must distinguish between effects on absorption rate and effects on extent of absorption. A reduction in only the absorption rate of a drug is seldom clinically important, whereas a reduction in the extent of absorption will be clinically important if it results in subtherapeutic serum levels of the drug (10).

Interactions between drugs proximal to or at the site of absorption can also occur because of effects on GI flora, intestinal motility, or gastric pH. Antibiotics can kill GI tract bacteria necessary for such processes as vitamin K synthesis; many antibiotics thus potentiate the action of warfarin (11).

Alterations in Protein Binding

The mechanisms by which drug interactions alter drug distribution include competition for plasma protein binding and displacement from tissue binding sites (12). Although competition for plasma protein binding can increase the free concentration (and thus the effect) of the displaced drug in plasma, the increase tends to be temporary owing to a compensatory increase in drug disposition. The clinical importance of protein binding displacement has probably been overemphasized; current evidence suggests that such interactions are unlikely to result in adverse effects. Displacement from tissue binding sites would tend to increase the blood concentration of the displaced drug (13). Such a mechanism is partially responsible for the elevation of serum digoxin concentration by concurrent quinidine therapy (14).

In the serum, acidic drugs generally bind to albumin and basic drugs to α_1-acid glycoprotein. Several drugs can bind to the same protein sites; the outcome of competition between compounds for binding sites depends on the relative drug affinities for these sites, drug concentrations, and the amount of available protein (15). Highly protein-bound drugs can have toxic effects if suddenly displaced from their binding sites by other drugs (4).

Changes in Drug Metabolism

The metabolism of drugs can be stimulated or inhibited by concurrent therapy. For example, starting phenobarbital can significantly decrease the half-life of quinidine. Similarly, rifampin reduces the half-life of conjugated estrogens. Induction (stimulation) of hepatic microsomal drug-metabolizing enzymes can be produced by drugs such as barbiturates, carbamazepine, glutethimide, phenytoin, primidone, and rifampin (16). Enzyme induction does not take place quickly; maximal effects usually occur after 7–10 days, and require an equal or longer time to dissipate after the enzyme inducer is stopped. Inhibition of metabolism generally takes place more quickly than enzyme induction, and may begin as soon as sufficient hepatic concentration of the inhibitor in achieved (17). However, if the half-life of the affected drug is long, it may take a week or more to reach a new steady-state serum level (18). Drugs that may inhibit hepatic microsomal metabolism of other drugs include allopurinol, chloramphenicol, cimetidine, ciprofloxacin, diltiazem, disulfiram, enoxacin, erythromycin, fluconazole, fluoxetine, isoniazid, ketoconazole, metronidazole, phenylbutazone, propoxyphene, quinidine, sulfonamides, and verapamil.

Many drugs can induce the synthesis of metabolic enzymes, particularly enzymes of the hepatic endoplasmic reticulum, and thereby enhance the breakdown of other drugs metabolized by this system (19).

Competition for Receptor Sites

Physicians must understand pharmacologic interactions between agonists and antagonists at specific receptor sites (17). For example, phenothiazines have α-adrenergic antagonist activity, and may block the effects of sympathomimetic amines like ephedrine in treating stress incontinence (20). Many examples of this type of competition are listed in Table 7–1.

Changes in Renal Excretion

The renal excretion of active drug can also be affected by concurrent drug therapy (8). Interactions that affect renal excretion of drugs will be clinically significant only when the drug or its active metabolite is appreciably eliminated by the renal route. The renal excretion of certain drugs that are weak acids or weak bases may be influenced by other drugs that affect urinary pH. This is due to changes in ionization of the drug, thus altering its lipid solubility and therefore its ability to be absorbed back into the blood from the kidney tubule. For some drugs, active secretion into the renal tubules is an important elimination pathway. This process may be affected by concurrent drug therapy, thus altering serum drug levels and pharmacologic response (21).

These changes include alterations in renal clearance, active tubular secretion, and passive tubular reabsorption. Drug clearance depends on serum protein binding and glomerular filtration rate. Drugs bound to protein do not get filtered, so coadministration of agents that displace such drugs from binding sites facilitates excretion by increasing the free fatty fraction (9).

Alterations in pH or Electrolyte Concentrations

Many medications, particularly diuretics, influence the pH and the electrolyte concentrations of body fluids. Furosemide may cause hypokalemia and thereby potentiate digoxin toxicity.

CLINICAL FACTORS

Not all drug interactions are hazardous. In fact, many types of interactions have been used to therapeutic advantage. Enzyme induction by phenobarbital has been used to reduce bilirubin levels in neonatal hyperbilirubinemia or excessive cortisol levels in patients with increased adrenocortical activity. Displacement of penicillin from plasma proteins by salicylates or inhibition of renal secretion by probenecid may increase serum and tissue antibacterial levels. Alteration of urinary pH to increase drug excretion may be useful in the treatment of some drug overdoses.

The potentially deleterious interactions may be classified by the severity and the frequency of occurrence. A few interactions are quite severe, and occur almost always when the two drugs are given concurrently. Interactions between MAOIs and sympathomimetic amines or between warfarin and phenylbutazone are obvious examples of therapeutic incompatibilities. In these cases, the course of action is clear. Interactions between drugs such as phenobarbital and phenytoin that are neither frequent nor severe are also rather simple to handle. The two drugs are usually used with the knowledge that dosage adjustments may be necessary. Unfortunately, many interactions fall in the less predictable class that may be severe but occur only in a few patients depending on the dosage regimen of each drug, the age, physiologic and pathologic conditions of the patient, and a host of other unknown variables.

Duration of therapy also is a critical factor. Enzyme induction requires several days to take effect and may not occur unless a drug is taken chronically. Inhibition of metabolism usually occurs rapidly. An increase in the half-life may not be immediately apparent, however, until a new steady-state plateau is reached, which requires six half-lives. Likewise, an interaction that involves competition for protein binding occurs immediately and is a transient effect, disappearing when the second drug is removed.

There are several general guidelines that indicate the types of patients and drugs most likely to be involved in drug interactions. The age of the patient is one of the most critical factors in determining the potential severity of an interaction (22). Examination of a large number of interactions that were fatal or nearly fatal shows that in the majority of the cases the age of the subject was more than 50 years. Infants, because of decreased metabolic and renal excretory functions, are also particularly susceptible to drug interactions.

TABLE 7–2. *Conditions most commonly involved in drug interactions*

Alcoholism
Diabetes
Extremes of age
Glaucoma
Hypertension
Peptic ulcer disease

TABLE 7–3. *Agents most commonly involved in drug interactions*

Anticoagulants
Anticonvulsants
Corticosteroids
Digitalis preparations
Oral contraceptives
Oral hypoglycemics
Quinidine
Sedative-hypnotics

Several disease states such as glaucoma, hypertension, ulcer, and diabetes predispose a patient to adverse reactions in general (Table 7–2). Patients taking chronic medication including corticosteroids, oral contraceptives, sedatives, and tranquilizers, or alcoholics are more susceptible as are patients taking doses at the upper limit of the dosage range of inherently toxic agents such as methotrexate. Drugs that must be titrated to the individual such as anticoagulants, anticonvulsants, digitalis, hypoglycemics, and quinidine are involved frequently in drug interactions (Table 7–3).

REFERENCES

1. Gibaldi M, Levy G: Pharmacokinetics in clinical practice: concepts. *JAMA* 1976;235:1864–1867.
2. Schwertz D: Basic principles of pharmacologic action. *Nurs Clin North Am* 1991;26:245–262.
3. Platt D: Pharmacokinetics of drug overdose. *Clin Lab Med* 1990; 10:261–269.
4. Feely J, Coakley D: Altered pharmacodynamics in the elderly. *Clin Geriatr Med* 1990;6:269–283.
5. Reed M, Besunder J: Developmental pharmacology: ontogenic basis of drug disposition. *Pediatr Clin North Am* 1989;36:1053–1074.
6. Gibaldi M, Levy G: Pharmacokinetics in clinical practice: applications. *JAMA* 1976;235:1987–1992.
7. Greenblatt D, Koch-Weser J: Clinical pharmacokinetics. *N Engl J Med* 1975;293:702–708.
8. LeSage J: Polypharmacy in geriatric patients. *Nurs Clin North Am* 1991;26:273–289.
9. Ariens E: Drug levels in the target tissue and effect. *Clin Pharmacol Ther* 1974;16:155–175.
10. Pagliaro L, Benet L: Pharmacokinetic data: clinical compilation of terminal half-lives, percent excreted unchanged, and changes of half-life in renal and hepatic dysfunction for studies in humans with references. *J Pharmacokinet Biopharmacol* 1975;3:333–383.

11. O'Malley K: Geriatric clinical pharmacology. *Clin Geriatr Med* 1990;6:229–234.
12. Koch-Weser J, Sellers E: Binding of drugs to serum albumin, part I. *N Engl J Med* 1976;294:311–316.
13. Koch-Weser J, Sellers E: Binding of drugs to serum albumin, part 2. *N Engl J Med* 1976;294:526–531.
14. Kelso T: Laboratory values in the elderly. Are they different? *Emerg Med Clin North Am* 1990;8:241–254.
15. Montamat S, Cusack B, Vestal R: Management of drug therapy in the elderly. *N Engl J Med* 1989;321:303–309.
16. Theodore W: Basic principles of clinical pharmacology. *Neurol Clin* 1990;8:1–13.
17. Vesell E: Factors causing interindividual variations of drug concentrations in blood. *Clin Pharmacol Ther* 1974;16:135–148.
18. Weise K: Receptor physiology: clinical implications. *Crit Care Clin* 1988;4:695–709.
19. Nightingale C, Carver P: Basic principles of pharmacokinetics. *Clin Lab Med* 1987;7:267–278.
20. Messerli F, Losem C: Antihypertensive therapy in the elderly. *Clin Geriatr Med* 1990;6:335–344.
21. Platt D: Pharmacokinetics of drug overdose. *Clin Lab Med* 1990; 10:261–269.
22. Wall R: Use of analgesics in the elderly. *Clin Geriatr Med* 1990; 6:345–364.

PART II

THE AUTONOMIC NERVOUS SYSTEM, NEUROTRANSMITTERS, AND DRUGS

CHAPTER 8

The Autonomic Nervous System

The autonomic nervous system is involved with the functions of almost all organs and tissues of the body (1,2). The toxicologist must therefore have a working knowledge of this system to understand the effects seen with many overdoses. This chapter reviews the autonomic nervous system, and subsequent chapters focus on the drugs that affect it.

The two major systems that integrate and control body functions are the nervous system and the endocrine system. The major difference between these two systems is in the mode of transmission of information (3). In the case of the endocrine system, transmission is largely chemical, via blood-borne hormones. The nervous system, on the other hand, relies primarily on rapid electrical transmission of information over nerve fibers. However, between nerve cells, and between nerve cells and their effector cells, signals are usually carried by chemical rather than electrical impulses (4). This chemical transmission takes place through the release of small amounts of transmitter or neuromediator substances from the nerve terminals into the region of the synapse (5–7).

Anatomically, the nervous system is divided into two major components: the central nervous system (CNS) and the peripheral nervous system (Table 8–1). The CNS, composed of the brain and spinal cord, is responsible for integrative functions related to both conscious and subconscious activities of the body (4). It is also ultimately responsible for the interpretation of, and reaction to, all information that the body receives from the environment (8).

The peripheral nervous system consists of all the nerve fibers that conduct information to (afferent) and from (efferent) the CNS and that lie outside the brain and spinal cord. Peripheral afferent fibers are involved with sensations such as pain, temperature, and touch, whereas peripheral efferent fibers are involved with the control of specific body functions. Efferent fibers are divided into two categories: somatic fibers, which control the function of skeletal muscle, and autonomic fibers, which control the activities of smooth muscles, cardiac muscles, and glands of excretion.

The conscious thoughts and voluntary muscle actions that demand most of a person's daily attention constitute only a small fraction of the body's activity. The maintenance of heart rate, blood pressure, bronchial tone, digestion, excretion, thermoregulation, visual accommodation, and procreation are performed by visceral organs largely or totally independent of voluntary control. Such involuntary processes are controlled in three ways: by an organ (autoregulation), by humoral messengers (endocrine regulation), and by neural communication. The nerve elements that regulate these visceral processes comprise the autonomic nervous system. The past decade has seen an explosion in our knowledge of autonomic pharmacology.

THE AUTONOMIC NERVOUS SYSTEM

The autonomic nervous system is also called the visceral, vegetative, or involuntary nervous system. It provides the innervation to the heart, blood vessels, glands, visceral organs, and smooth muscles of the body. The nerves of this system are widely distributed throughout the body, and regulate functions that are not under conscious control (9).

The autonomic nervous system is divided into two major branches—the sympathetic (adrenergic), and parasympathetic (cholinergic) branches (10) on the basis of anatomy, neurotransmitters, receptors, and physiologic effects (Table 8–2). A characteristic feature of the sympathetic and parasympathetic modulation is the reciprocal activities of the two nervous systems. Both systems consist of a preganglionic fiber, a ganglion, a postganglionic fiber, and a neuroeffector organ (4).

A distinctive feature of the motor innervation of the viscera is the break by a peripheral synapse in the path from the central axis to peripheral effectors. Making synaptic connections with axons originating in cells whose cell bodies are located in the CNS, the neurons that innervate these effectors lie entirely outside the CNS, grouped together in peripheral ganglia. There is always a ganglion interposed in the motor pathway. In the parasympathetic pathway, the ganglion is located within the target organ itself, and in the sympathetic pathway in a chain of separate ganglia outside the target organ (Fig. 8–1) (4,11).

TABLE 8–1. *The nervous system*

Central nervous system—integrative functions related to conscious and subconscious activity of the body
- Consists of
  - Brain
  - Spinal cord

Peripheral nervous system—conducts information to and from the CNS
- Peripheral afferent—pain, temperature, touch
- Peripheral efferent—specific body functions divided into:
  - Somatic fibers
    - Skeletal muscle
  - Autonomic fibers
    - Smooth muscle
    - Cardiac muscle
    - Glands of excretion

TABLE 8–2. *Division of the autonomic nervous system*

Sympathetic (Adrenergic)
- Secretes (mostly) norepinephrine
- Location
  - Most postganglionic sympathetic neurons
  - Exception: Sweat glands and certain blood vessels

Parasympathetic (Cholinergic)
- Secretes (mostly) acetylcholine
- Location
  - All preganglionic neurons
  - Postganglionic neurons of parasympathetic system

The peripheral sympathetic and parasympathetic nerve endings secrete two synaptic transmitter substances, norepinephrine and acetylcholine, respectively. In general, those fibers that secrete norepinephrine are adrenergic, and those that secrete acetylcholine are cholinergic. Epinephrine is a circulating hormone; that is, it is not released from postganglionic fibers but from the adrenal medulla (1,12,13). All preganglionic neurons are cholinergic in both the sympathetic and parasympathetic nervous system. Therefore, acetylcholine excites both sympathetic and parasympathetic preganglionic neurons. The postganglionic neurons of the parasympathetic system are also cholinergic. Most postganglionic sympathetic neurons are adrenergic except for sympathetic fibers to sweat glands and a few blood vessels (Table 8–3).

It is important to remember that the terms *sympathetic* and *parasympathetic* are anatomic ones and do not necessarily depend on the type of transmitter chemical released from the nerve endings nor on the kind of effect evoked by nerve activity. The traditional concept of a single neurotransmitter in each neuron has been abandoned in light of more recent evidence demonstrating the presence and release in individual neurons of a variety of substances capable of affecting or modifying neurotransmission (3).

The endogenous substances currently categorized as neurotransmitters are acetylcholine, dopamine, serotonin, norepinephrine, γ-aminobutyric acid (GABA), glycine, and glutamic acid (Table 8–4). Among the newer proposed transmitters are the cyclic nucleotides, such as cyclic AMP and cyclic guanosine monophosphate (GMP), which are considered secondary messengers because they appear to "translate" the presence of hormones into specific cellular effects, prostaglandins, histamine, and substance P. It is certain that other endogenous substances will be included within this category as research continues.

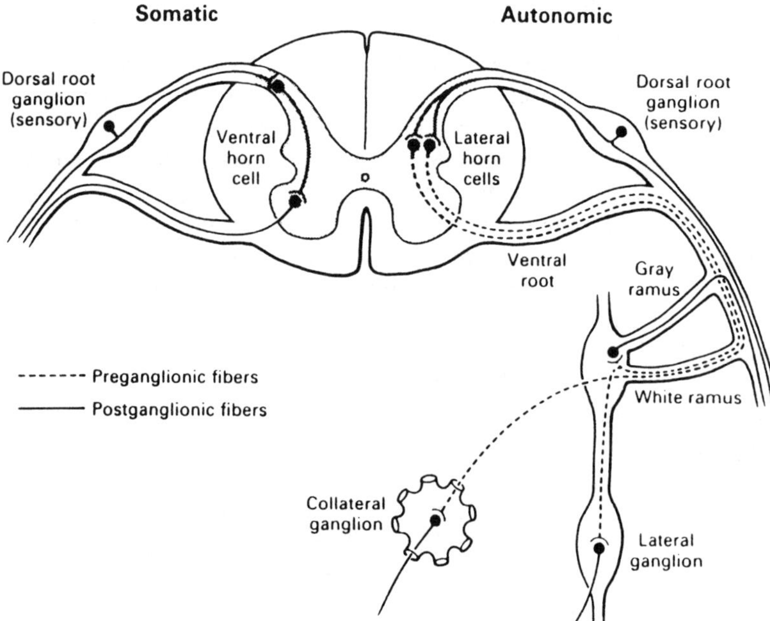

FIG 8–1. The spinal reflex arc of the somatic nerves (*left*) and the different arrangements of neurons in the sympathetic system (*right*). Preganglionic fibers coming out through white rami may make synaptic connections following one of three courses: (a) synapse in ganglia at the level of exit; (b) course up or down the sympathetic chain to synapse at another level; or (c) exit the chain without synapsing to an outlying collateral ganglion. Reproduced with permission from Barash PG, Cullen BF, Stoelting RK, eds. *Clinical anesthesia.* Philadelphia: Lippincott; 1989.

TABLE 8–3. *Division and actions of the autonomic nervous system*

Organ or tissue	Parasympathetic	Sympathetic
Eye	Constriction	Dilation
Blood vessels	Dilation	Constriction
Heart rate	Decrease	Increase
Intestine motility	Increase	Decrease
Salivation	Thin	Thick
Skin (pilomotor)	No effect	Contraction
Stomach acid secretion	Stimulation	Inhibition
Stomach motility	Increase	Decrease
Urinary bladder	Relaxation	Constriction

THE ROLE OF RECEPTORS

Virtually all hormones, drugs, and neurotransmitters released from postganglionic fibers initiate their biologic actions by binding to specific cellular recognition sites that are termed *receptors* (1,2,10,14,15). A receptor is a distinct molecule, usually a large protein or glycoprotein on the membrane of the receiving neuron synapse, into which the neurotransmitter chemical molecule fits (5–7).

Receptors for both endogenous humoral substances and exogenous drugs can be categorized into general classes based on the molecular mechanisms by which the receptors transduce signals (16). At least four distinct classes of receptors are identified on this basis: (a) ion channel receptors, (b) G proteins, or receptors linked to effector enzymes via guanine nucleotide binding proteins, (c) receptors with intrinsic tyrosine protein kinase activity, and (d) receptors for steroid hormones (1,2) (Table 8–5).

The activities of the first three types of receptors transduce information delivered extracellularly at the plasma membrane into ionic or biochemical signals within the cell, whereas the last receptor type is associated with the nuclear matrix, and is activated by steroid hormones that permeate cells (17). Although– receptors are generally associated with plasma membranes, they may be located at intracellular sites such as the endoplasmic reticulum, or even in the cytoplasm (e.g., steroid receptors) (1,2,18). The binding of the receptor is then followed by alterations of cellular metabolic events, such as enzyme activities or ion fluxes, that are ultimately expressed as characteristic physiologic or pharmacologic effects (19).

TABLE 8–4. *Neurotransmitters*

Primary messengers
- Acetylcholine
- Dopamine
- Norepinephrine
- γ-aminobutyric acid (GABA)
- Glycine
- Glutamic acid
- Histamine
- Serotonin
- Substance P

Secondary messengers
- Cyclic AMP
- Cyclic GMP

TABLE 8–5. *Types of receptors*

Ion-channel receptors
Receptors–G protein–effector
Tyrosine protein kinase receptors
Steroid hormone receptors

ION CHANNEL RECEPTORS (RECEPTOR–OPERATED CHANNELS)

Included in this superfamily of receptors and considered here are (a) the nicotinic acetylcholine receptor, (b) the GABA receptor, (c) the glycine receptor, and (d) glutamate receptors (Table 8–6) (17). By and large, these signaling systems are confined to excitable tissue of the CNS, the autonomic ganglia, and the neuromuscular junction (20).

Excitable cells are characterized by the presence of voltage-dependent sodium channels in their plasma membranes. Sodium ions are extremely hydrated and pass through the ion channels of the resting membrane much less easily than potassium ions. However, when the electrical potential across the membrane near a voltage-dependent sodium channel increases to a threshold value,

TABLE 8–6. *Ion-channel receptors involved in rapid propagation of electric impulses and the transfer of information across synapses throughout the nervous system*

Types of receptors
- Nicotinic acetylcholine receptor
  - All ganglia
  - Neuromuscular junction
  - Central nervous system
- GABA receptor
  - Major inhibitory neurotransmitter in CNS
  - Action occurs by activation of chloride channel
  - Benzodiazepines bind to receptor
- Glycine receptor
  - Major inhibitory neurotransmitter in brain stem and spinal cord
  - Action occurs by activation of chloride channel
  - Strychnine acts as competitive antagonist to glycine
- Glutamate receptor
- Also called excitatory amino acid receptors
- Modulates postsynaptic neuronal activity

Location of ion-channel receptors
- Excitable tissue of CNS
- Autonomic ganglia
- Neuromuscular junction

approximately −45 mV, the channel opens and sodium ions are free to cross. The channels spontaneously close after a short time, approximately 1 msec. For this reason they are often referred to as fast sodium channels (4).

Nicotinic Autylcholine Receptor

The best studied of the ion channel receptors is the nicotinic acetylcholine receptor (8). This receptor mediates the action of acetylcholine at excitable synapses in all ganglia, both sympathetic and parasympathetic, at neuromuscular junctions, and at sites in the CNS. Activation of this receptor depolarizes excitable membranes by increasing the permeability of the ion channel to sodium primarily but also to potassium.

For every ion there is a membrane potential at which the electrical force balances the chemical force. This potential is called "the equilibrium potential" for that ion. When an increase in membrane conductance for a particular ion occurs, the ion moves across the membrane and tends to displace the membrane potential in the direction of its equilibrium potential. For example, the equilibrium potential for K^+ is −90 mV. At rest, the cell membrane is highly permeable to K^+ ions. As a result, K^+ moves across the membrane, bringing the membrane potential toward the potassium equilibrium potential (21).

Some synapses, however, may operate by an opposite mechanism: a decrease in conductance. Synaptic depolarization (excitation) can be produced by decreasing a conductance, that is, closing K^+ channels that are open at rest. The decreased conductance raises the resistance of the membrane, thereby increasing the membrane time constant and slowing the potential response. The synaptic potential associated with this type of action tends to have a slow time course. In contrast, hyperpolarization may be produced by turning off an Na conductance (equilibrium potential +65 mV) (22).

The ganglionic and neuromuscular nicotinic receptors differ in their pharmacology. For example, nondepolarizing neuromuscular blocking drugs have variable effects in producing ganglionic blockade (21). Tubocurarine will block at both sites but acts predominantly as a true acetylcholine antagonist at the muscle nicotinic receptor and largely by noncompetitive channel blockade in the ganglia (23).

GABA Receptor

GABA is the major inhibitory neurotransmitter in the brain. GABA-mediated neuronal hyperpolarization results from increased membrane chloride conductance and is attributed to the activation of an integral chloride channel (24).

Benzodiazepines bind with high affinity to the receptor and increase GABA-stimulated ion current by increasing the frequency of channel opening (25). Barbiturates bind to a different site on the receptor and increase the mean open time of the chloride channel.

Glycine Receptor

Glycine is the principal inhibitory neurotransmitter in the spinal cord and brain stem. Like GABA, glycine inhibits neuronal firing by activating a chloride ion conductance that effectively hyperpolarizes excitable membranes (26).

Strychnine acts as a competitive antagonist of glycine binding and inhibits glycine-mediated but not GABA-mediated chloride conductances.

Glutamate Receptors

The glutamate receptors are also called the excitatory amino acid receptors and are responsible for most fast excitatory postsynaptic potentials in the brain and spinal cord. Although they are not directly involved in fast synaptic transmission, they modulate postsynaptic neuronal activity (27). Little is known about the molecular structure of the glutamate receptors.

G PROTEINS

Signal transduction by G proteins is a fundamental and widespread mechanism used by a wide variety of hormones, neurotransmitters, and autocrine and paracrine factors to regulate cellular function (28). G proteins modulate not only cAMP formation, but also intracellular Ca^{2+} mobilization, arachidonic acid release, and, very importantly, membrane potential (23). The G proteins are on the cytoplasmic face of the plasma membrane, thus facilitating interaction with both membrane-bound proteins and soluble components, such as guanine nucleotides (Table 8–7) (24).

G proteins consist of an α, a β, and a γ subunit. Although the structure of the β and γ subunits is very similar, the α subunit is species specific (24). Activation of the G protein is catalyzed by a conformational change in receptor structure caused by binding of an agonist, and involves the release of guanosine diphosphate (GDP) and the subsequent binding of guanosine triphosphate (GTP). Included in these receptors are the adrenergic, muscarinic acetylcholine, serotonergic, and dopaminergic receptors as well as a multitude of peptide receptors. About 80% of all known hormones and neurotransmitters elicit cellular responses by combining to specific receptors that are coupled to effector functions by G proteins (23).

There are at least five types of adrenergic receptors, known as β_1, β_2, α_1, α_{2a}, and α_{2b}. There are also at least five types of muscarinic acetylcholine receptors (M_1

TABLE 8–7. *Receptor–G protein–effector system*

Located on cytoplasmic face of plasma membrane 80% of known hormones and neurotransmitters use G proteins
Receptors influenced;
α-Adrenergic
α_1
α_{2a}
α_{2b}
β-Adrenergic
β_1
β_2
Dopaminergic
D_1 and D_2
Muscarinic acetylcholine
M_1–M_5
Serotonergic
Substance K
Angiotensin
Rhodopsin
Color opsins
G21 protein
Effector systems
Adenylate cyclase (cyclic AMP)
Phosphodiesterase
Phospholipase
K channel
Calcium channel

through M_5), two types of dopamine receptors (D_1 and D_2), and several types of histamine, and serotonin receptors (23).

All of the adrenergic receptors are coupled in cell membranes to guanine nucleoside binding proteins (G proteins) that serve as "transmembrane transducers," transforming the extracellular signal of catecholamine binding to an intracellular signal (8). G proteins can either directly alter the activity of transmembrane ion channels or can stimulate the synthesis of intracellular chemical second messenger molecules (28). Initially, G proteins were thought to couple autonomic receptors with their enzyme effector mechanisms. It is now clear that the activated G protein can directly interact with ion channels to mediate autonomic responses without involving cytoplasmic second messengers (29).

G proteins transduce extracellular stimulation into intracellular biochemical activity in a variety of systems. Signal transduction at muscarinic receptors involves at least three steps: agonist recognition, receptor activation of coupled G proteins, and G-protein stimulation or inhibition of intracellular effector mechanisms (24).

Second Messenger and the Role of Cyclic Adenosine Monophosphate

A key compound that is involved in the mediation of sympathetic effects is cyclic adenosine monophosphate (cAMP) (30–33). Cyclic AMP was identified as a chemical second messenger in 1959. It is the most thoroughly studied effector protein (4,34).

The sympathetics enhance the accumulation of cAMP by activating adenyl cyclase, an enzyme located on the internal surface of the plasma membrane (8). Adenyl cyclase converts adenosine triphosphate into cAMP. Cyclic AMP appears to activate a class of enzymes known as protein kinases, which phosphorylate a wide variety of important substrates (1,2). This action in turn creates an open pore through which sodium and potassium ions may flow to cause depolarization. Cyclic AMP is involved with β-adrenergic receptors, serotonin receptors, histamine receptors, and dopamine receptors.

TYROSINE KINASE RECEPTORS

Tyrosine kinase receptors are critical proteins in the control of cell growth and differentiation, but play a minor role in the area of toxicology (Table 8–8). They will not be further discussed in this text.

STEROID HORMONE RECEPTORS

Steroid hormone receptors are important in the regulation of diverse developmental and homeostatic processes. The mechanism of action of steroid hormones is attributable to their penetration into cells and their high affinity binding to intracellular receptors. The binding induces a structural change in the receptor, which facilitates its association with specific chromatin regions in the nucleus (20).

NEUROTRANSMISSION: GENERAL CONSIDERATIONS

Normal neuromuscular transmission begins with a nerve impulse that is conducted along the prejunctional neuron and reaches the motor nerve terminal. The site where two nerve endings meet or where a nerve meets the tissue that it innervates is a small gap that is termed the *synapse,* or *synaptic cleft* (35). This cleft separates the presynaptic membrane (the axon and axon terminal) from the postsynaptic membrane of the dendrite. The presynaptic terminal consists of mitochondria and numerous

TABLE 8–8. *Tyrosine kinase receptors*

Critical proteins in the control of cell growth and differentiation
Epidermal growth factor
Insulin
Macrophage colony stimulating factor
Platelet-derived growth factor
Insulin-like growth factor

synaptic vesicles. Transmitter chemical is stored in these vesicles before it is released and is capable of altering the permeability of the dendritic membrane of the next neuron, resulting in either a depolarization or hyperpolarization of the dendrites of that neuron. In the presynaptic membrane, regular rows of particles, believed to be calcium channels, line up along either side of the active zones; in the postsynaptic membrane, particles representing nicotinic acetylcholine receptors are concentrated near the edges of the postjunctional folds.

The impulse that reaches the prejunctional neuron then depolarizes the membrane, and calcium ions enter the prejunctional axoplasm and facilitate release of the excitatory or inhibitory chemical transmitter from storage vesicles into the junctional space. The neurotransmitter then diffuses across the junctional space and combines with receptors at the prejunctional membrane surface, resulting in permeability changes to small ions such as sodium and potassium. Depolarization (excitation) or hyperpolarization (inhibition) of the membrane then occurs and is followed by the effector response.

Sympathetic and Parasympathetic Nervous System

Many organs receive both sympathetic and parasympathetic fibers and are influenced in opposite ways by the two divisions of the autonomic nervous system (ANS) (36). In controlling bodily function under normal physiologic conditions, such as rest and/or restoration, the parasympathetic nervous system usually predominates; the sympathetic nervous system generally directs the response of the organism to various environmental stresses.

The parasympathetic division of the ANS, with its preganglionic cell bodies in the brain stem and the sacral cord, is also called the craniosacral division. The cells of the postganglionic fibers are near, on, or within the innervated organ. The sympathetic division of the ANS, with its preganglionic cell bodies in the thoracic and upper lumbar spinal cord, is also called the thoracolumbar division (37,38).

The activity of most organ systems reflects a balance of modulating influences between the sympathetic and parasympathetic nervous systems. Blockade of the sympathetic nervous system by drugs can be expected to result in an exaggeration of parasympathetic activity. Conversely, blockade of parasympathetic activity results in the exaggeration of sympathetic activity. When both pathways are blocked, the effect on the organ system depends on its inherent activity and on the pathway that normally dominates the organ system.

Parasympathetic (Cholinergic) Receptors

The terminals of cholinergic neurons contain large numbers of small membrane-bound vesicles concentrated near the synaptic portion of the cell membrane. These clear vesicles contain acetylcholine in high concentration and certain other molecules that may act as cotransmitters. Most of the acetylcholine is synthesized in the cytoplasm from choline and acetylcoenzyme A (acetyl-CoA) through the catalytic action of the enzyme choline acetyltransferase. Acetyl-CoA is synthesized in mitochondria, which are present in large numbers in the nerve ending. Choline is transported by a membrane carrier mechanism from the extracellular fluid into the neuron terminal. Vesicular storage of acetylcholine is accomplished by the packing of "quanta" of acetylcholine molecules in membranes cycled in from the neuronal surface. Release of a neurotransmitter occurs when an action potential reaches the terminal and triggers sufficient influx of calcium ions. It is believed that the increased Ca^{2+} concentration destabilizes the storage vesicles. Fusion of the vesicular membranes with the terminal membrane occurs, with exocytotic expulsion of several hundred quanta of acetylcholine molecules and cotransmitters into the synaptic cleft (10).

Inactivation of Acetylcholine

Acetylcholine is subjected to a number of inactivation processes following its release from the nerve endings. These include diffusion from the site of release, dilution in extracellular fluids, binding to nonspecific sites, and enzymatic destruction. For most cholinergic junctions, the most important inactivation process is the enzymatic hydrolysis of acetylcholine to acetate and choline (36). This reaction is catalyzed by the enzyme acetylcholinesterase, which is present in the terminal nerve ending itself and on the surface of the receptor organ. The choline that is formed is in turn transported back into the terminal nerve ending, where it is used again for synthesis of new acetylcholine. Pseudocholinesterase, a nonspecific enzyme, also hydrolyzes acetylcholine should any of it be transported into the plasma.

Types of Cholinesterases

Acetylcholinesterase is one of a family of enzymes that catalyze the hydrolysis of ester linkages. It differs from other members of the family in being almost completely specific for acetylcholine, which it hydrolyzes with great efficiency. For this reason, it is also termed "true," or specific cholinesterase (Table 8-9). Apart from neural structures, it also occurs in red blood cells, in the placenta, and in the motor endplate of skeletal muscle. Another member of this family of enzymes is butyrylcholinesterase, also called nonspecific cholinesterase or pseudocholinesterase, which is not specific for acetylcholine but hydrolyzes a great variety of esters in addition to acetylcholine. This enzyme is found in the plasma, in the liver, and in glial and other cells associated with nerve tissues (36).

TABLE 8–9. *Types of cholinesterase*

Acetylcholinesterase ("true" cholinesterase)—specific
- Located in
  - Neural structures
  - Red blood cells
  - Placenta
  - Motor end plate of skeletal muscle

Butyrylcholinesterase (pseudocholinesterase)—
- Nonspecific
  - Located in
    - Plasma
    - Liver
    - Glial cells

Location of Cholinergic Receptors

Cholinergic neurons are found in synapses in all autonomic ganglia, postganglionic parasympathetic fibers, a few sympathetic neuroeffectors (sweat glands), the neuromuscular junction or motor endplate of skeletal muscle innervated by the somatic or voluntary nervous system, and the adrenal medulla (Table 8–10). The CNS has a very extensive system of cholinergic neurons, whose axons are distributed widely throughout the brain and spinal cord. These pathways are important in the processes of memory and learning, in the control of extrapyramidal and vestibular function, and in analgesia (26).

Muscarinic and Nicotinic Receptors (Table 8–11)

Cholinergic neurons affect tissues by releasing the neurotransmitter acetylcholine, which stimulates acetylcholine receptors on the cell surface (39). These receptors are classified as nicotinic or muscarinic receptors on the basis of their response to the alkaloids nicotine and muscarine, respectively. The nicotinic receptors are widely distributed in tissues, and mediate the actions of acetylcholine at the neuromuscular junction of skeletal muscles, autonomic ganglia, and the CNS (26). Muscarine mimics the acetylcholine effects at the end organ of visceral smooth muscle of the gastrointestinal tract, urinary tract, uterus, bronchi, heart, vascular tissue, some secretory glands, and the CNS (37).

TABLE 8–10. *Cholinergic neurons*

All autonomic ganglia
Postganglionic parasympathetic fibers
Few sympathetic fibers—sweat glands
Neuromuscular junction of skeletal muscle
Adrenal medulla

TABLE 8–11. *Types of cholinergic receptors*

Muscarinic	Nicotinic
Postganglionic	Preganglionic
Visceral smooth muscle	Autonomic NS
Gastrointestinal tract	Voluntary NS
Urinary tract	Postganglionic
Uterus	Voluntary NS
Bronchi	Central NS
Heart	Adrenal medulla
Vascular tissue	

Muscarinic Receptors

Muscarinic receptors are key participants in many physiologic processes, such as nerve-to-nerve transmission, smooth muscle contraction, and exocrine and endocrine secretion. Muscarinic agonists and antagonists, popularly known as cholinergic and anticholinergic agents, have been used therapeutically for many years (26). Their usefulness has been limited by their low specificity, however, since muscarinic receptors are found in many tissues, and a therapeutic effect in one tissue is often accompanied by unwanted side effects in others (37,40).

All intracellular responses due to the stimulation of muscarinic receptors are thought to be mediated by G proteins, which bind guanine nucleotides and are part of the mechanism that transduces signals across the cell membrane (24).

Most smooth muscles contain muscarinic receptors that mediate muscle contraction (26). Muscarinic receptors may also antagonize the relaxing effects of a β-adrenergic receptor stimulation that occurs through increases in levels of intracellular cAMP and the opening of potassium channels (39,41).

Muscarinic Receptor Subtypes

Until recently, all muscarinic receptors were thought to be alike. However, at least three different pharmacologically identifiable types and at least five different molecular forms have now been identified (36). Tissues vary in their expression of muscarinic receptor subtypes with marked differences, for instance, between the heart and the gastrointestinal tract (GIT) (26). The recognition of muscarinic receptor subtypes is more than a pharmacologic curiosity, because it is now clear that these receptor subtypes may have different physiologic roles, may be coupled to different transduction mechanisms, and may be differentially regulated (17). Only recently, however, have muscarinic receptors been subdivided, and this has been made possible by the development of selective drugs (11). Accordingly, cholinergic antagonists selective for the GIT might relieve peptic symptoms without eliciting tachycardia at receptors in the heart (21).

Pirenzepine was the first selective muscarinic antagonist recognized, and pirenzepine-sensitive muscarinic receptors are therefore termed *M_1 receptors* (Table 8-12) (4). These receptors are generally found in the cerebral cortex and autonomic ganglia (42). Pirenzepine is used clinically to reduce gastric acid secretion, and although it was previously believed to act directly on acid-secreting cells, it is now apparent that it acts predominantly on ganglia in the stomach to inhibit neurally mediated gastric secretion (21).

Cardiac sinoventricular and atrioventricular nodes and cardiac muscle have M_2 receptors. Their stimulation decreases the cardiac rate by inhibiting the hyperpolarization-activated current that is involved in the generation of pacemaker activity (26).

Nicotinic Receptors

Nicotinic receptors are ion-channel receptors. As an example of receptor function, at the cellular level the nicotinic cholinergic receptor forms a chemically regulated channel for sodium ions. The subunits of this receptor-channel complex carry a recognition and binding site for acetylcholine, and on binding with acetylcholine the subunits change their configuration (27). This transducer function results in the opening of the previously closed channel, and the sodium ions flow into the cell, initiating depolarization. This is measured as an intercellular decrease (i.e., a shift toward zero) in the membrane's resting potential (−90 mV). Muscarinic receptors are a different family of acetylcholine receptors and do not form channels when activated.

Mechanism of Action

Acetylcholine released from the presynaptic terminal acts on nicotinic receptors in the postsynaptic membrane and is hydrolyzed by acetylcholinesterase in the synaptic cleft (24). The postsynaptic receptors are transmembrane proteins that, when activated, open to form aqueous pores in the membrane that are permeable to small cations. Two acetylcholine molecules are required to open a single channel (36). Each nicotinic receptor, therefore, has two binding sites for acetylcholine. When both sites are occupied by an agonist, a conformational change occurs in the molecule and a sodium channel is opened (43). If a sufficient number of postsynaptic nicotinic receptors are simultaneously occupied, the resulting inward sodium current initiates an action potential in the postsynaptic cell (27).

TABLE 8–12. *Types of muscarinic and nicotinic receptors*

Muscarinic receptors	
	M_1—Cerebral cortex
	Autonomic ganglia
	Involved in gastric acid secretion
	M_2—Cardiac atrioventricular node
	Cardiac sinoventricular node
	Stimulation decreases cardiac rate
Nicotinic receptors	
	N_1—Autonomic ganglia
	N_2—Skeletal muscle

Types of Nicotinic Receptors

The nicotinic receptors for acetylcholine are further subdivided into two groups: nicotinic I, found mainly in autonomic ganglia, and nicotinic II, located at the skeletal muscle end plate (4). There are drugs that selectively interfere with transmission in autonomic ganglia, called *ganglionic blocking agents*, and others that selectively interfere with neuromuscular transmission, called *neuromuscular blocking agents*. Although neuromuscular and ganglionic nicotinic receptors are not identical, the structure and function of the various nicotinic receptors are similar.

Although acetylcholine is the transmitter at both the nicotinic and muscarinic receptor sites, some agents display a degree of selectivity in blocking acetylcholine from nicotinic receptors at neuromuscular junctions or from those at autonomic ganglia. In addition, transmission in cholinergic neuroeffector junctions of skeletal muscle, viscera, autonomic ganglia, and heart differs with respect to the time limits of acetylcholine inactivation, which vary from milliseconds (motor end plate) to several seconds (heart) (36).

It is important to remember that cholinergic fibers to skeletal muscle and the nicotinic II receptors associated with the muscle end plate are part of the somatic nervous system, not the autonomic nervous system.

Muscarinic Receptors at Sympathetic Sites

In recent years it has been shown that sympathetic nerve terminals contain muscarinic receptors that can be activated by acetylcholine released from nerve fibers (39). This muscarinic activation inhibits the release of norepinephrine. Activation of muscarinic receptors can therefore powerfully modulate the positive inotropic, electrophysiologic, and metabolic effects of catecholamines acting on adrenergic receptors. These antagonistic effects of acetylcholine are directed at cAMP actions within the cell and not specifically at the β-adrenergic receptor (37).

Examples of Types of Cholinergic Compounds

Antimuscarinic Drugs

Antimuscarinic drugs compete with acetylcholine on smooth muscle receptors and only inhibit acetylcholine on nicotinic receptors at high concentrations. Atropine, for example, is a competitive antagonist to the muscarinic actions because it occupies the cholinergic receptor sites on autonomic effector cells and on the secondary muscarinic receptors of autonomic ganglion cells. *d*-Tubocurarine blocks transmission at both motor end plates and autonomic ganglia. Examples of other antimuscarinics are discussed in Chapter 10.

Botulinum Toxin

Botulinum toxin prevents the release of acetylcholine by all types of cholinergic fibers and thereby blocks transmission at the skeletal neuromuscular junction as well as at the autonomic cholinergic synapses (17). Only a minuscule amount of this toxin is necessary to bind irreversibly to their sites of action, producing an essentially irreversible blockade of all cholinergic junctions and resulting in anticholinergic symptoms (Chapter 73).

Acetylcholinesterase Inhibitors

Drugs that inhibit the enzyme acetylcholinesterase are called *anticholinesterase agents* or *acetylcholinesterase inhibitors*. They cause acetylcholine to accumulate at cholinergic receptor sites and thus produce effects equivalent to excessive stimulation of cholinergic receptors. On inhibition of acetylcholinesterase, the transmitter is removed principally by diffusion. Under these circumstances, the effects of released acetylcholine are potentiated and prolonged. Carbamates such as physostigmine, neostigmine, pyridostigmine (Antilirium), edrophonium (Tensilon), and the carbamate insecticides act in this manner. The organophosphate insecticides parathion, malathion, and others also act in this manner but at some point in time become irreversible.

Black Widow Spider Venom

Black widow spider venom causes a transient release of acetylcholine and a subsequent permanent block. This results in transient cholinomimetic effects that are followed by anticholinergic effects. This is further discussed in Chapter 76.

ADRENERGIC RECEPTORS

In the early 1900s, it was shown that preparations of ergot abolished the motor effects of sympathetic stimulation (44). In 1948, Ahlquist concluded that there were two distinct types of adrenergic receptors, α and β (1,2,44,45). α Receptors referred to those adrenergic receptors most sensitive to norepinephrine and least sensitive to isoproterenol, and β receptors referred to those showing the reverse pattern (1,2,46).

Adrenergic Neurotransmission

The bodies of the sympathetic preganglionic cells are located in the intermediate-lateral column of the gray matter of the thoracic and lumbar segments of the spinal cord. Their axons, the preganglionic fibers, make synaptic contact onto dendrites and cell bodies of the ganglion cells, providing a direct pathway to affect the output of postganglionic cells (10,19). Preganglionic fibers also make synaptic contacts with the intrinsic neurons, which in turn establish synaptic contact with the ganglion cells. The ganglion cells are also connected to each other by dendrodendritic contacts. The synaptic contact of preganglionic fibers with ganglionic cells and the dendrodendritic contact between ganglionic cells provide pathways for more complex processing and integration of information by the ganglia (46).

Termination of Adrenergic Neurotransmission

The actions of norepinephrine, epinephrine, and dopamine are terminated by various methods, including reuptake of the agonist into nerve terminals, dilution of the agonist by diffusion out of the junctional cleft, uptake at extraneuronal sites, metabolic transformation of the agonist, and actions on α inhibitory receptors (α_2 receptors) (Table 8–13) (9).

Although catecholamines can be inactivated by the enzymes monoamine oxidase and catechol *o*-methyltransferase, this is not usually how an action is terminated. Termination primarily occurs through the active process of catecholamine reuptake across the presynaptic nerve membrane back into the presynaptic nerve ending. The catecholamines are then stored again in the synaptic vesicles for reuse. This process differs from the hydrolysis that occurs with acetylcholine. A small portion of the released norepinephrine escapes into the plasma; this "free" norepinephrine provides the basis for relating plasma norepinephrine levels to the activity of sympathetic neurons (5–7).

The principle of agonist reuptake into the nerve terminal and then into the storage vesicles is of crucial importance because there are drugs that may block either the active reuptake process into the nerve terminal, thus potentiating the synaptic action of the transmitter, or the

TABLE 8–13. *Metabolism of catecholamines*

Reuptake of agonist into nerve terminals
Dilution of agonist by diffusion
Metabolic transformation
Monoamine oxidase (MAO)
Catechol *O*-methyltransferase (COMT)
Actions on α_2 receptors

reuptake of the transmitter from the intracellular fluid in the presynaptic nerve terminal back into the storage granule (synaptic vesicles), where it is stored and protected from monoamine oxidase. An example of the latter type of drug is reserpine. As a result of blockage by reserpine, norepinephrine may be metabolized by monoamine oxidase and the nervous system depleted of the transmitter, with the result of sedation and emotional depression. Cocaine and the tricyclic antidepressants are examples of the former type of drug; they block reuptake of norepinephrine from the synaptic cleft back into the nerve terminal, thus increasing its action at the synapse.

Some drugs are capable of blocking the enzyme monoamine oxidase, thereby increasing the norepinephrine concentration in the nerve terminal (3). Tranylcypromine (Parnate) is one such monoamine oxidase inhibitor. Some compounds (ephedrine) are capable of stimulating the postsynaptic norepinephrine receptor; others (such as phenoxybenzamine) are capable of blocking the receptor.

Monoamine Oxidase (MAO)

As previously mentioned, there are two major enzyme systems involved in the transformation of the catecholamines to inactivate degradation products. Oxidative deamination of epinephrine and norepinephrine is catalyzed by MAO. Adrenergic nerve ending contain large quantities of this enzyme, which is localized on the outer surface of mitochondrial membranes. Apparently, because of its intraneuronal localization, MAO plays more of a role in the regulation of the intraneuronal disposition of catecholamines than the destruction of circulating biogenic amines, which takes place in the liver. Inhibition of MAO leads to an increase in the tissue concentration of the catecholamines but has no appreciable effect on the responses to injected epinephrine or norepinephrine (36).

Catechol O-Methyltransferase (COMT)

The second major enzyme involved in the metabolism of the catecholamines is COMT. This enzyme is responsible for the inactivation of circulating catecholamines. Although the enzyme is widely distributed, highest concentrations are found in the liver and kidneys; lesser amounts are localized in the neuroeffector junction, especially in the tissues served by the adrenergic nerves. Sympathetic nerves contain very little COMT activity (9).

Sympathetic Cholinergic Fibers

The basic mechanism of release of acetylcholine by preganglionic sympathetic nerve terminals does not seem to be different from that described in other synapses, particularly at the motor nerve terminal of the neuromuscular junction. As in the neuromuscular junction, the stimulation of preganglionic nerve fibers induces an action potential that, when propagated to the fine nerve terminals, increases the permeability to Ca^{2+}. The entry of Ca^{2+} into the presynaptic nerve terminal favored by the Ca^{2+} electrochemical gradient increases the probability of release of acetylcholine present in the presynaptic vesicles.

Classification of Adrenergic Receptors

Although the use of the terms α and β *adrenoceptors* for describing catecholamine receptors is now generally accepted, adrenoceptors are much more complicated than what was first described (Tables 8–14 and 8–15) (2). The current concept is that there are subtypes of adrenergic receptors—α_1, α_2, β_1, and β_2—that are distinguished by the relative potencies of particular agonists and antagonists (16). Receptors are also subdivided morphologically as pre- and postsynaptic adrenoceptors (16). Morphologically, presynaptic receptors are located before the synapse, at the nerve terminal or nerve ending; a synonymous term is *prejunctional* (47). Postsynaptic or postjunctional receptors are located at the muscle cell (22). Another classification is based on pharmacologic or functional characteristics: α_1 receptors are located postsynaptically and cause stimulation, and α_2 receptors are located presynaptically and cause sympathetic inhibition (48).

Role of Cyclic AMP

Three of the four subtypes of adrenergic receptors are linked to the same biochemical effector, the adenyl cyclase system. This system generates cyclic AMP, which acts as a messenger provoking a series of reactions that leads to a physiologic response within the effector cell (14). The β receptors are thought to activate adenyl cyclase by a coupling protein that binds guanosine triphosphate. The β_1 and β_2 receptors stimulate adenyl cyclase, whereas the α_2 receptors inhibit it (5–7,10). The α_1 receptors appear to be coupled not to adenyl cyclase but rather to processes that regulate cellular calcium ion fluxes possibly mediated by increased phosphatidylinositol hydrolysis (1,2,10).

TABLE 8–14. *Adrenergic receptors (not absolute)*

α Receptor	β Receptor
Resistance vessels of	Heart
Skin	Skeletal muscle
Mucosa	Bronchi
Intestine	Metabolic effects
Kidney	Uterus

TABLE 8–15. *Differences between α- and β-adrenoceptor action*

	Action	
Organ	α receptor	β receptor
Heart		Increases heart rate Increases contractility Increases conduction velocity
Blood vessels	Constriction	Dilation
Bronchi		Dilation
Stomach	Contracts sphincter	Decreases motility
Intestine	Relaxation	Relaxation
Uterus	Contraction	Relaxation
Urinary bladder	Contraction	Relaxation
Eye	Pupil dilation	

Reprinted from *Med Clin North Am* 1968;52:1009–1016. With permission of WB Saunders Company.

α Adrenoceptors

α_1 Adrenoceptors

Peripheral α receptors located postsynaptically on the vascular smooth muscle cell are termed α_1 (46). These receptors are under the influence of the neurotransmitter norepinephrine, which is liberated from postganglionic adrenergic fibers by the nerve impulse (22). Stimulation of these receptors results in typical adrenergic effects.

α_2 Adrenoceptors

Receptors located presynaptically on the sympathetic nerve ending that inhibit peripheral neuronal neurotransmitter release are termed α_2 (45). These presynaptic autoregulatory α receptors are located peripherally and differ in their pharmacologic properties from postsynaptic α receptors mediating typical α-adrenergic effects (46). The peripheral α_2 receptors located at presynaptic sites on the nerve ending itself reduce the amount of norepinephrine released by nerve impulses when stimulated by norepinephrine in the synaptic cleft. When high concentrations of norepinephrine are present, subsequent nerve impulses release less norepinephrine (18). Thus, the presynaptic α_2 receptor forms part of a feedback loop that maintains the local level of sympathetic activity. Stimulation of the α_2 receptors therefore inhibits adenyl cyclase activity and in turn decreases cellular concentrations of cAMP (Table 8–16, Fig. 8–2) (45). Recent evidence suggests that postsynaptic α_2 adrenoceptors are not under direct neuronal control because of their extrasynaptic positions (22). This contrasts with the direct neuronal control over the postsynaptic α_1 adrenoceptors positioned within the synapse. Accordingly, postsynaptic α adrenoceptors are considered noninnervated. As such, they can be regarded as hormone receptors, predominantly, responsive to circulating catecholamines, especially epinephrine.

Although the exact function, distribution, and location of central α_2 receptors are currently under investigation, it is clear that they modulate autonomic nerve outflux from medullary brain structures (49). CNS α_2 adrenoceptors are found in the pontomedullary region where there are high densities of noradrenergic neurons and synapses. The major nuclei of this region, which are interconnected through several neuronal pathways, are: the vasomotor

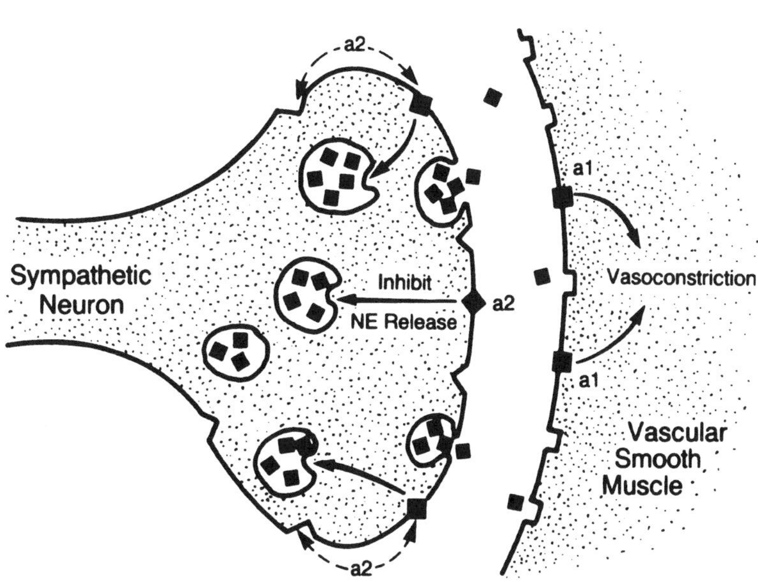

FIG. 8–2. Configuration of receptors. Schematic illustrating the suggested neuronal location of α_2 and vascular smooth muscle location of α_1 receptor prototypes. However, there is evidence for postsynaptic location in other organs for this α_2 receptor. Thus, the classification is functional rather than anatomic. Reprinted from *Life Sci* 1977;21:595–606. With permission of Pergamon Press.

TABLE 8–16. *Characteristics of α adrenoceptors*

Receptor type	Location	Function	Distribution
α_1	Postsynaptic	Raises intracellular calcium concentration	Myocardium vascular smooth muscle
α_2	Presynaptic (peripheral)	Inhibits norepinephrine release	Peripheral nervous system, cholinergic nerve endings
	Postsynaptic (central)	Inhibits adenyl cyclase	Central nervous system
	Nonsynaptic (platelet)		

center, the nucleus tractus solitarii, and the vagal nucleus. α_2 Adrenoceptors are present in all three nuclei. Stimulation of these postsynaptic receptor sites with lipophilic α agonists, clonidine or guanfacine, activates the inhibitory neuron to depress peripheral sympathetic nervous activity, which lowers both blood pressure and heart rate (50,51). So, stimulation of these receptors causes decreased sympathetic and increased parasympathetic nerve outflux from the CNS. This is a result of a decrease in cAMP by inhibition of adenyl cyclase. Drugs that inhibit α_2 receptors increase central epinephrine and norepinephrine turnover, resulting in increased sympathetic and decreased vagal nerve outflux from the CNS (Fig. 8–3) (20,46).

Originally it was thought that α_2 adrenoceptors were located exclusively presynaptically, but at present there is ample evidence for the existence of α_2 adrenoceptors outside noradrenergic terminal axons, on some organelles lacking synapses, and at postsynaptic sites (46,52–56). The important point is that the designation α_2 is based on pharmacologic studies and specific drugs and does not necessarily imply a presynaptic location (Table 8–17) (5–7,49,57).

Substances that decrease noradrenergic neurotransmission include purines (such as adenosine triphosphate and adenosine), prostaglandins of the E series, acetylcholine (by way of muscarinic receptors), dopamine, histamine, serotonin, morphine, and opioid peptides (54). Substances that facilitate noradrenergic neurotransmission include β-adrenoceptor agonists, acetylcholine (by way of nicotinic receptors), angiotensin, possibly prostaglandins of the F series, and thromboxane (51).

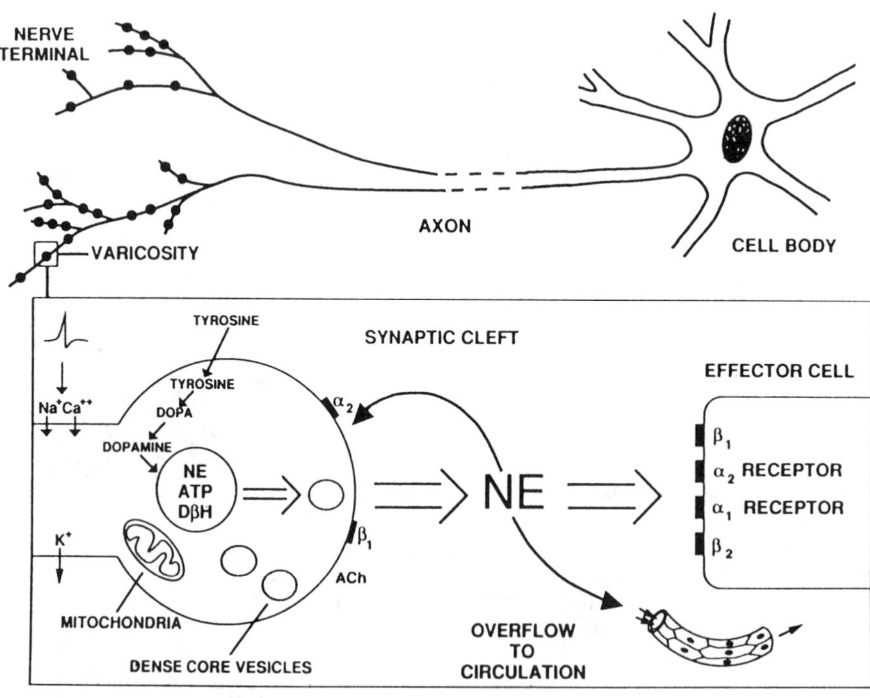

FIG. 8–3. The neuroeffector junction of a sympathetic postganglionic neuron. Norepinephrine (*NE*) released into the synaptic cleft adjacent to varicosities on adrenergic nerve endings may activate presynaptic α_2 receptors or various postsynaptic receptors located on the effector cells. (From Muldoon S, et al., *Int Anesthesiol Clin* 1989;27:263, with permission.)

TABLE 8–17. *Location and action of α receptors*

Location	Action
α_1 Receptors	
Smooth muscle	Contraction
Liver	Glycogenolysis
CNS	Increase in locomotor activity
α_2 Receptors	
Terminal noradrenergic axons	Inhibition of norepinephrine release
Cholinergic neurons	Inhibition
CNS	Sedation
Smooth muscle	Contraction
Platelets	Aggregation
Fat cells	Inhibition of lipolysis
Pancreatic islets	Inhibition of insulin release

β Adrenoceptors

Since 1967 it has been generally accepted that the β receptors are divided functionally into β_1 and β_2 (Table 8-18) (58). The β_1 receptors are located in the heart and mediate the positive inotropic effects; they are also located in the kidneys. The β_2 receptors mediate smooth muscle relaxation and are located in the vasculature, bronchi, and uterus (45). Actually, both receptor types appear to be present in these areas; for example, a small number of β_2 receptors appear to exist in the heart, and β_1 receptors are also present in the lung (10).

In physiologic terms, the β_1 receptors generally mediate the effects of the neuronally released neurotransmitter norepinephrine, whereas β_2 receptors that mediate vasodilation are not under neuronal control and generally respond to the hormone epinephrine, which is released from the adrenal medulla. Stimulation of β_1 receptors causes tachycardia and accentuation of cardiac contraction and atrioventricular conduction. The results of β_2 stimulation are bronchodilation, vasodilation, glycogenolysis, and fibrinolysis. Both β_1 and β_2 adrenoceptors activate adenyl cyclase (1,2,31–33).

The postsynaptic vascular β receptors are virtually β_2 subtypes, in which stimulation by appropriate agonists, including circulating epinephrine, causes modest vasodilation. Conversely, they are modestly vasoconstrictive when subject to blockade.

Selective β_1-adrenoceptor agonists are generally unavailable, although dobutamine is often characterized as a selective β_1- and α_1- adrenoceptor agonist. Both salbutamol and terbutaline are selective β_2-adrenoceptor agonists (23).

Dopamine Receptors

Dopamine is a central neurotransmitter and is also found in sympathetic nerve terminals and in the adrenal medulla (Table 8–19). Dopamine stimulates dopamine receptors in the brain and in vascular beds in the kidney, mesentery, and coronary arteries. Higher concentrations stimulate α and β receptors. The drug has little or no effect on β_2-adrenergic receptors. Dopamine promotes release of norepinephrine from synaptic terminals, and is also converted to norepinephrine in vivo. In high doses

TABLE 8–18. *Characteristics of β Adrenoceptors*

Receptor type	Location	Effect	Function	Distribution
β_1	Heart	Cardiac stimulation	Increases cyclic AMP	Peripheral nerve endings
	Kidney	Renin release		
	Fat	Lipolysis		
	Eye	Decreased aqueous humor production		
β_2	Bronchi	Bronchodilation	Increases cyclic AMP	Peripheral nerve endings
	Blood vessels	Vasodilation		
	Endocrine glands	Glycolysis, insulin release, lactic acid production		
	Uterus	Uterine relaxation		

TABLE 8–19. *Characteristics of dopamine receptors*

Location
- Blood vessels
  - Renal
  - Mesenteric
  - Coronary
  - Intracerebral

Effect
- Low doses
  - Renal/mesenteric vasodilation
- Intermediate doses
  - Myocardial contractility
- High doses
  - Vasoconstriction

within and above the therapeutic range, α-adrenergic effects become more prominent, and may result in increased peripheral resistance and renal vasoconstriction.

In the brain there are at least two types of dopamine receptors: the D_1 receptor (which is linked to adenyl cyclase) and the D_2 receptor. Dopamine is linked to fine motor coordination, emotion, memory, and neurohormonal balance. Peripherally, dopamine receptors are found in the renal and mesenteric vasculature, and cause vasodilation. In the CNS, dopamine is involved with fine skeletal muscle movement. It is also involved in the secretion of the posterior pituitary hormones. Another action is in the limbic system, where it is associated with the control of emotions.

Tachyphylaxis

When using catecholamines clinically, the phenomenon of tachyphylaxis, or decreased responsiveness to drug with time, is often seen. This may represent adaptation on the cellular level to excessive stimulus. The most commonly accepted and well-documented mechanism of decreased responsiveness in the face of high circulating catecholamine levels is that of receptor downregulation, defined as a decrease in the number of high affinity receptor sites available for Ca binding.

Increased adrenergic receptor density is seen in several clinical settings. Receptor upregulation, or increase in receptor density, has been demonstrated during use of β blocking agents such as propranolol. This phenomenon may be responsible for the rebound hypertension seen after sudden withdrawal of propranolol in clinical situations.

Agonists and Antagonists

Receptor agonists have an affinity for a receptor and, when combined with the receptor, transform it in such a way that a cellular response is initiated. A full agonist causes a maximal response, whereas a partial agonist causes a response that is qualitatively similar but always less in magnitude than that of a full agonist (5). A receptor antagonist interacts with the receptor but elicits no response on its own. By occupying the receptor, however, an antagonist may reduce the effect of an agonist (14). Through structural modifications, an agonist may become an antagonist by retaining its affinity for a receptor and losing its ability to initiate the reactions necessary for a response.

Methoxamine and phenylephrine are directly acting sympathomimetic amine agonists that selectively stimulate α_1 receptors (59). Clonidine is an α_2-selective agonist (47,60). Epinephrine and norepinephrine, having approximately equal potency at α_1 and α_2 receptors, are nonselective agonists (Table 8–20).

Among α-adrenergic antagonists, prazosin, terazosin, and corynanthine are considered α_1-selective. Prazosin is probably the most potent α_1-blocking agent currently available (5–7). Yohimbine and rauwolscine, both plant alkaloids, are specific α_2 antagonists (60). Phentolamine is generally equipotent at α_1 and α_2 receptors (61). It is therefore nonselective, so that both the postsynaptic receptor on the vascular smooth muscle cell and the presynaptic receptor on the peripheral nerve ending are blocked (59).

Among the β agonists, isoproterenol is nonselective, and dobutamine is selective for β_1 receptors (6). Propranolol is a nonselective β-adrenergic blocking agent, and metoprolol is a selective β_1 blocking agent (22).

TABLE 8–20. *Partial list of α- and β-adrenoceptor agonists and antagonists*

Receptor type	Agonists	Antagonists
α (nonselective)	Norepinephrine	Phentolamine
	Epinephrine	Tolazoline
α_1	Methoxamine	Prazosin
	Phenylephrine	Corynanthine
		Terazosin
α_2	Clonidine	Yohimbine
	Guanabenz	Rauwolscine
	Guanefesine	Piperoxan
	Methyldopa	
	Naphazoline	
	Oxymetazoline	
β (nonselective)	Isoproterenol	Nadolol
		Propranolol
		Timolol
β_1	Dobutamine	Acebutolol
	Tazolol	Alprenolol
	Prenalterol	Atenolol
		Metoprolol
		Practolol
β_2	Terbutaline	Butoxamine
	Salbutamol	
	Isoetharine	
	Fenoterol	
	Rimiterol	

REFERENCES

1. Abboud F: The sympathetic nervous system and α-adrenergic blocking agents in shock. *Med Clin North Am* 1968;52:1049–1060.
2. Abboud F: Concepts of adrenergic receptors. *Med Clin North Am* 1968;52:1009–1016.
3. Polinsky R: Clinical autonomic neuropharmacology. *Neurol Clin* 1990;8:77–91.
4. Pincus D, Magitsky L: Anatomy, physiology, and elementary pharmacology of the autonomic nervous system. *Int Anesthesiol Clin* 1989;27:219–233.
5. Hoffman B: Regulation of α- and β-adrenergic receptors in man. *Clin Endocrinol Metab* 1983;12:1–13.
6. Hoffman B, Lefkowitz R: α-Adrenergic receptor subtypes. *N Engl J Med* 1980;302:1390–1396.
7. Hoffman B, De Lean A, Wood C, et al: α-Adrenergic receptor subtypes. *Life Sci* 1979;24:1739–1746.
8. Towler S, Evers A: Anesthesia and chemical second messenger generation in the adrenergic nervous system. *Int Anesthesiol Clin* 1989;27:234–247.
9. Glusman S: Electrophysiology of ganglionic transmission in the sympathetic nervous system. *Int Anesthesiol Clin* 1989;27:273–282.
10. Casale T: The role of the autonomic nervous system in allergic diseases. *Ann Allergy* 1983;51:423–429.
11. Snyder S: Drug and neurotransmitter receptors. *JAMA* 1989;261:3126–3129.
12. Motulsky H, Insel P: Adrenergic receptors in man. *N Engl J Med* 1982;307:18–29.
13. Nadel J, Barnes P: Autonomic regulation of the airways. *Annu Rev Med* 1984;35:451–467.
14. Lefkowitz R, Caron M, Stiles G: Mechanisms of membrane receptor regulation. *N Engl J Med* 1984;310:1570–1579.
15. Lefkowitz R: β-Adrenergic receptors: recognition and regulation. *N Engl J Med* 1976;295:323–328.
16. Hughes A, Horstman D, Takemura H, et al: Inositol phosphate metabolism and signal transduction. *Am Rev Respir Dis* 1990;141:115–118.
17. Douglas J: Receptors on target cells. *Am Rev Respir Dis* 1990;141:S123–S126.
18. Brown R, Mann J: A clinical perspective on the role of neurotransmitters in mental disorders. *Hosp Community Psychiatry* 1985;36:141–150.
19. Axelrod J, Weinshilboum R: Catecholamines. *N Engl J Med* 1972:287:237–242.
20. Muldoon S, Cress L, Freas W: Presynaptic adrenergic effects of anesthetics. *Int Anesthesiol Clin* 1989;27:259–264.
21. Breslow M, Frankhauser M, Potter R, et al: Role of γ-aminobutyric acid in antipanic drug efficacy. *Am J Psychiatry* 1989;146:353–356.
22. Van Zwieten P: The role of adrenoceptors in circulatory and metabolic regulation. *Am Heart J* 1988;116:1384–1391.
23. Venter J, Fraser C: Receptor mechanisms. *Am Rev Respir Dis* 1990;141:99–105.
24. Gale K: GABA in epilepsy: The pharmacologic basis. *Epilepsia* 1992;30(Suppl.3):S1–S11.
25. Jones E: The γ-aminobutyric acid A ($GABA_A$) receptor complex and hepatic encephalopathy. *Ann Intern Med* 1989;110:532– 546.
26. Goyal R: Muscarinic receptor subtypes. *N Engl J Med* 1989;321:1022–1028.
27. Nijkamp F, Henricks P: Receptors in airway disease. *Am Rev Respir Dis* 1990;141:145–150.
28. Birnbaumer L, Brown A: G proteins and the mechanism of action of hormones, neurotransmitters, and autocrine and paracrine regulatory factors. *Am Rev Respir Dis* 1990;141:S106–S114.
29. Heusch G: Alpha adrenergic mechanisms in myocardial ischemia. *Circulation* 1990;81:1–13.
30. Sutherland E, Robison G: Metabolic effects of catecholamines. *Pharmacol Rev* 1966;18:145–161.
31. Wit A, Hoffman B, Rosen M: Electrophysiology and pharmacology of cardiac arrhythmias: part IX: cardiac electrophysiologic effects of β-adrenergic receptor stimulation and blockade: part A. *Am Heart J* 1975;90:521–533.
32. Wit A, Hoffman B, Rosen M: Electrophysiology and pharmacology of cardiac arrhythmias: part IX: cardiac electrophysiologic effects of β-adrenergic receptor stimulation and blockade: part B. *Am Heart J* 1975;90:665–675.
33. Wit A, Hoffman B, Rosen M: Electrophysiology and pharmacology of cardiac arrhythmias: part IX: cardiac electrophysiologic effects of β-adrenergic receptor stimulation and blockade: part C. *Am Heart J* 1975;90:795–803.
34. Epstein S, Levey G, Skelton C: Adenyl cyclase and cyclic AMP. *Circulation* 1977;43:437–450.
35. Polinsky RJ: Clinical autonomic neuropharmacology *Neurol Clin (US)* 1990;8:77–92.
36. Brodde OE. The functional importance of β_1 and β_2 adrenoceptors in the human heart. *Am J Cardiol* 1988;62:62-24C–29C.
37. Loeffelholz K, Pappano A: The parasympathetic neuroeffector junction of the heart. *Pharmacol Rev* 1985;37:1–24.
38. DeGramo B, Dronen S: Pharmacology and clinical use of neuromuscular blocking agents. *Ann Emerg Med* 1983;12:48–55.
39. Burnstock G: Autonomic neurotransmitters and trophic factors. *J Auton Nerv Syst* 1983;7:213–217.
40. Lepor H, Gup D, Shapiro E, et al: Muscarinic cholinergic receptors in the normal and neurogenic human bladder *J Urol* 1989;142:869–874.
41. Goldie R: Receptors in asthmatic airways. *Am Rev Respir Dis* 1990;141:151–156.
42. Lemanske R, Kaliner M: Autonomic nervous system abnormalities and asthma. *Am Rev Respir Dis* 1990;141;157–161.
43. Snyder S: Drug and neurotransmitter receptors. *JAMA* 1989;261:3126–3129.
44. Ahlquist R: A study of the adrenotropic receptors. *Am J Physiol* 1948;153:586–600.
45. Berthelsen S, Pettinger W: A functional basis for classification of α-adrenergic receptors. *Life Sci* 1977;21:595–606.
46. Colucci W: New developments in α-adrenergic receptor pharmacology: implications for the initial treatment of hypertension. *Am J Cardiol* 1983;51:639–643.
47. Doxey J, Smith C, Walker J: Selectivity of blocking agents for pre- and postsynaptic α adrenoceptors. *Br J Pharmacol* 1977;60:91–96.
48. Kobinger W: Central blood pressure regulation. *Chest* 1983;83(suppl.):296–299.
49. Starke K, Docherty J: α_1 and α_2 Adrenoceptors: pharmacology and clinical implications. *J Cardiovasc Pharmacol* 1981;3:S14–S23.
50. Weiss R, Tobes M, Wertz C, et al: Platelet α_2 adrenoceptors in chronic congestive heart failure. *Am J Cardiol* 1983;52:101–105.
51. Westfall T: Evidence that noradrenergic transmitter release is regulated by presynaptic receptors. *Fed Proc* 1984;43:1352–1357.
52. Langer S: Presynaptic regulation of catecholamine release. *Biochem Pharmacol* 1974;23:1793–1800.
53. Langer S: Presynaptic receptors and their role in the regulation of transmitter release. *Br J Pharmacol* 1977;60:481–497.
54. Bannister R: Clinical studies of autonomic function and dysfunction. *J Auton Nerv Syst* 1983;7:233–237.
55. Docherty J, Hyland L: Evidence for neuroeffector transmission through postjunctional α_2 adrenoceptors in human saphenous vein. *Br J Pharmacol* 1985;84:573–576.
56. Gross F: Central α adrenoceptors in cardiovascular regulation. *Chest* 1983;83(suppl):293–296.
57. DiJoseph J, Taylor J, Mir G, et al: α_2 Receptors in the gastrointestinal system: a new therapeutic approach. *Life Sci* 1984;35:1031–1042.
58. Lands A, Arnold A, McAuliff J, et al: Differentiation of receptor systems activated by sympathomimetic amines. *Nature (London)* 1967;214:597–598.
59. Goldberg M, Robertson D: Evidence for the existence of vascular α_2 adrenergic receptors in humans. *Hypertension* 1984;6:551–556.
60. Drew G: What do antagonists tell us about α adrenoceptors? *Clin Sci* 1985;68(Suppl. 10):15s–19s.
61. Jie K. Brummelen P, Vermey P: Identification of vascular postsynaptic α_1 and α_2 adrenoceptors in man. *Circ Res* 1984;54:447–452.

CHAPTER 9

Autonomic Nervous System Drugs

This chapter reviews the major autonomic nervous system drugs, *norepinephrine*, the neurotransmitter; *epinephrine*, the hormone secreted from the adrenal medulla; *dopamine*, an endogenous central nervous system (CNS) neurotransmitter; *isoproterenol*, a pure β agonist; and *dobutamine*, a pure β_1 agonist. All of these naturally occurring substances are commercially available as medications.

SYMPATHETIC AGONISTS

Sympathetic agonists vary in their action on the receptors. Among the catecholamines, norepinephrine acts mainly on α receptor sites and has little β-stimulating activity, except in the heart; epinephrine acts on β receptors in the heart and bronchial tree and on both α and β receptors in the blood vessels; isoproterenol is almost a pure β receptor agonist (1). Norepinephrine, its immediate precursor dopamine, and epinephrine are also neurotransmitters in the CNS (2). Dopamine serves two functions: it is a precursor of norepinephrine, and it is a neurotransmitter in the area of the brain involved in coordinating motor activity (3).

Norepinephrine

Norepinephrine is an endogenous catecholamine synthesized from tyrosine. It is formed by hydroxylation of dopamine, and is stored in vesicles in adrenergic nerve endings (4) (Table 9–1). Levophed is identical to the endogenous catecholamine. When sympathetic nerves are activated, norepinephrine is released from its stores, and stimulates α-adrenergic receptors (5,6). Norepinephrine is a neurotransmitter in the CNS and in sympathetic postganglionic nerves of the peripheral nervous system; it is also released from the adrenal medulla (7).

Norepinephrine acts predominantly by a direct effect on α-adrenergic receptors. The drug also directly stimulates β-adrenergic receptors of the heart (β_1-adrenergic receptors) but not those of the bronchi or peripheral blood vessels (β_2-adrenergic receptors). However, norepinephrine has less effect on β_1 receptors than does epinephrine or isoproterenol. It is believed that α-adrenergic effects result from inhibition of the production of cyclic AMP by inhibition of the enzyme adenyl cyclase, whereas β-adrenergic effects result from stimulation of adenyl cyclase activity (1). The main effects of therapeutic doses of norepinephrine are vasoconstriction and cardiac stimulation.

Release of norepinephrine into the synaptic cleft results in the stimulation of postsynaptic receptors that cause vasoconstriction at most vascular neuroeffector junctions. Presynaptic noradrenergic receptors serve as a feedback control system to inhibit further release of norepinephrine. The actions of norepinephrine are primarily terminated through an active neuronal uptake mechanism with subsequent intraneuronal metabolism.

In noradrenergic neurons, a portion of the norepinephrine is not stored in vesicles but exists in a protected form in the neuronal cytoplasm; this secondary pool is not released by nerve action potentials but may be expelled by the action of certain indirect-acting sympathomimetic drugs such as tyramine (7).

Several important transport mechanisms in the noradrenergic nerve terminal are potential sites of drug action. One of these, located in the terminal cell membrane, actively transports norepinephrine and similar molecules into the cytoplasm. It can be inhibited by such agents as the tricyclics and cocaine (8). A second high-affinity carrier for catecholamines is located in the wall of the storage vesicle itself, and can be inhibited by a different class of drugs, the reserpine alkaloids (6).

TABLE 9–1. *Norepinephrine*

α_1 and β_1 agonist
Endogenous catecholamine formed from dopamine
Adverse effects
Headache
Weakness
Dizziness
Tremor
Vasoconstriction
Palpitations
Bradycardia
Dysrhythmias
Tissue necrosis

Orally ingested norepinephrine is destroyed in the GI tract, and the drug is poorly absorbed after subcutaneous injection. After IV administration, a pressor response occurs rapidly. The drug has a short duration of action, and the pressor action stops within 1–2 minutes after the infusion is discontinued.

Adverse Effects

Norepinephrine may cause headache, weakness, dizziness, tremor, pallor, respiratory difficulty or apnea, and precordial pain. Norepinephrine may also cause restlessness, anxiety, and insomnia.

Norepinephrine can cause severe peripheral and visceral vasoconstriction, reduced blood flow to vital organs, decreased renal perfusion and therefore decreased urine output, tissue hypoxia, and metabolic acidosis. These effects are most likely to occur in hypovolemic patients.

Norepinephrine may cause palpitations and bradycardia as well as potentially fatal cardiac arrhythmias, including ventricular tachycardia, bigeminal rhythm, nodal rhythm, atrioventricular dissociation, and fibrillation. Bradycardia may be treated by administration of atropine. Arrhythmias are especially likely to occur in patients with acute myocardial infarction, hypoxia, or hypercapnia, or those receiving other drugs that may increase cardiac irritability such as cyclopropane or halogenated hydrocarbon general anesthetics.

Extravasation produces severe damage to contiguous structures. Except in extreme emergencies, norepinephrine should be administered only by central vein, with an infusion pump. Extravasation should be treated with local infiltration of phentolamine (9).

Epinephrine

Epinephrine is an endogenous compound formed from norepinephrine manufactured in and released from the adrenal medulla (Table 9–2) (8). It is a principal hormone of stress and produces widespread metabolic and hemodynamic effects. In contrast to norepinephrine, it acts at a site distant from where it is released. Many of the actions of epinephrine and norepinephrine are similar.

Epinephrine acts directly on both α- and β-adrenergic receptors of tissues innervated by sympathetic nerves except the sweat glands and arteries of the face (10). It is believed that β-adrenergic effects result from stimulation of the production of cyclic AMP by activation of the enzyme adenyl cyclase, whereas α-adrenergic effects result from inhibition of adenyl cyclase activity. The main effects of therapeutic parenteral doses of epinephrine are relaxation of smooth muscle of the bronchial tree, cardiac stimulation, and dilation of skeletal muscle vasculature.

β_1 Receptors are most sensitive to epinephrine and are affected by very low concentrations (11). Myocardial oxygen consumption increases and oxygen balance is thereby affected adversely. As the concentration of epinephrine increases, myocardial irritability occurs and is manifest by atrial and ventricular dysrhythmias (6).

Systemically absorbed epinephrine acts on β_1-adrenergic receptors in the heart, producing a positive chronotropic effect through the sinoatrial node and a positive inotropic effect on the myocardium. Cardiac output, oxygen consumption, and the work of the heart are increased, and cardiac efficiency is decreased (8).

Orally ingested epinephrine is rapidly metabolized in the GI tract and liver; pharmacologically active concentrations are not reached when the drug is given orally. Epinephrine is well absorbed after subcutaneous or intramuscular injection. Both rapid and prolonged absorption occur after subcutaneous injection of the aqueous suspension. After oral inhalation of epinephrine in the usual dosage, absorption is slight and the effects of the drug are restricted mainly to the respiratory tract. Absorption increases somewhat when larger doses are inhaled, and systemic effects may occur.

Adverse Effects

Epinephrine produces unpleasant subjective symptoms of CNS excitation, including anxiety, dread, vascular-type headaches, weakness, nausea, emesis, and dyspnea. Acute overdosage has been reported to produce transient apnea.

Accidental epinephrine overdosage is life-threatening. In adults, effects include myocardial infarction, ventricular tachycardia, extreme hypertension, cerebral hemorrhage, seizures, renal failure, and pulmonary edema. Bradycardia has also been observed (12).

TABLE 9–2. *Epinephrine*

Endogenous hormone formed from norepinephrine
Not a neurotransmitter
Formed from norepiphrine
Released from adrenal medulla
$\alpha_{1,2}$ **and** $\beta_{1,2}$ **agonist**
Adverse effects
Headache
Weakness
Excitation
Dread
Myocardial infarction
Ventricular tachycardia
Hypertension
Cerebral hemorrhage
Seizures
Renal failure
Pulmonary edema
Bradycardia

TABLE 9–3. *Isoproterenol*

Derivative of norepinephrine
Pure β agonist
Inotropic and chronotropic agent
Increases myocardial oxygen demand
Adverse effects
Dysrhythmias
Hypotension
Increased myocardial oxygen demand
Nervousness
Restlessness
Excitement
Asthenia

Toxicity associated with acute overdosage is treated symptomatically. Nonspecific β receptor antagonists such as propranolol are to be avoided, and more cardioselective agents should be tried. Esmolol may prove to be of great advantage in that it is cardioselective and very short-acting. Hypertension is treated symptomatically with short-acting antihypertensives, such as nitroprusside. Nitroglycerin has been employed to ameliorate myocardial ischemia (13).

Epinephrine is an α_1 agonist, and infiltration into local tissues or intra-arterial injection can produce severe vasospasm and tissue injury. If extravasation is followed by pallor and other signs of impaired local perfusion, phentolamine should be injected locally.

Isoproterenol

Isoproterenol is the synthetic isopropyl derivative of norepinephrine (Table 9–3). The terminal substituent confers both β_1 and β_2 receptor specificity. Isoproterenol does not affect the α-adrenergic receptors (12).

The principal therapeutic and adverse effects associated with isoproterenol relate to its inotropic, chronotropic, and peripheral vascular vasodilatory effects (8).

Isoproterenol relaxes bronchial, GI, and uterine smooth muscle by stimulation of β_2-adrenergic receptors. In addition, isoproterenol inhibits antigen-induced release of histamine and the slow-reacting substance anaphylaxis. In patients with bronchial constriction, usual doses of the drug may relieve bronchospasm, increase vital capacity, decrease residual volume in the lungs, and facilitate passage of pulmonary secretions when administered parenterally or by oral inhalation. However, arterial oxygen tension may be further reduced. Rebound bronchospasm may occur when the effects of isoproterenol end.

Isoproterenol acts on β_1-adrenergic receptors in the heart, producing a positive chronotropic effect through the sinoatrial node and a positive inotropic effect on the myocardium. Cardiac output is usually increased. Increased cardiac output is accompanied by an increase in stroke volume in some patients, but significant increases in stroke volume do not occur consistently. Isoproterenol also increases myocardial oxygen consumption and the work of the heart and decreases cardiac efficiency.

Isoproterenol causes intense tachycardia. It also produces a substantial increase in myocardial oxygen demand. Myocardial oxygen delivery decreases, because of shortened diastole and a decrease in diastolic blood pressure. Oxygen balance is so adversely affected that it is possible to induce myocardial infarction in the absence of coronary artery disease.

Adverse Effects

Arrhythmias, including premature ventricular contractions, ventricular tachycardia, ectopic ventricular beats, and fibrillation may occur in patients receiving isoproterenol, especially if the drug is given in large doses to patients with cardiogenic shock, acidosis, hypoxia, hypokalemia, or hyperkalemia, or to those whose hearts have been sensitized to this action by other drugs including digitalis or certain general anesthetics (8).

Serious adverse reactions to isoproterenol occur infrequently, especially when the drug is administered by oral inhalation. Most adverse effects subside rapidly when isoproterenol is discontinued or may abate while the drug is still in use.

Isoproterenol may cause nervousness, restlessness, insomnia, anxiety, tension, fear, or excitement. Rarely, sweating, weakness, dizziness, mild tremor, headache, flushing of the face or skin, nausea, vomiting, tinnitus, lightheadedness, or asthenia may occur. The drug has produced pulmonary edema in a patient intolerant to other sympathomimetic drugs.

Disturbances of cardiac rhythm and rate produced by isoproterenol may result in palpitation and ventricular tachycardia (7). Isoproterenol can cause potentially fatal ventricular arrhythmias in doses sufficient to increase heart rate above 130 beats/minute. Arrhythmias are most likely to occur in patients with cardiogenic shock; in those receiving other drugs that sensitize the heart to arrhythmias, including cardiac glycosides, cyclopropane, or halogenated hydrocarbon general anesthetics; or in those with acidosis, hypoxia, hypercapnia, hypokalemia, or hyperkalemia.

Dopamine

Dopamine is a central neurotransmitter and is also found in sympathetic nerve terminals and in the adrenal medulla (Table 9–4). Dopamine stimulates dopamine receptors in the brain and in vascular beds in the kidney, mesentery, and coronary arteries. Higher concentrations stimulate α and β receptors. The drug has little or no effect on β_2-

TABLE 9–4. *Dopamine*

Central neurotransmitter also found in adrenal medulla
Stimulates dopaminergic receptors in
Brain
Kidney
Mesentery
Coronary arteries
Higher doses stimulate α and β_1 receptors
Central nervous system dopamine
Fine motor movement
Secretion of posterior pituitary hormones
Control of emotions
Adverse effects
Dysrhythmias
Vasoconstriction
Hypotension
Nausea/Vomiting
Headache
Limb ischemia/gangrene

adrenergic receptors. Dopamine promotes release of norepinephrine from synaptic terminals and is also converted to norepinephrine in vivo. In high doses within and above the therapeutic range, α-adrenergic effects become more prominent and may result in increased peripheral resistance and renal vasoconstriction.

In the brain there are at least two types of dopamine receptors: the D_1 receptor (which is linked to adenyl cyclase) and the D_2 receptor. Dopamine is linked to fine motor coordination, emotion, memory, and neurohormonal balance. Peripherally, dopamine receptors are found in the renal and mesenteric vasculature and cause vasodilation. In the CNS, dopamine is involved with fine skeletal muscle movement. It is also involved in the secretion of the posterior pituitary hormones. Another action is in the limbic system where it is associated with the control of emotions.

Adverse Effects

Administration of dopamine is associated with CNS symptoms similar to those produced by epinephrine. Dopamine increases myocardial oxygen consumption and promotes dysrhythmias. Compared with other agents now available to treat various conditions, dopamine is more likely to evoke tachycardia and dysrhythmias (8).

Dopamine may cause ectopic heartbeats, tachycardia, angina, palpitation, vasoconstriction, hypotension, dyspnea, nausea, vomiting, and headache. Other less frequent adverse effects include cardiac conduction abnormalities, widened QRS complex, bradycardia, hypertension, azotemia, anxiety, and piloerection. Ventricular arrhythmias may occur with very high doses. Dopamine may cause elevations in serum glucose although the concentrations usually do not rise above normal limits.

Dopamine has been implicated in severe limb ischemia, gangrene, and amputation. Dopamine is more often associated with limb ischemia than other adrenergic compounds.

Extravasation of dopamine and other similar agents should be treated immediately by local infiltration with a solution of phentolamine (Regitine) 5–10 mg in 15 mL normal saline with a fine hypodermic needle (8).

Dobutamine

Dobutamine is a synthetic sympathomimetic drug that is structurally related to dopamine (Table 9–5). Unlike dopamine, dobutamine does not cause release of endogenous norepinephrine. Dobutamine has significant inotropic and minor chronotropic and vasopressor effects.

Dobutamine directly stimulates β_1 receptors and is considered a selective β_1 agonist, but the drug is complex (7). It is believed that the β-adrenergic effects result from stimulation of adenyl cyclase activity. In therapeutic doses, dobutamine also has mild β_2- and α_1-adrenergic agonist activity that is relatively balanced and result in minimal net direct effect on systemic vasculature.

Following intravenous (IV) administration, the onset of action of dobutamine occurs within 2 minutes. Peak plasma concentrations of the drug and peak effects occur within 10 minutes after initiation of an IV infusion. The plasma half-life of dobutamine is about 2 minutes.

Adverse Effects

The principal adverse effects of dobutamine include ectopic heartbeats, tachycardia, angina, chest palpitations, and hypertension. Precipitous decreases in blood pressure have been described on occasion. Blood pressure generally will return to baseline values following dosage reduction or discontinuance of the drug. Hypokalemia may occur rarely.

Serious or prominent CNS effects have not been described for dobutamine. Dobutamine is less likely to

TABLE 9–5. *Dobutamine*

β_1 receptor agonist
Mild β_2 and α_1 agonist activity
Structurally related to dopamine
Significant inotropic and minor chronotropic effects
Adverse effects
Ectopic heartbeats
Tachycardia
Angina pectoris
Palpitations
Hypertension
Hypotension
Hypokalemia

induce dysrhythmias than other catecholamines, but serious atrial and ventricular dysrhythmias can be induced or exacerbated, particularly in the context of myocarditis, electrolyte imbalance, or high infusion rates.

REFERENCES

1. Snyder S: Drug and neurotransmitter receptors. JAMA 1989;261:3126–3129.
2. Glusman S: Electrophysiology of ganglionic transmission in the sympathetic nervous system. *Int Anesthesiol Clin* 1989;27:273–282.
3. Van Zwieten P: The role of adrenoceptors in circulatory and metabolic regulation. *Am Heart J* 1988;116:1384–1391.
4. Axelrod J, Weinshilboum R: Calecholamines. *N Engl J Med* 1972;287:237–242.
5. Abboud F: The sympathetic nervous system and α-adrenergic blocking agents in shock. *Med Clin North Am* 1968;52:1049–1060.
6. Abboud F: Concepts of adrenergic receptors. *Med Clin North Am* 1968;52:1009–1016.
7. Notterman DA. Inotropic agents. *Crit Care Clin* 1991;7:583–613.
8. Polinsky R: Clinical autonomic neuropharmacology. *Neurol Clin (US)* 1990;8:77–92.
9. Pincus D, Magitsky L: Anatomy, physiology, and elementary pharmacology of the autonomic nervous system. *Int Anesthesiol Clin* 1989;27:219–233.
10. Muldoon S, Cress L, Freas W: Presynaptic adrenergic effects of anesthetics. *Int Anesthesiol Clin* 1989;27:259–264.
11. Snyder S: Drug and neurotransmitter receptors. *JAMA* 1989;261:3126–3129.
12. Durbin C: Neuromuscular blocking agents and sedative drugs. *Crit Care Clin* 1991;7:489–506.
13. Towler S, Evers A: Anesthesia and chemical second messenger generation in the adrenergic nervous system. *Int Anesthesiol Clin* 1989;27:234–247.

CHAPTER 10

Antimuscarinic Agents

Antimuscarinic agents act by competitively blocking acetylcholine at its parasympathetic effector site (the muscarinic site or postganglionic cholinergic nerve ending). Because most organs receive both sympathetic and parasympathetic nerves and because these tend to oppose each other, parasympathetic blockade in most organs results in sympathetic dominance and sympathomimetic effects. At therapeutic doses, antimuscarinics have little or no effect on cholinergic stimuli at skeletal muscle or ganglionic (nicotinic) receptors (1).

At autonomic ganglia and at the neuromuscular junction, where cholinergic transmission involves nicotinic receptors, atropine or other tertiary amine antimuscarinics produce a partial cholinergic block only at relatively high doses (2). However, quaternary ammonium antimuscarinics generally possess varying degrees of nicotinic blocking activity and may interfere with ganglionic or neuromuscular transmission at doses that block muscarinic receptors (3). At high doses, quaternary ammonium antimuscarinics may produce substantial ganglionic blockade with resultant adverse effects and, in overdosage, they may cause a curariform neuromuscular block.

Atropine is the prototype of the antimuscarinics, and many of the currently available antimuscarinics were developed as structural derivatives of atropine. However, other antimusarinics have been synthesized that have little structural similarity to atropine, and other drugs with a variety of structural characteristics also exhibit antimuscarinic activity.

Drugs are referred to as *antimuscarinics* because at usual doses they principally antagonize cholinergic stimuli at muscarinic receptors. Antimuscarinics have also been referred to as *anticholinergics* but this term is appropriate only when it describes the antagonism of cholinergic stimuli at any cholinergic receptor, whether muscarinic or nicotinic.

TYPES OF CHOLINERGIC RECEPTORS

There are three types of cholinergic receptors: muscarinic, nicotinic I, and nicotinic II (Table 10–1). Cholinergic receptor antagonists are classified based on their ability to selectively block one of these receptor types (4). Antimuscarinic drugs act at the peripheral and central muscarinic receptors. Ganglionic blocking agents selectively interfere with transmission in autonomic ganglia mediated through nicotinic I receptors. Neuromuscular blocking drugs act at nicotinic II receptors of the skeletal muscle end plate.

Atropine and other antimuscarinic drugs have a marked affinity for receptor sites that are activated through the postganglionic parasympathetic nerves. The alkaloid muscarine, derived from the mushroom *Amanita muscaria*, has a similar preference, and mimics the action of acetylcholine at these receptors. Thus, atropinic drugs are said to have antimuscarinic effects. The muscarinic receptors are found mainly at the following sites: sweat glands, salivary gland, and tear glands; mucus-secreting glands of the respiratory tract, the gastrointestinal tract, and the pancreas; involuntary muscle of the heart, bronchi, and intestine; and muscles of the iris and of accommodation.

CLINICAL USE

Antimuscarinics have been used principally in the treatment of peptic ulcer disease, irritable bowel syndrome, bradydysrhythmias, cardiac disorders, to dry secretions prior to surgery, certain disorders of the genitourinary system, bronchospasm, parkinsonian syndrome, and drug-induced extrapyramidal reactions.

TABLE 10–1. *Types of cholinergic receptors*

Type of receptor	Location of receptor	Blocking agent
Muscarinic	Parasympathetic nerve endings	Atropine
Nicotinic I	Autonomic ganglia	Ganglionic blocking agents
Nicotinic II	Skeletal muscle end plate (Striated muscle)	Neuromuscular blocking agents

Antimuscarinic drugs produce dilation of the pupil and cylcoplegia by rendering the pupillary sphincter and ciliary muscles insensitive to the effects of acetylcholine. Antimuscarinic medications that are administered ophthalmically (e.g., atropine sulfate, cyclopentolate hydrochloride, homatropine hydrobromide, scopolamine hydrobromide, and tropicamide) produce mydriasis and cycloplegia (5).

The tertiary amine antimuscarinics are readily absorbed from the gastrointestinal tract (GIT). Generally, those antimuscarinics having a quaternary ammonium group are incompletely absorbed from the GIT since they are completely ionized. They exhibit poor lipid solubility; they do not readily cross the blood–brain barrier and thus exhibit minimal CNS effects.

TYPES OF ANTIMUSCARINIC AGENTS

More than 600 pharmaceutical preparations, including the tricyclic antidepressants, major tranquilizers, antipsychotics, antiparkinsonism agents, belladonna alkaloids, ophthalmic solutions, and antihistamines, contain some form of natural or synthetic antimuscarinic agent (Table 10–2). Antimuscarinic toxicity is therefore widespread, and can be easily recognized. The anticholinergic agents are also called antimuscarinics because they competitively inhibit the muscarinic effects of acetylcholine.

ANTIHISTAMINES (TABLE 10-3)

The term *antihistamine* has been taken to indicate a compound that competitively antagonizes the H_1 receptors in areas such as the bronchi, GIT, blood vessels, and uterus (6). These H_1 blockers neither block the release of nor chemically inactivate histamine but rather prevent the action of histamine on the cell (2,7). Antihistamines are not blockers of H_2 receptors, which are located in the parietal cells of the stomach. These agents are discussed separately in Chapter 11.

TABLE 10–2. *Types of antimuscarinic compounds*

Antidepressants (cyclic)
Antihistamines
Antiparkinsonian agents
Antipsychotic agents
Antispasmodics
Belladonna alkaloids
Ophthalmic solutions
Plants and mushrooms
Jimson weed
Amanita muscaria

TABLE 10–3. *Antihistamines with selected trade names*

Parent compound	Derivatives
Ethylenediamine	Antazoline (Arithmin)
	Methapyrilene (Histadyl)
	Pyrilamine (Histalon, Neo-Pyramine)
	Tripelennamine (Pyribenzamine, PBZ)
Ethanolamine	Bromodiphenhydramine (Ambenyl)
	Carbinoxamine (Clistin, Rondec)
	Clemastine (Tavist)
	Dimenhydrinate (Dramamine, Dimate, Dimetabs, Dramocen, Eladryl, Hydrate, Marmine, Vertiban)
	Diphenhydramine (Benadryl, Benahist, Benylin, Dihydrex, Fenylhist, Noradryl)
	Diphenylpyraline (Hispril)
	Doxylamine (Decapryn)
	Phenyltoloxamine (Atrohist, Histaminic, Naldecon, Percogesic)
Propylamine	Brompheniramine (Bromamine, Bromphen, Dimetane, Spentane, Veltane)
	Chlorpheniramine (AL-R, Allerchlor, Chlor-Trimeton, Phenetron, Chloramate, Alermine, Ornade, Teldrin, Chloro-Amine, Chlorspan, Histrex, Trymegen)
	Dexbrompheniramine
	Dexchlorpheniramine (Polaramine)
	Dimethindene
	Pheniramine (Ru-Tuss D, Citra Forte)
	Pyrobutamine
	Triprolidine (Actidil)
Phenothiazine	Methdilazine (Tacaryl)
	Promethazine (Phenergan)
	Trimeprazine (Temaril)
Piperazine	Buclizine (Bucladin-S)
	Chlorcyclizine (Mantadil)
	Cyclizine (Marezine)
	Hydroxyzine (Vistaril)
	Meclizine (Antivert, Bonine)
Miscellaneous	Azatadine (Optimine)
	Cyproheptadine (Periactin)
	Orphenadrine (Disipal)
	Phenindamine (Nolahist)

ANTIPSYCHOTIC AGENTS

Among the antipsychotic medications, as with the antihistamines, there are significant differences in the amount of antimuscarinic activity between compounds. Trifluopromazine and thioridazine have substantial antimuscarinic activity whereas perphenazine, trifluoperazine, and haloperidol have considerably less antimuscarinic activity. Antipsychotic agents are discussed in Chapter 17.

ANTIPARKINSONISM AGENTS

The antiparkinsonism agents (Table 10–4) are used mainly in the prophylactic management of the side effects secondary to the major tranquilizers.

Benztropine

Benztropine resembles atropine in chemical structure, and its antimuscarinic effect is about equal to that of atropine. Benztropine also exhibits antihistaminic and local anesthetic properties (8–12). Although benztropine is successfully used to treat dystonia secondary to the major tranquilizers, it has also caused dyskinesia and dystonia in some individuals (13). This may result from a dopamine excess secondary to inhibition of dopamine reuptake.

Adverse reactions to benztropine are mainly extensions of its anticholinergic and antihistaminic effects. Dryness of the mouth, blurred vision, mydriasis, nausea, nervousness, tachycardia, or skin rash may occur. In high dosage or in particularly susceptible patients, mental confusion and excitement, weakness and inability to move certain muscle groups, and, occasionally, urinary retention and/or difficulty in urination may result. Constipation, numbness of the extremities, listlessness, depression, vomiting, paralytic ileus, hyperthermia, fever, heat stroke, and visual hallucinations have also been reported.

Orphenadrine

Orphenadrine (Norflex) is a tertiary amine antimuscarinic agent that may also have skeletal muscle relaxant properties, possibly through an atropine-like central action on cerebral motor centers or on the medulla.

Orphenadrine is used primarily to relieve the pain of local muscle spasm and lessen the symptoms of Parkinson's disease, but as an analog of the antihistamine diphenhydramine, excessive quantities can result in antimuscarinic toxicity. Some overdoses of this product have resulted in death.

TABLE 10–4. *Antiparkinsonism agents with selected trade names*

Benztropine (Cogentin)
Biperiden (Akineton)
Ethopropazine (Parsidol)
Orphenadrine (Norflex, Flexon, Norgesic)
Procyclidine (Kemadrin)
Trihexyphenidyl (Artane, Tremin, Trihexane)

Orphenadrine may reduce skeletal muscle spasm, possibly through an atropine-like central action on cerebral motor centers or on the medulla. The drug does not have direct skeletal muscle relaxant activity. It has been suggested that the drug may have analgesic activity that contributes to its effect in patients with skeletal muscle spasm. Orphenadrine also exhibits postganglionic anticholinergic effects and some antihistaminic and local anesthetic action. The antihistaminic activity of orphenadrine is less than that of diphenhydramine; in contrast to the sedative effect of diphenhydramine, orphenadrine produces slight CNS stimulation.

Orphenadrine is a highly lipid-soluble agent that has a half-life of approximately 14 hours. The potentially lethal dose of orphenadrine is 2 to 3 grams in adults, and death usually occurs within 3 to 5 hours as a result of respiratory insufficiency or cardiotoxic effects. Potentially lethal doses in young children are reported to be as low as 600 to 800 mg.

Ethopropazine

Ethopropazine is an antiparkinsonism agent derived from phenothiazine that has a strong atropine-like blocking agent. In addition to antimuscarinic action, the drug exhibits antihistaminic, local anesthetic, ganglionic blocking, and weak adrenolytic activity. Adverse reactions to ethopropazine are mainly extensions of its antimuscarinic effects.

Trihexyphenidyl

Trihexyphenidyl is a synthetic tertiary amine antimuscarinic antiparkinsonism agent that has atropine-like blocking action on parasympathetic innervated peripheral structures. The most frequently abused anticholinergic is trihexyphenidyl, and the dose of abuse ranges from 10 to 30 mg/d.

In common with other antimuscarinic agents, trihexyphenidyl produces an atropine-like blocking action on parasympathetic innervated peripheral structures, including smooth muscle. In addition, trihexyphenidyl exhibits a direct spasmolytic action on smooth muscle and exhibits weak mydriatic, antisialagogue, and cardiovagal blocking effects. The exact mechanism of action of trihexyphenidyl in parkinsonian syndrome is not understood but may result from blockade of efferent impulses and from central inhibition of cerebral motor centers. In small doses, trihexyphenidyl depresses the CNS but larger doses cause cerebral excitement resembling the signs of atropine toxicity.

Adverse effects of trihexyphenidyl may include dryness of the mouth, dizziness, blurred vision, nausea, and nervousness. Other adverse effects typical of those produced by antimuscarinic drugs include constipation, tachycardia, mydriasis, urinary hesitancy or retention, drowsiness, increased intraocular tension, weakness, vomiting, and headache. CNS stimulation, usually manifested by restlessness, agitation, confusion, delirium, and hallucination or euphoria, may occur with high dosage, or in persons with a history of hypersensitivity to other drugs, or in patients with arteriosclerosis. Isolated instances of rashes, dilatation of the colon, paralytic ileus, and suppurative parotitis secondary to dryness of the mouth have been reported. Angle-closure glaucoma has reportedly occurred in patients receiving prolonged therapy with trihexyphenidyl. Rarely, psychiatric disturbances such as delusion, amnesia, depersonalization, and a sense of unreality have been reported with trihexyphenidyl. The incidence and severity of adverse effects are generally dose-related.

ANTISPASMODICS

Dicyclomine is structurally related to the antimuscarinics and is often referred to as an antispasmodic or antimuscarinic-antispasmodic agent. Although the exact mechanism(s) of action of these drugs has not been established, they appear to act as nonselective smooth muscle relaxants. It has been suggested that they have a nonspecific direct action on smooth muscle. These drugs generally have little or no antimuscarinic activity, except at high doses, and little or no effect on gastric secretion. Because these drugs, like the antimuscarinics, have been used as adjunctive therapy for irritable bowel syndrome, they are generally included in discussions on antimuscarinics.

Several semisynthetic quaternary ammonium compounds are used for their atropinic effects; most are used as gastrointestinal antispasmodic agents. They are highly polar and lipid-soluble and are therefore poorly absorbed across biologic membranes. These compounds do not cross the blood–brain barrier, and thus lack CNS activity. The quaternary atropine-like drugs are not suitable for oral use, but are highly suited for aerosolization therapy (3). These and other antimuscarinic-antispasmodics are listed in Table 10–5.

PLANT ALKALOIDS

The genus *Datura* belongs to the family *Solanaceae*, which includes a great number of plants with hypnotic properties, among them the mandrake, deadly nightshade, and henbane (14). Tropane alkaloids, including scopolamine, hyoscyamine, norhyoscyamine, and atropine, have been isolated from these plants. There is great variation in the amounts and percentages of these alkaloids present, depending on the portion of the plant analyzed and the stage of maturation. Those plants of the genus *Datura* produce most cases of antimuscarinic plant poisoning in the United States.

TABLE 10–5. *Miscellaneous antimuscarinic agents with selected trade names*

Agent class	Drugs
Antispasmodic	Adiphenine (Trasentine) Clidinium bromide (Quarzan, Librax, Clindex) Dicyclomine (Bentyl) Methantheline bromide (Banthine) Methixene (Trest) Oxyphencyclimine (Daricon) Propantheline bromide (Pro-Banthine) Mepenzolate bromide (Cantil)
Synthetic belladonna alkaloids	Glycopyrrolate (Robinul) Homatropine (Dia-Quel, Homapin) Methscopolamine bromide (Pamine) Hexocyclium (Tral)
Ophthalmic solutions	Cyclopentolate (Cyclogyl) Eucatropine (Euphthalmine) Tropicamide (Mydriacyl)

The tropane alkaloids, often called belladonna alkaloids, include atropine (hyoscyamine), scopolamine (hyoscine), and ecgonine (cocaine). This group contains the large and commercially important family *Solanaceae*, which includes the medicinal belladonna, the poisonous jimson weed, and the food staples potato, tomato, eggplant, and pepper (Table 10-6).

Belladonna

Belladonna is a term applied to the various preparations of the naturally occurring solanaceous alkaloids. Belladonna leaf is derived from the dried leaf and flowering or

TABLE 10–6. *Plant alkaloids that have antimuscarinic activity*

Alkaloid	Plant (Common name)
Hyoscyamine	*Datura sarvolens* (angel's trumpet) *Datura stramonium* (jimson weed) *Hyoscyamus niger* (henbane) *Atropa belladonna* (deadly nightshade) *Lycium halimifolium* (matrimony vine)
Solanine	*Solanum dulcamara* (European bittersweet) *Solanum nigrum* (black nightshade) *Solanum tuberosum* (common potato) *Solanum pseudocapsicum* (Jerusalem cherry) *Solanum melongena* (eggplant) *Solanum gracile* (wild tomato)
Lycopersicon	(tomato)
Amanitin	*Amanita muscaria* (mushroom)

fruiting top of *Atropa belladonna.* Belladonna leaf contains several alkaloids, principally *l*-hyoscyamine and scopolamine. The pharmacologic activity of belladonna derives principally from its atropine content. *Atropa belladonna* is native to Europe and rare in the United States. Preparations of belladonna are marketed as Donnatal, Hyosophen, Bellalphen, Barbidonna, and Kinesed.

Belladonna leaf is used in the preparation of belladonna extract, belladonna extract tablets, and belladonna tincture; the alkaloid content of these preparations is expressed in terms of the alkaloids of belladonna leaf. Belladonna leaf itself is not used as a therapeutic agent because of the risk of overdosage of the alkaloids.

Atropine

Atropine (D,L-hyoscyamine), a naturally occurring tertiary amine is the main constituent of the traditional drug belladonna from which it was isolated in 1831. It is the prototype antimuscarinic drug. The drug may be prepared synthetically but is usually obtained by extraction from various members of the *Solanaceae* family of plants. As an example atropine is found in the plant *Atropa belladonna*, or deadly nightshade, and in *Datura stramonium*, also known as jimson weed. *Solanum dulcamara*, also known as bittersweet and climbing nightshade, is often inaccurately referred to by the lay public as deadly nightshade (5).

Many atropine-free medications have antimuscarinic pharmacologic properties. While the degree of anticholinergic activity varies between classes of agents and even among the various constituents of a pharmacologic class, the effects are generally not as pronounced as those with atropine.

Pharmacokinetics

In common with other tertiary ammonium products with antimuscarinic properties, atropine is effective when given topically, orally, or by injection. It is quickly and completely absorbed from mucosal surfaces and from the GIT. Its serum half-life in adults is about 3 hours, and may be much longer in young children and the elderly. It has a volume of distribution of 2 to 4 L/kg. The pharmacologic activity of atropine results almost completely from *l*-hyoscyamine; *d*-hyoscyamine has essentially no antimuscarinic activity. In general, atropine is more potent than scopolamine in its antimuscarinic action on the heart, bronchi, and intestinal smooth muscle.

Atropine is highly selective in its action, and the atropinic drugs do not readily inhibit nicotinic stimulation of autonomic ganglia. However, in large doses, atropine can inhibit nicotinic effects in the CNS, the spinal cord, and at voluntary muscle end plates (15).

Toxicity

Poisoning with atropine is uncommon but has been reported in children given atropine eye drops, in individuals who have ingested plants containing belladonna alkaloids, in errors in prescribing and dispensing, and in cases of deliberate self-poisoning (5).

The tissues most sensitive to atropine are the salivary, bronchial, and sweat glands. Secretion of acid by the gastric parietal cells is the least sensitive. Smooth muscle autonomic effectors and the heart are intermediate in responsiveness. Usually, atropine has no significant action on the skin vessels, but toxic doses cause vasodilation and marked flushing (5). A hot, dry, scarlatiniform appearance of the skin is characteristic of atropine poisoning.

In the doses usually used clinically, atropine has mild stimulant effects on medullary centers, especially the vagal nucleus, and a slower, longer-lasting sedative effect (15). The central vagal stimulant effect is frequently sufficient to cause bradycardia, which is later supplanted by tachycardia as the drug's antimuscarinic effects at the sinoatrial node become manifest.

Hyoscyamine

Hyoscyamine is a naturally occurring tertiary amine antimuscarinic. Hyoscyamine is one of the principal alkaloid components of belladonna. During the extraction of belladonna, a racemic mixture of *dl*-hyoscyamine (atropine) is formed. Hyoscyamine and its hydrobromide and sulfate salts are the *l*-isomer. Since hyoscyamine is one of the optical isomers comprising atropine, the pharmacokinetics of hyoscyamine (*l*-hyoscyamine) and atropine (*dl*-hyoscyamine) are generally considered similar.

Scopolamine

Scopolamine is a naturally occurring tertiary amine antimuscarinic. It is one of the principal antimuscarinic components of the belladonna alkaloids (16). The drug may be prepared synthetically but is usually obtained by extraction from various members of the *Solanaceae* genus of plants including *Datura metel* (datura herb), *D. stramonium* (jimson weed), *Hyoscyamus niger* (henbane), and *Scopolia carniolica.* Scopolamine (*l*-hyoscine) is a belladonna alkaloid and is among the oldest drugs in medicine.

The peripheral cholinergic blocking actions of scopolamine and atropine are similar; the two drugs differ mainly in their CNS effects. Unlike atropine and most other antimuscarinic agents, scopolamine, at usual dosages, produces CNS depression manifested as drowsiness, euphoria, amnesia, fatigue, and dreamless sleep. Higher doses of scopolamine produce CNS effects similar to those produced by toxic doses of other antimuscarinics. Pure scopolamine intoxications are extremely rare. Scopolamine is more potent than is atropine in its effect on the iris and the ciliary body, and on salivary, bronchial, and sweat glands. It is somewhat less effective as a bronchodilator, and it is weaker than atropine in its action on the heart and the intestinal tract. Its action is shorter lasting than that of atropine, and it has more side effects.

Unlike atropine and most other antimuscarinics, scopolamine, at usual dosages, produces CNS depression manifested as drowsiness, euphoria, amnesia, fatigue, and dreamless sleep (with a reduction in rapid eye movement). However, excitement, restlessness, hallucinations, or delirium may paradoxically occur, especially when scopolamine is used in the presence of severe pain. High doses of scopolamine produce CNS effects (e.g., restlessness, disorientation, irritability, hallucinations) similar to those produced by toxic doses of other antimuscarinics (10).

Although other antimuscarinics have been used in the prevention of motion sickness, it appears that scopolamine is the most effective. Scopolamine apparently corrects some central imbalance of acetylcholine and norepinephrine that may occur in patients with motion sickness. It has been suggested that antimuscarinics may block the transmission of cholinergic impulses from the vestibular nuclei to higher centers in the CNS and from the reticular formation to the vomiting center; these effects result in prevention of motion-induced nausea and vomiting.

Transdermal Scopolamine

A transdermal preparation is now available for treatment of motion sickness. The patches contain scopolamine 1.5 mg, of which 0.5 mg is gradually released over 3 days. After a used patch is discarded, a significant amount of scopolamine still remains, and antimuscarinic poisoning can develop if the discarded patch is ingested by a child (17).

Jimson Weed

Jimson weed (*Datura stramonium*), a member of the nightshade family, grows wild throughout the U.S. and is typically found in open, rich soil such as gardens and farms, in waste areas, and along roadsides. The plant is an annual that reaches 5 to 6 feet in height and has dark green leaves and a purple-green stem. In the spring, the plant has trumpet-shaped blue or white flowers; in the fall the plant produces an ovoid with spinous capsules that burst to release the black seeds (18). These are common annuals, and more than a dozen species occur across the country. Other common names include loco weed, devil's weed, thornapple and Jamestown weed (18).

References to jimson weed are found as far back as Homer's *Odyssey*. Early settlers in Jamestown, Virginia, were familiar with jimson weed as a potted herb and brought seeds from England. The plant was used in Jamestown to make tea for treating asthma. In the U.S., the plant was named Jamestown weed, which was eventually altered to jimson weed. Most cases of poisoning relate to ingestion or inhalation of extracts of *Datura stramonium*. The plant is also smoked in cigarettes and prepared as a powder (18).

In the United States, poisoning with jimson weed has shifted from accidental childhood poisonings to inadvertent overdoses in persons experimenting with mind-altering drugs. Recreational users usually ingest the seeds whole or make a tea with the leaves, but all parts of the plant are toxic. Intoxication with jimson weed is not uncommon in rural areas, especially among adolescents who may use the plant as a natural hallucinogen. As little as one-half teaspoonful of the seeds has been reported to cause death from cardiac and pulmonary arrest (18).

Datura stramonium has also been marketed as Asthmador, a preparation sold in health food stores as an asthma medication.

Anisotropine

Anisotropine is a synthetic antimuscarinic used as an adjunct in the treatment of peptic ulcer disease. Following oral administration, less than 10% of a dose is absorbed. This is because anisotropine is a quaternary ammonium drug that is completely ionized in the GIT.

Glycopyrrolate

Glycopyrrolate is a synthetic quaternary ammonium antimuscarinic. Glycopyrrolate, like other quaternary ammonium compounds is completely ionized in the GIT, resulting in incomplete absorption from the GIT.

Glycopyrrolate is used orally to control gastric acid output. It is a more effective antisialagogue than is atropine, and it can also prevent vagal reactions. The drug is often used for premedication for anesthesia and for bronchoscopy. It is available as glycopyrrolate methylbromide (Robinul).

Following IV administration of glycopyrrolate, the drug has an onset of action of about 1 minute. Following intramuscular (IM) or subcutaneous injection, pharmacologic effects are evident within 15–30 minutes, and peak within 30–45 minutes. The vagal blocking effects of the drug persist for 2–3 hours, and inhibition of salivation persists for up to 7 hours after parenteral administration of the drug. Following oral administration, the anticholinergic effects of glycopyrrolate may persist for up to 8–12 hours.

Homatropine

This is a semisynthetic product that is weaker than atropine, and is mainly used in ophthalmologic practice, where its short antimuscarinic action is an advantage. It is occasionally used as a drying agent in combination proprietary cough and cold products. Following topical application to the eye, homatropine hydrobromide blocks the responses of the sphincter muscle of the iris and ciliary muscle of the lens to cholinergic stimulation, thereby producing mydriasis and cycloplegia. Homatropine hydrobromide is a relatively short-acting mydriatic and cycloplegic agent, and has a shorter duration of action than atropine. The maximum mydriatic effect of homatropine hydrobromide occurs in about 10–30 minutes, and the maximum cycloplegic effect occurs in about 30–90 minutes. Mydriasis may last 6 hours to 4 days, and cycloplegia may persist 10–48 hours.

Propantheline

The pharmacologic actions of this compound are qualitatively identical with those of atropine, but in contrast to atropine, propantheline has a high ratio of ganglionic blocking to antimuscarinic activity. Moreover, an unusual toxicity with overdosage is the production of neuromuscular blockade resembling a curare-like action.

Hydrolysis of propantheline actually begins in the GIT. After a single oral dose, peak serum concentrations occur in about 1 hour. Plasma half-life of propantheline is approximately 2 hours. Propantheline bromide, like other quaternary ammonium drugs, is incompletely absorbed from the GIT since it is completely ionized. There is considerable interindividual variation in the extent of absorption following oral administration of the drug. Food appears to substantially decrease the extent of absorption of propantheline bromide. Propantheline bromide appears to undergo extensive metabolism in the upper small intestine prior to absorption.

Aerosolized Antimuscarinics

Only three antimuscarinics are currently available as inhalational agents in the U.S.: atropine sulfate, ipratropium bromide, and glycopyrrolate. The antimuscarinic drugs have a slower onset of bronchodilation than do the sympathomimetic aerosols, and they are less reliable as prophylactic agents for allergic and exercise-induced asthma (19). Progressive bronchodilation is produced by antimuscarinic drugs over a period of up to 2 hours, whereas most adrenergic bronchodilators attain a peak effect by 30 minutes. The evidence suggests that the adrenergic bronchodilators have a major effect on the more distal bronchioles, whereas the antimuscarinic agents act on the more centrally concentrated muscarinic receptors.

Atropine and ipratropium are potent bronchodilators, particularly in large bronchial airways, and are especially effective in reversing bronchoconstriction induced by parasympathetic stimulation. Antimuscarinics cause relaxation of smooth muscles of the bronchi and bronchioles with a resultant decrease in airway resistance. Antimuscarinics reduce the volume of secretions from the nose, mouth, pharynx, and bronchi.

The autonomic control of bronchoconstriction and the release of bronchoconstrictor substances from mast cells appear to be mediated by cyclic nucleotides. Antimuscarinics block acetylcholine-induced stimulation of guanyl cyclase and thus reduce tissue concentrations of cyclic guanosine monophosphate (cGMP), a mediator of bronchoconstriction.

Atropine Sulfate

Atropine sulfate is a tertiary amine that is well absorbed orally and by the aerosol route so that even the commonly used aerosol doses may produce toxicity in patients with an impaired ability to eliminate the drug.

Ipratropium

Ipratropium (Atrovent), the *N*-isopropyl derivative of atropine, was synthesized in the 1960s and has been available in Europe for many years. The aerosol route of administration provides the advantages of maximal concentration at the bronchial target tissue with reduced systemic effects (20).

Ipratropium is poorly absorbed when administered by mouth. It is readily soluble in water, and its solution is well suited for aerosol delivery into the respiratory tract. Following an inhaled dose, a small proportion is absorbed through the pulmonary epithelium, but the amount entering the circulation is negligible. The elimination half-life is similar for all routes of administration, being 3 to 4 hours.

The side effects that may occur with aerosolized atropine are less likely to be seen with the therapeutic dosage range of ipratropium.

TRICYCLIC ANTIDEPRESSANTS

The tricyclic antidepressants are described in Chapter 16.

MISCELLANEOUS COMPOUNDS

Other antimuscarinic agents include the synthetic relatives of the belladonna alkaloids, 17 ophthalmic solutions, and antispasmodic agents (Table 10–5).

CLINICAL MANIFESTATIONS OF INTOXICATION

The blocking of the action of acetylcholine on the muscarinic receptors results in the antimuscarinic syndrome:

"Hot as a hare, (blockade of sweat secretion),
Blind as a bat, (mydriasis and spasm of accommodation)
Dry as a bone, (blockade of salivary secretion),
Red as a beet, (cutaneous vasodilation),
Mad as a hatter." (cortical stimulation).

To some extent, adverse effects of antimuscarinics correlate with their structural class. Naturally occurring alkaloids possess the full range of antimuscarinic and antinicotinic activities of atropine and thus have the potential for producing adverse central and peripheral effects associated with atropine. Quaternary ammonium compounds are completely ionized at physiologic pH and are less soluble than tertiary amine compounds. As a result, quaternary ammonium compounds are relatively less active orally than tertiary amine compounds and exhibit fewer effects in the CNS and the eye.

The signs and symptoms of antimuscarinic poisoning can be divided into peripheral and central effects (Table 10–7). The classic presentation is rarely observed unless the toxic exposure is to a chemical with rather pure antimuscarinic properties. Many of the agents with antimuscarinic properties also exhibit other pharmacologic characteristics that tend to ameliorate or overshadow the antimuscarinic effects.

TABLE 10–7. *Signs and symptoms of antimuscarinic poisoning*

Peripheral effects
Sinus tachycardia
Mydriasis
Cycloplegia
Blurred vision
Vasodilation
Dry skin
Hyperpyrexia
Hypertension
Decreased secretions
Bronchi
Pharynx
Nasal
Salivary
Urinary retention
Decreased bowel motility
Central
Delirium
Anxiety
Hyperactivity
Hallucinations
Disorientation
Incoherence
Confusion
Paranoia
Restlessness
Seizure
Impairment of recent memory
Clonus
Hyperreflexia
Coma

Peripheral Manifestations of Toxicity

Peripheral toxicity may be manifested by sinus tachycardia; dilated and unreactive pupils; blurred vision; vasodilation and flushing; dry skin; hyperpyrexia; hypertension; decreased bronchial, pharyngeal, nasal, and salivary secretions; urinary retention; and decreased bowel motility. The intestinal inhibition that is induced by antimuscarinic drugs is temporary, because local mechanisms will usually reestablish some peristalsis after 1–3 days of antimuscarinic therapy.

Thermoregulatory sweating is suppressed by antimuscarinic drugs. The muscarinic receptors on eccrine sweat glands are innervated by sympathetic cholinergic fibers and are readily accessible to antimuscarinic drugs. In adults, body temperature is elevated by this effect only if large doses are administered, but in infants and children even ordinary doses may cause "atropine fever." The cutaneous flush that follows high doses of atropine is due to direct depression of arteriolar smooth muscle. Atropine is also a fairly potent local anesthetic and a histamine-1 receptor blocker in high doses.

The pupillary constrictor muscle is dependent on muscarinic-cholinergic activation. This activation is effectively blocked by topical atropine and other tertiary antimuscarinic drugs and results in unopposed sympathetic dilator activity and mydriasis. The second important ocular effect of atropine and other antimuscarinics is paralysis of the ciliary muscle, or cycloplegia. The result of cycloplegia is loss of the ability to accommodate; the fully atropinized eye cannot focus for near vision.

The relative sensitivity of physiologic functions, proceeding from the most sensitive, is as follows: secretions of the salivary, bronchial, and sweat glands; pupillary dilation, ocular accommodation, and heart rate; contraction of the detrusor muscle of the bladder and smooth muscle of the GIT; and gastric secretion and motility (Table 10-8).

Cardiac effects of antimuscarinics are dose-dependent. Average doses of antimuscarinics (0.4–0.6 mg of atropine)

TABLE 10-8. *Relative sensitivities of muscarinic physiologic function (descending order)*

Dry secretions
Mydriasis
Cycloplegia
Sinus tachycardia
Urinary retention
Decreased gastrointestinal motility
Decreased gastric acid secretion

may produce a slight decrease in heart rate attributable to central vagal stimulation that occurs before peripheral cholinergic blockade. Larger doses of antimuscarinics cause progressively increasing tachycardia by blocking normal vagal inhibition of the sinoatrial node.

In addition to blocking of the muscarinic receptor, atropine can block nicotinic cholinergic receptors at autonomic ganglion cells and the motor end plate of skeletal muscle, but only in doses far in excess of those employed clinically.

Central Nervous System Manifestations of Toxicity

Acute overdosage generally produces CNS stimulation with subsequent depression. These manifestations may resemble acute psychosis characterized by various neuropsychiatric signs and symptoms, including disorientation, incoherence, confusion, hallucinations (which are usually visual but may also be auditory or tactile), delusions, and paranoia. Disturbed speech and abnormal motor behavior such as ataxia, incoordination, agitation, and restlessness may also occur. In children antimuscarinic toxicity is commonly manifested as hyperpyrexia (21). Severe impairment of recent memory is a prominent symptom. Comatose patients may display clonic movements, hyperreflexia, and extensor plantar reflexes. Grand mal seizures are also a result of central antimuscarinic activity.

Typically, adults manifest CNS depression as somnolence, weakness, and coma after overdose; seizures are uncommon. Children manifest CNS stimulation as agitation, hallucinations, and ataxia; seizures are more common than in adults.

Manifestations of Severe Overdosage

In severe overdosage, CNS depression, circulatory collapse, and hypotension may occur. Coma and skeletal muscle paralysis may also occur and may be followed by death from respiratory failure. Death has also reportedly resulted from hyperpyrexia, especially in children. Additive adverse effects resulting from cholinergic blockade may occur when antimuscarinics are administered concomitantly with phenothiazines, amantadines, antiparkinsonism drugs, glutethimide, meperidine, tricyclic antidepressants, quinidine, disopyramide, antihistamines, or any other drug with prominent antimuscarinic effects (22).

Quaternary Ammonium Products

Poisoning caused by high doses of the quaternary antimuscarinic drugs is associated with all of the peripheral signs of parasympathetic blockade but few or none of the CNS effects of atropine. Quaternary ammonium antimuscarinics generally possess varying degrees of nicotinic blocking activity and may interfere with ganglionic or neuromuscular transmission at doses that block muscarinic receptors. At high doses, quaternary ammonium antimuscarinics may produce substantial ganglionic blockade with resultant impotence, and postural hypotension. In overdosage, a curariform neuromuscular block may ensue. Treatment of the antimuscarinic effects, if required, can be carried out with a quaternary cholinesterase inhibitor.

Systemic Manifestations after Ophthalmic Administration

Antimuscarinic eyedrops have caused systemic effects. After instillation of the compound into the conjunctival sac, systemic absorption may occur through the conjunctival capillaries by simple diffusion as well as through the nasal mucosa, oral pharynx, and gastrointestinal tract after passage through the lacrimal drainage system (23). Reactions to ophthalmic ointments are less frequent than reactions to eyedrops because of reduced absorption of ointments by the conjunctiva and lack of lacrimal duct passage. In some cases, atropine may produce an initial transitory central vagal stimulant action before the blocking effect is manifested. This is especially true when it is administered in large amounts. Symptoms noted after ophthalmic administration consist of restlessness, insomnia, ataxia, hallucinations, confusion (which at times progresses to supraventricular tachycardia), seizures, coma, and death (24,25). Agents that have caused these symptoms include atropine, scopolamine, homatropine, and cyclopentolate.

Ophthalmic Instillation in Children

There are several reported cases of anticholinergic psychosis following the administration of atropine sulfate and homatropine ophthalmic drops in children. The clinical picture tends to be a uniform one. Ataxia occurs early and can be so severe that the patient is unable to stand. Restlessness is a very prominent sign with periods of hyperactivity. These episodes of restlessness often alternate with periods of relative quiet in which the patient sits and stares, talking senselessly. Vivid visual hallucinations with an element of fear are noted frequently. Evidence of retrograde amnesia is often noted. Coma and convulsions have also been described. Reactions may subside in a few hours, although the majority of patients described needed 6–24 hours to recover.

Ophthalmic Instillation in Adults

Anticholinergic psychosis in adults following the administration of atropine and homatropine ophthalmic drops have also been reported. The signs and symptoms of these reactions are similar to those seen in children. Hallucinations, although usually visual, may also be auditory or tactile (23). The patient commonly claims to see animals, insects, or snakes. In addition, these hallucinations may evoke conversations with invisible people, smoking of imaginary cigarettes, or picking at nonexistent insects on clothing.

Ophthalmic Instillation in the Elderly

Clinicians should be aware that the elderly, especially nursing home patients, may be more vulnerable and subject to more significant complications from adverse reactions to anticholinergic ophthalmic drugs. Decreased renal function in the elderly may result in a decreased rate of elimination and accumulation of systemically absorbed anticholinergic ophthalmic medications. Several cases of changes in mental status associated with atropine, homatropine, cyclopentolate, and scopolamine ophthalmic medications have been described. In the elderly, especially nursing home residents, these reactions may be overlooked or misinterpreted as a progression of a patient's current diagnosis or new onset of dementia or psychosis (23).

LABORATORY ANALYSIS

In all cases of acutely altered mental status, blood should be obtained and analyzed for glucose, blood urea nitrogen, serum electrolytes, complete blood count, toxicologic screen, and arterial blood gas. Specific testing for antimuscarinics is usually of no value.

TREATMENT

The treatment of an acute overdose of an antimuscarinic agent consists of symptomatic and supportive therapy (Table 10–9). Removal of the material from the gastrointestinal tract should be attempted in the acute overdose, and should be followed by administration of activated charcoal and a cathartic. Fluid therapy and other standard treatments of shock should be administered as needed.

TABLE 10–9. *Treatment of antimuscarinic toxicity*

Condition	Treatment
Acute overdose	Monitor, prevent absorption
Ventricular ectopy	Lidocaine (1 mg/kg IV)
Seizure	Diazepam (5 to 10 mg IV)
Hyperthermia	Active cooling
Acute psychosis	Diazepam (5 to 10 mg IV) ?Physostigmine (1 to 2 mg IV)
Urinary retention	Urinary catheterization

In most cases, patients with anticholinergic syndrome will require only careful observation, and supportive care. However, it may be necessary to directly counteract this central and peripheral blockade by increasing the amount of acetylcholine available to compete with the antimuscarinic agent (20).

Patients with any evidence of cardiac dysrhythmias must be monitored. Ventricular ectopy in the absence of atrioventricular block may be treated with lidocaine. Because many of the antimuscarinic agents have a quinidine-like action, the use of procainamide, quinidine, or disopyramide should be avoided. Precautions against seizure must be undertaken. Hyperthermia is usually treated with cold packs, mechanical cooling devices, or sponging with tepid water. Diazepam may be administered to control excitement, delirium, or other symptoms of acute psychosis. Phenothiazines should not be used because they may contribute to antimuscarinic effects. If the patient is comatose, urinary catheterization should be performed to avoid urinary retention. Conjunctival application of pilocarpine may be used to counteract mydriasis.

Because most of the antimuscarinic agents are rapidly distributed to the tissues and have large volumes of distribution, little free drug is present in the plasma. Thus treatment modalities such as hemodialysis, hemoperfusion, and forced diuresis are of little benefit (26). In addition to supportive care, the intravenous use of physostigmine may be efficacious under certain circumstances.

Antidotal Therapy with Acetylcholinesterase Inhibitors

Anticholinesterase agents are antidotal agents that inhibit acetylcholinesterase, the enzyme that breaks down acetylcholine and allows acetylcholine to accumulate and to overcome the competitive inhibition of antimuscarinic agents (27). Some of these agents include physostigmine (Antilirium), neostigmine (Prostigmin), pyridostigmine (Mestinon), and edrophonium (Tensilon).

Physostigmine

Physostigmine belongs to a class of drugs known as acetylcholinesterase inhibitors (28). These anticholinesterases allow for the buildup of naturally generated acetylcholine, thereby reversing the effects of antimuscarinic overdose; thus, systemic administration of physostigmine salicylate produces generalized cholinergic responses including miosis, increased tonus of intestinal musculature, constriction of bronchi, and stimulation of secretion by salivary and sweat glands (29).

Physostigmine differs from other antimuscarinic compounds in that it is a tertiary amine, a nonionized lipophilic compound that can cross the blood–brain barrier and reverse both the peripheral and central effects of an antimuscarinic overdose (30). The other compounds are quaternary ammonium compounds, and, because they are charged molecules, they are not able to cross the blood–brain barrier and therefore will reverse only the peripheral antimuscarinic effects (29,31).

Indications for Use of Physostigmine

Treatment with physostigmine must be based on the presence of the antimuscarinic syndrome and not merely on a history of ingestion because the use of physostigmine is not without complications (Table 10–10) (32). Because of the potential for producing severe adverse effects, its use should be reserved for treatment of patients with extreme delirium or agitation who have the potential for inflicting injuries on themselves; for patients with severe, hemodynamically significant sinus tachycardia or supraventricular tachycardia; for patients with repetitive or long-lasting seizures; or for patients with extreme hyperthermia unresponsive to mechanical cooling (1). In other words, physostigmine should be used only in situations where a potential life-threatening emergency exists (33). Coma is not an indication for the use of physostigmine, other than to confirm a diagnosis.

When the drug is administered parenterally, it has an onset of action of 3–8 minutes and a duration of action of 30 minutes to 5 hours.

TABLE 10–10. *Use of physostigmine for antimuscarinic overdose*

Indications
Diagnostic
Therapeutic
Supraventricular dysrhythmias
Supraventricular
Seizures
Myoclonus
Hallucinations
Hypertension
Dosage
Adult: 1 to 2 mg IV, slowly
Child: 0.5 mg or 0.02 mg/kg IV, slowly
Cholinergic Side Effects
Bradycardia
Miosis
Increased secretions
Salivation
Lacrimation
Rhinorrhea
Pulmonary
Urination
Defecation
Seizures
Cardiac Side Effects
Shift of pacemaker from sinoatrial node to another site
Slowing of conduction through atrioventricular node
Prolonging of refractory period
Production of atrioventricular block
Asystole

Dosage

In adults, 1 to 2 mg of physostigmine may be administered intravenously. In children, a dose of 0.5 mg or 0.02 mg/kg may be administered intravenously. Physostigmine is available in 2-mL sterile vials containing 1 mg/mL (13). It should be diluted to 10 mL in dextrose in water or normal saline and given over 2–5 minutes (17). The half-life of physostigmine varies from 15 to 90 minutes, which may necessitate repeated doses for long-acting antimuscarinic compounds (34).

Contraindications to the Use of Physostigmine

Relative contraindications to the use of physostigmine are diabetes, glaucoma, asthma, heart block, coronary artery disease, gangrene, peptic ulcer disease, and ulcerative colitis. The absolute contraindications are mechanical obstruction of the gastrointestinal and genitourinary tracts (2). Physostigmine should be used with caution in patients with epilepsy, parkinsonian syndromes, or bradycardia. The drug should not be administered to patients receiving choline esters (e.g., methacholine, bethanechol) or depolarizing neuromuscular blocking agents (e.g., decamethonium, succinylcholine) (2).

Complications from Physostigmine

Adverse effects of parenterally administered physostigmine salicylate are chiefly those of exaggerated response to parasympathetic stimulation and include epigastric pain, miosis, salivation, sweating, lacrimation, dyspnea, and bronchospasm. The most common complications from the use of physostigmine are nausea and vomiting (35). If physostigmine is used in the absence of antimuscarinic overdose, patients may manifest the signs of cholinergic toxicity, including salivation, lacrimation, urination, defecation, gastrointestinal upset, and emesis. If cholinergic crisis occurs, an antimuscarinic agent may be necessary.

Stimulation of the CNS, restlessness, irregular pulse, palpitation, hallucinations, muscular twitching, and weakness may also occur. Seizures, collapse, and death from respiratory paralysis and/or pulmonary edema have occurred rarely. Rapid IV administration of physostigmine may produce bradycardia, hypersalivation leading to respiratory problems, or possibly seizures (35).

REFERENCES

1. Goldfrank L, Flomenbaum N, Lewin N. et al: Anticholinergic poisoning. *J Toxicol Clin Toxicol* 1982;19:17–25.
2. Richmond M, Seger D: Central anticholinergic syndrome in a child: a case report. *J Emerg Med* 1985;3: 453–456.
3. Ziment I, Au J: Anticholinergic agents. *Clin Chest Med* 1986;7:355–366.

4. Feldman M, Behar M: A case of massive diphenhydramine abuse and withdrawal from use of the drug. *JAMA* 1986;255:3119–3120.
5. Goetting M, Contreras E: Systemic atropine administration during cardiac arrest does not cause fixed and dilated pupils. *Ann Emerg Med* 1991;20:55–57.
6. Popa V: The classic antihistamines (H_1 blockers) in respiratory medicine. *Clin Chest Med* 1986;7:364–382.
7. Sankey R, Nunn A, Sills J: Visual hallucinations in children receiving decongestants. *Br Med J* 1984;288:1369.
8. Koppel C, Ibe K, Tenczer J: Clinical symptomatology of diphenhydramine overdose: an evaluation of 136 cases in 1982 to 1985. *Clin Toxicol* 1987;25:53–70.
9. Bratt K, Zagerman A: Dyskinesias after antihistamine use. *N Engl J Med* 1977;196:111–114.
10. Crowell E, Ketchum J: The treatment of scopolamine-induced delirium with physostigmine. *Clin Pharmacol Ther* 1978;8:409–414.
11. Hestand H, Teske D: Diphenhydramine hydrochloride intoxication. *J Pediatr* 1977;90:1017–1018.
12. Lavenstein B, Cantor F: Acute dystonia: an unusual reaction to diphenhydramine. *JAMA* 1976;236:291–292.
13. Howrie D, Rowley A, Krenzelok E: Benztropine-induced acute dystonic reaction. *Ann Emerg Med* 1986;15:594–596.
14. Hayman J: Datura poisoning—the angel's trumpet. *Pathology* 1985;17:465–466.
15. Amitai Y, Almog S, Singer R, et al: Atropine poisoning in children during the Persian Gulf crisis. *JAMA* 1992;268:630–632.
16. Thornton W: Sleep aids and sedatives. *JACEP* 1977;6:408–412.
17. Wilkinson J: Side effects of transdermal scopolamine. *J Emerg Med* 1987;5:389–392.
18. Vanderhoff B, Mosser K: Jimson weed toxicity: management of anticholinergic plant ingestion. *Am Fam Physician* 1992;46:526–530.
19. Runge J, Martinez J, Caravati E, et al: Histamine antagonists in the treatment of acute allergic reactions. *Ann Emerg Med* 1992;21: 237–242.
20. Kelly H, Murphy S: Should anticholinergics be used in acute severe asthma? *DICP Ann Pharmacother* 1990;24:409–416.
21. Magera B, Betlach C, Sweatt A, et al: Hydroxyzine intoxication in a 13-month-old child. *Pediatrics* 1981;67:280–283.
22. Clark R, Vance M: Massive diphenhydramine poisoning resulting in a wide-complex tachycardia: successful treatment with sodium bicarbonate. *Ann Emerg Med* 1992;21:318–321.
23. Barker D, Solomon D: The potential for mental status changes associated with systemic absorption of anticholinergic ophthalmic medications: concerns in the elderly. *DICP Ann Pharmacother* 1990;24:847–850.
24. Merli G, Weitz H, Martin J, et al: Cardiac dysrhythmias associated with ophthalmic atropine. *Arch Intern Med* 1986;146:45–47.
25. Adler A, McElwain G, Merli G, et al: Systemic effects of eye drops. *Arch Intern Med* 1982;142:2293–2294.
26. Worth D, Davison A, Roberts T, et al: Ineffectiveness of hemodialysis in atropine poisoning. *Br Med J* 1983;286:2023–2024.
27. Ullman K, Groh R: Identification and treatment of acute psychotic states secondary to the usage of over-the-counter sleeping preparations. *Am J Psychiatry* 1972;128:64–68.
28. Brashares Z, Conley W: Physostigmine in drug overdose. *JACEP* 1975;4:46–48.
29. Nattel S, Bayne L, Ruedy J: Physostigmine in coma due to drug overdose. *Clin Pharmacol Ther* 1979;25:96–102.
30. Granacher R, Baldessarini R: Physostigmine: its use in acute anticholinergic syndrome with antidepressant and antiparkinson drugs. *Arch Gen Psychiatry* 1975;32:375–379.
31. Janowsky D, Risch S, Heuy L: Central cardiovascular effects of physostigmine in humans. *Hypertension* 1985;7:140–145.
32. Levy R: Arrhythmias following physostigmine administration in jimson weed poisoning. *JACEP* 1977;6:107–108.
33. Hussey H: Physostigmine: value in treatment of central toxic effects of anticholinergic drugs. *JAMA* 1975;231:1066.
34. Lauwers L, Daelemans R, Baute L, et al: Scopolamine intoxications. *Intensive Care Med* 1983;9:283–285.
35. Rumack B: Anticholinergic poisoning: treatment with physostigmine. *Pediatrics* 1973;52:449–451.

ADDITIONAL SELECTED REFERENCES

Bailie G, Nelson M, Krenzelok E, et al: Unusual treatment response of a severe dystonia to diphenhydramine. *Ann Emerg Med* 1987;16:705–715.

Cockrell J: Acute hallucinogenic reaction to carbinoxamine maleate. *Clin Toxicol* 1987;25:161–167.

Furlanut M, Bettio I, Bertin G, et al: Orphenadrine serum levels in a poisoned patient. *Hum Toxicol* 1985;4:331–333.

Hooper R, Conner C, Rumack B: Acute poisoning from over-the-counter sleep preparations. *JACEP* 1979;8:98–100.

Kaplan M, Register D, Bierman A, et al: A nonfatal case of intentional scopolamine poisoning. *Clin Toxicol* 1974;7:509–512.

Krenzelok E, Anderson G, Mirick M: Massive diphenhydramine overdose resulting in death. *Ann Emerg Med* 1982;11:212–213.

Lacouture P, Lovejoy F, Mitchell A: Acute hypothermia associated with atropine. *Am J Dis Child* 1983;137:291–292.

Pentel P, Peterson C: Asystole complicating physostigmine treatment of tricyclic antidepressant overdose. *Ann Emerg Med* 1980;9:588–590.

Schuster P, Gabriel E, Kufferle B, et al: Reversal by physostigmine of clozapine-induced delirium. *Clin Toxicol* 1977;10:437–441.

Spaulding B, Choi S, Gross J, et al: The effect of physostigmine on diazepam-induced ventilatory depression: a double-blind study. *Anesthesiology* 1984;61:551–554.

CHAPTER 11

Antihistaminic Agents

Histamine was identified in 1911 as a potent vasoactive substance and was subsequently found to have many other physiologic activities. It was not until 60 years after its discovery that histamine's activities were shown to be mediated through two types of receptors. The allergy-related effects of histamine are mediated through its H_1 receptor and include smooth muscle contraction, increased vascular permeability, and pruritus (1). The H_2 receptors are located primarily in parietal cells in the stomach.

The H_2 antagonists have been in use since the 1970s and have become the most commonly employed method of decreasing acid production. Because of this, antihistamine ingestions are among the most common poisonings noted. The nonprescription status of many of the H_1 blockers as well as its ubiquitous presence in cough, cold, and sedative preparations account for the large number of both accidental and intentional ingestions (2).

It is now known that the histamine receptors are not as simple as originally thought. Three histamine receptors have now been isolated, and knowledge of their function can help predict the clinical features expected (Table 11–1)

The histamine-1 (H_1) receptor is responsible for coronary artery vasoconstriction, bronchoconstriction, cutaneous vascular permeability, and intestinal smooth muscle contraction. The H_2 receptor stimulates the ventricular and atrial isotropy, atrial chronotropy, coronary vasodilation, and gastric acid secretion. The H_3 receptors, on the other hand, inhibit central and peripheral nervous system neurotransmitter release and may inhibit histamine formation.

TABLE 11–1. *The histaminic receptors*

Histamine-1 receptor (H_1)
Bronchoconstriction
Coronary artery vasoconstriction
Cutaneous vascular permeability
Intestinal smooth muscle contraction
Histamine-2 receptor (H_2)
Atrial chronotropy
Coronary vasodilation
Gastric acid secretion
Ventricular and atrial isotropy
Histamine-3 receptor (H_3)
Inhibition of central and peripheral neurotransmitter release
Inhibition of histamine formation

H_1 ANTAGONISTS

H_1 receptor antagonists were discovered more than 50 years ago and have been in clinical use for more than 40 years. The first-generation H_1 receptor antagonists are known to be effective in the treatment of seasonal allergic rhinitis, but sedative and antimuscarinic side effects limit their use in many patients.

The H_1 antagonists are the major components of most over-the-counter sedatives and sleeping aids. These antihistamines have a number of actions including antimuscarinic, local anesthetic, antispasmodic and to treat motion sickness. Some antihistamines also demonstrate a quinidine-like effect on myocardial conduction, and some enhance the pressor action of norepinephrine. Part of the antiemetic and anti–motion-sickness actions of some antihistamines are a result of their central antimuscarinic and central nervous system depressant properties (2).

Traditional first-generation antihistamines are often classified according to these other groupings as amino alkyl ethers (diphenhydramine, clemastine), ethylenediamines (pyrilamine, tripelennamine), alkylamines (brompheniramine, chlorpheniramine, dexchlorpheni-

TABLE 11–2. *Selected first-generation antihistaminics*

Aminoalkyl ethers
Diphenhydramine
Clemastine
Ethylenediamines
Pyrilamine
Tripelennamine
Alkylamines
Brompheniramine
Chlorpheniramine
Dexchlorpheniramine
Triprolidine
Phenothiazines
Methdilazine
Promethazine
Trimeprazine

ramine, triprolidine), and phenothiazines (methdilazine, promethazine, trimeprazine) (Table 11–2) Several agents have widely varying added groupings. Cyproheptadine and its derivative, azatadine, contain a tricyclic nucleus with an attached piperidine side ring (3).

First-Generation Antihistaminics

Most of the clinical features of older antihistaminic poisoning are due to antimuscarinic toxicity, and the patient with this toxicity may present with a central or peripheral antimuscarinic syndrome (Chapter 10). Antimuscarinic poisoning is not a feature of the newer "second-generation" H_1 antihistaminics.

In general, the ethylenediamine derivatives have relatively weak central nervous system effects, but drowsiness may occur in some patients. Ethanolamine derivatives commonly cause central nervous system (CNS) depression. Propylamine derivatives cause less drowsiness and more CNS stimulation than the other antihistamines. These effects are frequently present when these drugs are used therapeutically, and they predominate when overdosage occurs.

Although antihistamines have relatively high therapeutic indexes, overdosage may result in death, especially in infants and children. Absorption of transdermal antihistamines as well as aerosol antihistamines has resulted in intoxication and organic psychosis in children.

Pharmacokinetics

The first-generation antihistamines, brompheniramine, chlorpheniramine, promethazine, diphenhydramine, and hydroxyzine are metabolized by the liver and thus may accumulate in patients with severe hepatic disease. The elimination half-lives of these agents are: diphenhydramine, about 8 hours; hydroxyzine, about 20 hours; promethazine, 10 to 14 hours; chlorpheniramine, 14 to 25 hours; and brompheniramine, about 25 hours. Total body clearances in adults range from 5 to 12 mL/kg/min, and apparent volumes of distribution are large (>4 L/kg).

Following oral administration of most first-generation agents, effects begin within 15 to 30 minutes and persist for 4 to 24 hours. Alkylamines, piperazines, and phenothiazines may have a considerably longer duration of action. The duration of action of an antihistamine cannot be predicted by its half-life and must be determined by assessment of clinical effects and duration of wheal suppression (4).

Actions Not Caused by Histamine Receptor Blockade

The older, first-generation H_1 receptor antagonists have many actions not ascribable to blockade of the actions of histamine (Table 11–3). The large number of these actions probably results from the similarity of the H_1 antagonist general structure to the structure of drugs that have effects at muscarinic cholinoceptor, α adrenoceptor, serotonin, and local anesthetic receptor sites. Some of these actions are of therapeutic value, and some are undesirable. The second-generation antihistamines that lack these effects are now available, and more are being investigated (2).

TABLE 11–3. *Additional effects of first-generation antihistaminics*

α-Blocking effect
Antiemetic effect
Antimuscarinic actions
Antiparkinsonism effect
Antiserotonin effect
CNS depression
Membrane-stabilizing effects (local anesthetic)

Antimuscarinic Actions

Many of the H_1 antagonists, especially those of the ethanolamine and ethylenediamine subgroups, have significant atropine-like effects on peripheral muscarinic receptors. This action may be responsible for some of the benefits reported for nonallergic rhinorrhea but also may cause urinary retention and blurred vision.

Local Anesthetic

Most of the H_1 antagonists are effective local anesthetics. They block sodium channels in excitable membranes in the same fashion as procaine and lidocaine. Diphenhydramine and promethazine are actually more potent as local anesthetics than is procaine. They are occasionally used to produce local anesthesia in patients allergic to the conventional local anesthetic drugs.

Sedation

A common effect of H_1 antagonists is sedation, but the intensity of this effect varies among chemical subgroups and among patients as well. The effect is sufficiently prominent with some agents to make them useful as "sleep aids" and unsuitable for daytime use. It is claimed that newer H_1 antagonists have little or no sedative action.

Nausea and Vomiting

Several H_1 antagonists have significant activity in preventing motion sickness. They are less effective against an episode of motion sickness already present. Certain H_1

antagonists, notably doxylamine (in Bendectin), have been used widely in the treatment of nausea and vomiting of pregnancy.

Antiparkinsonism Effects

Perhaps because of their antimuscarinic effects, some of the H_1 antagonists have significant acute suppressant effects on the parkinsonism-like symptoms associated with certain antipsychotic drugs.

Antiadrenoceptor Actions

Weak α receptor-blocking effects can be demonstrated for many H_1 antagonists, especially those in the phenothiazine subgroup. This action may cause orthostatic hypotension in susceptible individuals.

Antiserotonin Action

Strong blocking effects at serotonin receptors have been demonstrated for some H_1 antagonists, notably cyproheptadine. This drug is promoted as an antiserotonin agent and is discussed with that drug group. Nevertheless, it has a chemical structure that resembles the phenothiazine antihistamines and is a potent H_1 blocking agent.

Toxicity of First-Generation Agents (Table 11–4)

Antimuscarinic Effects

Many first-generation antihistamines have antimuscarinic actions. Antimuscarinic agents can produce both peripheral and central toxic effects. Peripheral manifestations include mydriasis, tachycardia, vasodilation, glaucoma; tightness of the chest; palpitations; headache; and urinary retention or dysuria, hyperpyrexia, decreased sweating, and decreased secretions, that are manifested as dryness of the mouth, throat, and nasal airway. Central effects include confusion, agitation, hallucinations, seizures, and coma. Antimuscarinic toxicity can be due to several classes of pharmacologic agents that include tricyclic antidepressants, phenothiazines, butyrophenones, antihistamines, belladonna alkaloids, and plant extracts. Monoamine oxidase inhibitors prolong and intensify the anticholinergic drying effects of antihistamines. The ethanolamine derivatives may show greater anticholinergic activity than the other classes of antihistamines. Astemizole, cetirizine, loratadine, and terfenadine have no significant anticholinergic activity.

Antimuscarinic toxicity is the subject of Chapter 10.

TABLE 11–4. *Toxicity of first-generation antihistaminics*

Antimuscarinic
Agitation
Coma
Confusion
Drying of secretions
Hallucinations
Hyperpyrexia
Mydriasis
Peripheral vasodilation
Seizures
Sinus tachycardia
Urinary retention
Cardiac effects
Sinus tachycardia
Hypertension
Ventricular arrhythmias
EKG changes
Bundle branch block
Nonspecific ST-T wave changes
Prolonged QT interval
Wandering pacemaker
Cardiogenic shock
Cardiac arrest

Cardiac Effects

Although cardiotoxicity is rare after ingestions of diphenhydramine and related antihistamines, they have been reported in severe overdoses. Tachycardia is the most common cardiac effect of antihistamine poisoning. Other cardiovascular changes have included hypertension, ventricular arrhythmias, and eventual cardiac arrest. Temporary EKG changes, such as prolonged QT interval, nonspecific ST-T changes, wandering pacemaker, and left bundle branch block may also be observed. Massive ingestions of diphenhydramine have been reported to cause widening of the QRS. Cardiogenic shock refractory to pharmacologic intervention has been reported secondary to ingestion of a massive amount of pyrilamine. Delayed-release preparations are available and should be considered when estimating the onset of drug effect.

Diphenhydramine has local anesthetic or membrane-stabilizing properties similar to those of lidocaine. Local anesthetics prevent conduction of nerve impulses by interacting with voltage-sensitive sodium channels along the neuronal membrane. Fast sodium channels are inhibited, increasing the threshold for electrical excitation of the neuron, prolonging the action potential, and slowing conduction. In higher concentrations, potassium channels along the membrane are also inhibited. Diphenhydramine and other antihistamines such as dimethindene, cyproheptadine, and antazoline have been studied as antiarrhythmics. All have been found to increase the duration of the action potential of the myocardium.

Diphenhydramine—A Prototypical First-Generation Antihistamine

Diphenhydramine is one of the classic first-generation antihistamines that is available in multiple formulations as a nonprescription antihistamine and hypnotic in doses not to exceed 50 mg. The FDA's approval of this drug as an over-the-counter drug has increased the availability of such products in the home. This important factor has contributed to the rise of diphenhydramine exposures (5).

The diphenhydramine component of Caladryl can be absorbed transdermally and can cause toxicity. Physicians should therefore be aware of the potential complications of topical diphenhydramine lotions.

Dimenhydrinate is an H_1 antagonist that is composed of equimolar concentrations of diphenhydramine and chlorotheophylline. Dimenhydrinate combats motion sickness and is readily available by prescription or on an over-the-counter basis. Although approximately half of the formulation of dimenhydrinate is chlorotheophylline, no published information is available on the bioavailability of chlorotheophylline as part of this medication. Its pharmacologic effects are believed to result from its diphenhydramine moiety.

Dimenhydrinate, like diphenhydramine, has CNS depressant, antimuscarinic, antiemetic, antihistaminic, and local anesthetic effects (6). Its margin of safety is excellent when used in the prescribed manner; this is reflected in the paucity of reports of toxicity. When used in higher-than-normal doses, altered sensorium and hallucinations have been reported. It is well absorbed orally, widely distributed into body tissues, crosses the placenta, is metabolized by the liver and is excreted in urine.

Pharmacokinetics

Diphenhydramine hydrochloride is well absorbed following oral administration, but apparently undergoes first-pass metabolism in the liver and only about 40–60% of an oral dose reaches systemic circulation as unchanged diphenhydramine. Diphenhydramine can be absorbed percutaneously following topical administration and rarely may result in systemic effects and toxicity (7). Following oral administration of a single dose of diphenhydramine, the drug appears in plasma within 15 minutes and peak plasma concentrations are attained within 1–4 hours. Therefore, following an overdose, toxic effects are observed quite rapidly. The estimated fatal dose of diphenhydramine in adults is 20 to 40 mg/kg (5,8).

Clinical Presentation

Deaths in children from diphenhydramine were reported soon after its introduction in 1946 (8). The usual temporal course has been one of muscle hyperactivity followed by seizures, fever, cardiorespiratory collapse, and death (5). The rapid absorption of diphenhydramine, combined with its lack of gastric irritability, allows early development of a potentially lethal dose. These characteristics separate diphenhydramine from other nonprescription drugs used in suicide attempts and make early recognition and appropriate therapy imperative (2).

Clinical presentation of patients ingesting toxic amounts of diphenhydramine is age-dependent (5). Children are remarkably susceptible to the antimuscarinic effects, and often present with CNS excitation including tremors, hyperpyrexia, and tonic-clonic seizures. Adults are more prone to have CNS depression including drowsiness, lethargy, ataxia, and coma (Chapter 10) (9).

Patients should be warned that simultaneous ingestion of alcohol or other CNS depressants increases somnolence. Other untoward effects include dizziness, lassitude, incoordination, fatigue, tinnitus, and diplopia (8). Paradoxically, euphoria, nervousness, irritability, insomnia, tremors, and increased tendency toward convulsions also may occur, especially in children and the elderly (2).

Treatment of First-Generation Antihistamine Overdose

Treatment including supportive care and proper gastrointestinal decontamination should begin promptly. The gastrointestinal tract should be evacuated with gastric lavage, followed by activated charcoal and sorbitol. Intravenous diazepam has been recommended for the treatment of seizures following a diphenhydramine overdosage. The induction of anesthesia with a short-acting barbiturate, thiopental, has been useful to control refractory seizures resulting from diphenhydramine ingestion (7,9). Because of the large volume of distribution, hemodialysis and hemoperfusion are not useful.

The use of physostigmine for antimuscarinic syndrome is controversial. It is generally reserved for hemodynamically significant supraventricular dysrhythmias, severe hallucinations, or intractable seizures when coupled with peripheral anticholinergic signs and symptoms. In an adult, physostigmine is administered in a 2-mg IV bolus; and in children, 0.5 mg intravenously over 5 minutes (3). For a further discussion of antimuscarinic overdose, see Chapter 10.

The treatment of choice for cardiac toxicity resulting from quinidine and other Class IA antiarrhythmics is sodium bicarbonate (7). The mechanism of action of hypertonic sodium bicarbonate in the treatment of cardiovascular toxicities is attributed to increases in the blood pH and extracellular sodium concentration, with a direct effect on phase O of the action potential (6). Since this is effective for other similar agents, this therapy may be tried with antihistamine overdose with severe cardiac manifestations (7,9).

Second-Generation H_1 Antagonists

In recent years, second-generation H_1 receptor antagonists have been developed that are clinically effective, safe, and convenient. Among these new H_1 receptor antagonists approved for use in the U.S. are terfenadine, astemizole, loratadine, and cetirizine (Table 11–5).

The second-generation antihistamines more strongly bind to the H_1 receptor, and have negligible affinity for nonhistamine receptors. They have been shown to lack antimuscarinic properties, as well as to lack significant CNS effects in contrast to the classic sedating antihistamines (10). This is because some structural modifications limit the ability of second-generation agents to cross the blood–brain barrier in appreciable amounts and as a result, in recommended doses they do not impair coordination or have other effects on the CNS in most patients.

Newer antihistamines also do not appear to have the drawback of tachyphylaxis, which is the development of tolerance with prolonged treatment. Because of these advantages, the newer H_1 receptor antagonists are supplanting the first-generation H_1 receptor antagonists in the treatment of allergic rhinitis and chronic urticaria. The affinity of second-generation agents for histamine receptors in the central and peripheral nervous systems is similar. Treatment of asthma is being investigated as an additional possible use of nonsedating antihistamines, an application not within the clinical scope of older agents.

Astemizole

Astemizole (Hismanal) belongs to a chemically heterologous class of agents of which terfenadine (Seldane), loratadine (Claritin), and acrivastine (Duact) are members. Astemizole binds to peripheral H_1 receptor sites with far greater affinity than does any other existing H_1 receptor antagonist (11).

Pharmacokinetics

After oral administration of astemizole, peak serum levels occur in 1 to 4 hours (12). Astemizole undergoes extensive first-pass metabolism in the liver to several active and inactive metabolites. Desmethylastemizole is the main active metabolite. Astemizole has a very high volume of distribution of 250 L/kg. Astemizole takes considerably longer to be eliminated from the body than the other second-generation antihistamines. This long duration of action occurs because of astemizole's high H_1 affinity and also because of the long half-life of both the parent drug (20 hours), and its active metabolite, desmethylastemizole (10 to 20 days). Astemizole is 96% protein-bound. The apparent elimination half-life of unchanged drug and metabolites is about 9.5 days (11).

TABLE 11–5. *Second-Generation Antihistaminics*

Acrivastine (Duact)
Astemizole (Hismanal)
Cetirizine (Reactine)
Loratadine (Claritin)
Terfenadine (Seldane)

Adverse Effects

Patients known to have conditions leading to QT prolongation may experience QT prolongation and/or ventricular arrhythmias with astemizole at recommended doses (12). The pathologic basis of astemizole cardiotoxicity is currently unknown. H_1 receptors are found in the heart, and may modulate atrioventricular conduction. Blockade of these receptors could then lead to prolongation of the QT interval and predisposition to reentry of cardiac conduction, resulting in torsade de pointes or ventricular tachycardia (11). It is advisable to avoid its use in patients who are taking medications that are reported to prolong QT intervals (including certain antiarrhythmics, certain tricyclic antidepressants, certain phenothiazines, certain calcium channel blockers such as bepridil, and terfenadine), patients with electrolyte abnormalities such as hypokalemia or hypomagnesemia, or those taking diuretics with potential for inducing electrolyte abnormalities (Table 11–6) (13).

Overdose

Substantial overdoses of astemizole can cause death, cardiac arrest, QT prolongation, torsade de pointes, and other ventricular arrhythmias. These events can also occur, although rarely, at doses close to the recommended dose.

Accidental astemizole ingestion in young children is dangerous because a few tablets may cause toxicity as well as the fact that the worst cardiac effects can appear

TABLE 11–6. *Medications that may increase cardiotoxicity of second-generation antihistaminics*

Medications reported to increase QT interval
Certain arrhythmics
Certain tricyclics
Certain phenothiazines
Certain calcium channel blockers
Patients with electrolyte abnormalities
Hypokalemia
Hypomagnesemia
Patients taking diuretics
Patients with hepatic dysfunction
Patients taking antifungals and antimicrobials
Ketoconazole
Itraconazole
Troleandomycin
Erythromycin
Clarithromycin

late and last long, probably because of the slow elimination of astemizole and metabolites. After overdosage, the cardiotoxic effects have included primarily ventricular conduction abnormalities and torsade de pointes in both adults and children. Overdose patients should be carefully monitored as long as the QT interval is prolonged or arrhythmias are present. In some cases, this has been up to 6 days.

Cetirizine (Reactine)

Cetirizine is the carboxylic acid metabolite of the first-generation H_1 receptor antagonist hydroxyzine. It has a protein binding of approximately 93%, and a time to peak concentration of 1 hour. Within 72 hours of a single dose of cetirizine, 70% of the medication appears unchanged in the urine (10). The serum half-life is approximately 7 hours in children and adults. Therapeutic dosing of cetirizine produces a low incidence of antimuscarinic and CNS adverse effects.

Acrivastine (Duact)

Acrivastine is well absorbed after oral administration; peak serum concentrations occur in 2 to 3 hours. About 16% of an oral dose is metabolized; most of the remainder is excreted unchanged by the kidneys.

Loratadine (Claritin)

Loratadine is well absorbed, and peak serum concentrations occur 1 to 2 hours after an oral dose. Loratadine also has an active major metabolite, descarboethoxyloratadine, The serum half-life of loratadine in adults is 8 to 11 hours, whereas that of the active metabolite is 17 to 24 hours. The half-life may be longer in elderly patients and those with liver disease. Both drugs are highly bound to plasma proteins, which contributes to difficulty in crossing the blood–brain barrier. About 60% of a dose of loratadine is eliminated in the feces; most of the remainder is recovered in the urine.

Loratadine in therapeutic doses does not cause antimuscarinic effects. In higher doses, sedation may occur. In vitro, loratadine has weak affinity for α-adrenergic and acetylcholine receptors. It penetrates poorly into the CNS and has low affinity for CNS H_1 receptors.

Terfenadine (Seldane)

Terfenadine is a specific, selective, histamine H_1 receptor antagonist. It is a nonsedating antihistamine chemically unrelated to astemizole. In recommended doses, terfenadine does not cause antimuscarinic effects. In these doses, it also does not interact with or potentiate the effects of alcohol, diazepam, or other CNS-active medications.

Unlike most other first-generation antihistamines, but like cyproheptadine, terfenadine appears to have a dual effect on histamine H_1 receptors. Evidence indicates that the drug exhibits a specific and selective antagonism of histamine H_1 receptors, and that the drug slowly binds to the H_1 receptor and forms a stable complex from which it subsequently slowly dissociates. These findings suggest that the prolonged and generally irreversible nature of terfenadine's antagonism of histamine results principally from the drug's slow dissociation from the H_1 receptors.

Pharmacokinetics

Terfenadine is completely absorbed from the gastrointestinal tract, and peak serum concentrations occur 1 to 2 hours after an oral dose. Less than 1% of the oral dose reaches the systemic circulation due to the extensive first-pass metabolism. The half-life is about 17 hours. Peak serum concentrations are approximately 1 to 2 ng/mL after a 60-mg dose. Two major metabolites of terfenadine have been identified; one, a carboxylic acid metabolite, has significant antihistaminic activity and is being studied as a therapeutic agent.

Adverse Reactions

In therapeutic doses, sedation and other CNS adverse effects do not occur in most patients taking terfenadine. In addition, this drug usually does not potentiate the sedative actions of CNS depressants or impair psychomotor performance. However, in an occasional patient, drowsiness, sedation, and other manifestations of CNS impairment occur when doses exceed the recommended amount (14).

Severe adverse reactions have been extremely rare even in patients taking massive overdoses of terfenadine. Unlike many older currently available antimuscarinics, terfenadine does not possess appreciable anticholinergic or antiserotonergic effects at usual antihistaminic doses in pharmacologic studies. Terfenadine also does not exhibit any appreciable α- or ß-adrenergic blocking activity or histamine H_2 receptor antagonism.

As with astemizole, terfenadine can also cause prolongation of the QT interval and ventricular arrhythmias after overdose or at excessive concentrations. Transient arrhythmias have occurred rarely in both adults and children. The disturbances in cardiac rhythm include an atypical ventricular tachycardia, torsade de pointes, and ventricular fibrillation.

The arrhythmogenic action of terfenadine appears to result from inhibition of the potassium channel, which slows repolarization; the active metabolite, terfenadine carboxylate, has no effect on potassium currents in vitro, and does not appear to have arrhythmogenic effects (15).

Drug Interactions

Use of recommended doses of astemizole or terfenadine in patients receiving drugs that inhibit hepatic metabolism (e.g., imidazole antifungals such as ketoconazole, itraconazole; macrolides such as troleandomycin, erythromycin, clarithromycin) also may prolong the QT interval and precipitate torsade de pointes. Therefore, concomitant use of terfenadine or astemizole in patients treated with such drugs is contraindicated. Furthermore, patients with severe hepatic dysfunction (e.g., hepatitis, alcoholic cirrhosis), those receiving other drugs that prolong the QT interval, and those susceptible to a prolonged QT interval (e.g., those with hypokalemia or congenital QT syndrome) also should not receive terfenadine or astemizole. Cardiac disturbances associated with terfenadine and astemizole also may occur with first-generation antihistamines.

Current data indicate that loratadine, cetirizine, and acrivastine, alone or in combination with other agents, do not prolong the QT interval. However, additional data are needed to determine the potential of these or other newer antihistamines to cause cardiac disturbances.

Treatment of Second-Generation Antihistaminic Overdosage

In the event of overdosage, supportive measures including gastric lavage, activated charcoal, and a cathartic should be employed. Other supportive measures should be administered as necessary.

With ventricular arrhythmias secondary to the antihistamines, Class Ia and III antiarrhythmic agents should be avoided. Temporary cardiac pacing is suggested in serious intoxications, and repeated DC cardioversion may become necessary.

The QTc interval of the ECG should be monitored, and the patient should not be discharged from the hospital until the QTc interval is normal. Until more information is available, all children who ingest astemizole should receive emergent medical evaluation and close cardiac monitoring for a minimum of 24 hours.

Torsade de pointes frequently terminates spontaneously. Effective regimens to suppress the arrhythmia in patients include discontinuation of the drug and institution of supportive measures, infusion of intravenous magnesium sulfate, and temporary rapid atrial or ventricular pacing. If pacing is not available, an alternative is the temporary cautious use of intravenous isoproterenol, which also decreases the QT interval. Magnesium corrects abnormal repolarization by a different mechanism; rather than the QT interval, sites of its action appear to be in the Na^+, K^+-ATPase system and potassium flux in the myocardial cell membrane. Magnesium is much safer than isoproterenol. Lidocaine, a Class 1B antiarrhythmic, also decreases the QT interval, and can be tried if necessary, but it has variable effectiveness.

TABLE 11–7. *H_2 receptor blocking agents*

Cimetidine (Tagamet)
Ranitidine (Zantac)
Famotidine (Pepcid)
Nizatidine (Axid)

H_2 ANTAGONISTS

H_2 blockers are among the more commonly prescribed medications in the U.S. They are also among the safest classes of drugs available. These agents are effective for treating and preventing both gastric and duodenal ulcers and are commonly prescribed for gastroesophageal reflux and stress ulcer prophylaxis in critically ill patients. Reports of adverse drug reactions due to these agents are rare considering their wide use in a variety of patients (16).

H_2 blockers specifically inhibit the effects of histamine on the H_2 subtype of histamine receptors on the parietal cells, thereby eliminating a major stimulus for acid secretion. The histamine receptors on the basolateral membrane of the acid-secreting parietal cell are of the H_2 type and thus are not blocked by conventional H_1 antihistamines. The four H_2 blocking drugs currently available in the U.S. are cimetidine, ranitidine, famotidine, and nizatidine (Table 11–7) (17). Ranitidine and cimetidine are currently the most widely used antiulcer medications. Ranitidine is about three times more potent than cimetidine, has little antiandrogenic activity, does not markedly inhibit hepatic drug-metabolizing enzymes, and causes fewer drug interactions than cimetidine. Larger doses than with cimetidine can be used in refractory patients because of the lower incidence of adverse reactions.

Mechanism of Action

The occupation of H_2 receptors by histamine, released from mast cells, activates adenylate cyclase, increasing intracellular concentrations of cyclic AMP. The increased levels of cyclic AMP activate the proton pump of the parietal cell, a hydrogen, potassium-ATPase, to secrete hydrogen ions against a large concentration gradient in exchange for potassium ions. H_2 blockers competitively and selectively inhibit the binding of histamine to H_2 receptors, thereby reducing both intracellular concentrations of cyclic AMP and the secretion of acid by the parietal cells (Fig. 11–1) (16)

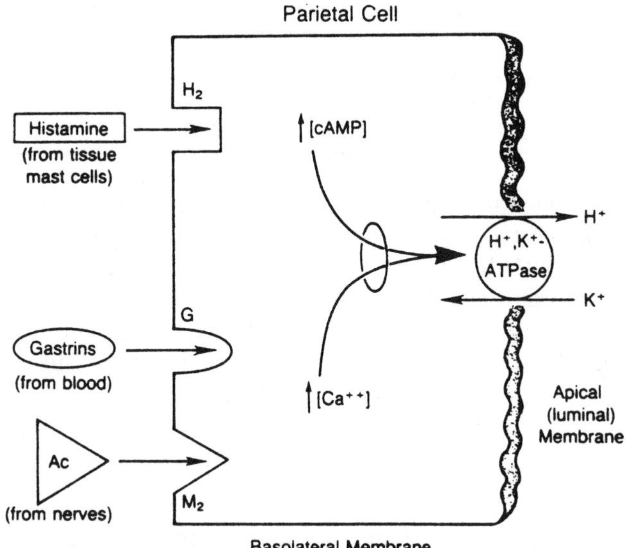

FIG. 11–1. Simplified model of a parietal cell, containing on its basolateral membrane separate receptors for histamine (*H_2*), gastrins (*G*), and acetylcholine (muscarinic-2 receptors, *M_2*). Histamine increases intracellular cyclic AMP (*cAMP*) concentrations, whereas gastrins and acetylcholine (*AC*) increase intracellular calcium. The proton pump (*H^+,K^+-ATPase*) is located on the apical membrane. (From Feldman M and Burton M, *N Engl J Med* 1990;323:1673, with permission.)

Clinical Indications

A common indication for acute, short-term H_2 antagonist use is prophylaxis against stress ulcerations. In addition, H_2 antagonists have been used for acute upper gastrointestinal bleeding, esophagitis, ulcers, gastritis, in the preoperative situation, as well as chronically for ulcers and esophagitis.

All of the available H_2 antagonists, cimetidine, ranitidine, famotidine, and nizatidine, indirectly suppress gastric acid and pepsin secretion by occupying H_2 receptors. Some evidence suggests that famotidine binding is noncompetitive, while the receptor binding of ranitidine, nizatidine, and cimetidine is competitive.

Evidence indicates that when all of the available drugs are given in appropriate doses, no differences in efficacy will be seen (16).

Adverse Reactions

H_2 blocking drugs are well tolerated, and adverse effects are reported in only 1–2% of cases. Although H_2 blockers have wide therapeutic indices, adverse reactions can occur in some patients. The most commonly reported adverse effects are diarrhea, dizziness, somnolence, headache, and rash. Others include constipation, vomiting, and arthralgia (18). Cimetidine is associated with the most adverse effects, while nizatidine seems to produce the fewest CNS reactions including mental status changes, delirium, psychosis, confusion, disorientation, hallucinations, hostility, irritability, obtundation, and agitation, which have been associated with H_2 blockers (19). Comparative studies of H_2 blockers have failed to detect differences in the incidence of CNS reactions among the various agents. Elderly and debilitated individuals, patients with impaired renal function, and those who require prolonged therapy with large doses are the most likely to experience effects.

Comparison of Agents

Of the four available H_2 antagonists, cimetidine is the least potent and famotidine the most potent. Although there is considerable variation in the clearance and elimination half-lives of H_2 blockers, their half-lives in serum range from 1.5 to 4 hours in normal subjects.

Ranitidine, although 4 to 10 times more potent than cimetidine, binds 5 to 10 fold less avidly to the cytochrome system (20). Famotidine and nizatidine do not bind notably to the cytochrome P-450 enzyme system, and thus have a limited potential for inhibiting the metabolism of other drugs.

Administration of the H_2 receptor blockers cimetidine, ranitidine, and nizatidine has been shown to increase blood alcohol concentrations that correspond to common social drinking. This has not been shown for famotidine.

Cimetidine (Tagamet)

Cimetidine was the first H_2 receptor antagonist to be developed and approved for clinical use (21). Cimetidine has also been used in a number of other clinical settings, including the treatment of chronic pruritus, prevention of adverse reactions to radiologic contrast media, dialysis pruritus, pain and itch associated with herpes zoster, cancer, and hypogammaglobulinemia (16).

Pharmacokinetics

Cimetidine is now available in oral, intramuscular, and intravenous forms. When taken orally, cimetidine is well absorbed from the gastrointestinal tract, reaches peak plasma concentrations in 1 to 2 hours, and has a half-life of 2 hours (22). A small portion of orally administered cimetidine is metabolized during the first pass through the liver, resulting in an average bioavailability of 60–70% when compared with intravenous injection. Approximately 50% to 60% is eliminated unchanged by the kidneys; the remainder is metabolized in the liver. Cimetidine is distributed throughout the body and is 15% to 20% bound to plasma proteins. The volume of distribution of cimetidine is 0.8 to 1.2 L/kg.

Drug Interactions

Cimetidine binds to receptors of the hepatic microsomal oxidase system and as a result, it reduces hepatic metabolism of several drugs, causing increased serum concentrations of phenytoin, anticoagulants, propranolol, lidocaine, metronidazole, diazepam, warfarin, quinidine, metroprolol, theophylline, and others (Table 11–8). Ketoconazole requires a relatively acidic environment in the stomach in order to dissolve, and thus the administration of an H_2 antagonist may markedly inhibit the absorption of ketoconazole (22).

Adverse Reactions

The overall incidence of adverse reactions is low (19). Untoward effects during short-term trials include diarrhea, dizziness, myalgia, and rash (which is usually transient). Cimetidine has rarely been reported to cause visual hallucinations, dysarthria, and alterations of consciousness in both adults and children. Cimetidine does not have an antimuscarinic action (17).

A number of adverse cardiovascular effects (Table 11–9) have been reported to be caused by cimetidine, including bradycardia, hypotension, and arrhythmias leading to cardiac arrest. Only bradycardia and hypotension have been consistently reported, and this seems to be a direct result of rapid intravenous administration of the drug.

Confusion and more severe CNS reactions have occurred, usually after ingestion of excessive doses, in elderly patients, or in those with renal impairment; these symptoms were reversed when the drug was discontinued. Some dementia-like symptoms may reflect interaction between cimetidine and concomitantly administered psychotropic drugs or may be primary side effects because cimetidine crosses the blood–brain barrier.

Toxicity

There are very limited reports of acute toxicity for cimetidine. Doses of up to 10 to 20 g have not been associated with great toxicity, except transient adverse effects similar to those encountered in normal clinical experience. There have been reports of severe CNS symptoms, including unresponsiveness, following ingestion of between 20 and 40 g of cimetidine. Death has been reported in adults following acute ingestion of more than 40 g of cimetidine (17).

Treatment

For the treatment of cimetidine overdosage, the usual measures to remove unabsorbed drug from the gastrointestinal tract, clinical monitoring, and supportive therapy should be employed. Studies in animals suggest that cimetidine overdosage may produce respiratory failure and tachycardia, which may be managed with assisted respiration and a ß-adrenergic blocking agent.

Famotidine (Pepcid)

Famotidine is the most potent of the currently available H_2 blockers. It is approximately eight to ten times more potent than ranitidine and its duration of action is 30% longer. Famotidine is eliminated mostly by the renal route, and patients with severe renal dysfunction may require reduced doses.

After oral doses, peak plasma levels occur in 1 to 3 hours, and activity persists for 10 to 12 hours. The plasma half-life is 2 to 4 hours. The oral bioavailability of famotidine is about 40% to 50%. The volume of distribution of famotidine is 1.1 to 1.4 L/kg.

There have been no documented interactions between famotidine and diazepam, phenytoin, procainamide, theophylline, and warfarin (23). To date, there has been no experience with an acute overdosage of famotidine. Doses of up to 640 mg/day have been given to patients with pathologic hypersecretory conditions with no serious adverse effects.

Treatment

In the event of overdosage, treatment should be symptomatic and supportive. Unabsorbed material should be removed from the gastrointestinal tract, the patient should be monitored, and supportive therapy should be employed.

Nizatidine (Axid)

The most recently approved H_2 blocker is nizatidine. The potency of this H_2 receptor antagonist in inhibiting gastric acid secretion is similar to that of ranitidine. The value of nizatidine in the management of acid-peptic disorders is comparable to that of ranitidine and cimetidine. The half-life of nizatidine is 1 to 2 hours. Because there is little first-pass hepatic metabolism of nizatidine, its bioavailability in normal subjects is close to 100%. The volume of distribution of nizatidine is 1.2 to 1.6 L/kg. Like cimetidine, the mean peak serum concentration after oral administration occurs in about 1 hour, and the plasma half-life is about 1.5 hours. Nizatidine has a duration of action of up to 10 hours. It is eliminated primarily by the kidneys; 90% of the administered dose (65% as unchanged drug) is recovered in the urine within 16 hours. Because nizatidine is excreted primarily by the kidneys, moderate to severe renal impairment significantly prolongs the half-life and

TABLE 11–8. *Drug interactions with cimetidine and ranitidine*

Increased serum concentrations of
Antiarrhythmics
Flecainide
Procainamide
Quinidine
Lidocaine
Anticoagulants
Coumarin
Antimicrobials
Metronidazole
Anti-seizure medications
Phenytoin
Carbamazepine
Benzodiazepines
Diazepam
Midazolam
Triazolam
Chlordiazepoxide
ß Blockers
Propranolol
Metoprolol
Calcium channel blockers
Nifedipine
Verapamil
Diltiazem
Local anesthetics
Lidocaine
Miscellaneous agents
Meperidine
Propafenone
Hydroxyzine
Chloroquine
Tricyclic antidepressants
Doxepin
Imipramine
Desipramine
Nortriptyline
Xanthines
Theophylline
Caffeine

decreases clearance (17). Nizatidine does not inhibit the cytochrome P-450 enzyme system, so drug interactions with this system do not occur (23).

Drug Interactions

Nizatidine may inhibit alcohol dehydrogenase in the gastric mucosa and may produce higher serum levels of alcohol, but this does not appear to be clinically significant. Like famotidine, nizatidine apparently does not interfere with hepatic metabolism of various other drugs, such as oral anticoagulants and theophyllines, which can accumulate in toxic amounts in patients taking cimetidine or, to a lesser extent, ranitidine (19).

Toxicity

If overdosage occurs, use of lavage and activated charcoal should be considered along with clinical monitoring and supportive therapy. Renal dialysis does not substantially increase clearance of nizatidine due to its large volume of distribution.

TABLE 11–9. *Adverse reactions to cimetidine*

Cardiovascular
Bradycardia
Hypotension
Central nervous system
Confusion
Dementia
Alteration of consciousness
Unresponsiveness
Miscellaneous
Diarrhea
Dizziness
Myalgia
Dermatitis
Dysarthria

Ranitidine (Zantac)

Ranitidine is approximately six times as potent as cimetidine in inhibiting gastric acid secretion. Although it is more potent than cimetidine in inhibiting gastric acid secretion, ulcers do not heal more quickly.

Ranitidine is well absorbed from the small intestine, and has a plasma half-life of approximately 2 to 3 hours. Bioavailability of ranitidine is 41% to 57%. The volume of distribution of ranitidine is 1.2 to 1.9 L/kg.

The effect of ranitidine on the pharmacokinetics of other drugs has been well studied (Table 11–8), and the results have demonstrated that ranitidine is very unlikely to inhibit hepatic drug metabolism. This is probably due to its lower binding affinity for drug-metabolizing enzymes. The particular pattern of CNS toxicity observed in adult patients treated with cimetidine has not been noted with ranitidine or famotidine therapy. Hypotension has been associated with the rapid infusion of ranitidine. There has been no experience to date with deliberate overdosage of ranitidine (17).

Drug Interactions

In contrast to cimetidine, ranitidine binds minimally to the hepatic mixed-function oxidase system, androgen receptors, or peripheral lymphocytes. Although ranitidine interacts with other medications less frequently than cimetidine, an increasing number of drug interactions is being reported. Interactions with nifedipine, warfarin, theophylline, and metoprolol have been observed. Mechanisms other than inhibition of P-450 hepatic drug metabolizing systems may be involved. Ranitidine may decrease the absorption of diazepam and reduce its plasma concentration by 25%; these drugs should be administered at least 1 hour apart. Ranitidine appears in breast milk and should be used with caution in nursing mothers (15).

Overdosage

There has been limited experience with overdosage. Reported acute ingestions of up to 18 g orally have been associated with transient adverse effects similar to those encountered in normal clinical experience. In addition, abnormalities of gait and hypotension have been reported.

Treatment

When overdosage occurs, the usual measures to remove unabsorbed material from the gastrointestinal tract, clinical monitoring, and supportive therapy should be employed.

REFERENCES

1. Kaiser H: H_1-receptor antagonist treatment of seasonal allergic rhinitis. *J Allergy Clin Immunol* 1990;86:1000–1003.
2. Simons F, Simons K: The pharmacology and use of H_1-receptor-antagonist drugs. *N Engl J Med* 1994;330:1663–1670.
3. Danze L, Langdorf M: Reversal of orphenadrine-induced ventricular tachycardia with physostigmine. *J Emerg Med* 1991;9:453–457.
4. Smith B, Ferguson D: Acute hydralazine overdose: marked ECG abnormalities in a young adult. *Ann Emerg Med* 1992;21:326–330.
5. Rinder C, D'Amato S, Rinder H, et al: Survival in complicated diphenhydramine overdose. *Crit Care Med* 1988;16:1161–1162.
6. Clark R, Vance M: Massive diphenhydramine poisoning resulting in a wide-complex tachycardia: successful treatment with sodium bicarbonate. *Ann Emerg Med* 1992;21:318–321.
7. Farell M, Heinrichs M, Tilelli J: Response of life threatening dimenhydrinate intoxication to sodium bicarbonate administration. *J Toxicol Clin Toxicol* 1991;29:527–535.
8. Goetz C, Lopez G, Dean B, et al: Accidental childhood death from diphenhydramine overdosage. *Am J Emerg Med* 1990;8:321–322.
9. Winn R, McDonnell K: Fatality secondary to massive overdose of dimenhydrinate. *Ann Emerg Med* 1993;22:1481–1484.
10. Simons F: Recent advances in H_1-receptor antagonist treatment. *J Allergy Clin Immunol* 1990;86:995–999.
11. Wiley J, Gelber M, Henretig F, et al: Cardiotoxic effects of astemizole overdose in children. *J Pediatr* 1992;120:799–802.
12. Hoppu K, Tikanoja T, Tapanainen P, et al: Accidental astemizole overdose in young children. *Lancet* 1991;338;538–540.
13. Saviuc P, Danel V, Dixmerias F: Prolonged QT interval and torsade de pointes following astemizole overdose. *J Toxicol Clin Toxicol* 1993;31:121–125.
14. Hansten P: Overview of the safety profile of the H_2-receptor antagonists. *DICP Ann Pharmacother* 1990;12:S38–S41.
15. Iberti TJ: Hemodynamic effects of H_2 receptor antagonists. *DICP Ann Pharmacother* 1990;24(suppl.):S35–S37.
16. Feldman M, Burton M: Histamine2 receptor antagonists. *N Engl J Med* 1990;323:1749–1755.
17. Keithley J: Histamine H_2-receptor antagonists. *Nurs Clin North* 1991;26:361–373.
18. Frankel D, Dolgin J, Murray B: Non-traumatic rhabdomyolysis complicating antihistamine overdose. *J Toxicol Clin Toxicol* 1993;31:493–496.
19. Cantu T, Korek J: Central nervous system reactions to histamine-2 receptor blockers. *Ann Intern Med* 1991;114:1027–1034.
20. DiPadova C, Roine R, Frezza M, et al: Effects of ranitidine on blood alcohol levels after ethanol ingestion. *JAMA* 1992;267:83–86.
21. Moore J: Achieving pH control in the critically ill patient: the role of continuous infusion of H_2-receptor antagonists. *DICP Ann Pharmacother* 1990;24(suppl.):S28–S30.
22. Dimand R: Use of H_2-receptor antagonists in children. *DICP Ann Pharmacother* 1990;24(suppl.):S42–S46.
23. Lipsy R, Fenerty B, Fagan T: Clinical review of histamine-2 receptor antagonists. *Arch Intern Med* 1990;150:745–751.

ADDITIONAL SELECTED REFERENCES

Bailie G, Nelson M, Krenzelok E, et al: Unusual treatment response of a severe dystonia to diphenhydramine. *Ann Emerg Med* 1987;16:705–715.

Cockrell J: Acute hallucinogenic reaction to carbinoxamine maleate. *Clin Toxicol* 1987;25:161–167.

Furlanut M, Bettio I, Bertin G, et al: Orphenadrine serum levels in a poisoned patient. *Hum Toxicol* 1985;4:331–333.

Hooper R, Conner C, Rumack B: Acute poisoning from over-the-counter sleep preparations. *JACEP* 1979;8:98–100.

Kaplan M, Register D, Bierman A, et al: A nonfatal case of intentional scopolamine poisoning. *Clin Toxicol* 1974;7:509–512.

Krenzelok E, Anderson G, Mirick M: Massive diphenhydramine overdose resulting in death. *Ann Emerg Med* 1982;11:212–213.

Lacouture P, Lovejoy F, Mitchell A: Acute hypothermia associated with atropine. *Am J Dis Child* 1983;137:291–292.

Pentel P, Peterson C: Asystole complicating physostigmine treatment of tricyclic antidepressant overdose. *Ann Emerg Med* 1980;9:588–590.

Schuster P, Gabriel E, Kufferle B, et al: Reversal by physostigmine of clozapine-induced delirium. *Clin Toxicol* 1977;10:437–441.

Spaulding B, Choi S, Gross J, et al: The effect of physostigmine on diazepam-induced ventilatory depression: a double-blind study. *Anesthesiology* 1984;61:551–554.

CHAPTER 12

α-Adrenergic Agonists

The adrenergic neuroeffector junction consists of the sympathetic neuron, which synthesizes, stores, and releases norepinephrine, and the effector cell. Sympathetic effector cells in different organs generally have a preponderance of one type of receptor. *Alpha* (α) refers to the receptors associated with most of the excitatory functions of the sympathetic nervous system, and *beta* (β) refers to receptors associated with most of the inhibitory functions (1). The myocardium is an important exception to this rule.

α Receptors are most abundant in the resistance vessels of the skin, mucosa, intestine, and kidney, and they cause vasoconstriction in these vascular beds. α-Adrenergic receptors classically mediate catecholamine effects, such as smooth muscle contraction. In contrast, smooth muscle relaxation and other β-adrenergic receptor-mediated responses to catecholamines are those for which isoproterenol is more potent than either epinephrine or norepinephrine. β Receptors are predominant in the heart, the arteries and arterioles of skeletal muscle, and the bronchi, where they cause cardiac excitation, vasodilation, and bronchial relaxation, respectively (See Table 8–14).

The α-adrenergic agents are adrenoceptor agonists or antagonists, and there are clinical uses for both. Although there are many α-adrenergic agents used in medicine, this chapter concentrates on those agents that may be taken as a purposeful or accidental overdose: clonidine, guanabenz, guanfacine, and methyldopa, which are antihypertensive α_2 receptor agonists; yohimbine, an α_2 receptor antagonist and a drug of abuse; prazosin, terazosin, and doxazosin, which are antihypertensive α_1 receptor antagonists; and phenoxybenzamine, tolazoline, and phentolamine, nonspecific α receptor antagonists (2).

α_1-ADRENERGIC AGONISTS

Phenylephrine

Phenylephrine is a sympathomimetic amine that is pharmacologically similar to methoxamine hydrochloride. Phenylephrine is considered an example of a directly acting, relatively pure α-adrenergic agonist. In therapeutic doses, the drug has no substantial stimulant effect on the β-adrenergic receptors of the heart (β_1-adrenergic receptors) but substantial activation of these receptors may occur when larger doses are given (3). Phenylephrine does not stimulate β-adrenergic receptors of the bronchi or peripheral blood vessels (β_2-adrenergic receptors). Because it is not a catechol derivative, it is not inactivated by catechol *O*-methyltransferase (COMT) and has a much longer duration of action than the catecholamines. Although toxicity from pure α-adrenergic agonists is rare, one may still encounter a rare reaction to drugs such as phenylephrine, as it occurs in over-the-counter nasal sprays, as well as in ophthalmic solutions.

Clinical Uses

Phenylephrine is applied topically to the nasal mucosa to relieve nasal congestion. In addition, phenylephrine is administered orally as a nasal decongestant in combination preparations in the treatment of coughs and colds. Phenylephrine is also an effective mydriatic and decongestant and is used to produce mydriasis without cycloplegia for examination of the intraocular structures. It is often given with an anticholinergic drug to achieve wider mydriasis. It is with this use that the physician may see toxicity secondary to phenylephrine.

Phenylephrine is indicated for the treatment of vascular failure, unresponsive to adequate fluid volume replacement. It is also indicated for the maintenance of an adequate level of blood pressure during spinal and inhalation anesthesia.

Mechanism of Action

It is believed that α-adrenergic effects result from the inhibition of the production of cyclic AMP by inhibition of the enzyme adenyl cyclase, whereas β-adrenergic effects result from stimulation of adenyl cyclase activity. Phenylephrine also has an indirect effect by releasing norepinephrine from its storage sites (1).

Pharmacokinetics

After ocular instillation of a 10% solution, maximal mydriasis is obtained in 60 to 90 minutes, and recovery occurs in about 6 hours. Phenylephrine is irregularly absorbed from and readily metabolized in the GI tract. Occasionally, enough phenylephrine may be absorbed after oral inhalation to produce systemic effects. Following oral administration, nasal decongestion may occur within 15 or 20 minutes, and may persist for 2–4 hours.

Toxicity

Phenylephrine may cause restlessness, anxiety, nervousness, weakness, dizziness, precordial pain or discomfort, tremor, respiratory distress, pallor or blanching of the skin, or a pilomotor response. Injections of the drug may be followed by paresthesia in the extremities or a feeling of coolness in the skin. Phenylephrine may cause necrosis or sloughing of tissue if extravasation occurs during intravenous administration or following subcutaneous administration.

Phenylephrine occasionally may cause systemic reactions with intraocular instillation, which may include tachycardia, hypertension and reflex bradycardia, angina, ventricular arrhythmias, myocardial infarction, cardiac failure, cardiac arrest, subarachnoid hemorrhage, particularly when a strong concentration is instilled repeatedly. Although the incidence of severe hypertensive responses to 10% phenylephrine eyedrops may be low, a pronounced increase in blood pressure can occur in neonates and elderly patients. Central nervous system toxicity is rarely observed with catecholamines or drugs such as phenylephrine (4).

The main effect of phenylephrine on the heart is bradycardia, which results from increased vagal activity occurring as a reflex to increased arterial blood pressure. Bradycardia occurs after parenteral administration of usual therapeutic doses, and may also result from overdosage via oral inhalation.

Overdosage of phenylephrine may cause hypertension, headache, seizures, cerebral hemorrhage, palpitation, paresthesia, or vomiting. Headache may be a symptom of hypertension.

Treatment

Hypertension may be relieved by administration of an α-adrenergic blocking agent such as phentolamine. Bradycardia may be treated by administration of atropine. To prevent sloughing of the skin, an α-adrenergic blocking agent can be used.

Methoxamine

Methoxamine acts pharmacologically like phenylephrine, since it is predominantly a direct-acting α-receptor agonist. It may cause prolonged increase in blood pressure due to vasoconstriction; it also causes a vagally mediated bradycardia. Methoxamine is available for parenteral use, but clinical applications are rare and limited to hypotensive states.

α_2-ADRENERGIC AGONISTS

Members of this important class of medications that act primarily on central adrenergic mechanisms to inhibit efferent sympathetic outflow are variously called centrally acting α or α_2 agonists, centrally acting sympatholytic agents, or centrally acting sympatholytics. The four α_2 agents available in the U.S. include clonidine, methyldopa, guanabenz, and guanfacine (5).

Because the actions of the centrally acting α_2 agents are so complex, the precise mechanism of action is not fully established. Currently, it is believed that stimulation of α_2 receptors in the vasomotor center of the brain stem is the principal factor. This action results in decreased central sympathetic tone, decreased brain turnover of norepinephrine, decreased central sympathetic outflow, decreased activity of the preganglionic sympathetic nerves, and reduced plasma levels of norepinephrine (6).

It is likely that centrally acting α_2 agonists have the potential to stimulate the peripheral α receptors that mediate vasoconstriction. This indicates that the overall effect of central sympatholytics on the blood pressure is a summation of central and peripheral actions. The peripheral vasoconstrictive effect appears to increase at higher plasma concentrations of the medications (7).

Clonidine

Clonidine (Catapres) is an imidazoline derivative originally synthesized as a sympathomimetic agent for use as a nasal decongestant (8). Clonidine is structurally similar to the α receptor blockers phentolamine and tolazoline and was one of the first drugs for which a central mechanism was recognized to be the most important factor in its hypotensive activity (9,10).

Clinical Use

Clonidine is primarily used as an antihypertensive agent. In this regard, it is frequently used for the management of hypertensive urgencies (Table 12–1): (9,10). Clonidine is useful in the prophylaxis of migraine headache, menopausal flushing, and dysmenorrhea by reducing the respon-

TABLE 12–1. *Medical uses of clonidine*

Antihypertensive agent
Migraine prophylaxis
Vascular headache prophylaxis
Menopause
Narcotic withdrawal

siveness of blood vessels to vasodilators or vasoconstrictors (11). Clonidine has also been used for detoxification of opiate-dependent individuals because it blocks the symptoms of narcotic withdrawal (9,10). The mechanism of action is thought to be an inhibition in the locus coeruleus through α_2-adrenergic receptors resulting in decreased noradrenergic activity in the central nervous system (CNS) (5). It is also thought that it is the noradrenergic activity that is responsible for the behavioral changes of opiate withdrawal (7,12). Because of this, clonidine has become a street drug used by opiate addicts during withdrawal or during periods of opiate scarcity. Lofexidine, a clonidine analog, is being investigated as a safe alternative in clinical settings. Clonidine has also been used in the treatment of alcohol and nicotine withdrawal (13).

Transdermal Clonidine

Recently clonidine was made available as a transdermal patch, which allows for a constant delivery of the drug over a 7-day period. This patch consists of clonidine, layered with mineral oil and a microporous polypropylene membrane that controls the rate of diffusion of the drug. Usually, a steady state is reached approximately 48 hours after the patch is applied. Toxicity has been noted in cases of irregular delivery or in children coming in contact with used patches (14).

To ensure a constant release of drug, the total drug content of the system is greater than the total amount of drug delivered. The amount of residual drug in the system after 7 days of use may vary from 20% to 75% and after 11 days may be as high as 40% (15). Clonidine patches have been reported to cause toxicity in a child sleeping with a treated adult. It has also been reported when disposed patches are chewed by toddlers (7).

Pharmacokinetics

Clonidine is rapidly absorbed by the oral route, and antihypertensive effects are noted 30 to 60 minutes after ingestion, peaking in 2 to 4 hours (9,10,15–17). Maximal effect on blood pressure occurs between 3 to 8 hours (13). Approximately 80% of an orally ingested dose of clonidine is absorbed with little first-pass metabolism. The volume of distribution of clonidine is 4l/kg. The half-life is between 10 to 16 hours, but that is prolonged to 18 to 40 hours in patients with renal insufficiency (2).

Mechanism of Action

Central Action

Clonidine appears to stimulate postsynaptic α_2-adrenergic receptors in the CNS, mainly in the medulla oblongata, and to cause inhibition but not blockade of sympathetic vasomotor centers (18,19). This results in decreased sympathetic outflux to the heart, kidneys, and peripheral vasculature (9). Cardiovascular reflexes remain intact, and normal homeostatic mechanisms and hemodynamic responses to exercise are maintained (20).

Peripheral Action

Peripherally, clonidine inhibits neuronal uptake of norepinephrine and stimulates α receptors (17,21). The peripheral effects are transient and are far overshadowed by the central hypotensive actions. In the therapeutic dose range, the peripheral α-adrenergic agonist effect of clonidine is not important. Yet, in the presence of high plasma concentrations of clonidine, such as in an overdose, a predominance of peripheral α agonistic activity may occur and may cause a pressor response. In a massive overdose, the vasoconstrictor effect may compete with or overcome the drug's central hypotensive mechanism (8).

Side Effects

Intimately connected with the desired circulatory effect are α_2-adrenergic side effects such as sedation and dryness of the mouth (22), the latter being at least partly due to α_2-adrenergic inhibition of cholinergic transmission to the salivary glands (23). Dizziness, lethargy, insomnia, hallucinations, depression, and delirium have also been reported (24,25) (Table 12–2).

Withdrawal Symptoms

The abrupt cessation of clonidine may precipitate withdrawal symptoms related to the drug's sympatholytic mechanism of action (10,26). The frequency and

TABLE 12–2. *Side effects of clonidine*

CNS depression
Delirium
Dizziness
Dryness of mouth
Hallucinations
Insomnia
Lethargy
Sedation

severity of symptoms appear to be greater in patients treated with high doses for long periods and in those with severe hypertension before treatment (27). This syndrome of adrenergic overactivity is manifested by rebound hypertension, tachycardia, tremor, flushing, insomnia, nausea, vomiting, palpitations, and cardiac dysrhythmias (Table 12–3) (28). Withdrawal from clonidine can begin as soon as 8 hours or up to 36 hours after the last dose and can last for 72 to 96 hours (29). The blood pressure may rise to values greater than those recorded before therapy is initiated. Death due to hypertensive encephalopathy has been reported (17). Concomitant β blocker therapy may predispose the patient to overshoot hypertension.

The exact mechanism of the withdrawal syndrome following discontinuance of clonidine and other α-adrenergic agonists has not been determined but may involve increased concentrations of circulating catecholamines, increased sensitivity of adrenergic receptors, enhanced renin-angiotensin system activity, decreased vagal function, failure of autoregulation of cerebral blood flow, and/or failure of central α_2-adrenergic receptor mechanisms that regulate sympathetic outflow from the CNS and modulate baroreflex function.

Because of the rather severe withdrawal symptoms, clonidine therapy should be terminated gradually, especially in a high-risk population (26). Nevertheless, withdrawal reactions have been reported even when the drug was slowly and gradually withdrawn (30).

An excessive rise in blood pressure after clonidine withdrawal can be reversed and symptoms relieved by resumption of clonidine (31,32). Withdrawal from centrally active α-adrenergic agonists has also been managed by combined administration of α- and β-adrenergic blocking agents such as phentolamine or prazosin with atenolol, labetalol, or propranolol. Mild withdrawal syndrome without elevated blood pressure has also been adequately treated with oral diazepam (13).

Toxicity

Acute clonidine ingestion is associated with significant morbidity necessitating hospitalization, intensive care observation, invasive monitoring, and artificial ventilation. While the triad of CNS depression, respiratory depression, and miosis usually prompts suspicion of narcotic overdose, the possibility of clonidine ingestion must also be considered. Accidental or intentional overdose with clonidine can result in severe toxicity with variable clinical presentation (Table 12–4) (10,33). Because of the rapid onset of hypotensive action, patients who have ingested overdoses of clonidine rapidly become symptomatic. Signs and symptoms of clonidine overdosage usually occur within 30 to 60 minutes after ingestion and may continue for 48 hours.

The most common features of overdose are CNS depression, hypotension, miosis, and bradycardia (19); prolonged coma has also been reported (34). Recurrent apnea is sometimes seen, especially in children (15). Central and presumably peripheral presynaptic cardiac α_2 adrenoceptors are involved in the bradycardic action of clonidine. Other symptoms include weakness, respiratory depression sometimes leading to apnea, cardiac conduction defects, cardiac dysrhythmias, hypothermia, and hypertension. In addition, peripheral actions include α_2 receptor stimulation and blockade of the neuronal reuptake of norepinephrine, resulting in hypertension (17,35,36). Hypertension may be transient, and may lead to hypotension even without therapy. Aggressive management of the initial hypertension therefore should only be undertaken when end-organ damage is evident because peripheral stimulation lasts transiently and the central effects predominate (17,36). Hypotension results from central presynaptic α_2 receptor stimulation in the cardiovascular center of the medulla oblongata. Other symptoms occurring less frequently include irritability, agitation, seizures, or paralytic ileus. Atrioventricular conduction delays have also been noted as well as first-, second-, and third-degree atrioventricular blocks (2,36).

TABLE 12–3. *Symptoms of clonidine withdrawal*

Cardiac dysrhythmias
Flushing
Hypertensive encephalopathy
Insomnia
Nausea
Palpitations
Rebound hypertension
Sinus tachycardia
Tremor
Vomiting

TABLE 12–4. *Symptoms of clonidine overdose*

Central nervous system
Agitation
Apnea
Coma
Impaired consciousness
Irritability
Miosis
Sedation
Seizures
Weakness
Cardiovascular
Atrioventricular blocks
Bradycardia
Cardiac dysrhythmia
Conduction defects
Hypertension (transient)
Hypotension

Laboratory Analysis

Methods for measuring clonidine concentration in body fluids are not widely available, and at present the usual toxicology screening tests will not detect clonidine (37). Although serum concentrations appear to correlate with the sedative effects of the drug, the correlation with blood pressure is poorly defined. An electrocardiogram should be obtained to evaluate cardiac rhythm and atrioventricular conduction. Typically, maximal therapeutic effect corresponds to clonidine concentrations less than 2 ng/mL.

Guanabenz and Guanfacine

Guanabenz (Wytensin) and guanfacine (Tenex) are guanidine derivatives that are centrally acting α_2-adrenergic agonists with pharmacologic properties and side effects that are similar to those of clonidine (38–40). The mode of action is stimulation of central α_2 receptors that cause suppression of the vasomotor center (5).

Guanabenz

Although guanabenz is not a true adrenergic blocking agent, the drug produces some postganglionic α- and β-adrenergic blockade, similar to guanethidine and decreases the response to peripheral sympathetic nerve stimulation. The affinity of guanabenz for the α_2-adrenergic receptor is greater than that for the α_1-adrenergic receptor. The central effects of the drug in the lower brain stem result in reduced peripheral sympathetic activity and a reduction in systolic and diastolic blood pressure. Guanabenz-induced bradycardia appears to result principally from central α_2-agonist effects, although a peripheral α_2-agonist effect on the heart may also be involved (1).

Pharmacokinetics

Guanabenz is rapidly absorbed after oral administration. Guanabenz undergoes substantial first-pass hepatic metabolism. Its onset of action is 1 to 2 hours, and peak plasma concentrations are achieved within 4 hours (41). Guanabenz has a duration of effect of 8 to 12 hours and a volume of distribution of 4 to 17 L/kg (38). It is 90% bound to human plasma protein (39). As with clonidine, sudden cessation of guanabenz therapy may result in withdrawal symptoms (40).

Clinical Use

Guanabenz has been shown to reduce the signs and symptoms of opiate withdrawal in individuals physically dependent on opiates. Guanabenz, like clonidine, appears to reduce the severity of opiate withdrawal symptoms by stimulating central presynaptic α_2-adrenergic receptors; the stimulation results in attenuation of rebound increases in noradrenergic activity in the CNS, which may be responsible for the behavioral symptoms of opiate withdrawal. Psychologic and/or physical dependence or addiction potential have not been associated with guanabenz administration (41).

Guanabenz Withdrawal

Like other centrally active α-adrenergic agonists, abrupt withdrawal of guanabenz may result in a rapid increase in systolic and diastolic blood pressure, and rebound increases in serum and urine catecholamine concentrations. Symptoms associated with abrupt withdrawal of guanabenz may result from sympathetic overactivity and may include nervousness, agitation, anxiety, insomnia, headache, dizziness, tingling in the hands, tremors, fatigue, malaise, flushing, sweating, chest pain, palpitations, nausea, vomiting, and abdominal pain. Following abrupt withdrawal of the drug, increased sympathetic activity and associated symptoms may occasionally occur without a substantial increase in blood pressure.

Toxicity

Signs and symptoms of guanabenz overdosage are similar to those following clonidine overdosage. Overdosage of guanabenz produces signs and symptoms that are mainly extensions of the usual pharmacologic and common adverse effects of the drug, including hypotension, respiratory depression, bradycardia, drowsiness, lethargy, irritability, miosis, and coma. Other effects occurring following overdosage of centrally active α_2-adrenergic agonists include tachycardia, hypertension, hypotonia, hypothermia, pallor, and arrhythmias.

Guanfacine (Tenex)

Pharmacokinetics

Guanfacine is rapidly and almost completely absorbed (90%) from the gastrointestinal tract. Guanfacine has a half-life of 15 to 20 hours, which is significantly longer than that of clonidine. With a plasma half-life of 15–20 hours, most patients need take the medication only once daily. The plasma half-life is not prolonged by increasing age, and is only slightly prolonged by renal insufficiency. It has a large volume of distribution (276 to 456 L) and, at therapeutic plasma concentrations, is 64% protein-bound. Guanfacine enters and leaves the CNS more slowly than clonidine (40).

Adverse Reactions

Adverse reactions noted with guanfacine are similar to those of other drugs of the central α_2-adrenoreceptor agonist class: dry mouth, sedation, weakness, dizziness, constipation, and impotence. While the reactions are common, most are mild and tend to disappear on continued dosing.

Drug Withdrawal

Development of tolerance to the drug as well as withdrawal reactions may be seen. Probably because of its longer duration of action, discontinuation phenomena seem to be very uncommon and are milder after abrupt cessation of guanfacine than with clonidine. Instead, a gradual recovery of pretreatment blood pressure occurs during a 2- to 4-day period following discontinuation of guanfacine treatment. Symptoms that may manifest and that are associated with withdrawal include headache, dizziness, hypertension, nausea, vomiting, palpitations, agitation, anxiety, and abdominal pain.

Toxicity

Symptoms of overdose and treatment are identical to those of clonidine.

Methyldopa

The mode of action of methyldopa (Aldomet) is also interference with central α adrenoceptors, although in a more complicated manner than is the case with clonidine. After oral ingestion of methyldopa, plasma concentrations reach a peak in approximately 3 to 6 hours. Methyldopa is a drug precursor in the sense that it needs to be converted to an active product. This occurs when it penetrates into the brain stem, where it is decarboxylated enzymatically to yield α-methyldopamine, which is in turn converted by enzymatic hydroxylation into α-methylnorepinephrine. α-Methylnorepinephrine, an α-adrenoceptor agonist, then stimulates central inhibitory α adrenoceptors in a manner similar to that of clonidine, causing a fall in arterial pressure.

Methyldopa does not appear to cause withdrawal reactions with any measurable frequency. This may be due to the active metabolite, which persists in nerve endings for some time and thus permits a gradual offset of effect.

Overdosage with methyldopa may produce acute hypotension, sedation, weakness, bradycardia, dizziness, light-headedness, constipation, diarrhea, nausea, and vomiting (Table 12–5) (42). Treatment is similar to that for clonidine overdosage.

TABLE 12–5. *Signs and symptoms of methyldopa overdose*

Central nervous system
Dizziness
Light-headedness
Sedation
Weakness
Cardiovascular
Hypotension
Bradycardia
Gastrointestinal
Constipation
Diarrhea
Nausea
Vomiting

Treatment of α_2 Agonist Overdose

General

Treatment must include the basics of overdose resuscitation and careful cardiovascular monitoring. If the patient has an altered mental status, 50% dextrose in water, thiamine, and naloxone should be administered (Table 12–6). In acute clonidine overdose an attempt should be made to empty the stomach by gastric lavage followed by administration of activated charcoal and a cathartic. Administration of ipecac for clonidine overdose is not advised because of the rapid onset of altered mental status (6).

If the patient is comatose, having seizures, or lacks the gag reflex, gastric lavage may be performed if an endotracheal tube with cuff inflated is in place to prevent aspiration of gastric contents. Supportive and symptomatic treatment should be initiated and an adequate airway established and maintained, using assisted respiration as necessary. Clinical monitoring of vital signs and fluid balance should also be initiated.

Use of Naloxone

Naloxone has been used with and without success (19,33,43,44). Although naloxone has been advocated in

Table 12–6. *Treatment of α_2 agonist overdose*

Indication	Treatment
Altered mental status	Dextrose and thiamine
Decreased respiration	Naloxone
Acute overdose	Lavage
	Charcoal and cathartic
Bradycardia with hypotension	Fluids
	Atropine
	Tolazoline
	Dopamine
Seizures	Diazepam

the treatment of α_2 agonist overdose due to an adrenergic–opioid interaction, its effectiveness has not been demonstrated. Because naloxone is relatively innocuous, and because α_2 agonist overdose closely resembles narcotic overdose, naloxane should be administered (45). The benefit of naloxone may be related to the fact that the α_2 agonist's inhibition of central sympathetic outflow is thought to be mediated by the release of an endogenous opioid. Seizures can be managed with intravenous diazepam (15).

Treatment of Hypotension

Blood pressure should be closely monitored after overdose because hypotension, if it occurs, will be detected within the first several hours after ingestion (46). Hypotension can initially be managed with intravenous fluids and by placing the patient in Trendelenburg's position (13). In most cases, hypotension associated with α_2 agonist overdose responds to intravenous fluids (6). Dopamine may be useful for severe hypotension (9,46).

Treatment of Bradycardia

Bradycardia, if not associated with hypotension, may not require treatment (2). Atropine has been used to control symptomatic bradycardia; however, multiple repeated doses are often necessary due to the long half-life of clonidine (17,21).

Treatment of Hypertension

The treatment of the paradoxical hypertension warrants special consideration (7). Aggressive therapy may result in a profound and prolonged hypotension necessitating the need for vasopressors. Intravenous nitroprusside delivered via an infusion pump in a monitored intensive care setting is the therapy of choice (16).

Use of Tolazoline

Tolazoline may be effective in reversing the hypotensive, bradycardic, and hypertensive effects of clonidine (17,21). Tolazoline, an imidazoline compound with a structure similar to that of clonidine, has both central and peripheral nonspecific α-adrenergic inhibitory effects (9,10). Tolazoline is similar to phentolamine. It is somewhat less potent than phentolamine, but is better absorbed from the gastrointestinal tract (16). Tolazoline penetrates into the brain and thereby reverses part of clonidine's CNS effects. It may be administered intravenously (0.5 to 1 mg/kg, up to 25 mg, in children, and 25 mg per dose in adults) every 5 to 10 minutes to a maximum of four doses. Tolazoline may be tried if fluids, atropine, and dopamine do not reverse hypotension and bradycardia (13).

Although tolazoline has been used with some success to reverse the effects of clonidine overdosage, use of tolazoline in guanabenz overdosage has not been studied, and additional information on the efficacy of α-adrenergic blockers in the treatment of guanabenz overdosage is necessary (38).

Tolazoline can be associated with toxic effects such as marked hypertension, cardiac dysrhythmias, and tachycardia. Because the cardiovascular responses of the drug are not always predictable, it should be reserved for those patients who do not respond to intravenous fluids, dopamine, or atropine (47).

Enhancing Elimination

Although forced diuresis has been suggested to enhance the elimination of α_2 agonists, there is no strong evidence that it increases urinary excretion, and it therefore should not be attempted. Dialysis and hemoperfusion are also not effective (9,10).

REFERENCES

1. Oster J, Epstein M: Use of centrally acting sympatholytic agents in the management of hypertension. *Arch Intern Med* 1991;151: 1638–1644.
2. Dire D, Kuhns D: The use of sublingual nifedipine in a patient with a clonidine overdose. *J Emerg Med* 1988;6:125–128.
3. Shepherd A, Kwan C, Brodie C, et al: Determination of alpha-adrenergic blocking activity. *Clin Pharmacol Ther* 1991;49:69–77.
4. Frishman W, Charlap S: Alpha-adrenergic blockers. *Med Clin North Am* 1988;72:427–439.
5. Doherty T: Alpha$_2$ antagonists. *Ann Emerg Med* 1989;18:710–711.
6. Heidemann S, Sarnaik A: Clonidine poisoning in children. *Crit Care Med* 1990;18:618–620.
7. Fiser D, Moss M, Walker W: Critical care for clonidine poisoning in toddlers. *Crit Care Med* 1990;18:1124–1128.
8. Roth A, Kalusi E, Felner S, et al: Clonidine for patients with rapid atrial fibrillation. *Ann Intern Med* 1992;116:388–390.
9. Anderson R, Hart G, Crumler C, et al: Clonidine overdose: report of six cases and review of the literature. *Ann Emerg Med* 1981;10: 107–112.
10. Anderson R, Hart G, Crumler C, et al: Oral clonidine loading in hypertensive urgencies. *JAMA* 1981;246:848–850.
11. Houston M: Oral clonidine loading in the treatment of hypertensive urgencies and emergencies. *Cardiovasc Rev Rep* 1985;6:1249–1252.
12. Javel A: Mixed substance abuse withdrawal treated by clonidine. *J Med Soc N J* 1983;80:1035–1036.
13. Wiley J, Wiley C, Torrey S, et al: Clonidine poisoning in young children. *J Pediatr* 1990;116:654–658.
14. Hamblin J: Transdermal patch poisoning. *Pediatrics* 1987;79:161.
15. Caravati E, Bennett D: Clonidine transdermal patch poisoning. *Ann Emerg Med* 1988;17:175–176.
16. Mendoza J, Medalle M: Clonidine poisoning with marked hypotension in a 2 1/2 year old child. *Clin Pediatr* 1979;18:123–127.
17. Mofenson H, Greensher J, Weiss T: Clonidine poisoning: is there a single antidote? *Clin Toxicol* 1979;14:271–275.
18. Augustine S, Tachikawa S, Lokhandwala M, et al: Central α-adrenergic control of blood pressure.*Chest* 1983;83(Suppl.):328–331.
19. Gremse D, Artman M, Boerth R: Hypertension associated with naloxone treatment for clonidine poisoning. *Pediatrics* 1986;108:776–778.
20. Korner P, Angus J, Lew M, et al: Characterization of the clonidine receptor site. *Chest* 1983;83:345–349.

21. Mathew P, Addy D, Wright N: Clonidine overdose in children. *Clin Toxicol* 1981;18:169–173.
22. Lowenstein J: Clonidine. *Ann Intern Med* 1980;92:74–77.
23. Conway T, Balson A: Concomitant abuse of clonidine and heroin. *South Med J* 1993;86:954–956.
24. MacFaul R, Miller G: Clonidine poisoning in children. *Lancet* 1977;1:1266–1267.
25. Brown M, Salmon D, Rendell M: Clonidine hallucinations. *Ann Intern Med* 1980;93:456–457.
26. Peters R. Hamilton B, Hamilton J, et al: Cardiac arrhythmias after abrupt clonidine withdrawal.*Clin Pharmacol Ther* 1983;34:435–439.
27. Collis M, Shepherd J: Antidepressant drug action and presynaptic α receptors. *Mayo Clin Proc* 1980;55:567–572.
28. Hamilton B, Mersey J, Hamilton J, et al: Withdrawal phenomena in subjects with essential hypertension on clonidine or tiamenidine. *Clin Pharmacol Ther* 1984;36:628–633.
29. Stiff J, Harris D: Clonidine withdrawal complicated by amitriptyline therapy. *Anesthesiology* 1983;59:73–74.
30. Reid J, Campbell B, Hamilton C: Withdrawal reactions following cessation of central α-adrenergic receptor agonists. *Hypertension* 1984;6(Suppl.II):71–75.
31. Ferguson R, Alvino E: Rebound hypertension after low-dose clonidine withdrawal. *South Med J* 1983;76:98.
32. Catapano M, Marx J: Management of urgent hypertensive: a comparison of oral treatment regimens in the emergency department. *J Emerg Med* 1986;4:361–368.
33. Banner W, Lund M, Clawson L: Failure of naloxone to reverse clonidine toxic effect. *Am J Dis Child* 1983;137:1170–1171.
34. Patnode R, Brouhard B, Travis L: Prolonged clonidine overdosage in a child. *J Pediatr* 1977;90:848–849.
35. Williams P, Krafeik J, Potter B, et al: Cardiac toxicity of clonidine. *Chest* 1977;72:784–785.
36. Neuvonen P, Vilska J, Keranen A: Severe poisoning in a child caused by a small dose of clonidine. *Clin Toxicol* 1979;14:369–374.
37. Farina P, Homon C, Chow C, et al: Radioimmunoassay for clonidine in human plasma and urine using a solid phase second antibody separation. *Therap Drug Monit* 1985;7:344–350.
38. Hall A, Smolinske S, Kulig K, et al: Guanabenz overdose. *Ann Intern Med* 1985;102:787–788.
39. Holmes B, Brogden R, Heel R, et al: Guanabenz: a review of its pharmacodynamic properties and therapeutic efficacy in hypertension. *Drugs* 1983;26:212–229.
40. Malini P, Strocchi E, Ambrosioni E, et al: Comparison of antihypertensive activity and tolerability of guanfacine and methyldopa. *Int J Clin Pharmacol Res* 1983;1:35–39.
41. Perrone J, Hoffman R, Jones B, et al: Guanabenz induced hypothermia in a poisoned elderly female. *J Toxicol Clin Toxicol* 1994;32:445–450.
42. Shnaps Y, Almog S, Halkin H, et al: Methyldopa poisoning. *J Toxicol Clin Toxicol* 1982;19:501–513.
43. Kulig K, Duffy J, Rumack B: Naloxone for treatment of clonidine overdose. *JAMA* 1982;247:1697.
44. Olsson J, Pruitt A: Management of clonidine ingestion in children. *J Pediatr* 1983;103:646–649.
45. Niemann J, Getzug T, Murphy W: Reversal of clonidine toxicity by naloxone. *Ann Emerg Med* 1986;15:1229–1231.
46. Artman M, Boerth R: Clonidine poisoning. *Am J Dis Child* 1983;137:171–174.
47. Frishman W, Eisen G, Lapsker J: Terazosin. *Med Clin North Am* 1988;72:441–447.

ADDITIONAL SELECTED REFERENCES

Buffum J: Pharmacosexology update: yohimbine and sexual function. *J Psychoactive Drugs* 1985;17:131–132.

Dunn F, Messerli F, Dreslinski G: Clonidine in hypertensive urgencies. *JAMA* 1982;247:1274–1275.

Houston M: Treatment of hypertensive emergencies and urgencies with oral clonidine loading and titration. *Arch Intern Med* 1986;146:586–589.

Louis W, Taylor H, McNeil J, et al: Clinical pharmacology of adrenergic adrenoreceptor blocking drugs. *Am Heart J* 1982;104:407–412.

Quart B, Guglielmo B: Prolonged diarrhea secondary to methyldopa therapy. *Drug Intell Clin Pharmacol* 1983;17:462.

Schaut J, Schnoll S: Four cases of clonidine abuse. *Am J Psychiatry* 1983;140:1625–1627.

Schieber R, Kaufman N: Use of tolazoline in massive clonidine poisoning. *Am J Dis Child* 1981;135:77–78.

Siegel G, Bonfiglo J, Ritschel W, et al: Investigation of clonidine and lofexidine for the treatment of barbiturate withdrawal in mice. *Vet Hum Toxicol* 1985;27:503–505.

CHAPTER 13

α-Adrenergic Blocking Agents

Although there are many α-adrenergic blocking agents, very few are encountered as an overdose. The ergot alkaloids were the first adrenergic blocking drugs to be investigated. The reason for the therapeutic use of these alkaloids in medicine today, though, is unrelated to α blockade (1).

All of the α blockers in clinical use inhibit the postsynaptic α_1 receptor and result in relaxation of vascular smooth muscle and vasodilation. However, the nonselective α blockers also can antagonize presynaptic α_2 receptors (2). This leads to increased release of neuronal norepinephrine. Although the α blockers effectively block the vasoconstricting effect of catecholamines, their use in hypertension, with the exception of prazosin and structural analogues, and labetalol, has been of little consequence (3).

α Blockers may be reversible or irreversible blockers of these receptors. Reversible antagonists may dissociate from the α receptor, whereas irreversible drugs do not. Phentolamine, tolazoline, prazosin, and labetalol are examples of reversible antagonists. Phenoxybenzamine forms a reactive ethyleneimonium intermediate that covalently binds to the α receptor site, resulting in irreversible blockade (3).

The rate of termination of the action of a reversible antagonist is largely dependent on the half-life of the drug as well as the rate at which it dissociates from its receptor: the shorter the half-life, the less time it takes until the effects of the drug are dissipated. However, the effects of an irreversible antagonist may persist long after the drug has been cleared from the plasma. In the case of phenoxybenzamine, the restoration of tissue responsiveness after extensive α-receptor blockade is dependent on synthesis of new receptors, which may take several days.

PHENOXYBENZAMINE (TABLE 13–1)

Phenoxybenzamine is a haloalkylamine that is structurally related to the nitrogen mustard alkylating agents used in cancer chemotherapy. Phenoxybenzamine produces an initial reversible competitive antagonism of adrenergic agonists at both α_1 and α_2 receptors that is similar to phentolamine (1). After the initial competitive phase, which is relatively short, the receptor blockade by phenoxybenzamine binds covalently, becoming more fully developed and leading to a persistent and irreversible blockade. It is somewhat selective for α_1 receptors but less so than prazosin.

In addition to the blockade of α receptors, high doses of phenoxybenzamine can inhibit responses to H_1 histamine, serotonin, and acetylcholine. Phenoxybenzamine, in addition, inhibits reuptake of released norepinephrine by presynaptic adrenergic nerve terminals.

Oral phenoxybenzamine has a rapid onset of action, with the maximal effect from a single dose seen in 1 to 2 hours. The gastrointestinal absorption is incomplete, and only 20% to 30% of an oral dose reaches the systemic circulation in active form. Although phenoxybenzamine has a low bioavailability, the drug is sufficiently absorbed from the gastrointestinal tract (GIT) to provide a therapeutic effect.

Intravenous phenoxybenzamine is initially started at 0.1 mg per minute and is then increased at increments of 0.1 mg per minute every 5 to 10 minutes until the desired hemodynamic effect is reached. The drug has a short duration of action of 3 to 10 minutes. The half-life of the drug is 24 hours (4).

The adverse effects of phenoxybenzamine derive from its α-receptor blocking action; the most important are postural hypotension, tachycardia, gastrointestinal disturbances, nasal stuffiness, and inhibition of ejaculation.

PHENTOLAMINE (TABLE 13–2)

Phentolamine is an imidazoline derivative that is equipotent at α_1 and α_2 receptors. Although virtually all the clinical effects of phenoxybenzamine are explicable in terms of α blockade, this is not the case with phentolamine, which also possesses several other properties, including a direct vasodilator action and sympathomimetic and parasympathomimetic effects.

At the H_1 and H_2 histamine receptor sites, phentolamine has both affinity and intrinsic activity. This is observed as a histamine-like effect on the stomach, caus-

TABLE 13–1. *α Blocking agents—phenoxybenzamine*

Effects
Antiacetylcholinergic
Antihistaminergic
Antiserotoninergic
Inhibits reuptake of norepinephrine
Irreversible inhibition of α receptors
Side effects
Gastrointestinal disturbances
Inhibition of ejaculation
Nasal stuffiness
Postural hypotension
Sinus tachycardia

ing secretion of both acid and pepsin. Phentolamine increases the motility of the intestine by a cholinomimetic action, which is the result of a direct effect on muscarinic receptors, and which is unrelated to its α blockade. Phentolamine has a sympathomimetic action on the heart, which appears to be the result of increased endogenous norepinephrine release due to blockade of presynaptic α_2 receptors and a reduction in negative feedback inhibition of neurotransmitter release.

Adverse effects are common with phentolamine and are attributable to cardiac and gastrointestinal stimulation. Tachycardia, anginal pain, cardiac arrhythmias, and episodes of hypotension may occur. Gastrointestinal stimulation may produce nausea, vomiting, abdominal pain, diarrhea, and exacerbation of peptic ulceration.

TOLAZOLINE (TABLE 13–3)

Tolazoline is a structural congener of phentolamine that has greater smooth muscle relaxant and histaminic action than phentolamine, but less α blocking activity (5,6). Although the drug inhibits responses to adrenergic

TABLE 13–2. *α Blocking agents—phentolamine*

Effects
Reversible inhibition of α receptors
H_1 and H_2 activity
Muscarinic activity
Sympathomimetic action (Blockade of α_2 cardiac receptors)
Adverse effects
Cardiac
Sinus tachycardia
Anginal pain
Cardiac arrhythmias
Hypotension
Gastrointestinal
Nausea
Vomiting
Abdominal pain
Diarrhea
Exacerbation of peptic ulceration

TABLE 13–3. *α Blocking agents—tolazoline*

Effects
Weak α blocking activity
Smooth muscle relaxant
Histaminic action
Sympathomimetic activity
Cholinergic activity
Adverse effects
Neurologic
Tingling
Flushing
Paresthesia
Headache
Dizziness
Blood dyscrasias
Agranulocytosis
Thrombocytopenia
Pancytopenia

stimuli by competitively blocking α-adrenergic receptors, this action of the drug is relatively transient, and α-adrenergic blockade is incomplete with usual doses (7). Tolazoline also possesses histamine-like, sympathomimetic, and cholinergic properties. The effect of tolazoline on the pulmonary vasculature has been attributed to its action on histamine receptors, but there is no conclusive evidence that it selectively dilates pulmonary, as opposed to systemic, vessels. Tolazoline also increases cardiac output.

Adverse Effects

Tolazoline causes increased pilomotor activity with goose flesh and piloerection. Tingling, chilliness, flushing, paresthesia, sweating, headache, and dizziness have occurred. Agranulocytosis, thrombocytopenia, and pancytopenia have been reported (8,9). Oliguria, hematuria, edema, hepatitis, and psychiatric reactions characterized by confusion or hallucinations have occurred rarely.

Treatment

Placing the patient in the supine position with the head down and administering intravenous infusion solutions is most important in the management of tolazoline-induced hypotension. If a vasopressor drug is necessary, a drug that has both central and peripheral action should be used (10).

PRAZOSIN

Prazosin (Minipress) is a quinazoline derivative used in the treatment of hypertension by reducing peripheral vascular resistance. Prazosin was originally introduced as a direct-acting vasodilator, but it now appears clear that it exerts its major effect by reversible blockade of postsynaptic α_1 receptors (11). Prazosin has a 5,000-fold greater affinity for the α_1 receptor than for the α_2 receptor (2,12,13). This may partially explain the relative absence of tachycardia seen with prazosin compared with that seen with phentolamine and phenoxybenzamine (14). High concentrations of prazosin could potentially also inhibit presynaptic α_2 receptors (4). This receptor selectivity allows norepinephrine to exert unopposed negative feedback (mediated by presynaptic α_2 receptors) on its own release; in contrast, phentolamine blocks both pre- and postsynaptic α receptors, with the result that reflex stimulation of sympathetic neurons produces greater release of transmitter onto β receptors and correspondingly greater cardioacceleration (15).

As a result of its vasodilating effects, prazosin produces both arterial and venous dilation. Unlike hydralazine, the antihypertensive effect of prazosin is accompanied by little or no increase in heart rate (13). This lack of reflex tachycardia is probably attributable to a number of reasons, one of which is that prazosin does not interrupt the α_2-adrenergic autoinhibition of norepinephrine release (16).

Prazosin is the most potent α_1 blocking drug currently available and has no α_2- or β-adrenergic activity. Also, unlike methyldopa and clonidine, prazosin appears to have no central action on blood pressure (17).

TABLE 13–4. *Side effects of prazosin*

Cardiac
Bradycardia
Postural hypotension
Tachycardia
Palpitations
Syncope
Neurologic
Dryness of mouth
Headache
Drowsiness
Lassitude
Nausea
Urinary frequency
First-dose phenomenon

Pharmacokinetics

After oral administration of prazosin, it is almost completely absorbed, with peak plasma levels achieved at 2 to 3 hours. The usual half-life of the drug is 2.5 to 4 hours, but may increase in patients with heart failure to 5 to 7 hours. Prazosin is extensively metabolized and because of this, only about 50% of the drug is available after oral administration. Prazosin is 97% bound to human plasma proteins and has an apparent volume of distribution of approximately 0.6 to 1 L/kg. Plasma concentrations generally do not correlate with therapeutic effects (14).

Side Effects

Commonly reported side effects of prazosin include drowsiness, headache, lassitude, dryness of the mouth, nausea, and urinary frequency with urgency (Table 13–4) (15). The major side effect of prazosin therapy in patients with hypertension is postural hypotension, which is usually most pronounced after the initial drug administration. This postural hypotension is accompanied by tachycardia and palpitations and occasionally proceeds to bradycardia and syncope (12). A "first-dose orthostatic hypotensive reaction" sometimes occurs, after the initial dose of prazosin, and may be severe. Syncope or other postural symptoms, such as dizziness, may occur. Subsequent occurrence with dosage increases is also possible (13). A similar effect can be anticipated if therapy is interrupted for more than a few doses. This "first dose phenomenon" may occur 30 to 90 minutes after the initial dose. Occasionally, bradycardia may be noted. The reason for this phenomenon may involve the rapid induction of venous and arteriolar dilation by a drug that elicits little reflex sympathetic stimulation and is believed to be due to an excessive postural hypotensive effect, although occasionally the syncopal episode has been preceded by a bout of severe supraventricular tachycardia with heart rates of 120–160 beats per minute. It is seen more widely when the drug is administered as a tablet rather than as a capsule, possibly related to the variable bioavailability or rates of absorption of the two formulations. Postural hypotension is not usually a problem during continued treatment.

Toxicity

Overdosage of prazosin has caused drowsiness and depressed reflexes, but no severe hypotension. Priapism has also been noted with prazosin overdose and is thought to be related to the sympatholytic effects from blockade of postsynaptic α-adrenergic receptors. This blockade appears to favor erection, which is parasympathetically mediated, and to inhibit ejaculation and detumescence, which are sympathetically mediated.

Treatment

If overdosage of prazosin causes hypotension, supportive therapy should be initiated. The patient should be kept in the supine position; if necessary, shock may be treated with plasma volume expanders and vasopressor drugs. Renal function should be monitored and supported as needed. Prazosin is not dialyzable because of its high degree of protein binding.

TERAZOSIN

Terazosin hydrochloride is a quinazoline-derivative postsynaptic α_1-adrenergic blocking agent. The drug is chemically and pharmacologically related to prazosin and doxazosin. It has more than 100 times the affinity for α_1 compared with α_2 receptors. Terazosin has a half-life of about 12 hours, which makes it an attractive once-a-day dosage (18). Following oral administration, terazosin is rapidly and almost entirely absorbed, and peak plasma concentrations occur within 1 to 2 hours. The bioavailability of the oral preparation is approximately 90%, with approximately 90% of the dose bound to plasma proteins (18).

Terazosin reduces peripheral vascular resistance and blood pressure as a result of its vasodilating effects; the drug produces both arterial and venous dilation. Terazosin reduces blood pressure in both supine and standing patients; the effect is most pronounced on standing blood pressure, and postural hypotension can occur. Terazosin generally causes no change in heart rate or cardiac output in the supine position. Cardiovascular responses to exercise are maintained during terazosin therapy.

Pharmacokinetics

Terazosin has been shown to undergo minimal hepatic first-pass metabolism, and nearly all of the circulating dose is in the form of parent drug. The plasma levels peak about 1 hour after dosing, and then decline, with a half-life of approximately 12 hours. The drug is highly bound to plasma proteins, and binding is constant over the clinically observed concentration range. Approximately 10% of an orally administered dose is excreted as parent drug in the urine, and approximately 20% is excreted in the feces. The remainder is eliminated as metabolites.

Adverse Effects

Adverse effects occurring most frequently during terazosin hydrochloride therapy for hypertension include dizziness, headache, asthenia, nasal congestion, peripheral edema, somnolence, nausea, and palpitations.

As previously mentioned, syncope has also been reported with other α-adrenergic blocking agents in association with rapid dosage increases or the introduction of another antihypertensive drug. This is called the first-dose phenomenon. While syncope is the most severe orthostatic effect of the drug, other less severe symptoms, such as dizziness, light-headedness, tachycardia, palpitations, and vertigo, also can be associated with terazosin-induced reductions in blood pressure.

DOXAZOSIN

Doxazosin (Cardura) mesylate is a quinazoline-derivative postsynaptic α_1-adrenergic blocking agent. The drug is chemically and pharmacologically related to prazosin and terazosin.

Effects of doxazosin on the cardiovascular system are mediated by the drug's activity at α_1-receptor sites on vascular smooth muscle. α_1-Adrenergic receptors also are located in nonvascular smooth muscle (e.g., bladder trigone and sphincters, GI tract and sphincters, prostate adenoma and capsule, ureters, uterus) and in nonmuscular tissues (e.g., central nervous system (CNS), liver, kidneys).

Adverse Effects

Adverse effects occurring most frequently during doxazosin mesylate therapy include dizziness, headache, drowsiness, lethargy, fatigue, nausea, edema, and rhinitis.

YOHIMBINE

Yohimbine is an indole alkylamine alkaloid that is chemically similar to reserpine and is the prototype of the α_2 blocking agents. It is a plant alkaloid derived from the bark of *Corynanthe johimbe*, *Rubaceae* and related trees, and has prominent CNS effects (19,20). It is a crystalline, odorless powder. When used as Yocon, it is supplied as a tablet that contains 5.4 mg of yohimbine hydrochloride.

Yohimbine acts by selectively blocking the central α_2 receptors (21) that cause the release of norepinephrine. Thus, yohimbine antagonizes α-adrenergic inhibition of adrenergic actions and reverses the effects of many centrally acting antihypertensive agents such as clonidine. Non-α_2 effects of yohimbine include local anesthetic actions and inhibition of monoamine oxidase (22).

The action of yohimbine on peripheral blood vessels resembles that of reserpine, though yohimbine is weaker and of shorter duration. Yohimbine's peripheral autonomic nervous system effect is to increase parasympathetic and decrease sympathetic activity (20).

Theoretically, yohimbine could be useful in autonomic insufficiency by promoting neurotransmitter release through presynaptic blockade of α_2 receptors. Yohimbine may improve symptoms in some patients with painful diabetic neuropathies. It has been suggested that yohimbine improves or enhances sexual function; however, evidence for this effect is limited (23).

Although yohimbine hydrochloride is available under the brand names Yohimex and Yocon and is suggested as a sympatholytic and mydriatic and for erectile dysfunction, its medical use is questionable (24). Yohimbine has no FDA sanctioned indications and is a drug of abuse (its street name is "yo-yo"). Although it has been promoted as an aphrodisiac for many years, in actuality it stimu-

TABLE 13–5. *Signs and symptoms of yohimbine overdose*

Anxiety
Hypertension
Increased motor activity
Irritability
Lacrimation
Mild hallucinations
Mydriasis
Penile erection
Salivation
Tachycardia
Tremors

lates erectile tissue without increasing sexual desire and thus is not a true aphrodisiac (25). The rationale for its use as an aphrodisiac is that erection is linked to cholinergic activity and to α_2-adrenergic blockade, which may theoretically result in increased penile inflow, decreased penile outflow, or both (22).

Yohimbine readily penetrates the CNS and produces a complex pattern of responses in lower doses than required to produce peripheral adrenergic blockade. These include antidiuresis, a general picture of central excitation including hypertension, tachycardia, mydriasis, lacrimation, salivation, diaphoresis, increased motor activity, irritability, priapism, and tremors. Sweating, nausea, and vomiting are common after parenteral administration of the drug. Mild hallucinations have also been noted (Table 13–5) (21).

Treatment

Treatment of yohimbine intoxication consists mainly of supportive care. Attempts to empty the stomach are usually of no benefit. Clonidine is the agent of choice for treating anxiety, hypertension, and other autonomic symptoms. Clonidine should be administered in an initial oral loading dose of 0.1 to 0.2 mg followed by several additional hourly doses of 0.1 mg (26).

REFERENCES

1. Oster J, Epstein M: Use of centrally acting sympatholytic agents in the management of hypertension. *Arch Intern Med* 1991;151:1638–1644.
2. Von Bahr C, Lindstrom B, Seideman P: α-Receptor function changes after the first dose of prazosin. *Clin Pharmacol Ther* 1982;32:41–47.
3. Shepherd A, Kwan C, Brodie C, et al: Determination of alpha-adrenergic blocking activity. *Clin Pharmacol Ther* 1991;49:69–77.
4. Frishman W, Charlap S: Alpha-adrenergic blockers. *Med Clin North Am* 1988;72:427–439.
5. Mathew P, Addy D, Wright N: Clonidine overdose in children. *Clin Toxicol* 1981;18:169–173.
6. Mofenson H, Greensher J, Weiss T: Clonidine poisoning: is there a single antidote? *Clin Toxicol* 1979;14:271–275.
7. Mendoza J, Medalle M: Clonidine poisoning with marked hypotension in a 2 1/2 year old child. *Clin Pediatr* 1979;18:123–127.
8. Anderson R, Hart G, Crumler C, et al: Clonidine overdose: report of six cases and review of the literature. *Ann Emerg Med* 1981;10:107–112.
9. Anderson R, Hart G, Crumler C, et al: Oral clonidine loading in hypertensive urgencies. *JAMA* 1981;246:848–850.
10. Hall A, Smolinske S, Kulig K, et al: Guanabenz overdose. *Ann Intern Med* 1985;102:787–788.
11. Cambridge D, Davey M, Massingham R: Prazosin, a selective antagonist of postsynaptic α adrenoceptors. *Br J Pharmacol* 1977;59: 514–515.
12. Brogden R, Hell R, Speight T, et al: Prazosin: a review of its pharmacological properties and therapeutic efficacy in hypertension. *Drugs* 1977;14:163–197.
13. Colucci W: α-Adrenergic receptor blockade with prazosin. *Ann Intern Med* 1982;97:67–77.
14. Baudouin S, Aitman T, Johnson A: Prazosin in the treatment of chronic asthma. *Thorax* 1988;43:385–387.
15. Itskovitz H, Krug K, Khoury S, et al: The long-term antihypertensive effects of prazosin and atenolol. *Am J Med* 1989;86:82–86.
16. Kobrin I, Stessman J, Yagil Y, et al: Prazosin-induced bradycardia in acute treatment of hypertension. *Arch Intern Med* 1983;143: 2019–2020.
17. Doherty T: Alpha$_2$ antagonists. *Ann Emerg Med* 1989;18:710–711.
18. Frishman W, Eisen G, Lapsker J: Terazosin. *Med Clin North Am* 1988;72:441–447.
19. Goldberg M, Hollister A, Robertson D: Influence of yohimbine on blood pressure, autonomic reflexes, and plasma catecholamines in humans. *Hypertension* 1983;5:772–778.
20. Goldberg M, Robertson D: Yohimbine: a pharmacological probe for study of the α_2 adrenoreceptor. *Pharmacol Rev* 1983;35:143–180.
21. Susset J, Tessier C, Wincze J, et al: Effect of yohimbine hydrochloride on erectile impotence: a double blind study. *J Urol* 1989;141: 1360–1363.
22. Lacomblez L, Bensimon G, Isnard F, et al: Effect of yohimbine on blood pressure in patients with depression and orthostatic hypotension induced by clomipramine. *Clin Pharmacol Ther* 1989;45: 241–251.
23. Berlin I, Crespo-Laumonnier B, Cournot A, et al: The alpha$_2$-adrenergic receptor antagonist yohimbine inhibits epinephrine-induced platelet aggregation in healthy subjects. *Clin Pharmacol Ther* 1991; 49:362–369.
24. Holmberg G, Gershon S: Autonomic and psychic effects of yohimbine hydrochloride. *Psychopharmacologia* 1961;2:93–106.
25. Charney D, Heninger G, Redmond D: Yohimbine-induced anxiety and increased noradrenergic function in humans: effects of diazepam and clonidine. *Life Sci* 1983;33:19–29.
26. Linden C, Vellman W, Rumack B: Yohimbine: a new street drug. *Ann Emerg Med* 1985;14:1002–1004.

ADDITIONAL SELECTED REFERENCES

Buffum J: Pharmacosexology update: yohimbine and sexual function. *J Psychoactive Drugs* 1985;17:131–132.

Dunn F, Messerli F, Dreslinski G: Clonidine in hypertensive urgencies. *JAMA* 1982;247:1274–1275.

Houston M: Treatment of hypertensive emergencies and urgencies with oral clonidine loading and titration. *Arch Intern Med* 1986;146:586–589.

Louis W, Taylor H, McNeil J, et al: Clinical pharmacology of adrenergic adrenoreceptor blocking drugs. *Am Heart J* 1982;104:407–412.

Quart B, Guglielmo B: Prolonged diarrhea secondary to methyldopa therapy. *Drug Intell Clin Pharmacol* 1983;17:462.

Schaut J, Schnoll S: Four cases of clonidine abuse. *Am J Psychiatry* 1983;140:1625–1627.

Schieber R, Kaufman N: Use of tolazoline in massive clonidine poisoning. *Am J Dis Child* 1981;135:77–78.

Siegel G, Bonfiglo J, Ritschel W, et al: Investigation of clonidine and lofexidine for the treatment of barbiturate withdrawal in mice. *Vet Hum Toxicol* 1985;27:503–505.

CHAPTER 14

β Receptor Agonists

The β receptors are divided into β_1 and β_2. The β_1 receptors are located primarily in cardiac tissue and the kidneys. The β_2 receptors mediate smooth muscle relaxation and are located in the vasculature, bronchi, and uterus (1). This is not absolute; β_1 receptors are present in the lung, and a small number of β_2 receptors are present in the heart (2,3). The β_1 receptors are under the control of the neurotransmitter norepinephrine, which is released from the sympathetic neuron. The β_2 receptors are not innervated and are under the control of circulating epinephrine.

Selectivity of the receptor effect is dose-dependent. The adrenergic neurotransmitters all favor β effect over α effect at low doses, whereas the α effect predominates at high doses.

β AGONISTS

Administration of β agonists produces direct and indirect stimulation of myocardial β_1 receptors. In addition, hemodynamic responses to β stimulation can result in changes in vagal and α-adrenergic activity (4). The characteristic dose-dependent increase in heart rate seen after the administration of nonselective β-adrenergic agonists has classically been attributed to stimulation of myocardial β_1 receptors. However, the identification of functional β_2 receptors in the myocardium has established a direct role for the receptors in mediating the increase in heart rate seen after both β_2 selective and nonselective β agonists.

Mechanism of Action

Both the β_1 and β_2 receptor subtypes are coupled to adenylate cyclase. Receptor activation results in stimulation of adenylate cyclase, increasing the rate of synthesis of cyclic adenosine monophosphate (cAMP). The receptors are coupled to the cyclase by a G protein. Increased cAMP synthesis activates cAMP-dependent protein kinase, which in turn phosphorylates target proteins (Fig. 14–1) (5). Phosphorylation alters target protein function, resulting in a variety of cellular responses. Oxygen consumption by the heart increases. Stimulating myocardial β_1 receptors also produces chronotropic effects. Automaticity is enhanced because diastolic (phase 4) depolarization of the sinoatrial node occurs more rapidly. The refractory period of the AV node is shortened. There is evidence that β-adrenergic stimulation increases the heterogeneity in the refractory period of different areas of the ventricular myocardium, and that this phenomenon may promote myocardial irritability.

In vascular and bronchial smooth muscle, activation of β_2 receptors also promotes formation of cAMP; the

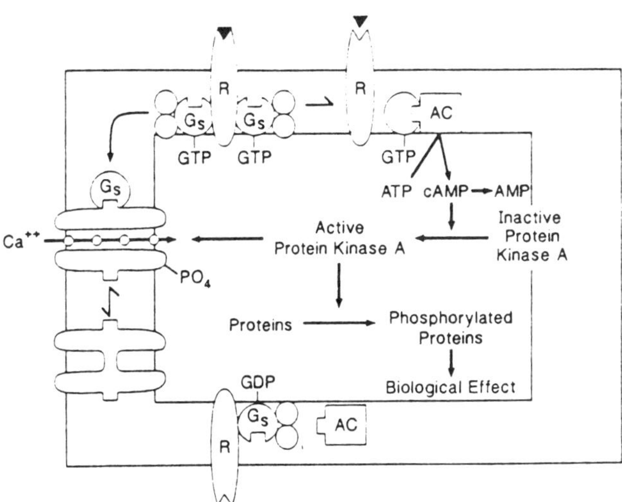

FIG. 14–1. Schematic representation of β-adrenergic signal transduction. The diagram shows the cascade activated by stimulation of β adrenoreceptors. The area between the lines represents the events occurring in the cytosol. Ligand(▼) binds to the β receptor (*top of panel*). The ligand/receptor complex activates the G protein (G_s), which in turn activates adenylate cyclase (*AC*).G_s may also interact directly with the calcium channel, increasing calcium entry into the cell (*left of panel*). Adenylate cyclase synthesizes cyclic adenosine monophosphate (*cAMP*) from adenosine triphosphate; cAMP activates protein kinase A. The kinase induces the biologic effect by phosphorylating specific target proteins including the calcium channel. Note the inactive G_s with guanosine 5′-diphosphate (GDP) bound to the α subunit (*bottom of panel*). (From Towler S and Evers A, *Int Anesthesiol Clin* 1989;27:239, with permission.)

resulting activation of cAMP-dependent protein kinase in those cells stimulates removal of calcium from the cytosol and promotes calcium uptake by the sarcoplasmic reticulum. This relaxes smooth muscle and causes the blood vessels to dilate.

β_2 AGONISTS

An important group of adrenoceptor agonist drugs, effective after oral administration, with a long duration of action and a significant degree of β_2 selectivity, is available (6). These agents differ structurally from epinephrine. When given by inhalation, these agents cause bronchodilation equivalent to that produced by isoproterenol. Bronchodilation is maximal by 30 minutes and persists for 3–4 hours.

Adrenergic agents with greater specificity for β_2 than β_1 receptors include isoetharine (Bronkometer, Bronkosol), metaproterenol (Alupent, Metaprel), terbutaline (Brethaire, Brethine, Bricanyl), albuterol (Proventil, Ventolin), bitolterol (Tornalate), and pirbuterol (Maxair) (Table 14–1) (7). Of these, isoetharine is the least selective for β_2 receptors. Other longer-acting and more selective drugs are preferred. These drugs are effective when administered by metered-dose inhaler.

General Pharmacokinetics

Many of the β_2 agonists can be administered in an oral form, or by inhalation. Following oral administration of β_2 agonists, the peak drug concentration in blood is achieved in 1 to 2 hours. Unlike the inhalation of β_2 agonists, which leads to bronchodilation despite barely measurable blood levels, the oral administration of these drugs is followed by blood concentration–dependent bronchodilation (8).

Actions

The β_2 agents are used as a bronchodilator in the symptomatic relief of bronchospasm in reversible, obstructive airway disease and as an agent in premature labor. The β_2-mediated positive inotropism is qualitatively the same as that produced by β_1 stimulation but quantitatively it appears to be less. This may be the function of either the agonist administered or the β_2 receptor density.

TABLE 14–1. *β_2 Agonists*

Albuterol (Proventil, Ventolin)
Bitolterol (Tornalate)
Isoetharine (Bronkometer, Bronkosol)
Metaproterenol (Alupent, Metaprel)
Pirbuterol (Maxair)
Terbutaline (Brethaire, Brethine, Bricanyl)

Administration of β_2 selective and nonselective agonists is associated with a dose-dependent increase in systolic blood pressure and a reduction in diastolic pressure, resulting in minimal changes in mean arterial blood pressure while the total peripheral resistance falls.

β_2 stimulation promotes an intracellular shift of potassium from serum, possibly via stimulation of Na-K-ATPase, and thereby appears to temporarily decrease both elevated and normal potassium concentrations (9). Epinephrine is more effective at producing hypokalemia than norepinephrine, because of the greater β_2 receptor activity of epinephrine. This results in a reduction in plasma potassium independent of renal potassium clearance and aldosterone and appears to be a predominant β_2 effect.

Side Effects

The side effects of β_2 agonists are due to stimulation of both β_1 and β_2 receptors. Palpitations and tachycardia are the most common, followed by small, dose-related increases in blood pressure. Tachycardia and flushing of the skin occur at high doses. Tachycardia can represent either a direct β_1 effect or a reflex tachycardia due to β_2 stimulation of the peripheral venules (10).

ALBUTEROL

Albuterol (Salbutamol, Proventil, Repetabs) is a synthetic sympathomimetic amine. It stimulates β-adrenergic receptors and has little or no effect on α receptors (11). Albuterol appears to have a greater stimulating effect on β_2-adrenergic receptors of the bronchial, uterine, and vascular smooth muscle than on other β_1-adrenergic receptors in the heart.

Albuterol is used as a bronchodilator in the symptomatic relief of bronchospasm in reversible, obstructive airway disease and as an agent in premature labor (Table 14–2). Oral or orally inhaled albuterol has a longer duration of action than isoproterenol, and only occasionally causes cardiac stimulation. The main effect following oral inhalation or oral administration of albuterol is bronchodilation resulting from relaxation of smooth muscles of the bronchial tree (12).

Albuterol will induce glycogenolysis and gluconeogenesis in the liver, and glycogenolysis, potassium uptake, and increased contractility in skeletal muscle. Because it is also a weak β_1 agonist, it may produce positive dromotropic, chronotropic, and inotropic effects in the heart (11). In contrast to isoproterenol, albuterol does not appear to decrease arterial oxygen tension. Albuterol may cause reflex tachycardia, especially with higher than usual doses (13).

TABLE 14–2. *Albuterol (and other β_2 agonists)*

Uses
- Bronchodilator
- Premature labor

Actions
- Predominant β_2 agonist
- Weak β_1 activity
- No α activity

Adverse effects
- Gastrointestinal
  - Nausea
  - Vomiting
  - Increased appetite
  - Unusual taste
  - Heartburn
- Neurologic
  - Dilated pupils
  - Headache
  - Vertigo
  - CNS stimulation
  - Irritable behavior
  - Insomnia
  - Weakness
  - Dizziness
  - Fine finger tremor
  - Tinnitus
- Cardiac
  - Angina pectoris
  - Dyspnea
  - Tachycardia
  - Palpitations
  - Peripheral vasodilation
  - ECG changes
- Metabolic
  - Stimulates Na-K-ATPase system
    - Hyperkalemia
  - Induces glycogenolysis and gluconeogenesis
    - Hyperglycemia

Both intravenous and orally inhaled forms of albuterol have been shown to decrease serum potassium concentrations, which makes the drug potentially useful in the treatment of conditions associated with hyperkalemia.

Pharmacokinetics

Oral

Albuterol is rapidly and well absorbed following oral administration. Albuterol is longer acting than isoproterenol by any route of administration in most patients because it is not a substrate for the cellular uptake processes for catecholamines nor for catechol *o*-methyltransferase (COMT). Maximum albuterol plasma levels are usually obtained between 2 and 3 hours after dosing, and the elimination half-life is 5 to 6 hours.

Peak plasma albuterol concentrations occur within 2.5 and 2 hours following administration of the conventional tablets and oral solution, respectively. Following administration of a single 4-mg dose of albuterol as an oral solution in healthy individuals, peak plasma drug concentrations of 18 ng/mL are attained.

Inhaled

Albuterol is absorbed gradually from the bronchi, with a portion of the swallowed fraction being absorbed from the gastrointestinal tract. Systemic concentrations are low following inhalation of recommended doses because inhaled doses are only 5% of those required orally.

Bronchodilation usually begins within 5 minutes following nebulization, with peak effect in approximately 1–2 hours, and generally persists 3–4 hours, but occasionally up to 6 hours or longer.

Extended Release

Albuterol extended-release tablets have been formulated to provide a duration of action of up to 12 hours. In addition, it has been shown that administration of a 4-mg albuterol extended-release tablet every 12 hours is bioequivalent to administration of a 2-mg albuterol tablet every 6 hours.

Following a single oral dose of albuterol as 4 mg every 12 hours as extended-release tablets, steady-state peak plasma albuterol concentrations average 5.4–6.5 ng/mL, and steady-state trough plasma concentrations average 3–4.8 ng/mL (14).

Metabolism

Albuterol is extensively metabolized in the liver, mainly to albuterol 4-O-sulfate, which has little or no β-adrenergic stimulating effect and no β-adrenergic blocking effect. Unlike isoproterenol, albuterol is not metabolized by the enzyme COMT and is not a substrate for catecholamine cellular uptake processes. Albuterol and its metabolites are rapidly excreted in urine and feces (15).

Adverse Effects

Nausea, vomiting, increased appetite, muscle cramps, increased or decreased blood pressure, ECG changes, sweating, dilated pupils, chest discomfort, angina, headache, vertigo, central nervous system (CNS) stimulation, hyperactivity, excitement, irritable behavior, insomnia, epistaxis, weakness, and dizziness may occur rarely. The most common adverse effects of albuterol are dose-related, and are characteristic of sympathomimetic agents, although certain cardiovascular effects appear to occur less frequently. Although infrequent, the principal adverse effects are tachycardia, palpitations, peripheral vasodilation, tremor, and nervousness. Inhalation of a selective β_2 agonist usually has only slight effects on heart rate in normal patients. When palpitations do occur, they are generally observed within 5 minutes after an inhaled dose. Death also has been reported in some patients receiving albuterol therapy.

One of the more common side effects of oral or inhaled albuterol is fine finger tremor, which may interfere with precise handwork. Skeletal muscle tremor resulting from β_2 receptor stimulation is more common with oral agents. A reduction in the dosage usually eliminates this reaction, and tolerance develops with continued use. Large doses of oral or intravenous albuterol can cause mild tachycardia and a slight fall in diastolic blood pressure, but equieffective doses may cause fewer cardiovascular side effects than with most other adrenergic bronchodilators. Thus, this drug usually is safe in patients with myocardial ischemia. With intravenous use, albuterol produces minimal arrhythmia, and is less likely to cause hypoxemia than isoproterenol and other nonselective β agonists. This and other β agonists may increase bronchial responsiveness when used in long-term maintenance therapy.

Unusual taste, heartburn, drowsiness, difficulty in micturition, cough, drying or irritation of the oropharynx, tinnitus, and rash may also occur (11).

Oral inhalation of albuterol may cause a small, transient increase in blood glucose concentration. Increased blood glucose and decreased serum potassium concentrations have occurred following inhalation via nebulization of higher than recommended doses of the drug (16). Large intravenous doses of albuterol have reportedly aggravated preexisting diabetes mellitus and ketoacidosis. In addition, albuterol and other β-adrenergic agonists may decrease serum potassium concentrations after intravenous administration; the decrease is usually transient, and supplemental potassium therapy is usually not required (10).

BITOLTEROL (TORNALATE)

Bitolterol is a synthetic sympathomimetic amine with little or no α effect. Bitolterol is a prodrug of colterol and has little or no bronchodilator activity until hydrolyzed in vivo to colterol (7). Colterol is structurally similar to albuterol. It has a greater stimulating effect on β_2 receptors than on β_1 receptors. Bitolterol relaxes bronchial smooth muscle and is usually administered by oral inhalation (6).

The pharmacologic effects of β-adrenergic drugs including bitolterol are attributable to stimulation of adenyl cyclase, the enzyme that catalyzes the conversion of ATP to cAMP. Increased cAMP levels are associated with relaxation of bronchial smooth muscle and with inhibition of release of mediators of immediate hypersensitivity. Bitolterol has a greater stimulating effect on β-adrenergic receptors of bronchial smooth muscle than on β-adrenergic receptors of the heart. The principal effect following oral inhalation of bitolterol is bronchodilation resulting from relaxation of smooth muscle of the bronchial tree. Bitolterol may cause some cardiac stimulations resulting in mild tachycardia or palpitations (4).

Although it has been suggested that most of a dose of an orally inhaled drug is actually swallowed, the bronchodilating action of orally inhaled sympathomimetic agents is believed to result from a local action of the portion of the dose that reaches the bronchial tree.

When inhaled, this prodrug is activated primarily by lung esterases to the active catecholamine, colterol. Its slightly longer duration of action compared with albuterol (about 5 hours compared with 4 hours for albuterol) may be due to its greater potency and/or to the relatively slow activation process.

Adverse Effects

Adverse nervous system effects of orally inhaled bitolterol generally are mild and transient. The most frequent adverse effect of bitolterol is tremor. Nervousness, headache, dizziness, and light-headedness reportedly occur (1). The frequency of bitolterol-induced adverse cardiovascular effects appears to be similar to or lower than that of other orally inhaled β-adrenergic agonists. Usual doses of bitolterol generally have been associated with mean maximum increases in heart rate of less than 10 beats/minute; however, increases in heart rate of 20–40 beats/minute have occurred in some patients. Ventricular premature contractions and flushing have occurred rarely in patients receiving the drug.

ISOETHARINE

Isoetharine is a synthetic sympathomimetic amine that is structurally similar to isoproterenol, but that has less β_1-adrenergic activity, and produces fewer adverse effects. It has little or no effect on α-adrenergic receptors. It is widely used in metered-dose inhaler form but is less effective than the newer selective β_2-adrenergic drugs. The onset of action is rapid, and the duration of action is relatively short (2 to 3 hours). Isoetharine is available only as a solution for nebulization in the United States.

Pharmacokinetics

Isoetharine hydrochloride and isoetharine mesylate are rapidly absorbed from the respiratory tract following oral inhalation. Bronchodilation occurs promptly after oral inhalation, peaks in 5–15 minutes, and persists 1–4 hours.

Adverse Effects

The most common adverse effects of isoetharine are dose-related and characteristic of sympathomimetic agents. The principal adverse effects that occur with excessive use of isoetharine are increased heart rate, palpitations, tremor, weakness, nausea, vomiting, headache, and increased or decreased blood pressure. Adverse CNS effects include anxiety, tension, restlessness, insomnia, dizziness, and excitement. Cough and bronchial irritation and edema may also occur. Occasionally, severe paradoxical bronchoconstriction has occurred hours after repeated excessive use of isoetharine oral inhalation and does not respond to other therapy until the sympathomimetic inhalations are withdrawn (14).

METAPROTERENOL

Metaproterenol stimulates β-adrenergic receptors of the sympathetic nervous system and has little or no effect on α-adrenergic receptors. The main effect of metaproterenol is relaxation of smooth muscle of the bronchial tree and the peripheral vasculature. Metaproterenol also can be used orally; therapy should be initiated with small doses, and the amount should be increased gradually. Although side effects are more common when metaproterenol is given orally, this route is generally safe, and the duration of action is 3 to 4 hours. Metaproterenol has a greater stimulating effect on the β_2-receptors and a lesser effect on the β_1-receptors than does isoproterenol. Metaproterenol has a less selective action on β_2-receptors than does albuterol (10).

Pharmacokinetics

Metaproterenol sulfate is well absorbed from the gastrointestinal (GI) tract, but only about 40% of an oral dose reaches systemic circulation as unchanged drug since it undergoes extensive metabolism on first pass through the liver. The drug is not metabolized by COMT or sulfatase enzymes in the GI tract.

The onset of action usually occurs within 1 minute after oral inhalation of the aerosol, within 5–30 minutes after nebulization, and within 15 minutes after oral administration. The peak effect is achieved within about 1 hour following oral inhalation or oral administration. Metaproterenol appears to be less rapidly metabolized than is isoproterenol, and its bronchodilating effect persists for at least 1 hour longer than that of equipotent doses of isoproterenol. Effects may persist for 4 hours or longer after a single dose of metaproterenol administered by inhalation or orally, but after long-term use the drug may have a shorter duration of action.

Adverse Effects

The principal adverse effects of metaproterenol are tachycardia, tremor, palpitations, hypertension, ECG changes, nervousness, headache, fatigue, malaise, dizziness, nausea, vomiting, bad taste, GI distress, throat irritation, cough, and exacerbation of asthma. The adverse effect profile in pediatric patients is similar; however, limited evidence suggests that the incidence of such effects may be higher in this patient population than in adults. It has been reported that some patients treated with metaproterenol had unspecified developed cramps in the muscles of the extremities, which responded to oral administration of potassium salts. Although rare, immediate hypersensitivity reactions can occur (10).

TERBUTALINE

Terbutaline sulfate is a synthetic sympathomimetic amine that is similar to isoproterenol and metaproterenol in chemical structure and in pharmacologic action. Terbutaline stimulates β-adrenergic receptors of the sympathetic nervous system, and has little or no effect on α-adrenergic receptors. The main effect of terbutaline is relaxation of smooth muscle of the bronchial tree and the peripheral vasculature.

Pharmacokinetics

About 33–50% of an oral dose of terbutaline sulfate is absorbed from the GI tract; the drug is well absorbed following subcutaneous administration. After subcutaneous administration, the drug has an onset of action within 15 minutes, peak effects occur within 30–60 minutes, and the duration of action ranges from 90 minutes to 4 hours. Following oral administration, a change in flow rate usually occurs within 30 minutes; substantial clinical improvement in pulmonary function occurs within 1–2 hours, and is maximal within 2–3 hours. The duration of action after oral administration ranges from 4 to 8 hours. Following oral inhalation, improvement in pulmonary function begins within 5–30 minutes, peaks within 1–2 hours in most patients, and generally persists 3–4 hours; in some patients, improvement may persist for up to 6 hours (13).

Adverse Effects

The most common adverse effects of terbutaline are dose-related and characteristic of sympathomimetic agents. The principal adverse effects of oral or subcutaneous terbutaline are an increase in heart rate, changes in blood pressure, nervousness, tremor, palpitations, and dizziness (4). Headzache, nausea, vomiting, anxiety, restlessness, lethargy, drowsiness, weakness, flushing, sweating, chest discomfort, and tinnitus have also been reported. Seizures, hypersensitivity vasculitis, and elevations in liver enzymes have been reported rarely in patients receiving terbutaline sulfate. Pain at the injection site may occur in some patients receiving terbutaline subcutaneously. Adverse effects with usual oral or subcutaneous doses are generally transient, and usually do not require treatment; however, the increase in heart rate may persist for a relatively long time.

Following oral inhalation, tachycardia, dysrhythmia, increased blood pressure, tremor or nervousness, drowsiness, headache, seizures, and nausea or digestive disorders may occur; seizures do not recur upon discontinuation of the drug. In addition, like other sympathomimetic agents, terbutaline may cause angina, dyspnea and wheezing, vertigo, stimulation, vomiting, insomnia, unusual taste, and drying or irritation of the oropharynx. ECG changes have also been reported (12).

PIRBUTEROL (MAXAIR)

Studies have demonstrated that pirbuterol has preferential effect on β_2-adrenergic receptors compared with isoproterenol. Although it is recognized that β_2-adrenergic receptors are the predominant receptors in bronchial smooth muscle, recent data indicate that there is a population of β_2 receptors in the human heart, existing in a concentration between 10–50%. The precise function of these, however, is not yet established.

Pirbuterol is not metabolized by COMT. The percentage of administered dose recovered as pirbuterol plus its sulfate conjugate does not change significantly over the range of 0.4 to 0.8 mg and is not significantly different from that after oral administration of pirbuterol. The plasma half-life measured after oral administration is about 2 hours

OVERDOSAGE OF β_2 AGONISTS (Table 14–3)

Excessive use of adrenergic aerosols is potentially dangerous. Overdosage of β_2 agonists may produce signs and symptoms typical of excessive sympathomimetic effects, including tachycardia, palpitations, arrhythmias, fatigue, dry mouth, nausea, headache, blood pressure changes, anxiety, restlessness, insomnia, tremor, weakness, dizziness, and excitation (14). In addition, overdosage of oral or the β agonists may produce angina, hypokalemia, hypertension, or hypotension. A significant drop in blood pressure may occur due to peripheral vasodilation.

Cardiovascular Effects

The cardiovascular and metabolic consequences of inhalational β agonist overdose are primarily due to β_2 adrenoceptor hyperactivity and therefore differ from the more familiar sympathomimetic toxidrome that results from both α- and β-adrenergic stimulation. Albuterol overdose may produce a modest decrease in mean arterial blood pressure, mainly as a result of a reduction in diastolic blood pressure due to vasodilation. The vasodilation accounts for the flushing that is commonly seen with the therapeutic use of albuterol.

Cardiac arrest and even fatalities may occur following excessive use of sympathomimetic amine oral inhalations.

TABLE 14–3. *Overdosage of β_2 agonists*

Cardiovascular
Tachycardia
Palpitations
Hypertension/Hypotension
Angina
Neurologic
Restlessness
Insomnia
Tremor
Weakness
Dizziness
Excitation
Headache
Fatigue
Insomnia
Metabolic
Hypokalemia
Hyperglycemia/Hypoglycemia

Hypokalemia

Alterations of glucose metabolism after intoxication by β sympathomimetics usually consist of hyperglycemia shortly after ingestion accompanied by hypokalemia, and expression of sympathomimetic activity (16). The hypokalemia is most likely due to a shift in potassium from the extracellular to the intracellular space without a significant change in the net potassium balance. This shift probably is due to β_2 stimulation of the membrane-bound Na-K-ATPase (6).

An alternate hypothesis is that β agonist-induced changes in carbohydrate metabolism result in hyperglycemia and insulin release, which may lead to the intracellular shift of potassium (11).

Miscellaneous

Acute overdose with β sympathomimetic agents may result in an elevation of blood glucose levels. The occurrence of hypoglycemia as an adverse reaction to sympathomimetics is less recognized and has been reported only in newborns of mothers treated with repeated doses of β sympathomimetics as well as in children (16). Hypoglycemia in infants and children may be secondary to depletion of hepatic glycogen stores due to the prolonged sympathomimetic effect on the liver. Another explanation may be the direct action of sympathomimetics on pancreatic β cells, leading to hyperinsulinemia that results in delayed hypoglycemia (16).

Tremors frequently are encountered with the use of β_2 stimulants in therapeutic doses as well as in poisonings. These tremors are due to the increased contractility of skeletal muscles caused by β_2 stimulation (11).

Tachypnea, probably due to stimulation of central adrenoceptors, and agitation have been reported in patients poisoned with β_2 stimulants (11).

Treatment

In an overdose with all β-adrenergic stimulating drugs, these drugs should be stopped, and supportive therapy provided. Currently, the management of patients with acute β sympathomimetic overdose is focused on the immediate alteration in the heart rate and in potassium and glucose levels, which usually resolve within several hours (16).

β_2 Overdosage, especially in children, usually is not severe, and in general does not require specific treatment. Occasionally, however, one may encounter a patient with toxicity that will require treatment.

Several reports have described the successful reversal of toxicity with β blockers, such as propranolol, yet the possibility that such agents can produce profound bronchospasm should be considered (11). Although the use of a selective β_1 blocker might offer the theoretical advantage of not inducing bronchospasm, studies comparing the cardioselective agents with the nonselective agent propranolol have shown that the former are less effective than propranolol in reversing the metabolic and cardiovascular effects of albuterol (1).

REFERENCES

1. Popa V: Beta-adrenergic drugs. *Clin Chest Med* 1986;7:313–329.
2. Louis W, McNeill J, Jarrott B, et al: β-Adrenoreceptor blocking drugs: current status and the significance of partial agonist activity. *Am J Cardiol* 1983;52:104A–107A.
3. Black C, Mann H: Intrinsic sympathomimetic activity: physiological reality or marketing phenomenon. *Drug Intell Clin Pharmacol* 1984; 18:554–559.
4. Brodde O: Beta_1- and beta_2-adrenoceptors in the human heart: properties, function, and alterations in chronic heart failure. *Pharmacol Rev* 1991;43:203–242.
5. Towler S, Evers A: Anesthesia and chemical second messenger generation in the adrenergic nervous system. *Int Anesthesiol Clin* 1989;27:234–247.
6. Reed M, Kelly H: Sympathomimetics for acute severe asthma: should only beta_2-selective agonists be used? *DICP Ann Pharmacother* 1990;24:868–873.
7. Burrows B, Lebowitz M: The beta-agonist dilemma. *N Engl J Med* 1992;326:560–561.
8. Cheung D, Timmers M, Zwinderman A, et al: Long-term effects of a long-acting beta2 adrenoceptor agonist, salmeterol, on airway hyperresponsiveness in patients with mild asthma. *N Engl J Med* 1992; 327:1198–1203.
9. Bodenhamer J, Bergstrom R, Brown D, et al: Frequently nebulized beta agonists for asthma: effects on serum electrolytes. *Ann Emerg Med* 1992;21:1337–1342.
10. Dennis K, Froman D, Morrison A, et al: β-blocker therapy: identification and management of side effects. *Heart Lung* 1991;20:459–463.
11. Ramoska E, Henretig F, Joffe M, et al: Propranolol treatment of albuterol poisoning in two asthmatic patients. *Ann Emerg Med* 1993; 22:1474–1476.
12. Spitzer W, Suissa S, Ernst P, et al: The use of beta-agonists and the risk of death and near death from asthma. *N Engl J Med* 1992;326: 501–506.
13. Frishman W, Murthy S, Strom J: Ultra-short acting beta adrenergic blockers. *Med Clin North Am* 1988;72:359–372.
14. O'Connor B, Aikman S, Barnes P: Tolerance to the nonbronchodilator effects of inhaled beta-2 agonists in asthma. *N Engl J Med* 1992;327: 1204–1208.
15. Pearlman D, Chervinsky P, LaForce C, et al: A comparison of salmeterol with albuterol in the treatment of mild to moderate asthma. *N Engl J Med* 1992;327:1420–1425.
16. Wasserman D, Amitai Y: Hypoglycemia following albuterol overdose in a child. *Am J Emerg Med* 1992;10:556–557.

ADDITIONAL SELECTED REFERENCES

Diamond G, Forrester J, Danzig R, et al: Acute myocardial infarction in man: comparative hemodynamic effects of norepinephrine and glucagon. *Am J Cardiol* 1971;27:612–616.

Dymowski J, Turnbull T: Glucagon and β blocker poisoning. *Ann Emerg Med* 1986;15:1118.

Frishman W: Pindolol: a new β adrenoceptor antagonist with partial agonist activity. *N Engl J Med* 1983;306:940–944.

Gibson D: Pharmacodynamic properties of β-adrenergic receptor blocking drugs in man. *Drugs* 1974;7:8–38.

Gibson D, Sowton E: The use of β-adrenergic receptor blocking drugs in dysrhythmias. *Prog Cardiovasc Dis* 1969;12:16–39.

Haddad L, Dimond K, Schweistris J: Phenol poisoning. *JACEP* 1979; 8:267–269.

Harrison D: The pharmacology and therapeutic use of β adrenergic receptor blocking drugs in cardiovascular disease. *Drugs* 1974;7:1–7.

Heel R, Brogden R, Speight T, et al: Atenolol: a review of its pharmacological properties and therapeutic efficacy in angina pectoris and hypertension. *Drugs* 1979;17:425–460.

Hiatt W, Fradl D, Zerbe G, et al: Selective and nonselective β blockade of the peripheral circulation. *Clin Pharmacol Ther* 1984;35:12–17.

Hong C, Yang W, Chiang B: Importance of membrane stabilizing effect in massive overdose of propranolol: plasma level study in a fatal case. *Hum Toxicol* 1983;3:511–517.

Kaplan N: The present and future use of β blockers. *Drugs* 1983;25(Suppl. 2):1–4.

Kelly H: Controversies in asthma therapy with theophylline and the 132-adrenergic agonists. *Clin Pharmacol* 1984;3:386–395.

Kristinsson J, Johannesson T: A case of fatal propranolol intoxication. *Acta Pharmacol Toxicol* 1977;41:190–192.

Mills G. Horn J: β Blockers and glucose control. *Drug Intell Clin Pharm* 1985;19:246–251.

Morelli H: Propranolol. *Ann Intern Med* 1973;78:913–917.

Theilen E, Wilson W: β-Adrenergic receptor blocking drugs in the treatment of cardiac arrhythmias. *Med Clin North Am* 1968;52:1017–1029.

Williams J: Glucagon and the cardiovascular system. *Ann Intern Med* 1969;71:419–423.

CHAPTER 15

β-Adrenergic Blocking Agents

The β-adrenergic blocking agents have come into increasing use in recent years, and their medical indications continue to expand. They have become the most commonly used drugs for a number of cardiovascular diseases. Because of this extensive use, inadvertent self-poisoning as well as deliberate overdosing with β-adrenergic blocking drugs is becoming an increasingly frequent and important problem.

THERAPEUTIC INDICATIONS FOR USE

Therapeutic indications for β-adrenergic blocking agents (Table 15–1) include exertion-induced angina pectoris; hypertension; atrial, nodal, or ventricular tachydysrhythmias (1); prophylaxis against reinfarction and sudden death after an acute myocardial infarction (2–4); alcohol and narcotic withdrawal; thyrotoxicosis; prophylaxis against migraine; obstructive cardiomyopathy; pheochromocytoma; essential tremor; anxiety; and dissecting aortic aneurysm (5). The β-adrenergic blocking agents share some indications with the centrally active α_2 agonist clonidine.

MECHANISM OF ACTION

All the β-adrenergic blocking agents competitively antagonize the action of catecholamines and other sympathomimetic agents at the β-adrenergic receptor (6). Nearly all the β-adrenergic blocking agents used clinically share with isoproterenol, the prototypical β receptor agonist, an isopropyl-substituted amine group thought to produce a high affinity for the β receptor (7).

TABLE 15–1. *Therapeutic indications for β-adrenergic blocking agents*

Angina pectoris
Anxiety
Dissecting aortic aneurysm
Essential tremor
Glaucoma
Hypertension
Infarction prophylaxis
Migraine prophylaxis
Obstructive cardiomyopathy
Pheochromocytoma
Substance withdrawal
Thyrotoxicosis
Ventricular tachydysrhythmias

When an adrenergic agonist combines with a receptor site, a response is elicited and the drug–receptor complex rapidly dissociates, leaving the receptor ready for further stimulation. The β receptor blocking agents are competitive antagonists, which means that the blocking agent occupies the same β receptor site as does the agonist isoproterenol but that the attachment results in little or no activation of adenyl cyclase or transmission of response to the tissue. This prolonged occupation of the receptor results in a reversible blockade (8). The result of β blockade is that higher concentrations of endogenous agonists or higher doses of exogenously administered agonists are required to induce the same β receptor-mediated response. This is important to remember when treating overdoses with β-adrenergic blocking agents (9).

Although all the β-adrenergic blocking agents competitively interact with β adrenoceptors, some are lipophilic, β_1 cardioselective, possess intrinsic sympathomimetic (partial agonist) activity, and have membrane-stabilizing properties (3,4,10,11). Differences in potency, route of elimination, half-life, and protein binding are also recognized (12). In equivalent doses, β-adrenergic blocking drugs are equally effective in the treatment of hypertension, angina, and dysrhythmias, but they may differ in other respects (10,11).

There are many β-adrenergic blocking drugs approved for use in the United States. The major differences among the available β-adrenergic blocking drugs are summarized in Table 15–2. Trade names for some of these drugs are listed in Table 15–3.

Route of Elimination

Broadly speaking, the β receptor blockers are divided into two groups: those that are largely metabolized by the liver, such as propranolol, practolol, and timolol; and those that are excreted predominantly unchanged by the kidneys, such as atenolol and nadolol (Table 15–4).

TABLE 15–2. *Differences among β-adrenergic blocking agents*

Cardioselectivity
Half-life
Intrinsic sympathomimetic activity
Lipophilicity
Membrane-stabilizing activity
Potency
Protein binding
Route of elimination

TABLE 15–4. *Metabolized and renally excreted β-adrenergic blocking agents*

Metabolized	Renally excreted
Acebutolol	Atenolol
Esmolol	Nadolol
Metoprolol	
Oxprenolol	
Propranolol	
Practolol	
Timolol	

Lipid Solubility

Drugs such as propranolol and metoprolol are highly lipid-soluble, and cross the blood–brain barrier easily. These drugs may therefore have more of an effect on the central nervous system (CNS) than drugs such as nadolol and atenolol, which are water-soluble and penetrate tissues less readily (Table 15–5).

Cardioselectivity

Certain β-adrenergic receptor blocking agents exhibit a higher affinity for β_1 than β_2 adrenoceptors. This property is called cardioselectivity and is a beneficial attribute of β receptor blocking agents in treating patients with bronchospastic disorders (13).

The nonselective cardiac β-adrenergic receptor blocking agents (Table 15–6) have both negative chronotropic and inotropic effects, may cause bronchospasm, and may impair glycogenolysis and the hyperglycemic response to epinephrine, thus predisposing the patient to hypoglycemia. They may also exert an adverse effect on the peripheral circulation: cold hands and feet as well as more severe forms of vasospasm have been described with these drugs. The cardioselective β-adrenergic blocking drugs antagonize β receptors in the heart at lower doses than those required for other tissue, and therefore do not produce bronchospasm or inhibit glycogenolysis at therapeutic doses.

Cardioselectivity of the β-adrenergic blocking drugs is not an "all or none" phenomenon. Pharmacologically, it is the relative ability of a blocking drug to block the effects of a marked sympathetic stimulus on the β_1 receptors while not affecting the influence of the stimulus on β_2 receptors. These agents begin to lose their β selectivity at high doses, and exert the same effects as the nonselective agents.

TABLE 15–3. *Partial listing of β-adrenergic blocking agents and their trade names*

Generic name	Trade name
Acebutolol	Sectral
Atenolol	Tenormin
Betaxolol	Betalol
Bisoprolol	Zebeta
Carteolol	Cartrol
Esmolol	Brevibloc
Labetalol	Trandate, Normodyne
Levobunolol	Betagan
Metoprolol	Lopressor
Nadolol	Corgard
Penbutolol	Levatol
Pindolol	Visken
Propranolol	Inderal
Sotalol	Betapace
Timolol	Timoptic, Blocadren

Membrane-Stabilizing Activity

Membrane-stabilizing activity refers to the ability of certain drugs to interact with sodium channels, thereby impeding the depolarization of excitable tissues (14). These drugs are considered to stabilize the cellular membrane, which results in depression of myocardial cells. Local anesthetics, quinidine, the tricyclic antidepressants, and β-adrenergic blocking agents with membrane-stabilizing activity (Table 15–7) all share this property, which is unrelated to competitive inhibition of catecholamines. This property is also described as quinidine-like, and causes an effect similar to that of a local anesthetic, decreasing the reduction in the rate of rise in the cardiac action potential without affecting the overall duration of the spike or the resting potential (8,15). The membrane-stabilizing properties of these compounds come into play at doses greater than those used in clinical practice.

TABLE 15–5. *Solubility of β-adrenergic blocking agents*

Lipid-soluble	Water-soluble
Acebutolol	
Alprenolol	Atenolol
Labetalol	Nadolol
Metoprolol	Practolol
Oxprenolol	Sotalol
Propranolol	Timolol

TABLE 15–6. *Cardioselective and nonselective β-adrenergic blocking drugs*

Nonselective	Cardioselective
Alprenolol	Acebutolol
Carteolol	Atenolol
Labetalol	Betaxolol
Levobunolol	Esmolol
Nadolol	Metoprolol
Oxprenolol	Practolol
Penbutolol	
Pindolol	
Propranolol	
Sotalol	
Timolol	

TABLE 15–8. *β-Adrenergic blocking drugs with and without intrinsic sympathomimetic activity*

With intrinsic sympathomimetic activity	Without intrinsic sympathomimetic activity
Acebutolol	Atenolol
Alprenolol	Betaxolol
Carteolol	Labetalol
Oxprenolol	Metoprolol
Pindolol	Nadolol
Practolol	Propranolol
	Sotalol
	Timolol

Intrinsic Sympathomimetic Activity

Because almost all β blockers are chemical relatives of isoproterenol, it is not surprising that some have intrinsic sympathomimetic or partial agonist activity (Table 15–8). (11). These drugs cause a slight to moderate activation of the β receptors in addition to preventing the access of natural or synthetic catecholamines to the receptor site (6,16,17). There is no strong evidence that β blocking drugs with intrinsic sympathomimetic activity are inherently safer than those without it.

SELECTED β-ADRENERGIC BLOCKING AGENTS

Acebutolol (Sectral)

Acebutolol is a β_1 selective adrenoceptor blocking agent. It also has some partial intrinsic sympathomimetic activity (Table 15–9). (18). Acebutolol also has a membrane-stabilizing effect on the heart, which is similar to that of quinidine but occurs only at high plasma concentrations, and usually is not apparent at dosages used clinically.

The pharmacologic effects of acebutolol result from both the unchanged drug and its major metabolite, diacetolol. Diacetolol is equipotent to acebutolol and has a greater β_1 blocking activity than the parent drug.

Acebutolol is completely absorbed from the gastrointestinal tract (GI) and undergoes extensive first-pass hepatic metabolism, but its major metabolite is also active. Following oral administration, peak plasma levels of acebutolol occur within 2.5 hours. Peak plasma concentrations of diacetolol occur at 4 hours (19). The pharmacologic half-life of acebutolol is about 8 hours.

As with other β blockers, there has been a lack of correlation and wide interindividual variation between plasma acebutolol and/or diacetolol concentration and blood pressure reduction.

Most adverse effects of acebutolol are mild, do not require discontinuance of the drug, and tend to decrease with time. The most common adverse effects of acebutolol are nervous system and GI effects. The most common adverse nervous system effects are fatigue, dizziness,

TABLE 15–7. *β-Adrenergic blocking drugs with and without membrane-stabilizing activity*

With membrane-stabilizing activity	Without membrane-stabilizing activity
Acebutolol	Atenolol
Alprenolol	Betaxolol
Labetalol	Carteolol
Metoprolol	Nadolol
Oxprenolol	Practolol
Penbutolol	Sotalol
Pindolol	Timolol
Propranolol	

TABLE 15–9. *Summary of β-adrenergic blocking drugs*

Name	Lipophilic	β_1	ISA	MSA
Acebutolol*	–	+	+	+
Alprenolol	+	–	+	+
Atenolol*	–	+	–	–
Betaxolol*	–	+	–	–
Carteolol*	–	–	+	–
Esmolol*	–	+	0	0
Labetalol*	+	–	–	+
Levobunolol*	0	–	0	0
Metoprolol*	+	+	–	+/–
Nadolol*	–	–	–	–
Oxprenolol	+	–	++	+
Penbutolol*	+	–	+	+
Pindolol*	+	–	+++	+
Practolol	–	+	++	–
Propranolol*	++	–	–	++
Sotalol*	–	–	–	–
Timolol*	–	–	–	–

* indicates FDA approval.

+ = effect; – = no effect; 0 = effect not known.

ISA, intrinsic sympathomimetic activity; MSA, membrane-stabilizing activity.

and headache. Insomnia, mental depression, and unusual dreams have also been reported. As with other β blockers, symptomatic bradycardia, advanced atrioventricular (AV) block, intraventricular conduction defects, hypotension, acute cardiac failure, seizures, and in susceptible individuals, bronchospasm and hypoglycemia might occur with acebutolol overdosage. There have been some deaths reported following the overdose of acebutolol (18).

Antinuclear antibodies, sometimes associated with generally persistent arthralgias and myalgias, may develop in patients receiving acebutolol. The frequency of this reaction appears to be greater than that occurring with propranolol.

Alprenolol

Alprenolol closely resembles propranolol in its pharmacologic properties. It differs from propranolol only in that it has significant intrinsic sympathomimetic activity. The half-life of alprenolol is approximately 2 hours, and its maximum effects occur 1 to 3 hours after oral ingestion.

Atenolol (Tenormin)

Like metoprolol, low doses of atenolol selectively inhibit cardiac and lipolytic β_1 receptors while having little effect on β_2 receptors (20). At high doses of more than 100 mg/day, this selectivity of atenolol for β_1 receptors usually diminishes. Atenolol does not exhibit the intrinsic sympathomimetic activity seen with pindolol or the membrane-stabilizing activity possessed by propranolol or pindolol. Only about 50% to 60% of an oral dose of atenolol is absorbed (21).

Peak plasma concentrations of 1 to 2 μg/mL are achieved 2 to 4 hours after oral administration of a single 200-mg dose of atenolol (21). The elimination half-life in patients with normal renal function is approximately 6 to 7 hours, and the volume of distribution is 0.56 L/kg. About 5% to 15% of atenolol is bound to plasma proteins (21). Because of its low lipid solubility, atenolol penetrates poorly into the central nervous system. Because of the long half-life, in the event of overdose supportive measures may be needed for an extended period (20).

Betaxolol (Betalol)

Betaxolol is structurally similar to metoprolol and displays cardioselectivity. Its only approved use is to reduce elevated intraocular pressure by topical administration. It is one of the most potent and selective β-adrenergic blocking agents currently available. It does not exhibit intrinsic sympathomimetic activity and does not have substantial membrane-stabilizing activity. It also causes no change in the size of the pupils.

Betaxolol may cause more local irritation than timolol. Although it is safer than a nonselective β blocker, β_1 selectivity is not absolute and bronchospasm has occurred occasionally in patients with asthma or chronic obstructive lung disease. Bradycardia, syncope, and sinus arrest have occurred rarely.

Carteolol

Carteolol (Cartrol) is a long-acting, nonselective, β-adrenergic receptor blocking agent with intrinsic sympathomimetic activity (ISA) and without significant membrane-stabilizing (local anesthetic) activity. It has a long duration of action, and is used for once-daily treatment of systemic hypertension.

Esmolol (Brevibloc)

Esmolol is an ultrashort-acting, cardioselective β blocker that has therapeutic potential in the control of supraventricular arrhythmias, postoperative hypertension, and possibly, acute myocardial ischemia. Esmolol is a parenterally administered β-adrenergic blocking agent that has a rapid distribution half-life of about 2 minutes and a short elimination half-life of about 9 minutes. Its cardioselectivity, titratability, rapid onset, and 9-minute elimination half-life provide a margin of acute safety not found with currently available intravenous β blockers or calcium blockers.

Esmolol doses required in adults are generally 100 to 200 μg/kg/min. Doses up to 300 μg/kg/min are rarely needed but have been administered safely in adults.

Esmolol is metabolized rapidly by erythrocyte esterases. An unidentified plasma factor is required for the full expression of this esterase activity, and there may be some drug metabolism by tissue esterases. Unlike most ester-containing drugs, esmolol is not metabolized by plasma cholinesterase. The hydrolysis of esmolol results in the formation of a weakly active acid metabolite and methanol. The amount of methanol formed is within the normal range seen in humans and therefore is clinically insignificant (22). Even patients receiving continuous doses of esmolol for up to 24 hours have not been noted to have significant methanol concentrations.

Labetalol (Trandate, Normodyne)

Labetalol possesses neither cardioselectivity nor partial agonist activity (23). It does possess weak membrane-stabilizing properties at high doses. In addition, labetalol exhibits α-adrenergic blocking activity and is able to inhibit the reuptake of norepinephrine into nerve terminals (24). It is the only agent in this class that blocks both α_1 and β receptors, but it is 4 to 16 times more potent at β than at α receptors (25). These properties yield a drug that hemodynamically resembles a combination of propranolol and prazosin (25). Because it undergoes significant first-pass metabolism, its bioavailability is 30% to 40% (26). Labetalol is approximately 50% bound to plasma proteins, and has a volume of distribution of 11 L/kg. Intravenous labetalol is available for use in patients who require rapid control of severe hypertension.

Metoprolol (Lopressor)

Metoprolol has no intrinsic sympathomimetic activity and has only weak membrane-stabilizing activity. Metoprolol is rapidly and almost completely absorbed from the GI tract (27). After an oral dose, about 50% of the drug appears to undergo first-pass metabolism in the liver. Following a single oral dose, metoprolol appears in the plasma within 10 minutes, and peak plasma concentrations are reached in about 90 minutes. Elimination of metoprolol appears to follow first-order kinetics and occurs mainly in the liver; the time required for the process apparently is independent of dose and duration of therapy (22).

Most adverse effects of metoprolol are mild and transient and occur more frequently at the onset of therapy than during prolonged treatment. The most frequent adverse effects are dizziness, fatigue, insomnia, and gastric upset (28–30).

Nadolol (Corgard)

Nadolol is noncardioselective and lacks both intrinsic sympathomimetic activity and membrane-stabilizing properties (31). It is distinguished from other β-adrenergic blocking drugs on the basis of its long plasma half-life, which is about 20 to 24 hours, the longest of the β blockers. Plasma concentrations of nadolol reach their peak between 3 to 4 hours after administration. Unlike propranolol and metoprolol, most nadolol is not metabolized; about 75% of the amount absorbed is excreted unchanged by the kidneys. The drug is 30% bound to plasma protein and has a large volume of distribution of 2 L/kg (31).

Through its myocardial β_1 blocking action, nadolol decreases resting heart rate, inhibits exercise-induced increases in heart rate, and decreases cardiac output at rest and during exercise.

Limited information is available on nadolol overdosage. In general, overdosage of nadolol may be expected to produce effects that are mainly extensions of pharmacologic effects, including symptomatic bradycardia, hypotension, bronchospasm, and acute cardiac failure.

Oxprenolol

Oxprenolol has approximately the same β-adrenergic blocking potency as propranolol but less local anesthetic activity and less membrane-stabilizing action. Like alprenolol, it has significant intrinsic sympathomimetic activity (32). Oxprenolol may be used interchangeably with alprenolol.

Penbutolol (Levatol)

Penbutolol is an oral β-adrenergic blocking drug recently approved by the FDA for once-daily treatment of systemic hypertension. Penbutolol is a nonselective β-blocker with mild partial agonist activity.

Penbutolol is almost completely absorbed from the tract, reaching peak plasma concentrations 1 to 3 hours after ingestion. Penbutolol has an elimination half-life of about 5 to 6 hours. The peak effect is between 1.5 and 3 hours after oral administration. The duration of effect exceeds 20 hours during a once-daily dosing regimen. During chronic administration of penbutolol, the duration of antihypertensive effects permits a once-daily dosage schedule.

Pindolol (Visken)

Pindolol is noncardioselective, acts as a weak adrenergic agonist, and has weak membrane-depressant activity. It is absorbed almost completely from the tract, and achieves peak plasma concentrations within 1 hour of administration. Approximately 13% of a dose of pindolol undergoes first-pass metabolism, and the rest is excreted by the kidney. It has a relatively short half-life. The intrinsic sympathomimetic activity of pindolol may be blocked by other β blockers. Because of its intrinsic sympathomimetic activity, it does not decrease cardiac contractility or resting cardiac output as much as other β-adrenergic blocking drugs.

Practolol

Practolol has cardioselectivity, partial agonist activity, and no membrane-stabilizing effect. It is associated with a unique, serious, delayed adverse reaction known as oculocutaneous syndrome. This syndrome consists of a sclerosing peritonitis, psoriasiform rash, secretory otitis media, pleurisy, ocular involvement, and pericarditis. These symptoms have not been reported with other β blockers (10). Practolol is no longer available for general use in the United States.

Propranolol (Inderal)

Propranolol is the prototype of the β-adrenergic blocking drugs and was the first to come into wide clinical use. It remains the β-adrenergic blocking drug most commonly used in clinical medicine. Of all the β-adrenergic blocking drugs, propranolol seems consistently to produce the most severe picture with overdosage (33). Self-induced poisoning with propranolol is increasing in frequency as the therapeutic indications for this medication continue to grow.

Propranolol is noncardioselective, and has no intrinsic sympathomimetic activity, although it does induce membrane-depressant effects (11). In the usual dose range for propranolol this membrane-depressant effect is of little importance, but with massive ingestion this effect may be clinically manifested (34,35). Propranolol is extremely lipid-soluble, and crosses the blood–brain barrier rapidly, concentrating in brain tissue.

After oral administration, propranolol is completely absorbed from the tract, but it undergoes substantial first-pass metabolism by the liver. Propranolol is more than 90% bound to plasma proteins. Propranolol appears in the plasma within 30 minutes, and peak plasma levels are reached in 60 to 90 minutes after oral administration of the conventional tablets. The bioavailability of propranolol in tablet form, or in solution is equivalent. The volume of distribution is 3 to 5 L/kg (8), and the plasma half-life is 3 to 6 hours. Following oral administration of extended-release tablets, peak blood concentrations are reached approximately 6 hours after administration (26). Following intravenous administration, the onset of action is almost immediate.

There is considerable interpatient variation in the relationship of plasma concentrations and therapeutic effect, but therapeutic plasma concentrations are usually 50 to 100 ng/mL (26). Propranolol is metabolized to 4-hydroxypropranolol, an active metabolite that is present in almost equal amounts. Several other β-adrenergic blocking drugs, including oxprenolol and alprenolol, appear to have kinetics similar to those of propranolol.

Sotalol

Sotalol has both β-adrenoreceptor blocking and cardiac action potential duration prolongation, Class III antiarrhythmic properties. Sotalol is therefore a noncardioselective β blocker that has neither partial agonist nor membrane-depressant properties.

Because it prolongs the duration of the action potential, it has the properties of an antidysrhythmic agent, and may induce ventricular tachydysrhythmias (36,37). This appears as a prolonged QT interval. Because of this action, sotalol has been reported as a cause of torsade de pointes-type ventricular tachycardia. Like other antiarrhythmic agents, sotalol tablets can provoke new or worsened ventricular arrhythmias in some patients, including sustained ventricular tachycardia or ventricular fibrillation, with potentially fatal consequences (38). Because of its effect on cardiac repolarization (QTc interval prolongation), torsade de pointes, a polymorphic ventricular tachycardia with prolongation of the QT interval and a shifting electrical axis is the most common form of proarrhythmias associated with sotalol tablets, occurring in high-risk patients. The risk of torsade de pointes progressively increases with prolongation of the QT interval, and is also worsened by reduction in heart rate and reduction in serum potassium.

Timolol (Timoptic)

Timolol is noncardioselective, has no demonstrable membrane-stabilizing properties, and has no intrinsic sympathomimetic activity (39–42). It is less lipid-soluble than propranolol or metoprolol; thus it penetrates the brain to a low degree and causes few side effects in the central nervous system. Timolol is 10% to 60% bound to plasma proteins, depending on the assay method employed (43). Timolol is approved for treatment of glaucoma, and reduces intraocular pressure without changing the pupil size. Although it is used locally, because of its absorption through the nasal mucosa systemic side effects have been reported (44–46). Orally administered timolol is completely absorbed from the tract. Peak plasma levels of the drug are reached usually within 1 to 2 hours after oral administration, and the drug has a half-life of 3 to 4 hours (43).

β BLOCKER TOXICITY

The β-adrenergic blocking drugs are relatively safe when properly administered, and there is a wide gap between therapeutic and toxic doses. In general, adverse effects of β-adrenergic blocking drugs appear to be an extension of their pharmacologic properties (10,11). Because all the β-adrenergic blocking drugs are rapidly absorbed from the tract, the first critical signs of overdosage can appear 20 minutes after ingestion but are more commonly seen within 1 to 2 hours after ingestion, and sudden deterioration with cardiovascular collapse is common.

The principal manifestations of massive overdosage are bradycardia, hypotension, lowered cardiac output, left ventricular failure, respiratory depression, and cardiogenic shock (Table 15–10). Bradycardia is caused by the slowing of spontaneous diastolic depolarization in cardiac conducting tissue, an effect that is prominent in the sinoatrial node and that accounts for the reduction in sinus rate. Not all seriously ill patients have a bradycardia, and sinus tachycardia and tachydysrhythmias have been reported in overdoses of practolol and sotalol. In massive overdoses, sudden rapid deterioration with cardiovascular collapse is common. Death is usually due to asystole (32).

Changes in mental and neurologic status have been reported in patients treated with highly lipid-soluble drugs (47). This may be due either to direct toxicity or to

TABLE 15–10. *Symptoms of toxicity from β-adrenergic blocking drugs*

Cardiovascular
Sinus bradycardia
Hypotension
Prolonged atrioventricular conduction
Bundle branch block
Asystole
Sinus tachycardia (rare)
Cardiogenic shock
Congestive heart failure
Central nervous system
Loss of consciousness
Delirium
Psychosis
Hallucinations
Coma
Seizures
Respiratory
Bronchospasm (rare)
Acute pulmonary edema
Respiratory arrest
Metabolic
Hypoglycemia
Masking of hypoglycemia
Miscellaneous
Peripheral cyanosis

reduced cerebral blood flow. Grand mal seizures may occur especially with propranolol, which is highly lipid-soluble and thus gains access to the central nervous system easily. Other central nervous system symptoms are also attributed to the drug's high lipid solubility and ability to cross the blood–brain barrier. These symptoms include sedation, fatigue, psychosis, hallucinations, coma, and respiratory depression. Peripheral cyanosis has also been reported (48,49).

Because mobilization of liver glycogen is a β receptor function, β-adrenergic blocking drugs may retard recovery from hyperglycemia. If glycogen is reduced, they may prolong recovery from hypoglycemia because alternative glycogen stores cannot be mobilized. Hypoglycemia has been reported in diabetic patients on insulin who have taken β-adrenergic blockers, and cases of spontaneous hypoglycemia have also been reported (48,49). Masking of hypoglycemia is more common.

Bronchospasm is a rare complication of overdosage with β-adrenergic blocking drugs, except in patients who already have bronchospastic disease.

The usual electrocardiographic manifestations of β blockade include first-degree atrioventricular heart block and sinus bradycardia (32). With massive intoxication, disappearance of P waves, intraventricular conduction defects, and asystole may be seen. The widening of the QRS complex appears to be related to the membrane-depressant effect of some of the β-adrenergic blocking drugs (50). It has been estimated that, for this change to appear in humans, the plasma concentration must be 50 to 100 times that needed for β blockade. Not all seriously ill patients have a bradycardia. Sinus tachycardia and tachydysrhythmias have been reported in overdoses of practolol and sotalol, respectively (51–53).

LABORATORY ANALYSIS

Although plasma drug concentrations can be measured, they do not always reflect the degree of β-adrenergic blocker intoxication. Moreover, certain compounds yield active metabolites that may not be easily detected in plasma assays. Because of the variability in patient sensitivity, the degree of β blockade cannot be accurately related to the β blocker's plasma concentration. Severity of intoxication can be judged only by clinical findings. In addition, because the effects of β-adrenergic blocking drugs on the body last longer than their chemical half-life in plasma, intensive care may have to be continued for several days.

TREATMENT

All patients should be carefully observed by cardiac monitoring, and venous access should be readily available, even if they are clinically stable on presentation (Table 15–11). All overdoses with β-adrenergic blocking drugs can be treated in a similar fashion. The major goals of treatment are to quickly remove any ingested tablets, to counteract life-threatening cardiovascular and pulmonary effects, and to treat CNS disturbances.

If the ingestion is recent, lavage should be initiated, and should be followed by administration of activated charcoal and a cathartic. Intravenous diazepam should be used to treat seizure activity. Hemodialysis and hemoperfusion have not been shown to enhance excretion of β-adrenergic blocking drugs. In the pharmacologic therapy for overdoses with β-adrenergic blocking drugs, patients are symptomatic as a result of a competitive antagonism

TABLE 15–11. *Treatment of overdoses of β-adrenergic blocking drugs*

Indication	Treatment
Acute ingestion	Lavage Charcoal and cathartic
Hypotension or bradycardia, asystole	Sympathomimetics (epinephrine,dopamine)
Bradycardia or hypotension, asystole	Atropine
Bradycardia or hypotension, asystole	Glucagon
Hypotension	Fluids
Bradycardia or hypotension, asystole	Pacemaker

of the drug with the receptor. To be effective, large doses of selected agents are usually necessary (54).

Current therapy of hypotension, conduction defects, and bradycardia requires maintenance of optimal filling pressures with volume expansion, inotropic support, and atropine. Severe bradycardia should initially be treated with atropine. If there is an inadequate response, sympathomimetics should be administered.

Sympathomimetics

Inotropic support may include glucagon or large doses of a drug that competitively challenges the blocked β receptor adenyl cyclase-mediated transmission. Epinephrine may be given intravenously as needed for bradycardia or hypotension (or both). Epinephrine is a good choice in that it has maximal β effect on the myocardium as well as peripheral vasoconstrictor effects. The dose of epinephrine administered may be inadequate, however, because the β receptors are being competitively blocked. It is for this reason that larger doses than what might be normally recommended are necessary (54). This is similar to the use of larger doses of atropine than usually required to overcome the competitive block seen with the organophosphates and other acetylcholinesterase inhibitors.

Other sympathomimetic agents such as dopamine, isoproterenol, dobutamine, and norepinephrine are usually administered as intravenous infusions, and are not effective if a bolus of epinephrine is not effective. Bradycardia may be resistant to the traditional drugs such as epinephrine, atropine, isoproterenol, dopamine, and dobutamine, even in large doses. In addition, although isoproterenol is often thought of as the agent of choice, a great disadvantage to its use is that it has vasodilator properties and may reduce diastolic blood pressure.

Epinephrine may cause severe hypertension and reflex bradycardia in patients taking nonselective β blockers. Nonselective β blockers appear to pose the highest risk of adverse interaction with epinephrine, and the extent of the interaction appears to be partly dependent on the dose of epinephrine (55).

Other Methods

Intravenous atropine may be given to reduce unopposed vagal activity. A temporary transvenous pacemaker may be inserted if heart block or severe bradycardia cannot be readily controlled by pharmacologic means. The rarely reported occurrence of significant bronchospasm after overdose with β-adrenergic blocking drugs may be treated with epinephrine and aerosol β receptor agonists. Aminophylline, which acts independently of β-adrenergic receptors and produces an accumulation of cyclic AMP, may also be used.

Glucagon

Glucagon is considered the agent of choice for overdoses of β-adrenergic blocking drugs by many clinicians, and should be available in all emergency departments (Table 15–12) (56). Glucagon is a naturally occurring polypeptide hormone produced by the α cells of the pancreatic islets (32,57–60). This hormone has been known to have inotropic and chronotropic effects on the heart when administered in pharmacologic doses (61–64). Its action stems from its ability to increase cyclic AMP by stimulation of adenyl cyclase (65).

There are numerous substances, both endogenous and exogenous, known to influence cyclic AMP synthesis. Exogenous agents with actions mediated through cyclic AMP include methylxanthines and sympathomimetic amines. Endogenous hormones, which include catecholamines and glucagon, also utilize cyclic AMP as an intermediary (66). Glucagon is thought to activate the adenylate cyclase system in the myocardium at a different site than that activated by isoproterenol (67).

The effects of glucagon are not blocked by β-adrenergic blocking drugs (10,11,63), and unlike other positive inotropic agents it has the advantage of not increasing cardiac irritability (52,53,57,68). Glucagon does not inhibit phosphodiesterase, the enzyme responsible for the degradation of cyclic AMP, nor are the actions related to a vagolytic mechanism or the release of endogenous catecholamines (61).

Glucagon is the drug of choice for initial treatment of myocardial depression and hypotension in overdoses with β-adrenergic blockers because the inotropic response is not affected by even high degrees of β receptor blockage (57). Catecholamines are less likely to be effective, and are more often associated with complications such as arrhythmias due to the high doses required to overcome β blockade (50). Although both catecholamines and glucagon stimulate adenyl cyclase, no additive effect is noted

TABLE 15–12. *Glucagon and its properties*

Produced by α cells of pancreas
Has inotropic and chronotropic properties
Activates cAMP

Uses
- Gastrointestinal procedures
- Hypoglycemia
- β Blocker overdose
- Calcium channel overdose

Dosage: 50 μg/kg (3–10 mg IV) followed by 0.07 mg/kg/hr

Side effects
- Nausea
- Vomiting
- Hyperglycemia
- Hypokalemia
- Phenol toxicity (from diluent)

(52,61,69–71). Glucagon is therefore considered superior to the sympathomimetic agents in that it has no dysrhythmia-producing properties, and its effects are sustained over a long period of time (57).

The recommended dosage of glucagon is 50 μg/kg as an initial intravenous dose or 3 to 10 mg infused over 1 to 2 minutes with subsequent continuous infusion of 2 to 5 mg/hour or 0.07 mg/kg/hour (52,57). The onset of glucagon's effects is within 1 to 3 minutes, with peak activity occurring within 5 to 7 minutes and persisting for 15 to 20 minutes (57,61). The serum half-life of glucagon is 3 to 6 minutes (61).

When given parenterally, glucagon has few side effects; the most important side effects are hyperglycemia and nausea (53). The nausea is usually transient, lasting only 1 to 2 minutes in most cases. Vomiting may also occasionally occur. Hyperglycemia rarely requires the administration of insulin. Lesser effects are hypokalemia and hypocalcemia. Potassium concentrations should be monitored frequently during glucagon therapy because of the possible intracellular shifts of potassium that may occur (57). Glucagon has not been found to be arrhythmogenic (61). Glucagon has successfully reversed hypotension and dysrhythmias in patients unresponsive to other pharmacologic therapies (69,70,72).

The diluent provided with glucagon is 0.2% phenol. Phenol, which is chemically related to benzene, denatures proteins, and is considered a general protoplasmic poison. Venous thrombosis has also resulted from some phenol injections. If large doses of glucagon are necessary, the glucagon should be reconstituted with 5% dextrose instead of the diluent provided (73). Glucagon is stable in dextrose solutions but will precipitate if mixed with solutions containing sodium, potassium, or calcium chloride.

WITHDRAWAL OF β-ADRENERGIC BLOCKING DRUGS

Abrupt discontinuation of therapy with β-adrenergic blocking drugs has led to a syndrome resembling rebound adrenergic hyperactivity (Table 15–13) (15,74). The characteristics and pharmacokinetics of the β blocker that is discontinued, the presence of cardioselectivity and intrinsic sympathomimetic activity, and the dose, duration of treatment, and tapering schedule are all factors that may contribute to the frequency and severity of the withdrawal syndrome. The clinical signs and symptoms associated with abrupt withdrawal of β blockers include nervousness, restlessness, anxiety, palpitations, abdominal cramps and pain, anorexia, nausea, vomiting, insomnia, headaches, vivid dreams, malaise, fatigue, tremor, diaphoresis, tachycardia, excessive salivation, and an excessive cardiovascular morbidity and mortality. Withdrawal symptoms may begin within 1 to 2 days or be delayed for several weeks following cessation of the β blockers, depending on the particular β blocker. There are no controlled studies demonstrating that slow withdrawal of these drugs prevents the withdrawal syndrome. In addition, some researchers have failed to confirm the existence of β blocker withdrawal (75).

TABLE 15–13. *β Blocker withdrawal*

Mild
Abdominal cramps
Anxiety
Insomnia
Nausea
Nervousness
Restlessness
Vomiting
Severe
Acute coronary insufficiency
Encephalopathy
Hypertension
Hyperthyroidism
Myocardial infarction
Sudden death
Tachyarrhythmias

Abrupt cessation of most of the β blockers has been associated with morbid cardiovascular events including severe hypertension, encephalopathy, marked sympathetic overactivity, hyperthyroidism, tachyarrhythmias, myocardial infarction, acute coronary insufficiency, accelerated or unstable angina in predisposed patients, or sudden death (76,77).

β blocker withdrawal syndromes usually resolve following readministration of the β blocker, at a dose smaller than the previously administered dose. Either oral or parenteral administration is appropriate, depending on the urgency of the situation and the severity of the symptoms and signs of withdrawal. Treatment of medical problems should not be overlooked.

REFERENCES

1. Singh B, Jewitt D: β-Adrenergic receptor blocking drugs in cardiac arrhythmias. *Drugs* 1974;7:426–461.
2. Mueller H, Ayres S: The role of propranolol in the treatment of acute myocardial infarction. *Prog Cardiovasc Dis* 1977;19:405–412.
3. Shand D: Clinical pharmacology of the β blocking drugs: implications for the postinfarction patient. *Circulation* 1983;67(Suppl.I):2–5.
4. Shand D: Pharmacokinetic properties of the β-adrenergic receptor blocking drugs. *Drugs* 1974;7:39–47.
5. Tinker J: β-Adrenergic agonists and antagonists. *Contemp Anesthesiol Pract* 1983;7:97–112.
6. McDevitt D, Shanks R, Prichard B: The clinical pharmacology of β-adrenergic blocking drugs. *J R Coll Physicians* 1976;11:21–34.
7. Louis W, McNeill J, Jarrott B, et al: β-Adrenoreceptor blocking drugs: current status and the significance of partial agonist activity. *Am J Cardiol* 1983;52:104A–107A.
8. Conolly M, Kersting F, Dollery, C: The clinical pharmacology of β-adrenergic blocking drugs. *Prog Cardiovasc Dis* 1976;19:203–234.
9. Shanks R: The properties of β-adrenoceptor antagonists. *Postgrad Med J* 1976;52(Suppl.4):14–20.

10. Ahlquist R: Adrenergic β blocking agents. *Prog Drug Res* 1976; 20:2743.
11. Ahlquist R: Present state of α and β adrenergic drugs: part III: β-blocking agents. *Am Heart J* 1977;93:117–120.
12. Crowe D: The β and calcium channel blockers. *Top Emerg Med* 1986;8:26–33.
13. McDevitt D: Clinical significance of cardioselectivity. *Drugs* 1983;25(Suppl. 2):219–226.
14. McDevitt D: β-Adrenoceptor blocking drugs and partial agonist activity: is it clinically relevant? *Drugs* 1983;25:331–338.
15. Black C, Mann H: Intrinsic sympathomimetic activity: physiological reality or marketing phenomenon? *Drug Intell Clin Pharmacol* 1984;18:554–559.
16. Wood A: Pharmacologic differences between blockers. *Am Heart J* 1984;108:1070–1077.
17. Dollery C, Paterson J, Conolly M: Clinical pharmacology of β receptor blocking drugs. *Clin Pharmacol Ther* 1969;10:765–798.
18. Sangster B, Wildt D, Dijk A: A case of acebutolol intoxication. *Clin Toxicol* 1983;20:69–77.
19. Bodenhamer J, Bergstrom R, Brown D, et al: Frequently nebulized beta agonists for asthma: effects on serum electrolytes. *Ann Emerg Med* 1992;21:1337–1342.
20. Brown H, Carruthers G, Johnston G, et al: Clinical pharmacologic observations on atenolol, a β-adrenoceptor blocker. *Clin Pharmacol Ther* 1976;20:524–534.
21. Cheung D, Timmers M, Zwinderman A, et al: Long-term effects of a long-acting beta2 adrenoceptor agonist, salmeterol, on airway hyperresponsiveness in patients with mild asthma. *N Engl J Med* 1992;327:1198–1203.
22. Frishman W, Murthy S, Strom J: Ultra-short acting beta adrenergic blockers. *Med Clin North Am* 1988;72:359–372.
23. MacCarthy E, Bloomfield S: Labetalol: a review of its pharmacology, pharmacokinetics, clinical uses and adverse effects. *Pharmacotherapy* 1983;3:193–219.
24. Brogden R, Heel R, Speight T, et al: Labetalol: a review of its pharmacology and therapeutic use in hypertension. *Drugs* 1978;15: 251–270.
25. Carter B: Labetalol. *Drug Intell Clin Pharmacol* 1983;17:704–712.
26. Burrows B, Lebowitz M: The beta-agonist dilemma. *N Engl J Med* 1992;326:560–561.
27. Anthony T, Jastremski M, Elliott W, et al: Charcoal hemoperfusion for the treatment of a combined diltiazem and metoprolol overdose. *Ann Emerg Med* 1986;15:1344–1348.
28. Wallin C, Hylting J: Massive metoprolol poisoning treated with prenalterol. *Acta Med Scand* 1983;214:253–255.
29. Shore E, Cepin D, Davidson M: Metoprolol overdose. *Ann Emerg Med* 1981;10:524–527.
30. Smit A, Mulder P, Jong P, et al: Acute renal failure after overdose of labetalol. *Br Med J* 1986;293:1142–1143.
31. Frishman W: Nadolol: a new β adrenoceptor antagonist. *N Engl J Med* 1981;305:678–682.
32. Khan M, Miller M: β-Blocker toxicity—the role of glucagon. *South Afr Med J* 1985;67:1062–1063.
33. Langerfelt J, Matell C: Attempted suicide with 5.1 g of propranolol. *Acta Med Scand* 1976;199:517–518.
34. Shand D: Propranolol. *N Engl J Med* 1975;293:280–285.
35. Shand D: Pharmacokinetics of propranolol: a review. *Postgrad Med J* 1976;52(Suppl 4):22–25.
36. Kontopoulos A, Manoudis F, Filindris A, et al: Sotalol-induced torsade de pointes. *Postgrad Med J* 1981;57:321–323.
37. Totterman K, Turto H, Pellinen T: Overdrive pacing as treatment of sotalol-induced ventricular tachyarrhythmias (torsade de pointes). *Acta Med Scand* 1982;668:28–33.
38. Hohnloser S, Woosley R: Drug therapy: sotalol. *N Engl J Med* 1994;331:31–38.
39. Frishman W: Atenolol and timolol: two new systemic β-adrenoceptor antagonists. *N Engl J Med* 1982;306:1456–1462.
40. Aronow W, Ferlinz J, Del Vicaro M, et al: Effect of timolol versus propranolol on hypertension and hemodynamics. *Circulation* 1976;54:47–51.
41. Boger W, Puliafito C, Steinert R, et al: Long-term experience with timolol ophthalmic solution in patients with open-angle glaucoma. *Am J Ophthalmol* 1978;85:259–267.
42. Boger W, Steinert R, Puliafito C, et al: Clinical trial comparing timolol ophthalmic solution to pilocarpine in open-angle glaucoma. *Am J Ophthalmol* 1978;86:8–18.
43. Ramoska E, Henretig F, Joffe M, et al: Propranolol treatment of albuterol poisoning in two asthmatic patients. *Ann Emerg Med* 1993;22:1474–1476.
44. Fraunfelder F: Ocular β-blockers and systemic effects. *Arch Intern Med* 1986;146:1073–1074.
45. Munroe W, Rindone J, Kershner R: Systemic side effects associated with the ophthalmic administration of timolol. *Drug Intell Clin Pharmacol* 1985;19:85–89.
46. Swenson E: Severe hyperkalemia as a complication of timolol, a topically applied β-adrenergic antagonist. *Arch Intern Med* 1986;146: 1220–1221.
47. Dimsdale J, Newton R, Joist T: Neuropsychological side effects of beta-blockers. *Arch Intern Med* 1989;149:514–525.
48. Kotler M, Berman J, Rubenstein A: Hypoglycemia precipitated by propranolol. *Lancet* 1966;2:1389–1390.
49. Mackintosh T: Propranolol and hypoglycemia. *Lancet* 1967;1: 104–105.
50. Shanks R: Clinical pharmacology of vasodilatory β-blocking drugs. *Am Heart J* 1991;121:1006–1011.
51. Montagna M, Groppi A: Fatal sotalol poisoning. *Arch Toxicol* 1980;43:221–226.
52. Frishman W, Jacob H, Eisenberg E, et al: Clinical pharmacology of the new β-adrenergic blocking drugs: part 8: self-poisoning with β-adrenoceptor blocking agents: recognition and management. *Am Heart J* 1979;98:798–811.
53. Frishman W: β Adrenoceptor antagonists: new drugs and new indications. *N Engl J Med* 1981;305:500–505.
54. Kosinski E, Malindzak G: Glucagon and isoproterenol in reversing propranolol toxicity. *Arch Intern Med* 1973;132:840–843.
55. Gandy W: Severe epinephrine-propranolol interaction. *Ann Emerg Med* 1989;18:98–99.
56. Love J, Leasure J, Mundt D, et al: A comparison of amrinone and glucagon therapy for cardiovascular depression associated with propranolol toxicity in a canine model. *J Toxicol Clin Toxicol* 1992;30:399–412.
57. Parmley W, Glick G, Sonnenblick E: Cardiovascular effects of glucagon in man. *N Engl J Med* 1968;279:12–17.
58. Prasad K: Effect of glucagon on the transmembrane potential, contraction, and ATPase activity of the failing human heart. *Cardiovasc Res* 1972;6:684–695.
59. Smitherman T, Osborn R, Atkins J: Cardiac dose response relationship for intravenously infused glucagon in normal intact dogs and men. *Am Heart J* 1978;96:363–371.
60. Wilkinson J: β Blocker overdoses. *Ann Emerg Med* 1986;15:982.
61. Ehgartner G, Zelinka M: Hemodynamic instability following intentional nadolol overdose. *Arch Intern Med* 1988;148:801–802.
62. Nord H, Fontanes A, Williams J: Treatment of congestive heart failure with glucagon. *Ann Intern Med* 1970;72:649–653.
63. Peterson C, Leeder S, Sterner S: Glucagon therapy for β blocker overdose. *Drug Intell Clin Pharmacol* 1984;18:394–398.
64. Lucchesi B: Cardiac actions of glucagon. *Circ Res* 1968;22:777–787.
65. Vukmir R, Paris P, Yealy D: Glucagon: prehospital therapy for hypoglycemia. *Ann Emerg Med* 1991;20:375–379.
66. Wilson J, Nelson R: Glucagon as a therapeutic agent in the treatment of asthma. *J Emerg Med* 1990;8:127–130.
67. Kenyon C, Aldinger G, Joshipura P, et al: Successful resuscitation using external cardiac pacing in beta adrenergic antagonist-induced bradysystolic arrest. *Ann Emerg Med* 1988;17:711–713.
68. Timmis G, Ramos R, Parikh J. et al: The unique cardiotonic properties of glucagon. *Mich Med* 1973;21:353–357.
69. Weinstein R: Recognition and management of poisoning with β-adrenergic blocking agents. *Ann Emerg Med* 1984;13:1123–1131.
70. Weinstein R, Cole S, Knaster H, et al: β Blocker overdose with propranolol and with atenolol. *Ann Emerg Med* 1984;14:161–163.
71. Salzberg M, Gallagher E: Propranolol overdose. *Ann Emerg Med* 1980;9:26–27.
72. Ward D, Jones B: Glucagon and β toxicity. *Br Med J* 1976;2:151.
73. Illingworth R: Glucagon for β blocker poisoning. *Practitioner* 1979;223:683–685.
74. Myers J, Horwitz L: Hemodynamic and metabolic response after abrupt withdrawal of long-term propranolol. *Circulation* 1978;58: 196–203.

75. Lindenfeld R, Levine S, Pontiel M, et al: Adrenergic responsiveness after abrupt propranolol withdrawal in normal subjects and in patients with angina pectoris. *Circulation* 1980;62:704–710.
76. Alderman E, Coltart J, Wettach G, et al: Coronary artery syndromes after sudden propranolol withdrawal. *Ann Intern Med* 1974;81: 625–627.
77. Houston M, Hodge R: Beta-adrenergic blocker withdrawal syndromes in hypertension and other cardiovascular diseases. *Am Heart J* 1988;116:515–522.

ADDITIONAL SELECTED REFERENCES

Diamond G, Forrester J, Danzig R, et al: Acute myocardial infarction in man: comparative hemodynamic effects of norepinephrine and glucagon. *Am J Cardiol* 1971;27:612–616.

Dymowski J, Turnbull T: Glucagon and β blocker poisoning. *Ann Emerg Med* 1986;15:1118.

Frishman W: Pindolol: a new β adrenoceptor antagonist with partial agonist activity. *N Engl J Med* 1983;306:940–944.

Gibson D: Pharmacodynamic properties of β-adrenergic receptor blocking drugs in man. *Drugs* 1974;7:8–38.

Gibson D, Sowton E: The use of β-adrenergic receptor blocking drugs in dysrhythmias. *Prog Cardiovasc Dis* 1969;12:16–39.

Haddad L, Dimond K, Schweistris J: Phenol poisoning. *JACEP* 1979;8: 267–269.

Harrison D: The pharmacology and therapeutic use of β-adrenergic receptor blocking drugs in cardiovascular disease. *Drugs* 1974;7:1–7.

Heel R, Brogden R, Speight T, et al: Atenolol: a review of its pharmacological properties and therapeutic efficacy in angina pectoris and hypertension. *Drugs* 1979;17:425–460.

Hiatt W, Fradl D, Zerbe G, et al: Selective and nonselective β blockade of the peripheral circulation. *Clin Pharmacol Ther* 1984;35:12–17.

Hong C, Yang W, Chiang B: Importance of membrane stabilizing effect in massive overdose of propranolol: plasma level study in a fatal case. *Hum Toxicol* 1983;3:511–517.

Kaplan N: The present and future use of β blockers. *Drugs* 1983;25(Suppl. 2):1–4.

Kelly H: Controversies in asthma therapy with theophylline and the 132-adrenergic agonists. *Clin Pharmacol* 1984;3:386–395.

Kristinsson J, Johannesson T: A case of fatal propranolol intoxication. *Acta Pharmacol Toxicol* 1977;41:190–192.

Mills G. Horn J: β Blockers and glucose control. *Drug Intell Clin Pharmacol* 1985;19:246–251.

Morelli H: Propranolol. *Ann Intern Med* 1973;78:913–917.

Theilen E, Wilson W: β-Adrenergic receptor blocking drugs in the treatment of cardiac arrhythmias. *Med Clin North Am* 1968;52:1017–1029.

Williams J: Glucagon and the cardiovascular system. *Ann Intern Med* 1969;71:419–423.

PART III

DRUGS USED IN PSYCHIATRY

CHAPTER 16

Cyclic Antidepressants

One of the most serious types of poisoning, and one that appears to be increasing in frequency in both adults and children, is that due to cyclic antidepressants (1–3). This group of drugs comprises the monocyclic, bicyclic, tricyclic, and tetracyclic compounds as well as the newer agents that inhibit 5-hydroxytryptamine (5-HT) (4). Most of the newer antidepressants are difficult to categorize according to structure and activity, and there are now numerous types of chemical structures as well as functional differences among many of the antidepressants. In this chapter the term *tricyclic* refers to any of the cyclic compounds as well as the noncyclic triazobipyridine derivative trazodone (5–7). The newer selective inhibitors of serotonin uptake (SSUIs) are discussed separately within this chapter, but their toxicity profile is quite different (Table 16–1).

The true tricyclics are the most well known of the cyclic compounds; this group comprises imipramine (8,9), amitriptyline, doxepin (7,10), trimipramine, nortriptyline (11), protriptyline, desipramine, and others. These compounds are structurally similar to the phenothiazines and were first noted during the clinical investigation of phenothiazines in the early 1960s (12,13). The antidepressant properties of these compounds were discovered at that time (14). The rationale for the treatment of depression with tricyclics was a fortuitous discovery (12,13). Imipramine was originally developed as an antipsychotic medicine, but it was noted that patients taking imipramine experienced significant relief of their depression.

The tricyclics have a relatively narrow therapeutic margin, and toxic doses are only 3 to 4 times greater than therapeutic doses. These compounds are therefore particularly dangerous in the context of overdose. Tricyclic overdoses commonly result in hospitalizations because of their potential for causing severe cardiovascular complications. As a result, they account not only for many lives lost but also for untold millions of dollars spent on hospitalizations and intensive care monitoring (12,13).

Cyclic antidepressants are among the most frequently prescribed medications in the U.S. (15) and are also one of the most common causes of drug overdose, accounting for as much as 25% of all serious ingestions (16–18). Their high potential for causing death results from their profound effects on the myocardium and the central nervous system (CNS) (19) and accounts for 20% to 25% of all drug-related deaths (20–26). Although some recent reports indicate that mortality has decreased, antidepressants are still a leading cause of death due to poison exposure in the U.S. (27). It is ironic that the individuals for whom these medications are prescribed are also at greatest risk for overdosage because they are either suicide prone and depressed or young children being treated for nocturnal enuresis (28–30). Because of the complex central and peripheral toxic effects of these drugs, the clinician who treats the overdosed patient may have to manage a number of complex problems, such as hypotension, coma with respiratory arrest, convulsions, complex dysrhythmias, and myocardial depression (16,31,32). Because of these potential complications, a thorough understanding of the action of these drugs is important (33–38).

The true tricyclic antidepressant (TCA) drugs have a three-ring nucleus consisting of a seven-membered central ring bound by two benzene rings (17). They may be categorized as follows: (a) dibenzocycloheptadiene derivatives (nortriptyline and amitriptyline); (b) dihydrodibenzepine derivatives (imipramine, desipramine, and chlorimipramine); (c) dibenzoxepine derivatives (doxepin); and (d) dibenzocycloheptatrine derivatives (protriptyline). Chemical alterations of the basic three-ring molecule have led to the development of similar drugs. Although there

TABLE 16–1. *Relative toxicity associated with overdose of antidepressants*

Antidepressant	Toxicity of overdose
MAOIs	High
Classic TCA	Very high
Amoxapine	Very high
Maprotiline	Very high
Trazodone	Low
Bupropion	Low
Fluoxetine	Low
Sertraline	Low
Paroxetine	Low
Venlafaxine	Low

are numerous preparations on the market, there is actually little difference in the acute toxicity of these products (Table 16–2). The older "second-generation" tricyclics, such as doxepin, were developed as an attempt to produce a less toxic alternative, but there were no real advantages to these agents. Recently, however, antidepressants have been developed that are radically different in structure and function. These appear to have pharmacodynamic characteristics that offer significant advantages. These drugs will also be discussed in this chapter.

TABLE 16–2. *Commonly used cyclic-type compounds and their trade names*

Compound	Trade name(s)
Amitriptyline	Amitid Amitril Elavil Endep Antipress Etrafon Limbitrol Perphenyline Triavil
Imipramine	Imavate Janimine Presamine K-Pramine Tofranil
Doxepin	Adapin Sinequan
Nortriptyline	Aventyl Pamelor
Desipramine	Norpramine Pertofrane
Amoxapine	Asendin
Protriptyline	Vivactil
Trimipramine	Surmontil
Trazodone	Desyrel
Maprotiline	Ludiomil
Fluoxetine	Prozac
Sertraline	Zoloft
Paroxetine	Paxil

MECHANISM OF ACTION

The major hypothesis of the biogenic amine theory of affective illness is that major depressive disorders arise from a functional decrease of certain biogenic amines, such as norepinephrine, dopamine, or serotonin, at functionally important synapses in the brain (39,40). Even where neurotransmitter levels may be high, the sensitivity of the postsynaptic receptor is thought to be abnormally low as a result of agonist-induced receptor desensitization (19). Thus, decreased central neuronal activity may arise from either an actual decrease in synaptic transmitter or a decrease in sensitivity of the postsynaptic receptor for the transmitter.

The apparent mode of action of the antidepressants is thought to be through an increase in the activity of central neurotransmitter systems (Table 16–3). This in turn is thought to be related to their abilities to block the reuptake of norepinephrine and serotonin from within the synaptic cleft into the presynaptic terminal (14). Blockade of amine reuptake leads to increasing synaptic levels of transmitter with secondary effects.

The tricyclics therefore appear to reduce depression by inhibiting the reuptake of norepinephrine, serotonin, and other amines (17). This prolongs the action of these amine neurotransmitters by allowing them to remain at the receptors, thus increasing CNS transmission. The

TABLE 16–3. *Biochemical activity of selected older and newer antidepressants*

	Inhibition of reuptake			Receptor affinity				
Drug	Norepinephrine	Serotonin	Dopamine	α_1-Adrenergic	α_2-Adrenergic	H_1 Histaminergic	Muscarinic	D_2 Dopaminergic
Older drugs								
Amitriptyline	±	++	0	+++	±	++++	++++	0
Nortriptyline	++	±	0	+	0	+	++	0
Imipramine	+	+	0	++	0	+	++	0
Desipramine	+++	0	0	+	0	0	+	0
Clomipramine	+	+++	0	++	0	+	++	0
Trimipramine	+	0	0	++	±	+++	++	+
Doxepin	++	+	0	++	0	+++	++	0
Newer drugs								
Maprotiline	++	0	0	+	0	++	+	0
Amoxapine	++	0	0	++	±	±	0	++
Fluoxetine	0	+++	0	0	0		0	0
Trazodone	0	+	0	++	±	±	+	0
Bupropion	±	0	++	0	0		0	0
Mianserin	0	0	0	++	++	+++	0	0
Alprazolam	0	0	0	0	0	0	0	0

*0 (Zero) denotes no effect, ± an equivocal effect, ++ a moderate effect. +++ a large effect, and ++++ a maximal effect.

actual antidepressant effects seem to be related to down-regulation of presynaptic receptors and enhanced neurotransmitter release (41).

PHARMACOKINETICS

Tricyclics may be tertiary or secondary amines. There is a significant difference between these two types of amines in that tertiary amines are metabolized by *N*-demethylation to the corresponding secondary amines by the hepatic microsomal enzymes (42–44). These secondary amines are pharmacologically active and contribute to both therapeutic and toxic effects. The tertiary amines therefore show dual toxicity (45). On the other hand, the secondary amines are metabolized in the liver by aromatic hydroxylation and glucuronidization to compounds that have neither the therapeutic nor the toxic effects of the tricyclics (36). Tertiary amines are therefore toxic in the parent form as well as in metabolite form, whereas secondary amines are only toxic in the parent form (46).

For example, imipramine is a tertiary amine and is partially metabolized to desipramine, its active secondary amine. Amitriptyline is also a tertiary amine that is metabolized to its active secondary amine nortriptyline. Because the demethylation reaction is not reversible, patients treated with the secondary tricyclics are only exposed to these products and not to the tertiary or parent compound (Table 16–4).

In general, secondary amines such as desipramine are more potent inhibitors of norepinephrine uptake, whereas tertiary amines such as imipramine exert more potent effects on the uptake of 5-hydroxytryptamine. Because the tertiary amines are broken down to secondary amines, they have both actions.

Absorption

Tricyclics are rapidly absorbed from the gastrointestinal tract in therapeutic doses, and after oral administration their plasma concentrations reach their peak within 2 to 4 hours. Although absorption of the tricyclics is complete, the amount of tricyclic that is bioavailable is substantially less than that administered because of a significant first-pass effect. Because of their high lipid solubility, tricyclics are rapidly distributed to body tissues and fat, leaving only a small amount of the drug in the blood. In an overdose, they are absorbed more slowly because, owing to their antimuscarinic effects, they decrease peristalsis and delay gastric emptying. Delayed absorption of oral doses of the tricyclics, with peak serum concentrations reached up to 12 hours after ingestion, has been noted (47).

TABLE 16–4. *Tertiary and secondary amine tricyclics*

Tertiary amine	Secondary amine
Amitriptyline	Nortriptyline
Imipramine	Desipramine
Doxepin	Nordoxepin

Protein Binding

The tricyclics are approximately 85% to 98% protein-bound to alpha acid glycoproteins and lipoproteins (17); that is, free drug concentrations are 2% to 15% (5,48). The bound tricyclic is pharmacologically inactive but equilibrates between bound and unbound states in milliseconds. There is a direct relationship between protein binding and pH in that the more alkalotic the patient, the greater the degree of protein binding, with a consequent decrease in free or active drug concentrations at drug receptor sites (17).

Metabolism

Metabolism occurs by demethylation, oxidation, aromatic hydroxylation, and glucuronidization by the microsomal enzyme system in the liver (14,17,42–44). Demethylation of the tertiary tricyclics, such as amitriptyline and imipramine, yields the pharmacologically active secondary amines, nortriptyline and desipramine respectively (49). After hepatic metabolism, a small fraction of cyclic antidepressants enter an enterohepatic cycle with less than 5% of the ingested dose excreted into the bile. Another 5% to 16% is excreted in gastric juices (17,47,50).

Volume of Distribution

The volume of distribution of the tricyclics is large and varies with the particular drug; the range is from 8 L/kg (for amitriptyline) to 34 L/kg (for desipramine). This large volume of distribution reflects the vast tissue distribution of the drugs. The large volume of distribution and the high degree of protein binding make the tricyclics virtually inaccessible to hemodialysis or hemoperfusion. Because of the high lipid solubility of these drugs, concentrations in tissue may be 10 times greater than those in the plasma. Concentrations in myocardial tissue have been reported to be as much as 50 to 200 times higher than in plasma (47).

ACTIONS

The tricyclics have four major actions when taken in therapeutic amounts (Tables 16–5 and 16–6). In the United States, they are approved by the FDA as antide-

TABLE 16–5. *Actions of the tricyclics*

Antidepressant (blocks the reuptake of 5-hydroxytryptamine and norepinephrine)
Antidysrhythmic (Class Ia type)
Antihistaminic (H_1 and H_2 antagonist)
Antienuretic (antimuscarinic action)
α Blocking

pressant agents. They have also been used in children for enuresis. Although approved in Europe for dysrhythmias and peptic ulcer disease, the tricyclics are not approved in the United States for those indications. Other uses not approved by the FDA include treatment for migraine, chronic pain, attention deficit disorder, anorexia nervosa, insomnia, panic attacks, phobias, and bulimia (19,51).

Antidepressant Effect

As mentioned earlier, the tricyclics are antidepressants owing to their ability to block the reuptake of norepinephrine and 5-hydroxytryptamine in the central nervous system. In patients with endogenous depression, an effect can be seen in 2 to 3 weeks. The tricyclics do not appear to offer mood elevation or euphoria to nonendogenously depressed individuals; therefore, these compounds have not appeared as drugs of abuse.

Antidysrhythmic Effect

Therapeutic doses of tricyclics produce electrocardiographic changes similar to those seen with quinidine, procainamide, and disopyramide; thus, the tricyclics are considered antidysrhythmic agents of the Class Ia type (17,52–55). Imipramine, for example, is attractive as a potential antidysrhythmic drug because it has a long half-life that would permit twice-daily dosing (52,56). Although effective as antidysrhythmic agents and used in Europe for this purpose, the tricyclics are not approved for such use in the United States.

Antihistaminic Effect

The tricyclics have antihistaminic effects, exhibiting potent inhibition of both H_1 and H_2 receptors (Table 16-7): (14). Some of the tricyclics, notably doxepin, amitriptyline, and trimipramine, are the most potent histamine antagonists currently available; they are more potent than cimetidine. Trimipramine has been used in Europe for duodenal ulcers and has been shown to be effective (57,58). Tricyclics have also been beneficial for gastric ulcers (59). As an example of its potent H_1 blocking activity, doxepin has an affinity 800 times greater than diphenhydramine (47). Although these drugs are effective as histamine antagonists, they have not been approved for this use in the United States.

Antienuresis Effect

The tricyclics have been used in the pediatric age group for enuresis (60). The mechanism of action of the tricyclics in the treatment of enuresis is not known but may involve inhibition of urination as a result of anticholinergic activity. This therapy poses a problem in that children have small fat stores, which makes more free and active drug available and creates the potential for toxicity (34,61). The indications for the tricyclics have increased in the pediatrics age group. These now include hyperkinesis, school phobia, and sleep disorders (17).

SIDE EFFECTS OF THERAPEUTIC AMOUNTS

It is estimated that 5% to 10% of patients placed on long-term therapy with tricyclic agents experience significant side effects, including antimuscarinic effects such as dryness of the mouth, tachycardia, and urinary retention (Table 16-8) (62–65). Although these problems can be bothersome, a tolerance develops to them. Sweating, a paradoxical response, occurs by an unknown mechanism. Weakness, fatigue, and sedation have also been noted; these are possibly due to the anticholinergic actions causing drowsiness. Muscle tremors may occur in 10% to

TABLE 16–6. *Comparison of the actions of the tricyclics*

Compound	Orthostatic hypotension	Antimuscarinic action	Quinidine-like action	Adrenergic side effects
Amitriptyline	+++++	+++++	+	+
Doxepin	+++	+++	+/−	0
Imipramine	++++	++++	+	+++
Nortriptyline	++	++	+	+++
Desipramine	++	++	+	+++++
Maprotiline	+	+	+	+++++
Trazodone	+	+	−	0

Reprinted from *Med Clin North Am* 1986;70:1185–1201, with permission of WB Saunders Company.

TABLE 16–7. *Side effects of blockade of histamine H_1 receptors*

Potentiation of central depressant drugs
Sedation, drowsiness
Weight gain
Hypotension

20% of patients receiving the drug. On occasion, periods of confusion may be noted while the dosage is being increased; this abates when the medication is withheld for 1 day. Orthostatic hypotension is a significant side effect of tricyclic therapy that is unrelated to the age of the patient or to the duration of use of the drug. This action is due to a receptor blockade. Obstructive jaundice, when seen, is an idiosyncratic reaction (also noted with phenothiazines) that improves after discontinuance of the medication.

As with the phenothiazines, extrapyramidal symptoms may occur in patients receiving tricyclics (Table 16-8). In addition, a persistent fine tremor may develop in any age group, and parkinsonism is most commonly seen in geriatric patients receiving high doses. Other extrapyramidal side effects include rigidity, akathisia, dystonia, oculogyric crisis, opisthotonus, dysphagia, and chorea (15). Another relatively rare idiosyncratic reaction is the syndrome of inappropriate antidiuretic hormone secretion with resultant hyponatremia, lethargy, and seizures (17,66).

In the healthy adult the tricyclics do not cause clinically important adverse cardiovascular effects except for postural hypotension, which can occur at therapeutic levels. Postural hypotension may result from the α blocking action of the tricyclics and is more likely to occur in the presence of existing cardiovascular disease (Table 16-9) (66,67). Some patients with ventricular dysrhythmias have even shown improvement during treatment for their psychiatric disorder (52,53). The patients at greatest risk for cardiac problems are those with preexisting bundle branch block, who have an increased risk for developing high grades of atrioventricular block.

At therapeutic doses, the quinidine-like effect can result in increased PR, QRS, and QT intervals, inversion or flattening of T waves, and heart block. These changes, however, are usually not clinically significant and will often resolve with time (47).

TABLE 16–8. *Side effects of therapeutic amounts of tricyclics*

Antimuscarinic
Sweating
Headache
Weakness
Fatigue
Muscle tremors
Cardiac toxicity
Seizures
Obstructive jaundice
Extrapyramidal
Muscular rigidity
Akathisia
Dystonia
Oculogyric crisis
Opisthotonus
Chorea
Dysphagia
Parkinsonism
Postural hypotension
Inappropriate secretion of antidiuretic hormone
Hyponatremia
Lethargy
Seizures

TRICYCLIC WITHDRAWAL

A withdrawal syndrome has been described that is associated with abrupt discontinuance of tricyclics (68). The syndrome is considered mild and consists of akathisia (69) (which may be related to a sudden decrease in dopamine concentration at the receptor site), nausea, vomiting, diarrhea, chills, headache, and malaise. No treatment is necessary for this condition except to replace the discontinued medicine if warranted.

TOXICITY OF CYCLIC ANTIDEPRESSANTS

Most patients who have overdosed with tricyclics have no more than transient minor toxic effects, although serious toxic effects can certainly occur. After a significant overdose the patient may progress from a state of alertness and lucidity to unconsciousness, usually within a short period of time. This rapid clinical presentation is typical of cyclic antidepressant poisoning (70). It is well established that a relatively well appearing patient can rapidly deteriorate over 30 to 120 minutes and become lethargic or comatose, or have seizures (47). Typically, a patient intoxicated with tricyclics becomes symptomatic within a 3- to 4-hour period, but symptoms may begin as early as 20 to 30 minutes after ingestion (23,24). Most

TABLE 16–9. *Side effects of blockade of α_1-adrenergic receptors*

Potentiation of antihypertensive effect of
Prazosin
Terazosin
Doxazosin
Labetalol
Postural hypotension
Dizziness
Reflex tachycardia

patients who develop a dysrhythmia or conduction abnormality do so within 1 to 2 hours after ingestion. Myoclonus and grand mal seizures may also be noted shortly after ingestion. Generally, patients wake up within 24 hours even after a severe overdose of cyclic antidepressant (70).

Toxicity of the tricyclics is caused by a number of different mechanisms: (a) the antimuscarinic (anticholinergic) actions, (b) the blocking of the reuptake of norepinephrine, (c) the membrane-stabilizing or quinidine-like action on the myocardium, and (d) miscellaneous actions (Table 16–10) (71,72). The signs and symptoms of tricyclic intoxication can also be placed in three categories: atropine-like, neurologic, and cardiovascular.

Antimuscarinic (Anticholinergic Action)

Muscarinic receptors are found in the peripheral autonomic nervous system and are the predominant acetylcholine receptors in the brain (47). Because of an atropine-like action, the tricyclics bind to the muscarinic receptor in a competitive fashion. When acetylcholine is released it cannot bind to the receptor and is destroyed by the enzyme acetylcholinesterase, resulting in parasympathetic paralysis. This is the mechanism of action for any of the antimuscarinic compounds (see Chapter 10). Although some of the cyclic antidepressants have strong antimuscarinic effects through competitive antagonism of muscarinic acetylcholine receptors, they have no effect on nicotinic receptors. Although they are described as anticholinergics, in reality, they are antimuscarinics (47). Cardiac and smooth muscle, exocrine gland, and brain tissue are the most markedly affected by the tricyclics; there is little effect on autonomic ganglia or motor endplates (73).

The antimuscarinic effect of these drugs varies widely, with tertiary cyclic antidepressant having a greater effect than secondary amines.

Peripheral Antimuscarinic Effects

Peripheral effects include supraventricular tachycardia, hyperpyrexia, mydriasis, vasodilation, urinary retention, decreased gastrointestinal motility, and decreased secretions (Table 16–11) (74).

TABLE 16–10. *Major toxicity of the tricyclics*

Action	Manifestations
Antimuscarinic	Atropine-like effects
Blocking of reuptake of norepinephrine	Sympathomimetic effects
Membrane stabilization	Quinidine-like effects
α-Adrenergic blocking action	Hypotension
Miscellaneous	Coma, bradycardia

Central Antimuscarinic Effects

The central antimuscarinic effects include anxiety, delirium, disorientation, hallucinations, hyperactivity, seizures, myoclonus, choreoathetosis, coma, and, possibly, death (Table 16-11) (75). Coma usually occurs within 6 hours of the ingestion and may last for 24 hours, in some cases simulating brain death with complete loss of brainstem and cerebral function (76,77). CNS depression may cause ventilatory failure and contribute to aspiration pneumonia, and seizures, agitation, and marked muscle activity can lead to rhabdomyolysis and acute renal failure (78). Many of these symptoms result from an imbalance of acetylcholine and dopamine, with a resultant decrease in acetylcholine relative to dopamine in the basal ganglia. Myoclonus results from the decrease in serotonin uptake and subsequent increase in serotonin at the synapse.

Many of the movement disorders associated with these drugs are often inaccurately classified as seizures. Recognizing the movements as chorea, athetosis, or myoclonus may be important in helping to establish the correct diagnosis as well as initiating proper treatment.

Antimuscarinic effects, although common after tricyclic overdose, are not the primary mechanism by which the tricyclics are lethal.

Blocking of the Reuptake of Norepinephrine

The second action of the tricyclics is an exaggeration of the beneficial mechanism of action—the central and

TABLE 16–11. *Peripheral and central antimuscarinic effects of tricyclics*

Peripheral
Tachycardia
Hypertension
Hyperpyrexia
Mydriasis
Vasodilation
Supraventricular dysrhythmias
Urinary retention
Decreased secretions
Central
Anxiety
Confusion
Disorientation
Myoclonus
Choreoathetosis
Hallucinations
Seizures
Medullary paralysis
Death

TABLE 16–12. *Side effects of blockade of reuptake of norepinephrine*

Tremors
Tachycardia
Erectile and ejaculatory dysfunction
Blockade of the antihypertensive effects of guanethidine
Augmentation of pressor effects of sympathetic amines
Decreased myocardial contractility
Hypotension
Bradycardia
Hyperthermia

peripheral blockage of the reuptake of norepinephrine (79). In contrast to many metabolic processes in which the actions of pharmacologically active substances are terminated by enzymatic transformation of the substance into less active metabolites, reuptake of the neurotransmitter back into the vesicle, rather than metabolism, is the major mechanism by which an action is terminated at the adrenergic site for compounds such as norepinephrine, epinephrine, and dopamine. This action occurs by means of an active pump mechanism. The norepinephrine is again stored intraneuronally until released again by the next stimulus; this is the reuptake mechanism.

The tricyclics block this reuptake of norepinephrine both centrally and peripherally, resulting in increased neurotransmitter action at the receptor site. Such an action causes potentiation of transmitter action. Blocking of the reuptake of the neurotransmitter also eventually leads to local or generalized norepinephrine depletion because the neurotransmitter is metabolized once it is in the bloodstream. This eventually causes decreased myocardial contractility, hypotension, and bradycardia (Table 16–12).

Membrane-Stabilizing Action

The most dangerous action of the tricyclics is the membrane-stabilizing action, sometimes referred to as the quinidine-like effect. Membrane stabilizers depress excitability in nerve and muscle tissue, including the heart, and depress both conduction and contractility of the myocardium (80,81). This occurs through direct depression of the myocardium caused by interference with the sodium-potassium pump. This is believed to be due to an inhibition of the adenosine triphosphate phosphohydrolase enzyme, which is the enzyme involved in the maintenance of sodium and potassium balance across the myocardial cell membrane. This slowing of sodium flux into cells results in altered repolarization and conduction (79). Interruption of ionic balance across the cell therefore leads to myocardial depression and conduction defects. This is because slowing of phase 0 depolarization of the action potential results in slowing of conduction through the His-Purkinje system and myocardium

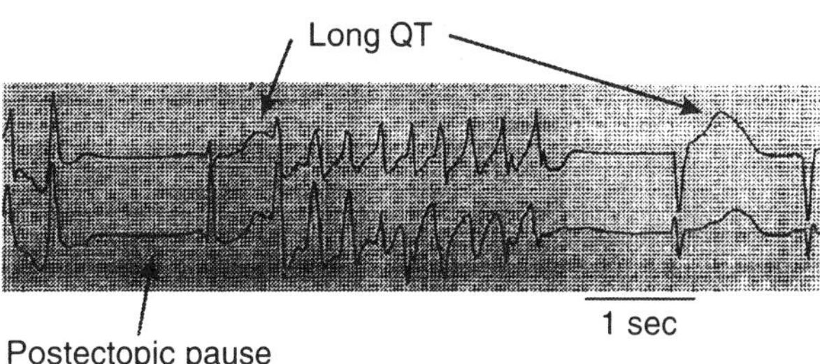

FIG. 16–1. A self-limited episode of torsade de pointes ventricular tachycardia recorded on a two-channel Holter monitor during treatment with a drug that prolongs the QT interval. The typical pattern of initiation is shown. A normal postectopic pause follows a brief episode of tachycardia *(left)*. The sinus beat that terminates the pause has a very long QT interval, which is interrupted after the peak of the T wave by the first beat of torsade de pointes. Note that the beat that follows the episode (and which is paced) also has a markedly prolonged QT interval.

(54,55). Slow impulse conduction is responsible for QRS prolongation and atrioventricular block and contributes to ventricular dysrhythmias and hypotension. Cardiotoxicity is manifested by decreased myocardial contractile force, increased PR interval, and pronounced intraventricular conduction delays, all of which predispose the patient to reentry and ventricular dysrhythmias (20–22).

Because of slowed conduction in the ventricles, a widened QRS may be noted. This is a sensitive indicator of toxicity and toxic blood levels (12,13,17,76,77). An increased QT interval may predispose the patient to torsade de pointes (84) which is seen during treatment with drugs that prolong the QT interval (54,55). The mechanism of torsade is thought to be increased temporal dispersion of ventricular depolarization. Drug-induced torsade de pointes is typically triggered by a premature ventricular beat on the terminal position of the T wave and often occurs after a sinus pause (Fig. 16–1) (82–84). This rhythm is more likely to occur at slow heart rates and has been observed when therapeutic doses of tricyclics are administered. Torsade de pointes is unlikely to occur with tachycardia associated with tricyclic overdose. In addition to torsade, myocardial depression, hypotension, bradycardia, and asystole have been noted (Table 16–13) (85).

Widened QRS Duration

The QRS duration in the limb leads of an electrocardiogram is an important prognostic indicator of toxicity (12,14,21,76). It has been found that patients with a QRS duration of less than 0.10 second are not likely to experience seizures or ventricular dysrhythmias (16,86). Those with a QRS duration of 0.10 second or more have a greater incidence of seizures, and those with a QRS duration that exceeds 0.16 second are likely to experience

TABLE 16–13. *Membrane-stabilizing (quinidine-like) cardiovascular effects of tricyclics*

Primary
Increased refractory period
Decreased conduction velocity
Decreased ventricular automaticity
Secondary
Increased PR interval
Increased QT interval
Increased QRS duration
Predisposition to reentry
Hypotension
Rightward deviation of T40-ms axis

ventricular dysrhythmias (16). Other studies have shown that the QRS interval might not be a reliable indicator of toxicity (87).

Inhibition of the sodium current slowing of phase 0 depolarization is the most important toxic effect of the tricyclics on the cardiac action potential. This effect on the depolarization rate is also rate dependent. At rapid heart rates depolarization is depressed, and the QRS complex becomes prolonged. Thus sinus tachycardia may aggravate the conduction abnormality. Although a potentially toxic patient can present with a normal QRS interval, the interval may widen with time and an increasing QRS interval should be considered as a sign of worsening toxicity. It should be remembered that the prognostic value of the ECG has not been studied for newer agents. Of these agents, maprotiline should probably be approached as a typical cyclic antidepressant (27).

Terminal 40 ms on ECG

The terminal 40-ms axis of the frontal plane QRS vector has also been looked at as a marker for the occurrence of cyclic antidepressant overdose (21). It has been postulated that the rightward deviation of the T40-ms axis may be due to the quinidine-like effects of cyclic antidepressants on the distal conduction system on the right side of the heart (89). Although this may be useful in the emergency evaluation of an overdose patient, a terminal 40-ms axis of less than 120 does not eliminate the possibility of cyclic antidepressant toxicity. In addition, there is no correlation between the T40-ms axis and plasma cyclic antidepressant concentrations (19). The presence of a terminal 40-ms axis between 120 and 270 in an unknown overdose patient should lead to a high index of suspicion that the patient is toxic from cyclic antidepressants (Fig. 16–2) (89).

It has been postulated that cyclic antidepressant induces a rightward deviation of the 140-ms axis because the right ventricular conduction system is more susceptible than the left to cyclic antidepressant induced conduction inhibition. A rightward terminal vector, best seen as an R wave in lead aVr is a valuable tool for recognizing early or unsuspected cyclic antidepressant toxicity (27).

Summary of Membrane-Stabilizing Effects of the ECG

The membrane-stabilizing effects of the cyclic antidepressants, which block the inward sodium channels, result in altered repolarization and conduction. This effect occurs distal to the atrioventricular node, producing a depression of the His-Purkinje conduction system and a direct negative inotropic effect (47). The quinidine-like effect results in the following abnormalities: ST-T wave changes, prolongation of the QT and PR intervals, prolongation of the QRS complex, bundle branch block, especially right, atrioventricular conduction blocks, and right axis deviation of 130° to 270° in the terminal 40 ms frontal plane QRS axis (T40-ms).

Early cyclic antidepressant-induced ECG changes include a rightward terminal vector and QT prolongation, followed by progressive QRS increase, followed by superimposed ventricular ectopy, followed by ventricular tachycardia, followed by resolution of ectopy and development of a slow, very wide idioventricular rhythm, which is the usual preterminal rhythm. The appearance

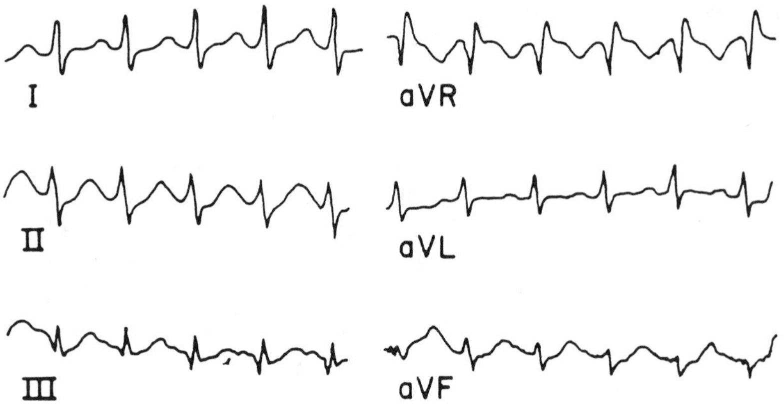

I

aVR

II

aVL

III

aVF

FIG. 16–2. ECG from a TCA overdose patient. A T40-ms axis falling between 120° and 270° requires a negative T40-ms deflection in lead I and a positive T40-ms deflection in lead aVR. (From Wolfe TR, et al., *Ann Emerg Med* 1989;4: 36/349, with permission.)

and disappearance of ventricular dysrhythmias is presumably due to their reentrant origin (90).

Cardiotoxic Effects

Cardiovascular toxic reactions account for most fatalities from tricyclic overdosage and are the most difficult to treat; they are therefore the major adverse action of the tricyclics. Owing to the antimuscarinic action, there may be a sinus tachycardia and other evidence of a hyperdynamic state (Table 16–14). Sinus tachycardia is considered one of the most sensitive early indicators of tricyclic toxicity (14,55,91,92). Sinus tachycardia may contribute to cardiotoxicity, but is rarely the cause of life-threatening sequelae (27). Mild hypertension may also be produced. The antimuscarinic effects are not thought to be responsible for ventricular conduction blocks because cholinergic innervation of the ventricle is sparse. Attempts to improve conduction through the atrioventricular node with atropine, therefore, are usually ineffective because of the distal AV conduction block produced by the cyclic antidepressants (47).

Because of the blockage of the reuptake of norepinephrine, there may also be a sinus tachycardia, hypertension, an associated increase in cardiac output, and ventricular dysrhythmias (93). Hypotension may be noted and is caused by the α blocking action of the tricyclics or, over a longer period of time, by the depletion of norepinephrine with subsequent metabolism of the catecholamine. Hypotension may at times be severe and, when combined with marked bradycardia and heart block, may lead to cardiac arrest. Hypotension may also aggravate tricyclic-induced dysrhythmias by impairing myocardial perfusion or causing systemic acidosis and appears to herald other more dangerous complications such as life-threatening arrhythmias and pulmonary edema (17,94).

TABLE 16–14. *Summary of cardiotoxic effects*

Sinus tachycardia
Antimuscarinic effect
Blocking reuptake of norepinephrine
Secondary to hypotension
Hypertension
Antimuscarinic effect
Blocking reuptake of norepinephrine
Hypotension
Depletion of norepinephrine
Direct myocardial depression
α Blocking action of TCAs
Sinus bradycardia
Depletion of norepinephrine
Membrane-stabilizing effect
Widened QRS
Membrane-stabilizing effect
Rightward axis deviation
Membrane-stabilizing effect
Bundle branch block
Membrane-stabilizing effect

Toxic doses of the tricyclics are capable of producing various rate and rhythm disturbances, including sinus tachycardia, sinus bradycardia, supraventricular and ventricular tachycardia, wandering atrial pacemaker, atrial and ventricular flutter and fibrillation, partial or complete atrioventricular block, bundle branch blocks, intraventricular blocks, ectopic beats, and asystole (55). The most frequent dysrhythmias noted are supraventricular tachycardia, conduction defects, ventricular ectopic beats, and ventricular tachycardia or fibrillation. Sometimes differentiating supraventricular dysrhythmias with aberrant conduction from ventricular dysrhythmias may be difficult, as recent studies suggest (95).

Continuous infusion of imipramine in animals has resulted in a progression of electrocardiographic changes similar to that seen in humans (20). These changes are typically seen in order and consist of sinus tachycardia, intraventricular conduction defects (with right bundle branch block occurring more frequently than left bundle branch block), ventricular dysrhythmias including ventricular tachycardia and ventricular fibrillation, and atrioventricular conduction defects that eventually lead to bradycardia and cardiac arrest (96,97). First-degree atrioventricular block and intraventricular conduction delay in tricyclic antidepressant poisoning do not cause hemodynamic abnormalities and are not life-threatening (98,99). The importance of these conduction abnormalities lies in their being the most reliable premonitory signs of severe tricyclic antidepressant poisoning, heralding the increased probability of subsequent dysrhythmias, heart block, cardiac arrest, and sudden death (13,25).

Owing to the complex pharmacokinetics of the tricyclics, many instances of delayed complications including dysrhythmias, conduction blocks, coma, and death have been reported. The recurrence of symptoms and rebound of plasma concentrations may be due to the release of the tissue-bound supply of the tricyclic.

Children may be at an increased risk of tricyclic cardiotoxicity because they have smaller lipid compartments than adults and tend to have less tricyclic stored in the fat and more available free drug. In addition, children appear to have a low capacity for drug binding to albumin, which also increases the amount of available free drug (100).

Significant ECG indicators of cyclic antidepressant toxicity include QRS prolongation, QTc prolongation, and rightward axis deviation (89). Even though the absence of these indicators does not preclude complications, their presence generally correlates with developing cardiovascular toxicity, possibly leading to refractory myocardial depression, ventricular tachycardia, or fibrillation and death (48). The most prudent way to evaluate the initial ECG then is to consider that positive findings are consistent with cyclic antidepressant overdose, but that a lack of findings should never rule out the possibility of serious toxicity (47).

Other Effects (Table 16–15)

Seizures

Generalized seizures may be noted after a serious tricyclic overdose. The epileptogenic potential of cyclic antidepressants has been suggested to be related to the inhibition of reuptake of certain brain monoamines (101). Although many times seizures are usually short-lived and often resolve without specific treatment, seizures have also been associated with abrupt cardiovascular deterioration and death. This phenomenon may be related to the metabolic acidosis produced by the seizure. The acidosis could worsen the cardiac toxicity due to enhanced sodium-channel blockade. For this reason, sodium bicarbonate should be administered to patients who have seizures with the understanding that it does not directly affect the seizure activity itself but may avert cardiovascular collapse (47). The CNS status is not a reliable predictor of seizures because patients have ranged from awake and alert, to comatose (102). As with other medical disorders, hypoxia, hypoglycemia, and other metabolic and structural causes of seizures must first be ruled out (17).

Pseudoseizures

Pseudoseizures such as myoclonus, tremor, chorea, and choreoathetosis may occur in many of the serious overdoses (17). Myoclonus may be related to tricyclic blockade of amine neurotransmitter uptake, which then increases serotonin at peripheral synapses. Coarse myoclonic jerking may precede seizure activity and may be difficult to differentiate, but patients experiencing myoclonus usually remain awake (14). An imbalance of dopamine and acetylcholine in the central nervous system may produce tremor and chorea.

TABLE 16–15. *Miscellaneous effects of the TCAs*

Grand mal seizures
Pseudoseizures
Myoclonus
Tremor
Chorea
Choreoathetosis
Anion gap metabolic acidosis
Hyperthermia/hypothermia
Coma
Pulmonary complications
Pulmonary edema
Atelectasis
Aspiration pneumonitis

Acidemia

The patient overdosed on tricyclics may experience hypotension, hypoventilation, or seizures that may lead to acidemia (54). Vigorous management is required to treat the acidemia because it could lead to cardiac arrest.

Hyperthermia and Hypothermia

Both hypothermia and hyperthermia in tricyclic overdose have been reported (34–36). Hyperthermia is a result of the blocking of the reuptake of norepinephrine, increased muscular generation of heat from seizures, myoclonus, or agitation combined with impaired heat loss from decreased sweating due to cholinergic blockade (54). Hypothermia may be seen in patients with severe poisoning and is thought to be due to a combination of low cardiac output, peripheral vasodilation, and low external temperature.

Coma

Coma resulting from tricyclic overdose is generally of short duration. Although coma may be accompanied by other signs of tricyclic poisoning, this is not always the case, and coma may be the sole symptom. Respiratory failure in tricyclic overdose can occur from CNS depression, seizures, upper airway obstruction, aspiration, and pulmonary edema.

Pulmonary

Pulmonary abnormalities have received little attention compared with the cardiac and neurologic sequelae of cyclic antidepressant overdose, yet a significant number of patients with cyclic antidepressant overdose requiring admission to the intensive care unit will manifest some pulmonary complication such as pulmonary edema, atelectasis, or aspiration pneumonitis (103).

A high incidence of aspiration pneumonia in cyclic antidepressant ingestion is not unexpected since these patients have a multitude of risk factors for aspiration such as a high incidence of seizures, deep coma with concomitant loss of gag reflex, manipulation of the hypopharynx for gastric lavage and intubation, and repetitive administration of activated charcoal and cathartics in the face of decreased gut motility, all leading to potential gastroesophageal reflux (103,104).

LABORATORY ANALYSIS FOR TRICYCLIC OVERDOSE (TABLE 16–16)

Electrocardiogram

A 12-lead electrocardiogram should be immediately obtained looking for evidence of cardiovascular effects,

TABLE 16–16. *Laboratory analysis for TCA overdose*

Electrocardiogram
Plasma assay (qualitative)
Serum electrolytes
Arterial blood gases
Chest roentgenogram

including sinus tachycardia and bundle branch block (88). A limb lead QRS duration of more than 0.10 second identifies patients at greatest risk for seizures, and a QRS duration of less than 0.16 second identifies patients at greatest risk for developing ventricular dysrhythmias or hypotension (16). Although there appears to be a positive correlation between the QRS duration and the development of significant symptoms, (12,13,16,20–22,76,77), a QRS interval of less than 0.10 second cannot be used as the sole indicator of safety (105). This finding alone therefore does not exclude the risk of significant toxic events, including seizures and ventricular dysrhythmias (106).

Plasma Assays

Plasma assays of tricyclics are not a routine procedure in most hospitals, but they can be performed in larger institutions (107,108). The tricyclics are among the most difficult drugs to analyze, and unpredictable losses of the compound can occur if scrupulous care is not taken with the specimen (109). It is only recently that methods have become available to measure the tricyclics at the low concentrations that occur in serum. In addition, to measure tricyclic concentrations accurately a laboratory must also assay the pharmacologically active metabolites, which may also contribute to toxicity and in some cases are more toxic than the parent compound (110).

Although thin-layer chromatography can detect the tricyclics, it is not a quantitative method. The most widely used methods are gas chromatography with a nitrogen detector, high-performance liquid chromatography with an ultraviolet absorbance detector, and gas chromatography combined with mass spectrometry (5,6,111). Radioimmunoassays are also available but have certain drawbacks that limit their usefulness (112).

In general, tests for serum tricyclic concentrations are not helpful in the acute ingestion because they are relatively time-consuming and because the plasma concentrations may be small (in the nanogram range) while tissue levels may be toxic (43). In addition, the results of laboratory tests are not as helpful in determining treatment as is the interpretation of the patient's signs and symptoms (113). Laboratory studies can be useful, however, in confirming a diagnosis or in following the hospital course of a tricyclic-intoxicated patient. Highly elevated serum cyclic antidepressant levels in acute overdose patients have been previously associated with severe clinical toxicity but, in general, there is not a direct correlation between cyclic antidepressant levels and ECG or clinical findings (88).

Value of Quantitative Blood Levels

Under therapeutic conditions the concentration of a tricyclic drug in plasma is low, usually between 20 to 500 ng/mL depending on the specific tricyclic (5–7,31,107). In acute intoxications, tricyclic concentrations greater than 1,000 ng/mL (for imipramine) are associated with severe toxicity, including electrocardiographic widening of the QRS of more than 100 msec, development of serious dysrhythmias, and coma (13,31,76,77). High concentrations may remain high for several days, particularly if the patient overdosed with a tertiary tricyclic antidepressant (49). Marked differences in steady-state plasma concentrations of the tricyclics occur even in patients treated therapeutically with equal oral doses. This variation has been shown to be the result of individual differences in the rate of drug metabolism and the apparent volume of distribution. Therefore, wide variations in toxic plasma concentrations may also occur. Some investigators have reported that falsely low laboratory values have been obtained if Vacutainer tubes are used for blood drawing because of the chemical in the rubber stopper (46).

Although serious toxic complications may occur more frequently when the combined plasma concentration of the antidepressant (amitripytline) and its main metabolite exceeds 1,000 μg/L, serious toxic complications can be seen at lower plasma concentrations. Alert patients can have plasma concentrations exceeding 1,000 μg/L without later developing any toxic complications. Thus, the often difficult and time-consuming quantitative analysis of cyclic antidepressant is unlikely to contribute to the immediate clinical management of the patient (113). The qualitative detection of a cyclic antidepressant drug may, however, be vitally useful in circumstances where the diagnosis may be uncertain or is complicated by other factors (16,114).

Miscellaneous Tests

In addition to the previously mentioned laboratory analyses, serum electrolyte and arterial blood gas determinations should be performed to judge the acid-base status of the patient.

SECOND-GENERATION ANTIDEPRESSANTS

The past decade has witnessed the development of second-generation antidepressants. These agents were marketed as "safer" antidepressants secondary to atypical pharmacology and a lower incidence of toxicity (39,115).

Those new antidepressant agents that do not have the receptor interactions typical of tricyclic drugs do not cause antimuscarinic effects, cardiac conduction and slowing, weight gain, or changes in blood pressure. Others, such as maprotiline and amoxapine, are more like standard tricyclic drugs.

Amoxapine

Amoxapine (Asendin), a dibenzoxapine (116), resembles imipramine and other tricyclics in both structure and pharmacology (115). Although amoxapine has potent antidepressant properties, it is a metabolite of the antipsychotic drug loxapine and appears to have less cardiotoxic effects than the tricyclics (57,63,111). There are prominent manifestations of CNS depression and seizures associated with an overdose (101).

Side Effects

Amoxapine, like imipramine, is a potent inhibitor of neuronal norepinephrine reuptake but has little potency as an inhibitor of the neuronal uptake of serotonin (111). Amoxapine has been shown to have neuroleptic activity nearly as potent as thioridazine (117). One of its primary metabolites, 7-hydroxyamoxapine, has significant dopamine blocking effect and has neuroleptic activity approximately equal to haloperidol (58,59,101). In psychomotor systems, amoxapine treatment is associated with many of the movement disorders classically associated with neuroleptic treatment. These extrapyramidal side effects have been ascribed to the dopamine-receptor blockade by the 7-hydroxyamoxapine metabolite (117). These include dystonia, akathisia, parkinsonism, neuroleptic malignant syndrome, tardive dyskinesia, and chorea (see Chapter 17). Ocular dystonia in the form of oculogyric crisis has been also ascribed to amoxapine (Table 16–17) (58,117).

Pharmacokinetics

Amoxapine is rapidly absorbed and reaches peak blood concentrations within 1 to 2 hours after oral administration. Amoxapine is metabolized to 8- and 7-hydroxyamoxapine. The latter has significant dopamine receptor blocking activity. Amoxapine has a half-life of 8 hours, and its active metabolite has a half-life of 30 hours (101).

Although amoxapine has somewhat less antimuscarinic effect than other cyclic antidepressants, the clinical features of amoxapine poisoning are reported to be similar to those suggested for classical cyclic antidepressant overdose (118).

TABLE 16–17. *Side effects of blockade of dopamine (D2) receptors*

Extrapyramidal movement disorders
Dystonia
Akathisia
Parkinsonism
Neuroleptic malignant syndrome
Tardive dyskinesia
Oculogyric crisis
Endocrine changes
Sexual dysfunction (males)

Overdosage

Amoxapine poisoning has produced severe acidosis, cardiac dysrhythmias, heart block, hypotension, renal failure, coma, and cardiorespiratory arrest (Table 16–18) (101). Overdosage with large doses, is characterized primarily by central nervous system toxicity, including an extremely high incidence of treatment-resistant seizures, coma, hypotension, and respiratory depression (14,57–59,116). Many reports of cardiotoxicity of amoxapine include sinus tachycardia due to the agent's marked antimuscarinic effects. Conduction disturbances and arrhythmias are usually not noted because of amoxapine's lack of quinidine-like activity. In addition, a substantial number of cases of amoxapine overdose have been accompanied by acute renal failure, and some of these patients have required dialysis (119). The specific pathophysiologic cause of the acute renal failure is unclear, although the hypotension, rhabdomyolysis, and direct nephrotoxicity appear to be the most likely explanations. Because of conflicting reports concerning the

TABLE 16–18. *Toxicity of second-generation antidepressants*

Drug	Overdose symptoms
Amoxapine	Acute renal failure Cardiac dysrhythmias Cardiorespiratory arrest Coma Heart blocks Hypotension Metabolic acidosis Seizures Sinus tachycardia
Maprotiline	Seizures Metabolic acidosis Fewer cardiac effects than amoxapine
Trazodone	Drowsiness Hypotension Ataxia Priapism
SSUIs	Sinus tachycardia Nausea Vomiting Dizziness Tremor

cardiotoxic nature of amoxapine, no firm statement can be made regarding its cardiac toxicity.

Maprotiline

Maprotiline (Ludiomil), marketed in 1981, is the only tetracyclic antidepressant approved for clinical use in the United States and belongs to the class of anthracenes. The pharmacology of maprotiline is similar to that of the tricyclics in that it blocks the reuptake of norepinephrine at the neuronal membrane and has antimuscarinic activity (62). Maprotiline differs from the first-generation tricyclics in that it has little or no effect on the reuptake of serotonin or dopamine. Maprotiline does not inhibit monoamine oxidase (120).

Pharmacokinetics

Maprotiline is well absorbed following oral administration and has a biologic half-life of 43 hours (39). The drug is highly bound (88%) to serum proteins and has a volume of distribution of 23 L/kg. It is largely metabolized into its demethylated derivatives, which are later excreted into the urine and bile. Its extremely long half-life is of significance because toxic effects may be prolonged in overdosage and in elderly patients who may be slower to metabolize drugs.

Toxicity

Although initially there appeared to be fewer cardiotoxic effects noted with overdosage of maprotiline, high doses comparable to those commonly prescribed are likely to be associated with a cardiac risk similar to that of the first-generation tricyclics (57,58). More prominent CNS effects, including a greater incidence of seizures, have been associated with maprotiline. In addition, metabolic acidosis and hypokalemia have also been noted. Maprotiline-induced seizures may occur without previous history of seizure disorder, antimuscarinic symptoms, or cardiac conduction or rhythm disturbances (61). There have also been reports of seizures occurring during therapeutic use (60,62,116). The drug's relatively long half-life has been implicated as the possible cause of the increased incidence of seizures (120).

BICYCLIC ANTIDEPRESSANTS

Trazodone

Trazodone (Desyrel) is a bicyclic-type antidepressant. This drug exerts its antidepressant effect by interfering with serotonin reuptake and does not significantly interfere with the adrenergic nervous system. It is therefore relatively devoid of toxic cardiovascular effects.

Trazodone (Desyrel) is chemically and structurally unrelated to the tricyclic, tetracyclic, or other known antidepressant agents. It is the first triazolopyridine derivative, a new class of antidepressant (17,116).

Pharmacokinetics

Trazodone is rapidly and completely absorbed within the digestive tract after oral administration. Plasma concentrations reach their peak within 2 hours, and the half-life is 6 to 11 hours (39). It is extensively metabolized, and less than 1% of an oral dose is excreted unchanged.

Actions

Trazodone does not appear to influence the reuptake of dopamine or norepinephrine within the central nervous system; at the same time it has been shown to block selectively the reuptake of serotonin at the presynaptic neuronal membrane (57,58,62). It also has little clinical antimuscarinic activity. Desirable central therapeutic effects may therefore be obtained with doses too small to produce any cardiovascular effects. The efficacy of trazodone appears to be equal to that of the tricyclics, and there also appears to be a lower incidence of cardiotoxic effects, antimuscarinic effects, and lethal overdoses (121).

Side Effects

Although trazodone has little antimuscarinic effects, it will sometimes cause dry mouth and constipation by other mechanisms. CNS manifestations such as delirium and seizures have been reported (122–124). Priapism is a troublesome adverse reaction and may have an onset between 6 and 14 days after treatment at therapeutic doses. Although this side effect is relatively uncommon, patients should be warned to present themselves to an emergency room if a nonsexual erection should occur and persist for more than 1 hour. Surgery has been required in some of these cases.

Overdosage

Compared with other agents, overdosage with trazodone alone has been reported to be relatively benign (14,39,116,125). In an overdose its effects are comparable to those of the benzodiazepines. With the exception of drowsiness and minor antimuscarinic effects, trazodone overdoses have not been associated with significant toxicity. The primary manifestations are hypotension, central nervous system effects, and gastrointestinal effects. Like the tricyclics and phenothiazines, trazodone is a moderately potent α-adrenergic blocking agent, and hypotension may occur because of this action. Drowsiness, ataxia, nausea, vomiting, and dryness of the mouth may also be seen. CNS depression has been noted to progress to coma in some cases. Seizures, death, and the type of cardiovascular toxicity described for the other tricyclic agents are extremely rare (39,125).

THE SELECTIVE SEROTONIN UPTAKE INHIBITORS

The selective serotonin uptake inhibitors (SSUIs) block the uptake of serotonin (5 hydroxytryptamine, 5-HT) in the presynaptic cleft and have minimal affinity for other neurotransmitters. Currently there are three approved selective serotonin uptake inhibitors in the U.S., fluoxetine (Prozac), sertraline (Zoloft), and paroxetine (Paxil). There are few chemical structural similarities among these three agents. These agents minimally affect the uptake of dopamine and norepinephrine.

These agents are generally better tolerated than tricyclic antidepressants. They are not commonly associated with cardiac adverse effects. Psychomotor, sedative, and antimuscarinic adverse effects have been noted with the SSUIs but to a lesser degree when compared with tertiary TCAs.

Fluoxetine

Fluoxetine is a phenylpropylamine derivative, bicyclic antidepressant that differs structurally and chemically from currently available first-generation cyclic antidepressants, tetracyclic agents, and monoamine oxidase inhibitors. Since its introduction in 1988, fluoxetine has become the most frequently prescribed antidepressant in the U.S.

Actions

Fluoxetine is a selective serotonin uptake inhibitor. Receptor binding studies reveal fluoxetine displaying weak affinity for muscarinic, histaminic, opioid, dopaminergic, γ-aminobutyric acid, and benzodiazepine receptors. The low muscarinic potency explains the reduced antimuscarinic phenomena (126).

Pharmacokinetics

Fluoxetine is well absorbed from the GIT following oral administration and has bioavailability of at least 60% to 80%. Peak plasma concentrations occur within 6 to 12 hours after an oral dose.

Fluoxetine is primarily metabolized in the liver to norfluoxetine which also is a potent and selective serotonin reuptake blocker. Fluoxetine has a large V_d, and has extensive protein binding (126). The elimination half-life of fluoxetine averages 2 to 5 days, and that of norfluoxetine averages 8 to 14 days. The active metabolite retains selectivity for serotonin reuptake blockade (126).

Side Effects

Fluoxetine generally does not cause antimuscarinic effects such as dry mouth, dizziness, blurred vision, sedation, and weight gain, which are encountered commonly with cyclic antidepressants, yet adverse CNS and GI effects occur relatively frequently with fluoxetine therapy (127). Nausea appears to be the most common side effect, with most patients experiencing mild nausea early in treatment, with relief after several weeks. Nervousness, dizziness, insomnia, headache, tremor, fatigue, drowsiness, and anxiety have also been reported (126). The most common adverse effect related to the CNS is headache and tremor. Seizures, in patients with no prior history of seizure disorder, have been reported in patients taking fluoxetine. Akathisia, parkinsonian symptoms, and acute dystonic reactions have been described with fluoxetine (128). The drug is relatively safe in that it does not appear to cause significant clinical symptoms in doses 10 to 20 times therapeutic (Table 16–19) (127).

Fluoxetine has been implicated in an increased incidence of violent suicidal ideation. Although there is no conclusion to be made at this time, it would be prudent to admit and observe patients who admit to violent suicidal thoughts.

Sertraline

Sertraline is a selective inhibitor of serotonin reuptake, increasing concentrations of the neurotransmitter in the CNS. Sertraline does not bind to α- or β-adrenergic, dopaminergic, histaminic, or muscarinic cholinergic receptors (129).

TABLE 16–19. *Side effects of blockade of serotonin uptake*

Gastrointestinal disturbances
Nausea
Increase or decrease in anxiety (dose-dependent)
Nervousness
Dizziness
Tremor
Extrapyramidal side effects
Akathisia
Parkinsonian syndrome
Acute dystonia
Sexual dysfunction
Interaction with:
L-tryptophan
Monoamine oxidase inhibitors
Fenfluamine

Sertraline reaches maximum plasma concentrations between 5 and 8 hours after an oral dose. Sertraline is extensively metabolized in the liver, mainly to *N*-desmethylsertraline, which has little activity, and eliminated in urine and feces. It has an elimination half-life of 26 hours. Sertraline is 98% protein-bound, with a volume of distribution of approximately 20 L/kg.

Like fluoxetine, sertraline appears to stimulate the CNS, in contrast to the tricyclic antidepressants, which usually have a sedating effect. The most frequent adverse effects of sertraline have included headache, tremor, nausea, diarrhea, insomnia, agitation, and nervousness. Sertraline is slowly absorbed from the GIT and the maximum plasma concentration is higher if it is administered with food. The steady-state plasma concentration sertraline can be achieved after 1 week (129). Sertraline plasma clearance is 40% lower in elderly than in younger individuals. Because sertraline is metabolized in the liver, it should be used with caution in patients with severe renal impairment.

Paroxetine (Paxil)

The antidepressant action of paroxetine is linked to potentiation of serotonergic activity in the central nervous system resulting from inhibition of neuronal reuptake of serotonin and has only very weak effects on norepinephrine and dopamine neuronal reuptake. Paroxetine has little affinity for other receptors. Paroxetine also differs structurally from other selective serotonin-reuptake inhibitors.

Paroxetine has a volume of distribution of approximately 17 L/kg, and is 95% protein-bound. Its major route of elimination is via hepatic metabolism, with an elimination half-life of approximately 24 hours. Paroxetine has no clinically active metabolite.

No deaths were reported following the acute overdosage with paroxetine alone or in combination with other drugs and/or alcohol during premarketing clinical trials. Signs and symptoms of overdosage include nausea, vomiting, drowsiness, sinus tachycardia, and dilated pupils. There were no reports of ECG abnormalities, coma, or convulsions following overdosage with paroxetine alone.

Drug Interactions

There are a variety of drug interactions associated with the various antidepressants, including the monoamine oxidase (MAO) inhibitors. Some of these are noted in Table 16-20, and a more extensive list is presented in Chapter 7.

TABLE 16–20. *Drug interactions among antidepressants*

Antidepressant	Severity of interaction
MAOIs	Lethal with serotonin selective reuptake inhibitor
Classic TCA	Intermediate
Amoxapine	Intermediate
Maprotiline	Intermediate
Trazodone	Low
Bupropion	Low
Fluoxetine	Lethal with MAOIs
Sertraline	Lethal with MAOIs
Paroxetine	Lethal with MAOIs
Venlafaxine	Lethal with MAOIs

Overdosage of the Selective Serotonin Uptake Inhibitors

Fluoxetine appears to have a benign effect on the cardiovascular system (126). A large number of patients who overdose may not develop symptoms, although tachycardia, drowsiness, tremor, nausea, and vomiting have been noted (128). Although fluoxetine has a wide safety margin, the potential for lethality exists. The ingestion of fluoxetine at doses greater than 500 mg when combined with ethanol may result in tachycardia, hypertension, and a decreased level of consciousness (127).

There have been relatively few acute overdoses, especially of large amounts (128). Based on the available information, acute ingestion of 40 to 600 mg of fluoxetine is generally well tolerated and appears to produce symptoms that reflect extension of the drug's pharmacologic actions and adverse effects. In most of the patients who have ingested a maximum of 1.5 g, the clinical course has been relatively benign when ingested alone. However, isolated deaths from fluoxetine have been reported (127).

Patients who have ingested large amounts of SSUIs, or have clinical evidence of toxicity, or overdose with an SSUI in combination with alcohol or other drugs should be admitted to a monitored hospital unit for a minimum of 24 hours (128). Supportive care is the only indicated intervention for acute fluoxetine overdose (128).

TREATMENT OF ANTIDEPRESSANT OVERDOSE

The following discussion concerns the older TCAs and the second-generation compounds, because the toxicity profile of the SSUIs has been discussed and does not involve the serious cardiac and hemodynamic problems associated with the older antidepressants.

The older cyclic antidepressant overdoses are medical emergencies and should be treated accordingly. Advanced life support measures are critical to successful treatment outcomes and should be implemented as soon as possible because life-threatening cardiovascular and CNS events may develop in dramatic fashion (74,130).

All patients suspected of cyclic antidepressant overdose need to be aggressively and rapidly evaluated. A history of only a small quantity of pills ingested should not diminish one's level of concern in evaluating the patient because the degree of toxicity from the same dose of drug can vary greatly among individuals (47). Because cyclic antidepressants are rapidly absorbed, it is not unusual to observe rapid loss of consciousness and severe toxicity within 60 minutes (131).

Airway management should be aggressive and follow the same general guidelines for any toxic patient, but it is particularly important to assist ventilation in cyclic antidepressant overdose patients with altered levels of consciousness and elevated CO_2. A Foley catheter should be placed when toxicity is apparent to allow rapid assessment of urine output and to protect against antimuscarinic urinary retention. Rectal temperatures should be taken frequently to watch for the development of hyperthermia (54).

It is difficult to predict the severity of an acute intoxication on the basis of the amount of ingested drug. Therefore, as stated earlier, it is prudent to consider the ingestion of any quantity of these drugs potentially toxic and to treat it as such (Table 16–21). Good supportive care is essential. Several studies have shown that the toxicity of the tricyclics is exaggerated by factors that increase cardiac work; thus, efforts should be made to minimize conditions such as fluid overload, seizures, agitation, and extremes of blood pressure.

Patients are most at risk before or soon after admission to the hospital, when plasma concentrations of the drug are maximal. Most patients brought to the emergency department after tricyclic overdose who subsequently die do so within the first few hours (14,123). The rapid decline in plasma concentration indicates that, within 2 to 3 hours of the overdose, redistribution from plasma to tissues is exceeding absorption. Toxicity also diminishes during this time. Life-threatening complications in serious tricyclic overdose almost always develop within 2 hours of the patient's presentation to the emergency department (131).

TABLE 16–21. *Summary of treatment for tricyclic overdose*

Gastric lavage
Activated charcoal
Cathartic
Alkalinization Sodium bicarbonate, 0.5 to 2.0 mEq/kg
Respiratory alkalosis to pH 7.50 to 7.55
Phenytoin, 15–20 mg/kg IV (for ventricular dysrhythmias, conduction disturbances, or seizures)
Lidocaine, 1 mg/kg (for ventricular dysrhythmias)
β-Adrenergic blocking drugs (not recommended)
Bretylium (not recommended)
Calcium (not recommended)
Diazepam (for seizures)
Fluids (for hypotension)
Norepinephrine (for refractory hypotension)
Pacemaker (for refractory bradycardia or hypotension)

Prevention of Absorption

Any patient with a history of tricyclic overdose should be placed on a cardiac monitor with a patent intravenous line in place. Lavage should also be performed even late after an ingestion because of the decreased peristalsis and delayed absorption associated with antimuscarinics (21). If the patient is alert with an intact gag reflex and appears to be in no immediate danger of losing consciousness, gastric lavage can be performed (14). Rapid loss of consciousness is a hallmark finding in most cyclic antidepressant overdoses, and the potential for it to develop, in conjunction with the vagal effects associated with emesis, contraindicate the use of syrup of ipecac–induced emesis as a means of gastric emptying in cyclic antidepressant overdose (132).

Activated charcoal effectively binds tricyclics, and therefore 50 to 100 g of activated charcoal should be administered after adequate gastric emptying has been obtained (14). Because of the enterohepatic recirculation and gastric resecretion, the use of multiple-dose activated charcoal every 2 to 4 hours may be effective in adsorbing the material that is recirculated (7,23,133).

Continuous nasogastric suction has been advocated to remove any additional drug that is resecreted into the stomach; some studies have shown a removal of 5% to 15% of an ingested dose because of such resecretion. The clinical effectiveness of this method has still not been shown and it is therefore not recommended.

As mentioned earlier, respiratory depression or failure should be vigorously treated with intubation and mechanical ventilation because acidosis of any kind may precipitate fatal cardiac dysrhythmias (17).

Physostigmine

Considerable controversy has arisen over the years as to the use of physostigmine (Antilirium) (134). Many believe that there is essentially no justification for the use of physostigmine in the setting of cyclic antidepressant toxicity (27). Although physostigmine is not considered a first-line drug for any of the problems associated with the tricyclics, it has a theoretical role in the treatment of some of the tricyclic-associated disorders (52,53,135), yet its routine use in this overdose setting is discouraged.

Mechanism of Action

Physostigmine is a cholinergic drug that hydrolyzes the enzyme acetylcholinesterase, which is responsible for the metabolism of acetylcholine. It is considered a reversible carbamate acetylcholinesterase inhibitor. After an overdose of a tricyclic, the receptor is bound by the drug, so that when acetylcholine is released it cannot bind with the receptor. Physostigmine inhibits the acetylcholinesterase, thereby allowing more acetylcholine to be available and to displace competitively the antimuscarinic drug (136,137).

Other acetylcholinesterase inhibitors are available, including neostigmine (Prostigmin), pyridostigmine (Mestinon), and edrophonium (Tensilon). Although these compounds are successful in reversing the peripheral antimuscarinic effects of the tricyclics, they do not cross the blood–brain barrier because they are all quaternary ammonium-charged compounds. Physostigmine is a tertiary amine and can cross the blood–brain barrier to reverse both the peripheral and the central antimuscarinic effects (17).

Clinical Indications for Use

Physostigmine may be indicated in the diagnosis of antimuscarinic overdose and may be effective in reversing dysrhythmias that are the result of vagal blockade (138). Dysrhythmias that develop from the direct effect of the antidepressant action on the myocardium are probably not affected. Supraventricular dysrhythmias that are hemodynamically significant—seizures, myoclonus (especially when violent), hallucinations (when severe), and hypertension (when marked)—are all considered indications for the use of physostigmine (Table 16–22). Because the ventricles do not have significant cholinergic innervation, beneficial effects in treating ventricular dysrhythmias with physostigmine are not expected.

TABLE 16–22. *The use of physostigmine for tricyclic overdose*

Indications
Diagnostic
Therapeutic
Supraventricular dysrhythmias
Seizures
Myoclonus
Hallucinations
Hypertension
Dosage
Adult: 1 to 2 mg IV slowly
Child: 0.5 mg or 0.02 mg/kg IV slowly
Muscarinic side effects
Bradycardia
Miosis
Increased secretions
Urination
Defecation
Seizures
Cardiac side effects
Shift of pacemaker from sinoatrial node to another site
Slowing of conduction through atrioventricular node
Prolonged refractory period
Atrioventricular block
Asystole

Dosage

The dosage of physostigmine is 1 to 2 mg intravenously, administered slowly. In children, a dose of 0.5 mg or 0.02 mg/kg may be administered intravenously (139). Physostigmine has a short half-life; consequently it may reverse symptoms of tricyclic overdose for only 30 to 45 minutes (17). Because physostigmine is rapidly metabolized, the dose may need to be repeated.

Contraindications to Use

Relative contraindications to the use of physostigmine include asthma, gangrene, and mechanical obstruction of the gastrointestinal tract or genitourinary tract. Caution should be exercised because physostigmine can precipitate seizures when administered too rapidly or cause a cholinergic crisis consisting of bradycardia, miosis, increased secretions, urination, and defecation if given to a patient who has not ingested an antimuscarinic compound (Table 16–22) (140). Physostigmine may also have undesirable effects in a quinidine-like overdose because it can shift the pacemaker from the sinoatrial node to another atrial site, slow conduction through the atrioventricular node, prolong the refractory period, produce atrioventricular blocks, and cause asystole (Table 16–22) (140). Its use has therefore greatly diminished over the last few years, and it should not be considered a first-line drug. It has been suggested that physostigmine be administered to patients to make them alert enough that steps can be taken to induce vomiting. This is a potentially dangerous procedure because the duration of action of physostigmine is short and the patient may lose consciousness before or during vomiting. In addition, coma is not a life-threatening condition and often may be preferable in violent, uncontrollable patients who may harm themselves. Hence, coma alone should not be an indication for the use of physostigmine (91,92,141).

Physostigmine has not been shown to be very effective in treating widened QRS complexes and associated dysrhythmias; in fact, physostigmine may even induce sinus bradycardia, complete heart block, asystole, or hypotension (53).

Alkalinization

Alkalinization of the patient has long been advocated in Europe and Australia, and in the United States (142). The effectiveness of this therapy has been confirmed in both animals and humans (79,143–145). Similar therapy has been used to treat quinidine toxicity.

Clinical Indications

Administration of sodium bicarbonate parenterally to cause metabolic alkalosis, or induction of hyperventilation (142,143) to cause respiratory alkalosis has been shown to be effective for treating ventricular dysrhythmias, specifically ventricular tachycardia and fibrillation, as well as conduction disturbances and bundle branch blocks, seizures, and hypotension due to decreased cardiac contractility (Table 16–23) (14,79,146–148). Alkalinization may be useful regardless of whether blood pH is low or normal (27,79).

Dosage of Sodium Bicarbonate

Alkalinization of the patient to a blood pH of 7.50 to 7.55 is suggested as a first-line approach to treatment (148). The optimal dose of sodium bicarbonate has not been established, but roughly 0.5 to 2 mEq/kg intravenously is effective. If the patient is experiencing controlled respirations, hyperventilation may be induced instead (143–146,148). If sodium bicarbonate is used, the addition of potassium chloride (20 to 40 mEq/L) is useful in compensating for the potential fall in serum potassium that occurs with acute alkalinization. Whereas bicarbonate boluses are effective immediately, the efficacy of continuous bicarbonate maintenance infusions has been questioned, and to be effective large amounts of sodium and fluid must be given (27).

Mechanism of Action

The mechanism by which alkalinization is effective for the tricyclics is still unclear. The ability of sodium bicarbonate to reverse cardiac abnormalities appears to be related to both a direct effect of sodium and to the alkalosis produced by it (47). The increase in extracellular sodium ion appears to partially overcome sodium-channel blockade, counteracting the primary cause of altered conduction, but some investigators postulate that it is due to the increased protein binding that occurs in an alkaline environment, which reduces the amount of free or active drug (143–147).

TABLE 16–23. *Indications for alkalinization procedures*

Widened QRS interval
QRS > 0.10 sec
Ventricular dysrhythmias
Ventricular fibrillation
Ventricular tachycardia
Seizures
To correct acidemia
Hypotension
If due to membrane-stabilizing effect

Increasing plasma pH increases cyclic antidepressant protein binding, decreasing the amount of biologically active free drug. Because the amount of drug in the blood is small, the clinical significance of this effect is unclear. Possibly of more significance is that increases in pH have been shown to enhance the recovery of sodium channels blocked by cyclic antidepressants (149). It is thought that alkalinization alters the cyclic antidepressant ionization, which facilitates the drug's egress from the receptor site on the sodium channel (47). It may be that the effects of increasing the extracellular sodium concentration and of increasing the blood pH are distinct and additive actions and that both mechanisms operate (79,148).

Although the rationale for the use of sodium bicarbonate is still unclear, that alkalinization is effective is beyond question and its use is encouraged (149). Sodium bicarbonate appears to be more commonly used than hyperventilation for the production of alkalemia, but hyperventilation has an advantage in that it does not predispose the patient to the hazards of sodium overload, which may then make the patient more vulnerable to pulmonary edema (143).

Sodium bicarbonate reverses the cardiac manifestations regardless of heart rate or blood pH (79,148). It is usually effective immediately after administration, and, although its effects are not long lasting, repeated administration is usually effective. If the patient is intubated, ventilatory prophylaxis ensuring a slight respiratory alkalosis and hypocapnia may be sufficient (150). Although hyperventilation can be used to rapidly increase serum pH as a temporizing measure, this should be limited to allow the administration of as much sodium bicarbonate as can be safely tolerated by the patient. The prophylactic efficacy of alkalosis in patients who have ingested tricyclics but have no QRS prolongation or other signs of toxicity has not been well studied (21).

TREATMENT OF RHYTHM DISTURBANCES

Lidocaine

There is much debate concerning whether lidocaine or phenytoin is the best drug for the ventricular dysrhythmias associated with an overdose of tricyclics (151,152). Lidocaine can be useful in low to moderate doses because it has little effect on atrioventricular conduction (14,147). Care should be exercised when high doses are administered because lidocaine also has the ability to decrease atrioventricular conduction, cause sinoatrial nodal arrest, and, at times, seizures. Lidocaine can be administered relatively rapidly and can therefore control the dysrhythmias in a shorter period of time than phenytoin, which makes it highly recommended for quick control. Toxic doses of lidocaine should be avoided, because at very high concentrations Type Ib agents such as lidocaine can cause conduction abnormalities.

Phenytoin

The use of phenytoin is another reasonable form of therapy for tricyclic overdose because this drug has both antidysrhythmic and anticonvulsant activity, enhances atrioventricular and intraventricular conduction, and decreases ventricular automaticity (148,153,154). It is contraindicated in patients with severe bradycardia, second- and third-degree blocks, asystole, and ventricular fibrillation. The recommended dosage of phenytoin in an adult is 15 to 20 mg/kg (usually 1 g) intravenously, not exceeding 25 to 50 mg/min. This is the main drawback to the use of phenytoin: it may take 20 to 40 minutes to administer (Table 16–24). Phenytoin is not approved by the FDA for use as an antidysrhythmic agent, although such use is generally accepted.

β Blockers

The use of β-adrenergic blockers, although initially thought to be of benefit for the tachydysrhythmias, is not appropriate because these drugs decrease atrioventricular conduction and have some quinidine-like membrane effects (151). In animals, the β-adrenergic blockers have also been shown not to counteract the cardiac effects and electrocardiographic changes associated with the tricyclics. In addition, it is not wise to administer a drug that may precipitate or aggravate hypotension and cardiac failure induced by the ingested drug (151). Furthermore, using β-adrenergic blockers for treatment of tricyclic antidepressant toxicity may be hazardous because increased catecholamines may be necessary to counteract the depressant actions of tricyclics on the heart rate and contractility. Since severe catecholamine depletion and α-adrenergic blockage may exist, β blockade may further compromise an already incompetent sympathetic nervous system. If used, it should be with extreme caution. If the patient has high grade of atrioventricular block, evidence of depressed myocardial contractility, or asthma, propranolol is absolutely contraindicated (148).

TABLE 16–24. *Use of phenytoin for tricyclic overdose*

Actions
Enhances atrioventricular conduction
Enhances intraventricular conduction
Decreases ventricular automaticity
Contraindications
Severe bradycardia
Second- and third-degree blocks
Asystole
Ventricular fibrillation
Dosage
Adult: 1 g, not more than 25 to 50 mg/min
Child: 15 to 20 mg/kg over 20 to 30 minutes

Bretylium

Bretylium causes an initial release of norepinephrine from peripheral adrenergic nerve terminals, resulting in eventual adrenergic blockade and hypotension. This initial action is similar to the effects of the tricyclics, and because of this bretylium should not be used routinely. It should only be used for refractory ventricular fibrillation or tachycardia.

Calcium

Calcium, although generally not used for tricyclic overdose, has the theoretical benefit of increasing atrioventricular conduction, increasing intraventricular conduction, shortening the QT interval, and increasing contractility. Although calcium administration is not suggested, its usefulness should be kept in mind if all other agents have been tried without success.

TREATMENT OF SEIZURES

Seizures secondary to the tricyclics should be first treated with bicarbonate (Table 16–25).This is not so much an attempt to stop the seizure as to reverse the metabolic acidosis that will ensue. Diazepam should be administered to control the seizure. Intractable seizures are more often seen with amoxapine and maprotiline overdoses and may require the use of anticonvulsants other than diazepam. Paralysis and general anesthesia may be required for status epilepticus. If seizure prevention is necessary, phenytoin can be given in a loading dose. Physostigmine has also been reported to be effective for seizures secondary to antimuscarinic drugs,

TABLE 16–25. *Summary of treatment by symptoms and signs*

Bradydysrhythmias	Fluids Trendelenburg's position Atropine Pacemaker
Hypotension	Trendelenburg's position Fluid challenge Norepinephrine or dopamine Sodium bicarbonate
Sinus tachycardia	None unless markedly symptomatic
Torsade de pointes	Overdrive pacing
Ventricular dysrhythmias	Sodium bicarbonate Lidocaine or phenytoin
Widened QRS	Sodium bicarbonate

although as stated earlier this is not considered a first-line drug.

Seizures should be treated promptly to prevent acidemia because this condition may increase the amount of free drug. Therefore, concomitant with the use of diazepam, seizures due to tricyclic antidepressants should be vigorously treated with bicarbonate to correct the metabolic component of the acidosis.

TREATMENT OF HYPOTENSION

Blood pressure support may be required in view of the hypotensive effect of the tricyclics. Hypotension is a serious manifestation of tricyclic overdose and may be the harbinger of cardiac arrest (144). Fluids and bicarbonate should be administered (17). If there is no response to Trendelenburg's position or to bicarbonate and saline challenge of 10 to 20 mL/kg, pressor agents should be used. Because myocardial depression contributes to altered blood pressure, Swan-Ganz catheterization should be considered for refractory hypotension. This could then differentiate between vasodilation and myocardial depression.

Dopamine is often ineffective in the setting of hypotension secondary to cyclic overdose. The uptake of dopamine is presumably prevented by cyclic antidepressant-induced catecholamine uptake blockade, but perhaps more importantly, dopamine requires presynaptic norepinephrine for its largely indirect pressor activity. Because presynaptic norepinephrine stores are depleted after cyclic antidepressant poisoning, any indirect pressor, that is, one that acts by triggering the release of endogenous norepinephrine, would be ineffective (27).

Norepinephrine or phenylephrine–direct-acting sympathetic agents—rather than an indirectly acting agent (which may first have to be taken up by the cells before it will function)—should be administered. Drugs such as metaraminol, ephedrine, and dopamine may have attenuated effectiveness as pressor agents because the tricyclics block their reuptake into the adrenergic neuron. An exaggerated response may occur with norepinephrine; vasopressors should therefore be reserved for refractory hypotension, and low doses should be used initially because the effect of further sensitizing the myocardium may induce or worsen dysrhythmias.

The prolonged QTc interval produced can predispose to the development of torsade de pointes. This has been successfully treated with overdrive pacing in rare cases. Isoproterenol may also be effective against bradyarrhythmias and torsade de pointes, but it has the potential to exacerbate hypotension and should be used cautiously (17,148). Intravenous magnesium sulfate may also successfully abolish this dysrhythmia. Unlike isoproterenol, magnesium sulfate is not known to precipitate dysrhythmias and hypotension (49).

DELAYED TOXICITY

Tricyclic overdose is widely believed to be associated with late sudden cardiac dysrhythmias. Deaths from cardiac dysrhythmia have been reported to occur as long as 5 days after ingestion (151). Most patients who developed these late cardiac complications have had severe overdoses that previously required treatment. In addition, these cases did not occur after a 24-hour period of electrocardiographic normalization (118). Recent reports concerning delayed complications after tricyclic overdose do not support the development of delayed complications after a symptom-free period of 24 hours (1,2,16,55,155). Late complications do not appear to occur in properly treated patients who do not have obvious early evidence of toxicity (118). To date, there are no reports in the literature of delayed complications or fatalities in cyclic antidepressant overdose patients who were without major signs of toxicity, had normal bowel activity after 6 hours of observation, and were given appropriate initial treatment, including activated charcoal (156).

In the patient who is awake and alert after an acute overdose and who does not develop any clinical signs of tricyclic overdose after 6 hours, delayed dysrhythmias are unlikely (16). In the previously symptomatic patient, an observation period of 12 to 24 hours after recovery appears to be adequate (156).

Therapeutic Agents To Avoid

Type Ia agents and Type Ic agents slow phase 0 upslope and should be avoided (17,27). Forced diuresis is also contraindicated because excretion of the tricyclics is not enhanced with diuresis and because of the possibility of worsening the patient's condition through fluid overload (154,157). Although it is theoretically possible that acidification of the urine will enhance the excretion of the tricyclics, the increase in urine output is minimal and there is a possibility of increasing the risk from systemic tricyclic toxicity. Although dialysis and hemoperfusion have been reported to be effective (154,158–161), they should not be attempted because the volume of distribution is so large that there is no significant retrieval of material (17,33,158,162). Charcoal hemoperfusion binds almost all the drug passing through the device but is limited in usefulness because most of the ingested drug is located in the body tissue pool, not in the blood. The degree of protein binding also precludes a satisfactory removal of the drug (Table 16–26) (154).

SUMMARY OF EFFECTS, TREATMENT, AND RECOMMENDATIONS

Sinus tachycardia is a sensitive indicator of tricyclic antimuscarinic effect but an insensitive marker of the

TABLE 16–26. *Drugs and procedures contraindicated*

Class Ia antidysrhythmias
Quinidine
Procainamide
Disopyramide
Forced diuresis
Dialysis
Hemodialysis
Peritoneal dialysis
Hemoperfusion

development of serious toxicity. These dysrhythmias are due to the antimuscarinic effects of the tricyclics in conjunction with the blocking of the reuptake of norepinephrine. Unless they cause severe hemodynamic changes, they need not be treated (Table 16–16).

Although the sinus tachycardia that is frequently present, in general, requires no specific treatment, it has been shown that the effects of amitriptyline on conduction are rate-dependent. It is hypothesized that at higher heart rates, cyclic antidepressants are less able to leave sodium channels, resulting in a greater cumulative sodium-channel blockade. A slowing of the heart rate may result in decreased sodium-channel blockade and improvement in conduction. It should be kept in mind that sinus tachycardia with QRS prolongation may be difficult to distinguish from ventricular tachycardia. Supraventricular tachydysrhythmias, in contrast to sinus tachycardia, are relatively uncommon with tricyclic intoxication.

Ventricular tachydysrhythmias are caused by increased sympathetic activity in conjunction with the direct depressant quinidine-like action of the tricyclics. Sodium bicarbonate (0.5 to 2 mEq/kg) is suggested as a first-line drug to raise the arterial pH to 7.50 to 7.55 (148). Antidysrhythmic therapy should then be instituted with either lidocaine or phenytoin. Propranolol, quinidine, procainamide, disopyramide, and physostigmine should be avoided. What may appear to be ectopy may actually be intermittent aberrance due to depressed conduction.

Torsade de pointes can be treated with temporary overdrive pacing. It is not clear whether bicarbonate is effective for this condition. Bundle branch blocks are one of the more serious disturbances and occur because of the quinidine-like action of the tricyclics. Sodium bicarbonate (0.5 to 2 mEq/kg) or hyperventilation is suggested. Phenytoin may also be effective. Although QRS prolongation alone is not compromising, it is a marker for patients at highest risk of developing seizures, dysrhythmias, or hypotension.

Bradydysrhythmias are a result of the direct myocardial depressant quinidine-like effect of the tricyclics in conjunction with depletion of neurotransmitter at the myocardium and are difficult to treat. Sodium bicarbonate may be effective for this condition, but a temporary transvenous pacemaker may be lifesaving. Atropine is often unsuccessful in severe cases of cyclic antidepressant toxicity, as the muscarinic receptors are blocked. Although often unsuccessful, a temporary pacemaker should be considered for Mobitz II heart block and complete heart block. The finding of bradycardia, rather than tachycardia, usually indicates a later course or a massive overdose, unless the patient is taking a pharmacologic β-adrenergic blocking agent.

Hypotension occurs as a result of the direct depressant quinidine-like effect of tricyclics in conjunction with a depletion of neurotransmitter and the α-adrenergic blocking action of the tricyclics (94). Sodium bicarbonate (0.5 to 2 mEq/kg) or hyperventilation are recommended treatments in conjunction with fluid therapy. Care must be taken not to administer excessive amounts of fluids in these patients because depressed myocardial contractility makes them particularly susceptible to fluid overload and the development of heart failure and pulmonary edema.

Norepinephrine, a direct-acting sympathomimetic, is reserved for the refractory cases because an exaggerated response may ensue. An indirectly acting agent must enter the adrenergic neuron by the same uptake mechanism as the neurotransmitter, and consequently its uptake will be blocked by the tricyclic.

Generalized seizures have been associated with increased mortality in tricyclic overdose and have been noted immediately before cardiac arrest (103). Seizure may cause significant metabolic acidemia, thereby increasing unbound tricyclic in the circulation and contributing to the development of fatal dysrhythmias.

Asymptomatic Patients

In the asymptomatic individual, methods for prevention of absorption should be attempted (115). The patient should be placed on a cardiac monitor and observed for a period of at least 6 to 8 hours (16). If the patient remains completely asymptomatic, has no electrocardiographic changes, has a normal 12 lead electrocardiogram, and has been given psychiatric clearance, then he or she may be discharged (163). Patients demonstrating an isolated sinus tachycardia that resolves with volume repletion or time, and in whom no further signs of toxicity develop, can be medically cleared for psychiatric disposition (22). If an isolated sinus tachycardia does not resolve, the patient should be admitted (90).

The QRS interval must be weighed with the presence or absence of mental status changes, dysrhythmias, seizures, blood pressure stability, and other ECG changes in serial ECGs to determine whether toxicity is likely (49). This includes all patients with QRS prolongation, but also those without conduction defects if vital sign abnormalities, altered mental status, significant antimuscarinic symptoms, seizures, or other evidence of toxicity is evident (27).

Symptomatic Patients

For the symptomatic individual or in one with a widened QRS interval (indicating bundle branch block), admittance to the intensive care unit is recommended so that monitoring can be continued (115,163). After the patient is awake and alert and shows no evidence of cardiovascular symptoms, monitoring should be continued for 12 to 24 hours after apparent recovery (1,2, 22,54,155,163).

Future Treatment

The successful use of digoxin-specific Fab fragments for antidotal treatment of digoxin overdoses raises the possibility that cyclic antidepressant-specific Fab may be effective in the treatment of cyclic antidepressant overdose.

Fab are antigen-specific peptides prepared by papain digestion of IgG. Both digoxin-specific and phencyclidine-specific Fab have been shown to significantly alter the pharmacokinetics of the respective drug studied and to decrease the amount of drug available for tissue toxicity (164). In the future, monoclonal antibodies directed against a specific cyclic antidepressant may provide reversal of toxicity (19,47).

REFERENCES

1. Goldberg R, Capone R: Cardiac complications following tricyclic antidepressant overdose. *JAMA* 1985;254:1772–1775.
2. Goldberg M, Park G, Spector R, et al: Lack of effect of oral activated charcoal on imipramine clearance. *Clin Pharmacol Ther* 1985;38:350–353.
3. Sullivan J, Rumack B, Peterson R: Management of tricyclic antidepressant toxicity, *Top Emerg Med* 1979;1:65–71.
4. Watson W, Leighton J, Guy J, et al: Recovery of cyclic antidepressants with gastric lavage. *J Emerg Med* 1989;7:373–377.
5. Hollister L: Tricyclic antidepressants. *N Engl J Med* 1978; 299:1106–1109.
6. Hollister L: Monitoring tricyclic antidepressant concentration. *JAMA* 1979;241:2530–2533.
7. Hollister L: Doxepin hydrochloride. *Ann Intern Med* 1974;81:360–363.
8. Hong W, Mauer P, Hochman R, et al: Amitriptyline cardiotoxicity. *Chest* 1974;66:304–306.
9. Moir D, Cornwell W, Dingwall-Fordyce I, et al: Cardiotoxicity of amitriptyline. *Lancet* 1972;2:561–564.
10. Janson P, Watt J, Hermos J: Doxepin overdose. *JAMA* 1977; 237;2632–2633.
11. Stinnett J, Valentine J, Abrutyn E: Nortriptyline hydrochloride overdosage. *JAMA* 1968;204:69–71.
12. Biggs J: Clinical pharmacology and toxicology of antidepressants. *Hosp Pract* 1978;13:79–84.
13. Biggs J, Spiker D, Petit J, et al: Tricyclic antidepressant overdose. *JAMA* 1977;238:135–138.
14. Fromer D, Kulig K, Rumack B: Tricyclic antidepressant overdose: a review. *JAMA* 1987;257:521–526.
15. Yang K, Dantzker D: Reversible brain death. A manifestation of amitriptyline overdose.*Chest* 1991;99:1937–1038.
16. Boehnert M, Lovejoy F: Value of the QRS duration versus the serum drug level in predicting seizures and ventricular arrhythmias after an acute overdose of tricyclic antidepressants. *N Engl J Med* 1985; 313:474–479.
17. Braden N, Jackson J, Watson P: Tricyclic antidepressant overdose. *Pediatr Clin North Am* 1986;33:287–297.
18. Bramble M, Lishman A, Diffey B: An analysis of plasma levels and 24-hour ECG recordings in tricyclic antidepressant poisoning: implications for management. *Q J Med* 1985;56:357–366.
19. Shannon M, Lovejoy F: Pulmonary consequences of severe tricyclic antidepressant ingestion. *J Toxicol Clin Toxicol* 1987;25:443–461.
20. Callaham M: Tricyclic antidepressant overdose. *JACEP* 1979; 8:413–425.
21. Callaham M: Antidepressant toxicity. *Ann Emerg Med* 1986;15:1036–1038.
22. Callaham M: Admission criteria for tricyclic antidepressant ingestion. *West J Med* 1982;137:425–429.
23. Manoguerra A: Tricyclic antidepressants. *Crit Care Quart* 1982;4:43–54.
24. Manoguerra A, Weaver L: Poisoning with tricyclic antidepressant drugs. *Clin Toxicol* 1977;10:149–158.
25. Petit J, Spiker D, Ruwitch J, et al: Tricyclic antidepressant plasma levels and adverse effects after overdose. *Clin Pharmacol Ther* 1976;21:47–51.
26. Fauman M: Tricyclic antidepressant prescription by general hospital physicians. *Am J Psychiatry* 1980;137:490–491.
27. Smilkstein M: Reviewing cyclic antidepressant cardiotoxicity: wheat and chaff. *J Emerg Med* 1990;8:645–648.
28. Herson V, Schmitt B, Rumack B: Magical thinking and imipramine poisoning in two school-aged children. *JAMA* 1979;241:1926–1927.
29. Hayes T, Panitch M, Barker E: Imipramine dosage in children: a comment on "Imipramine and Electrocardiographic Abnormalities in Hyperactive Children." *Am J Psychiatry* 1975;132:546–547.
30. Saraf K, Gittelman-Klein R, Groff S: Imipramine side effects in children. *Psychopharmacologia* 1974;37:265–274.
31. Cram L, Reisby N, Ibsen I, et al: Plasma levels and antidepressive effect of imipramine. *Clin Pharmacol Ther* 1975;19:318–324.
32. Greenblatt D, Koch-Weser J, Shader R: Multiple complications and death following protriptyline overdose. *JAMA* 1974;229:556–557.
33. Crome P, Hampel G, Vale J, et al: Hemoperfusion in treatment of drug intoxication. *Br Med J* 1978;1:174–178.
34. Crome P, Newman B: The problem of tricyclic antidepressant poisoning. *Postgrad Med J* 1979;55:528–532.
35. Crome P, Newman B: Fatal tricyclic antidepressant poisoning. *J R Soc Med* 1979;72:649–653.
36. Crome P, Ali C: Clinical features and management of self-poisoning with newer antidepressants. *Med Toxicol* 1986;1:411–420.
37. Crome P: Poisoning due to tricyclic antidepressant overdosage: clinical presentation and treatment. *Med Toxicol* 1986;1:261–285.
38. Burks J, Walker J, Rumack B, et al: Tricyclic antidepressant poisoning. *JAMA* 1974;230:1405–1407.
39. Coccaro E, Siever L: Second generation antidepressants: a comparative review. *J Clin Pharmacol* 1985;25:241–260.
40. Montgomery S: Development of new treatments for depression. *J Clin Psychiatry* 1985;46:3–6.
41. Hulten B, Heath A, Knudsen K, et al: Amitriptyline and amitriptyline metabolites in blood and cerebrospinal fluid following human overdose. *J Toxicol Clin Toxicol* 1992;30:181–201.
42. Gram L: Metabolism of tricyclic antidepressants. *Dan Med Bull* 1974;21:218–231.
43. Gram L: Factors influencing the metabolism of tricyclic antidepressants. *Dan Med Bull* 1977;24:81–88.
44. Gram L, Reisby N, Ibsen I, et al: Plasma levels and antidepressive effect of imipramine. *Clin Pharmacol Ther* 1976;19:318–324.
45. Christiansen J, Gram L: Imipramine and its metabolites in human brain. *J Pharm Pharmacol* 1973;25:604–608.
46. Amsterdam J, Brunswick D, Mednels J: The clinical application of tricyclic antidepressant pharmacokinetics and plasma levels. *Am J Psychiatry* 1980;137:653–662.
47. Krishel S, Jackimczyk K: Cyclic antidepressants, lithium, and neuroleptic agents. *Emerg Clin North Am* 1991;9:53–86.
48. Moody J: Some aspects of the metabolism of tricyclic antidepressants. *Postgrad Med J* 1976;52:59–61.
49. Groleau G, Jotte R, Barish R: The electrocardiographic manifestations of cyclic antidepressant therapy and overdose: a review. *J Emerg Med* 1990;8;597–605.
50. Knapp H, Hanenson I, Walle T, et al: Studies on the disposition of amitriptyline and other tricyclic antidepressant drugs in man as it relates to the management of the overdosed patient. *Adv Biochem*

Psychopharmacol 1973;7:95–105.

51. Richelson E: Tricyclic antidepressants—drugs for other diseases. *Arch Intern Med* 1982;142:231–232.
52. Bigger J, Giardina E, Kantor S, et al: Cardiac antiarrhythmic effects of imipramine hydrochloride. *N Engl J Med* 1977;296:206–208.
53. Bigger J, Kantor S, Glassman A, et al: Is physostigmine effective for cardiac toxicity of tricyclic antidepressant drugs? *JAMA* 1977;237:1311.
54. Pentel P, Benowitz N: Tricyclic antidepressant poisoning: management of arrhythmias. *Med Toxicol* 1986;1:101–121.
55. Pentel P, Sioris L: Incidence of late arrhythmias following tricyclic overdose. *Clin Toxicol* 1981;18:543–548.
56. Glassman A: Bigger J: Cardiovascular effects of therapeutic doses of tricyclic antidepressants—a review. *Arch Gen Psychiatr* 1981;38: 815–820.
57. Nitter L, Haraldsson A, Holck P, et al: The effect of trimipramine on the healing of peptic ulcer: a double-blind study. *Scand J Gastroenterol* 1977;12:39–41.
58. Wetterhus S, Aubert E, Berg C, et al: The effect of trimipramine on symptoms and healing of peptic ulcer: a double-blind study. *Scand J Gastroenterol* 1977;12:33–38.
59. Mangla J, Pereira M: Tricyclic antidepressants in the treatment of peptic ulcer disease. *Arch Intern Med* 1982;142:273–275.
60. Siomopoulos V, Seneczko L: Heterocyclic antidepressants in nonpsychiatric disorders. *Am Fam Pract* 1984;29:203–208.
61. Winsberg B, Goldstein S, Yepes L, et al: Imipramine and electrocardiographic abnormalities in hyperactive children. *Am J Psychiatry* 1975;132:542–545.
62. Rudorfer M, Golden R, Potter W: Second-generation antidepressants. *Psychiatr Clin North Am* 1984;7:519–534.
63. Alexander C, Nino A: Cardiovascular complications in young patients taking psychotropic drugs. *Am Heart J* 1969;78:757–769.
64. Stewart R: Tricyclic antidepressant poisoning. *Am Fam Physician* 1979;19:136–144.
65. Ostrow D: The new generation antidepressants: promising innovations or disappointments? *J Clin Psychiatry* 1985;46:25–30.
66. Abbott R: Hyponatremia due to antidepressant medications. *Ann Emerg Med* 1983;12:708–710.
67. Veith R, Raskind M, Caldwell J, et al: Cardiovascular effects of tricyclic antidepressants in depressed patients with chronic heart disease. *N Engl J Med* 1982;306:954–959.
68. Stern S, Mendels J: Withdrawal symptoms during the course of imipramine therapy. *J Clin Psychiatry* 1980;41:66–67.
69. Sathananthan G, Gershon S: Imipramine withdrawal: an akathisia-like syndrome. *Am J Psychiatry* 1973;130:1286–1287.
70. Hulten B, Heath A, Knudsen K, et al: Severe amitriptyline overdose: relationship between toxicokinetics and toxicodynamics. *J Toxicol Clin Toxicol* 1992;30:171–179.
71. Mayron R, Ruiz E: Phenytoin: does it reverse tricyclic antidepressant-induced cardiac conduction abnormalities? *Ann Emerg Med* 1986;15:876–880.
72. McAlpine S, Calabro J, Robinson M, et al: Late death in tricyclic antidepressant overdose revisited. *Ann Emerg Med* 1986;15:1349–1352.
73. Henry J, Volans G: Psychoactive drugs. *Br Med J* 1984; 289:1291–1294.
74. Steel C, O'Duffy J, Brown S: Clinical effects and treatment of imipramine and amitriptyline poisoning in children. *Br Med J* 1967;3:663–667.
75. Noble J, Matthew H: Acute poisoning by tricyclic antidepressants: clinical features and management of one hundred patients. *Clin Toxicol* 1969;2:403–421.
76. Spiker D, Wiess A, Chang S, et al: Tricyclic antidepressant overdose: clinical presentation and plasma levels. *Clin Pharmacol Ther* 1975;18:539–546.
77. Spiker D, Biggs J: Tricyclic antidepressants. *JAMA* 1976;236: 1711–1712.
78. Flomenbaum N, Price D: Recognition and management of antidepressant overdoses: tricyclics and trazodone. *Neuropsychobiology* 1986;15:46–51.
79. Sasyniuk B, Jharmandas V, Valois M: Experimental amitriptyline intoxication: treatment of cardiac toxicity with sodium bicarbonate. *Ann Emerg Med* 1986;15:1052–1059.
80. Vohra J, Burrows G, Sloman G: Assessment of cardiovascular side effects of therapeutic doses of tricyclic antidepressant drugs. *Aust N Z J Med* 1975;5:7–11.
81. Vohra J, Burrows G, Hunt D, et al: The effect of toxic and therapeutic drugs on intracardiac conduction. *Eur J Cardiol* 1975;3: 219–227.
82. Michelson E, Freifus L: Newer antiarrhythmic drugs. *Med Clin North Am* 1988;72:275–319.
83. Tobis J, Aronow W: Effect of amitriptyline antidotes on repetitive extrasystole threshold. *Clin Pharmacol Ther* 1980;27:6026.
84. Tobis J, Das B: Cardiac complications in amitriptyline poisoning. *JAMA* 1976;235:1474–1476.
85. Kantor S, Bigger J, Glassman A, et al: Imipramine-induced heart block: a longitudinal case study. *JAMA* 1975;231:1364–1366.
86. Shannon M: Duration of QRS disturbances after severe tricyclic antidepressant intoxication. *J Toxicol Clin Toxicol* 1992;30:377–386.
87. Emermon C, Connors A, Burma G: Level of consciousness as a predictor of complications following tricyclic overdose. *Ann Emerg Med* 1987;16:326–330.
88. Caravati E, Bossart P: Demographic and electrocardiographic factors associated with severe tricyclic antidepressant toxicity. *J Toxicol Clin Toxicol* 1991;29:31–43.
89. Wolfe T, Caravati E, Rollins D: Terminal 40-ms frontal plane QRS axis as a marker for tricyclic antidepressant overdose. *Ann Emerg Med* 1989;18:348–351.
90. Tokarski G, Young M: Criteria for admitting patients with tricyclic antidepressant overdose. *J Emerg Med* 1988;6:121–124.
91. Rumack B: Anticholinergic poisoning: treatment with physostigmine. *Pediatrics* 1973;52:449–451.
2. Rumack B: Physostigmine use in drug overdose questioned. *JACEP* 1975;4:555–556.
93. Raisfeld I: Cardiovascular complications of antidepressant therapy: interactions at the adrenergic neuron. *Am Heart J* 1972;83:129–133.
94. Shannon M, Merola J, Lovejoy F: Hypotension in severe tricyclic antidepressant overdose. *Am J Emerg Med* 1988;6:439–442.
95. Langou R, Van Dyke C, Tahan S, et al: Cardiovascular manifestations of tricyclic antidepressant overdose. *Am Heart J* 1980; 100:458–464.
96. Dumovic P, Burrows G, Vohra J, et al: The effect of tricyclic antidepressant drugs on the heart. *Arch Toxicol* 1976;35;255–262.
97. Gaultier M, Boissier J, Barceix A, et al: The cardiotoxicity of imipramine in man. *Eur Soc Study Drug Toxicol* 1965;6:174–178.
98. Marshall A, Moore K: Pulmonary disease after amitriptyline overdosage. *Br Med J* 1973;1:716–717.
99. Marshall J, Forker A: Tricyclic antidepressant overdose: clinical and cardiovascular features. *Nebr Med J* 1980;65:77–80.
100. Robinson D, Barker E: Tricyclic antidepressant cardiotoxicity. *JAMA* 1976;236:2089–2090.
101. Miles M, Grenwood R, Hussy B: Diagnostic pitfalls associated with amoxapine overdose: a case report. *Am J Emerg Med* 1990;8:335–337.
102. Ellison D, Pentel P: Clinical features and consequences of seizures due to cyclic antidepressant overdose. *Am J Emerg Med* 1989;7:5–10.
103. Roy T, Ossoria M, Cipolla L, et al: Pulmonary complications after tricyclic antidepressant overdose. *Chest* 1989;96:852–856.
104. Varnall R, Godwin J, Richardson M, et al: Adult respiratory distress syndrome from overdose of tricyclic antidepressants. *Radiology* 1989;170:667–670.
105. Foulke G, Albertson T: QRS interval in tricyclic antidepressant overdosage: inaccuracy as a toxicity indicator in emergency settings. *Ann Emerg Med* 1987;16:160–163.
106. Poklis A, Soghoian D, Crooks C, et al: Evaluation of the Abbott ADx total serum tricyclic immunoassay. *J Toxicol Clin Toxicol* 1990;28:235–248.
107. Asberg M: Plasma nortriptyline levels—relationship to clinical effects. *Clin Pharmacol Ther* 1974;16:215–229.
108. Hackett L, Dusci L: The use of high-performance liquid chromatography in clinical toxicology: tricyclic antidepressants. *Clin Toxicol* 1979;15:55–61.
109. DeVane C: Monitoring cyclic antidepressants. *Clin Lab Med* 1987;7:551–566.
110. Rossi G: Pharmacology of tricyclic antidepressants. *Am J Pharmacol* 1976;148:37–45.
111. Rudorfer M: Tricyclic antidepressant plasma levels in overdose. *JAMA* 1981;245:703–704.
112. Jatlow P: Therapeutic monitoring of plasma concentrations of tricyclic antidepressants. *Arch Pathol Lab Med* 1980;104:341–344.
113. Lavoie F, Gansert G, Weiss R: Value of initial ECG findings and

plasma drug levels in cyclic antidepressant overdose. *Ann Emerg Med* 1990;19:696–700.
114. Hulten B, Adams R, Askenasi R, et al: Predicting severity of tricyclic antidepressant overdose. *J Toxicol Clin Toxicol* 1992;30:161–170.
115. Munger M, Effron B: Amoxapine cardiotoxicity. *Ann Emerg Med* 1988;17:274–278.
116. Wedin G, Oderda G, Klein-Schwartz W, et al: Relative toxicity of cyclic antidepressants. *Ann Emerg Med* 1986;15:797–804.
117. Nosko M, McLean D, Chin W: Loss of brainstem and pupillary reflexes in amoxapine overdose: a case report. *J Toxicol Clin Toxicol* 1988;26:117–122
118. Merigian K, Hedges J, Kaplan L, et al: Plasma catecholamine levels in cyclic antidepressant overdose. *J Toxicol Clin Toxicol* 1991;29:177–190.
119. Miles M, Grenwood R, Hussy B: Diagnostic pitfalls associated with amoxapine overdose: a case report. *Am J Emerg Med* 1990;8:335–337.
120. Peverini R, Ashwal S, Petry E: Maprotiline poisoning in a child. *Am J Emerg Med* 1988;6:247–249.
121. Larkin G, Graeber G, Hollingsed M: Experimental amitriptyline poisoning: treatment of severe cardiovascular toxicity with cardiopulmonary bypass. *Ann Emerg Med* 1994;23:480–486.
122. Kulig K, Rumack B, Sullivan J, et al: Amoxapine overdose—coma and seizures without cardiotoxic effects. *JAMA* 1982;248:1092–1094.
123. Kulig K: Management of poisoning associated with "newer" antidepressant agents. *Ann Emerg Med* 1986;15:1039–1045.
124. Lesar T, Kingston R, Dahms R, et al: Trazodone overdose. *Ann Emerg Med* 1983;12:221–223.
125. Ali C, Henry J: Trazodone overdosage: experience over 5 years. *Neuropsychobiology* 1986;15:11–15.
126. Pary R, Tobias C, Lippmann S: Fluoxetine: prescribing guidelines for the newest antidepressant. *South Med J* 1989;82:1005–1009.
127. Borys D, Setzer S, Ling L, et al: The effects of fluoxetine in the overdose patient. *J Toxicol Clin Toxicol* 1990;28:331–340.
128. Borys D, Setzer S, Ling L, et al: Acute fluoxetine overdose: a report of 234 cases. Am *J Emerg Med* 1992;10:115–120.
129. Kaminski C, Robbins M, Weibley R: Sertraline intoxication in a child. *Ann Emerg Med* 1994;23:1371–1374.
130. Starkey I, Lawson A: Poisoning with tricyclic and related antidepressants—a ten-year review. *Q J Med* 1980;49:33–49.
131. Banahan B, Schelkum P: Tricyclic antidepressant overdose: conservative management in a community hospital with cost-saving implications. *J Emerg Med* 1990;8:451–454.
132. Rinder H, Murphy J, Higgins G: Impact of unusual gastrointestinal problems on the treatment of tricyclic antidepressant overdose. *Ann Emerg Med* 1988;17:1079–1081.
133. Gard H, Knapp D, Walla T, et al: Qualitative and quantitative studies on the disposition of amitriptyline and other tricyclic antidepressants in man as it relates to the management of the overdosed patient. *Clin Toxicol* 1973;6:571–584.
134. Granscher R, Baldessarini R: Physostigmine. *Arch Gen Psychiatry* 1975;32:375–379.
135. Slovis T, Ott J, Teitelbaum D, et al: Physostigmine therapy in acute tricyclic antidepressant poisoning. *Clin Toxicol* 1971;4:451–459.
136. Brashares Z, Conley W: Physostigmine in drug overdose. *JACEP* 1975;4:46–48.
137. Lum B, Follmer C, Lockwood R, et al: Experimental studies on the effects of physostigmine and of isoproterenol on toxicity produced by tricyclic antidepressant agents. *J Toxicol Clin Toxicol* 1982;19: 51–65.
138. Goldberger A, Curtis G: Immediate effects of physostigmine on amitriptyline-induced QRS prolongation. *J Toxicol Clin Toxicol* 1982;19:445–454.
139. Spoerke D, Hall A, Dodson C, et al: Mystery root ingestion. *J Emerg Med* 1987;5:385–388.
140. Pentel P, Peterson C: Asystole complicating physostigmine treatment of tricyclic antidepressant overdose. *Ann Emerg Med* 1980;9: 588–590,
141. Bessen H, Niemann J: Improvement of cardiac conduction after hyperventilation in tricyclic antidepressant overdose. *Clin Toxicol* 1986;23:537–546.
142. Nattel S: Physostigmine in coma due to drug overdose. *Clin Pharmacol Ther* 1979;25:96–102.
143. Kingston M: Hyperventilation in tricyclic antidepressant poisoning. *Crit Care Med* 1979;7:550–551.
144. Brown T, Leversha A: Comparison of the cardiovascular toxicity of three tricyclic antidepressant drugs: imipramine, amitriptyline, and doxepin. *Clin Toxicol* 1979;14:253–256.
145. Brown T, Barker G, Dunlop M, et al: The use of sodium bicarbonate in the treatment of tricyclic antidepressant-induced arrhythmias. *Anaesth Intensive Care* 1973;14:203–210.
146. Hoffman J, McElroy C: Bicarbonate therapy for dysrhythmia and hypotension in tricyclic antidepressant overdose. *West J Med* 1981;134:60–64.
147. Hedges J, Baker P, Tasset J, et al: Bicarbonate therapy for the cardiovascular toxicity of amitriptyline in an animal model. *J Emerg Med* 1985;3:253–260.
148. Pentel P, Benowitz N: Efficacy and mechanism of action of sodium bicarbonate in the treatment of desipramine toxicity in rats. *J Pharmacol Exp Ther* 1984;230:12–19.
149. Hoffman J, Votey S, Bayer M, et al: Effect of hypertonic sodium bicarbonate in the treatment of moderate-to-severe cyclic antidepressant overdose. *Am J Emerg Med* 1993:11:336–341.
150. Slovis C, Murray L, Segar D: Emergency management of cyclic antidepressant overdose: an effective and organized approach. *Emerg Med Rep* 1993;14:115–124.
151. Freeman J, Loughhead M: β Blockade in the treatment of tricyclic antidepressant overdosage. *Med J Aust* 1973;1:1233–1235.
152. Freeman J, Mundy G, Beattie R, et al: Cardiac abnormalities in poisoning with tricyclic antidepressants. *Br Med J* 1969;2:610–611.
153. Uhl J: Phenytoin: the drug of choice in tricyclic antidepressant overdose? *Ann Emerg Med* 1981;10:270–274.
154. Hagerman G, Hanashiro P: Reversal of tricyclic antidepressant-induced cardiac conduction abnormalities by phenytoin. *Ann Emerg Med* 1981;10:82–86.
155. Greenland P, Howe T: Cardiac monitoring in tricyclic antidepressant overdose. *Heart Lung* 1981;10: 856–859.
156. Fasoli R, Glauser F: Cardiac arrhythmias and ECG abnormalities in tricyclic antidepressant overdose. *Clin Toxicol* 1981;18:155–163.
157. Harthorne W, Marcus A, Kaye M: Management of massive imipramine overdosage with mannitol and artificial dialysis. *N Engl J Med* 1963;268:33–36.
158. Baake O, Iversen B, Willassen Y: Charcoal hemoperfusion in nortriptyline poisoning. *Lancet* 1978;1:388–389.
159. Diaz-Buxo J, Farmer C, Chandler J: Hemoperfusion in the treatment of amitriptyline intoxication. *Trans Am Soc Artif Intern Organs* 1978;24:699.
160. Marbury T, Mahoney J, Fuller L, et al: Treatment of amitriptyline overdose with charcoal hemoperfusion. *Kidney Int* 1977;12:458–461.
161. Pederson R, JorgensonOelsen A, et al: Charcoal hemoperfusion and antidepressant overdose. *Lancet* 1978;1:719–722.
162. Pentel P, Bullock M, Devane C: Hemoperfusion for imipramine overdose: elimination of active metabolites. *J Toxicol Clin Toxicol* 1982;19:239–248.
163. Tokarski G, Young M: Criteria for admitting patients with tricyclic antidepressant overdose. *J Emerg Med* 1988;6:121–124.
164. Hursting M, Opheim K, Raisys V, et al: Tricyclic antidepressant specific Fab fragments alter the distribution and elimination of desipramine in the rabbit: a model for overdose treatment. *J Toxicol Clin Toxicol* 1989;27:53–66.

ADDITIONAL SELECTED REFERENCES

Boakes A, Laurence D, Teoh P, et al: Interactions between sympathomimetic amines and antidepressant agents in man. *Br Med J* 1973;1:311–315.
Cain N, Cain R: A compendium of antidepressants. *Clin Toxicol* 1979; 14:545–574.
Collis M, Shepherd J: Antidepressant drug action and presynaptic α receptors, *Mayo Clin Proc* 1980;55:567–572.
Crocker J, Morton B: Tricyclic antidepressant drug toxicity. *Clin Toxicol* 1969;2:397–402.
Desautels S, Filteau C, St Jean A: Ventricular tachycardia associated with administration of thioridazine hydrochloride. *Can Med Assoc J* 1964;99:1030–1031.
El-Hage A, Balazs T, West W: Protective effects of clonidine and verapamil in experimental amitriptyline poisoning in rabbits. *J Toxicol Clin Toxicol* 1982;19:321–335.

Goldfrank L, Flomenbaum N, Lewin N: Anticholinergic poisoning. *J Toxicol Clin Toxicol* 1982;19:17–25.

Goldfrank L, Melinek M: Locoweed and other anticholinergics. *Hosp Physician* 1979;8:18–26,39.

Hudson C: Tricyclic antidepressants and alcoholic blackouts. *J Nerv Ment Dis* 1981;169:381–382.

Hussey H: Physostigmine: value in treatment of central toxic effects of anticholinergic drugs. *JAMA* 1975;231:1066.

Kleber H, Weissman M, Rounsaville B, et al: Imipramine as treatment for depression in addicts. *Arch Gen Psychiatry* 1983;40:649–653.

Lepor S: Antidepressant drug overdose. *Emergency* 1983;15:36–39.

Lindstroem F, Flodmark O, Gustafsson B: Respiratory distress syndrome and thrombotic, nonbacterial endocarditis after amitriptyline overdose. *Acta Med Scand* 1977;202:203–212.

Lundberg G: Antidepressant drugs as a cause of death: a call for caution and data. *JAMA* 1982;248:1879.

Meador-Woodruff J, Grunhaus L: Profound behavioral toxicity due to tricyclic antidepressants. *J Nerv Ment Dis* 1986;174:628–629.

Smith R, O'Mara K: Tricyclic antidepressant overdose. *J Fam Pract* 1982;15:247–253.

Thompson T, Cardoni A: Tricyclic antidepressant overdose: case report and review of the literature. *Poison Inf Bull* 1977;2:1–9.

Thorstrand C: Cardiovascular effects of poisoning with tricyclic antidepressants. *Acta Med Scand* 1974;195:505–514.

Uhlenhuth E: Depressives, donors, and antidepressants. *JAMA* 1982;248:1879–1880.

Woodhead R: Cardiac rhythm in tricyclic antidepressant poisoning. *Clin Toxicol* 1979;14:499–505.

CHAPTER 17

Neuroleptic–Antipsychotic Agents

The introduction of antipsychotic agents in 1954 revolutionized the treatment of psychosis (1). The use of antipsychotic agents has provided for rapid treatment and rehabilitation of many patients who formerly would have been hospitalized for long periods and suffered prolonged or lifelong difficulty (2).

Of all the psychotropic drugs, the neuroleptic agents are the most important in psychiatry. Major chemical classes of neuroleptic agents are the phenothiazines, butyrophenones, and thioxanthenes, and there are miscellaneous agents such as loxapine, molindone, and clozapine (3). The phenothiazines evolved from the aniline dyes and antihistamines, and the butyrophenones evolved from the meperidine-like analgesics. These agents are used primarily to treat psychotic disorders in adults and children. They are called neuroleptic agents because of their ability to cause a change in affect, with emotional quieting, psychomotor slowing, disinterest in surroundings, and decreased aggression and impulsivity. These drugs have a marked effect on thought disturbances associated with paranoid ideation, delusions, anxiety, and agitation (4). These drugs do not merely sedate or calm patients, they exert a selective antischizophrenic action.

CLINICAL USES

Neuroleptic agents are widely used in various settings, including treatment of acute nausea and vomiting, as an adjunct to narcotic analgesia, for intractable hiccups, for relief of severe itching, for treatment of acute intermittent porphyria, as antitussive agents, and for sedation (4,5). In psychiatric patients, neuroleptic agents are employed in the treatment of acute and chronic schizophrenia, organic mental disorders, anxiety disorders, mixed anxiety-depressive illness, and anxiety-agitation accompanying dementia (Table 17–1). These drugs are associated with a wide variety of side effects (5).

Neuroleptic drugs are grouped into five categories: phenothiazines, thioxanthenes, butyrophenones, indoles, and dibenzoxapines. Widespread use of phenothiazines over several decades has made clinicians most familiar with this group of agents (6).

TABLE 17–1. *Uses of neuroleptic agents*

Antipsychotic agent
Treatment of nausea and vomiting
Preanesthetic medication
Adjunct to narcotic analgesia
Relief of itching
Antitussive agent
Sedation

The phenothiazine tranquilizers are not a homogeneous group of drugs, and, although they share many structural similarities, enough variation exists to "affect" their spectrum of adverse effects and perhaps the toxicity seen in overdose. There are more than 20 phenothiazine derivatives available for clinical use. They have a basic three-ring structure and can be categorized into three major classes: the aliphatic derivatives, of which chlorpromazine and triflupromazine are the most widely used; the piperazine group, which includes fluphenazine, prochlorperazine, and trifluoperazine; and piperidine derivatives, which include thioridazine and mepazine (Table 17–2) (6). The thioxanthenes are derivatives of the phenothiazines. The butyrophenones are structurally unrelated to the phenothiazines, but their pharmacologic actions are similar. Clozapine is an example of a dibenzodiazepine, related chemically to the antipsychotic loxapine (7).

The physical, chemical, pharmacologic, and toxicologic properties of the various phenothiazines are generally similar, but the relative potencies and the nature of their toxicity depend on the chemical substitutions. Piperazine derivatives, for example, are more potent as antiemetics, antipsychotics, and extrapyramidal syndrome inducers than the aliphatic and piperidine derivatives, but they have less potent hypotensive, antimuscarinic, and sedative actions (5).

The pharmacology of the antipsychotic agents is complex because the drugs may affect many different sites in the body (8). The major pharmacologic action of the phenothiazines is on the central and autonomic nervous systems, the cardiovascular system, the endocrine glands, and body metabolism (9).

TABLE 17–2. *The neuroleptic agents*

Compound	Derivatives (Trade names)
Butyrophenones	Haloperidol (Haldol)
	Droperidol (Innovar, Inapsine)
Phenothiazines	Aliphatic
	Chlorpromazine (Thorazine, Chloramead)
	Promazine (Sparine, Prozine)
	Promethazine (Phenergan)
	Triflupromazine (Vesprin)
	Piperidine
	Mesoridazine (Serentil, Lidanar)
	Piperacetazine (Quide)
	Thioridazine (Mellaril)
	Piperazine
	Acetophenazine (Tindal)
	Butaperizine (Repoise)
	Carphenazine (Prokethazine)
	Fluphenazine (Prolixin, Permitil)
	Perphenazine (Trilafon, Etrafon, Triavil)
	Prochlorperazine (Compazine)
	Thiethylperazine (Torecan)
	Trifluoperazine (Stelazine)
Thioxanthenes	Chlorprothixene (Taractan)
	Thiothixene (Navane)
Dibenzoxapine	Loxapine (Loxitane, Daxolin)
Dihydroindolone	Molindone (Moban, Lidone)
Miscellaneous	Methoxypromazine
	Pipamazine

Mechanism of Action

The dopamine hypothesis of schizophrenia, which states that an increase in dopaminergic activity in the mesolimbic system is relevant to the etiology of schizophrenia, has served as a useful model for schizophrenia for more than 30 years (5,8). The neuroleptic agents are antidopaminergics to varying degrees. Dopamine is one of the two principal catecholamines in the brain. Receptors for dopamine occur most prominently in the reticular formation of the brainstem, the hypothalamus, the limbic system, and the basal ganglia (9). Blocking of the postsynaptic dopamine receptor site in the limbic system and basal ganglia is thought to account for the antipsychotic activity of the neuroleptic agents. Receptor blockade results in decreased enzyme activity with decreased cell firing and increased production rate of dopamine metabolites.

At least two different dopamine antagonist receptors have been identified, D_1 and D_2 (10). Some of the D_1 receptors are linked to adenylate cyclase, and haloperidol binding preferentially labels the D_2 receptor. Both receptors are thought to be blocked by antipsychotics. Some investigators hypothesize that D_1 receptors are primarily responsible for efficacy whereas D_2 receptors are responsible for extrapyramidal symptoms and perhaps efficacy (11). Although the inhibitory effect of the neuroleptics on classical D_2 receptors appears to correlate very well with antipsychotic dosage, this effect alone cannot explain all the clinically relevant differences between these drugs (8). Recently, multiple D_2 receptors have been identified. It is possible that atypical antipsychotics may preferentially interact with different isoforms of the D_2 receptor. Neuroleptics are not completely specific for D_1 and D_2 dopamine receptors (10).

Miscellaneous Actions

Other important physiologic properties of the neuroleptics are peripheral cholinergic blockade (antimuscarinic), α-adrenergic blockade, membrane-stabilizing activity, blocking of the reuptake of norepinephrine in the peripheral synapses, serotonergic action, and antihistaminic (H_1 receptor) action (Table 17–3). Each of the neuroleptic agents differs in the degree of pharmacologic activity (Table 17–4). The effects of the neuroleptics on the autonomic nervous system are therefore complex and unpredictable because the drugs exert varying degrees of effects on many areas of the autonomic nervous system.

The phenothiazines act as potent central antiemetics by depressing the chemoreceptor trigger zone in the medulla. These drugs effectively antagonize centrally induced emesis but have no effect on emesis caused by gastrointestinal irritation or vestibular stimulation. The piperazines have a potent antiemetic effect, and thioridazine, a piperidine derivative, has no antiemetic properties.

Because dopaminergic neurons in the basal ganglia act to inhibit cholinergic neurons, blockade of the dopaminergic receptors results in an excess cholinergic stimulation. This can result in side effects, such as acute dystonia, akathisia, or a Parkinson-like presentation.

At therapeutic doses, neuroleptics may induce orthostatic hypotension due to peripheral α blockade and direct vasodilation. In overdoses, the drug may also exhibit a direct myocardial depressant effect. A lowering

TABLE 17–3. *Pharmacologic actions of neuroleptic agents*

- Antidopaminergic
  - Greater effects on D_2 receptors
  - Results in excess cholinergic stimulation
- Antimuscarinic
- α-Adrenergic blockade
- Antihistaminic (H_1 receptor)
- Antiemetic
  - Central depression of chemoreceptor trigger zone
- Blockade of reuptake of norepinephrine
- Lowers seizure threshold
- Membrane stabilization
- Serotonergic

TABLE 17–4. *Comparison of effects of phenothiazines*

Compound	Antiemetic	Antimuscarinic	Extrapyramidal	Hypotensive	Sedative
Aliphatic					
Chlorpromazine	+++	+++	++	+++	+++
Promazine	++	+++	++	+++	+++
Triflupromazine	+++	+++	++	++	++
Piperidine					
Mesoridazine	+	++	+	++	+++
Piperacetazine	+	+	++	++	+
Thioridazine	+	+++	+	++	+++
Piperazine					
Acetophenazine	+	+	++	+	++
Carphenazine	+	+	+++	+	++
Fluphenazine	+	+	+++	+	+
Perphenazine	+++	++	+++	+	+
Prochlorperazine	+++	+	+++	+	++
Trifluoperazine	+++	+	+++	+	+

of the seizure threshold occurs with some of the major tranquilizers.

PHARMACOKINETICS

The neuroleptics can be administered by intravenous, intramuscular, oral, and rectal routes. Intramuscular absorption is variable, and some neuroleptics may cause profound hypotension when administered by this route. The neuroleptics are highly plasma protein bound (more than 90%) and lipophilic. These agents also have a large volume of distribution (more than 20 L/kg), which accounts for the large amount of these agents within tissues (5). The neuroleptics are metabolized extensively in the liver by glucuronidization and sulfoxidation. There are many metabolites formed, some of which are pharmacologically active. Typically, plasma concentrations reach their peak within 2 to 4 hours of oral administration, and there is little correlation among dose, serum concentration, and antipsychotic effect (12).

TOXIC EFFECTS

Neuroleptic agents are usually quite safe when taken in significant overdose, although abnormal electrocardiograms (EKGs) and sudden death of patients receiving standard therapeutic doses have been reported. Deaths have been most frequently reported in cases of overdose with thioridazine (13) and mesoridazine (a metabolite of thioridazine) (14,15) or when phenothiazines are taken in excessive amounts together with decongestants, antihistamines, or tricyclic agents. Deaths have been attributed to cardiac dysrhythmias (16), vasodilation, hypotension, hyperpyrexia, and aspiration. Cardiotoxicity and CNS toxicity account for the vast majority of side effects.

Toxicity of the neuroleptic agents can be broadly categorized into three major presentations: acute or chronic overdose, extrapyramidal manifestations, and neuroleptic malignant syndrome.

Acute or Chronic Overdose

An acute or chronic overdose of neuroleptic agents may produce both cardiovascular and CNS toxicity. The cardiovascular effects are complex because the drugs exert both direct cardiac toxicity, described as a local anesthetic effect, as well as indirect actions on the heart and vasculature (17). The indirect actions include peripheral vascular effects as well as a combination of autonomic changes. A peripheral antimuscarinic effect may be evident in neuroleptic overdose resulting in dry mouth, decreased gastric motility, dry mucous membranes, and urinary retention.

Cardiac Complications

Cardiovascular symptoms result from the antimuscarinic effects, quinidine-like effects, and α-adrenergic blocking activity these drugs have on the heart (Table 17–5) (18). Mild hypertension has also been reported. EKG changes are variable, depending on the drug involved (19). At low doses, most neuroleptics exhibit an

TABLE 17–5. *Cardiovascular complications of the neuroleptics*

Antimuscarinic effects
Sinus tachycardia
Hypertension
Quinidine-like effects
Widened QRS
Rightward axis deviation
Ventricular dysrhythmias
α-Blocking effects
Orthostatic hypotension

antiarrhythmic effect similar to effects caused by quinidine or procainamide. This may be manifested as prolongation of PR, QRS, and QT intervals or as nonspecific ST-T wave changes. Toxic doses of antipsychotics may be arrhythmogenic and may cause development of conduction defects or ventricular arrhythmias. The most common cardiovascular complication is orthostatic hypotension (19). The hypotension seen with the neuroleptics may be due to the α-adrenergic blocking activity in combination with the quinidine-like action on the myocardium (18).

The incidence of serious complications or deaths resulting from neuroleptic overdose is quite low. Death from cardiac complications is of two types, both of which are considered rare. The first is death from acute overdose (20) and the second is the sudden death of patients receiving standard doses of neuroleptic agents (12,21). The cardiovascular manifestation of neuroleptic intoxication may include dysrhythmias such as atrioventricular dissociation, supraventricular tachycardia, ventricular tachycardia, ventricular fibrillation, and torsade de pointes (12). The neuroleptics also have a negative inotropic effect on the myocardium. Thioridazine (Mellaril) and mesoridazine (Serentil) are especially apt to cause cardiotoxicity (18). Most reported ventricular dysrhythmias have occurred in patients taking these drugs as long-term therapy rather than after an acute overdose.

Eye Effects

Although mydriasis may be expected, miosis may also be seen. This is observed most often in the severely poisoned patient, and may serve as a clinical clue to the severity of the overdose. Miosis represents an overriding of the atropine effect by the α-adrenergic blocking effect of these agents.

Neurologic Effects

Neurologic symptoms in overdose include a depressive state characterized by psychomotor slowing, emotional quieting, and affective indifference (Table 17–6). This depressive state can be preceded by a period of agitation, hyperactivity, or seizures. Patients can also exhibit drowsiness, lethargy, suppression of reflexes, and coma of any grade, which may be accompanied by respiratory depression (2). Sedation is the most common side effect from most major tranquilizers. It can be a problem during the initial phase of treatment, but tolerance usually develops with chronic therapy (18).

The neuroleptics may also lower the seizure threshold and induce a discharge pattern associated with seizure disorders. Overt seizures may occur in patients with a history of seizure disorder. Seizures are uncommon but may be seen, especially with newer agents, such as loxapine.

TABLE 17–6. *Neurologic symptoms of neuroleptic overdose*

CNS Stimulation
Agitation
Hyperactivity
Seizures
CNS Depression
Psychomotor slowing
Emotional quieting
Drowsiness
Lethargy
Sedation
Coma
Hyperthermia

Hyperthermia or Hypothermia

Neuroleptics have a poikilothermic effect; that is, they interfere with temperature regulation in the hypothalamus. Depending on environmental conditions, hyperthermia or hypothermia may occur. Hypothermia is most often seen with haloperidol and hyperthermia with a phenothiazine. This poikilothermy is thought to occur because the dopaminergic receptor blockade in the hypothalamus impairs the body's thermoregulatory control mechanism, making the patient less adaptable to environmental thermal stress. Patients may present with mild hypothermia that will usually respond to external passive rewarming.

Laboratory

Rapid urine screening for phenothiazines can be accomplished with either ferric chloride or a urinalysis strip test (Phenistix) testing. Ten to 15 drops of 10% ferric chloride mixed with 1 mL of urine will produce a deep burgundy color if phenothiazines are present (2). This must be distinguished from the dark purple reaction seen with aspirin. Determination of serum levels of neuroleptics is usually not very helpful in the immediate management of the overdosed patient.

An EKG should be obtained on all suspected neuroleptic ingestions because conduction blocks and dysrhythmias may occur (18).

Treatment

The treatment of overdose with a neuroleptic agent is mostly supportive. Monitoring and support of respiratory and cardiovascular function are of primary importance. Immediate discontinuance of the agent, initiating measures to reduce the patient's fever, hydration, and vigorous monitoring of vital signs, neurologic status, fluid status, and renal function are necessary. Lavage, even long after ingestion, may be effective because the antimuscarinic effect of these agents delays gastric emptying and because neuroleptics are water-soluble and therefore slowly absorbed from the gastrointestinal tract. Activated charcoal and a cathartic should follow lavage.

Hypotension is treated by placing the patient in the Trendelenburg position and administering a fluid challenge. If hypotension is refractory to these measures, a pure α-adrenergic pressor agent such as norepinephrine should be started.

Pressor agents with mixed α and β effects should be avoided because neuroleptics cause α blockade and administration of mixed α and β pressors could result in unopposed β stimulation with peripheral vasodilation and worsening hypotension. After acute neuroleptic overdoses, the potential for cardiac dysrhythmias, particularly ventricular tachydysrhythmias, should be considered, and patients should be monitored for at least 48 hours.

Phenytoin or lidocaine should be used for treatment of ventricular dysrhythmias. Drugs such as quinidine or procainamide should not be given because they will add to the quinidine effect of the neuroleptics. Although there are no controlled studies with the use of sodium bicarbonate, it would appear reasonable to attempt its use for evidence of major cardiac manifestations. The indications for use would be the same as for the cyclic antidepressants. A pacemaker may be of value in the treatment of ventricular dysrhythmias that are unresponsive to antidysrhythmic drugs. Diazepam or lorazepam may be used for initial control of seizures.

Disposition

Most patients who overdose with neuroleptic drugs are asymptomatic and may be safely discharged after they have been lavaged and observed for a few hours (22).

Patients with hypotension or new conduction delays should be admitted and monitored. Patients with an altered mental status that does not clear during a few hours of observation in the emergency department (ED) should be admitted. Children who ingest haloperidol and are asymptomatic should be admitted because they are prone to development of hypertension.

Because of the large volume of distribution and extensive tissue binding of these agents, hemodialysis, hemoperfusion, and forced diuresis are ineffective in enhancing elimination.

Extrapyramidal Manifestations

Acute dystonic reactions, parkinsonism, and akathisia are extrapyramidal syndromes that may appear after antipsychotic drug therapy (23). These signs occur with an acute ingestion or are side effects of long-term treatment. They may be noted within 20 minutes after ingestion of a single therapeutic dose, be delayed in onset up to 72 hours or more, or appear intermittently (21). These reactions often resemble symptoms of Parkinson's disease. Acute dystonic reactions, sometimes referred to as dyskinetic reactions, are involuntary tonic contractions of muscles that may occur suddenly and intermittently. Normal mentation is maintained (24).

An additional problem that can be seen with long-term use of neuroleptics is denervation hypersensitivity (25). When the receptors are continually blocked, they may become more sensitive to stimulation. This coupled with an increased production of dopamine in the brain can lead to hyperkinesthetic side effects, such as tardive dyskinesia.

Pathogenesis

Extrapyramidal symptoms are the result of the disruption of the dopaminergic–cholinergic balance in the corpus striatum neurons, which results in dopamine blockade with a compensatory increase in acetylcholine activity and cholinergic dominance (24). In the extrapyramidal system, especially the basal ganglia, acetylcholine is an excitatory transmitter and dopamine is an inhibitory transmitter (26). Under normal conditions, the cholinergic–dopaminergic system maintains physiologic balance, which results in coordinated neuromuscular activity (27). When a patient takes a therapeutic dose of a neuroleptic, blockade of the dopamine receptors occurs, especially in the nitrostriatal system (28). The acetylcholine neurotransmitters become dominant and overactive after sudden withdrawal of the dopaminergic inhibition, which leads to an acute dystonic reaction (23).

Neuroleptics vary considerably in their ability to elicit such reactions. Neuroleptics with antidopaminergic activity far in excess of their antimuscarinic potency are responsible for the greatest incidence of dystonic side effects. Piperazine phenothiazines such as trifluoperazine and fluphenazine, and butyrophenones such as haloperidol, are associated with a high incidence of such side effects. In contrast, thioridazine has a low incidence of extrapyramidal reactions (25). Young children tend to be prone to extrapyramidal signs and to have generalized manifestations, whereas adolescents and adults tend to have signs localized to the face and trunk. Nonneuroleptic compounds have also caused acute dystonic reactions, probably as a result of dopamine blocking effects of the compounds (23). Nonphenothiazine antiemetics such as metoclopramide (Reglan) and trimethobenzamide (Tigan) have also produced dystonic reactions. Antihistamines and antiparkinsonism agents, although used to treat acute dystonic reactions, have also been reported to cause these reactions (29–32).

Clinical Features

Acute Dystonic Reactions

Acute dystonic reactions may be sudden in onset and consist of bizarre muscular spasms. The muscles of the head and neck are predominantly affected. Involvement of pharyngeal muscles may lead to dysarthria, dysphagia, sialorrhea, and grimacing (Table 17–7). The neck muscles are also frequently affected; thus opisthotonus and torticollis can occur and may be associated with oculogyric crisis or spasm of the external ocular muscles with painful upward gaze persisting for minutes to hours (33).

Akathisia is a feeling of anxiety or inner tension manifested by motor restlessness and the inability to sit still. It is believed to be related to excessive cholinergic stimulation secondary to dopaminergic receptor blockade. Akathisia usually occurs within 2 months of the initiation of therapy and affects women more often than men. Elderly patients are also predisposed. Parkinsonism may also be noted as motor retardation, depression, mask-like facial expression, tremor at rest, "pill-rolling" movements of the fingers, rigidity, salivation, and a shuffling gait. Treatment of the disorder usually includes lowering the neuroleptic dose and treating with an antimuscarinic drug (23).

Tardive Dyskinesia

Chronic use of neuroleptic drugs may result in neurotoxic syndromes of tardive dyskinesia or perioral tremor (Rabbit syndrome). Development of tardive dyskinesia is one of the most distressing complications of antipsychotic drug use due to its resistance to therapy (25). Chronic dopaminergic receptor inhibition is thought to result in a denervation hypersensitivity with subsequent overactivity of the nigrostriatal pathways in the basal ganglia and resultant choreiform movements of the buccolingual muscles. Haloperidol (Haldol) and fluphenazine (Prolixin) are the agents most commonly implicated.

Tardive dyskinesia may be noted by involuntary repetitive movements of the mouth and tongue although the trunk and extremities can also be involved. The movements increase during anxiety and stop during sleep. Therapy of tardive dyskinesia is difficult. Neuroleptic-induced dyskinetic reactions are generally of late onset, and may persist even after drug elimination (25).

TABLE 17–7. *Extrapyramidal signs from neuroleptic agents*

Akathisia
Buccolingual incoordination
Dysphagia
Grimacing
Oculogyric crisis
Opisthotonus
Parkinsonism
Sialorrhea
Torticollis

Treatment of Extrapyramidal Reactions

Treatment consists of either restoring dopaminergic function by discontinuing the neuroleptic, giving the patient antimuscarinic medication to alleviate the enhanced cholinergic function, or both. Dystonic reactions are reversed rapidly with several agents. Resolution of symptoms after administration of these agents is not only therapeutic but also establishes the diagnosis when a clear history of recent drug ingestion is not available.

The extrapyramidal symptoms in most cases respond to intravenous diphenhydramine (Benadryl, 25 to 50 mg) or benztropine (Cogentin, 1 to 2 mg). These agents are generally successful in 2 to 5 minutes (34). The recommended route of administration for these agents is intravenous or intramuscular, although oral administration has shown good results. The almost immediate relief of symptoms after the initial treatment has been thought to obviate the need for continued outpatient treatment, but relapses of dyskinesia may occur. For this reason at least 48 to 72 hours of outpatient treatment is necessary (23,24). Trihexyphenidyl (Artane, Tremin) is not suggested for immediate treatment because it is not available in an injectable form. Outpatient therapy of trihexyphenidyl may consist of 2-mg doses twice daily.

Neuroleptic Malignant Syndrome

An uncommon but potentially life-threatening adverse effect of antipsychotic agents, called the neuroleptic malignant syndrome, was first described in 1968 (35–37). It is the rarest and least known of the complications of neuroleptic drug therapy (38). The infrequent recognition of this disorder may be due to a lack of awareness of it on the part of many physicians (39). Neither duration of neuroleptic therapy nor toxic overdoses have been associated with the development of neuroleptic malignant syndrome (35).

Signs and Symptoms

Neuroleptic malignant syndrome is a life-threatening idiosyncratic disorder that may develop after major tranquilizer exposure (40). Although specific diagnostic criteria remain controversial, four clinical findings are present: (a) hyperthermia above 40°C, (b) altered or fluctuating level of consciousness, (c) a "lead pipe" muscular rigidity, and (d) autonomic nervous system disturbances that may be manifested as fluctuating blood pressure, tachycardia, diaphoresis, incontinence, and dysrhythmias (35).

The clinical features of this syndrome may evolve over 24 to 72 hours (Table 17–8) (41). The autonomic instability has been described as labile hypertension, profound vasoconstriction, tachycardia, and severe diaphoresis (38). The hyperthermia is secondary to severe muscle contraction, which produces excessive body heat that cannot be efficiently dissipated because vasoconstriction reduces heat transfer (22). This fever is often accompanied by hypertension, tachycardia, mental status changes, and extrapyramidal effects such as dysarthria, dysphasia, and muscle rigidity. Temperatures higher than 41°C may create irreversible cell damage affecting many tissues and organs, including brain, muscle, and kidney (6). Mortality attributable to cardiac or respiratory failure may reach 20% and is related to the duration and severity of symptoms (28,42–44), so that early recognition and prompt treatment are top priorities. In severe cases, death occurs as a result of respiratory or renal failure. Occasionally, renal failure is due to rhabdomyolysis, which occurs after a long period of muscle rigidity produces myoglobinuria.

The mortality rate has decreased significantly in past years due to increased awareness and early diagnosis of this syndrome. The clinical course is variable, but is usually 5 to 10 days in duration despite neuroleptic termination. The course of neuroleptic malignant syndrome may be prolonged for several days to weeks when depot neuroleptics have been administered (27).

The syndrome typically begins with diffuse muscle rigidity often accompanied by extrapyramidal symptoms of tremor, dysarthria, or dysphagia (6). Hyperpyrexia follows and is usually attended by a decreasing level of consciousness (35). Many of these findings are identical to those in heat stroke; temperatures higher than 42°C have been noted. Most complications of neuroleptic malignant syndrome are produced by the severe hyperthermia. Other complications in the course of neuroleptic malignant syndrome are frequent and include principally acute respiratory failure, thromboembolism, and acute renal failure (11).

TABLE 17–8. *Signs and symptoms of neuroleptic malignant syndrome*

Muscle rigidity
Extrapyramidal effects
Tremor
Dysarthria
Dysphagia
Autonomic instability
Hyperthermia
Labile hypertension
Vasoconstriction
Pallor
Sialorrhea
Tachycardia
Diaphoresis
Altered level of consciousness

The differential diagnosis may include malignant hyperthermia, "lethal catatonia," heat stroke, the central antimuscarinic syndrome, and infection (37). Although this syndrome resembles malignant hyperthermia, the most striking difference between the two is that malignant hyperthermia occurs only minutes and rarely hours after drug administration, whereas neuroleptic malignant syndrome develops in days or longer (38).

Neuroleptic malignant syndrome is considered a disturbance of dopamine function within the central nervous system that affects both the basal ganglia and the hypothalamus (28). The onset of neuroleptic malignant syndrome is not related to the duration of drug administration and can occur soon after the first dose of a drug or after prolonged treatment (11). Both oral and intramuscular administration of neuroleptic drugs can initiate the syndrome.

The syndrome has been reported with use of the phenothiazines (fluphenazine, piperacetazine, chlorpromazine), the butyrophenones (haloperidol), and the thioxanthenes (chlorprothixene) (38). The agents most frequently associated with neuroleptic malignant syndrome are fluphenazine, which is usually given in depot form, and oral haloperidol. These two drugs account for more than 90% of cases (39).

Laboratory

Although laboratory findings are abnormal, they are nonspecific (Table 17–9). Diagnostic measures should include complete blood count, urinalysis, Sequential Multiple Analysis—12-channel biochemical profile (SMA-12), a computed tomographic (CT) scan, electroencephalogram (EEG), and a lumbar puncture. Laboratory evaluation may be significant for leukocytosis, with or without a left shift; an elevation of creatine phosphokinase (CPK); and an increase in hepatic aminotransferases (aspartate aminotransferase [AST] and alanine aminotransferase [ALT]), alkaline phosphatase, and lactate dehydrogenase (LDH) (39). The increase in CPK may reflect myonecrosis after intense and sustained skeletal muscle contraction. Myoglobinuria following excessive rigidity of skeletal muscles may lead to impairment of

TABLE 17–9. *Laboratory abnormalities associated with neuroleptic malignant syndrome*

Elevation of
White blood count
Creatine phosphokinase
Aminotransferases
AST
ALT
Alkaline phosphatase
Lactic dehydrogenase
Myoglobinuria

renal function (35). Computed tomography reveals no acute changes, and standard cerebrospinal fluid analysis reveals no abnormalities.

Prophylaxis for neuroleptic malignant syndrome is difficult because the syndrome is related to individual intolerance rather than toxic overdose (11).

Treatment

Treatment includes discontinuing the agent and immediately initiating measures to reduce the patient's fever (6). This can be done with cooling blankets, ice bags, antipyretic agents, and alcohol sponge baths (Table 17–10). It is helpful to review all medications for "hidden" dopamine antagonists such as metoclopramide (Reglan), phenothiazines such as Compazine, and piperazines such as hydroxyzine (Vistaril). Vigorous monitoring of the vital signs, cardiovascular function, neurologic status, fluid status, and renal function should also be attempted. Intubation and mechanical ventilation may be necessary, and intensive-care monitoring of the fluid and electrolyte balance is indicated. Pharmacologic therapy is directed at altering the central nervous system (CNS) dopaminergic to cholinergic ratio. Originally, antimuscarinics were recommended for this purpose, but they are now considered ineffective (6,42). Specific drug treatment for neuroleptic malignant syndrome is controversial because there are numerous reports of successful treatment but no well-controlled large studies. Pharmacologic agents that have been suggested include bromocriptine, dantrolene, and amantadine and sodium nitroprusside (45).

Bromocriptine. Bromocriptine (Parlodel) is an ergot alkaloid and a dopamine agonist that acts postsynaptically. It has been shown to act within hours and to reverse both hyperpyrexia and muscle rigidity. It is available only in oral form, in tablets of 2.5 mg, so it must be given early, before the patient loses the gag reflex. The dosage to treat neuroleptic malignant syndrome has ranged from 7.5 to 60 mg/day. In high doses, the most common notable side effects are hypotension and dyskinesia. Side effects are frequent, and include mental changes such as confusion with occasional psychosis, nausea, vomiting, hiccups, and dyskinesias (1,6,45).

TABLE 17–10. *Treatment of neuroleptic malignant syndrome*

Discontinue incriminating medicine(s)
Active fever reduction
Cooling blankets
Ice bags
Antipyretic agents
Vigorous supportive care
Agents possibly effective:
Bromocriptine
Dantrolene
Amantadine
Sodium nitroprusside

Dantrolene. Dantrolene (Dantrium), a skeletal muscle relaxant, has also been reported to be successful in a few cases (37), especially in patients with severe muscle rigidity (38). It appears to act directly on the muscle to block heat production. This is accomplished by dissociation of the excitation–contraction coupling mechanism in peripheral muscle through inhibiting the release of calcium from the sarcoplasmic reticulum. Dantrolene does not affect the rate of acetylcholine synthesis or release, nor does it have an effect on the electrical activity at the myoneural junction. It has little effect on cardiac or intestinal smooth muscle at the suggested doses (11).

Dantrolene is used primarily in the treatment of the spasticity of multiple sclerosis and cerebral palsy, but it has also become a treatment of choice for malignant hyperthermia.

Dantrolene may be given in divided doses of 1.0 to 2.5 mg/kg every 6 hours either orally or parenterally. Few adverse reactions are noted as long as the maximal dose of 10 mg/kg is not administered (45). It can also be given orally 50 to 200 mg/day once the patient has been stabilized. Rapid resolution of symptoms (usually within 24 hours) is possible if treatment is begun early, though the usual course is 5 to 10 days. Optimal treatment consists of the concomitant use of bromocriptine and dantrolene because the effects of these drugs may be synergistic (6,28).

Amantadine. Amantadine (Symmetrel), a dopamine agonist that acts presynaptically, may be administered orally as 100 mg two or three times daily. Amantadine has been used with a combination of carbidopa and levodopa to increase synaptic dopamine availability. If amantadine is abruptly withdrawn it may worsen or precipitate neuroleptic malignant syndrome.

Sodium nitroprusside. Sodium nitroprusside (Nipride) has also been used to successfully treat the severe hypertension and consequently the severe hyperthermia. In patients in whom peripheral vasoconstriction rather than muscle rigidity is dominant, infusion of nitroprusside may be beneficial by lowering the patient's temperature through increasing heat loss from the skin by increasing the flow of blood to vessels near the skin surface (6). Approximately 50% of patients will suffer a recurrence of neuroleptic malignant syndrome upon reintroduction of the same agent.

REFERENCES

1. Olmsted T: Neuroleptic malignant syndrome: guidelines for treatment and reinstitution of neuroleptics. *South Med J* 1988;81:888–891.
2. Baldessarini R, Cohen B, Teicher M: Significance of neuroleptic dose and plasma level in the pharmacological treatment of psychosis. *Arch Gen Psychiatry* 1988;45:79–91.
3. Garza-Trevino E, Hollister L, Overall J, et al: Efficacy of combinations of intramuscular antipsychotics and sedative-hypnotics for control of psychotic agitation. *Am J Psychiatry* 1989;146:1598–1601.

4. Rivera-Calimlim L: The pharmacology and therapeutic application of the phenothiazines. *Ration Drug Ther* 1977;11:1–8.
5. Knight M, Roberts R: Phenothiazine and butyrophenone intoxication in children. *Pediatr Clin North Am* 1986;33:299–309.
6. Harpe C, Stoudemire A: Aetiology and treatment of neuroleptic malignant syndrome. *Med Toxicol* 1987;2:166–176.
7. Bablenis E, Weber S, Wagner R: Clozapine: a novel antispychotic agent. *DICP* 1989;23:109–115.
8. Meltzer H, Nash J: Effects of antipsychotic drugs on serotonin receptors. *Pharmacol Rev* 1991;43:587–604.
9. Wysowski D, Baum C: Antipsychotic drug use in the United States, 1976–1985. *Arch Gen Psychiatry* 1989;46:929–932
10. Farde L, Wiesel F, Halldin C, et al: Central D_2-dopamine receptor occupancy in schizophrenic patients treated with antipsychotic drugs. *Arch Gen Psychiatry* 1988;45:71–76.
11. Legras A, Hurel D, Dabrowski G, et al: Protracted neuroleptic malignant syndrome complicating long-acting neuroleptic administration. *Am J Med* 1988;85:875–878.
12. Coyle J: The clinical use of antipsychotic medications. *Med Clin North Am* 1982;66:993–1009.
13. Burgess K, Stevenson I: Fatal thioridazine cardiotoxicity. *Med J Aust* 1979;2:177–178.
14. Donlon P, Tupin J: Successful suicides with thioridazine and mesoridazine. *Arch Gen Psychiatry* 1977;34:955–957.
15. Desautels S, Filteau C, St Jean A, et al: Ventricular tachycardia associated with administration of thioridazine hydrochloride (Mellaril). *Can Med Assoc J* 1964;90:1030–1031.
16. Alexander C, Nino A: Cardiovascular complications in young patients taking psychotropic drugs. *Am Heart J* 1969;78:757–769.
17. Ban T, St Jean A: The effect of phenothiazines on the EKG. *Can Med Assoc J* 1964;91:537–540.
18. Vertrees J, Siebel G: Rapid death resulting from mesoridazine overdose. *Vet Hum Toxicol* 1987;29:65–67.
19. Wilt J, Minema A, Johnson R, et al: Torsade de pointes associated with the use of intravenous haloperidol. *Ann Intern Med* 1993;119: 391–394.
20. Lumpkin J, Watanabe A, Rumack B, et al: Phenothiazine-induced ventricular tachycardia following acute overdose. *JACEP* 1979;8: 476–478.
21. Tri T, Combs D: Phenothiazine-induced ventricular tachycardia. *West J Med* 1975;123:412–416.
22. Taylor N, Schwartz H: Neuroleptic malignant syndrome following amoxapine overdose. *J Nerv Ment Dis* 1988;176:249–251.
23. Demetropoulos S, Schauben J: Acute dystonic reactions from "street valium." *J Emerg Med* 1987;5:293–297.
24. Corre K, Niemann J, Bessen H, et al: Extended therapy for acute dystonic reactions. *Ann Emerg Med* 1984;13:194–197.
25. Richardson M, Haugland G, Craig T: Neuroleptic use, parkinsonian symptoms, tardive dyskinesia, and associated factors in child and adolescent psychiatric patients. *Am J Psychiatry* 1991;148: 1322–1328.
26. Lee A: Drug-induced dystonic reactions. *JACEP* 1977;6:351–354.
27. Epperly T, McGlaughlin V, Leo K: A hazardous side effect of neuroleptics: diagnosis and treatment, *Geriatrics* 1990;45:58–62.
28. Granato J, Stein B, Ringel A, et al: Neuroleptic malignant syndrome: successful treatment with dantrolene and bromocriptine. *Ann Neurol* 1983;14:89–90.
29. Baile G, Nelson M, Krenzlok E, et al: Unusual treatment response of a severe dystonia to diphenhydramine. *Ann Emerg Med* 1987;16: 705–708.
30. Lavenstein B, Cantor F: Acute dystonia: an unusual reaction to diphenhydramine. *JAMA* 1976;236:216.
31. Howrie D, Rowley A, Krenzelok E: Benztropine-induced acute dystonic reaction. *Ann Emerg Med* 1986;15:595–596.
32. Brait K, Zagerman A: Dyskinesias after antihistamine use. *N Engl J Med* 1976;296:111.
33. Lee A: Treatment of drug-induced dystonic reactions. *JACEP* 1979;8:453–457.
34. Ott D, Goeden S: Treatment of acute phenothiazine reaction. JACEP 1979;8:471–472.
35. Wells AJ, Sommi RW, Crismon ML: Neuroleptic rechallenge after neuroleptic malignant syndrome: case report and literature review. *Drug Intell Clin Pharm* 1988;22:475–480.
36. Blue M, Schneider S, Noro S, et al: Successful treatment of neuroleptic malignant syndrome with sodium nitroprusside. *Ann Intern Med* 1986;104:56–57.
37. May D, Morris S, Stewart R, et al: Neuroleptic malignant syndrome: response to dantrolene sodium. *Ann Intern Med* 1983;98:183–184.
38. Goulon M, Rohan-Chabot P, Elkharrat D, et al: Beneficial effects of dantrolene in the treatment of neuroleptic malignant syndrome: a report of two cases. *Neurology* 1983;33:516–518.
39. Henderson V, Wooten G: Neuroleptic malignant syndrome: a pathogenetic role for dopamine receptor blockade? *Neurology* 1981;31: 132–137.
40. Joshi P, Capozzoli J, Coyle J: Neuroleptic malignant syndrome: life threatening complication of neuroleptic treatment in adolescents with affective disorder. *Pediatrics* 1991;87:235–239.
41. Keck P, Pope H, Cohen B, et al: Risk factors for neuroleptic malignant syndrome. *Arch Gen Psychiatry* 1989;46:914–918.
42. Mueller P, Vester J, Fermaglich J: Neuroleptic malignant syndrome. *JAMA* 1983;249:386–388.
43. Niemann J, Stapczynski J, Rothstein R, et al: Cardiac conduction and rhythm disturbances following suicidal ingestion of mesoridazine. *Ann Emerg Med* 1981;10:585–588.
44. Smego R, Durack K: The neuroleptic malignant syndrome. *Arch Intern Med* 1982;142:1183–1185.
45. Ellison J, Jacobs D: Emergency psychopharmacology: a review and update. *Ann Emerg Med* 1986;15:962–968.

ADDITIONAL SELECTED REFERENCES

Ambani L, Van Woert M, Bowers M: Physostigmine: effects on phenothiazine-induced extrapyramidal reactions. *Arch Neurol* 1973;29:444–446.

Barry D, Meyskens F, Becker C: Phenothiazines and sudden infant death syndrome. *Pediatrics* 1982;70:75–78.

Black J, Richelson E: Antipsychotic drugs: prediction of side effect profiles based on neuroreceptor data derived from human brain tissue. *Mayo Clin Proc* 1987;62:369–372.

Craig D, Rosen P: Abuse of antiparkinsonian drugs. *Ann Emerg Med* 1981;10:98–100.

Cummingham D, Challapalli M: Hypertension in acute haloperidol poisoning. *J Pediatr* 1979;95:489–490.

Hollister L, Kosek J: Sudden death during treatment with phenothiazine derivatives. *JAMA* 1965;192:93–96.

Kahn A, Blum D: Phenothiazines and sudden infant death syndrome. *Pediatrics* 1982;70:75–78.

Klawans H: The pharmacology of tardive dyskinesias. *Am J Psychiatry* 1973;130:82–86.

Kobayashi R: Drug therapy of tardive dyskinesia. *N Engl J Med* 1977;296:257–260.

Rainey J, Nesse R: Psychobiology of anxiety and anxiety disorders. *Psychiatr Clin North Am* 1985;8:133–144.

Weisdorf D, Kramer J, Goldberg A, et al: Physostigmine for cardiac and neurologic manifestations of phenothiazine poisoning. *Clin Pharmacol Ther* 1978;24:663–668.

CHAPTER 18

Monoamine Oxidase Inhibitors

Monoamine oxidase (MAO) is a complex flavin-containing enzyme found principally on the outer mitochondrial membranes. Monoamine oxidase is one of the two main enzymes involved in the oxidative deamination of monoamines (1); the other enzyme is catechol *o*-methyl transferase (COMT) (2). Monoamine oxidase functions via oxidative deamination to inactivate more than 15 monoamines formed in the body, some of which serve important roles as synaptic neurotransmitters or neuromodulators, e.g., epinephrine, norepinephrine, dopamine, and 5-hydroxytryptamine (5HT) (3). As a result, the concentration of endogenous epinephrine, norepinephrine, dopamine, and serotonin increases in storage sites throughout the nervous system. It is thought that the increase in the concentration of monoamines in the central nervous system (CNS) is the basis for the antidepressant activity of these agents, but their exact mechanism of action is unknown. The monoamine oxidase inhibitors (MAOIs) are valuable antidepressants that have for the most part been supplanted by the tricyclic antidepressants in the treatment of endogenous depression (4).

HISTORY

Isoniazid and its close relative iproniazid were introduced for the treatment of tuberculosis in 1951. Iproniazid was soon demonstrated to inhibit the enzyme monoamine oxidase and in 1957 (5) it was first used for the treatment of depression (6). Although iproniazid was efficacious, its toxicity required its withdrawal from the market. It has since been replaced by MAOIs without the hepatotoxicity associated with iproniazid (5) and during the 1960s they were the principal pharmacologic modality for the treatment of endogenous depression (3). They are now used less frequently than the tricyclic antidepressants because of their detrimental interactions with a wide variety of foods. Although MAOIs have historically been relegated to the position of agents of second choice in the treatment of depression, current evidence establishes their value in atypical depression as well as refractory and bipolar depression.

TYPES OF MONOAMINE OXIDASE

Monoamine oxidase has been divided into two subtypes, MAO-A and MAO-B, on the basis of the different substrate specificities of the two forms (7). The substrates for MAO can also be divided into three broad categories on the basis of the affinity of the two isoenzymes for them, namely MAO-A specific, MAO-B specific, and mixed substrates for which the two enzyme forms have approximately equal affinity (Table 18–1) (2,3).

The concentration of MAO is especially high in the liver, the kidneys, the stomach, the intestinal walls, and the brain. MAO-A is the dominant enzyme occurring in the intestinal mucosa and many other sites, whereas MAO-B is present in the human brain (8).

The substrates for MAO-A are epinephrine, norepinephrine, metanephrine, and serotonin, whereas the substrates for MAO-B are phenylethylamine, tyramine, and benzylamine (3). Substrates for mixed A and B are tyramine, dopamine, and tryptamine. In the gastrointestinal tract (GIT) and the liver, MAO-A is thought to provide protec-

TABLE 18–1. *Types of monoamine oxidase*

MAO-A
Found in
Liver
Kidneys
Stomach
Intestinal walls
Substrate
Norepinephrine
Metanephrine
Serotonin
MAO-B
Found in
Brain
Substrate
Phenylethylamine
Tyramine
Benzylamine
Mixed MAO-A and MAO-B
Substrate
Tyramine
Dopamine
Tryptamine

tion from tyramine-induced reactions caused by certain foods (1). Because intestinal MAO consists mainly of the A form, as a result of monoamine oxidase inhibition, tyramine escapes oxidative deamination in the intestines and liver, leading to increased release of catecholamines from nerve endings and the adrenal medulla (9). The liver, kidneys, and lungs contain high MAO content. This appears to serve a defensive function where circulating monoamines would then be inactivated. In particular, they appear to form the first line of defense against monoamines absorbed from foods, such as tyramine and β-phenylethanolamine, which would otherwise produce an indirect sympathomimetic response resulting in a precipitous rise in blood pressure (8).

USE

The MAOIs are used for the treatment of neurotic and atypical depression as well as agoraphobia, eating disorders, obsessive-compulsive disorders, and posttraumatic stress disorders (4). Monoamine oxidase inhibitors currently available in the U.S. are the antidepressants tranylcypromine (Parnate), phenelzine (Nardil), and isocarboxazid (Marplan), the antimicrobial furazolidone (Furoxone), the antineoplastic procarbazine (Matulane), and the antihypertensive pargyline (Eutonyl) used for the treatment of moderate to severe hypertension that is resistant to other pharmacologic modalities. The antituberculosis drug isoniazid inhibits monoamine and diamine oxidase, and interactions have also been reported with this drug and food (4,10). Selegiline is an MAOI recently approved for the treatment of Parkinson's disease.

PHARMACOKINETICS

The MAOIs are generally classified in two main categories: hydrazines and nonhydrazines (Table 18–2). Currently available hydrazines include isocarboxazid and phenelzine, and currently available nonhydrazines include pargyline and tranylcypromine. The MAOIs are rapidly and completely absorbed from the gastrointestinal tract. They are metabolized in the liver and excreted by the kidneys.

TABLE 18–2. *The monoamine oxidase inhibitors*

Generic name	Trade name(s)
Hydrazines	
Isocarboxazid	Marplan
Phenelzine	Nardil
Nonhydrazines	
Tranylcypromine	Parnate
Pargyline	Eutonyl, Eutron

Mechanism of Action

Monoamine oxidase is an enzyme found mainly in mitochondrial membranes in nerve tissue and in the liver, lungs, and other organs (Fig. 18–1) (7). The MAOIs now marketed for use are relatively nonselective. Inhibition of MAO results in an increase in the concentration of various amines throughout the body. In other words, the MAOIs exert their effects by delaying the metabolism of sympathomimetic amines and by increasing the store of releasable norepinephrine in postganglionic sympathetic neurons.

Isocarboxazid, phenelzine, and pargyline bind irreversibly to MAO. These compounds appear to attack and inactivate the flavin group after their oxidation to reactive intermediaries by MAO. This causes an irreversible inhibition of MAO. Tranylcypromine binds reversibly to the enzyme (11). This drug bears a close resemblance to dextroamphetamine, which is a weak inhibitor of MAO (4). Tranylcypromine retains some of the sympathomimetic characteristics of the amphetamine, which may be due to some degree of metabolism to an amphetamine-like compound (4,10). The ability of these drugs to bind to MAO appears to be due to their structural similarity to the enzyme's natural substrates. Because some of them bind

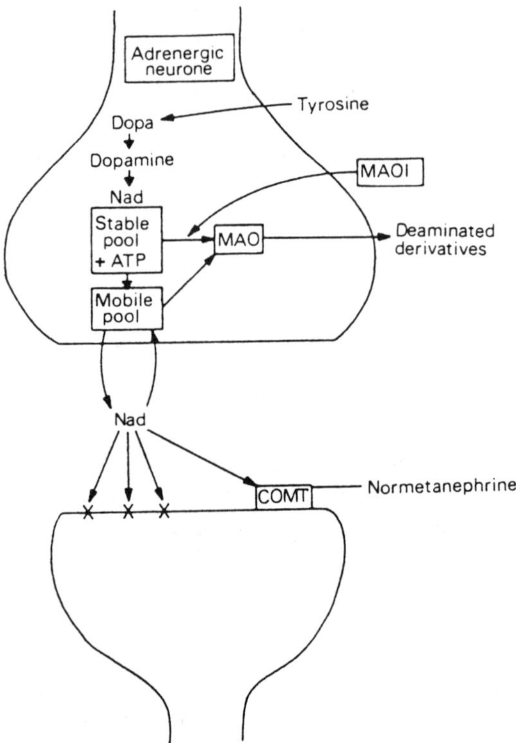

FIG. 18–1. Representation of the adrenergic neuron and the site of activity of the monoamine oxidase inhibitors, to increase the stable and mobile pools of norepinephrine. COMT, catechol *o*-methyl transferase; MAO, monoamine oxidase; MAOI, monoamine oxidase inhibitor; Nad, noradrenaline (norepinephrine). (From Stack C et al., *Br J Anaesth* 1988;60:224, with permission.)

to MAO in an irreversible manner, despite the discontinuation of MAOI therapy, enzyme inhibition may persist for several weeks until enzyme stores are repleted (12,13).

The MAOIs also have pharmacologic properties that are unrelated to their ability to inhibit MAO. Phenelzine and tranylcypromine appear to be capable of stimulating the release of norepinephrine from sympathetic nerve endings (11). MAOIs also have sympatholytic activity that is due to their ability to reduce the amount of norepinephrine released from postganglionic sympathetic neurons (14).

Side Effects

There is no clear evidence that any of the available MAOIs is more effective or has fewer side effects than the others (2). Tranylcypromine is known for being a better stimulant, perhaps because of the similarity between its structure and the amphetamines; however, its stimulant effect is neither reliable nor predictable (1).

The main side effects of the MAOIs include orthostatic hypotension, insomnia, weight gain, and on occasion, interference with orgasm and sexual function.

The major side effects of chronic MAO inhibition will relate to a general reduction in sympathetic outflow, producing a lower resting blood pressure, and a decrease in the ability of the sympathetic system to respond to stimuli, resulting in such conditions as orthostatic hypotension. In addition, there is the risk of a marked potentiation of indirectly acting sympathomimetic agents with a precipitous rise in blood pressure (3).

Drug Interactions

MAO-A Inhibitors

The MAOIs prolong and intensify the effects of other drugs and interfere with the metabolism of various substances (13). It is the diversity and number of substances as well as the unpredictability of the development of adverse effects that has contributed to the unpopularity of the MAOIs as therapeutic agents (12).

The interactions fall into two categories: (a) exacerbation or prolongation of the normally occurring actions of the drug (sedation or coma caused by alcohol, anesthetics, or opiate analgesics, or atropine-like central toxicity caused by tricyclics); and (b) hypertensive crisis attributable to the release and potentiation of catecholamines (Table 18–3) (12). The most important reaction is the latter, the so-called "cheese effect." Because relatively small amounts of aged cheese, which is particularly high in tyramine, could produce a hypertensive crisis in individuals treated with MAOIs, the term "cheese effect" was coined, although other foods such as red wine, chocolate, and yeast products can also induce this side effect. This term refers to the acute sympathomimetic effects: severe hypertension, tachycardia, headache, and vomiting that may occur when MAOIs are combined with dietary or pharmacologic ingestion of tyramine or certain other monoamines (8). The mechanism of this effect is displacement of norepinephrine from nerve terminals by ingested amines. This adverse reaction is dependent on the metabolism of dietary tyramine by intestinal MAO-A. Selective inhibition of MAO-B does not result in the "cheese effect."

Hypertensive crises have sometimes led to death. These crises usually occur within several hours after the ingestion of a contraindicated substance. They are char-

TABLE 18–3. *Substances that interact with MAOIs*

Drugs
Amphetamine
Caffeine
Cocaine
Dopamine
Ephedrine
Epinephrine
Levodopa
Mephenteramine
Metaraminol
Methyldopa
Methylphenidate
Norepinephrine
Phenylephrine
Phenylpropanolamine
Pseudoephedrine
Reserpine
Tryptophan
Foodstuffs
Alcohol (beer, wine)
Amine-containing foods
Avocado
Broad beans
Canned figs
Caviar
Cheese (natural or aged)
Chicken livers
Chocolate
Pickled herring
Snails
Sour cream
Soy sauce
Yeast extracts
Substances that inhibit hepatic drug-metabolizing enzyme
Anesthetics (general and local)
Antiparkinsonism agents
Barbiturates
Benzodiazepines
Chloral hydrate
Diuretics
Hypoglycemia agents
Opiate analgesics
Thyroid extract
Tricyclic agents

Adapted with permission from *Psychiatr Clin North Am* 1984;7:625–637. WB Saunders Company.

acterized by occipital headache, palpitations, neck stiffness or soreness, nausea, vomiting, mydriasis, and photophobia (Table 18–4). The toxic effects of the MAOIs are greater when they interact with indirectly acting amines, such as amphetamine and tyramine, than with directly acting amines, such as epinephrine and phenylpropanolamine (5).

MAOIs can interact with any protein food that contains decarboxylating bacteria because these produce amines by conversion of amino acids to amines (6). Certain foods containing tyramine, such as natural or aged cheese, pickled herring, canned figs, chocolate, large quantities of coffee, citrus fruits, chicken liver, yeast, bananas, avocados, and snails, may interact with MAOIs to cause hypertensive crisis. Yet, tyramine is formed from protein degradation by bacteria; consequently, any meat can become dangerous if not consumed while fresh. In many cases, food and beverage restrictions have occurred on the basis of a single reported adverse reaction, cases in which tyramine levels were not analyzed and may have represented reactions to spoiled foods (12).

Ingestion of fava (or Italian green, or broad) beans produces a hypertensive crisis secondary to the pressor effects of dopamine found in the bean pod (3). Broad beans should not be confused with the usual green bean or lima bean, which are safe.

In addition to tyramine, hypertensive reactions have been reported with ephedrine, metaraminol, methylamphetamine, phenylpropanolamine, phenylephrine, levodopa, and dopamine (Table 18–3) (6). Many fermented foods contain tyramine as a by-product formed by the bacterial breakdown of the amino acid tyrosine; it can also be formed by the parahydroxylation of phenylethylamine or dehydroxylation of DOPA and dopamine.

Fresh fish and vacuum-packed pickled fish or caviar contain only small amounts of tyramine and are safe if eaten promptly or refrigerated only for short periods; longer storage may not be safe, and overripe, fermented, smoked, and otherwise aged fish, meat, or any spoiled food may contain large amounts of tyramine and could be dangerous (6).

Wine generally does not contain tyramine and is probably safe if taken in small amounts, but reactions have been reported, presumably due to amines formed by contaminating organisms introduced during fermentation. Domestic beer appears to be safe, but imported beer should be avoided unless specific brands are known to be safe. Caffeine and chocolate are safe for most patients, unless ingested in large amounts. Yeast used in baking is safe, but extracts and tablets should not be used as dietary supplements.

TABLE 18–4. *Signs and symptoms of MAO–drug/food interactions*

Exacerbation of normally occurring actions
Associated with
Alcohol
Anesthetics
Opiates
Atropine
Sedation
Coma
Antimuscarinic activity
"Cheese effect" (exaggerated sympathomimetic effects)
Associated with tyramine-like products
Cardiac dysrhythmias
Cerebrovascular accident
Hypertension
Mydriasis
Nausea/vomiting
Neck stiffness
Occipital headache
Palpitations
Photophobia
Pulmonary edema

MAO-B Inhibitors

In the 1960s, an irreversible MAOI was developed that was based on the structure of methamphetamine, yet lacked the "cheese effect." This substance was isopropyl-methyl-propargylamine, also known as selegiline (Deprenyl, Eldepryl) (1). Selegiline hydrochloride is a highly potent, irreversible inhibitor of MAO that demonstrates selective inhibition of MAO-B. Although MAO-A is also inhibited by selegiline, it does it at much higher concentrations. A discussion of selegiline will follow.

Types of Reactions

Clinical presentations of hypertensive syndromes vary in severity, depending largely on the amount of exogenous amine ingested and the previous degree of MAOI inhibition achieved in the patient (13). Hypertension with cerebrovascular accident, cardiac dysrhythmias, and pulmonary edema have been observed as an exaggerated response to sympathomimetic amines after ingestion of an MAOI (6). Hypertension is related to varying degrees of α-adrenergic vasoconstriction and β-adrenergic cardiac stimulation. These are the most serious adverse reactions associated with MAOI therapy (5,15). Hypotension is more common when MAOIs are used with CNS depressant-like narcotics and anesthetics. Malignant hyperthermia is a unique feature of the toxicity of MAOIs. This syndrome has been seen especially after combined use of MAOIs and other antidepressant drugs such as imipramine, amitriptyline, and amphetamine, and mortality has been high.

Almost all of the fatalities in patients taking MAOIs have resulted from the ingestion of cheese. The hypertensive crisis is a dose-related phenomenon and aged cheeses have the highest tyramine content, whereas cottage and cream cheese have no detectable content.

Much of the published data on the tyramine content in foods were collected more than a decade ago. Recent changes in the processing of foods, more reliable methods of analysis, and development of more specific MAOIs currently undergoing clinical trials have prompted a reevaluation (9).

ACUTE TOXICITY

Acute poisoning with MAOIs is uncommon but potentially serious. In general, acute overdose produces effects that are extensions of common adverse reactions. Serious toxic symptoms rarely develop in less than 12 hours, and sometimes do not develop until 24 hours after an overdose, even though the MAOIs are rapidly absorbed from the gastrointestinal tract. During the latent phase after ingestion of an acute overdose, endogenous catecholamines accumulate in the brain and elsewhere as the result of MAO enzyme inhibition.

The pharmacologic basis for the delayed onset of toxic signs and symptoms after MAOI overdose is unclear. Initial reversible binding of the drugs to MAO, cumulative effects, or the time required to achieve significant enzyme inhibition with subsequent alterations of MAO substrate stores and metabolism may be responsible for delayed toxicity (1).

The overdose of a MAOI can induce a complex array of hypermetabolic signs, including hyperpyrexia, tachycardia, generalized muscle rigidity, tachypnea, metabolic acidosis, hypoxemia, and hypercapnia (Table 18–5) (16). An acute overdose of MAOI does not usually produce a hypertensive crisis unless the patient deliberately provokes the interaction.

TABLE 18–5. *Symptoms of acute MAOI intoxication*

Symptoms
Mild
Irritability
Anxiety
Flushing
Diaphoresis
Drowsiness
Dizziness
Ataxia
Moderate
Altered mental status
Hyperpyrexia
Hypertension
Tachycardia
Tachypnea
Severe
Severe hyperpyrexia
Seizures
Central nervous system depression
Coma
Cardiorespiratory depression
Malignant hyperthermia
Muscle rigidity

Early mild clinical features of poisoning may be consistent with neuromuscular hyperactivity and include irritability, anxiety, flushing, and sweating. Drowsiness, dizziness, and ataxia may also occur. In moderate intoxication, an altered mental status as well as hyperpyrexia, hypertension, tachycardia, and tachypnea may be noted (4). Severe intoxication may be characterized by CNS depression, coma, severe hyperpyrexia, and seizures. Although seizures may be grand mal type, myoclonus may also be noted. Decorticate or decerebrate rigidity may alternate with flaccid paralysis. Muscle rigidity may be so marked that respiration is seriously embarrassed. Dystonic-like reactions, including grimacing and writhing movements of the trunk and limbs, have also been described.

Malignant hyperthermia is also associated with MAOIs (13). The pathophysiologic abnormality appears to be an increase in sarcoplasmic concentrations of calcium ion, which leads to sustained contracture of the muscle, uncoupling of oxidative phosphorylation in the mitochondria, and accelerated glycolysis by activation of phosphorylase kinase.

LABORATORY ANALYSIS

Laboratory confirmation of MAOI overdose by drug assay is difficult because of the low concentrations of MAOIs in biologic samples and lack of availability of assay procedures.

TREATMENT

Supportive Care

Treatment for MAOI overdose consists mainly of supportive care as well as more specific therapy aimed at significant autonomic dysfunction (Table 18–6). Because there may be delayed and severe toxicity, monitoring of the patient in the intensive care unit is necessary for a full 24 hours (13,15).

Dietary precautions should be instituted, and medications should be prescribed cautiously. The rectal temperature should be monitored closely. If the patient presented in a timely fashion from the ingestion, the stomach should be emptied by gastric lavage. This should be followed with activated charcoal and a cathartic (16).

Mild to moderate CNS excitation and muscular irritability may be treated with diazepam. In addition, diazepam or phenytoin (or both) may be used if seizures develop. Sedative-hypnotic agents should be used with caution because they may potentiate the CNS depression that often develops later in the course. Narcotics also should be avoided because they may lead to exaggerated CNS and cardiorespiratory depression (4).

TABLE 18–6. *Treatment of MAOI overdose*

Condition	Treatment
Acute overdose	Supportive care Lavage Charcoal and cathartic Dietary precautions
Muscle irritability	Diazepam
Seizures	Diazepam Phenytoin
Hypertension	Phentolamine Sodium nitroprusside Labetalol
Hyperthermia	Antipyretic agents Cooling blankets Sponge baths Dantrolene Bromocriptine
Hypotension	Volume expansion Military antishock trousers Vasopressors
Cardiac dysrhythmias	Lidocaine Phenytoin Procainamide

Treatment of Hypertension

Various antihypertensive agents can be recommended. Phentolamine, an α-adrenergic blocking agent, has been used (13,15). Phentolamine may precipitate or exacerbate angina, tachyarrhythmias are common, and extreme gastrointestinal stimulation can be unpleasant (4). Nifedipine capsules chewed and placed under the tongue have also been effective and safe and have the advantage that the patient may begin therapy at the first sign of a reaction. Sodium nitroprusside may also be used. Labetalol, an antihypertensive agent that competitively inhibits both α- and β-adrenergic receptors, has also been suggested for treatment of the acute hypertension secondary to MAOI overdose (16). It may be administered intravenously in a dosage of 20 mg over 5 minutes. Because MAOI overdose may cause a sudden rapid fall in blood pressure, α blockers should be used cautiously.

Treatment of Hyperthermia

Antipyretic agents such as acetaminophen or salicylates, cool compresses, sponge baths, and hypothermic blankets may be effective treatment for mild to moderate hyperthermia (4). Dantrolene relaxes skeletal muscle directly to block heat production. This drug inhibits the release of calcium ions from the sarcoplasmic reticulum by action on transverse tubular membrane-sarcoplasmic reticulum coupling or by direct action on the sarcoplasmic reticulum. Dantrolene in a dose of 2.5 mg/kg can be administered intravenously every 6 hours for 24 hours (16). Bromocriptine, an ergot alkaloid and dopamine agonist, has also been used for hyperthermia and muscle rigidity (4).

Treatment of Hypotension

Hypotension unresponsive to volume expansion may be treated with military antishock trousers and vasopressors. A direct-acting α-adrenergic blocking agent is preferable to an indirect pressor because the former does not require the release of intracellular amines.

Treatment of Cardiac Dysrhythmias

Cardiac dysrhythmias are usually difficult to treat. Lidocaine, phenytoin, and procainamide appear to be safe choices for the treatment of ventricular tachydysrhythmias. Bretylium should be avoided. Atropine, epinephrine, and temporary pacing may be used to treat bradydysrhythmias.

Methods to Enhance Excretion

Although MAOI excretion is enhanced by urinary acidification, there is no evidence that forced acid diuresis is effective in reducing the severity of an overdose (4). The usefulness of extracorporeal measures such as hemodialysis or hemoperfusion in the treatment of MAOI overdose remains to be demonstrated.

SELEGILINE

Selegiline (Eldepryl), a selective MAOI, has recently been approved by the Food and Drug Administration as an adjunct to carbidopa/levodopa (Sinemet) therapy in the management of Parkinson's disease (8). It is indicated for patients who show deterioration in the quality of the response to carbidopa/levodopa. Under the name Deprenyl, selegiline has been in use for several years, mainly in Europe (17). In the United States, interest in selegiline increased after discovery of its ability to completely antagonize the effects of 1-methyl-4-phenyl-1,2,5,6-tetrahydropyridine (MPTP), a "designer drug" that causes the symptoms of Parkinson's disease (18).

MPTP is a protoxin that is converted to toxic derivatives by MAO that acts specifically in the substantia nigra to cause a Parkinson's-like syndrome in humans (19). MPTP may cause neuronal damage by free radical production. Blockage of the oxidation of MPTP by MAO-B inhibitors, such as selegiline, has a protective effect on MPTP-induced Parkinson's disease by inhibiting MAO-B, the enzyme that metabolizes dopamine, and thereby prolongs the action of dopamine (20). Normally, MAO-B converts MPTP to MPP+, a toxic metabolite (1). This step can be eliminated with the use of selegiline, thereby preventing toxicity from MPTP (8). By decreasing the breakdown of dopamine, selegiline also may act as an antioxidant with a resultant slowing of disease progression. Selegiline does not inhibit the oxidation of tyramine (19). Because selegiline primarily inhibits MAO-B, it is not associated with symptoms of sympathetic crisis (3). Therefore, selegiline in the currently recommended dose can be administered with L-dopa, and dietary restrictions are not necessary. In the typical dosages used in this disorder, between 5 and 15 mg per day, approximately 90% of MAO-B is inhibited. When daily doses exceed 20 mg, selegiline tends to lose selectivity for MAO-B and begins to inhibit MAO-A, thus increasing the risk of potentiating the cheese effect (18). Low (less than 15 mg) doses of deprenyl, although they have efficacy in Parkinson's disease, fail to produce clear antidepressant effects, and they are associated with an even more dangerous toxic interaction characterized by altered mental status, hyperpyrexia, and hyperreflexia when administered in combination with fluoxetine or meperidine (20). In daily doses of 30 mg or more, deprenyl inhibits both subtypes of MAO inhibitor and is an effective antidepressant (18).

Pharmacokinetics

Selegiline is rapidly absorbed from the gastrointestinal tract and readily crosses the blood–brain barrier. The duration of MAO-B inhibition in the brain is unknown (9). Selegiline is metabolized to *l*-amphetamine and *l*-methamphetamine, among other metabolites; the amphetamines apparently do not contribute to the drug's therapeutic effect, but may play a role in its toxicity (17). After oral administration of 5 mg, maximum plasma concentrations ranging from 33 to 45 ng/mL are attained in one half to 2 hours, with an elimination half-life of 40 hours (18). Peak blood levels occur 30 minutes to 2 hours after a single dose (17).

Adverse Effects

At the recommended dosage of 5 mg twice daily, selegiline has relatively few adverse effects. In patients receiving levodopa, selegiline may precipitate or exacerbate such effects as chorea, confusion, or hallucinations (9). These effects can usually be minimized by decreasing the dosage of levodopa (1).

No reports of interactions between selegiline and other drugs have emerged from the extensive clinical experience with this drug (18). Selegiline therapy is relatively free from major side effects. The most common adverse effects due to interaction with L-dopa are associated with dopaminergic excess because selegiline can effectively increase dopamine by inhibiting its metabolism. These include dyskinesia, hallucinations, confusion, agitation, anxiety, and dry mouth. These adverse effects frequently resolve when the dose of L-dopa is reduced. Selegiline has no effect on renal, hepatic, and cardiac function (18).

The main metabolites of selegiline are L-amphetamine and L-methamphetamine. The levo amphetamine derivative has 3 to 4 times less activity than the dextroamphetamine derivative (8). These do not contribute to the drug's efficacy but may cause insomnia or other amphetamine-like symptoms (18).

Selegiline appears to be a very safe drug, with its toxicity limited mainly to exacerbation of the adverse reactions of levodopa. If selegiline does induce levodopa side effects, they often become evident within the first 24 to 48 hours of its administration and will usually resolve in 1 to several days after reducing levodopa dosage (8).

REFERENCES

1. Tetrud J, Langston W: Protective and preventive therapeutic strategies: monoamine oxidase inhibitors. *Neurol Clin* 1992;10:541–552.
2. Stack C, Rogers P, Linter S: Monoamine oxidase inhibitors and anaesthesia: a review. *Br J Anaesth* 1988;60:222–227.
3. Wells D, Bjorksten A: Monoamine oxidase inhibitors revisited. *Can J Anaesth* 1989;36:64–74.
4. Linden C, Rumack B, Strehlke C, et al: Monoamine oxidase inhibitor overdose. *Ann Emerg Med* 1984;13:1137–1144.
5. Smookler S, Bermudez A: Hypertensive crisis resulting from an MAO inhibitor and an over-the-counter appetite suppressant. *Ann Emerg Med* 1982;11:482–484.
6. Brown C, Bryant S: Monoamine oxidase inhibitors: safety and efficacy issues. *Drug Intell Clin Pharm* 1988;22:232–235.
7. Jones A, Pare C, Nicholson W, et al: Brain amine concentrations after monoamine oxidase inhibitor administration. *Br Med J* 1972;1:17–19.
8. Koller W, Giron L: Selegiline HCl: selective MAO-type B inhibitor. *Neurology* 1990;40:58–60.
9. Schulz R, Antonin K, Hoffman E, et al: Tyramine kinetics and pressor sensitivity during monoamine oxidase inhibition by selegiline. *Clin Pharmacol Ther* 1989;46:528–536.
10. Youdim M, Aronson J, Blau K, et al: Tranylcypromine (Parnate) overdose: measurement of tranylcypromine concentrations and MAO inhibitory activity and identification of amphetamines in plasma. *Psychol Med* 1979;9:377–382.
11. Bieck P, Firkusny L, Schick C, et al: Monoamine oxidase inhibition by phenelzine and bromfaromine in healthy volunteers. *Clin Pharmacol Ther* 1989;45:260–269.
12. Blackwell B, Schmidt G: Drug interactions in psychopharmacology. *Pyschiatr Clin North Am* 1984;7:625–637.
13. Ciocatto E, Fagiano G, Bava G: Clinical features and treatment of overdosage of monoamine oxidase inhibitors and their interaction with other psychotropic drugs. *Resuscitation* 1972;1:69–72.
14. Kalaria R, Mitchell M, Harik S: Monoamine oxidases of the human brain and liver. *Brain* 1988;111:1441–1451.
15. Abrams J, Schulman P, White W: Successful treatment of a monoamine oxidase inhibitor–tyramine hypertensive emergency with intravenous labetalol. *N Engl J Med* 1985;305:52.
16. Kaplan R, Feinglass N, Webster W, et al: Phenelzine overdose treated with dantrolene sodium. *JAMA* 1986;255:642–644.
17. Calesnick B: Selegiline for Parkinson's disease. *Am Fam Physic* 1990;41:589–591.
18. Robin D: Selegiline in the treatment of Parkinson's disease. *Am J Med Sci* 1991;302:392–395.
19. Walsh R, Gladis M, Roose S, et al: Phenelzine vs placebo in 50 patients with bulimia. *Arch Gen Psychiatry* 1988;45:471–475.
20. Langston J: Selegiline as neuroprotective therapy in Parkinson's disease: concepts and controversies. *Neurology* 1990;40:61–69.

ADDITIONAL SELECTED REFERENCES

Henry J, Volans G: Psychoactive drugs. *Br Med J* 1984;289:1291–1294.

Pope H, Jonas J, Hudson J, et al: Toxic reactions to the combination of monoamine oxidase inhibitors and tryptophan. *Am J Psychiatry* 1985; 142:491–492.

Shepherd J: β-Adrenergic blockade in the treatment of MAOI self-poisoning. *Lancet* 1974;2:1021.

CHAPTER 19

Lithium

Lithium ion is a monovalent alkali metal cation that is chemically similar to other monovalent cations, such as sodium and potassium (1), and that sometimes acts like a divalent cation, such as magnesium and calcium (2,3). Lithium has no known physiologic function and is present only in trace amounts in the body (4). As a metallic ion, lithium is not metabolized (5). The term as used in this chapter refers to the nonprotein-bound lithium ions or lithium salts (6).

Lithium is one of the oldest and most effective psychotropic drugs (4,7–9). and is administered exclusively by the oral route. Lithium is available in the U.S. in three forms. The standard formulation and the most common lithium product is lithium carbonate, which contains 8.12 mEq of lithium per 300-mg tablet or capsule. This salt is the most common because it is the most stable (10) and has the highest concentration of lithium suitable for tablets or capsules. Lithium citrate contains 8.12 mEq of lithium per 5 cc and is primarily used by patients in institutions who are unable or unwilling to swallow tablets or capsules. It is not as frequently used (11). Slow-release lithium carbonate is available in two forms. The sustained-release preparations (Lithobid) are useful for those patients who cannot tolerate large differences in peak and trough lithium levels (12). The salt of citrate is available as a liquid. Other lithium salts include the chloride, sulfate, gluconate, glutamate, and acetate, although these are not used to any great extent (Table 19–1).

TABLE 19–1. *Lithium compounds*

Lithium carbonate
Eskalith
Lithonate
Lithane
Lithotabs
Lithobid
Lithium citrate
Cibalith-S

USES

As early as 1871 lithium was prescribed as an effective treatment for manic-depressive disorder. In the past, lithium was also used as a salt substitute but was removed from the market after deaths were attributed to its consumption (9,13). Lithium bromide was once used as a hypnotic and sedative (14). In 1949 it was again discovered that lithium was useful as treatment for manic-depressive psychoses because it terminates the manic and hypomanic phases of this bipolar affective disorder (14,15). It is still considered the treatment of choice for this disorder and is also used for prophylaxis (1,16). Furthermore, there is evidence that some patients with major depressive disorders show an antidepressant response to lithium (14,17). Lithium may also be therapeutic in a diverse group of clinical problems, including premenstrual syndrome, neutropenia, cluster headaches, and certain movement disorders (18).

Affective illness is divided into two subtypes: unipolar and bipolar. A bipolar psychosis is characterized by both manic and depressive episodes in the same person, and unipolar psychosis is characterized by more recurrent depressions and fewer recurrent manic states (19). Lithium exerts a true and specific antimanic action in that euphoria, expansiveness of mood, overactivity, flight of ideas, and other symptoms of mania are suppressed (20).

PHARMACOKINETICS

The pharmacokinetics of lithium is of particular interest because lithium is not bound to plasma proteins, lipid, or tissue. Lithium is not metabolized but is almost entirely eliminated in urine. Although lithium has a volume of distribution of 0.7 L/kg, which is about the same as that of total body water, it is not distributed evenly throughout the water phase (21). The initial distribution of lithium has a half-life of 6 hours but lithium has an elimination half-life of up to 24 hours (22). This is critical to understanding differences between acute and chronic toxicity.

Lithium is a highly water-soluble ion that is well absorbed from the gastrointestinal tract. Absorption is complete within 8 hours, with peak serum levels in 1 to 3 hours after a therapeutic oral dose (1). Slow-release preparations peak at 4 to 12 hours. Absorption can also be significantly delayed in an acute overdose (23). Because in some respects it is distributed in a fashion similar to that of sodium and potassium, it shares some of the properties of extracellular sodium and intracellular potassium with some important differences (1).

Lithium is initially distributed into extracellular fluid and then gradually accumulates in varying amounts in tissues. Lithium crosses cell boundaries at a relatively slow rate. This slow entry into and exit from the intracellular space accounts for the delay of 6 to 10 days in achieving a full therapeutic response to lithium (3,14,24) and also accounts for the lag in onset of symptoms in the acute overdose (16).

Because the main route of lithium excretion is through the kidneys, its elimination in the urine is of decisive importance for the safe use of this drug. One third to two thirds of a dose is cleared in the urine within 6 to 12 hours, the remainder being excreted over 10 to 14 days. This prolonged excretion pattern may be related to tissue storage (25). There is a prolongation of the half-life due to decreased renal excretion in patients with renal impairment (2). In addition, the aging kidney, which has a reduced number of functioning nephrons, has an impaired ability to excrete lithium, and furthermore the drug may injure the kidney. Of equal importance is the maintenance of normal salt and fluid intake when this drug is administered.

MECHANISM OF ACTION

The action mechanism of lithium is not fully understood. It may act by at least two nonindependent mechanisms: (a) as an imperfect substitute for other monovalent or divalent cations such as sodium, potassium, or magnesium in basic ion-transport mechanisms that affect cellular membrane properties, or (b) by altering the cellular microenvironment by interfering with hormonal activation of adenyl cyclase, which then reduces the concentration of cyclic AMP, or by interfering with the effect of cyclic AMP (26).

Lithium is also thought to inhibit the release of norepinephrine and serotonin, to increase reuptake of norepinephrine, and possibly to increase synthesis and turnover rate of serotonin (1).

SIDE EFFECTS

Although lithium is widely acknowledged as an effective and specific therapy for bipolar affective disorders, its therapeutic index is notoriously low (9,11). Lithium intoxication is a dose-related phenomenon that occurs when more lithium is ingested than can be excreted. Lithium intoxication is a potentially serious condition that can lead to death or permanent disability (9).

TABLE 19–2. *Side effects from lithium therapy*

Neurologic
Cerebellar
Incoordination
Dysarthria
Ataxia
Nystagmus
Dysphoria
Slowed reaction time
Lack of spontaneity
Tremor of hands
Gastrointestinal
Abdominal pain
Diarrhea
Irritation
Nausea
Vomiting
Renal
Acute renal failure
Incomplete renal tubular acidosis
Nephrogenic diabetes insipidus
Nephrotic syndrome
Polydipsia
Polyuria
Cutaneous
Folliculitis
Pretibial ulcerations
Psoriasis
Acne
Hormonal (elderly patients)
Antidiuretic hormone
Growth hormone
Luteinizing hormone
Parathyroid hormone
Testosterone
Thyroid-stimulating hormone
Thyrotropin-stimulating hormone
Miscellaneous
Cardiac rhythm disturbances (rare)

Three main types of unwanted lithium effects can be distinguished: (a) transient effects at low serum concentrations; (b) permanent side effects at low serum concentrations; and (c) toxic effects from an acute or chronic overdose. The first type is represented by transient minor side effects occurring at the beginning of therapy at low serum concentrations. These effects take place primarily in three physiologic systems: the neurologic and neuromuscular, gastrointestinal, and renal systems (Table 19–2).

Neurologic

Neurologic symptoms include cerebellar malfunctions such as incoordination, dysarthria, and ataxia. Lithium has been reported as a cause of nystagmus. The most common form is horizontal gaze-evoked nystagmus, although downbeat nystagmus has also been noted (11).

The majority of patients suffer side effects at therapeutic doses, although most classify them as mild. Neurologic side effects of dysphoria, slowed reaction time, lack of spontaneity, and intellectual inefficiency are common complaints early in the course of treatment. These symptoms will often resolve spontaneously or improve with a decreased dosage. A tremor of the hands is the most frequent adverse side effect and may fluctuate with anxiety (11). The tremor is more severe in patients with essential tremor or in those treated with other antipsychotic medications (11).

Gastrointestinal

Gastrointestinal symptoms include gastric irritation, abdominal pain, nausea, vomiting, and diarrhea and are common side effects seen also with the initiation of lithium therapy. These symptoms are usually transient; however, they may be the first sign of toxic reactions in patients receiving long-term therapy (25).

Renal

The kidneys provide the only route of lithium excretion, and reductions in glomerular filtration rate and/or enhanced proximal tubular reabsorption promote lithium retention that may result in toxicity. Therefore, lithium has the potential to impair its own excretion, with increased risk of toxic serum concentrations (2,27).

Renal side effects may be nephrogenic diabetes insipidus with polyuria and polydipsia. This occurs because lithium reduces the effect of antidiuretic hormone on the collecting tubule cell. Other renal disorders include inappropriate salt wasting, incomplete distal renal tubular acidosis, nephrotic syndrome, and acute renal failure (15,28).

Cutaneous

Many cutaneous side effects have also been associated with lithium therapy. These include folliculitis, pretibial ulcerations, psoriasis, and acne. These symptoms are inconvenient rather than dangerous (29–31).

The permanent side effects represent minor but persistent findings at low serum concentrations. The most dangerous side effects are from lithium intoxication or poisoning associated with an accumulation of lithium to serum concentrations greater than 1.5 mEq/L.

Cardiovascular

Cardiovascular symptoms are uncommon from therapeutic levels of lithium (32). Conduction and rhythm abnormalities are rare and may be secondary to an underlying cardiac disease, or the use of cardiac drugs. Sinus node dysfunction has been reported in association with therapeutic lithium levels and has resolved after discontinuation of therapy.

Hormonal

Elderly patients taking lithium for recurrent affective disorder are at more risk of toxicity and possibly myxedema than are younger patients (32). Thyroid function tests before initiation of therapy and periodic monitoring during lithium therapy in elderly patients are necessary (33). Thyroid-stimulating hormone, testosterone, luteinizing hormone, thyrotropin-releasing hormone, antidiuretic hormone, growth hormone, and parathyroid hormone have been found to be affected by lithium therapy (12). When stimulated by lithium, parathyroid hormone increases the serum calcium and lowers the serum phosphorus (27).

LITHIUM INTOXICATION

Lithium intoxication can result from acute overdose or from a long-term nonpurposeful accumulation (34). This may be secondary to decreased excretion of lithium in a patient receiving optimum subtoxic therapeutic doses who is experiencing reduced sodium or water intake or concurrent illness (35,36). Most poisonings have occurred over weeks to months of intake, not from episodes of single ingestion (9).

The clinical course of lithium overdose is influenced by the drug's distribution kinetics. Although the volume of distribution of lithium is equal to or a little greater than the total water volume, the tissue distribution of lithium is delayed and varies with the different organs: lithium diffusion is fast for the liver and the kidneys but slow for the brain, in which equilibrium with serum concentration is reached after 8 or 10 days (21). This slow rate of distribution explains the observation that, after an acute overdose, the severity of intoxication does not correlate well with serum concentrations: patients may be asymptomatic with relatively high serum concentrations (3). In patients who become intoxicated during the course of long-term administration of lithium, there is a better correlation between serum lithium concentrations and the onset of neurologic signs. Routine monitoring of serum lithium levels therefore can reduce the incidence of lithium intoxication but will not prevent serious sequelae from acute overdoses.

There are three basic types of lithium overdosage: acute, chronic, and a mixed acute and chronic presentation. Symptoms associated with both acute and chronic toxicity are very similar but the dramatic nature of their onset is the primary difference. Acute overdoses, in the absence of other co-ingestants, manifest toxicity after sufficient distribution of the lithium has occurred. In chronic cases, subacute intoxication insidiously progresses to a toxidrome of characteristic mental, neurologic, and gastrointestinal signs and symptoms (37).

Acute Intoxication

In general, acute ingestions are not as severe as the chronic and mixed varieties but no case of lithium intoxication should be looked upon complacently. In acute poisoning, the peak cerebrospinal fluid levels may be delayed for up to 24 hours, accounting for the lack of symptoms in the presence of extraordinarily high serum levels. Presumably, this is due to slow attainment of equilibrium of lithium between the serum and central nervous system (CNS). Also, with severe intoxication, symptoms commonly progress despite dramatic reductions in serum lithium concentrations (25).

In the acute overdose, slow intracellular diffusion may protect the patient from severe adverse reactions for a number of hours. Also, the lithium blood concentration may continue to rise for up to 1 week after absorption (38). Symptoms rarely occur quickly, even when massive doses are ingested (14). A common scenario is that of a patient who is initially alert and oriented with a normal urine output but whose condition deteriorates within 24 to 48 hours to a critical state.

Acutely poisoned patients usually present with GI symptoms (Table 19–3) (23). The immediate high concentration of lithium in the stomach often induces vomiting within 1 hour of ingestion, but as lithium is rapidly absorbed significant amounts can still reach the circulation (5).

The acute neurologic effects of lithium may last for days to weeks and may be followed by persistent sequelae. Most frequently, these include cerebellar signs such as dysarthria, tremor, rigidity, and increased deep tendon reflexes. Long-lasting choreoathetosis, nystagmus, and ataxia suggest damage to the basal ganglia. Deficits in short-term memory may also be permanent (39). Impairment of neurologic deficits usually occurs within 6 to 12 months, but significant improvement after this period is rare.

Chronic Intoxication

Chronic lithium poisoning is likely to be more common than acute intentional poisoning episodes, and is underreported because it may not be recognized, has an insidious onset, and may be assumed to be part of the underlying psychological illness.

The most common mode of lithium overdose results from weeks to months of ingestion of maintenance therapy. The diagnosis may therefore be difficult (33). In addition, various factors enter into chronic intoxication. Conditions affecting fluid and electrolyte balance, such as gastroenteritis or vomiting from any cause, diuretic treatment, dietary intake low in sodium, and decreased fluid intake, commonly precede intoxication (Table 19–4). In the presence of sodium deficiency secondary to vomiting, diarrhea, diuretics, or low-salt diet, volume contraction occurs. Under these conditions, the lithium ion is selectively reabsorbed in the renal tubules and may accumulate to toxic levels. A cycle is then set up that further exacerbates both the lithium toxicity and renal insufficiency (40).

Certain drugs decrease the clearance of lithium (Table 19–5). Diuretics such as hydrochlorothiazide act in this manner, as do the prostaglandin inhibitors such as aspirin, indomethacin, and other nonsteroidal anti-inflammatory drugs.

TABLE 19–3. *Signs and symptoms of acute lithium intoxication*

Delay in onset of symptoms of
Nausea
Vomiting
Dysarthria
Tremor
Muscle rigidity
Decreased deep tendon reflexes
Long-lasting effects include
Choreoathetosis
Nystagmus
Ataxia
Short-term memory loss

TABLE 19–4. *Conditions affecting lithium toxicity*

Decreased elimination and increased toxicity
Fluid and electrolyte imbalance
Gastroenteritis
Diuretic therapy
Vomiting
Low sodium intake
Decreased fluid intake
Concurrent drug therapy (see Table 19–5)
Increased elimination and decreased therapeutic concentrations
Acute phase of therapy
Increased sodium intake
Concurrent drug therapy (see Table 19–5)

TABLE 19–5. *Medications that can alter lithium elimination*

Decreased elimination and increased toxicity
Diuretics
Chlorthalidone (Hygroton)
Furosemide (Lasix)
Spironolactone (Aldactone)
Hydrochlorothiazide (HydroDIURIL)
Nonsteroidal anti-inflammatory agents
Ibuprofen (Motrin, Ruten, Advil)
Indomethacin (Indocin)
Phenylbutazone (Butazolidin)
Salicylates
Antihypertensives
Methyldopa (Aldomet)
Antipsychotics
Haloperidol (Haldol)
Thioridazine
Miscellaneous
Carbamazepine (Tegretol)
Phenytoin (Dilantin)
Tetracyclines
Increased elimination and decreased therapeutic concentrations
Xanthines
Aminophylline
Caffeine
Theophylline
Chlorpromazine (Thorazine)
Osmotic diuretics

The prodromes of chronic intoxication are mainly gastrointestinal and cerebrovascular, and precede full intoxication by several days to 1 week. Mild reactions that may be associated with serum concentrations between 1.5 and 2.0 mEq/L are nausea, vomiting, diarrhea, malaise, drowsiness, muscular weakness, thirst, polyuria, polydipsia, fatigue, fine hand tremor, and mild incoordination (Table 19–6). Some of these symptoms may be confused with the spontaneous advent of a depressive phase of a manic disorder.

When serum concentrations reach 2.0 to 2.5 mEq/L, anorexia, blurred vision, slurred speech, dryness of the mouth, abdominal pain, weight loss, lethargy, dizziness, and nystagmus may occur. Moderate to severe toxic reactions that are usually associated with serum concentrations of 2.5 to 3.0 mEq/L include ataxia, hyperactive deep tendon reflexes, choreoathetoid movements (16), seizures, confusion, syncope, and electrocardiographic changes (24,38). Most investigators believe that lithium cardiotoxic effects are related to cation shifts with intracellular lithium ion accumulation, which prevents potassium from reentering the cell (32). The intracellular potassium depletion prolongs the repolarization period. T wave flattening has been the electrocardiographic abnormality reported most commonly with lithium therapy (41). These changes are usually reversible, occurring within 5 days of starting treatment and disappearing within 3 to 5 days of discontinuation. Their clinical significance, if any, is unclear. First-degree atrioventricular block has also been reported (42).

TABLE 19–6. *Signs of lithium intoxication*

Mild (serum concentration, 1.5 to 2.0 mEq/L)
Neurologic
Malaise
Drowsiness
Weakness
Fine hand tremor
Mild incoordination
Sedation
Confusion
Gastrointestinal
Anorexia
Nausea
Vomiting
Diarrhea
Thirst
Metabolic
Polyuria
Moderate (serum concentration, 2.0 to 2.5 mEq/L)
Neurologic
Blurred vision
Slurred speech
Lethargy
Dizziness
Nystagmus
Gastrointestinal
Dryness of mouth
Abdominal pain
Weight loss
Moderate to severe (serum concentration, 2.5 to 3.0 mEq/L)
Neurologic
Ataxia
Increased deep tendon reflexes
Choreoathetosis
Seizures
Confusion
Dysarthria
Restlessness
Syncope
Cardiac
EKG changes
T wave flattening
First-degree AV block
Severe (serum concentration, more than 3.0 mEq/L)
Generalized seizures
Oliguria
Circulatory failure
Coma
Death

Patients with moderate to severe lithium intoxication are frequently azotemic but rarely experience overt renal failure. Very severe adverse reactions associated with concentrations of more than 3.0 mEq/L include generalized seizures (43), oliguria, acute circulatory failure, stupor, coma, irreversible brain damage, and death.

Long-Term Sequelae

In chronic poisoning, the patient may remain unresponsive long after serum levels have dissipated to the

TABLE 19–7. *Persistent sequelae from lithium intoxication*

Basal ganglia damage
Dysarthria
Spasticity
Tremor
Cerebellar damage
Ataxia
Nystagmus
Dementia
Polyuria

normal therapeutic range due to the persistence of lithium in the cerebrospinal fluid. Lithium intoxication can therefore result in persistent neurologic sequelae including dementia, cerebellar ataxia, polyuria, dysarthria, spasticity, nystagmus, and tremor. Permanent damage of the basal ganglia and cerebellar connections, despite effective lowering of lithium concentration by hemodialysis, has also been noted (Table 19–7) (44).

LABORATORY DETERMINATIONS

The initial laboratory examination should include a coma screen, measurements of serum lithium concentration, serum electrolytes, blood urea nitrogen, creatinine, a complete blood count, calcium, magnesium, an electrocardiogram, and urinalysis (Table 19–8) (24,41). It has been found that a markedly elevated serum lithium concentration is associated with a reduced anion gap (45). This may be a helpful clue to the diagnosis in the comatose patient with no history of ingested substance. Electrocardiographic changes are nonspecific and may include a reversible flattening or inversion of the T waves, first-degree atrioventricular block, and sinus node dysfunction (46).

Serum Lithium Concentrations

Lithium concentrations are most frequently determined by flame photometry or atomic absorption spectrometry (12). A steady-state lithium concentration in the range of 0.8 to 1.2 mEq/L is considered therapeutic (11,14,24). Somewhat lower serum concentrations, between 0.6 and 1.0 mEq/L, are necessary for prophylaxis. Clinical response to lithium, however, varies from patient to patient, and a good response may be seen at serum concentrations less than 0.5 mEq/L (29). The categorization of degree of toxicity based on serum lithium levels is only a rough guide, as there is often a poor correlation between the level and the severity of symptoms (12). Patients on chronic therapy can have large intracellular stores of lithium that may not be reflected by the serum lithium level, and it is probably the intracellular concentration of lithium that results in its therapeutic and toxic effects. True toxicity seldom occurs below 1.5 mEq/L. Serum lithium concentrations of 1.5 to 2.5 mEq/L often indicate slight to moderate intoxication; concentrations of 2.5 to 3.5 mEq/L often indicate severe intoxication. Concentrations greater than 4.0 mEq/L often indicate potentially lethal intoxication (Table 19–6).

A single 300-mg dose of lithium carbonate or 600-mg dose of a sustained-release preparation can be expected to raise the serum concentration by 0.2 to 0.4 mEq/L (10) in a 70-kg person. This relation does not always hold true, however, and serum concentrations may not necessarily coincide with the severity of the clinical symptoms. The concentration may be in the normal range and still be associated with clinical toxicity, especially in the acute overdose. Thus, the relation between serum concentration and toxicity is only an indirect one because toxicity depends on the intracellular concentration. In some cases of lithium intoxication, the patient's condition can worsen to the point of death while the lithium serum levels are diminishing.

The therapeutic range is based on drawing the blood sample 12 hours after the last dose of lithium. Serum levels drawn significantly earlier or later are of limited value because of the elimination and distribution characteristics of lithium (12).

TABLE 19–8. *Laboratory determinations for lithium overdose*

Blood urea nitrogen
Calcium
Complete blood count
Creatinine
Electrocardiogram
Magnesium
Serum electrolytes
Anion gap
Serum lithium concentration
Toxicology screen
Urinalysis

TREATMENT

The severe and sometimes persistent effects of lithium underline the importance of both rapid and adequate treatment of lithium toxicity and also prevention by good education for patients and their families concerning the signs and symptoms of incipient intoxication (22).

The management of lithium intoxication is still controversial (Table 19–9). Because there is no specific treatment, it is largely supportive and depends on the patient's clinical condition and the serum lithium concentration. General supportive measures consist of maintaining blood pressure and airway and correcting dehydration and electrolyte imbalance. At the same time, care must be taken to avoid iatrogenic fluid and electrolyte disorders (24). Mere withdrawal of the drug does not always prevent serious complications or death.

TABLE 19–9. *Treatment of lithium intoxication*

Discontinue drug
Prevent further absorption (acute ingestion)
Gastric lavage (acute ingestion)
Charcoal and cathartic (acute ingestion)
Whole bowel irrigation (acute ingestion)
Institute supportive measures
Correct fluid and electrolyte losses
Hemodialysis
Controversial treatments
Forced saline diuresis
Aminophylline
Alkaline diuresis
Diuretics

Even though all patients with very elevated serum lithium levels do not suffer severe morbidity, procedures that promote excretion of lithium should be initiated early to prevent CNS toxicity and possible renal failure.

Supportive Care

In the acute ingestion, gastric lavage is necessary and should be followed by administration of activated charcoal and a cathartic. Charcoal is not of value in adsorbing electrically charged drugs such as lithium; however, it should be given to adsorb other drugs that may have been in the possession of patients with psychiatric disorders (3). Those patients chronically intoxicated with lithium will not benefit from this procedure (33).

Although lithium is usually rapidly absorbed, both sustained-release tablets and the large amounts of lithium ingested in overdose can significantly delay absorption (23). Whole bowel irrigation (WBI) has been suggested as a way of decontaminating the gut after a significant overdose. It has been stated that overdose of lithium is ideally suited to management with WBI because it is often sustained-release and because lithium is not adsorbed by charcoal (47,48). WBI may not be of as much benefit for ingestions of standard lithium preparations. Sodium polystyrene sulfonate, a cation exchange resin, has been investigated as an agent that might decrease the gastrointestinal absorption of lithium (49,50). There are no conclusions that can be made concerning this agent at this time (51,52).

Because more than half the lithium in the body is excreted within 24 hours, discontinuing the drug in many instances may be the only action required. Recovery takes place gradually over 4 to 5 days in uncomplicated cases. Mild intoxication usually responds to this therapy along with correction of fluid and electrolyte abnormalities. Since virtually all patients are dehydrated or sodium depleted, normal saline can be given until the intravascular volume is repleted. This is necessary even in elderly patients who may have poor cardiac reserve. However, once the glomerular filtration rate is normalized, the beneficial effects of sodium administration on the lithium ion clearance diminish. Because more than 98% of ingested lithium is excreted in the urine, patients with serum lithium concentrations less than 2.5 mEq/L who are not stuporous and have relatively well-maintained neurologic functioning can be initially treated with rapid intravenous infusion of normal saline in an attempt to rehydrate the patient and prevent hyponatremia. Sodium loading increases the sodium content of the glomerular filtrate. This is presumably then reabsorbed in preference to lithium in the proximal convoluted tubule (33).

Forced saline diuresis, aminophylline, sodium bicarbonate, urea, acetazolamide, and furosemide have all been recommended in the treatment of mild to moderate lithium toxicity (3). There are no controlled studies that have demonstrated clinical improvement from any of these treatment modalities (24,53).

Although diuresis had been suggested for increasing the clearance of lithium, it may be that forced diuresis is not actually attained but rather that large amounts of fluid merely rehydrate the patient. The glomerular filtration rate and the lithium clearance are restored through rehydration rather than through an acceleration of the usual renal clearance (8,9).

Acutely overdosed or chronically toxic patients who do not initially appear to need dialysis should be maintained on normal saline infusion to correct hypovolemia, to guarantee good urine output, and to allow elimination of lithium.

Hemodialysis (Table 19–10)

Hemodialysis is now accepted as the treatment of choice for serum lithium concentrations in excess of 3.5 mmol/L or in a clinically unstable patient (7,34). Lithium is easily removed by dialysis, but because of its slow movement between compartments its intracellular concentration falls slowly, and serum concentrations may rise after dialysis as further lithium moves out of the intracellular compartment (21). Dialysis is the only treatment modality that consistently and effectively increases lithium clearance. Peritoneal dialysis clears 15 mL/min, in addition to any renal clearance, whereas hemodialysis clears 50 mL/min (54). Due to the redistribution of lithium from tissues, prolonged and repeated dialysis is required to prevent serum lithium levels from rising (5).

TABLE 19–10. *Dialysis and lithium treatment*

Acute toxicity
Prevents lithium entry into the brain
Decreases onset of severe toxicity
Chronic toxicity
Enhances elimination of lithium from brain
Lengthy dialysis

Because lithium is located in the extracellular space, its concentrations in plasma can be lowered rapidly by dialysis. Although hemodialysis is the treatment of choice in severe lithium intoxication, patients who have taken a single acute overdose must be distinguished from those who have been taking the drug on a long-term basis. In the acute overdose, hemodialysis prevents lithium diffusion into the brain and the onset of severe toxicity (5). In the long-term overdose, hemodialysis enhances elimination of lithium from brain but must be continued for a long period of time.

Hemodialysis significantly increases serum lithium clearance. However, simply removing lithium from the serum does not guarantee clinical improvement. In fact, in some patients, neurologic status deteriorates as lithium levels fall. Because lithium crosses cell membranes and the blood–brain barrier slowly, intracellular lithium can cause continued toxicity despite falling levels in the serum. After dialysis is completed, lithium levels may rebound as the intracellular lithium equilibrates with the extracellular fluid. Hence, repeated dialysis may be needed (7,21,23). The reason is that, even though lithium is distributed throughout body water, as the extracellular concentration falls rapidly with removal, the intracellular concentration is still high and takes longer to equilibrate, hence a rebound effect. A plasma lithium concentration less than 1 mEq/L 6 to 8 hours after cessation of dialysis has been considered evidence of adequate treatment (9,55).

Indications for Dialysis (Table 19–11)

It is best not to settle on rigid criteria but instead to base an informed decision concerning hemodialysis on the patient's condition, serum lithium level, the time since the ingestion, and whether it is an acute or chronic episode. Although the usefulness of dialysis is controversial, it should be performed if the serum lithium concentration is between 2.0 and 4.0 mEq/L and the patient's clinical condition is poor or if the serum concentration is greater than 4 mEq/L regardless of the patient's condition (3,24,56). Hemodialysis may need to be carried out for 8 to 12 hours because of the large tissue storage pool of lithium (41) and should be repeated 6 to 8 hours later if indicated. Because blood concentrations may rise for some time after an acute overdose, and because clinical symptoms may worsen during this time, some patients who do not initially appear to be ill may require dialysis after 2 to 3 days of hospitalization. Current recommendations state that hemodialysis should be continued until lithium concentrations are consistently below 1 mEq/L after equilibrium has been established (22).

Hemodialysis only removes lithium from the extracellular compartment. Because lithium partitions into the intracellular space, it will not be removed from that compartment. For this reason, one should not expect dramatic neurologic recovery during or immediately after hemodialysis. Multiple runs of dialysis may be necessary to deplete intracellular lithium (54).

Intensive care monitoring should be considered in all patients with severe toxic reactions. This measure is indicated in the presence of cardiac dysrhythmias, obtundation, or difficulty with fluid and electrolyte management.

TABLE 19–11. *Indications for hemodialysis*

Based on		
Condition of patient		
Serum lithium level		
Time since ingestion		
Acute versus chronic ingestion		
Lithium level	Patient condition	Dialysis
2.0–4.0 mEq/L	Poor[a]	Yes
>4.0 mEq/L	Normal	Yes
Long dialysis may be necessary		
Repeat dialysis may be necessary		
Rebound phenomenon may occur		

[a]Cardiac dysrhythmias, CNS depression, and abnormalities in fluid and electrolytes

REFERENCES

1. Heng M: Lithium carbonate toxicity. *Arch Dermatol* 1982;118: 246–248.
2. Myers J, Morgan T, Carney S, et al: Effects of lithium on the kidney. *Kidney Int* 1980;18:601–608.
3. Goldfrank L, Flomenbaum N, Weisman R: Management of overdose with psychoactive medications. *Emerg Med Clin North Am* 1984; 2:63–76.
4. Murray J: Lithium therapy for mania and depression. *J Gen Psychol* 1984;112:5–33.
5. Amdisen A: Clinical features and management of lithium poisoning. *Med Toxicol* 1988;3:18–32.
6. Sansone M, Ziegler D: Lithium toxicity: a review of neurologic complications. *Clin Neuropharmacol* 1985;8:242–248.
7. Fenves A, Emmett M, While M: Lithium intoxication associated with acute renal failure. *South Med J* 1984;77:1472–1473.
8. Hansen H: Renal toxicity of lithium. *Drugs* 1981;22:461–476.
9. Hansen H, Amdisen A: Lithium intoxication. *Q J Med* 1978;47: 123–144.
10. Saran B, Gaind R: Lithium. *Clin Toxicol* 1973;6:257–269.
11. Lesar T, Tollefson G: Lithium therapy. *Postgrad Med J* 1984; 75:269–286.
12. Frings C: Lithium monitoring. *Clin Lab Med* 1987;7:545–550.
13. Doyal L, Morton W: The clinical usefulness of lithium as an antidepressant. *Hosp Commun Psychol* 1984;35:685–691.
14. DePaulo J: Lithium. *Psychiatr Clin North Am* 1984;7:587–599.
15. Bear R, Sugar L, Paul M: Nephrotic syndrome and renal failure secondary to lithium carbonate therapy. *Can Med Assoc J* 1985; 132:735–736.
16. Cohen W, Cohen N: Lithium carbonate, haloperidol, and irreversible brain damage. *JAMA* 1974;230:1283–1287.
17. Campbell M, Perry R, Green W: Use of lithium in children and adolescents. *Psychosomatics* 1984;25:96–106.
18. Potter W, Rudorfer M, Manji H: The pharmacologic treatment of depression. *N Engl J Med* 1991;325:633–642.
19. Cole J: The drug treatment of anxiety and depression. *Med Clin North Am* 1988;72:815–830.
20. Corbett J, Jacobson D, Thompson H, et al: Downbeating nystagmus

and other ocular motor defects caused by lithium toxicity. *Neurology* 1989;39:481–487.
21. Jaeger A, Sauder P, Kopferschmitt J, et al: Toxicokinetics of lithium intoxication treated by hemodialysis. *Clin Toxicol* 1986;23:501–517.
22. Tinter R: Lithium intoxication. *Br Med J* 1991;302:1267–1269.
23. Krishel S, Jackimczyk K: Cyclic antidepressants, lithium, and neuroleptic agents. *Emerg Med Clin North Am* 1991;9:53–86.
24. Mateer J, Clark M: Lithium toxicity with rarely reported ECG manifestations. *Ann Emerg Med* 982;11:208–211.
25. Simard M, Gumbiner B, Lee A, et al: Lithium carbonate intoxication: a case report and review of the literature. *Arch Intern Med* 1989; 149:36–46.
26. Fyro B, Petterson U, Sedvall G: The effect of lithium treatment on manic symptoms and levels of monoamine metabolites in cerebrospinal fluid of manic-depressive patients. *Psychopharmacologia* 1975;44:99–103.
27. Rose S, Klein-Schwartz W, Oderda G, et al: Lithium intoxication with acute renal failure and death. *Drug Intell Clin Pharm* 1988; 22:691–694.
28. Kalina K, Burnett G: Lithium and the nephrotic syndrome. *J Clin Psychopharmacol* 1984;4:148–150.
29. Hwang S, Tuason V: Long-term maintenance lithium therapy and possible irreversible renal damage. *J Clin Psychiatry* 1980;41:11–19.
30. Schou M: Lithium in psychiatric therapy and prophylaxis. *J Psychiatr Res* 1968;6:67–95.
31. Schou M, Amdisen A, Trap-Jensen J: Lithium poisoning. *Am J Psychiatry* 1968;125:112–116.
32. Brady H, Horgan J: Lithium and the heart: unanswered questions. *Chest* 1988;93:166–169.
33. Santiago R, Rashkin M: Lithium toxicity and myxedema coma in an elderly woman. *J Emerg Med* 1990;8:63–66.
34. Jacobsen D, Aasen G, Frederichsen P, et al: Lithium intoxication: pharmacokinetics during and after terminated hemodialysis in acute intoxications. *Clin Toxicol* 1987;25:81–94.
35. Demers R, Heninger G: Pretibial edema and sodium retention during lithium carbonate treatment. *JAMA* 1970;214:1845–1848.
36. Demers R, Rivenbark J: Lithium intoxication and its clinical management. *South Med J* 1982;75:738–739.
37. Smith S, Ling L, Halstenson C: Whole-bowel irrigation as a treatment for acute lithium overdose. *Ann Emerg Med* 1991;20:536–539.
38. Kondziela J: Extreme lithium intoxication without severe symptoms. *Hosp Commun Psychol* 1984;35:727–728.
39. Bosse G, Arnold T: Overdose with sustained-release lithium preparations. *J Emerg Med* 1992;10:719–721.
40. Gelenberg A, Kane J, Keller M, et al: Comparison of standard and low serum levels of lithium for maintenance treatment of bipolar disorder. *N Engl J Med* 1989;321:1489–1493.
41. Sugarman J: Management of lithium intoxication. *J Family Pract* 1984;18:237–239.
42. Martin C, Piascik M: First-degree A-V block in patients on lithium carbonate. *Can J Psychiatry* 1985;30:114–116.
43. Massey E, Folger W: Seizures activated by therapeutic levels of lithium carbonate. *South Med J* 1984;77:1173–1175.
44. Bejar J: Cerebellar degeneration due to acute lithium toxicity. *Clin Neuropharmacol* 1985;8:379–381.
45. Kelleher S, Raciti A, Arbert J: Reduced or absent serum anion gap as a marker of severe lithium carbonate intoxication. *Arch Intern Med* 1986;146:1839–1840.
46. Montalescot Y, Levy Y, Farge D, et al: Lithium causing a serious sinus node dysfunction at therapeutic doses. *Clin Cardiol* 1984;7:617–620.
47. Favin F, Klein-Schwartz W, Oderda G, et al: In vitro study of lithium carbonate adsorption by activated charcoal. *J Toxicol Clin Toxicol* 1988;26:443–450.
48. Smith S, Ling L, Halstenson C: Whole-bowel irrigation as a treatment for acute lithium overdose. *Ann Emerg Med* 1991;20:536–539.
49. Belanger D, Tierney M, Dickinson G: Effect of sodium polystyrene sulfonate on lithium bioavailability. *Ann Emerg Med* 1992;21: 1312–1315.
50. Tomaszewski C, Musso C, Pearson J, et al: Lithium absorption prevented by sodium polystyrene sulfonate in volunteers. *Ann Emerg Med* 1992;21:1308–1311.
51. Perrier D, Martin P, Favre H, et al: Very severe self-poisoning lithium carbonate intoxication causing a myocardial infarction. *Chest* 1991;100:863–865.
52. Fein S, Paz V, Pao N, et al: The combination of lithium carbonate and an MAOI in refractory depressions. *Am J Psychiatry* 1988;145: 249–250.
53. Parfrey P, Ikeman R, Anglin D, et al: Severe lithium intoxication treated by forced diuresis. *Can Med Assoc J* 1983;29:979–980.
54. Jaeger A, Sauder P, Kopferschmitt J, et al: When should dialysis be performed in lithium poisoning? A kinetic study in 14 cases of lithium poisoning. *J Toxicol Clin Toxicol* 1993:31:429–447.
55. Gomolin I, Brandt J: Treatment of severe lithium intoxication. *Can Med Assoc J* 1984;130:847.
56. Goetting M: Acute lithium poisoning in a child with dystonia. *Pediatrics* 1985;76:978–980.

ADDITIONAL SELECTED REFERENCES

Bowers M, Heninger G: Lithium: clinical effects and cerebrospinal fluid acid monamine metabolites. *Commun Psychopharmacol* 1977;1:135–145.

Danielson D, Jick H, Porter J, et al: Drug toxicity and hospitalization among lithium users. *J Clin Psychopharmacol* 1984;4:108–110.

Erwin C, Gerber C, Morrison S, et al: Lithium carbonate and convulsive disorders. *Arch Gen Psychiatry* 1973;28: 646–648.

Fava G, Molnar G, Block B, et al: The lithium loading dose method in a clinical setting. *Am J Psychiatry* 1984;141:812–813.

Fawcett J, Clark D, Gibbons R, et al: Evaluation of lithium therapy for alcoholism. *J Clin Psychiatry* 1984;45:494–499.

Hesketh J: Effects of potassium and lithium on sodium transport from blood to cerebrospinal fluid. *J Neurochem* 1977;28:597–603.

Judd L, Huey L: Lithium antagonizes ethanol intoxication in alcoholics. *Am J Psychiatry* 1984;141:1517–1521.

King J, Aylard P, Hullin R: Side effects of lithium at lower therapeutic levels: the significance of thirst. *Psychol Med* 1985;15:355–361.

Lackroy G, Van Pragg H: Lithium salts as sedatives. *Acta Psychiatr Scand* 1971;47:163–173.

Louie A, Meltzer H: Lithium potentiation of antidepressant treatment. *J Clin Psychopharmacol* 1984;4:316–321.

Lyles M: Deep venous thrombophlebitis associated with lithium toxicity. *J Natl Med Assoc* 1984;76:633–634.

Prockop L, Marcus D: Cerebrospinal fluid lithium: passive transfer kinetics. *Life Sci* 1972;11:859–868.

Rosen P, Stevens R: Action myoclonus in lithium toxicity. *Ann Neurol* 1983;13:221–222.

Spring G: Hazards of lithium prophylaxis. *Dis Nerv System* 1974;35: 351–354.

Walevski A, Radwan M: Choreoathetosis as toxic effect of lithium treatment. *Eur Neurol* 1986;25:412–415.

Yassa R, Archer J, Cordoza S: The long-term effect of lithium carbonate on tardive dyskinesia. *Can J Psychiatry* 1984;29:36–37.

Yung G: A review of clinical trials of lithium in medicine. *Pharmacol Biochem Behav* 1984;21(Suppl. 1):51–55.

PART IV

CARDIAC DRUGS

CHAPTER 20

Antiarrhythmic Agents

Several attempts have been made to classify antiarrhythmic drugs according to their effects on isolated myocardial tissues (1). The most frequently used system was originated by Vaughan Williams (2). In this system the antiarrhythmic agents have traditionally been divided into four distinct classes on the basis of mechanism of action (Table 20–1) (3). Compounds that do not fall into any one class have also been described and are considered "miscellaneous" agents (4).

Class I consists of the sodium channel blockers, all of which behave like local anesthetics. This is the largest group of antiarrhythmic drugs. Class I agents are frequently subdivided according to their effects on action potential duration: *Class IA* lengthens the duration, *Class IB* shortens or has no effect on it, and *Class IC* has no effect on it but promotes greater sodium current depression than the other two groups. It is important to recognize that this subclassification of sodium channel blockers ignores many differences among co-classified drugs and overlapping properties of drugs assigned to different groups (2). Drugs that reduce adrenergic activity in the heart constitute *Class II*. *Class III* is composed of drugs that prolong the effective refractory period by some mechanism other than blockade of sodium channels. *Class IV* consists of calcium channel blockers (1).

Although it is commonly accepted that antiarrhythmics are classified based on the particular physiologic effect they exert on myocardial cells, not all agents within a class will produce the same effect in any one individual. A particular drug may have more than one antiarrhythmic effect or even extra cardiac effects, and its pharmacologic actions may be modified by various physiologic factors.

Arrhythmias are caused by abnormal pacemaker activity or abnormal impulse propagation. Thus, the aim of therapy of the arrhythmias is to reduce ectopic pacemaker activity and modify critically impaired conduction. The major mechanisms for accomplishing these goals are sodium channel blockade, blockade of sympathetic autonomic effects in the heart, prolongation of the effective refractory period, and calcium channel blockade.

ACTION POTENTIAL AND "CHANNELS"

The action potential of excitable cardiac cells is the result of the movement of ions, particularly sodium and calcium. It is thought that there are movable macromolecules that function as gates that allow ions to cross excitable membranes. Each ion channel has one gate that controls activation and another gate that controls inactivation. Each ion (sodium, calcium, chloride, or potassium) has a transmembrane flux that is regulated by the opening and closing of these gates.

The changes in transmembrane potential that occur during the action potential of cardiac cells are divided into five phases: phase 0, rapid depolarization; phase 1, early repolarization; phase 2, plateau; phase 3, rapid repolarization; and phase 4, diastole (Fig. 20–1) (5).

When cardiac cells in normal atrial and ventricular contractile tissues are stimulated sufficiently to alter membrane permeability for sodium, a "fast" channel allows rapid sodium ionic influx during phase 0 depolarization of the action potential. This is seen as a rapid upstroke of the action potential. This current is dependent on the extracellular sodium concentration and can be blocked by type I antidysrhythmics, such as quinidine and procainamide. During phase 0, when the interior of the cell becomes less negative, or depolarized, from approximately −90 mV to −40 mV, the membrane conductance for sodium rapidly increases. At this point, the fast sodium channel becomes inactivated, but not before it activates a second inward current. Because the rates of activation and inactivation of this second inward current are several orders of magnitude slower than those of the fast inward current, and because these channels are approximately 100 times more selective for calcium than for sodium, this channel is termed the "slow" inward current or the calcium channel. The plateau phase or phase 2 is largely dependent on a slow inward current through calcium-specific channels. The slow channels are not entirely calcium-mediated, however.

The fast channel forms the basis for the depolarization of most normal conducting tissues in the heart: atrial and ventricular muscle, His-Purkinje fibers, atrial internodal pathways, and anomalous tracts in the pre-excitation syn-

TABLE 20–1. *Classes of antiarrhythmics (based on Vaughan Williams)*

Class I
Class IA
Block fast sodium channel
Prolong repolarization
Prolong refractory period
Prolong action potential
Includes
Quinidine
Procainamide
Disopyramide
Class IB
Block fast sodium channel
Little effect of conduction
Prolong refractory period
Shorten action potential
Includes
Lidocaine
Tocainide
Mexiletine
Class IC
Potent sodium channel blockers
Slow conduction velocity
Little effect on repolarization
Little effect on action potential
Includes
Flecainide
Encainide
Lorcainide
Class II
Counteracts sympathetic stimulation
Includes
β-adrenergic blockers
Class III
Prolongs action potential
Prolongs refractory period
Prolongs repolarization
Includes
Bretylium
Amiodarone
Class IV
Prolongs conduction through AV node
Lengthening of PR interval
Includes
Calcium channel blockers
Miscellaneous
Adenosine

dromes. In such fast response fibers, the slow channel effect is greatly overshadowed by the rapid channel activity. Thus, the slow channel, the charge carrier for which is largely calcium, is slowly activated at a threshold potential of −35 mV, compared with the −65 mV for the rapid channel, and has a long time constant of inactivation; it therefore contributes to the maintenance of the plateau phase of the action potential.

In fast-channel tissues, such as the atrial and ventricular contractile tissues and the His-Purkinje system, electrical excitability results primarily from transmembrane sodium flux. These tissues have high diastolic potentials and rapid rates of phase 0 depolarization (fast conduction velocities) and recover excitability coincident with repolarization (have short refractory periods).

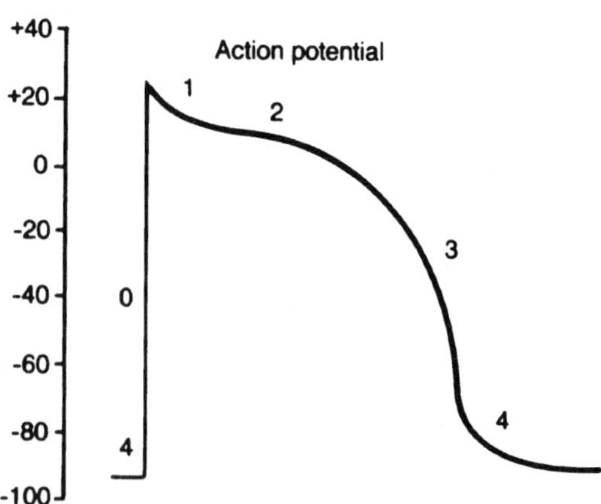

FIG.20–1. The action potential of cardiac muscle. Adapted with permission from Antman E, et al: Calcium channel blocking agents in the treatment of cardiovascular disorders. *Ann Intern Med* 1980;93:875–885. American College of Physicians.

Antiarrhythmic Agents and "Proarrhythmias"

Antiarrhythmic drugs have the potential to exacerbate existing or induce new arrhythmias (Table 20–2). These "proarrhythmic" effects may include hemodynamically significant bradyarrhythmias or conduction blocks, accelerated ventricular response during atrial fibrillation with or without ventricular pre-excitation, increased frequency of ventricular premature beats, new or accelerated sustained ventricular tachycardia, ventricular fibrillation, and polymorphic ventricular tachycardia, including torsade de pointes (1)

All antiarrhythmic drugs with the exception of β-adrenoceptor antagonists have been reported to worsen arrhythmias in some patients, more commonly in those with impaired left ventricular function and sustained ventricular arrhythmias (6).

Proarrhythmic responses typically occur within the first four days of the start of therapy (7). A mechanism underlying a proarrhythmia that has been proposed is antiarrhythmic drug-induced depression of conduction in abnormal cardiac myocardium, thereby allowing normal

TABLE 20–2. *Proarrhythmic effects of antiarrhythmics*

Bradydysrhythmias
Conduction blocks
Atrial fibrillation with accelerated ventricular response
Ventricular premature beats
Ventricular tachycardia
Ventricular fibrillation
Polymorphic ventricular tachycardia
Torsade de pointes

myocardium to recover excitability and promoting reentry. This mechanism has been previously referred to as "incessant reentry" and is most commonly associated with type IC agents, which have the most potent sodium-channel blocking effects.

CLASSES OF COMPOUNDS

CLASS I

Class I agents have a local anesthetic effect on both myocardial and nerve cell membranes. The primary effect of these agents is to slow the rate of rise in the action potential. These agents have been subdivided based on their effect on the duration of the action potential (8).

Subclasses IA, IB, IC

Subclasses IA, IB, and IC further divide this class according to major differences among the drugs. Quinidine, procainamide, and disopyramide are agents with Class IA action. These drugs not only block the fast sodium channels but also prolong both repolarization and the refractory period of isolated cardiac tissue. In clinical use, they may cause a measurable increase in the QRS duration and the QT interval (2).

In contrast to Class IA agents, Class IB agents have little effect on conduction and work primarily by prolonging the effective refractory period, thus reducing excitability. Drugs with IB action are only moderately potent sodium channel inhibitors, and act to shorten AP duration (2). Therefore, they exert little effect on the PR, QRS, or QT interval. Lidocaine and the more recently developed orally active congeners, tocainide and mexiletine, belong to this group (3).

Drugs with Class IC actions, flecainide, encainide, and lorcainide, are newer and more potent sodium channel inhibitors that slow conduction velocity with little effect on repolarization. Agents with Class IC action increase the PR and QRS intervals. QT is prolonged as well, but only to the degree that QRS prolongation is seen.

To reiterate, Class IA agents prolong the action potential duration whereas Class IB agents shorten the duration of the action potential and Class IC agents have little or no effect on the duration of the action potential (8).

Class I Agents and Torsade de Pointes

Pause-dependent torsade de pointes is a morphologically distinct, polymorphic ventricular tachycardia associated with a prolonged QT interval and a prominent u wave preceding the commencement of the arrhythmia (see Fig. 16–1 (9). Torsade de pointes, therefore, has been described as a complication of therapy with virtually all antiarrhythmic agents that prolong the QT interval (10). Among antiarrhythmic agents, this arrhythmia is most commonly precipitated by Class IA antiarrhythmic drugs (11).

When torsade de pointes occurs with Class IA agents, it tends to occur at low therapeutic or even subtherapeutic concentrations of these agents often relatively early in therapy, when sodium channels may be only slightly affected, but significant numbers of potassium channels might be blocked in certain susceptible individuals (12).

Class IA

Quinidine

Quinidine is an alkaloid obtained from various species of *Cinchona* or their hybrids. Quinidine is the dextrorotatory isomer of quinine and was among the first drugs observed to possess antiarrhythmic activity. Quinidine is available commercially in at least three forms: the sulfate, gluconate, and polygalacturonate. The quinidine content varies with each of the forms (2).

Actions and Uses

Quinidine is a broad-spectrum antiarrhythmic most commonly used to terminate atrial flutter and fibrillation (3). Quinidine exhibits electrophysiologic effects characteristic of Class IA antiarrhythmic agents with an intermediate rate of attachment and dissociation from transmembrane sodium channels. Like other Class I antiarrhythmic agents, quinidine is believed to combine with fast sodium channels in their inactive state and thereby inhibit recovery after repolarization in a time- and voltage-dependent manner, which is associated with subsequent dissociation of the drug from the sodium channels.

Quinidine is regarded as a myocardial depressant because it decreases myocardial excitability and conduction velocity, and may depress myocardial contractility. In addition to depressing cardiac automaticity and conduction, quinidine possesses antimuscarinic and vasodilatory properties that may modify the direct myocardial effects of the drug (3).

Quinidine possesses α adrenoceptor-blocking properties that can cause vasodilation and a reflex increase in sinoatrial nodal rate (Table 20–3). These effects are most prominent after intravenous administration. Quinidine

TABLE 20–3. *Additional actions of Class IA antiarrhythmics*

α–Adrenoceptor blocking properties
Antimalarial effects (quinidine)
Antipyretic effects (quinidine)
Oxytocic effects (quinidine)
Antimuscarinic actions (all)

also has antimalarial, antipyretic, and oxytocic properties. Quinidine has antimuscarinic actions in the heart that inhibit vagal effects. This can overcome its direct membrane effect and lead to increased sinus rate and increased atrioventricular conduction.

Pharmacokinetics

Quinidine is usually administered orally and is rapidly absorbed from the gastrointestinal tract. Plasma protein binding varies widely, ranging from 50% to 95% (2). The apparent elimination half-life of quinidine ranges from 4 to 10 hours in healthy persons with a usual mean value of 6 to 7 hours. The half-life may be prolonged in elderly persons. Quinidine is hydroxylated in the liver, but 20% is excreted unchanged in the urine. Its half-life is about 6 hours and may be longer in patients with congestive heart failure or hepatic or renal disease (3).

Laboratory

Plasma levels of quinidine can be measured and values vary according to the assay employed. Therefore, plasma quinidine concentrations are quite variable among individuals. Traditionally, plasma concentrations for effective use of quinidine have been reported to range from 2 to 5 μg/mL; concentrations of greater than 5 μg/mL are associated with toxicity. This information is based on less specific analytic methods, which quantitate metabolites as well as intact quinidine. However, with the use of more specific assays plasma quinidine concentrations will be lower. Therefore, clinicians requesting serum quinidine determinations should be aware of the method of analysis. Because there is a wide individual variation in response to quinidine therapy, the physician should carefully consider patient response and evidence of toxicity along with blood levels in determining optimal quinidine therapy. In healthy fasting individuals, mean peak plasma quinidine concentrations are attained 1–2 hours after oral administration of a single 200-mg dose of quinidine sulfate (11).

Drug Interactions

Quinidine metabolism is inhibited by cimetidine and induced by phenytoin, phenobarbital, and rifampin, with the latter agents leading to reduced, subtherapeutic quinidine concentrations (2).

Clinical digoxin toxicity has been described in a large number of patients receiving quinidine and digoxin concurrently. This interaction is dependent on quinidine dosage, and in some patients may appear only as the dosage is increased to higher levels.

Adverse Reactions

Adverse reactions to quinidine include hypotension due to its action as an α-adrenergic antagonist, a high incidence of gastrointestinal symptoms, tinnitus at high plasma levels, rare thrombocytopenia, and in usual cases, conduction block in patient with preexisting conduction system disease.

A small percentage of patients given quinidine develop a syndrome called quinidine syncope, characterized by recurrent light-headedness and episodes of fainting. The symptoms are a result of a drug-induced rapid, torsade de pointes, resembling ventricular fibrillation, which usually terminates spontaneously but may recur incessantly or become sustained. It is associated with a striking prolongation of the QT interval.

Overdosage

Overdosage of quinidine has produced ataxia, respiratory depression or distress, apnea, vomiting, diarrhea, vertigo, headache, paresthesia, and quinidine concentrations exceeding the therapeutic range of 2 to 5 μg/mL (Table 20–4) (1). More serious manifestations include severe hypotension, syncope, anuria, absence of P waves, broad-

TABLE 20–4. *Toxicity of Class IA compounds*

Anticholinergic
Dry mouth
Blurred vision
Constipation
Urinary retention
Neurologic
Cinchonism (Quinidine)
Tinnitus
Headache
Nausea
Disturbed vision
Hallucinations
Ataxia
Paresthesia
Vertigo
Irritability
Seizures
Coma
Gastrointestinal
Nausea
Vomiting
Diarrhea
Cardiovascular
Hypotension
Syncope
Widening of QRS
Widening of PR and QT intervals
Ventricular arrhythmias
Torsade de pointes
Miscellaneous
Lupus-like syndrome (Procainamide)
Arthralgia
Arthritis
Pleuritis
Pericarditis
Parenchymal pulmonary disease
Respiratory arrest

ening of the QRS complex, PR and QT intervals, ventricular arrhythmias, extrasystoles, heart block, heart failure, irritability, lethargy, respiratory depression, hallucinations, generalized seizures, coma, and death (4). Signs of cinchonism may also occur which consist of ringing in ears, headache, nausea and disturbed vision, and may appear in sensitive patients after a single dose of the drug.

Treatment will be discussed with the rest of the Class IA compounds.

Procainamide

Procainamide is an antiarrhythmic agent whose cardiac actions appear to be similar to those of quinidine. Procainamide is regarded as a myocardial depressant because it decreases myocardial excitability and conduction velocity, and may depress myocardial contractility. Procainamide differs structurally from procaine in the replacement of the ester group of procaine with an amide group. Procainamide has local anesthetic properties equal to but more sustained than those of procaine. Procainamide produces less CNS stimulation than does procaine.

Procainamide, like disopyramide and quinidine, also possesses antimuscarinic properties which may modify the direct myocardial effects of the drug. The most important difference between quinidine and procainamide is the less prominent antimuscarinic action of procainamide. Therefore, the directly depressant actions of procainamide on sinoatrial and atrioventricular nodes are not as effectively counterbalanced by drug-induced vagal block as in the case of quinidine. Procainamide also has ganglionic blocking properties and thus more potent negative inotropic effects than quinidine. In patients with preexisting ventricular dysfunction, procainamide may induce severe congestive heart failure.

Pharmacokinetics

Approximately 75–95% of a dose of procainamide hydrochloride is usually absorbed from the intestine, but a few patients may absorb less than 50% of an oral dose. Oral absorption of procainamide is slowed by delayed gastric emptying, decreased intestinal motility, presence of food in the GI tract, decreases in intestinal pH, or decreased splanchnic blood flow. Sustained-release preparations are also available. Extended-release tablets containing procainamide are formulated to provide a sustained and relatively constant rate of release and absorption of the drug throughout the small intestine.

Procainamide undergoes both glomerular filtration and renal tubular secretion and in normal subjects, the kidney removes over 50% of an administered dose of procainamide (2). In addition, the principal metabolite of procainamide, *N*-acetylprocainamide (NAPA), a compound with Class III antiarrhythmic activity, is primarily eliminated by glomerular filtration and renal tubular secretion. The pharmacokinetics of procainamide and NAPA, therefore, will be altered in clinical situations in which renal function is diminished, such as renal failure and advanced age. Procainamide is acetylated in the liver, to form NAPA. Acetylation of procainamide is related to genetic acetylator phenotype. The rate of acetylation is genetically determined and varies among individuals; however, it is constant for each person. In normal subjects, the mean half-life of procainamide is 3.4 hours; NAPA half-life is 6 hours. Because the half-life of NAPA is considerably longer than that of procainamide, it accumulates more readily. Thus, it is important to measure plasma levels of both procainamide and NAPA especially in patients with circulatory or renal impairment (11).

Adverse Effects

The incidence of adverse effects associated with long-term procainamide therapy limits its usefulness. Common adverse effects include hypotension, bradycardia, and QRS prolongation.

The most troublesome adverse effect of procainamide is a syndrome resembling lupus erythematosus and usually consisting of arthralgia and arthritis. In some patients, pleuritis, pericarditis, or parenchymal pulmonary disease also occurs. Renal lupus is rarely induced by procainamide. During long-term therapy, serologic abnormalities such as increased antinuclear antibody titer occur in approximately 90% of patients, 50% of whom develop a lupus-like syndrome (3). Cessation of the drug at this time will usually not result in further difficulty. Continuation of the drug may lead to pleural effusion and a potentially lethal cardiac tamponade (2).

Laboratory

The usefulness of measuring plasma levels of procainamide is limited because of its genetically determined hepatic conversion to its active metabolite, NAPA. When each is given as the sole agent, the therapeutic ranges are 4 to 8 µg/mL for procainamide and 7 to 15 µg/mL for NAPA. Plasma levels above 10 µg/mL are increasingly associated with toxic findings, which are seen occasionally in the 10 to 12 µg/mL range, more often in the 12 to 15 µg/mL range, and commonly in patients with plasma levels greater than 15 µg/mL.

If available, procainamide and NAPA plasma levels may be helpful in assessing the potential degree of toxicity and response to therapy. NAPA plasma concentrations may represent more than 50% of the total drug in the plasma (2).

Overdosage

Acute overdosage of procainamide has produced hypotension, widening of the QRS complex, junctional tachycardia, intraventricular conduction delay, oliguria, lethargy, confusion, nausea, and vomiting. Treatment will be discussed with the rest of the Class IA compounds.

Disopyramide

Disopyramide, like other Class I antiarrhythmic agents, combines with fast sodium channels. Disopyramide is a drug better suited for long-term therapy than procainamide in that it has little associated chronic toxicity. In the U.S., disopyramide is only available for oral use. Its cardiac antimuscarinic effects are even more marked than those of quinidine, which may modify the direct myocardial effects of the drug.

Pharmacokinetics

Following oral administration of immediate-release disopyramide, it is rapidly and almost completely absorbed, and peak plasma levels are usually attained within 2 hours. Disopyramide is distributed throughout the extracellular body water and is not extensively bound to tissues. Its half-life of elimination, usually 6 to 8 hours, is lengthened to as much as 15 hours in cardiac patients. Disopyramide's oral bioavailability is 90% (2). Between 20% and 50% of disopyramide is bound to plasma proteins but since binding sites become saturated with increasing dosage, this results in a nonlinear rise in free drug levels. As a result, measurements of total plasma concentration may be misleading. Therapeutic levels range from 2 to 4 μg/mL (3).

Adverse Actions

Noncardiac side effects are common, most frequently caused by the drug's antimuscarinic effects, and include dry mouth, dry eyes, blurred vision, constipation, urinary retention in male patients with prostatic hypertrophy, and worsening of preexisting glaucoma (3). These effects may require discontinuance of the drug. Congestive heart failure has also been reported (8).

Laboratory

Plasma disopyramide concentrations necessary to produce a therapeutic response vary depending on the type of cardiac arrhythmia, the severity and duration of the arrhythmia, and the sensitivity of the patient to the drug. Plasma disopyramide concentrations of approximately 2–4 μg/mL are generally required to suppress ventricular arrhythmias; some patients require up to 7 μg/mL to suppress and prevent the recurrence of refractory ventricular tachycardia. Toxicity is generally associated with plasma disopyramide concentrations greater than 9 μg/mL. Because of concentration-dependent protein binding, it is difficult to predict the concentration of the free drug when total drug is measured (11).

Overdosage

Overdosage of disopyramide has produced antimuscarinic effects, loss of consciousness, hypotension, respiratory arrest, episodes of apnea, cardiac conduction disturbances, arrhythmias, widening of the QRS complex and QT interval, bradycardia, congestive heart failure, asystole, and seizures. Death has occurred following overdosage.

TREATMENT OF OVERDOSE OF CLASS IA DRUGS

Management of overdosage of Class IA antiarrhythmics (Table 20-5) includes symptomatic treatment with EKG and blood pressure monitoring. The patient's airway should be protected and ventilation and perfusion should be supported. The patient's vital signs, blood gases, and serum electrolytes should be meticulously monitored and maintained within acceptable limits. Gastric lavage, supportive therapy, and if necessary, cardiac glycosides, diuretics, vasopressors and sympathomimetics, intra-aortic balloon counterpulsation, and mechanically assisted respiration may be used. If progressive atrioventricular (AV) block occurs, endocardial pacing should be instituted. Hypotension may be treated, if necessary, with metaraminol or norepinephrine after adequate fluid volume replacement. Heart block may be treated with a pacemaker. Tachydysrhythmias should respond to phenytoin or lidocaine.

Intravenous sodium infusions of sodium lactate have reportedly reduced the cardiotoxic effects of some of the Class IA compounds. Alkalinization of the urine may decrease excretion of Class IA antiarrhythmics and should be avoided.

TABLE 20–5. *Treatment of overdose of Class IA antiarrhythmics*

Sign/Symptom	Treatment
Acute overdose	Gastric lavage Activated charcoal Cathartic
AV Block	Endocardial pacing
Hypotension	Volume replacement Sympathomimetics Sodium bicarbonate
Tachydysrhythmias	Phenytoin Lidocaine Sodium bicarbonate

Class IA antiarrhythmics which prolong the QRS and QTc intervals are contraindicated. Because marked CNS depression may occur even in the presence of convulsions, CNS depressants should not be administered.

Class IB

Lidocaine

The cardiac actions of lidocaine appear to be similar to those of phenytoin. Unlike quinidine and procainamide, lidocaine has little effect on autonomic tone and generally does not produce a substantial fall in blood pressure, decreased myocardial contractility, or diminished cardiac output in usual doses.

The electrophysiologic characteristics of the subgroups of Class I antiarrhythmic agents are related to quantitative differences in their rates of attachment to and dissociation from transmembrane sodium channels, with Class IB agents exhibiting rapid rates of attachment and dissociation. Lidocaine is a potent suppressor of abnormal cardiac activity, yet it appears to act exclusively on the sodium channel. Its interaction with this channel differs substantially from that of Class IA antiarrhythmics. Whereas Class IA antiarrhythmics mostly block sodium channels in the activated state, lidocaine blocks both activated and inactivated sodium channels (13). As a result, a large fraction of the unblocked sodium channels become blocked during each action potential in Purkinje fibers and ventricular cells, which have long plateaus. During diastole, most of the sodium channels in normally polarized cells become drug-free. Since lidocaine may shorten the action potential duration, diastole may be prolonged, thereby extending the time available for recovery. As a result, lidocaine has few electrophysiologic effects in normal cardiac tissue. In contrast, depolarized (inactivated) sodium channels remain largely blocked during diastole, and more may become blocked. Thus, lidocaine suppresses the electrical activity of the depolarized, arrhythmogenic tissues while minimally interfering with the electrical activity of normal tissues (14). These factors appear to be responsible for the fact that lidocaine is a very effective agent for suppressing arrhythmias associated with depolarization as with ischemia and digitalis toxicity, but it is relatively ineffective against arrhythmias occurring in normally polarized tissues such as with atrial flutter and fibrillation. At therapeutic plasma concentrations, lidocaine has little effect on AV node conduction and His-Purkinje conduction in the normal heart. Specialized conducting tissues of the atria are less sensitive to the effects of lidocaine than are those of ventricular tissues. Unlike the drugs with Class IA effects, it is very unlikely that Class IB compounds cause torsade de pointe; thus, they can be used safely in patients with a history of this condition or long QT syndrome (2).

Pharmacokinetics

Although lidocaine hydrochloride is absorbed from the gastrointestinal tract, it passes into the hepatic portal circulation and only a very small percentage of the oral dose reaches systemic circulation unchanged. Thus, lidocaine must be given parenterally. Because lidocaine chiefly undergoes hepatic metabolism, patients with impaired hepatic blood flow secondary to shock or congestive heart failure are more prone to its toxic effects (3). Following IV administration of a bolus dose of 50–100 mg of lidocaine hydrochloride, the drug has an onset of action within 45–90 seconds and a duration of action of 10–20 minutes.

Laboratory

Plasma lidocaine concentrations of approximately 1–5 μg/mL are required to suppress ventricular arrhythmias. Toxicity has been associated with plasma lidocaine concentrations greater than 5 μg/mL (13).

Toxicity

Lidocaine is a CNS depressant and produces sedative, analgesic, and anticonvulsant effects. With high doses, seizures may result from depression of inhibitory influences on motor pathways; severe overdosage may cause respiratory arrest because of motor nerve paralysis and/or inadequate medullary blood flow. Lidocaine also suppresses the cough and gag reflexes (13). In large doses, especially in patients with preexisting heart failure, lidocaine may cause hypotension, partly by depressing myocardial contractility, yet lidocaine is the least cardiotoxic of the currently used antiarrhythmic drugs.

Adverse effects of the drug mainly involve the CNS, are usually of short duration, and are dose-related. The first neurologic manifestations are headache, hallucinations, nystagmus, myoclonia, and decreased consciousness. Other adverse CNS reactions may also be manifested by paresthesias, tremor, nausea and vomiting of central origin, and a myriad of other neurologic abnormalities (Table 20–6). Muscle twitching or tremors, seizures, unconsciousness, coma, and respiratory depression and arrest may also occur (13). Seizures occur mostly in elderly or otherwise vulnerable patients and are dose-related, usually short-lived, and respond to intravenous diazepam. In general, if plasma levels above 9 μg/mL are avoided, lidocaine is extremely well tolerated. Hypersensitivity to lidocaine is rare and may be characterized by skin lesions, urticaria, edema, and anaphylactoid reactions.

Cardiovascular toxicity is partly due to sodium channel blockage which is responsible for dysrhythmia, shortening of conduction time with sinus bradycardia,

TABLE 20–6. *Toxicity of Class IB antiarrhythmics*

Neurologic
Headache
Hallucinations
Nystagmus
Myoclonia
Decreased level of consciousness
Slurred speech
Drowsiness
Dizziness
Disorientation
Confusion
Tremulousness
Psychosis
Euphoria
Visual disturbances
Seizures
Respiratory arrest
Decreased gag reflex
Decreased cough reflex
Cardiovascular
Hypotension
Heart block
Cardiovascular collapse
Bradycardia
Gastrointestinal (Oral agents)
Nausea
Vomiting
Constipation
Anorexia
Liver function test (LFT) abnormalities
Miscellaneous
Pulmonary fibrosis (Tocainide)
Agranulocytosis (Tocainide)

widening of the QRS complex, and vascular collapse. Although usual doses of lidocaine generally produce no adverse cardiovascular effects, patients with high plasma concentrations of the drug may develop hypotension, arrhythmias, heart block, cardiovascular collapse, and bradycardia which may lead to cardiac arrest. Cardiac arrest, however, is usually secondary to respiratory arrest.

Clinical toxicity correlates with plasma and cerebrospinal fluid (CSF) levels of lidocaine (13). Toxicity is increased by acidosis and decreased by alkalosis. There is no specific treatment of overdose and management is symptomatic. Treatment is discussed below.

Tocainide

Tocainide (Tonocard) is a Class IB agent, and it is a primary amine analog of lidocaine with similar electrophysiologic properties. The drug was synthesized during a search for oral pharmaceutical agents with lidocaine-like electrophysiologic effects that could be used for long-term treatment of ventricular arrhythmias (8). Since tocainide is a primary amine, this modification is associated with resistance to first-pass metabolism following oral administration, a problem associated with the oral administration of lidocaine.

Tocainide exhibits electrophysiologic effects characteristic of Class IB antiarrhythmic agents. Tocainide acts by decreasing the duration of the AP and the refractory period and by reducing automaticity (3). Tocainide is similar to lidocaine in that the PR, and QT intervals are not prolonged. Like lidocaine, tocainide's cardiac actions appear to be mediated via a dose-dependent decrease in sodium and potassium conductance, resulting in an increase of the effective refractory period relative to the duration of the action potential and suppression of automaticity in the His-Purkinje system by inhibition of spontaneous phase 4 depolarization of the ventricles during diastole. Like other Class I antiarrhythmic agents, tocainide is believed to combine with fast sodium channels in their inactive state and thereby inhibit recovery after repolarization in a time- and voltage-dependent manner which is associated with subsequent dissociation of the drug from the sodium channels. Evidence indicates that the dose-dependent, tocainide-induced decrease in sodium conductance is more pronounced in ischemic tissue than in healthy tissue.

Unlike quinidine, procainamide, or disopyramide, which possess antimuscarinic properties that may modify direct myocardial effects of the drugs, tocainide, like lidocaine, appears to have little effect on autonomic tone.

Pharmacokinetics

Tocainide hydrochloride is rapidly and almost completely absorbed from the GI tract following oral administration. After oral administration of tocainide, the peak serum concentrations are reached in 30 to 120 minutes (8). Unlike lidocaine, tocainide first-pass hepatic metabolism is negligible, and the bioavailability is near 100% (8). Approximately 50% of the drug is protein-bound, and nearly 40% is cleared unchanged in the urine (8). The therapeutic half-life of tocainide is between 8 and 20 hours. The apparent volume of distribution of tocainide hydrochloride at steady state is reportedly about 1.5–4 L/kg.

Side Effects

Adverse reactions to tocainide occur frequently, generally involve the nervous system and GI tract, and are usually mild, transient, and reversible following reduction in dosage or discontinuance of the drug. Some of the side effects of tocainide have limited its usefulness. These effects usually involve the CNS, with vertigo, lethargy, tremors, paresthesias, ataxia, and personality and sleep disorders noted. Gastrointestinal side effects include nausea, vomiting, and abnormalities noted in liver function tests. These are predominantly neurologic, including tremor, blurred vision, and lethargy. Nausea is also a common effect (3).

A very serious reaction to tocainide therapy is the incidence of severe reactions such as pulmonary fibrosis and agranulocytosis (2).

Laboratory

There appears to be considerable interpatient variation in the relationship of plasma tocainide hydrochloride concentrations and therapeutic effect, but therapeutic plasma concentrations of the drug are usually 3–10 µg/mL. There is no clearly defined relationship between plasma tocainide hydrochloride concentration and severity of intoxication (4).

Toxicity

In general, overdosage of tocainide may be expected to produce effects that are extensions of common adverse reactions, particularly those involving the nervous system and gastrointestinal tract. Treatment will be discussed below.

Mexiletine

Mexiletine (Mexitil) is a Class IB antiarrhythmic. The drug originally was developed as an anticonvulsant and anorexic agent. Chemically, the drug resembles lidocaine, and like tocainide demonstrates good oral absorption. Mexiletine will decrease the rate of rise in phase 0 of the AP and shorten the AP duration (8). Mexiletine affects the cardiac transmembrane potential, thus reducing excitability and automaticity (3).

Pharmacokinetics

Mexiletine is well absorbed from the gastrointestinal tract and peak blood levels are reached in 2 to 3 hours (1). The absorption rate of mexiletine is reduced in clinical situations such as acute myocardial infarction in which gastric emptying time is increased. Narcotics, atropine, and magnesium-aluminum hydroxide have also been reported to slow the absorption of mexiletine. Metoclopramide has been reported to accelerate absorption.

The bioavailability of mexiletine approaches 90%. Peak plasma concentrations are achieved 2 to 4 hours after oral administration. It is 50–60% bound to plasma protein, with a volume of distribution of 5–7 L/Kg. Plasma half-life normally varies from 10 to 16 hours (8). Whereas urinary pH does not normally have much influence on elimination, marked changes in the urinary pH influence the rate of excretion; acidification accelerates excretion, while alkalinization retards it.

Adverse Effects

The negative effects of mexiletine on cardiac contractility are minimal. Like lidocaine, mexiletine does not prolong the PR, QRS, or QT intervals. Noncardiac side effects develop in a great percent of patients requiring cessation of the drug in many patients (3). Gastrointestinal side effects include nausea, vomiting, constipation, and anorexia. The most common effects are neurologic, which include tremors, dizziness, ataxia, paresthesias, blurred vision, agitation, and seizures (15).

Laboratory

Mexiletine plasma levels of at least 0.5 µg/mL are generally required for therapeutic response. An increase in the frequency of central nervous system adverse effects has been observed when plasma levels exceed 2.0 µg/mL. Although therapeutic concentrations are reported as 0.5 to 2.0 µg/mL, toxicity has been reported over a wide range of concentrations and may occur at concentrations as low as 1.5 µg/mL (16). Toxicity will develop in most patients at concentrations exceeding 3.0 µg/mL (8).

Toxicity

Symptoms associated with overdosage include nausea, hypotension, sinus bradycardia, paresthesia, seizures, intermittent left bundle branch block, and temporary asystole.

TREATMENT OF OVERDOSE OF CLASS IB DRUGS

Treatment of overdosage generally involves symptomatic and supportive care. In acute overdose of orally ingested agents, the stomach should be emptied immediately by gastric lavage. If the patient is comatose, having seizures, or has lost the gag reflex, gastric lavage may be performed if an endotracheal tube with cuff inflated is in place to prevent aspiration of gastric contents. Appropriate therapy should be instituted if hypotension, respiratory depression or arrest, or seizures occur, including patency of the airway and adequate ventilation. For the treatment of severe seizures, small IV doses of diazepam or an ultrashort-acting barbiturate may be administered. If the patient is anesthetized, a short-acting neuromuscular blocking agent such as succinylcholine may be given intravenously.

Acidification of urine does not significantly alter tocainide excretion, but forced alkalinization decreases excretion. If circulatory depression occurs, IV fluids and vasopressors such as ephedrine or metaraminol may be used if necessary.

Class IC

Encainide (Enkaid)

Encainide is a very potent local anesthetic-type antiarrhythmic agent, structurally related to procainamide and flecainide in that the drugs are benzamide derivatives (2). Like other Class IC antiarrhythmic agents, encainide slows intracardiac conduction at low concentrations, has relatively small effects on refractoriness, and generally has little effect on repolarization. The principal effect of encainide on cardiac tissue appears to be a concentration-dependent inhibition of the transmembrane influx of extracellular sodium ions via fast sodium channels, as indicated by a decrease in the maximal rate of depolarization of phase 0 of the action potential (17). Encainide does not appear to possess substantial agonist or antagonist adrenergic, cholinergic, histaminergic, or serotonergic properties.

Pharmacokinetics

Encainide hydrochloride is rapidly and almost completely absorbed from the GI tract following oral administration (11). The absolute bioavailability of commercially available encainide depends principally on a patient's genetically determined ability to metabolize the drug (oxidizer phenotype) and with acute versus chronic administration of the drug (17). Consequently, the observed effects are a somewhat complex aggregate that depend on the relative proportions of unchanged drug and its metabolites.

Toxicity

Limited information is available on the acute toxicity of encainide. In general, overdosage of encainide may be expected to produce effects that involve cardiac conduction and function as well as the nervous system. Possible effects may include increases in QRS and QT intervals and AV dissociation; a variety of conduction disturbances, arrhythmogenic effects, hypotension, bradycardia, asystole, and seizures (Table 20–7).

TABLE 20–7. *Toxicity of Class IC antiarrhythmics*

Cardiac
Proarrhythmic effects
Increase QT interval
Widened QRS duration
AV dissociation
Second-degree block
Third-degree block
Bradycardia
Asystole
Neurologic
Dizziness
Blurred vision
Headache
Nausea

Like other antiarrhythmic agents, encainide can worsen existing arrhythmias or cause new arrhythmias. The arrhythmogenic effects of the drug may range from an increased frequency of ventricular premature complexes to the development of more severe and potentially fatal ventricular tachyarrhythmias. Effective 1991, encainide has only been available in the U.S. for qualifying patients via restricted distribution through their physician.

Flecainide

Flecainide (Tambocor) is a fluorinated benzamide derivative and is a Class IC agent, approved for oral treatment of ventricular arrhythmias. Flecainide is a local anesthetic-type antiarrhythmic agent and is at least as effective and more potent on a weight basis than most currently available antiarrhythmic agents in preventing and/or suppressing experimentally induced arrhythmias (18). Flecainide prolongs conduction in all cardiac tissues, particularly in the His-Purkinje system and ventricular myocardium, with relatively minor effects on repolarization (19).

Flecainide decreases ventricular conduction and increases the ventricular refractory period, primarily by blocking sodium channels. The dissociation of flecainide from sodium channels is slow as compared to lidocaine or quinidine (20).

Pharmacokinetics

Following oral administration, the absorption of flecainide is nearly complete; the bioavailability of flecainide being approximately 95%. Food or antacid does not affect absorption. Peak plasma flecainide concentrations usually occur within 2–3 hours after oral administration. The apparent plasma half-life averages about 20 hours and is quite variable after multiple oral doses. A specific advantage of flecainide is its very slow elimination (2). Because of the long elimination half-life of flecainide and the possibility of markedly nonlinear pharmacokinetics at very high doses, treatment for an extended period of time may be necessary. Urinary alkalinization will reduce renal clearance and result in elevated plasma concentrations of the drug (21).

Two major metabolites are pharmacologically active. These metabolites are less potent than the parent drug (22). The actual contribution of these metabolites to the antiarrhythmic effect is low, and therapeutic monitoring of these metabolites is not necessary (8).

Adverse Effects

Flecainide has a proarrhythmic effect and this may occur within the "therapeutic range" (23). As for other antiarrhythmic drugs, flecainide may pose a higher risk for adverse rhythm effects in elderly patients with sick sinus syndrome (18). Side effects of flecainide include sinus node dysfunction and second- or third-degree AV block (2). This occurs most often in patients with a history of sustained ventricular tachycardia. Because of this, this drug is currently reserved for treatment of severe ventricular tachyarrhythmias, when the risk–benefit ratio is likely to be favorable. Other side effects of flecainide include dizziness, blurred vision, headache, and nausea. Gastrointestinal disorders occur, but are generally less severe than with other antiarrhythmics. These agents may also prove useful in patients with supraventricular arrhythmias, who are less prone to proarrhythmic toxicity (8).

Laboratory

Based on premature ventricular contraction (PVC) suppression, it appears that plasma levels of 0.2 to 1.0 μg/mL may be needed to obtain the maximal therapeutic effect. It is more difficult to assess the dose needed to suppress serious arrhythmias (23). Plasma levels above 0.7–1.0 μg/mL are associated with a higher rate of cardiac adverse experiences such as conduction defects or bradycardia. The relation of plasma levels to proarrhythmic events is not established (18).

Moricizine

Moricizine was first synthesized in the then Soviet Union in 1964 and was approved by the FDA in 1990 to treat documented life-threatening ventricular arrhythmias (15). It is chemically unrelated to any currently approved antiarrhythmic drug, and despite having a phenothiazine structure, it lacks dopamine-antagonist activity and the behavioral and autonomic actions of neuroleptic phenothiazines (15).

It has proved difficult to subclassify moricizine within the group of Class I antiarrhythmic agents. On the basis of available data, moricizine does not fit readily into any of the subclasses of sodium-channel blocking agents. Although controversy has surrounded the classification of moricizine, the electrophysiologic effects suggest that the drug is best considered in the IC group of antiarrhythmic agents with potent local anesthetic activity and myocardial membrane stabilizing effects (6).

Pharmacokinetics

Orally administered moricizine is almost completely absorbed from the gastrointestinal tract. Its bioavailability is approximately 30% to 40%, resulting primarily from a first-pass effect (6). Peak plasma concentrations of moricizine occur in 1 to 2 hours (15). The apparent volume of distribution after oral administration is very large. Moricizine is approximately 95% bound to plasma proteins. This binding interaction is independent of moricizine plasma concentration. Moricizine has been shown to induce its own metabolism. Some moricizine is also recycled through enterohepatic circulation (4). The plasma half-life of moricizine is 1.5–3.5 hours following single or multiple oral doses in patients with ventricular ectopy (15).

Drug Interactions

Moricizine increases the plasma concentrations of theophylline by approximately 50% by decreasing the elimination half-life of theophylline. Therefore, plasma theophylline concentrations should be monitored when these drugs are used concomitantly (16).

Adverse Effects

The adverse cardiovascular effects of moricizine include the worsening of arrhythmias, conduction disturbances, and heart failure. A disturbing incidence of proarrhythmic responses has been noted with moricizine.

Laboratory

The antiarrhythmic and electrophysiologic effects of moricizine are not related in time course or intensity to plasma moricizine concentrations or to the concentrations of any identified metabolite, all of which have short half-lives of 2 to 3 hours (16).

Overdosage

Overdosage with moricizine may produce emesis, lethargy, coma, syncope, hypotension, conduction disturbances, exacerbation of congestive heart failure, myocardial infarction, sinus arrest, arrhythmias, including junctional bradycardia, ventricular tachycardia, ventricular fibrillation and asystole, and respiratory failure (Table 20–8) (16). Treatment is discussed below.

TREATMENT OF OVERDOSE OF CLASS IC DRUGS

Treatment of Class IC overdosage generally involves symptomatic and supportive care, with EKG and blood pressure monitoring and frequent neurologic evaluation.

Following acute ingestion of drugs in this class, the stomach should be emptied immediately by gastric lavage, followed by activated charcoal and a cathartic. Limited data suggest that IV sodium bicarbonate may be useful for the management of cardiac toxicity associated with overdosage of drugs in this class. Supportive treatment may include IV administration of inotropic agents or cardiac

TABLE 20–8. *Signs and symptoms of moricizine toxicity*

Gastrointestinal
Nausea
Emesis
Neurologic
Lethargy
Coma
Syncope
Cardiac
Hypotension
Conduction disturbances
Exacerbation of congestive heart failure
Myocardial infarction
Sinus arrest
Arrhythmias
Junctional bradycardia
Ventricular tachycardia
Ventricular fibrillation
Asystole
Respiratory
Respiratory failure

stimulants such as dopamine or dobutamine and circulatory assistance which may require intra-aortic balloon counterpulsation, if necessary, as well as transvenous pacing. It is not known whether hemodialysis or peritoneal dialysis would enhance the elimination of these drugs.

CLASS II

Class II agents are capable of counteracting sympathetic stimulation of the heart. These agents may directly compete with receptors, as with β-receptor blockers, or interfere with norepinephrine release from sympathetic nerves such as guanethidine.

The β blockers are discussed in Chapter 15.

CLASS III

Class III agents include bretylium and amiodarone. These agents prolong the AP and the effective refractory period without appreciable effect on the rate of rise of the AP. These agents mainly prolong repolarization, prolong the PR and QRS intervals as well as the QT interval (3).

Bretylium

Bretylium is an adrenergic blocking agent that is used as an antiarrhythmic agent. Bretylium affects cardiac electrical activity by three mechanisms: (a) indirectly by an initial sympathomimetic effect, (b) directly by an antifibrillatory effect, and (c) directly by altering the transmembrane AP; the result of this is a prolongation of the AP and effective refractory period without altering depolarization or conduction velocity.

Bretylium selectively accumulates in sympathetic ganglia and their postganglionic adrenergic neurons where it inhibits norepinephrine release by depressing adrenergic nerve terminal excitability. Bretylium also suppresses ventricular fibrillation and ventricular arrhythmias. Bretylium induces a chemical sympathectomy-like state which resembles a surgical sympathectomy. Catecholamine stores are not depleted by bretylium, but catecholamine effects on the myocardium and on peripheral vascular resistance are often seen shortly after administration because bretylium causes an early release of norepinephrine from the adrenergic postganglionic nerve terminals. Subsequently, bretylium blocks the release of norepinephrine in response to neuron stimulation. Peripheral adrenergic blockade regularly causes orthostatic hypotension but has less effect on supine blood pressure.

Pharmacokinetics

Bretylium is incompletely and erratically absorbed from the gastrointestinal tract. Bretylium is eliminated intact by the kidneys. No metabolites have been identified following administration of bretylium.

Side Effects

Hypotension is the most frequent adverse effect of bretylium and often occurs within the first hour of therapy. Vertigo, dizziness, lightheadedness, faintness, and syncope are symptoms of postural hypotension. The initial release of norepinephrine may worsen arrhythmias caused by cardiac glycoside toxicity.

Treatment

If bretylium is overdosed and symptoms of toxicity develop, administration of nitroprusside or another short-acting intravenous antihypertensive agent should be considered for the treatment of the hypertensive response. Long-acting drugs that might potentiate the subsequent hypotensive effects of bretylium should not be used. Hypotension should be treated with appropriate fluid therapy and pressor agents such as dopamine or norepinephrine. Dialysis is not useful in the treatment of bretylium overdose.

Amiodarone

Amiodarone (Cordarone) is an iodinated benzofuran derivative that differs structurally and pharmacologically from other currently available antiarrhythmic agents. The antiarrhythmic and electrophysiologic actions of amiodarone are complex and also differ from those of currently available antiarrhythmic agents (24).

Although amiodarone has been classified as a Class III agent, it is now clear that amiodarone has actions that fit all the four classes: blockade of the fast sodium current (Class I); blockade of the slow calcium current (Class II);

TABLE 20–9. *Effects of amiodarone*

Blockade of sodium channel—Class I
β Blocker—Class II
Blockade of delayed outward potassium currents—Class III
Blockade of slow calcium current—Class IV
α-Adrenergic receptor blockade
Inhibition of sodium-potassium ATPase pump
Unique pharmacokinetics
Poor gastrointestinal absorption
Slow onset of action
Very long half-life (10–100 days)
Active metabolites
Large volume of distribution (150 L/kg)

blockade of delayed outward potassium currents causing prolonged repolarization (Class III); and noncompetitive β-adrenergic antagonism (Class II) (Table 20–9). In addition, other effects include inhibition of the Na-K ATPase pump. Amiodarone is a unique Class III agent, therefore, because it is a calcium channel, β and α blocker that contains iodine.

Amiodarone was originally intended for angina treatment, but has been shown to be effective for treating supraventricular arrhythmias, especially Wolff-Parkinson-White syndrome as well as some ventricular arrhythmias. Amiodarone also has antianginal effects. This may result from its noncompetitive α and β adrenoceptor-blocking properties as well as from its apparent ability to block calcium influx in coronary arterial smooth muscle.

Amiodarone causes peripheral vascular dilatation, presumably through its α adrenoceptor-blocking and calcium channel-inhibiting effects (25). In some patients, this may be beneficial; rarely, it may require discontinuance of the drug (12).

The principal effect of amiodarone on cardiac tissue is to delay repolarization by prolonging the AP duration and effective refractory period. It increases the ventricular fibrillation threshold without altering the membrane resting potential. The drug also appears to inhibit transmembrane influx of extracellular sodium ions via fast sodium channels, as indicated by a decrease in the maximal rate of depolarization of phase O of the AP (26). Amiodarone has a broad spectrum of actions on the heart (2). It is a very effective blocker of sodium channels, but unlike quinidine it has a low affinity for activated channels, combining instead almost exclusively with channels in the inactivated state (12). Thus, the sodium-blocking action of amiodarone is most pronounced in tissues that have long action potentials, frequent action potentials, or less negative diastolic potentials. The drug has also been shown to be a powerful inhibitor of abnormal automaticity (24).

Pharmacokinetics

Amiodarone has unique pharmacokinetic properties in that it is poor and variably absorbed with a very slow onset of action, very long half-lives of elimination, active metabolites, a complex pattern of tissue distribution and tissue actions, and poor correlation between gross cardiac accumulation and cardiac effects (2).

The pharmacokinetic profile of amiodarone after a single dose is best described by use of a three-compartment model: the central compartment, a peripheral compartment with which equilibrium is reached in days, and a deep compartment with a high affinity for lipid-soluble compounds, for which equilibrium is reached in weeks or months. Early electrophysiologic effects, including changes in sinus and atrioventricular node properties may be evident within several days.

Amiodarone is extremely lipid-soluble, with a volume of distribution of approximately 150 L/kg. The plasma half-life with long-term administration is long and variable, ranging from 9 to 100 days. This long half-life may lead to antiarrhythmic or toxic effects for as long as 30 days after discontinuation of the drug (8). In addition, amiodarone also has an active metabolite, desethylamiodarone (DEA), which has a more variable pharmacokinetic profile than its parent compound. It takes 15–30 days to load the body stores with sufficient amiodarone to estimate the drug's efficacy.

Plasma concentrations of 1.0 to 2.5 μg/mL are clinically effective (8). Therapeutically effective serum concentrations are in the range of 0.2 to 7 μg/mL and there is a strong correlation between concentration and improvement in hemodynamic function (12).

Side Effects

Pulmonary fibrosis has been recognized in the last few years as a serious problem associated with amiodarone treatment. The benzofuran portion of the amiodarone molecule is structurally similar to that of nitrofurantoin and other compounds that cause lung damage, and is suspected to be the cause of this complication (Table 20–10) (25). Amiodarone-induced pulmonary toxicity may result from pulmonary interstitial pneumonitis or from hypersensitivity pneumonitis (11).

TABLE 20–10. *Toxicity of amiodarone*

Pulmonary
Pulmonary fibrosis
Dyspnea
Nonproductive cough
Miscellaneous
Corneal deposits of microcrystals
Elevated aminotransferases
Photosensitivity
Bluish discoloration of skin
Peripheral neuropathy
Overdosage
Nausea
Vomiting
Sinus bradycardia
Hypotension
QT prolongation

Other dose-related side effects, including tremor, anorexia, emesis, nausea, elevated hepatic aminotransferases, photosensitization, bluish discoloration of the skin, and peripheral neuropathy, typically respond to dose reduction and rarely require drug withdrawal (24).

Factors predisposing patients to amiodarone toxicity include advanced age, higher amiodarone doses, lower pretreatment diffusion capacity, and, perhaps, elevated serum amiodarone metabolite concentrations (11).

The serious side effects of the drug limit its usefulness and make it a drug of last resort for treating refractory arrhythmias (12).

Drug Interactions

Increased plasma concentrations of digoxin, quinidine, procainamide, NAPA, phenytoin, flecainide, diltiazem, and theophylline have been reported in patients treated with amiodarone. The anticoagulant effects of warfarin are potentiated, which may lead to a serious coagulopathy. Although amiodarone is a highly effective antiarrhythmic agent, its toxicity limits its clinical usefulness.

Adverse Effects

Amiodarone is deposited in tissue and can be found in virtually every organ. The most readily detected deposits are those in the cornea, which appear as yellowish-brown microcrystals within a few weeks after initiation of therapy. These corneal deposits rarely cause visual symptoms except for occasional halos in the peripheral visual fields, most prominent at night. Only infrequently does reduction of visual acuity occur, requiring discontinuance or reduction of amiodarone dosage. Skin deposits result in photodermatitis in about 25% of patients, and these patients must avoid exposure to the sun. In a small percentage of patients, a grayish-blue skin discoloration develops.

Overdose

Limited information is available on the acute toxicity of amiodarone. In general, overdosage may produce effects such as sinus bradycardia and/or heart block, hypotension, and QT prolongation (Table 20–10). Nausea is likely to occur with ingestions of greater than 1 g of the drug. In patients with sinus or atrioventricular nodal disease, amiodarone may produce symptomatic bradycardia or heart block. It may also precipitate heart failure in susceptible patients.

Because the onset of toxicity may be delayed, EKG monitoring may be necessary for several days following acute ingestion of the drug (10).

Treatment of Overdose

Management of amiodarone overdosage generally involves symptomatic and supportive care, with EKG and blood pressure monitoring. Following recent acute ingestion, the stomach should be emptied by gastric lavage, followed by activated charcoal and a cathartic.

Administration of IV fluids and placement of the patient in Trendelenburg's position is recommended for the initial treatment of hypotension. An inotropic agent or vasopressor should be given for hypotension accompanied by signs of inadequate tissue perfusion.

Amiodarone-induced bradycardia generally is not fully responsive to atropine, therefore IV administration of a β-adrenergic agonist or the use of a transvenous pacemaker may be necessary.

Attempts at extracorporeal removal of the drug by hemoperfusion or hemodialysis are not effective, and therefore not recommended.

CLASS IV

The calcium channel blockers are Class IV antiarrhythmic agents. They act by prolonging conduction through the AV node, and their major EKG effect is lengthening of the PR interval. They are discussed in Chapter 22.

MISCELLANEOUS COMPOUNDS

Adenosine (Adenocard)

Adenosine is an endogenous nucleoside that is present in all cells of the body and is formed as a product of the enzymatic breakdown of either ATP or adenosylhomocysteine through at least three enzymatic pathways. Adenosine is not a new drug, and much of what is known about the effects of adenosine was obtained in the 1930s.

The precise function of endogenous adenosine is unknown, but the actions of adenosine tend to maintain the balance between oxygen delivery and oxygen demand in the heart and other organs. During periods of hypoxia or ischemia, the production of adenosine by cardiac myocytes increases (Table 20–11). Consequently, adenosine can be seen as a locally acting metabolite that has a homeostatic role in protecting the heart against hypoxia (4).

TABLE 20–11. *Adenosine*

Endogenous nucleoside (A_1 adenosine receptor)
Increases with hypoxia/ischemia
Actions inhibited by methylxanthines
Causes hyperpolarization of atrial myocytes
Ineffective when given as infusion
Half-life: 10 seconds
Side effects (transient)
Dyspnea
Flushing
Chest discomfort/pain
Transient AV block

Uses

Adenosine produces transient AV nodal conduction delay after IV administration and thus is effective in terminating supraventricular tachycardias involving the AV node. Adenosine is a potent dilator of coronary arteries and is capable of decreasing cardiac oxygen consumption by its antiadrenergic and negative chronotropic actions.

Actions

All the cellular electrophysiologic effects of adenosine are competitively and reversibly antagonized by methylxanthines and are thought to be mediated by the specific A_1 adenosine receptor. Stimulation of the A_1 receptor on the cell surface is thought to influence both the adenosine-sensitive potassium channels and cyclic AMP production by means of an inhibitory guanine nucleotide-binding protein (G_I). The actions of ATP on AV nodal conduction are thought to be mediated primarily by hydrolysis to adenosine.

The principal electrophysiologic actions of adenosine on supraventricular tissues, the sinoatrial node and atrium, are mediated by the stimulation of a specific time-independent outward potassium current that is identical to that stimulated by acetylcholine. The stimulation of this membrane current is accompanied by the hyperpolarization of atrial myocytes, a decrease in the duration of the atrial action potentials, and a decrease in the diastolic depolarization (phase 4) of the pacemaker cells of the SA node (7).

The effects of adenosine on sinus rate and AV nodal conduction are different when the agent is administered as a continuous intravenous infusion (4). Under these circumstances, there is a dose-dependent sinus tachycardia, and AV nodal conduction is unaffected. This difference is presumably related to a higher local concentration of adenosine at the AV node after bolus administration, as well as the fact that after a bolus dose, the direct AV nodal effects precede and are therefore unopposed by the effects of sympathetic stimulation. As a consequence, adenosine is ineffective in the management of supraventricular tachycardias when given as an infusion rather than as a bolus dose.

Adenosine does not significantly alter blood pressure, and to date there have been no reports of hemodynamic collapse associated with its use (27).

Pharmacokinetics

Intravenously administered adenosine is removed from the circulation very rapidly. Following an intravenous bolus, adenosine is taken up by erythrocytes and vascular endothelial cells. The half-life of intravenous adenosine is estimated to be less than 10 seconds. In the range of physiologic concentrations, the half-life of adenosine in plasma is as short as 0.6 to 1.5 seconds, because of both its deamination to inosine in the plasma and its uptake by red cells (28). Because of such a short half-life, it is thought that adenosine exerts its effect during the first pass through the cardiac circulation and is most effective when given rapidly and close to the central circulation. Adenosine enters the body pool and is primarily metabolized to inosine and adenosine monophosphate.

It is the very short half-life of adenosine that provides the intravenously administered compound with its principal advantage over other antiarrhythmic agents in the management of tachycardia.

Side Effects

Adenosine given as a bolus dose through a peripheral vein is associated with dose-related symptoms of dyspnea, flushing, and chest discomfort or pain. The chest pain may radiate in different directions: toward the ears, shoulders, ulnar aspect of the upper and lower arms, back, or upper abdomen. It may reproduce the pain of cardiac ischemia in patients with chronic stable angina and may mimic that of duodenal ulcer. These effects are short-lived, lasting an average of 5 to 20 seconds (28).

Transient AV block, induced during the administration, sometimes can be prolonged. All of these effects are transient and usually require no intervention (7).

Drug Interactions

Drug interactions include theophylline, which antagonizes its effects through receptor blockade, and dipyridamole, which enhances the effects of adenosine through inhibition of cellular reuptake (7).

Overdose

Because the half-life of adenosine is so short, the adverse effects are generally rapidly self-limiting and symptoms of overdose may be treated symptomatically, if treatment is necessary at all (7). Treatment of any prolonged adverse effects should be individualized and be directed toward the specific effect, due to the extremely short half-life, and by stopping the infusion (28).

REFERENCES

1. Nolan P, Raehl C: Antiarrhythmic agents. *Crit Care Clin* 1991;7: 507–520.
2. Woosley R, Funck-Bretano C: Overview of the clinical pharmacology of antiarrhythmic drugs. *Am J Cardiol* 1988;61:61A–69A.
3. Karkal S, Stapczynski J, Podrid P: Update on antiarrhythmic drugs. *Emerg Med Rep* 1989;10:41–48.
4. Woosley R: Antiarrhytmic drugs. *Annu Rev Pharmaocol Toxicol* 1991;31:427–455.
5. Artman E, et al: Calcium channel blocking agents in the treatment of cardiovascular disorders. *Ann Intern Med* 1980;93:875–885.
6. Powell A, Gold M, Brooks R, et al: Electrophysiologic response to moricizine in patients with sustained ventricular arrhythmias. *Ann Intern Med* 1992;116:382–387.

7. McCabe J, Adhar G, Menegazzi J, et al: Intravenous adenosine in the prehospital treatment of paroxysmal supraventricular tachycardia. *Ann Emerg Med* 1992;21:358–361.
8. Kelner M: Newer cardiac agents: antiarrhythmics and antianginal agents. *Clin Lab Med* 1987;7:567–585.
9. Michelson E, Freifus L: Newer antiarrhythmic drugs. *Med Clin North Amer* 1988;72:275–319.
10. Mattioni T, Zheutlin T, Sarmiento J, et al: Amiodarone in patients with previous drug-mediated torsade de pointes. *Ann Intern Med* 1989;111:574–580.
11. Nolan P, Raehl C: Antiarrhythmic agents. *Crit Care Clin* 1991; 7:507–520.
12. Lazzara R: Amiodarone and torsade de pointes. *Ann Intern Med* 1989;111:549–551.
13. Jonville A, Barbier P, Blond M, et al: Accidental lidocaine overdosage in an infant. *J Toxicol Clin Toxicol* 1990;28:101–106.
14. Derlet R, Albertson T, Tharratt R: Lidocaine potention of cocaine toxicity. *Ann Emerg Med* 1991;20:135–138.
15. Clyne C, Estes N, Wang P: Moricizine. *N Engl J Med* 1992;327: 255–260.
16. Damle R, Levine J, Matos J, et al: Efficacy and risks of moricizine in inducible sustained ventricular tachycardia. *Ann Intern* Med 1992; 116:375–381.
17. Koppel C, Oberdisse U, Heinemeyer G: Clinical course and outcome in class IC antiarrhythmic overdose. *J Toxicol Clin Toxicol* 1990;28: 433–444.
18. Zeigler V, Gillette P, Hammill B, et al: Flecainide for supraventricular tachycardia in children. *Am J Cardiol* 1988;62:41D–43D.
19. Cheng C, Kim S, Ruffy R: Flecainide acetate for treatment of bypass tract mediated reentrant tachycardia. *Am J Cardiol* 1988;62:23D–28D.
20. Anderson J, Jolivette D, Fredell P: Summary of efficacy and safety of flecainide for supraventricular arrhythmias. *Am J Cardiol* 1988;62: 62D–66D.
21. Starmer F, Lancaster A, Lastra A, et al: Cardiac instability amplified by use-dependent Na channel blockade. *Am J Physiol* 1992;262: H1305–H1310.
22. Kim S, Smith P, Ruffy R: Treatment of atrial tachyarrhythmias and preexcitation syndrome with flecainide acetate. *Am J Cardiol* 1988; 62:29D–34D.
23. Hellestrand K: Intravenous flecainide acetate for supraventricular tachycardias. *Am J Cardiol* 1988;62:16D–22D.
24. Middlekauff H, Wiener I, Saxoin L, et al: Low-dose amiodarone for atrial fibrillation: time for a prospective study. *Ann Intern Med* 1992;116:1017–1020.
25. Bonati M, D'Arrano V, Galletti F, et al: Acute overdosage of amiodarone in a suicide attempt. *J Toxicol Clin Toxicol* 1983;20:181–186.
26. Van Zwieten P: The role of adrenoceptors in circulatory and metabolic regulation. *Am Heart J* 1988;116:1384–1391.
27. Roden D: Risks and benefits of antiarrhythmic therapy. *N Engl J Med* 1994;331:785–791.
28. Camm A, Garratt C: Adenosine and supraventricular tachycardia. *N Engl J Med* 1991;325:1621–1629.

CHAPTER 21

Digitalis Glycosides

Glycosides that have positive inotropic actions on the heart occur widely in nature and can be prepared synthetically. The cardiac glycosides consist of a group of chemically and pharmacologically related substances derived from various plants (Table 21–1); each comprises a characteristic steroid molecule coupled with one or more types of sugar molecules.

Cardiac glycosides of medicinal importance are obtained from *Digitalis purpurea* (digitoxin, digitalis, gitalin), from *Digitalis lanata* (digoxin, digitoxin, lanatoside C, deslanoside, acetyldigitoxin), *Strophanthus gratus* (ouabain), and *Acocanthera schimperi* (ouabain) (1).

The term *digitalis* is generally used to designate any of the steroid glycoside compounds that exert typical positive inotropic and electrophysiologic effects on the heart (2). There are more than 300 compounds with this property. Powdered digitalis leaf has been superseded by purer preparations, including digoxin, digitoxin, ouabain, lanatoside C, deslanoside, and medigoxin; only the first two of these are widely prescribed. Commercially available digitalis preparations are listed in Table 21–2. Even though the frequency of digitalis intoxication appears to be decreasing, life-threatening toxicity continues to occur in patients who take overdoses by mistake or with suicidal intent.

Although uncommon, digitalis toxicity also can arise from accidental ingestion of cardiac glycoside-containing plants such as oleanders, foxglove, lily of the valley, and red squill. The yew plant also contains an arrhythmogenic alkaloid that although chemically unrelated, has actions similar to digitalis (3).

TABLE 21–1. *Common plants containing cardiac glycosides*

Plant	Common name
Asclepias fruticosa	Balloon cotton
Digitalis purpurea	Foxglove
Plumeria rubra	Frangipani
Calotropis procera	King's crown
Convallaria majalis	Lily of the valley
Nerium oleander	Oleander
Cryptostegia grandifloria	Ruber vine
Cerbera manghas	Sea mango
Urginea maritima	Squill
Thevetia peruviana	Yellow oleander

PHARMACOKINETICS

Digoxin

Digoxin is the most commonly used cardiac glycoside primarily because it may be administered by various routes. Digoxin is 60% to 85% absorbed from the gastrointestinal tract (Table 21–3) (4–6). After oral administration, the onset of action occurs in 30 minutes to 2 hours; and the drug reaches its peak plasma concentration in 3 to 8 hours. Digoxin has a volume of distribution of 7 to 10 L/kg. Approximately 23% of digoxin is bound to plasma proteins (6). Fifteen percent undergoes hepatic transformation, and 85% is excreted unchanged by the kidney (7). Digoxin is excreted exponentially and has an average half-life in patients with normal renal function of 36 hours, which results in a daily loss of about 37% of body stores. Renal excretion of digoxin is proportional to the glomerular filtration rate and hence to the creatinine clearance rate. The elimination half-life of digoxin is therefore greater in patients with impaired

TABLE 21–2. *Commercially available digitalis preparations*

Compound	Trade names
Digoxin	Lanoxin Lanoxicaps Novodigoxin
Digitoxin	Crystodigin Digitaline Purodigin

TABLE 21–3. *Differences in pharmacokinetics between digoxin and digitoxin*

Parameter	Digoxin	Digitoxin
Oral absorption	75% to 90%	90% to 100%
Plasma protein binding	25%	90%
Metabolism (M) compared to excretion (E)	E > M	M > E
Half-life	1.6 days	7 days
Volume of distribution	7–10 L/kg	0.5 L/kg
Enterohepatic recirculation	No	Yes

renal function and may be up to 4 to 6 days for patients with severely compromised renal function (8). In previously undigitalized patients with normal renal function, institution of daily maintenance therapy of digoxin without a loading dose results in development of steady-state concentrations after four to five half-lives or about 7 days.

Distribution

The distribution phase of digoxin from the blood is relatively slow, with a half-life of about 30 minutes following intravenous or oral administration of the drug. This means that initially, very high concentrations of digoxin can be measured in the serum. The practical implication of this slow distribution phase is that initial levels measured close to the time of administration may be erroneously interpreted as potentially toxic.

Bioavailability

Variation among digoxin tablets in bioavailability, and therefore in steady-state serum digoxin concentrations, was a cause of digitalis intoxication until quite recently. This was not due so much to differences in digoxin content as to differences in the dissolution rate of the tablets (9). This was partly a result of differences in digoxin particular size or in "inert" additives that had an effect on disintegration and dissolution rates within the intestinal lumen (10–12).

Digitoxin

Oral absorption of digitoxin is considered virtually 100% (4,6,13). This drug undergoes substantial enterohepatic circulation that is about fourfold that of digoxin (4). It is mostly metabolized by the liver, whereas digoxin is mostly excreted by the kidney. The volume of distribution of digitoxin is approximately 0.54 L/kg. The maximum effect is attained in 4 to 12 hours. Digitoxin is 95% protein-bound to serum albumin and has a half-life of 5 to 7 days (13). Administration of daily maintenance doses of digitoxin results in gradual digitalization with establishment of a final steady-state concentration after 3 to 4 weeks.

Digitoxin gives rise to intoxication less frequently than digoxin because its excretion is independent of renal function. Nevertheless, if intoxication does occur the signs and symptoms may persist for up to a week owing to the long half-life (14).

Although the elimination of digitoxin is appreciably different from that of digoxin in that most of the body load of digitoxin is metabolized by the liver, the elimination is not prolonged in patients with hepatic insufficiency, probably owing to the high capacity of the metabolizing system. Unlike digoxin, the elimination of digotoxin is not affected by renal insufficiency, and therefore it has been suggested as the cardiac glycoside of choice in patients with various degrees of renal insufficiency (3).

Oleander

The dogbane family (*Apocynaceae*) contains many species, including the ornamental shrubs yellow oleander (*Thevetia peruviana*) and common oleander (*Nerium oleander*). Both are widely cultivated in tropical and subtropical regions (15). The latter is more common in the United States. The plant is a flowering shrub valued for its colorful flowers, dense green foliage, and hardy nature (16). It is common to many areas of the United States as a garden plant, and it is used widely in hedges and freeway medians (17).

All parts of the oleander plant are toxic, including the sap, leaves, blossoms, stems, seeds, honey, and berries. Most poisonings occur in children (18) and when the stems have been used as skewers or stirrers for outdoor picnics. Inhalation of oleander smoke has also caused toxicity. Boiling or drying the plant does not inactivate the toxins (19).

Even today, oleander is still used therapeutically in some parts of the U.S. In areas where folk medicine is common, oleander is purported to have a variety of curative powers, including use as an abortifacient and in the treatment of leprosy, ringworm, malaria and venereal disease (15). Acute oleander poisoning is not uncommon in tropical and subtropical parts of the world including the U.S. (17).

The glycosides associated with oleander include oleandrin, digitoxigenin, and nerium from *Nerium oleander*, and thevetin A and B and thevetoxin from *Thevetia peruviana* (18). These glycosides account for the plants' cardiotoxic effects (19). The similarities in activity and aglycone ring structure between these oleander glycosides and digoxin also allow a cross-reactivity in radioimmunoassays for digoxin (18).

Potential hyperkalemia, a well-known complication of acute digoxin toxicity, also characterizes severe oleander poisoning. In addition to cardiotoxicity, other constitutional symptoms after exposure include mucous membrane irritation, nausea, vomiting, cramping abdominal pain, dizziness, and weakness (15).

CLINICAL USES OF CARDIAC GLYCOSIDES

Cardiac glycosides are used principally in the prophylactic management and treatment of heart failure and to control the ventricular rate in patients with atrial fibrillation or flutter (Table 21–4) (20). Although there may be a common belief that digoxin effectively restores sinus rhythm in patients with recent onset of atrial fibrillation, this is not the case (21). Digoxin is used in atrial fibrillation to establish a ventricular rate that will produce an

TABLE 21–4. *Clinical uses of digitalis preparations*

Congestive heart failure
Atrial fibrillation
Atrial flutter
Paroxysmal atrial tachycardia
Atrioventricular functional rhythm
Supraventricular tachycardia

improved cardiac output (21). It has also been used to treat and prevent recurrent paroxysmal atrial tachycardia (22).

ACTIONS

All cardiac glycosides produce the same qualitative therapeutic effect on the heart. This includes an increase in the force of contraction, an increase in the refractory period of the atrioventricular node, and an effect on the sinoatrial node and conduction system by way of the autonomic nervous system (Table 21–5) (2).

The main pharmacologic property of cardiac glycosides is their ability to increase the force and velocity of myocardial systolic contraction by a direct action on the myocardium (4). Digitalis and the other cardiac glycosides can alter electrophysiologic properties such as automaticity, conduction, refractoriness, and excitability of the various specialized conduction tissues, including the sinoatrial node, specialized tissues within the atrium, and atrioventricular, junctional, and Purkinje fibers (5,6).

Mechanical Effects

The effects of digitalis can be separated into mechanical and electrophysiologic actions. The mechanical effect is caused by increased intracellular calcium, which augments the force of a myocardial contraction and leads to a positive inotropic state (2,23).

Electrophysiologic Effects

The electrophysiologic actions are varied. The chronotropic effect of digitalis is mediated primarily through an increase in vagal tone, which decreases the rate of sinoatrial node depolarization. In addition, digitalis increases the refractory period of the atrioventricular node and the His-Purkinje system accounting for the decreased ventricular response in atrial fibrillation. Increased phase 4 depolarization (as a result of Na influx) leads to the appearance of new or latent pacemakers, which increases automaticity. This sodium influx also lowers the resting membrane potential threshold, which in turn increases excitability (24).

TABLE 21–5. *Cardiac actions of digitalis*

Negative chronotropism
Positive inotropism
Slowing of sinus node impulse formation
Enhancement of intra-atrial conduction
Slowing of conduction velocity
Increase in rate of spontaneous depolarization

Summary of Effects

The effects of digoxin on these tissues may be to a different degree and sometimes in an opposite direction. For example, digitalis acts to cause negative chronotropic effects as well as positive inotropic effects. The negative chronotropic effect is reflected clinically as slowing of the heart rate, whereas the positive inotropic effect is reflected clinically as increased force of contraction of the cardiac muscle (2). The negative chronotropic effect is due to an increase in vagal tone, prolongation of the refractory periods of the atrioventricular node and bundle of His, and slowing of the conduction velocity, although myocardial automaticity is increased. Digitalis can also slow sinus node impulse, hyperpolarize cells in the atrium, and enhance intra-atrial conduction (6). The sinus slowing that accompanies digitalis therapy is therefore attributed to both a direct effect of the drug on impulse initiation by the sinus pacemaker cells and a cholinergic action mediated by the vagus nerve (25).

Some of the pharmacologic properties of digitalis contribute to the relatively high incidence of cardiotoxic reactions (26). This is attributable to the widespread use of cardiac glycosides coupled with the narrow margin between therapeutic and toxic doses and toxic and lethal doses.

Digitalis and the Action Potential

The transmembrane resting potential of cardiac cells is maintained by sodium and potassium gradients, which are in turn dependent on the integrity of the active sodium-potassium-activated adenosine triphosphatase (Na-K ATPase) pump. Because of the size of pores of the cells, the membrane is freely permeable to potassium and chloride ions (which are small), relatively impermeable to sodium, and essentially impermeable to organic anions (which are present as large protein molecules). The concentrations of sodium and chloride are much higher in the extracellular fluid than in the intracellular fluid, and the concentrations of potassium and organic acids are much higher in the intracellular fluid than in the extracellular fluid (27).

As a consequence of this ionic imbalance, there is an electrical potential across the membrane. This electrical potential may reach 50 to 90 mV, with the inside of the membrane negative in relation to the outside. Such a difference in potential exists in every cell of the body and is referred to as the resting potential of the cell. When the neuron becomes less negative in relation to the extracellular fluid, the axon is said to be depolarized. When the axon is depolarized by a few millivolts, the permeability of the membrane is altered so that the membrane becomes rapidly more permeable to sodium (28).

Sodium conductance is activated first because of its greater voltage sensitivity. The sodium channel is about 20 times more selective for sodium than for potassium, and therefore sodium flows inward down the ion's electrochemical gradient. The consequent addition of positive charge to the inner membrane results in depolarization. After about 1 msec, the sodium conductance turns off, or inactivates. Inactivation proceeds much more slowly than does activation and persists transiently even after the membrane has been repolarized (29).

Before the sodium conductance inactivates, the potassium conductance has activated. The potassium channels favor potassium over sodium by about 100:1, so that potassium flows outward down its electrochemical gradient. The inner membrane surface loses positive charge, and the membrane is repolarized.

Digitalis exerts a positive inotropic effect on cardiac muscle by directly binding to the membrane Na-K ATPase pump (4,30). This enzyme is required for active transport of sodium across myocardial cell membranes (27). By impairing active transport of these ions the increase in intracellular sodium causes a net influx of calcium, which results in an increased concentration of calcium in the sarcoplasm (3). The subsequent rise in intracellular calcium allows an increase in the number of actin–myosin interactions, thereby increasing the force of myocardial contraction (1). Because ATPase appears to be essential to couple metabolic energy to the active cation transport mechanism at the cell surface, the digitalis-poisoned myocardium cannot extrude the sodium gained or recover the potassium lost during each action potential. This results in a slower rate of rise of the action potential, a slower conduction velocity with resultant conduction delays, and an increase in spontaneous depolarization. This mechanism can explain the re-entrant tachydysrhythmias, the enhanced ventricular ectopic activity, and the depression of the atrioventricular conduction that are seen with toxic concentrations of digitalis. In addition, toxicity results in part from loss of intracellular potassium associated with the inhibition of Na-K ATPase (30).

The Na-K ATPase Pump

To reiterate, digoxin effectively inhibits Na-K ATPase or the sodium pump on the cardiac cell membrane. With high affinity and specificity, free digoxin reversibly binds onto Na-K ATPase, causing a conformational change (28). The inhibitory site is located on the extracellular aspect of the α subunit of the pump. In this way, digoxin prevents ATP from binding onto the pump (4,31,32).

Normally, Na-K ATPase pumps two K ions into the cell for every three Na ions it pumps out. Inhibition of this pump results in an accumulation of intracellular Na ions, which stimulates the Na-Ca exchanger. The Na-Ca exchanger functions as a mediator for the trans-sarcolemmal movement of Ca ion in exchange for Na ion (25). This movement tends toward an equilibrium at which any increase in intracellular Na favors Na extrusion and simultaneous Ca entry into the cell through Na-Ca exchange. The consequence of an increased influx of Ca is an associated increase in slow inward current during the action potential, which is responsible for an enhanced myocardial contractile force.

Effects of Electrolytes

Both hypo- and hyperkalemia can exacerbate digitalis cardiotoxicity. Hypokalemia, especially at serum levels less than 2.5 mEq/L, inhibits the Na-K ATPase activity and adds to the pump inhibition induced by toxic levels of digitalis. In addition, hypokalemia enhances myocardial automaticity and is potentially arrhythmogenic. The net effect of hypokalemia is intensification of digitalis-related tachydysrhythmias. In contrast, hyperkalemia, especially at serum levels exceeding 5.4 mEq/L, leads to hyperpolarization of myocardial cells, especially in conductive tissue such as the atrioventricular (AV) node, aggravating digitalis-induced bradydysrhythmias and conduction delays.

Digitalis and the Autonomic Nervous System

The actions of digitalis on the autonomic nervous system are also important clinically and play a major role in determining the clinical pharmacodynamic effects of the drug (2). At therapeutic concentrations, the predominant effect is activation of vagal tone which depresses conduction through the AV node and results in a negative chronotropic effect (3). At toxic concentrations, there appears to be activation of sympathetic tone. This may contribute to the dysrhythmogenic effects of digoxin. Therefore, digitalis causes cardiac dysrhythmias not only by mechanisms that result from its inhibition of Na-K ATPase but also by mechanisms that result from its neural effects, such as augmentation of activity on vagal and sympathetic nerves (14).

DRUG INTERACTIONS

Calcium Antagonists

Certain calcium antagonists interact with digitalis to produce potentially undesirable electrophysiologic effects. Although many of the calcium channel blockers have been identified as potentially increasing the serum digoxin level, convincing evidence of clinical significance has been documented only for verapamil (29). Verapamil can raise the serum digoxin level via changes in renal and extrarenal clearance. Moreover, verapamil also reduces AV nodal conduction. These combined effects can lead to dramatic elevated digoxin levels, with resulting bradysystolic manifestations of cardiac toxicity (3,6).

Quinidine

The administration of quinidine to patients taking digoxin causes a significant increase in serum digoxin concentrations, with steady-state concentrations increasing by two to three times (33). The increase in serum digoxin concentration is due to a decrease in the apparent volume of distribution for digoxin caused by quinidine (30,34–36). This is because quinidine displaces digoxin from tissues by decreasing the affinity of receptor sites on Na-K ATPase membranes for digoxin (4,34,37). Thus the decrease in volume of distribution may reflect in part a decrease in the affinity of tissue receptors for digoxin (38). Quinidine also appears to cause a decrease in the rate of digitalis elimination or the clearance of digoxin (30,37).

Other Drug Interactions

Other drug interactions facilitate digoxin toxicity through various mechanisms and are especially relevant in chronic digitalis intoxication. For example, antacids, cholestyramine, colestipol, and sulfasalazine decrease digoxin absorption (Table 21–6) Patients receiving digoxin and one or more of these agents may develop acute digitalis toxicity if they abruptly stop taking the other agent and do not have their maintenance digoxin dose reduced (3). Examples of drug interactions also include antibiotic suppression of gut bacteria that normally metabolized digoxin, and slowed movement of the medication through the gastrointestinal tract by anticholinergic agents (29). Hypoxia, hypokalemia, alkalosis, as well as the sympathomimetic effects of β agonists or theophylline therapy may add to the neuroexcitatory effects of digoxin, which in turn may cause arrhythmias characteristic of digoxin toxicity (29). Antiadrenergic agents such as clonidine, methyldopa, and β blockers can predispose to bradydysrhythmias when used concomitantly with digoxin, especially individuals with underlying sinus node disease. Amiodarone exhibits a dose-related property of elevating serum digoxin levels via inhibition of renal tubular secretion of the glycoside (3).

TABLE 21–6. *Interactions with digoxin*

Drug/Condition	Effect
Amiodarone	Increases digoxin level
Verapamil	Increases digoxin level
Quinidine	Increases digoxin level
Antacids	Decreases digoxin level
Cholestyramine	Decreases digoxin level
Sulfasalazine	Decreases digoxin level
Hypoxia	Increases digoxin effect
Hypokalemia	Increases digoxin effect
Alkalosis	Increases digoxin effect
Clonidine	Increases bradydysrhythmias
Methyldopa	Increases bradydysrhythmias
β Blockers	Increases bradydysrhythmias

DIGITALIS IN THE ELDERLY

Digitalis is one of the most commonly prescribed drugs among this group of patients and it is second only to diuretics as the most frequently used cardiovascular drug (39). A major pharmacokinetic factor contributing to the increased predisposition to digoxin toxicity in the elderly relates to the change in volume of distribution of digoxin with aging (29). Older persons have a decrease in muscle mass and an increase in fat mass. This smaller volume of distribution leads to higher serum digoxin levels (39).

The principal route of elimination of digoxin is by renal excretion. The normal age-related decrease in renal clearance and the loss of renal function due to chronic disease are probably the major factors that increase the risk of toxicity in the elderly. In addition, optimal binding of free digoxin to its receptor requires the presence of Na, Mg, and ATP, and is inhibited by extracellular K. Unfortunately, elderly patients who depend on digoxin for their heart problems are too often the same population who, because of K or Mg deficiency, tend to be particularly sensitive to the toxic effects of the drug (40).

PLASMA DIGITALIS CONCENTRATIONS

The technology to measure serum digoxin concentrations was discovered in 1967 with the production of antibodies to digoxin (41). Radioimmunoassay uses antibodies of high affinity and specificity for cardiac glycosides and permits the rapid and accurate determination of serum digitalis concentrations (20,31,42). A specific plasma concentration may be therapeutic or toxic in an individual patient, however, depending on factors other than dosage, such as serum electrolytes; acid-base balance; type, severity, and duration of cardiac disorder; thyroid status; autonomic nervous system tone; and concurrently administered drugs (10,20,26). Increased serum digoxin concentrations are sometimes seen without toxicity in patients with atrial dysrhythmias or hyperkalemia (which may be protective) and in infants and children (20). Serum digoxin concentration may also be falsely high in acute poisoning; therefore this measurement by itself lacks usefulness in the initial assessment of acute poisoning.

Because digoxin follows a two-compartment model of distribution, caution must be exercised in interpreting the serum digoxin concentration in the setting of acute overdose. Normally, digoxin is absorbed into the plasma with levels peaking in 30 to 90 minutes. Following this, digoxin is redistributed into the tissue compartment with a distribution half-life of 30 to 60 minutes. However, after an acute overdose this redistribution may be prolonged (24). At steady state, only about 1% of the body load of digoxin is located in the bloodstream; the remainder is found in various tissues (3). A serum digoxin concentration should be performed at least 6 to 8 hours after the ingestion to ensure steady-state sampling after the rapid initial phase of drug redistribution into body tissues. When determined earlier than this, serum digoxin concentrations may give a false impression of severity.

With digoxin, impairment of renal function is associated with high serum concentrations at any given dose (20,32). Plasma digitoxin concentrations correlate poorly with renal function.

In radioimmunoassay, digoxin and oleander glycoside cross-react. This causes an increase in the digoxin concentration after ingestion of oleander. Because the degree of cross-reactivity is unknown (16), digoxin radioimmunoassays reveal only the presence of the oleander glycoside, not the degree of toxicity (43).

Digoxin-Like Immunoreactive Substance

A digoxin-like immunoreactive substance that causes false-positive digoxin immunoassays has been found in adults with renal insufficiency who are not taking digoxin (44), pregnant women (45), and neonates, fetuses, and infants less than 2 months of age (46). This substance may be produced by the infant before as well as after birth. This has raised concern about the reliability of the present method of digoxin measurements from the serum or plasma of neonatal patients (44). This substance may not simply interfere in the digoxin immunoassay but may be a hormone of interest in various responses to stress or disease (46).

TOXICITY

Acute vs. Chronic Toxicity

Acute toxicity occurs after a large overdose of digitalis by either accidental ingestion as in the case of many pediatric poisonings, or by intentional overdose. Chronic toxicity can develop by many mechanisms, but commonly occurs in the setting of decreasing renal function without a comparable decrease in digoxin dose (41).

Two of the most significant determinants of susceptibility to digitalis poisoning are the age of the patient and the presence or absence of preexisting heart disease. Except for premature infants and neonates, infants and children are more tolerant than adults to the therapeutic and toxic actions of cardiac glycosides. Similarly, young adults are more tolerant than old adults. In addition, the clinical picture associated with acute ingestion of digitalis often is different from that seen with toxicity associated with excessive therapeutic use. Young adults and children may demonstrate bradycardia with various degrees of entrance and exit blocks at the atrioventricular junction, whereas older patients with heart disease have ventricular dysrhythmias. It is important, therefore, to distinguish between acute poisoning in a nondigitalized individual and the gradual development of intoxication in a patient taking the drug for heart failure. Patients without heart disease tend to tolerate high levels of serum digoxin, and the dysrhythmias encountered are most often disturbances of conduction. Patients with underlying heart disease have the greatest problems with ventricular ectopy and the worst prognosis.

Acute Toxicity

In acute digitalis overdose one should attempt to estimate the amount ingested and the time since exposure. Although the lethal dose varies with age and underlying cardiac status, in general, an acute ingestion of more than 10 to 20 mg in a previously healthy adult can prove fatal. In older patients with underlying heart disease or hypokalemia, smaller doses can be life-threatening (3). Hard data to support the diagnosis are nonspecific, as even EKG and serum digitalis levels are frequently inconclusive (40).

The molecular mechanism of digitalis intoxication is an extension of its therapeutic action. Alterations in cardiac rhythm as well as extracardiac manifestations of digitalis action, such as gastrointestinal and CNS symptoms, are dose-related. Serum concentration may correlate with chronic toxicity, but there is considerable overlap between therapeutic and toxic concentrations. The single oral lethal dose of cardiac glycosides is approximately 20 to 50 times the usual daily maintenance dose. Massive acute doses of digitalis poison the membrane-bound NaK-ATPase throughout the body. In acute intoxication, the most pronounced feature may be hyperkalemia, because of the digitalis blockade of the ATP-dependent sodium/potassium pump.

Few children become ill with life-threatening symptoms after an acute overdose of digoxin. Those who do either have taken massive overdoses or have severe preexisting cardiac disease (47).

Chronic Toxicity

The diagnosis of digitalis toxicity can be elusive. It presents as a myriad of nonspecific symptoms that vary depending on the patient's overall health. Chronic digitalis toxicity may occur for a number of reasons. It may simply be an error in dosage, or, more commonly, a change in the pharmacokinetics may have occurred secondary to drug interactions, increases in bioavailability, decrease in renal clearance, or a change in the distribution of digitalis. Another common reason for chronic digitalis toxicity is that there has been a change in sensitivity or pharmacodynamics, such that there is an alteration in the response of the heart to a stable plasma digoxin concentration as in hypokalemia, hypercalcemia, myocardial disease, or thyrotoxicosis.

A major reason for the continuing morbidity and mortality from digitalis intoxication, especially that of the more common chronic form of the syndrome, is the difficulty of rapid diagnosis. Early manifestations are subtle and nonspecific and may simulate exacerbation of underlying congestive heart failure or a variety of other illnesses. Underlying disease states such as renal insufficiency, pulmonary disease, and hypothyroidism also increase the likelihood of toxicity (1). Renal insufficiency results in compromised digoxin excretion, and digoxin is metabolized more slowly during the hypometabolic state of hypothyroidism (3).

Factors that may precipitate toxic reactions include an increasing severity of myocardial disease; electrolyte disturbance such as hypokalemia (30), hypercalcemia, and hypomagnesemia; hypoxia; and hepatic disease (Table 21–7). A common cause of digoxin intoxication is reduced renal elimination of the drug, which may be insidious. Some patients who have certain anaerobic bacteria in the colon may require large doses of digoxin to achieve adequate serum digoxin concentrations because the organism reduces the lactone ring of the glycoside (48). When these patients are treated with antibiotics that abolish this organism, such as erythromycin or tetracycline, the serum digoxin concentrations can rise to toxic levels because bacterial inactivation is abruptly removed. Patients with pulmonary disease, especially chronic obstructive lung disease, are more sensitive to the effects of digitalis. This increase in sensitivity is not well understood but may be related to hypoxemia and pH changes caused by ventilatory dysfunction (49).

TABLE 21–7. *Factors increasing the likelihood of toxic reactions to digoxin*

Age of patient
Degree of heart disease
Electrolyte disturbances
Hypokalemia
Hypomagnesemia
Hypercalcemia
Hypoxia
Hepatic disease
Renal disease
Antibiotic therapy
Pulmonary disease

Signs of intoxication do not typically occur in a regular sequence, and subjective signs of toxicity are frequently less easily recognized in infants and children than in adults. Toxicity may be manifested by gastrointestinal, CNS, psychic, visual, and cardiac symptoms.

Gastrointestinal Symptoms

Gastrointestinal symptoms are frequent in both acute and chronic digitalis intoxication (6). The commonly recognized GI symptoms of digoxin toxicity are anorexia, nausea, and vomiting, but diarrhea and abdominal pain can be a part of the syndrome and are usually present early in the course of an overdose (29) and may not be recognized (5). Nausea and vomiting may be mediated through increased vagal activity or induced by a direct effect of digitalis on the chemoreceptor trigger zone in the area postrema of the medulla (21). Because this area is not protected by the blood–brain barrier, the symptoms tend to occur at a much lower digitalis level than other CNS symptoms (40) and are seen with both intravenous and oral preparations (6).

Gastrointestinal symptoms precede cardiac manifestations of digoxin toxicity in most patients, yet, in elderly patients who frequently have GI complaints for other reasons, it is often difficult to discern symptoms of toxicity (29).

Central Nervous System Symptoms

CNS toxicity occurs more frequently than is generally recognized. Fatigue, malaise, drowsiness, and generalized muscle weakness are the most common CNS signs of intoxication in addition to confusion, disorientation, drowsiness, agitation, bad dreams, and rarely, seizures (Table 21–8) (49). Neurologic manifestations that have been reported include visual and auditory hallucinations, paranoid ideation, trigeminal neuralgia, depression (50), headaches, delirium, and dizziness, irritability, vertigo, syncope, apathy, lethargy, delusions and opisthotonus. These CNS manifestations may occur at levels of serum digoxin that are in the therapeutic range (29,50–52).

TABLE 21–8. *CNS disturbances associated with digitalis intoxication*

Neurologic
Agitation
Dizziness
Drowsiness
Fatigue
Headache
Irritability
Lethargy
Malaise
Weakness

TABLE 21–9. *Psychic disturbances associated with digitalis intoxication*

Amnesia
Aphasia
Confusion
Depression
Disorientation
Hallucinations
Visual
Auditory
Paranoid ideation
Trigeminal neuralgia
Seizures
Syncope
Vertigo

Clinicians will likely encounter neuropsychiatric manifestations more frequently in chronic digitalis intoxication (Table 21–9) (3,51,52).

Visual Symptoms

Visual disturbances caused by toxic doses of cardiac glycosides are partly due to effects on the retina, in which the cones are affected more than the rods. Color vision is commonly affected, and objects may appear to be yellow or green and, less commonly, brown, red, blue, or white (6,53). Blurred vision, photophobia, and perceived halos or borders on objects may also occur (Table 21–10). In addition, transient amblyopia and scotoma may occur. Other visual symptoms include "snowy" vision, flashing or flickering of lights, sparks, bright spots of various colors, decreased visual acuity and amblyopia. It has been noted that in elderly patients, cloudy or blurry vision is more common than changes in color vision. Visual symptoms occasionally may be a precursor of more severe manifestations (29).

Cardiac Symptoms

Cardiac manifestations are the most frequent and most dangerous sign of digitalis intoxication (Table 21–11) (6). Digitalis is capable of producing almost every known cardiac dysrhythmia (20,54,55). Nevertheless, some disorders such as intraventricular block evidenced by a wide QRS interval and atrial fibrillation are rarely seen. No dysrhythmia is unique to digitalis poisoning, but cardiotonic glycosides are by far the most likely cause of nonparoxysmal nodal tachycardia, atrial tachycardia with atrioventricular dissociation, and bidirectional ventricular tachycardia. The cardiac dysrhythmias induced by digitalis are nonspecific, and electrocardiographically identical dysrhythmias may be induced by underlying heart disease, drugs other than digitalis, or numerous extracardiac aberrations (30). The cardiac manifestations of digitalis intoxication differ in the patient with underlying heart disease and chronic intoxication compared with the patient with a relatively normal myocardium and acute intoxication (Table 21–12) (5).

TABLE 21–10. *Visual disturbances associated with digitalis intoxication*

Distorted color vision
Blurred vision
Halos around lights
Photophobia
Scotoma

TABLE 21–11. *Cardiac manifestations of digitalis intoxication*

Acute intoxication
Atrioventricular conduction disturbances
First-degree block
Sinus impulse formation disturbances
Sinus bradycardia
Sinus arrest
Sinoatrial block
Second-degree atrioventricular block (Mobitz type I)
Third-degree atrioventricular block
Chronic intoxication
Paroxysmal atrial tachycardia with block
Nonparoxysmal junctional tachycardia
Bidirectional ventricular tachycardia
Atrioventricular dissociation
Second-degree atrioventricular block (Mobitz type I)
Ventricular tachycardia
Ventricular fibrillation

TABLE 21–12. *Symptoms of acute compared with chronic digoxin overdose*

Parameter	Acute overdose (normal heart)	Chronic overdose (diseased heart)
Serum digoxin concentration	Increased	Increased or therapeutic
Serum potassium concentration	Normal to high	Normal to low
Noncardiac manifestations	Nausea, vomiting	Anorexia, nausea, vomiting, ocular disturbances, CNS disturbances

Adapted with permission from *Am J Hosp Pharm* 1978;35:268–277. American Society of Hospital Pharmacists.

Cardiac Manifestations From Acute Intoxication

In an otherwise healthy patient with acute intoxication, ventricular dysrhythmias or ectopy are uncommon. It is well recognized that, in contrast to adults, children without intrinsic heart disease will often tolerate an acute overdose of digitalis with few clinical effects (29). The healthy myocardium responds to an excess of digitalis by developing atrioventricular conduction disturbances with evidence of first-degree atrioventricular block (6,54). Infants, young children, and healthy adults with digitalis intoxication therefore respond in this manner (30). Disturbances of sinus impulse formation take the form of an inappropriate sinus bradycardia, sinus arrest, or sinoatrial block. First-degree atrioventricular block is also common. The acute overdose is further characterized by second- or third-degree atrioventricular block in the presence of normal or abnormal sinus rhythm. These effects result primarily from increased vagal activity (30). Rarely, and usually as a result of higher doses, ventricular arrhythmias or ectopy may occur.

Cardiac Manifestations From Chronic Intoxication

There are no protean rules to the EKG manifestations of digitalis intoxication. Some patients develop ventricular ectopy and tachycardia, whereas others present with varying degrees of blocks and progress to asystole without ever having a tachydysrhythmia (6). No cardiac dysrhythmia is unique to digitalis poisoning, and the same dysrhythmia may arise from preexisting cardiac disease, other concomitantly administered drugs, or even noncardiac processes. In older individuals with chronic digitalis intoxication, characteristic dysrhythmias result from both enhanced myocardial automaticity and impaired conduction (28). Classically, this electrophysiologic combination manifests as nonparoxysmal junctional tachycardia with AV block, which many authorities believe is virtually diagnostic of digitalis toxicity. AV dissociation with accelerated junctional rhythm and nonparoxysmal atrial tachycardia with AV block (often mislabeled as paroxysmal atrial tachycardia with block) are less common but are likewise highly suggestive of digitalis toxicity (6).

Additional dysrhythmias that are highly suggestive of toxic reactions to long-term administration of digitalis include bidirectional ventricular tachycardia, atrioventricular dissociation usually with acceleration of the junctional focus, and other rhythms. Second-degree block usually manifests as Wenckebach period. Mobitz type II block is also uncommon in digitalis toxicity. Atrial fibrillation or atrial flutter with rapid atrioventricular conduction are not usually seen with long-term digitalis intoxication. Although atrial fibrillation or flutter with rapid ventricular rates is rarely seen in cases of intoxication, atrial fibrillation and flutter with ventricular bigeminy or high-degree atrioventricular block does suggest a diagnosis of toxicity (40). Abrupt regularization of the ventricular response of atrial fibrillation suggests the development of an accelerated junctional rhythm or tachycardia and should make one suspect the presence of digoxin excess (56).

Fascicular tachycardias usually represent digoxin toxic rhythms. The fascicular tachycardia will characteristically have a narrow or incomplete right bundle branch block QRS pattern (<0.12 sec) and either right or left axis deviation or a beat to beat alternating axis in the frontal plane (40).

Of note, digoxin rarely causes a regular, wide complex unimorphic ventricular tachycardia and the presence of such a rhythm should make one consider other etiologies, most commonly chronic coronary artery disease.

Premature ventricular contractions, often multifocal, are the most frequent isolated rhythm disturbance, although premature atrial contraction and premature junctional contractions are also common. Ventricular bigeminy or bidirectional ventricular tachycardia are highly indicative of chronic digitalis toxicity (3).

LABORATORY TESTS

Initial laboratory studies should include serum digoxin, potassium, magnesium, calcium, and creatinine concentrations as well as blood urea nitrogen. An electrocardiogram should also be obtained (Table 21–13). Therapeutic plasma concentrations of digoxin are generally 0.5 to 2.0 ng/mL. In adults, toxicity is usually but not always associated with steady-state digoxin plasma concentrations greater than 2 ng/mL (Table 21–14) (5,57).

TABLE 21–13. *Laboratory tests in digoxin intoxication*

Serum digoxin concentration
Serum potassium concentration
Serum magnesium concentration
Serum calcium concentration
Serum creatinine concentration
Blood urea nitrogen
Electrocardiogram

TABLE 21–14. *Therapeutic and toxic concentrations of digoxin and digitoxin*

Drug	Therapeutic	Toxic
Digoxin	0.5 to 2.0 ng/mL	>2.0 ng/mL
Digitoxin	15 to 30 ng/mL	>45 ng/mL

Potassium and Magnesium

Binding of digoxin to ATPase is affected by serum potassium levels. Hyperkalemia depresses digoxin binding whereas hypokalemia has the opposite effect, in part accounting for the fact that hypokalemia increases the frequency and severity of digoxin-induced dysrhythmias. Inhibition of ATPase produces an increase in intracellular sodium concentration. Because of this, exchange of extracellular sodium for intracellular calcium is reduced, and the concentration of intracellular calcium rises. It is this rise in intracellular calcium that is ultimately responsible for both enhanced contractility and the manifestations of digoxin toxicity.

In general, relative hyperkalemia is protective against, and hypokalemia may exacerbate, an abnormal rhythm induced by digitalis intoxication (Table 21–15). Because cardiac glycosides inhibit the Na-K ATPase pump, acute cardiac glycoside intoxication often leads to a release of intracellular potassium into the extracellular space, which results in high or even fatal elevations of serum potassium (58,59). The hyperkalemia results from poisoning of the membrane-bound Na-K ATPase system not only in the myocardium but in all body tissues (58,60). Hyperkalemia with serum potassium concentrations sometimes exceeding 13 mEq/L have been reported (19,43,61). The resulting decrease in intracellular potassium concentration reduces the normal resting membrane potential (6). The myocardial cells lose their ability to function as pacemaker cells, and asystole results. Ultimately there is a complete loss of cardiac electrical activity. Increased renal excretion of potassium may result from hyperkalemia, and thus some patients may appear to be hyperkalemic while having a total body deficit of potassium.

Hypokalemia is often a problem in chronic digitalis intoxication because of concurrent use of a diuretic, not as a direct result of the digitalis. In this setting of hypokalemia there is increased binding of digoxin with the NaK-ATPase molecule enhancing the electrophysiologic consequences of this effect (56). Hypokalemia predisposes patients to ventricular ectopy and tachydysrhythmias because depletion of myocardial potassium reduces the threshold for depolarization of ectopic pacemakers. Magnesium is a necessary cofactor for maintenance of the sodium-potassium pump. As a result, hypomagnesemia may cause a decrease in tissue potassium stores (29). Hypomagnesemia has a similar potential for exacerbating digitalis cardiotoxicity. Hypomagnesemia increases myocardial digoxin uptake, decreases cellular Na-K-ATPase activity, and can cause intracellular hypokalemia refractory to potassium replacement (3,5,6).

Patients with hypomagnesemia, hypokalemia, or both may become cardiotoxic even with "therapeutic" digitalis levels.

TABLE 21–15. *Selected electrolytes and associated digitalis toxicity*

Electrolyte	High concentration	Low concentration
Potassium	Protective	Increased toxicity
Magnesium	Protective	Increased toxicity
Calcium	Increased toxicity	Protective

Calcium

Chronic digitalis intoxication may be exacerbated by rapid infusions of calcium, and intoxication may occur at low serum digoxin concentrations when hypercalcemia is present. This is probably because calcium administration decreases the serum potassium concentration. Hypocalcemia appears to be protective against dysrhythmias resulting from digitalis toxicity (6).

TREATMENT OF DIGITALIS INTOXICATION

Treatment of acute cardiac glycoside ingestion begins with basic life support measures, including airway control and circulatory support (Table 21–16) (7). Gastric lavage should be performed, and activated charcoal and a cathar-

TABLE 21–16. *Treatment of digitalis intoxication*

Indication	Modality
Acute ingestion	Lavage
Acute ingestion	Charcoal and cathartic
Symptomatic	Atropine
Bradycardia	
Atrioventricular block	
Sinus exit block	
Second-degree block	
Third-degree block	
Ventricular abnormalities	Phenytoin
Bigeminy	
Tachycardia	
Premature contractions	
Ventricular abnormalities	Lidocaine
Bigeminy	
Tachycardia	
Premature contractions	
Hypokalemia	Potassium
Symptomatic and unresponsive	Pacemaker
Bradycardia	
Atrioventricular block	
Second-degree block	
Third-degree block	
Severe hyperkalemia	Hemodialysis
Ventricular abnormalities	Antibody therapy
Tachycardia	
Fibrillation	
Symptomatic and unresponsive	
Bradycardia	
Second-degree block	
Third-degree block	
Severe hyperkalemia	
Significant ingestion	

tic should be administered (60). In patients with heart block or sinus bradycardia, vomiting or placement of a lavage tube may lead to increased vagal tone and worsening of the rhythm or asystole (6). Therefore, some authorities recommend omitting gastric evacuation and proceeding to immediate charcoal administration. At this time, however, gastric emptying is still recommended (40). If a conduction disturbance is noted or if there is great potential for this disturbance, atropine should be administered intravenously before the performance of lavage.

Supportive Measures

There is no effective means for increasing digitalis excretion or metabolism. Forced diuresis and dialysis have been studied as methods of quickly expelling digitalis from the bloodstream. However, elimination of the toxin is not enhanced by forced diuresis. It may even complicate the situation through exacerbation of electrolyte imbalances. Dialysis does not significantly remove digitalis from the body due to the drug's high volume of distribution which means that the majority of the drug is tissue-bound and thus not available for removal (7,43,60,62–66). The only indication for dialysis in digitalis toxicity is to remove potassium in the setting of acute digitalis-induced hyperkalemia (5,62).

Toxic manifestations of digoxin rapidly disappear when the drug is withdrawn, so that in the vast majority of patients digitalis cardiotoxic reactions can be handled by simply discontinuing the drug. Because digoxin is eliminated from the body by first-order kinetics, with 30% of the residual drug in the body being eliminated each day, if renal function is normal, toxic symptoms will usually disappear within 24 hours and often sooner (67). On the basis of this first-order elimination, by obtaining a minimum of two serum digoxin concentration values the time scale for recovery can be predicted.

Dysrhythmias such as paroxysmal atrial tachycardia with atrioventricular block, atrioventricular junctional rhythm with slow rate, and atrial fibrillation or flutter with slow ventricular rate induced by digitalis can usually be treated by stopping the drug. Further management of digitalis intoxication includes close attention to the metabolic state with correction of hypoxemia, acid-base disturbances, and alterations in potassium metabolism.

The choice of therapy for digoxin toxicity should depend on the presence or absence of symptoms and hemodynamic disturbances, the nature of associated arrhythmias, and the overall clinical status of the patient. If an asymptomatic patient has a high serum digoxin level, there is usually no danger in simply discontinuing the medication and monitoring the patient. Similarly, the patient with GI symptoms but no evidence of cardiac arrhythmia by EKG or cardiac monitoring can probably be safely treated by discontinuation of the medication and measures to relieve symptoms.

Atropine

Atropine is the initial treatment of choice in digitalis-poisoned patients who are hemodynamically compromised by sinus bradycardia, high-degree AV block, and sinus exit block (6,68). The action of atropine depends on its ability to block vagal activity and by so doing to increase impulse formation and conduction rate at the sinoatrial and atrioventricular nodes. However, because these effects are only partially vagally mediated, atropine does not consistently abolish AV blocks and bradydysrhythmias in digitalis toxicity (22,63). Atropine is likely to be more successful in reducing block in acute poisoning than in chronic poisoning. As a general rule, however, the drug is not effective, and electrical pacing may be attempted if more aggressive treatment is indicated for a slow rate (29).

Phenytoin

Phenytoin, historically, has been used for the treatment of premature ventricular contractions, ventricular tachycardia, and AV nodal block (14). Its mechanism of action is similar to that of lidocaine in the treatment of ventricular arrhythmias. It was suggested that phenytoin could improve AV nodal conduction unlike lidocaine. Its use, however, is limited by the need to infuse phenytoin slowly and the widespread experience with lidocaine (6,41).

Phenytoin is the drug of choice in treating ventricular dysrhythmias in the presence of atrioventricular blocks (14). It depresses enhanced ventricular automaticity without affecting intraventricular conduction and also reverses digitalis-induced prolongation of atrioventricular conduction. Phenytoin has been used effectively in reversing digitalis-induced ventricular dysrhythmias, including bigeminy, unifocal and multifocal premature ventricular contractions, and ventricular tachycardia (7,69). Phenytoin increases the membrane potential toward normal and enhances atrioventricular and interventricular conduction. It remains effective in the presence of acid-base imbalance and electrolyte imbalance such as hyperkalemia. It should be dosed in 100-mg boluses slowly IV every 5 minutes until signs of phenytoin toxicity develop, the arrhythmia is suppressed, or 1 g has been given (40). Phenytoin is not approved by the FDA for use as an antidysrhythmic agent; however, its use has been generally accepted.

Lidocaine

Lidocaine may be useful in managing digitalis-induced ventricular tachydysrhythmias, premature contractions, and bigeminy (14). In this respect it is similar to phenytoin but has essentially no effect on alterations of atrial activity and does not improve conduction through the atrioventricular node. Lidocaine may be given as a bolus of 1.0 mg/kg and followed by a constant infusion of 1 to 4 mg/min. Because lidocaine does not affect atrioventricular conduction, it can be used in the presence of atrioventricular block (6).

Magnesium

It is well documented that magnesium may abort toxic arrhythmias of digoxin toxicity, even in patients with normal magnesium levels (43). Thus, attention to a potential magnesium deficit should be as important as monitoring of serum potassium (29). Although precisely how intravenous magnesium is effective in digitalis poisoning remains unknown, in digitalis intoxication magnesium appears either to block the transient inward current of calcium or to antagonize calcium at cellular binding sites (70). Some investigators have shown that magnesium in adequate doses specifically counteracts the ventricular irritability caused by excessive amounts of digitalis. Magnesium may also be useful in counteracting the hyperkalemia associated with digitalis by blocking the egress of potassium from the cells (5).

The dosage of magnesium for adults is 2 g of 10% magnesium sulfate intravenously over 20 minutes (5). Because the effect of the magnesium bolus injection may be transient secondary to rapid renal clearance in those with normal kidneys, the initial dose should be followed by an infusion of 1 to 2 g/hr. Carefully monitor the patient for clinical and laboratory evidence of hypermagnesemia. Magnesium concentrations should be checked every 2 hours and a dose titrated to maintain 4 to 5 mEq/L.

Potassium

Potassium is an excellent agent for the prompt suppression of the ventricular dysrhythmias secondary to chronic digitalis intoxication associated with hypokalemia (14). The cation may be administered intravenously in the form of potassium chloride at a rate of 0.5 mEq/min as a solution in saline or 5% dextrose containing 50 to 60 mEq of potassium per liter.

Potassium is contraindicated in the presence of renal failure or hyperkalemia. Potassium infusion in acute massive digoxin overdose is also contraindicated because massive efflux of potassium is noted after the acute overdose (63), so that as a blind maneuver it is potentially hazardous in the face of high-normal to high serum potassium concentrations.

Treatment of Hyperkalemia

Hyperkalemia after an acute digoxin overdose may be life-threatening. Initial attempts at controlling hyperkalemia consist of administration of bicarbonate, glucose, and insulin to drive potassium intracellularly. In addition, Kayexalate may be used for long-term control of hyperkalemia if not well controlled. Although calcium is usually considered a mainstay in the treatment of life-threatening hyperkalemia, it has been shown to prolong PQ intervals and the QRS duration, which could worsen digitalis-induced cardiac abnormalities. Therefore, calcium is contraindicated in digitalis intoxication. Magnesium will halt digitalis-induced flow of potassium out of the cell. Also, magnesium is effective in certain digitalis-toxic dysrhythmias refractory to lidocaine and phenytoin (40).

This serious problem may not respond to methods that are normally effective, such as calcium administration, glucose and insulin administration, or bicarbonate infusion. This is because the Na-K ATPase pump has been "poisoned" by the digoxin (71). Potassium concentrations in hyperkalemic patients must be controlled by other measures, such as the use of resins or hemodialysis. Although such measures may lower serum potassium concentrations, they may be ineffective in reestablishing membrane potentials because of the poisoning of the Na-K ATPase pump. In stable patients, sodium polystyrene sulfonate (Kayexalate) may help reduce serum potassium concentrations. Sodium polystyrene sulfonate (1 g per milliequivalent of excess potassium in the serum) may be administered with 70% sorbitol either orally or as a retention enema. This resin complex acts to lower serum potassium by exchange of a cation (sodium or hydrogen) for potassium, for which the resin has a high affinity. The time needed for therapeutic effect is slow. Fragment antigen-binding (Fab) antibody therapy has also been shown to lower serum potassium concentrations quickly and is the agent of choice for life-threatening hyperkalemia (see below) (49).

Cardiac Pacemaker

Although pacemaker insertion is relatively safe, myocardial cells poisoned by cardiac glycosides may not respond to electrical stimulation (72). Current indications for temporary transvenous ventricular pacing for digoxin overdose include sinus bradycardia, exit block, or high-degree atrioventricular block unresponsive to atropine and associated with signs and symptoms of inadequate organ perfusion (72). Because cardiac glycosides lower the threshold for pacemaker-induced extrasystole, placement of a pacemaker may produce life-threatening dysrhythmias (6).

Cardioversion

Cardioversion should be performed only when necessary because it may induce ventricular fibrillation in the digitalis-intoxicated patient. When necessary, it should be done at the lowest energy setting possible (7,43).

Bile Acid Resins

Because of the extensive enterohepatic recirculation of digitoxin, nonabsorbed substances such as cholestyramine (73,74), colestipol (75), kaolin, nonabsorbable antacids, and activated charcoal may interrupt this mechanism (13,14,60). Although many of these agents have been used to increase the enterohepatic elimination of digitoxin, the results have often been unimpressive (22). Cholestyramine has been administered as a 4-g dose orally every 8 hours for 3 days (73,74). Nevertheless, cholestyramine has no advantages over activated charcoal, which is preferred because of its lack of side effects (73).

Digitalis Antibody Therapy (Digibind)

For several decades in the past no significant advance was made in the treatment of severe digoxin intoxication and accepted treatment did not offer optimal results for the severely intoxicated patient (76). Treatment was directed toward either inhibiting the absorption of the drug or counteracting its cardiac effects (77). The availability of digoxin antibodies led to the development of a radioimmunoassay to measure serum digoxin concentrations; this assay is now used routinely to determine patient compliance and digoxin toxicity (78,79). Shortly after this development it was postulated that antibodies to digoxin could be used to reverse its pharmacologic and toxic effects (80). Probably the most dramatic breakthrough in the treatment of severe digoxin intoxication occurred in the mid 1970s, when a report appeared describing the use of immunotherapy to reverse the signs of toxicity and hasten the elimination of the offending agent (67,81–84).

Mechanism of Action

Digitalis has a relatively low molecular weight and is therefore not immunogenic. It is rendered antigenic by coupling it to a carrier protein. As early as 1967 it was shown that whole antibody from the serum of animals bound digoxin, but the large size of the molecule and the lack of purity precluded its use (85). The whole antibody to digoxin was also antigenic in its own right and had a prolonged half-life in the body because the intact antibody–digoxin complex was too large to enter the glomerular filtrate (86,87). To promote more rapid excretion as well as decreased antigenicity, the antibody produced in sheep was digested with papain to yield three fragments. Two of these are called the Fab fragments, and they retain the antigen-binding properties of the molecule (88). The other portion, which is not used, is the "c" fragment (Fc). This is the portion involved in complement activation and other effector functions. Each Fab segment has one combining site of the parent antigen molecule (77,83–85). They are smaller than the parent antigen and have intact binding affinity and specificity for digoxin when separated from nonspecific antigen fragments (83,84). This results in more rapid distribution, a shorter elimination time, and lower immunogenicity than the parent antigen (64).

The Fab–digoxin complex is small enough to allow rapid clearance that, coupled with the absence of c fragment, results in minimal antigenic stimulus to the patient (85). The Fab segments, which have a molecular size of 50,000 daltons, bind free digoxin, which has a molecular size of 781 daltons, and render it inactive (83). The affinity of digoxin-specific Fab for digoxin is greater than the affinity of digoxin for Na-K ATPase (89).

Because the interaction of cardiac glycosides is reversible, a concentration gradient is established that results in a progressive efflux of membrane-bound digoxin. Because the interaction of digoxin with its cellular receptors is also reversible, the reduction in free digoxin results in progressive removal of digoxin from receptor sites as the drug–receptor equilibrium is displaced in the direction of dissociation (1). The dissociation of the cardiac glycoside from its cellular receptor and its subsequent bonding to the high-affinity Fab antibody results in rapid reversal of the cardiac rhythm disturbances. In other words, after intravenous administration of Fab, any free digoxin is bound intravascularly (90). Fab antibodies then diffuse into the extracellular space and bind any free digoxin (91). Because of the reduction in concentration, there is an efflux of free intracellular digoxin into the extracellular fluid, where it is also immediately bound (92). Digoxin molecules dissociate from the membrane receptors and are removed from the site of action by binding to Fab (48). In patients with good renal function, the digoxin–Fab complex appears to be eliminated fairly rapidly by glomerular filtration; the elimination half-life is about 16 to 20 hours (79,85), and complete elimination of the digoxin–antibody complex may require a week or longer (86). In the presence of renal failure a prolonged elimination time may lead to breakdown of the bound complex requiring administration of additional Fab fragments (24).

Fab and Hemodialysis

Hemodialysis is not an effective means of reducing serum digoxin concentrations in a renal failure patient who receives digoxin-immune Fab (73,83). The inability to effectively remove the complex is more likely a function of molecular size than of a large volume of distribution, because the molecular weight of the Fab fragment is 50,000 daltons and conventional hemodialysis is probably ineffective in removing a drug whose molecular weight exceeds 500 (80).

Fab and Serum Digoxin Levels

Fab antibodies interfere with digitalis immunoassay measurements, although serum digoxin concentrations do not decrease but rather rise dramatically (57,79). These high concentrations, however, reflect the amount of digoxin bound in an inactive form to the antibody fragment that is consistent with the dissociation of digoxin from its membrane site (85). Free digoxin decreases rapidly to undetectable concentrations after Fab administration (93,94). The antidysrhythmic effect of the antibody can be dramatic, with complete reversal of potentially lethal problems seen in as little as 30 minutes (80,85,87).

The use of purified, digoxin-specific Fab antibodies therefore provides a new and exciting therapeutic approach in the management of advanced digoxin intoxication. The glycosides' high potency requires that only a relatively small amount of foreign antibody protein be administered, thereby reducing the likelihood of developing serum sickness.

Indications for Fab Therapy

Common symptoms of digitalis intoxication including anorexia, nausea, vomiting, fatigue, malaise, and visual changes are not severe enough to warrant the use of digoxin-specific antibody fragments (56,86). Fab therapy should be reserved for those cases in which there is a life-threatening situation or the potential for such (84). Manifestations of life-threatening toxicity include severe ventricular dysrhythmias, such as ventricular tachycardia or ventricular fibrillation, or progressive bradydysrhythmias, such as severe sinus bradycardia or second- or third-degree heart block not responsive to atropine or pacemaker (24). Fab therapy is indicated in patients with digitalis-induced hyperkalemia (>5.5 mEq/L) who have concurrent signs and symptoms of severe digitalis intoxication (4,79,84,86). In addition, histories of ingestions of more than 10 mg of digoxin in previously healthy adults or 4 mg in previously healthy children (92), or of ingestion causing steady-state serum concentrations greater than 10 ng/mL, often result in cardiac arrest and would warrant serious consideration for Fab therapy (41). In patients with elevated serum digoxin concentrations but with no signs of toxicity, Fab therapy is unwarranted (79).

Since the advent of digoxin-specific Fab antibodies, there has been a marked reduction in mortality rates. This treatment constitutes an effective and highly specific means of reversing advanced, life-threatening digitalis intoxication. The FDA approved digoxin-specific Fab antibodies for clinical use, and the preparation is marketed as Digibind (89). True nonresponders to Fab treatment are uncommon, and lack of response to an adequate dose of Fab fragments should raise a question as to whether the clinical signs and symptoms are actually caused by digitalis toxicity (24).

Occasionally, one may wish to remove only part of the total digitalis body load to alleviate signs and symptoms of toxicity while maintaining "therapeutic concentrations" to control severe heart failure or a fast ventricular response to atrial fibrillation in non-life-threatening situations (23). The calculation of this partial neutralizing dose is empiric, as there are no studies available to evaluate this concept (41).

Although antibodies to a large number of drugs have been produced, their use therapeutically is likely to be limited (48). The immense problems in manufacturing, purifying, and administering large quantities of antibodies are such that this technique is restricted to the very few drugs that cause serious toxicity when taken in milligram amounts (79).

Dosage

Digibind is available in 40-mg vials of lyophilized powder which must be reconstituted with 4 mL of sterile water prior to administration. Care should be taken not to shake the reconstituted vials because the solution will foam. Once reconstituted, the solution should be administered or discarded within 4 hours because it does not contain a preservative (41).

The dosage of Fab must be determined according to the severity of the poisoning and the quantity of glycoside in the body (Table 21–17) (95). Eighty milligrams of Fab bind 1 mg of glycoside. Each vial binds approximately 0.6 mg of digoxin. In most cases, however, the quantity of glycoside is not known precisely and can therefore only be estimated (91). The calculated quantity of Fab is dissolved in physiologic saline to give a concentration of 2 to 4 mg/mL and is infused over 30 minutes. In chronic intoxication, clinicians may use the serum digitalis concentration to estimate the Fab dose. However, one must obtain the serum concentration at least 8 hours after the last dose (3).

Fab should be infused intravenously over 30 minutes through a 0.22-micron filter. Although minimal dilutions have not been established, a solution more concentrated than 10 mg/mL may be necessary in children or fluid-restricted patients in order to avoid fluid overload (86).

Fab should be administered in a 5% dextrose or normal saline solution. Compatibility of Fab fragments with other agents such as potassium has not been established and should, therefore, be avoided. If clinically indicated, Fab can be given as an IV bolus injection. Within 1 minute of IV administration in most patients, free digoxin levels become unmeasurable (3).

If neither the quantity ingested nor the serum digoxin concentration can be determined, an initial dose of 800 mg of Fab (20 vials) is recommended for both children

TABLE 21–17. *Fab antibody dosage calculation chart*

Approximate Digibind dose for reversal of single-ingestion digoxin overdose

Number of tablets or capsules of digoxin ingested				Digibind dose	
0.05 mg capsules	0.125 mg tablets or 0.1 mg capsules	0.25 mg tablets or 0.2 mg capsules	0.5 mg tablets	mg	vials
25	12–13	6	3	85	2
50	25	12–13	6	170	4.25
100	50	25	12–13	340	8.5
200	100	50	25	680	17
300	150	75	37–38	1000	25
400	200	100	50	1360	34

Estimated adult dose in vials (v) from serum digoxin concentration (ng/mL)

Patient weight (kg)	Serum digoxin concentration (ng/mL)						
	1	2	4	8	12	16	20
40	0.5v	1v	2v	3v	5v	6v	8v
60	0.5v	1v	2v	5v	7v	9v	11v
70	1.0v	2v	3v	5v	8v	11v	13v
80	1.0v	2v	3v	6v	9v	12v	15v
100	1.0v	2v	4v	8v	11v	15v	19v

Estimated pediatric dose in mg from serum digoxin concentration (ng/mL)

Patient weight (kg)	Serum digoxin concentration (ng/mL)						
	1	2	4	8	12	16	20
1	0.5 mg	1.0 mg	1.5 mg	3.0 mg	5 mg	6 mg	8 mg
3	1.0 mg	2.0 mg	5.0 mg	9.0 mg	13 mg	18 mg	22 mg
5	2.0 mg	4.0 mg	8.0 mg	15.0 mg	22 mg	30 mg	40 mg
10	4.0 mg	8.0 mg	15.0 mg	30.0 mg	40 mg	60 mg	80 mg
20	8.0 mg	15.0 mg	30.0 mg	60.0 mg	80 mg	120 mg	160 mg

Courtesy of Burroughs Wellcome Company, Research Triangle Park, North Carolina.

and adults and should be adequate to treat most life-threatening overdoses (86). Readministration of Fab, at a dose guided by clinical judgment, may be necessary if toxicity persists or recurs. Following the administration of Fab, reversal of toxicity is seen within approximately 30 minutes to 4 hours, with a mean response time of approximately 90 minutes. The accumulated evidence demonstrates that an inadequate dose of Fab is the single clear factor associated with recrudescence (90).

Fab therapy has also been effective in cases of digitoxin poisoning. In addition, the cross-reactivity between the glycosides in oleander and in digoxin noted in radioimmunoassay may mean that treatment of oleander poisoning with digoxin-specific Fab antibody could be effective (15,17).

Although the average wholesale price of one 40-mg vial of Digibind is expensive, it appears to be cost-effective because of the lessened intensive care unit (ICU) time necessary, in addition to its ethical benefit of saving lives. Cost should not be a factor in the use of this agent when life-threatening situations arise (8,41).

Side Effects of Fab Therapy

The manufacturer states that since allergy testing may delay urgently needed therapy, it is not routinely required before the treatment of life-threatening digitalis toxicity (24) yet it seems appropriate to perform skin testing in high-risk individuals, those with a known allergy to sheep protein, or those previously treated with digoxin-immune Fab (94). No serious adverse reactions have occurred from Fab therapy, yet the possibility exists. This may be especially true in patients who are subsequently exposed to antibody therapy in the future (79). Although allergic manifestations have not been reported, the production of Fab from ovine antibodies imparts the potential to produce anaphylactic, hypersensitivity, or febrile reactions (88).

Clinically important side effects related to treatment include worsening of heart failure, increased ventricular rate of patients with atrial fibrillation, or clinically important hypokalemia (24).

If Fab antibodies are given to a patient with chronic digoxin toxicity, there may be a significant decrease in the serum potassium concentration after the administration of Fab (23). The inhibition of the membrane-bound sodium pump by digitalis results in a loss of intracellular potassium to the extracellular space, whence it is excreted by the kidney, causing elevated serum potassium concentrations but an overall depletion. When toxicity is rapidly reversed by Fab, the total-body potassium deficit is reflected as hypokalemia. This should prompt clinicians to monitor their patient's serum potassium concentrations serially, beginning immediately after the administration of Fab (47).

Until digoxin can be reinstituted, inotropic agents such as dopamine and dobutamine have been used successfully in the post-Fab infusion period. Additional supportive measures may include diuretics, peripheral vasodilators, or antiarrhythmic agents for management of supraventricular dysrhythmias (86). Patients need to be closely monitored following Fab administration for hypokalemia, resolution of toxicity, recrudescence of heart failure or a return of a fast ventricular response to atrial fibrillation, and/or allergic manifestations (41).

Other Agents

Propranolol

β Blockers have also been proposed for the treatment of digitalis-induced arrhythmias because of their ability to decrease automaticity. Extreme caution must be observed in this situation because β blockers may also potentiate the toxic effects of digitalis on the sinoatrial (SA) and AV nodes (41).

Propranolol has been successful in terminating ventricular premature beats secondary to digitalis intoxication. Its use should be limited to controlling ectopy and tachydysrhythmias (92). It is contraindicated in the presence of blocks, such as atrial tachycardia with block, because its net effect is to decrease automaticity and to slow conduction velocity, thereby inducing bradycardia (70). Propranolol cannot be thought of as a first-line drug and should not be used unless lidocaine and phenytoin have been ineffective.

Bretylium, Procainamide, and Quinidine

Bretylium should be avoided because it may worsen dysrhythmias by stimulating the release of catecholamines, which have been shown to aggravate digitalis-induced dysrhythmias (6,7). Procainamide and quinidine should also be avoided (70).

SUMMARY

Conventional measures such as the administration of lidocaine or phenytoin for control of ventricular dysrhythmias, the use of atropine or transvenous pacemakers for symptomatic bradycardia, restoration of potassium balance and, most important, the allowance of time for excretion of digoxin or metabolism of digitoxin are at present the best recommendations for most patients with digitalis intoxication (72). Fab therapy should be reserved for the severely intoxicated patient. Elderly patients with severe cardiac disease and patients with severe suicidal poisoning are at greatest risk of mortality (23,29).

REFERENCES

1. Koren G, Soldin S: Cardiac glycosides. *Clin Lab Med* 1987;7: 587–606.
2. Powis D: Cardiac glycosides and autonomic neurotransmisslon. *J Auton Pharmacol* 1983;3:127–154.
3. Karkal S, Ordog G, Wasserberger J: Digitalis intoxication: dealing rapidly and effectively with a complex cardiac toxidrome. *Emerg Med Rep* 1991;12:29–39.
4. Doherty J, Straub K, Murphy M, et al: Digoxin-quinidine interaction. *Am J Cardiol* 1980;45:1196–1200.
5. Reisdorff E, Clark M, Walters B: Acute digitalis poisoning: the role of intravenous magnesium sulfate. *J Emerg Med* 1986;4:463–469.
6. Sharff J, Bayer M: Acute and chronic digitalis toxicity: presentation and treatment. *Ann Emerg Med* 1982;11:327–331.
7. Drake C: Cardiac drug overdose. *Am Fam Physician* 1982;25: 181–187.
8. Mauskopf J, Wenger T: Cost effectiveness analysis of the use of digoxin immune Fab (Ovine) for treatment of digoxin toxicity. *Am J Cardiol* 1991;68:1709–1714.
9. Cohen A, Kroon R, Schoemaker R, et al: Influence of gastric acidity on the bioavailability of digoxin. *Ann Intern Med* 1991;115: 540–545.
10. Smith T, Haber E: Digitalis (first of four parts). *N Engl J Med* 1973;289:945–952.
11. Smith T, Haber E: Digitalis (second of four parts). *N Engl J Med* 1973;289:1010–1015.
12. Smith T, Haber E: Digitalis (third of four parts). *N Engl J Med* 1973;289:1063–1069.
13. Baciewicz A, Isaacson M, Lipscomb G: Cholestyramine resin in the treatment of digitoxin toxicity. *Drug Intell Clin Pharmacol* 1983; 17:57–59.
14. Cady W, Rehder T, Campbell J: Use of cholestyramine resin in the treatment of digitoxin toxicity. *Am J Hosp Pharmacol* 1979;36: 92–94.
15. Shumaik G, Wu A, Ping A: Oleander poisoning: treatment with digoxin-specific Fab antibody fragments. *Ann Emerg Med* 1988;17: 732–735.
16. Radford D, Gillies A, Hinds J, et al: Naturally occurring cardiac glycosides. *Med J Aust* 1986;144:540–544.
17. Clark R, Selden B, Curry S: Digoxin-specific Fab fragments in the treatment of oleander toxicity in a canine model. *Ann Emerg Med* 1991;20:1073–1077.
18. Ansford H, Morris H: Fatal oleander poisoning. *Med J Aust* 1981; 1:360–361.
19. Osterloh J, Herold S, Pond S: Oleander interference in the digoxin radioimmunoassay in a fatal ingestion. *JAMA* 1982;247:1596–1597.
20. Smith T: New advances in the assessment and treatment of digitalis toxicity. *J Clin Pharmacol* 19885;25: 522–528.
21. Falk R, Leavitt J: Digoxin for atrial fibrillation: a drug whose time has gone? *Ann Intern Med* 1991;114:573–575.
22. Smith T, Willerson J: Suicidal and accidental digoxin ingestion.*Circulation* 1971;44:29–36.
23. Clarke W, Ramoska E: Acute digoxin overdose: use of digoxin-specific antibody fragments. *Am J Emerg Med* 1991;6:465–470.
24. Smith T: Review of clinical experience with digoxin immune Fab (Ovine). *Am J Emerg Med* 1991;9:1–6.

25. Rosen M, Wit A, Hoffman B: Electrophysiology and pharmacology of cardiac arrhythmias: part IV: cardiac antiarrhythmic and toxic effects of digitalis. *Am Heart J* 1975;89:391–399.
26. Ordog G, Benaron S, Bhasin V, et al: Serum digoxin levels and mortality in 5,100 patients. *Ann Emerg Med* 1987;16:32–39.
27. Watanabe A: Digitalis and the autonomic nervous system. *J Am Coll Cardiol* 1985;5:35A–42A.
28. Armstrong C, Cota G: Calcium ion as a cofactor in Na channel gating. *Proc Natl Acad Sci* 1991;88:6528–6531.
29. Wofford J, Ettinger W: Risk factors and manifestations of digoxin toxicity in the elderly. *Am J Emerg Med* 1991;9:11–15.
30. Bigger J: Digitalis toxicity. *J Clin Pharmacol* 1985;25:514–521.
31. Mason D, Zelis R, Lee G: Current concepts and treatment of digitalis toxicity. *Am J Cardiol* 1971;27:546–559.
32. Mason D: Digitalis pharmacology and therapeutics: recent advances. *Ann Intern Med* 1974;80:520–530.
33. Fenster P, Hager W, Perrier D, et al: Digoxin-quinidine interaction in patients with chronic renal failure. *Circulation* 1982;66:1277–1279.
34. Ball W, Tse-eng D, Wallick E, et al: Effect of quinidine on the digoxin receptor in vitro. *J Clin Invest* 1981;68:1065–1074.
35. Chen T, Friedman H: Alteration of digoxin pharmacokinetics by a single dose of quinidine. *JAMA* 1980;244:669–762.
36. Leahey E, Bigger J, Butler V, et al: Quinidine-digoxin interaction: time course and pharmacokinetics. *Am J Cardiol* 1981;48:1141–1146.
37. Belz G, Doering W, Aust P, et al: Quinidine-digoxin interaction: cardiac efficacy of elevated serum digoxin concentration. *Clin Pharmacol Ther* 1982;31:548–554.
38. Hager W, Mayersohn M, Graves P: Digoxin bioavailability during quinidine administration. *Clin Pharmacol Ther* 1981;30:594–599.
39. Tsang P, Gerson B: Understanding digoxin use in the elderly patient. *Clin Emerg Med* 1990;19:479–491.
40. Propp D, Hogan T, Mattimore J: Nausea, dyspnea, and heart block in an 86-year old patient with congestive heart failure. *Ann Emerg Med* 1988;17:261–267.
41. Allen N, Dunham G: Treatment of digitalis intoxication with emphasis on the clinical use of digoxin immune Fab. *DICP Ann Pharmacother* 1990;24:991–998.
42. Hobson J, Zettner A: Digoxin serum half-life following suicidal digoxin poisoning. *JAMA* 1973;223:147–150.
43. Haynes B, Bessen H, Wightman W: Oleander tea: herbal draught of death. *Ann Emerg Med* 1985;14:350–353.
44. Valdes R, Graves S, Brown B, et al: Endogenous substance in newborn infants causing false positive digoxin measurements. *J Pediatr* 1983;102:947–950.
45. Friedman H, Abramowitz I, Nguyen T, et al: Urinary digoxin-like immunoreactive substance in pregnancy. *Am J Med* 1987;83:261–264.
46. Spiehler W, Fisher W, Richards R: Digoxin-like immunoreactive substance in postmortem blood of infants and children. *J Forensic Sci* 1985;30:86–91.
47. Woolf A, Wenger T, Smith T, et al: The use of digoxin-specific Fab fragments for severe digitalis intoxicaton in children. *N Engl J Med* 1992;326:1739–1744.
48. Woolf A: Revising the management of digitalis poisoning. *J Toxicol Clin Toxicol* 1993;31;275–276.
49. Smith H, Janz T, Erker M: Digoxin toxicity presenting as altered mental status in a patient with severe chronic obstructive lung disease. *Heart Lung* 1992;21:78–80.
50. Walker A, Cody R, Greenblatt D, et al: Drug toxicity in patients receiving digoxin and quinidine. *Am Heart J* 1983;105:1025–1028.
51. Closson R: Visual hallucinations as the earliest symptom of digoxin intoxication. *Arch Neurol* 1983;40:386.
52. Volpe B, Soave R: Formed visual hallucinations as digitalis toxicity. *Ann Intern Med* 1979;91:865–866.
53. Chuman M, LeSage J: Color vision deficiencies in two cases of digoxin toxicity. *Am J Ophthalmol* 1985;100:682–685.
54. Fisch C, Knoebel S: Recognition and therapy of digitalis toxicity. *Prog Cardiovasc Dis* 1970;13:71–95.
55. Fisch C: Digitalis intoxication. *JAMA* 1971;216:1770–1773.
56. Marchlinski F, Hook B, Callans D: Which cardiac disturbances should be treated with digoxin immune Fab (Ovine) antibody? *Am J Emerg Med* 1991;9:24–28.
57. Banner W, Bach P, Burk B, et al: Influence of assay methods on serum concentrations of digoxin during Fab fragment treatment. *J Toxicol Clin Toxicol* 1992;30:259–267.
58. Doherty J: Digitalis glycosides. *Ann Intern Med* 1973;79:229–238.
59. Doherty J: Digoxin antibodies and digitalis intoxication. *N Engl J Med* 1982;307:1398–1399.
60. Ekins B, Watanabe A: Acute digoxin poisonings: review of therapy. *Am J Hosp Pharmacol* 1978;35:268–277.
61. Reza M, Kovick R, Shine K, et al: Massive intravenous digoxin overdosage. *N Engl J Med* 1974;291:777–778.
62. Warren S, Fanestil D: Digoxin overdose: limitations of hemoperfusion-hemodialysis treatment. *JAMA* 1979;242:2100–2101.
63. Hansteen V, Jacobsen D, Knudsen K, et al: Acute, massive poisoning with digitoxin: report of seven cases and discussion of treatment. *Clin Toxicol* 1981;18:679–692.
64. Hess T, Riesen W, Scholtysik G, et al: Digotoxin intoxication with severe thrombocytopenia: reversal by digoxin-specific antibodies. *Eur J Clin Invest* 1983;13:159–163.
65. Lai K, Swaminathan R, Pun C, et al: Hemofiltration in digoxin overdose. *Arch Intern Med* 1986;146:1219–1220.
66. Mathieu D, Gosselin B, Nolf M, et al: Massive digitoxin intoxication: treatment by Amberlite XAD-4 resin hemoperfusion. *J Toxicol Clin Toxicol* 1983;19:931–950.
67. Gibb J, Adams P, Parnham A: Plasma digoxin: assay anomalies in Fab-treated patients. *Br J Clin Pharmacol* 1983;16:445–447.
68. Duke M: Atrioventricular block due to accidental digoxin ingestion treated with atropine. *Am J Dis Child* 1972;124:754–756.
69. Rumack B, Wolfe R, Gilfrich H: Phenytoin (diphenylhydantoin) treatment of massive digoxin overdose. *Br Heart J* 1974;36: 405–408.
70. French J, Thomas R, Siskind A: Magnesium therapy in massive digoxin intoxication. *Ann Emerg Med* 1984;13:562–566.
71. Murphy D, Bremner F, Haber E, et al: Massive digoxin poisoning treated with Fab fragments of digoxin-specific antibodies. *Pediatrics* 1982;70:472–473.
72. Taboulet P, Baud F, Bismuth C, et al: Acute digitalis intoxication—is pacing still appropriate? *J Toxicol Clin Toxicol* 1993;31;261–273.
73. Henderson R, Solomon C: Use of cholestyramine in the treatment of digoxin intoxication. *Arch Intern Med* 1988;148:745–746.
74. Pieroni R, Fisher H: Use of cholestyramine resin in digitoxin toxicity. *JAMA* 1981;245:1939–1940.
75. Payne V, Secter R, Noback R: Use of colestipol in a patient with digoxin intoxication. *Drug Intell Clin Pharmacol* 1981;15:902–903.
76. Cohen S: Antibody therapy of digoxin intoxication. *Pediatrics* 1982; 70:494.
77. Leikin J, Vogel S, Graff J, et al: Use of Fab fragments of digoxin-specific antibodies in the therapy of massive digoxin poisoning. *Ann Emerg Med* 1985;14:175–178.
78. Goldman R: The use of serum digoxin levels in clinical practice. *JAMA* 1974;229:331–332.
79. Rollins D, Brizgys M: Immunological approach to poisoning. *Ann Emerg Med* 1986;15:1046–1051.
80. Clifton G, McIntyre W, Zannikos P, et al: Free and total serum digoxin concentrations in a renal failure patient after treatment with digoxin immune Fab. *Clin Pharm* 1989;8:441–445.
81. Gibson T: Comparison of XAD-4 and charcoal hemoperfusion for removal of digoxin and digitoxin. *Kidney Int* 1980;18:S101–S105.
82. Gibson T: Hemoperfusion of digoxin intoxication. *Clin Toxicol* 1980; 17:501–513.
83. Smith T, Butler V, Haber E, et al: Treatment of life threatening digitalis intoxication with digoxin-specific Fab antibody fragments. *N Engl J Med* 1982;307:1357–1362.
84. Smith T, Haber E: Digoxin intoxication: the relationship of clinical presentation to serum digoxin concentration. *J Clin Invest* 1970;49: 2377–2386.
85. Wenger T, Butler V, Haber E, et al: Treatment of 63 severely digitalis-toxic patients with digoxin-specific antibody fragments. *J Am Coll Cardiol* 1985;5:118A–123A.
86. Martiny S, Phelps S, Massey K: Treatment of severe digitalis intoxication with digoxin-specific antibody fragments: a clinical review. *Crit Care Med* 1988;16:629–635.
87. Smolarz A, Roesch E, Lenz E, et al: Digoxin-specific antibody (Fab) fragments in 34 cases of severe digitalis intoxication. *Clin Toxicol* 1985;23:327–340.
88. Kirkpatrick C: Allergic histories and reactions of patients treated with digoxin immune Fab (Ovine) antibody. *Am J Emerg Med* 1991;9: 7–10.

89. Kaufman J, Leiken J, Kendzierski D, et al: Use of digoxin Fab immune fragments in a seven day old infant. *Pediatr Emerg Care* 1990;6:118–121.
90. Wenger T: Experience with digoxin immune Fab (Ovine) in patients with renal transplant. *Am J Emerg Med* 1991;9:21–23.
91. Ujhelyi M, Robert S, Cummings D, et al: Influence of digoxin immune Fab therapy and renal dysfunction on the disposition of total and free digoxin. *Ann Intern Med* 1993;119:273–277.
92. Woolf A, Wenger T, Smith T, et al: Results of multicenter studies of digoxin-specific antibody fragments in managing digitalis intoxication in the pediatric population. *Am J Emerg Med* 1991;9:16–20.
93. Taboulet P, Baud F, Bismuth C: Clinical features and management of digitalis poisoning—rationale for immunotherapy. *J Toxicol Clin Toxicol* 1993;31:247–260.
94. Hansell A: Effect of therapeutic digoxin antibodies on digoxin assays. *Arch Pathol Lab Med* 1989;113:1259–1262.
95. Zucker A, Lacina S, DasGupta D, et al: Fab fragments of digoxin-specific antibodies used to reverse ventricular fibrillation induced by digoxin ingestion in a child. *Pediatrics* 1982;70:468–471.

ADDITIONAL SELECTED REFERENCES

Cohn J: Indications for digitalis therapy.*JAMA* 1974;229:1911–1914.

Das G: Digoxin-quinidine interaction. *Am J Cardiol* 1982;49:495.

Doering W: Is there a clinically relevant interaction between quinine and digoxin in human beings? *Am J Cardiol* 1981;48:975–976.

Gullner H, Stinson E, Harrison D, et al: Correlation of serum concentrations with heart concentrations of digoxin in human subjects. *Circulation* 1974;50:653–655.

Henry D, Lawson D, Lowe J, et al: The changing pattern of toxicity to digoxin. *Postgrad Med J* 1981;57:358–362.

Koch-Weser J, Greenblatt D: Influence of serum digoxin concentration measurements on frequency of digitoxicity. *Clin Pharmacol Ther* 1975; 16:284–288.

Mooradian A, Wynn E: Pharmacokinetic prediction of serum digoxin concentration in the elderly. *Arch Intern Med* 1987;147:650–653.

Schaumann W, Kaufmann B, Neubert P, et al: Kinetics of the Fab fragments of digoxin antibodies and of bound digoxin in patients with severe digoxin intoxication. *Eur J Clin Pharmacol* 1986;30:527–533.

CHAPTER 22

Calcium Channel Blockers

Calcium ions play a critical role in numerous essential biologic processes, and the importance of calcium as a messenger system cannot be overstated (1). Calcium has a central role in mediating the contraction of all forms of muscle, the secretion of exocrine, endocrine, and neuroendocrine products, the metabolic processes of glycogenolysis and gluconeogenesis, the transport and secretion of fluids and electrolytes, and the growth of cells (2,3). In particular, calcium catalyzes enzymatic reactions that split high-energy phosphate bonds and are involved in the electrical activation of excitable cells, hemostasis, and metabolism of bone (Table 22–1) (4). In terms of clinical effects that relate to calcium channel blockers, calcium ion influx is primarily involved in the genesis of the cardiac action potential (2), facilitates the intracardiac conduction of electrical impulses (5), promotes contraction of cardiac and smooth muscle cells, and may also cause irreversible cellular injury of anoxic tissue (2,4).

CALCIUM ANTAGONISM

Several inorganic cations, such as cobalt and manganese, function as general calcium antagonists (4). These agents are effective in blocking a wide variety of calcium-dependent processes, but they are considered nonselective agents (6). This nonselectivity of action arises from the ability of these cations to substitute for calcium at various calcium-binding sites. The calcium channel blockers are different in action in that they selectively act on calcium as it relates to the "slow" channel of an action potential.

TABLE 22–1. *The role of calcium in biologic processes*

Electrical activation of excitable cells
Enzymatic reactions
Glycogenolysis
Gluconeogenesis
Hemostasis
Metabolism of bone
Genesis of cardiac action potential
Promotes contraction of smooth muscle
Secretion of exocrine, endocrine, and neuroendocrine products
Transport and secretion of fluid and electrolytes
Causes irreversible cellular injury of anoxic tissue

GENERAL OVERVIEW OF CALCIUM CHANNEL BLOCKERS

Calcium channel blockers have three main sites of action: myocardial muscle, vascular smooth muscle, and the cardiac conduction system. All three systems share the need for calcium to assist with contraction or to regulate nerve impulse propagation. In myocardial muscle, increasing cytoplasmic calcium concentration increases the force of contraction (4,7).

In vascular smooth muscle, calcium initially binds to a small protein, calmodulin, which then activates myosin kinase to produce contraction (8). A second mechanism capable of initiating contraction exists in vascular smooth muscle (9). This mechanism is modulated by α_1 receptors and is independent of calcium channel blockade (2,10).

In the cardiac conduction system, sodium ions are rapidly conducted to the intracellular space when a critical transmembrane potential is achieved, followed by a second, slower influx of calcium ions (8). This influx of calcium ions contributes to the plateau (phase 2) of the cardiac action potential (1,4,7).

Calcium channel blockers impede the movement of calcium ions into vascular smooth muscle and cardiac muscle. All of the calcium channel blockers currently available in the United States, except for verapamil and diltiazem, are dihydropyridines. Verapamil and diltiazem are more likely to suppress cardiac contractility and slow cardiac conduction; the dihydropyridines are more potent vasodilators (4).

Uses of Calcium Channel Blockers

Introduced almost 30 years ago for the treatment of angina, calcium channel blockers are now successfully used for a wide variety of medical conditions including angina pectoris, hypertension, myocardial infarction,

TABLE 22–2. *Uses of the calcium channel blockers*

Stable and unstable angina
Vasospastic angina
Acute myocardial infarction
Congestive heart failure
Hypertrophic cardiomyopathy
Dysrhythmias
Paroxysmal atrial tachycardia
Atrial fibrillation
Atrial flutter
Systemic hypertension
Pulmonary hypertension
Raynaud's phenomenon

arrhythmias, migraine headache, heart failure, stroke, Raynaud's phenomenon, and primary pulmonary hypertension (Table 22–2).

THE ROLE OF CALCIUM IN THE ACTION POTENTIAL

Calcium has important roles in the excitation–contraction coupling process of heart and vascular smooth muscle cells and in the electrical discharge of the specialized conduction cells of the heart (11). The membranes of these cells contain numerous channels that carry a slow inward current and that are selective for calcium.

The calcium channel blockers are organic compounds that produce electromechanical uncoupling in heart muscle by selectively blocking the slow inward current of cardiac action potential. By inhibiting calcium influx, the calcium channel blockers inhibit the contractile processes of cardiac and vascular smooth muscle. This in turn leads to a negative inotropic effect as well as a reduction in cardiac work and myocardial oxygen demand. The effect of calcium channel blockade of the sinoatrial and atrioventricular nodes is to block or decrease impulse conduction by increasing the effective and functional refractory periods of these nodal cells. This is due to the inhibition of coupling of actin and myosin, two proteins necessary for muscular contraction of myocardial and vascular smooth muscle (12).

In skeletal muscle, most of the calcium ion required for electromechanical coupling is derived from intracellular stores within the sarcoplasmic reticulum. In cardiac and smooth muscle, most of the calcium ions reach the intracellular site from transmembrane calcium ion flow. As a result, the calcium channel blockers can only affect cardiac and smooth muscle (5).

Calcium and Smooth Muscle

The normal cell membrane is relatively impermeable to calcium so that a steep calcium gradient is maintained. In the relaxed state the calcium concentration outside cells is about 5,000 to 10,000 times greater than that within cells, which allows calcium ions to enter through voltage-dependent channels in the cell membranes (13). Intracellular calcium levels are reduced through energy-dependent membrane pumps that promote calcium efflux (4).

At the onset of muscle contraction, extracellular calcium enters the cell through "calcium channels." The rapid influx of calcium also stimulates release of stored calcium from the sarcoplasmic reticulum, further increasing intracellular calcium (8). Intracellular calcium binds to the calmodulin molecule located on the actin filament, causing a change in the configuration of troponin so that actin now comes in contact with the myosin filament, producing contraction (Fig. 22–1) (1,12,14).

To maintain the smooth muscle fibers in a noncontracted state, these fibers must extrude calcium ions, a process that requires energy. It has been suggested that extracellular concentrations of sodium ions play a central role in this extrusion: Sodium entering the cell moves down an electrochemical gradient, and the energy thereby released is tapped to transport calcium ions out of the cell (14). A change in the ratio of intracellular to extracellular sodium ions, therefore, can alter the concentration of calcium ions within the cell (4,15).

Calcium and the Heart Muscle

In the resting myocardial cell, the extracellular and intracellular calcium gradients are maintained by both cell membranes and efficient pumping systems, thereby maintaining the constancy of the environment. It is this gradient of free ionized calcium that contributes to the propagation of the action potential and determines the contractile state of the heart. The calcium channel blockers therefore exert their pharmacologic effects primarily through calcium antagonism at the cell membrane of these excitable tissues, thereby inhibiting the transmembrane influx of extracellular calcium (4,15). They do not modify calcium intake, binding, or exchange by cardiac microsomes, nor do they have an effect on calcium-activated ATPase or cause a change in serum calcium concentrations (10).

The "Slow" Channel

The slow channel is responsible for excitation–contraction coupling. It is the selective inhibition of the slow channel activity in cardiac muscle that characterizes the fundamental property of the calcium channel blockers (5,12). From the standpoint of their overall cardiocirculatory effects, their main loci of actions are therefore on the sinoatrial and atrioventricular nodes in the heart and in the systemic and coronary circulation in the periphery (16).

The electrical activity of the sinoatrial and atrioventricular nodal cells has a slowly rising action potential

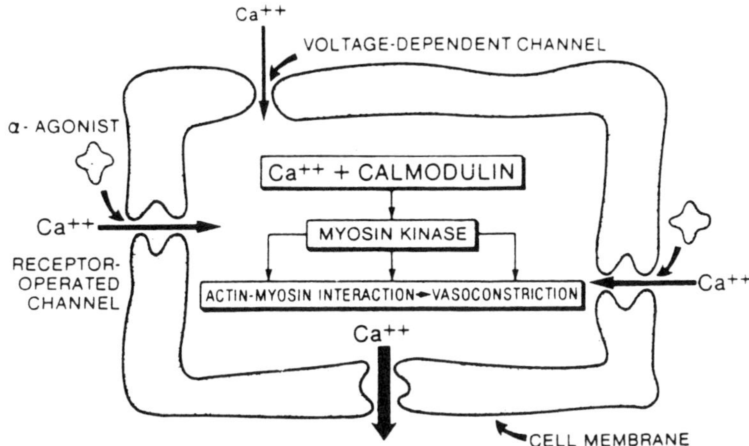

FIG. 22–1. Calcium ion–dependent regulation of muscle tone in vascular smooth muscle. Calcium ions (Ca^{2+}) entry can occur in response to electrical stimulation through the voltage-dependent channel, or receptor activation through the adrenergic receptor–mediated channel, or both. On entry into the cell, the cellular-free calcium ions bind to the calcium binding protein calmodulin. This calmodulin–calcium ion complex, in turn, activates myosin kinase, which causes the phosphorylation of myosin's light chain. Phosphorylation then activates the binding of actin to myosin and leads to contraction. Intracellular calcium ion levels are reduced through energy-dependent membrane pumps that promote calcium efflux, which involves sodium/calcium countertransport.

and a reduced rate of conduction and is especially dependent on the slow current, which accounts for the effectiveness of the calcium channel blockers (2). The rest of the specialized conduction system is dependent on the fast current. Slow channel-dependent tissues, such as the sinoatrial and atrioventricular nodes, therefore have low diastolic potentials, slow rates of phase 0 depolarization (slow conduction velocities), spontaneous phase 4 depolarization (automaticity), and delayed recovery of excitability outlasting the duration of the action potential (long refractory periods). The effects of slow-channel blocking agents are thus most evident in the sinoatrial node, atrioventricular node, and diseased fast-channel tissues (11,16).

THE CALCIUM CHANNEL BLOCKERS

The Older Calcium Channel Blockers

The commonly used older calcium channel blockers are (a) verapamil, a papaverine derivative; (b) diltiazem, a benzothiazepine; and (c) nifedipine, the prototype of the dihydropyridine group (13). Newer agents have been introduced, almost exclusively of the dihydropyridine group (4,17,18).

The introduction of sustained-release formulations of the calcium channel blockers brings new problems and risks in overdose not encountered in standard formulations. Their growing availability increases the possibility of accidental and intentional exposure. Three calcium channel blockers are available in the United States in sustained-release preparations: verapamil (Calan SR and Isoptin SR), diltiazem (Cardizem SR), and nifedipine (Procardia XL).

Although each drug may act as a calcium channel blocker, there are also significant differences in their clinical indications (Table 22–3) and their effects (Table 22–4) (19). Although the calcium channel blockers share the same general mechanism of action, they are chemically unrelated. The structural dissimilarity among the broad group of compounds that block calcium transfer within the heart or the vascular smooth muscle, or both, has suggested that some of them might have pharmacologic properties independent of their slow channel blocking actions. Each of the calcium channel blockers differs in apparent mode of action, time course of action, concentration–effect relation, and pharmacologic action in different tissues (14).

TABLE 22–3. *Comparison of indications for use of older calcium channel blockers*

Indication	Verapamil	Diltiazem	Nifedipine
Vasospastic angina	+	+	+
Effort angina	0	+	+
Supraventricular tachycardia	+	0	0
Left ventricular failure	0	0	+
Malignant hypertension	0	0	+
Migraine prophylaxis	+	0	0

Adapted with permission from *Emerg Med* 1984;5:31. Cahners Publishing Company.

TABLE 22–4. *Comparison of effects of older calcium channel blockers*

Effect	Verapamil	Diltiazem	Nifedipine
Hypotension	+	+	+
Flushing	+	–	++
Headache	+	+	++
Peripheral edema	+	+	+
Palpitations	+	+	+
Chest pain	+	+	+
Conduction disturbances	++	+	–
Heart failure	+	–	+/–
Bradycardia	++	+	–

Adapted with permission from Krebs R: Adverse reactions with calcium antagonists. In *Hypertension* 5 (Suppl. 11):11-125–11-129. American Heart Association.

Verapamil's most potent activity is electrophysiologic, and nifedipine's effects are hemodynamic; diltiazem acts like a less potent combination of the two (1). All three cause an increase in coronary blood flow, with nifedipine having a greater effect than verapamil or diltiazem. All cause vasodilation of vascular smooth muscle, although diltiazem dilates coronary vessels with less potent effects on blood flow in the other vascular beds. Verapamil and nifedipine appear to be roughly equivalent in the various vascular beds (20,21).

β Blocking agents reduce blood pressure by decreasing cardiac output and renin secretion, and peripheral vascular resistance is either unchanged or slightly increased. Calcium channel blockers, on the other hand, produce vasodilation and reduce the elevated peripheral vascular resistance. Furthermore, calcium channel blockers have no adverse renal effects and produce minimal undesirable effects on serum lipids (6).

The bioavailability of each compound is relatively low owing to extensive first-pass metabolism in the liver (17). Nifedipine has the shortest half-life, and verapamil has the longest half-life and partially active metabolites (2). Because the calcium channel blockers mainly are metabolized in the liver, daily dosages have to be reduced in patients with concomitant hepatic diseases. Dosage adjustment also may be needed in elderly patients who may be hypersensitive to the drugs or may metabolize them more slowly (14).

Verapamil, diltiazem, and nifedipine are of markedly dissimilar structures, which probably is partly responsible for their different cardiovascular effects. Thus, verapamil has the greatest chronotropic and inotropic depressant actions while nifedipine has the least, with diltiazem's effect being intermediate. In contrast, nifedipine is the most potent vasodilator of the three, and the vasodilation is often accompanied by reflex tachycardia. Because their pharmacologic actions are varied, observations regarding one drug may not be generalizable to the group as a whole.

An initial reflex increase in heart rate usually occurs with the dihydropyridines (nifedipine, nicardipine, isradipine, and felodipine); verapamil and diltiazem cause little or no change in heart rate. Verapamil and diltiazem can, however, slow atrioventricular conduction and should be used with caution in patients also taking a β blocker; dihydropyridines generally do not affect atrioventricular conduction and can be used with a β blocker, which decreases reflex tachycardia.

Verapamil (Isoptin, Calan)

Verapamil, a papaverine derivative (22), was introduced as a smooth muscle relaxant with potent peripheral and coronary vasodilator properties (23). It was originally thought to be an adrenergic blocking agent because its myocardial effects were opposite those resulting from catecholamine action. Verapamil is the prototype of Class IV antidysrhythmic agents (20,24).

The effects of verapamil consist of negative inotropic and chronotropic actions (25). Of the three older calcium channel blockers, it has the most profound influence on the calcium current of the sinoatrial and atrioventricular nodes and thus is the most useful in the treatment of supraventricular tachycardia, which is often caused by reentry through the atrioventricular node (2,5). Verapamil has also been shown to inhibit a second slow current carried by the sodium ion (24).

Actions

Verapamil is a calcium channel blocker with antianginal, antidysrhythmic, and antihypertensive properties (23). Verapamil has a greater affinity for the calcium "slow" channels in the cardiac conducting system than vascular tissue (26). This is clinically evidenced by its effect of slowing conduction through the atrioventricular node (20,24).

Verapamil acts on vascular smooth muscle, causing coronary and peripheral vascular arterial dilatation. Unlike its action in the myocardial cell, in vascular smooth muscle the transmembrane influx of calcium binds directly to a regulatory protein, calmodulin, without requiring the release of calcium from the sarcoplasmic reticulum (27). Calmodulin then activates the enzyme myosin kinase to initiate contraction (2,5).

Verapamil blocks the slow inward transmembrane calcium influx but does not affect the intracellular mobilization of calcium from the sarcoplasmic reticulum. Verapamil is more active in cells that have the least sarcoplasmic reticulum and are dependent on transmembrane calcium influx for intracellular events (9). Skeletal muscle is richest in sarcoplasmic reticulum and is not affected by verapamil. Myocardial muscle has significantly less sarcoplasmic reticulum. Vascular smooth muscle has the least and is therefore most susceptible to calcium channel blockade (24).

The most prominent clinical effect of verapamil is depression of sinoatrial rate and conduction through the atrioventricular node. Conduction at the atrioventricular node is delayed by prolonging the A-H interval and the atrioventricular node refractory period. On the surface EKG, verapamil's effect on the atrioventricular node is manifested by a dose-dependent prolongation of the PR interval. No change in the QRS or QTc intervals occurs (9). Although verapamil directly suppresses the sinoatrial node rate, this effect is easily overcome in most patients by reflex stimulation (10). In contrast, the effect of delayed atrioventricular node conduction is significant and results in prolongation of the PR interval. This accounts for verapamil's efficacy in slowing or converting most supraventricular tachydysrhythmias (28).

Pharmacokinetics

After oral administration of verapamil, absorption is rapid and virtually complete (24). The first-pass effect through the hepatic portal circulation causes 60% to 70% of the oral dose to be biotransformed; thus, bioavailability of verapamil ranges from 20% to 35% (1,29). To be effective, an oral dose must be 10 to 20 times more than the recommended intravenous dose. Plasma concentrations reach their peak within 1 to 2 hours after oral administration (8). Sustained-release verapamil peak plasma concentrations are between 4 and 8 hours but can be delayed with the presence of food (30). The duration of effect is greater than 14 hours for sustained-release verapamil. In patients with hepatic dysfunction or cirrhosis, the serum half-life of verapamil is increased to 14 to 16 hours, and plasma levels may reach five times those seen in normal patients at the same doses (9).

The steady-state volume of distribution ranges from 4.5 to 7 L/kg, and approximately 90% of the drug is bound to plasma proteins (12). The plasma half-life of verapamil in adults is approximately 3 to 7 hours and may be longer in children. Norverapamil, an active metabolite, achieves plasma concentrations approximately equal to those of verapamil within 4 to 6 hours after administration (17,20).

The onset of action of intravenous verapamil is almost immediate, with the maximal effect on atrioventricular node conduction occurring in 3 to 5 minutes (15). The slowing of atrioventricular node conduction lasts up to 6 hours because of preferential binding of the drug at atrioventricular nodal tissues.

Serum Levels

Therapeutic serum concentrations are reported to range from 80 to 300 ng/mL (25). While seldom used in maintenance therapy, plasma levels may be useful in determining toxicity. After chronic oral doses of 480 mg/day, verapamil levels peak at 323 ng/mL and norverapamil levels at 255 ng/mL (9). A single, immediate-release dose of 80 mg of verapamil produces an average peak plasma concentration of 39 ng/mL (30). Early signs of toxicity are more likely at levels > 300 ng/mL and may be heralded by prolongation of the PR interval (9).

Adverse Effects

Reports concerning verapamil's side effects and associated acute intoxication are scarce (17). Side effects result from the drug's action on the conducting tissue of the heart and peripheral smooth muscle (Table 22–5). Constipation, headache, dizziness, hepatic dysfunction (23), hypotension, fatigue, prolonged atrioventricular conduction, and decreased cardiac output have been noted (17,31).

Because insulin release by the islet cells of the pancreas is triggered by the intracellular accumulation of calcium, overdose with a calcium channel blocker could lead to a hyperglycemic state (9). There are some reports of impaired carbohydrate metabolism associated with verapamil (28). Reports document hyperglycemia in nondiabetic patients with acute intoxication of verapamil, some requiring intravenous insulin infusions (27).

The most significant adverse cardiovascular effects are hypotension, bradydysrhythmias, conduction disturbances, and left ventricular failure, which is normally transient and mild. Sinus bradycardia is usually not manifested in therapeutic doses except in patients with underlying disease in their conduction system (9). Severe hypotension has been noted most often in patients concurrently taking β blockers, so that caution must be exercised when administering calcium channel blockers to such patients (15,20,31–33). The most frequently observed benign cardiac effects are first- or second-degree atrioventricular block (Wenckebach period) and atrioventricular junc-

TABLE 22–5. *Adverse effects of verapamil*

Adverse effects
Noncardiac
Constipation
Headache
Dizziness
Hepatic dysfunction
Fatigue
Hyperglycemia
Cardiac
Hypotension
Bradydysrhythmias
Conduction disturbances
Left ventricular failure
First-, second-, and third-degree block

tional rhythm (30). Although verapamil rarely produces clinically important changes in the rate of sinoatrial node discharge or recovery time, it may reduce the resting heart rate and produce sinus arrest in patients with sinoatrial node disease (9). Verapamil is an uncommon but potentially lethal cause of poisoning (8,9).

Drug Interactions

Chronic verapamil treatment can increase serum digoxin levels by 50% to 75% during the first week of therapy, and this may result in digoxin intoxication. This digoxin interaction has not yet been shown with diltiazem (14).

Verapamil and diltiazem need to be used with some caution in elderly patients who are receiving β blockers because heart block or heart failure may be precipitated. Cimetidine may reduce verapamil clearance and increase its elimination half-life. Verapamil may result in a lowering of serum lithium levels in patients receiving chronic oral lithium therapy (14).

Nifedipine (Procardia)

Nifedipine, a dihydropyridine derivative, has a greater affinity for vascular tissue than for cardiac tissue and has its marked effects against vascular spasm and hypertension with no atrioventricular nodal interference (3). At the doses used clinically, therefore, it does not have a depressant effect on the sinoatrial or atrioventricular conduction in the heart (1). This is in contrast to both verapamil and diltiazem, which produce sinoatrial and atrioventricular node depression. Nifedipine causes relaxation of blood vessels and therefore is a coronary vasodilator that increases coronary flow (1). Because it has no important myocardial depressant actions or electrophysiologic effects in therapeutic doses, the drug has found primary clinical application in disorders associated with abnormal or inappropriate vasoconstriction (5).

Pharmacokinetics

Approximately 90% of an oral dose of nifedipine is rapidly absorbed from the gastrointestinal tract. Of the total oral dose, 65% to 75% reaches systemic circulation unchanged because nifedipine is metabolized to some extent on first pass through the liver. In patients with normal renal and hepatic function, the plasma half-life is 2 to 5 hours. Nifedipine has no active metabolites. The protein-binding of nifedipine is greater than 95% (3).

Onset of action after oral administration is within 20 minutes, with a peak effect between 1 and 2 hours. A sublingual preparation is available, and has an onset of action of 3 minutes and a peak at 20 minutes (34). Therapeutic concentrations of nifedipine are reported to be in the range of 25 to 100 ng/mL (25). It is unclear how the plasma level correlates with the toxicity of nifedipine.

Adverse Effects

The adverse effects of nifedipine are related to its potent vasodilation and include flushing, headache, hypotension, fatigue, peripheral paresthesias and dysesthesia, palpitations, peripheral edema, and syncope (Table 22–6) (17,35). Caution should be used when administering nifedipine together with β blockers (31). When administered with digoxin it may increase digoxin levels by 50%. Nifedipine interferes with glucose tolerance in both diabetic and normal patients (5,26).

TABLE 22–6. *Adverse effects of nifedipine*

Fatigue
Flushing
Headache
Hypotension
Peripheral paresthesias
Palpitations
Peripheral edema
Syncope

Diltiazem (Cardizem)

Diltiazem is a benzothiazepine derivative. Like the other calcium channel blockers, it causes a dose-dependent inhibition of the slow inward calcium current in normal cardiac tissue. Diltiazem prolongs atrioventricular node conduction time and slows the sinoatrial node rate without the reflex changes seen with verapamil (1). This is because diltiazem exerts only a minimal effect on blood vessels elsewhere in the body. Both verapamil and diltiazem are equivalent in their slowing of atrioventricular node conduction, but diltiazem causes less prolongation of the atrioventricular node refractory period than verapamil (36). Diltiazem is also a potent vasodilator of coronary vessels. It has a stronger depressant action on sinoatrial node discharge than does verapamil and can cause significant bradycardia or sinus arrest in patients with sick sinus syndrome.

Pharmacokinetics

Approximately 80% of an oral dose of diltiazem is rapidly absorbed from the gastrointestinal tract. The onset of action of oral diltiazem is within 15 minutes, with peak effect within 1 to 2 hours. It has a plasma half-life of 4 to 9 hours. Diltiazem also undergoes significant first-pass metabolism by the liver, with 40% of an oral dose reaching the systemic circulation (11). The mean volume of distribution is approximately 5 L/kg (3). Whereas the therapeutic plasma level of diltiazem is 50 to 200 ng/mL, there is no correlation between plasma levels and toxicity in limited studies, making the clinical usefulness of plasma levels questionable. Diltiazem has one active metabolite, desacetyl diltiazem, which has 25% to 50% of the original activity (3).

TABLE 22–7. *Adverse effects of diltiazem*

Atrioventricular block
Flushing
Headache
Hepatic dysfunction
Hypotension
Sinus bradycardia

Adverse Effects

Diltiazem offers benefits similar to verapamil without the severity of its complications and, because of this, has become a well-accepted treatment for angina. Due to diltiazem's increasing popularity and availability, its toxicity has been seen with escalating frequency in emergency departments, yet diltiazem has a wide therapeutic index and is the best tolerated of the three agents (Table 22–7) (37). Minor side effects with diltiazem are of low incidence, and are primarily constipation, nausea, and edema (36). The major and potentially most serious side effects are vasodilation resulting in headache, flushing, occasional hypotension, and depression of atrioventricular nodal conduction, the last of which may result in a sinus bradycardia or various degrees of atrioventricular block and asystole (21). Hepatic dysfunction has also been reported. Caution should be exercised when administering diltiazem to patients taking β blockers or with preexisting hypotension. Although diltiazem is widely used in the treatment of a variety of cardiovascular disorders, there are only a few reports of overdose of this drug (37). Of the few cases reported, bradycardia and hypotension were the main presenting complaints (36).

The Newer Calcium Channel Blockers

Newer agents—nicardipine, nimodipine, felodipine, and amlodipine—have been introduced to the market in the last two years. Like their counterparts, they also inhibit transmembrane ion flux through calcium "slow" channels and cause vasodilation of vascular smooth muscle. All of these agents are structurally related to nifedipine and, therefore, possess greater activity on vascular smooth muscle than on cardiac muscle or cardiac conducting tissue; however, their affinities for specific vascular tissues impart to them distinctive characteristics (Table 22–8) (10). Other newer agents are also discussed.

Although nicardipine can have a profound hypotensive effect, its coronary vascular selectivity limits the reflex tachycardia commonly seen with nifedipine at normal doses.

Although there are no published reports of overdose with these calcium channel blockers, hypotension is a common adverse reaction. One would expect an overdose to have similar findings, as with other calcium channel blockers, except for the profound atrioventricular node conduction disturbances seen with verapamil and diltiazem.

Nicardipine

Nicardipine (Cardene) is a dihydropyridine calcium channel blocking agent that is structurally related to amlodipine, felodipine, nifedipine, and nimodipine.

Nicardipine is administered orally and is rapidly absorbed from the gastrointestinal tract. The drug is rapidly and extensively metabolized in the liver. The terminal plasma half-life of 8 to 9 hours may be markedly prolonged in patients with severe liver disease.

Nicardipine has been shown to have more vascular smooth muscle selectivity than nifedipine, with minimal negative inotropic properties and no effect on atrioventricular node conduction. Its effect on vascular smooth muscle is more pronounced on coronary vasculature,

TABLE 22–8. *Pharmacologic effects of the calcium channel blockers*

	Heart rate								
	Acute	Chronic	Conduction SA node	Conduction AV node	Myocardial contractility	Peripheral vasodilator	Cardiac output	Coronary Blood flow	Myocardial O_2 demand
Diltiazem	↓	↓	↓	↓	↓	↓	V	↑	↓
Verapamil	↑	↓	↓	↓	↓↓	↓	V	↑	↓
Nifedipine	↑	↑ –	–	↑–	↓	↓↓	↑–	↑	↓
Nicardipine	↑	↑–	–	↑–	–	↓↓	↑–	↑	↓
Nitrendipine	↑	↑–	–	↑–	↓	↓↓	↑–	↑	↓

↓ = Decrease; ↑ = increase; – = no change; V, variable; SA, sinoatrial; AV, atrioventricular.

increasing coronary blood flow and limiting infarct size to a higher degree than other calcium channel blockers (3).

The most common adverse effects of nicardipine have been flushing, headache, pedal edema, asthenia, palpitations, and dizziness. Compared with verapamil, nicardipine appears less likely to cause constipation or atrioventricular block and more likely to cause edema or reflex tachycardia.

Nimodipine

Nimodipine's (Nimotop) vascular smooth muscle selectivity is directed at cerebral vasculature due to its lipid solubility and ability to cross the blood–brain barrier (3). Nimodipine is indicated for the improvement of neurologic outcome by reducing the incidence and severity of ischemic deficits in patients with subarachnoid hemorrhage from ruptured congenital aneurysms who are in good neurologic condition.

Pharmacokinetics and Metabolism

In humans, nimodipine is rapidly absorbed after oral administration, and peak concentrations are generally attained within 1 hour. The terminal elimination half-life is approximately 8 to 9 hours but earlier elimination rates are much more rapid, equivalent to a half-life of 1–2 hours; a consequence is the need for frequent dosing. Nimodipine is more than 95% bound to plasma proteins. Because of a high first-pass metabolism, the bioavailability of nimodipine averages 13% after oral administration.

Overdosage

There have been no reports of overdosage from the oral administration of nimodipine. Symptoms of overdosage would be expected to be related to cardiovascular effects such as excessive peripheral vasodilation with marked systemic hypotension.

Isradipine

Isradipine (DynaCirc) is a 1,4-dihydropyridine-derivative calcium channel blocking agent that binds to calcium channels with high affinity and specificity and inhibits calcium flux into cardiac and smooth muscle. It was approved in 1991 for the treatment of hypertension. Like nicardipine and nifedipine, isradipine is a more potent vasodilator than verapamil or diltiazem. Reflex tachycardia is minimal with isradipine, and myocardial oxygen requirements generally do not increase.

Isradipine is 90–95% absorbed and is subject to extensive first-pass metabolism, resulting in a bioavailability of about 15% to 24%. Serum concentrations of the drug reach a peak in about 1–2 hours. Isradipine is completely metabolized prior to excretion, and no unchanged drug is detected in the urine (14).

Like other dihydropyridine calcium channel blockers, isradipine is less likely than verapamil to cause constipation, but may cause flushing, headache, tachycardia, dizziness, and ankle edema, especially in the first week of use.

Although there is no well-documented experience with isradipine overdosage, as with other dihydropyridines, gross overdosage would result in excessive peripheral vasodilation with subsequent marked and probably prolonged systemic hypotension.

Nitrendipine

The need for frequent administration and the relatively high incidence of adverse effects associated with nifedipine administration has prompted the development of newer dihydropyridine calcium channel blocking agents. Nitrendipine is a new calcium channel blocker belonging to the dihydropyridine subgroup. Nitrendipine differs from nifedipine in having a long plasma half-life, allowing once-daily dosage (14).

The difference between nitrendipine and nifedipine in relaxing vascular smooth muscle is their duration of action. The maximal effect of nitrendipine occurs 1 to 2 hours after an oral dose, and the elimination half-life is about 12 hours. Blood pressure is maximally reduced for 4 hours and remains below pretreatment levels for 6 to 8 hours.

Similar to nifedipine, the hypotensive effect is associated with reflex increase in heart rate and cardiac output, both of which decrease with time (6).

Felodipine

Felodipine (Plendil) is an extended-release preparation of a dihydropyridine calcium channel blocker that was recently marketed in the United States for oral treatment of hypertension.

Felodipine is well absorbed from the gastrointestinal tract, but due to extensive first-pass metabolism, systemic bioavailability is only about 20%. Plasma concentrations reach a peak in 2.5 to 5 hours, and the drug has a mean terminal half-life of about 24 hours. Plasma concentrations may be higher in patients more than 65 years old and those with hepatic dysfunction.

Adverse Effects

Like other dihydropyridine calcium channel blockers, felodipine frequently causes an initial tachycardia, which usually subsides after the first few weeks of treatment. Dose-dependent adverse effects include peripheral edema, headache, flushing, and postural dizziness, presumably related to peripheral vasodilation. As with nicardipine, gingival hyperplasia has been reported with felodipine. Negative inotropic effects have not been reported with felodipine. Calcium channel blockers do not affect serum lipid concentrations.

Amlodipine

Amlodipine (Norvasc) is another dihydropyridine calcium channel blocker that has been approved for once-daily oral treatment of hypertension, chronic stable angina, and vasospastic angina. Amlodipine inhibits calcium ion influx across cell membranes selectively, with a greater effect on vascular smooth muscle cells than on cardiac muscle cells. Amlodipine is a peripheral arterial vasodilator that acts directly on vascular smooth muscle to cause a reduction in peripheral vascular resistance and reduction in blood pressure. Amlodipine inhibits the transmembrane influx of calcium ions into vascular smooth muscle and cardiac muscle in that amlodipine binds to both dihydropyridine and nondihydropyridine binding sites. The contractile processes of cardiac muscle and vascular smooth muscle are dependent upon the movement of extracellular calcium ions into these cells through specific ion channels.

Pharmacokinetics

Amlodipine is absorbed slowly from the gastrointestinal tract; serum concentrations reach a peak 6 to 12 hours after an oral dose. Steady-state plasma levels of amlodipine are reached after 7 to 8 days of consecutive daily dosing. Absolute bioavailability has been estimated to be between 64% and 90%. Approximately 90% of the circulating drug is bound to plasma proteins. Elimination from the plasma is biphasic, with a terminal elimination half-life of about 30–50 hours. Metabolism is slower, and plasma concentrations may be higher in older patients

Overdosage

Overdosage might be expected to cause excessive peripheral vasodilation with marked hypotension and possibly a reflex tachycardia.

Bepridil

Bepridil (Vascor) is a calcium channel blocker chemically unrelated to verapamil, nifedipine, or other drugs in this class. Unlike previously available calcium channel blockers, bepridil is an anti-anginal agent that inhibits slow calcium as well as fast sodium channels, interferes with calcium binding to calmodulin, and blocks both voltage- and receptor-operated calcium channels.

Pharmacokinetics

After oral administration, more than 90% of the dose is absorbed, and more than 99% is bound to plasma proteins. The drug is extensively metabolized in the liver. The time to peak bepridil plasma concentration is about 2 to 3 hours. Elimination of bepridil is biphasic, with a distribution half-life of about 2 hours. The terminal elimination half-life following the cessation of multiple dosing averages 42 hours (38).

Adverse Effects

Adverse effects of bepridil have included dizziness, nausea, dyspepsia, headache, tremor, asthenia, diarrhea, and nervousness (Table 22–9). Agranulocytosis has occurred.

Bepridil hydrochloride has Class 1 antiarrhythmic properties and, like other such drugs, can induce new arrhythmias, including ventricular tachycardia and ventricular fibrillation. In addition, because of its ability to prolong the QT interval, bepridil can cause torsade de pointes type ventricular tachycardia. Bepridil hydrochloride has been associated with the usual range of proarrhythmic effects characteristic of Class 1 antiarrhythmics including increased premature ventricular contraction rates, new sustained ventricular tachycardia, and ventricular fibrillation that is more difficult than previously to convert to sinus rhythm.

TABLE 22–9. *Adverse effects of Bepridil*

Neurologic
Nausea
Dizziness
Headache
Tremor
Nervousness
Gastrointestinal
Dyspepsia
Diarrhea
Cardiac
Torsade de pointes
Ventricular tachycardia
Ventricular fibrillation
Miscellaneous
Agranulocytosis

TABLE 22–10. *Signs and symptoms of overdosage with calcium channel blockers*

Cardiovascular
Hypotension
Bradydysrhythmias
Congestive heart failure
First-, second-, and third-degree heart block
Bundle branch block
Neurologic
Dizziness
Syncope
Mental confusion
Miscellaneous
Anuria
Hyperglycemia
Metabolic acidosis

OVERDOSAGE OF CALCIUM CHANNEL BLOCKERS

The increasing popularity of the calcium channel blockers as therapeutic agents has led to an increase in overdoses, both accidental and intentional (Table 22–10). In overdose, calcium channel blockers have presented a picture of rapid onset of symptomatology, yet the appearance of symptoms with a sustained-release formulation may be delayed as long as 12 to 24 hours, leading to a false sense of security.

Acute overdose may be manifested by symptomatic hypotension due to peripheral vasodilation, bradydysrhythmias due to depression of cardiac nodal tissues, and left ventricular decompensation due to negative inotropism. Suppression of the sinus node may lead to a slow ventricular escape rhythm. In addition, first-, second-, and third-degree atrioventricular block and bundle branch block have been noted (22). Hypotension is most likely to occur in patients with poor left ventricular function in whom peripheral vasodilation and negative inotropic effects cannot be compensated. Patients with a high risk of profound bradycardia are those with prior evidence of sick sinus syndrome or atrioventricular conduction delay. Cardiac arrest and other cases of severe myocardial depression have been noted as a result of intentional or accidental overdosage. Other clinical manifestations of overdose include mental confusion, syncope, anuria, and coma. Although most reported cases are nonfatal, fatalities have been reported. Fatalities with sustained-release formulations have been reported less frequently, probably due to the more recent availability of this product (39,40).

Verapamil

Because more experience has been gained with overdose of verapamil and because certain differences exist between verapamil and the other calcium channel blockers, verapamil overdose is discussed separately. Overdosage of verapamil should be treated as serious, and observation should be maintained for at least 48 hours. This is especially true for the sustained-release preparation.

Although clinical presentation of verapamil overdose can vary, certain consistencies exist. Initial nausea and vomiting are common. Mental status changes can range from alert and oriented to comatose; but most striking is the number of patients who are alert initially despite severe hypotension, only to become unresponsive 1 to 2 hours after hospital admission. This may be particularly true of the sustained-release formulation and may be caused by delayed peak blood levels not found with the regular formulation. Regardless of the preparation ingested, the requirement for a pacemaker appears to correlate with significant toxicity, and despite the resumption of a suitable cardiac rate, a high proportion of paced patients die from progressive, recalcitrant hypotension. Severe metabolic acidosis and hyperglycemia have also been reported with verapamil overdose. If bradycardia or second- or third-degree atrioventricular block occurs, intravenous atropine should be administered. If bradycardia and atrioventricular block do not respond to vagal blockade, isoproterenol may be administered with caution. Fixed second- or third-degree atrioventricular block should be treated with cardiac pacing. Hypotension may be treated with fluids and a vasopressor agent such as dopamine or norepinephrine (8).

Patients who die generally do so within 72 hours of admission; those who survive typically experience no harmful long-term sequelae. Delayed pharmacodynamic consequences may occur with the sustained-release formulation.

TREATMENT OF OVERDOSAGE

Supportive Care

The management of the calcium channel blocker ingestion begins with attention to airway protection and maintenance of adequate oxygenation (9). Simultaneous cardiac monitoring, intravenous access, and a fluid challenge should also occur during the initial assessment (Table 22–11). If the half-life of the ingested drug is short, intoxication usually responds promptly to withdrawal of the drug.

Methods to prevent absorption in acute ingestion should be attempted and aggressive gastric decontamination procedures would be prudent in a suspected ingestion involving a sustained-release calcium channel blocker. Ipecac-induced emesis is not indicated because it may produce vagal stimulation and theoretically worsen a cal-

TABLE 22–11. *Treatment of calcium channel blocker overdose*

Indication	Agent
History of ingestion	Intravenous line (sodium chloride)
History of ingestion	Cardiac monitor
History of ingestion	Gastric lavage
History of ingestion	Charcoal and cathartic Whole bowel irrigation
Symptomatic bradycardia or atrioventricular blocks	Atropine
Symptomatic bradycardia, atrioventricular blocks, or hypotension	Calcium chloride Glucagon Sodium chloride
Significant hypotension	Sympathomimetics Glucagon
Symptomatic refractory bradycardia or atrioventricular blocks	Transvenous pacemaker

cium channel blocker overdose (30). Prevention of delayed toxic effects should be a primary goal of therapy. The increased tablet size of sustained-release formulations and their resistance to disintegration in the stomach may interfere with adequate removal by gastric lavage (16). Activated charcoal should therefore also play a major role in decontamination.

Whole bowel irrigation has been suggested as a possibly effective method of decontamination in both sustained-release formulation ingestion as well as late patient presentation.

Calcium Salts

Although calcium has been used empirically as the "antidote" for acute intoxication, there is limited experience to date in the proper use of either calcium or sodium (41).

The tissues most responsive to an elevated serum calcium concentration in calcium channel blocker intoxication are myocardium and vascular smooth muscle, whereas cardiac conduction tissues appear to require the addition of sodium for partial reversal of calcium channel blocker–induced depression (41). For these reasons, both calcium infusion and sodium chloride infusion may be helpful in calcium channel blocker overdose (42).

Both calcium chloride and calcium gluconate (43) have been used in single and infusion doses to reverse the untoward bradycardia and hypotension of the calcium channel blockers (17,41,44,45). Calcium chloride [5 to 10 mL of 10% solution or 10 mg/kg (46)] or calcium gluconate (10 to 20 mL of 10% solution) may be injected over 5 minutes. If the response is temporary the dose may be repeated, or calcium mixed with 5% dextrose and water and titrated to the patient's response may be given by infusion. When calcium salts are compared, calcium chloride provides three times more calcium per volume. Further, when compared with the gluconated salt, calcium chloride produces a more predictable increase in extracellular ionized calcium and a greater positive inotropic effect when equimolar amounts of calcium are administered (30).

In summary, the reported cardiovascular response to intravenous calcium in severe calcium channel blocker poisoning has varied. The regulation of free intracellular ionized calcium is important to vascular tone, resistance, and blood pressure. Calcium enters the cell through calcium-permeable channels in the plasma membrane, and calcium is released from intracellular sites in which it is normally stored, that is, sarcoplasmic reticulum, mitochondria, and inner surface of the plasma membrane. Because the pharmacologic action of verapamil specifically blocks extracellular calcium, there is little reason to believe that administration of calcium, except possibly in massive doses, would increase intracellular calcium concentration and thus affect cardiac contractility.

Adrenergic Agents

Although dopamine is the inotropic agent most frequently used for the overdose of verapamil, its use is disappointing in increasing the blood pressure after a verapamil overdose. In addition to its positive inotropic effect, dopamine also has a mild positive chronotropic effect. Dopamine may increase systemic vascular resistance at high doses when its predominant α-adrenergic effect occurs (9).

The use of β agonists has been questioned in the treatment of verapamil overdose. β_1 Stimulation will accelerate sinoatrial node discharge rate, enhance atrioventricular node conduction, and improve myocardial contractility (40). β_2 Stimulation, which occurs at higher doses of isoproterenol, will worsen hypotension, decrease perfusion, and increase myocardial oxygen consumption. These β_2 effects are all potential mitigating factors in considering the use of isoproterenol. Dobutamine is known to increase cardiac contractility without significantly changing heart rate or pulmonary vascular pressures. One potential drawback to the use of dobutamine is its potential to decrease systemic vascular resistance at high doses. This action may be minimal in severe verapamil overdoses in which the patient is already maximally vasodilated (16). The failure of dobutamine for inotropic support suggests that the hypotensive effect of calcium channel blocker toxicity is not due to myocardial depression but to peripheral vasodilation (6).

α_1 Agonists are capable of stimulating smooth muscle contraction by a receptor-mediated pathway independent of calcium channels. It appears that α_1 stimulation may increase the calcium sensitivity of the contractile apparatus in vascular smooth muscle. The use of epinephrine or norepinephrine should therefore be considered early in the course of severe calcium channel blocker overdoses associated with severe hypotension. The α_1 agonist effects of these agents appear to make them well suited pharmacologically for the treatment of vasodilatory shock in verapamil overdose.

Atropine and Pacemaker

Resuscitation of bradycardia associated with third-degree atrioventricular block usually is treated with atropine and pacemaker insertion. However, atropine has been uniformly ineffective in the few cases in which it has been used to treat bradycardia and third-degree atrioventricular block in calcium channel blocker toxicity. Because the predominant action of atropine is through vagally mediated inhibition at the sinoatrial node, it is unlikely that it would be effective in reversing atrioventricular nodal conduction delay and block. Although there may be only a partial response or no response to atropine, atropine should be administered for symptomatic bradycardia or a fixed second- or third-degree atrioventricular block.

A fixed high-degree atrioventricular block, symptomatic sinus bradycardia, or asystole may be indications for placement of a temporary pacemaker (21). When needed, the time course for electrical pacing is typically 24 to 48 hours, which makes the use of an external pacer a realistic alternative. Any patient who either presents with or deteriorates to asystole should have a pacer placed without delay.

Glucagon

Glucagon has been used as a bolus agent to reverse myocardial depression and hypotension in β blocker overdoses. Glucagon is a polypeptide hormone that promotes glycogenolysis and hyperglycemia, but also has chronotropic and inotropic cardiovascular effects. Its postulated mechanism of action is through glucagon-specific receptors on the cell membrane mediated by cAMP (26). Activation results in alterations of calcium ion fluxes across the cell membrane, totally independent of α- and β-adrenergic receptors (9).

Glucagon has little toxicity, and although it is not extensively used in calcium channel blocker overdoses, there may be a future role in calcium channel blocker overdose (3).

The recommended dosage of glucagon is 50 μg/kg as an initial intravenous dose or 3 to 10 mg infused over 1 to 2 minutes with subsequent continuous infusion of 2 to 5 mg/hour or 0.07 mg/kg/hour. The onset of glucagon's effects is within 1 to 3 minutes, with peak activity occurring within 5 to 7 minutes and persisting for 15 to 20 minutes. The serum half-life of glucagon is 3 to 6 minutes.

4-Aminopyridine

The specific antidote for verapamil and other calcium channel blocker toxicity may be 4-aminopyridine (Pymodine). This drug is marketed in Europe where it is used to reverse the nondepolarizing neuromuscular blockade to agents such as Pavulon. Its ability to facilitate transsynaptic transmission is attributable to its direct effect on enhancing transmembrane calcium influx at calcium channels directly opposing verapamil's action. It also indirectly enhances calcium influx by blocking potassium channels in excitation (9).

4-Aminopyridine is presently available in the United States only for experimental use. In Europe, where its use for human treatment is accepted, the usual dose to reverse neuromuscular blockade is 0.3 to 0.5 mg/kg (9).

Extracorporeal Removal

The calcium channel blockers and their active metabolites are not effectively removed by forced diuresis, hemodialysis, or hemoperfusion.

REFERENCES

1. Conti C, Mazzullo J, Meyers F: All calcium channel blockers are not created equal. *Emerg Med Rep* 1984;5: 29–34.
2. Karlsberg R: Calcium channel blockers for cardiovascular disorders. *Arch Intern Med* 1982;142:452–455.
3. Erickson F, Ling L, Grande G, et al: Diltiazem overdose: case report and review. *J Emerg Med* 1991;9:357–366.
4. Braunwald E: Mechanism of action of calcium channel blocking agents. *N Engl J Med* 1982;307:1618–1627.
5. Antman E, Stone P, Muller J, et al: Calcium channel blocking agents in the treatment of cardiovascular disorders: part 1: basic and clinical electrophysiologic effects. *Ann Intern Med* 1980;93:875–885.
6. Lam Y: Calcium metabolism, calcium-channel blocking agents, and hypertension management. *Drug Intell Clin Pharm* 1988;22:659–671.
7. Donovan P, Propp D: Calcium and its role in cardiac arrest: understanding the controversy. *J Emerg Med* 1985;3:105–116.
8. MacDonald D, Alguire P: Case report: fatal overdose with sustained release verapamil. *Am J Med Sci* 1992;303:115–117.
9. Horowitz B, Rhee K: Massive verapamil ingestion: a report of two cases and a review of the literature. *Am J Emerg Med* 1989;7:624–631.
10. Kuhn M: Verapamil in the treatment of PSVT. *Ann Emerg Med* 1981; 10;538–544.
11. Chaffman M, Brogden R: Diltiazem. *Drugs* 1985;29:387–454.
12. McGoon M, Vlietstra R, Holmes D, et al: The clinical use of verapamil. *Mayo Clin Proc* 1982;57:495–510.
13. Chan L, Schrier R: Effects of calcium channel blockers on renal function. *Annu Rev Med* 1990;41:289–302.
14. Frishman W, Stroh J, Greenberg S, et al: Calcium channel blockers in systemic hypertension. *Med Clin North Am* 1988;72:449–499.
15. Young G: Calcium channel blockers in emergency medicine. *Ann Emerg Med* 1984;13:712–722.
16. Singh B, Nademanee K, Baky S: Calcium antagonists: clinical use in the treatment of arrhythmias. *Drugs* 1983;25:125–153.
17. Crowe D: The β and calcium channel blockers. *Top Emerg Med* 1986;8:26–33.
18. Mauritson D, Winniford M, Walker S, et al: Oral verapamil for paroxysmal supraventricular tachycardia. *Ann Intern Med* 1982;96:409–412.
19. Krebs R: Adverse reactions with calcium antagonists. *Hypertension* 1983;5:11-125–11-129.

20. McAllister R: Clinical pharmacology of slow channel blocking agents. *Prog Cardiovasc Dis* 1982;25:83–102,
21. Snover S, Bocchino V: Massive diltiazem overdose. *Ann Emerg Med* 1986;15:1221–1224.
22. Candell J, Valle V, Soler M, et al: Acute intoxication with verapamil. *Chest* 1979;75:200–201.
23. Brodsky S, Cutler S, Weiner D, et al: Hepatotoxicity due to treatment with verapamil. *Ann Intern Med* 1981;94:490–491.
24. Enyeart J, Price W, Hoffman D, et al: Profound hyperglycemia and metabolic acidosis after verapamil overdose. *J Am Coll Cardiol* 1983; 2:1228–1231.
25. Kelner M: Newer cardiac agents: antiarrhythmics and antianginal agents. *Clin Lab Med* 1987;7:567–585.
26. McMillan R: Management of acute severe verapamil intoxication. *J Emerg Med* 1988;6:193–196.
27. Rosansky S: Verapamil toxicity—treatment with hemoperfusion. *Ann Intern Med* 1991;114:340–341
28. Spiller H, Meyers A, Ziewmba T, et al: Delayed onset of cardiac arrhythmias from sustained-release verapamil. *Ann Emerg Med* 1991; 20:201–203.
29. Koike Y, Shimamura K, Shudo I, et al: Pharmacokinetics of verapamil in man. *Res Commun Chem Pathol Pharmacol* 1979;24:37–47.
30. Krick S, Gums J, Grauer K, et al: Severe verapamil (sustained release) overdose. *DICP Ann Pharmacother* 1990;24:705–706.
31. Lewis J: Adverse reactions to calcium antagonists. *Drugs* 1983;25: 196–222.
32. Krebs R: Adverse reactions with calcium antagonists. *Hypertension* 1983;5(Suppl.II):125–129.
33. Lander R: Verapamil/β blocker interaction. *Mo Med* 1983;80:626–629.
34. Lown B: The future clinical role of nifedipine. *Am J Cardiol* 1979;44:839–841.
35. Zangerie K, Wolford R: Syncope and conduction disturbances following sublingual nifedipine for hypertension. *Ann Emerg Med* 1985;14:1005–1006.
36. Humbert V, Munn N, Hawkins R: Noncardiogenic pulmonary edema complicating massive diltiazem overdose. *Chest* 1991;88:258–260.
37. Roberts D, Honcharik N, Sitar D, et al: Diltiazem overdose: pharmacokinetics of diltiazem and its metabolites and effect of multiple dose charcoal therapy. *J Toxicol Clin Toxicol* 1991;29:45–52.
38. Dustan H: Calcium channel blockers: potential medical benefits and side effects. *Hypertension* 1989;13:I-137–I-140.
39. Gelbke H, Schlicht H, Schmidt G: Fatal poisoning with verapamil. *Arch Toxicol* 1977;37:89–94.
40. Immonen P, Linkola A, Waris E: Three cases of severe verapamil poisoning. *Int J Cardiol* 1981;1:101–105.
41. Moroni F, Mannaioni P, Dolara A, et al: Calcium gluconate and hypertonic sodium chloride in a case of massive verapamil poisoning. *Clin Toxicol* 1980;17:395–400.
42. Dolan D: Intravenous calcium before verapamil to prevent hypotension. *Ann Emerg Med* 1991;20:588–589.
43. Silva O, Melo R, Filho J: Verapamil acute self poisoning. *Clin Toxicol* 1979;14:361–367.
44. Strubelt O, Diederich K: Experimental investigation on the antidotal treatment of nifedipine overdosage. *Clin Toxicol* 1986;24:135–149.
45. Lipman J, Jardine I, Roos C, et al: Intravenous calcium chloride as an antidote to verapamil-induced hypotension. *Intensive Care Med* 1982;8:55–57.
46. Passal D, Crespin F: Verapamil poisoning in an infant. *Pediatrics* 1984;73:543–545.

ADDITIONAL SELECTED REFERENCES

Dominic J, Bourne D, Tan T, et al: The pharmacology of verapamil: part III: pharmacokinetics in normal subjects after intravenous drug administration. *J Cardiovasc Pharmacol* 1981;3:25–38.

Giannini A, Houser V, Loiselle R, et al: Antimanic effects of verapamil. *Am J Psychiatry* 1984;141:1602–1603.

Hughes W, Ruedy J: Should calcium be used in cardiac arrest? *Am J Med* 1986;81:285–294.

Pedrinelli R, Fouad F, Tarazi R, et al: Nitrendipine, a calcium entry blocker. *Arch Intern Med* 1986;146:62–65.

Raftery E: Cardiovascular drug withdrawal syndromes: a potential problem with calcium antagonists? *Drugs* 1984;28:371–374.

Schiffl H, Ziupa J, Schollmeyer P: Clinical features and management of nifedipine overdosage in a patient with renal insufficiency. *Clin Toxicol* 1984;22:387–395.

Secher C, Brofeldt S, Mygind N: Intranasal verapamil in allergen-induced rhinitis. *Allergy* 1983;38:565–570.

Zaloga G, Malcolm D, Holaday J, et al: Verapamil reverses calcium cardiotoxicity. *Ann Emerg Med* 1987;16:637–639.

PART V

CORROSIVE AGENTS

CHAPTER 23

Alkalis

Corrosive agents consist of certain acids and alkalis as well as other compounds and are responsible for significant immediate and long-term morbidity (1). They are among the most dangerous commercial products found in the home (2,3). These substances are used widely as raw materials and for cleaning, curing, extracting, and preserving in industry as well as in the home.

TABLE 23–1. *Sources of alkalis*

Lye (Sodium, potassium, calcium, and lithium hydroxide)
Ammonium hydroxide
Calcium hydroxide
Calcium oxide
Lithium hydroxide
Sodium carbonate
Sodium hydroxide
Potassium carbonate
Potassium hydroxide
Lime
Calcium oxide
Disinfectants
Quaternary ammonium compounds
Sodium hypochlorite (Clorox)
Calcium hypochlorite
Phosphates
Potassium permanganate
Hexachlorobenzene
Phenol
Pine oil
Toilet bowl cleaners (Vanish, Saniflush, Vansol)
Sodium metasilicate
Soda ash
Paint removers
Sodium hydroxide
Methylene chloride
Phenols
Cresols
Hair dyes, tints, and bleaches
Ammonia
Hydrogen peroxide
Automatic dishwasher detergents (Electrosol, Cascade)
Trisodium phosphate
Sodium metasilicate
Sodium carbonate
Portland cement
Calcium oxide
Low-phosphate detergents
Sodium metasilicate

Corrosive agents are so called because of the extensiveness of denaturization that they cause in tissue protein (4). The corrosive agents include sodium metals and lyes, phenols and cresols, and white phosphorus (Chapter 26) (Table 23–1). The various corrosive agents, and the percentage of ingredients that they contain are listed in Table 23–2 (1).

This chapter will discuss burns from sodium metals and lyes, lime, low-phosphate laundry detergent, dishwashing detergent, Clinitest tablets, and pool chlorinating substances. A discussion of the mechanism of toxicity of alkalis will follow.

SODIUM METALS AND LYES

Alkalis are substances that dissociate in water to yield an excess of hydroxyl ions, producing a pH above 7.0. The strong corrosive alkalis that are termed lyes include sodium, potassium, calcium, ammonium, lithium, and barium hydroxide; sodium and potassium carbonate; phosphates; and sodium metal. Lye tends to be odorless and tasteless and therefore causes most pediatric caustic injuries (5).

Sources of lye or strong corrosive alkalis include lime, Clinitest tablets, bleaches, disinfectants, oven cleaners, drain cleaners, toilet bowl cleaners, and the other agents listed in Table 23–1 (4). Although modern household products are less concentrated than products sold in previous years, highly concentrated, industrial-strength alkali products are still available (6–8).

Potassium Hydroxide and Sodium Hydroxide

Potassium hydroxide (caustic potash) and sodium hydroxide (caustic soda) are commonly available as white lumps, rods, or pellets. They are two of the strongest alkalis and are extremely corrosive (Table 23–3).

Potent liquid lye, commonly available as a drain cleaner, has greatly extended the spectrum of potential injuries caused by caustic ingestion. These agents produce a more severe injury than that produced by powder or granular alkaline agents or by nonalkaline corrosive

TABLE 23–2. *Common household corrosives*

Type of corrosive	Examples of products	Major caustic ingredient (%)
Acids	Mister Plumber (liquid)	Sulfuric acid (99.5%)
	SnoBol (liquid)	Hydrochloric acid (15%)
	Lysol (liquid)	Hydrochloric acid (8.5%)
	Cost Cutter (liquid)	Hydrochloric acid (9.55%)
	Sani-flush (granular)	Sodium bisulfate (75%)
	Vanish (granular)	Sodium bisulfate (75%)
Bleach	Clorox	Sodium hypochlorite (5.25%)
	Peroxide	Hydrogen peroxide (3.0%)
	Minute Mildew Remover	Calcium hypochlorite (48%)
	Tilex Instant Mildew Stain Remover	Sodium hypochlorite (5%), Sodium hydroxide (1%)
Detergents	Oxydol	Sodium tripolyphosphate (25%–49%)
	Electrasol	Sodium tripolyphosphates (20%–40%)
	Calgonite	Sodium phosphates (<50%)
	Cascade	Phosphates (25%–50%)
	Comet Cleanser	Trisodium phosphate (14.5%)
	Polident Powder	Sodium tripolyphosphate (<15%)
Alkali	Drano (liquid)	Sodium hydroxide (9.5%)
	Drano Professional (liquid)	Sodium hydroxide (32.0%)
	Liquid-Plumr	Sodium hydroxide (0.5%–2%); sodium hypochlorite (5%–10%)
	Dow Oven Cleaner (liquid)	Sodium hydroxide (4%)
	Crystal Drano (granular)	Sodium hydroxide (54%)
Thermal/ Alkali	Clinitest	Sodium hydroxide (233 mg)
	Efferdent	Sodium hydroxide 50% (0.5%–1%)

From Moore WR: Caustic ingestions: pathophysiology, diagnosis, and treatment. *Clin Pediatr* 1986;25:193.

TABLE 23–3. *Products that contain sodium or potassium hydroxide*

Alkaline batteries
Clinitest tablets
Detergents
Drain cleaners (Draino, Liquid Plumr)
Oven cleaners (Easy-off)
Paint removers

liquids. Solid lye tends to stick to the mucosa, and rarely injures the gastrointestinal tract (GIT) beyond the proximal esophagus unless ingested as a tablet or put in a capsule in a suicide attempt (9).

Lithium Hydroxide (Lithium Hydrate)

Lithium hydroxide is a white, strongly alkaline powder that forms an irritating dust; it has been used to absorb carbon dioxide from the air in space capsules. Lithium hydride and related compounds react vigorously on contact with moisture to generate lithium hydroxide and hydrogen gas, which may ignite spontaneously.

Calcium Hydroxide (Calcium Hydrate, Slaked Lime, Hydrated Lime)

Calcium hydroxide is a white powdered or granular solid that is used in making mortar, plaster, cement, and whitewash. It is a typical lye and may cause major burns.

Lime (Calcium Oxide, Quicklime, Burnt Lime, Unslaked Lime)

Lime is a substance found in various cements and is converted by water, with the evolution of heat, to calcium hydroxide, which is an alkali with a pH of 11 to 13 (10). The mixture of compounds will set to a hard product by the admixture of water. Hydration of this mixture will yield calcium hydroxide from the lime content, and sodium and potassium hydroxide from the corresponding alkali oxides (11). The pH of the mixture is usually about 12. The material is hazardous, especially in its fresh form, and perspiration and skin moisture may be sufficient to initiate the reaction (12). The resultant burn, which is both thermal and chemical, is often serious because the material may remain in contact with the skin for a prolonged period. Hardening of cement causes any residual surface calcium hydroxide to react with carbon dioxide from the atmosphere and become a relatively inert material.

Cement burns result from prolonged direct contact of the material with the skin or contact with wet saturated clothing that remains on the skin. Cement burns usually occur on the lower extremities because the individual has walked or knelt in the wet cement (13). The knees, pretibial areas, and ankles are the areas most often affected. Some of these burns have resulted in deep necrotic ulcerations, sometimes requiring extensive hospitalization and skin grafts (10,12).

Concrete, a mixture of sand and gravel that is added to wet cement, is abrasive as well as caustic. In addition to these dermatologic problems, cement often contains hexavalent chromate salts as a contaminant, and these can cause an allergic dermatitis in cement handlers who have become sensitive to this metallic salt (10).

LOW-PHOSPHATE LAUNDRY DETERGENT

Modern synthetic detergents are used in large quantities as household and industrial cleaners (14). Many of the older detergents contained phosphates, which by themselves have only a moderate toxicity (15). The new, low-phosphate detergents contain active chemicals such as carbonates or metasilicates that react with metals in water to "soften" the water. Large quantities of high concentrations of these reactive anions are necessary for this purpose (16). They have also been shown to be potent emetics, thus compounding the potential for injury if ingested (17).

Most commercially available nonphosphate detergents are highly alkaline, with pH values of 10.5 to 12.0. They commonly contain combinations of sodium metasilicate, sodium borate, sodium silicate, and sodium carbonate (Table 23–4). Sodium metasilicate is the most alkaline and corrosive substance found in such products; a weak solution has a pH of approximately 12.5.

Highly alkaline nonphosphate chemicals have caustic effects similar to the commonly recognized alkalis, with corrosive esophagitis, severe gastric erosion, permanent injury, and death as consequences of ingestion (16). In addition, alkaline soap solutions administered as an enema have produced inflammatory colitis and have resulted in severe serosanguineous fluid loss, rectal gangrene, colonic stricture, and even death (18). Recently, low-phosphate and nonphosphate detergents have been balanced with other builders to reduce their alkalinity (19).

TABLE 23–4. *Active chemicals in low-phosphate laundry and dishwasher detergents*

Sodium borate
Sodium carbonate
Sodium metasilicate
Sodium silicate
Sodium sulfate
Trisodium polyphosphate

Dishwashing Detergent

Granular automatic dishwashing detergents have been regarded as caustic substances secondary to the alkaline builders, such as salts of carbonates, silicates, and phosphates. A limited number of case reports and literature reviews support their potential to result in caustic damage, especially when ingested (17).

Recently, liquid automatic dishwashing detergent has become commercially available. At full-strength concentrations, the pH of these products ranges from 11.8 to 12.7. The high pH of liquid automatic dishwashing detergents and their association with the granular products resulted in significant concern about their caustic potential (20). Although one might expect more toxicity from the liquid automatic dishwashing detergents, this is apparently not the case. The most likely reason for the lack of significant toxicity lies in the amount of inherent titratable alkalinity of the alkaline builders in the liquid automatic dishwashing detergents. In this case, titratable alkalinity is defined as the amount of hydrochloric acid needed to neutralize an alkaline substance. For example, although phosphates may have the same pH as nonphosphate alkaline builders, they are truly more alkaline because more hydrochloric acid is required to neutralize the nonphosphates than the phosphates. Similarly it would require more acid to neutralize sodium or potassium hydroxide than a nonphosphate alkaline detergent builder, even if they had the same pH.

CLINITEST TABLETS

Clinitest tablets, which are used commonly by diabetics to check their urine, are alkaline agents that cause significant thermal as well as caustic injury to the esophagus (21). Clinitest tablets are white with green-blue flecks of copper sulfate, citric acid, sodium hydroxide, and sodium carbonate (22,23). In contrast to liquid forms of caustics, Clinitest tablets contain 45% to 50% potassium or sodium hydroxide, copper sulfate, citric acid, and sodium carbonate. Individuals who have ingested Clinitest tablets develop thermal burns from the heat of the sodium hydroxide hydration. Accidental ingestion of Clinitest tablets by adults is more common than suicidal ingestion because the tablets may be mistaken for an oral medication (22,23). A single tablet is considered extremely dangerous, and may cause a devastatingly deep burn that may progress to stricture formation. The ingested tablet mixes with saliva in the mouth and usually sticks in the upper third of the esophagus because of thermal coagulation of the mucosa. Because of this, ingestion of Clinitest tablets results in a high incidence of major morbidity (19).

POOL CHLORINATING SUBSTANCES

Pool chlorinating solution is a concentrated concoction of sodium hypochlorite prepared by adding chlorine to a solution of sodium hydroxide. The resulting solution contains sodium hypochlorite and excess sodium hydroxide to maintain its stability. The solution has a pH between 13.2 and 13.5. Thus, it combines the hydrolytic activity of sodium hydroxide toward fats and proteins with the strong oxidizing potential of the hypochlorite (24).

Household liquid bleach, which has a negligible corrosive effect on soft tissues, is also composed of sodium hypochlorite, but its concentration is 3% to 6%, and its pH is approximately 11. Therefore, it is to be expected that pool chlorinating solution is considerably more corrosive to soft tissues than bleach is.

MECHANISM OF TOXICITY OF CORROSIVE ALKALIS

Many different corrosive agents have been reported to be responsible for chemical injuries, but readily available household alkali compounds are the most frequently ingested corrosives. In order of severity, the most significant alkali burns result from liquid lye products, followed by granular lye, and then by other products such as Clinitest tablets and disc batteries.

Lyes are extremely corrosive and penetrating as a function of their ability to saponify lipids and to cause soap formation with subsequent epithelial sloughing and dehydration of tissue cells (25). The term *liquefaction necrosis* is often associated with lye injury because a soft, gelatinous, friable, often brownish eschar is produced (26,27). As these organic complexes penetrate further into the body, they carry unattached alkali molecules and continue to destroy tissue. Hemorrhage, thrombosis, and a marked inflammatory response with significant edema are seen within the first 24 hours of injury. Depending on the extent of the burn, inflammation may extend through the muscle layer, and perforation may occur. Tissue destruction with lye is more intense than with acids (28).

The age distribution of alkaline ingestors exhibits a bimodal pattern. The majority of patients are children aged 1 to 5 years who accidentally ingest improperly stored caustic solutions. The second, smaller group consists of adults in their 20s and 30s. This group is more likely to have ingested a caustic substance as a suicide attempt (1). Although the distribution of caustic ingestion has changed, with suicide attempts or gestures becoming more prevalent, most injuries still occur as accidents in children (9).

Four factors may determine whether a corrosive effect may be observed: pH, concentration, viscosity, and titratable alkalinity. Maintaining pH at a constant value and increasing concentration and viscosity have been demonstrated to increase the corrosive effects of alkaline substances (29).

TABLE 23–5. *Toxic effects of corrosive alkalis*

Form	Effects
Solid (crystalline)	Liquefaction necrosis of oropharynx, glossopharynx, palate, proximal esophagus
Effects	More rapid pain
	Promotes reflex expectoration
	Deep penetration
	Vascular thrombosis
	Perforation
Liquid	Liquefaction necrosis of distal esophagus, stomach

The closer to 14 the pH measures, the more destructive the caustic agent (30). The critical pH that causes esophageal stricture and ulcer is approximately 12.5. Most lye solution concentrations and commercial lye products have a pH of 14 (32). Nonlye solutions known to cause esophageal ulceration have a pH in the range of 12.5 to 13.5, but most cases of deep ulcer developing into stricture formation involve lye solutions of pH 14 (31). A pH less than 11.4 is rarely associated with more than superficial mucosal burns (26,30). This is true for common household bleach, for example.

Caustic material ingested accidentally or in a suicide attempt produces a wide array of injuries to the proximal gastrointestinal tract. The form (liquid or solid), pH, concentration, and chemical nature of the ingested material are important in the caustic agent's ability to damage delicate mucosa (Table 23–5).

There are multiple points of normal anatomic narrowing in the esophagus. These are the cricopharyngeal area, the impression of the aortic arch, the left main stem bronchus, and the area of the lower esophageal sphincter or diaphragmatic hiatus (27). These are also the most common points of stasis for ingested material passing through the esophagus and therefore the areas where ingested corrosive agents cause the most significant burns (Table 23–6) (32).

Small quantities of alkali are sufficient to produce major esophageal injuries without even reaching the stomach. The gastric mucosa, however, is not preferentially resistant to alkaline destruction, and the neutraliz-

TABLE 23–6. *Anatomic points of narrowing*

Cricopharyngeal area
Impression of aortic arch
Left mainstem bronchus
Lower esophageal sphincter (diaphragmatic hiatus)

ing potential of the total gastric acid is insufficient when compared with even relatively small volumes of strong alkalis.

Solid Caustic Agents

Solid crystalline caustics tend to adhere to moist surfaces and cause pain rapidly (27,30,33). This tendency results from the greater amount of initial pain experienced when swallowing solid lye, which promotes reflexive expectoration of the substance (34). The oropharyngeal, glossopharyngeal, palatal, and proximal esophageal mucosa are usually involved, and deep, irregularly arranged burns may be produced (35). The limited areas of involvement show deeper penetration, with vascular thrombosis, ulceration, and frequently perforation (5).

Liquid Caustic Agents

In 1967, lye in a liquid state was first marketed in the U.S. as a drain cleaner. Although the solid alkali compounds may cause deeper injury, the more solid compounds stick to the buccal and hypopharyngeal mucosa, thereby precluding severe esophageal or gastric injury (36). These extremely concentrated substances in liquid form produce severe tissue destruction, so that the consequences of its ingestion are death or long-term morbidity, not isolated or segmental strictures as when flakes or solid pellets of sodium hydroxide are ingested (37). In contrast, the less concentrated, but more easily swallowed liquid drain cleaners cause severe esophageal and stomach injury (9).

High-density liquid caustics, because of their easy passage down the esophagus, usually pass rapidly through the oropharynx and upper esophagus and cause more significant damage to the lower esophagus and stomach (27,30, 35). There may therefore be minimal injury to the mouth and oropharynx with liquid caustics (Table 23–5) (26).

When the liquid alkaline agent reaches the pharynx, the cricopharyngeal muscle develops spasm and the esophagus propels the lye into the stomach. The pylorus immediately closes, and the stomach churns the lye with a to-and-fro motion between the stomach and esophagus until the lye is neutralized or gastric atony ensues.

Factors that have contributed to the decrease in the overall incidence and severity of injuries have been legal intervention by the government, which has prohibited high concentrations of certain agents from the retail consumer, and the Safe Packaging Act, which has made the bottles more difficult for children to open (38). Even with the protective legislation, caustic ingestion continues to occur.

The work-up and treatment of oral ingestion of alkaline substances are discussed in Chapter 25.

REFERENCES

1. Wason S, Karkal S: Coping swiftly and effectively with caustic ingestions. *Emerg Med Rep* 1989;10:25–32.
2. Leape L, Ashcraft K, Scalpelli D, et al: Hazard to health—liquid lye. *N Engl J Med* 1971;284:578–581.
3. Maull K, Osmand A, Mauli C: Liquid caustic ingestions: an in vitro study of the effects of buffer, neutralization, and dilution. *Ann Emerg Med* 1985;14:1160–1162.
4. Jelenko C: Chemicals that "burn." *J Trauma* 1974;14:65–72.
5. Sugawa C, Lucas C: Caustic injury of the upper gastrointestinal tract in adults: a clinical and endoscopic study. *Surgery* 1989;106:802–807.
6. Adam J, Birck H: Pediatric caustic ingestion. *Ann Otol Rhinol Laryngol* 1982;91:656–658.
7. Ashcraft K, Padula R: The effect of dilute corrosives on the esophagus. *Pediatrics* 1974;53:226–232.
8. Edmonson M: Caustic alkali ingestions by farm children. *Pediatrics* 1987;79:413–416.
9. Meredith W, Kon N, Thompson J: Management of injuries from liquid lye ingestion. *J Trauma* 1988;28:1173–1180.
10. Skiendzielewski J: Cement burns. *Ann Emerg Med* 1980;9:316–318.
11. Early S, Simpson R: Caustic burns from contact with wet cement. *JAMA* 1985;254:528–529.
12. Stewart C: Chemical skin burns. *Am Fam Physician* 1985;31:149–157.
13. Tosti A, Peluso A, Varotti C: Skin burns due to transit-mixed Portland cement. *Contact Dermatitis* 1989;21:58.
14. Mercurius-Taylor L, Jayaraj A, Clark C: Is chronic detergent ingestion harmful to the gut? *Br J Indust Med* 1984;40:279–281.
15. Scott J, Jones B, Eisele D, et al: Caustic ingestion injuries of the upper aerodigestive tract. *Laryngoscope* 1992;102:1–8.
16. Scharph L, Hill I, Kelly R: Relative eye-injury potential of heavy-duty phosphate and non-phosphate laundry detergents. *Food Cosmet Toxicol* 1972;10:829–837.
17. Einhorn A, Horton L, Altieri M, et al: Serious respiratory consequences of detergent ingestions in children. *Pediatrics* 1989;84:472–474.
18. Kirchner S, Buckspan G, O'Neill J, et al: Detergent enema: a cause of caustic colitis. *Pediatr Radiol* 1977;6:141–146.
19. Wason S: The emergency management of caustic ingestions. *J Emerg Med* 1985;2:175–182.
20. Krenzelok E: Liquid automatic dishwashing detergents: a profile of toxicity. *Ann Emerg Med* 1989;18:60–63.
21. Burrington J: Clinitest burns of the esophagus. *Ann Thorac Surg* 1975;20:401–404.
22. O'Conner H, Grant A, Axon A, et al: Fatal accidental ingestion of Clinitest in an adult. *J R Soc Med* 1984;77:963–965.
23. Lacouture P, Gaudreault P, Lovejoy F: Clinitest tablet ingestion: an in vitro investigation concerned with initial emergency management. *Ann Emerg Med* 1986;15:143–146.
24. Rao V, Hearn W: Death from pool chlorine—an unusual case. *J Forens Sci* 1988;33:812–815.
25. Penner G: Acid ingestion: toxicology and treatment. *Ann Emerg Med* 1980;9:374–379.
26. Howell J: Alkaline ingestions. *Ann Emerg Med* 1986;15:820–825.
27. Buntain W, Cain W: Caustic injuries to the esophagus: a pediatric overview. *South Med J* 1981;74:590–593.
28. Friedman E, Lovejoy F: The emergency management of caustic ingestions. *Emerg Med Clin North Am* 1984;2:77–86.
29. Chen Y, Ott D, Thompson J, et al: Progressive roentgenographic appearance of caustic esophagitis. *South Med J* 1988;81:724–728.
30. Ulin L: Caustic ingestions. *Curr Top Emerg Med* 1981;3:1–5.
31. Vancura E, Clinton J, Ruiz E, et al: Toxicity of alkaline solutions. *Ann Emerg Med* 1980;9:118–122.
32. Tucker J, Yarington C: The treatment of caustic ingestion. *Otolaryngol Clin North Am* 1979;12:343–351.
33. Wasserman R, Ginsburg C: Caustic substance injuries. *J Pediatr* 1985;107:169–174.
34. Zargar S, Kochhar R, Nagi B, et al: Ingestion of corrosive acids: spectrum of injury to upper gastrointestinal tract and natural history. *Gastroenterology* 1989;97:702–707.
35. Cello J, Fogel R, Boland R: Liquid caustic ingestion. *Arch Intern Med* 1980;140:501–504.
36. Kochhar R, Mehta S, Nagi B, et al: Corrosive acid-induced esophageal intramural pseudodiverticulosis: a study of 14 patients. *Clin Gastroenterol* 1991;13:371–375.

37. Sarfati E, Jacob L, Servant J, et al: Tracheobronchial necrosis after caustic ingestion. *J Thorac Cardiovasc Surg* 1992;103:412–413.
38. Christesen H: Caustic ingestion in adults—epidemiology and prevention. *J Toxicol Clin Toxicol* 1994;32:557–568.

ADDITIONAL SELECTED REFERENCES

Davis L, Raffensperger J, Novak G: Necrosis of the stomach secondary to ingestion of corrosive agents. *Chest* 1972;62:48–51.

Ellis E, Brouhard B, Lynch R, et al: Effects of hemodialysis and dimercaprol in acute dichromate poisoning. *J Toxicol Clin Toxicol* 1982;19: 249–258.

Fitzpatrick K, Moylan J: Emergency care of chemical burns. *Postgrad Med J* 1985;78:189–194.

Hardin J: Caustic burns of the esophagus. *Am J Surg* 1956;91:742–748.

Michel L, Grillo H, Malt R: Esophageal perforation. *Ann Thorac Surg* 1982;33:202–210.

Oakes D, Sherck J, Mark J: Lye ingestion. *J Thorac Cardiovasc Surg* 1982; 83:194–204.

Okonek S, Bierbach H, Atzpodien W: Unexpected metabolic acidosis in severe lye poisoning. *Clin Toxicol* 1981;18:225–230.

CHAPTER 24

Acids

The occurrence of acid ingestion injuries in the U.S. is less common than those caused by alkali products, as greater use is made of the latter (1). The mildly alkaline pH of the esophagus, as well as its squamous epithelial covering, also provides relatively greater resistance to acid than to alkali (2). In contrast to lye, strong acids have an offensive odor and a bitter taste, and hurt the lips, buccal mucosa, and hypopharynx, resulting in rapid expulsion if taken accidentally (3).

Acids are found in swimming pool cleaners, toilet bowl cleaners, batteries, metal cleaners, antirust agents, and disinfectants (4,5). Automobile battery acid is usually about 28% sulfuric acid. Toilet bowl cleaners frequently contain sodium bisulfate, which forms sulfuric acid in water (6). Similar products containing hydrochloric or phosphoric acids are also marketed. Soldering fluxes are often solutions or pastes of zinc chloride and hydrochloric acid. Gun barrel cleaning fluid may contain about 5% nitric acid (Table 24–1) (6–9).

Although the following substances are acids, they also have additional actions that classify them as reducing substances, salt-forming agents, and desiccants (10). Some low-molecular-weight organic acids present a hazard similar to that of the mineral acids (11). These organic acids include formic, acetic, lactic, and trichloroacetic acids and metabolic competitors such as oxalic acid, mono-, di-, and trichloroacetic acids, and reducing agents (Table 24–2).

This chapter discusses the reducing agent *hydrochloric acid*; the salt-forming agents *picric acid, acetic acid, dichloroacetic acid, trichloroacetic acid, formic acid,* and *tannic acid*; the desiccant *sulfuric acid*; the metabolic competitors *oxalic acid* and *monochloroacetic acid*; and *boric acid.*

REDUCING AGENTS

The reducing agents produce their effect by binding free electrons in tissue proteins, thereby producing protein denaturization (6). Reducing substances include hydrochloric acid, nitric acid, and the alkyl mercuric agents.

TABLE 24–1. *Sources of acids*

Swimming pool cleaners
Sodium bisulfite
Toilet bowl cleaners
Sodium bisulfite
Hydrochloric acid
Phosphoric acid
Batteries
Sulfuric acid
Metal cleaners
Nitric acid
Drain cleaners
Hydrochloric acid
Sulfuric acid
Antirust agents
Hydrofluoric acid
Oxalic acid
Disinfectants
Soldering flux
Hydrochloric acid
Gun barrel cleaning fluid
Nitric acid

TABLE 24–2. *Miscellaneous chemicals that burn*

Reducing agents
Hydrochloric acid
Nitric acid
Alkyl mercury agents
Metabolic competitors
Monochloroacetic acid
Trichloroacetic acid
Oxalic acid
Hydrofluoric acid
Organic acids
Formic acid
Boric acid
Vesicants
Cantharides (Spanish fly)
Dimethylsulfoxide
Mustard gas
Lewisite
Miscellaneous
Mace

Hydrochloric Acid

Hydrochloric acid is one of the most common acids, and is a solution of hydrogen chloride in water (10). Concentrated hydrochloric acid is usually 38% hydrogen chloride; technical muriatic acid is usually 32%. Concentrated solutions of this reducing acid cause rapid conversion of surface protein to the chloride salt (6). The resulting coagulum overlies a shallow ulcer. The process continues as long as active acid remains in contact with the nondenatured protein (12).

Alkyl Mercuric Agents

The many actions of the alkyl mercuric agents include skin irritation. This can progress to severe skin lesions and burns, which have been reported with both ethyl and methyl mercuric compounds (2). The metallic mercury within the blister fluid can also be absorbed. These compounds are discussed further in Chapter 61.

SALT-FORMING AGENTS

This group of agents (Table 3) produces its detrimental effects by forming salts with proteins (6). Among the protoplasmic poisons are the alkaloidal acids such as tungstic, picric, sulfosalicylic, tannic, acetic, dichloroacetic, trichloroacetic, and formic acids (13).

Salt-forming agents have wide industrial use. Most have pungent odors, frequently with a suffocating effect. Often they occur in crystalline form. When in contact with tissues, the material combines with a variety of functional groups to form additional products or to initiate polymerization. These agents form an eschar with some sparing of the underlying supporting structures. They are frequently absorbed, producing hepatic toxicity or nephrotoxicity.

TABLE 24–3. *Salt-forming agents*

Acetic acid
Dichloroacetic acid
Formic acid
Picric acid
Sulfosalicylic acid
Tannic acid
Trichloroacetic acid
Tungstic acid

Picric Acid (Trinitrophenol, Carbazotic Acid, Picronitric Acid)

Picric acid is a yellow crystalline solid used in the manufacture of explosives, fireworks, electric batteries, textiles, and colored glass (Table 24–4). Antiseptic solutions have been employed medically in 0.5% to 3% concentration. Picric acid and its salts are toxic by inhalation, ingestion, and percutaneous absorption.

TABLE 24–4. *Uses and toxicity of picric acid*

Uses
Explosives
Fireworks
Electric batteries
Textiles
Colored glass
Toxic effects
Burns
Gastroenteritis
Hemorrhagic nephritis
Intravascular hemolysis
Acute hepatitis
Hyperthermia
Uncoupling of oxidative phosphorylation
Stupor
Coma
Death

Poisonings may manifest as severe gastroenteritis, hemorrhagic nephritis with anuria, intravascular hemolysis, acute hepatitis, progressive stupor, coma, and death. Picric acid is similar to dinitrophenol in that it accelerates body metabolism.

Acetic Acid

Vinegar and dilute acetic acid are about 4% to 6% acetic acid. Essence of vinegar is 14% acetic acid. Glacial acetic acid (100%) is highly corrosive, and its ingestion has produced penetrating lesions of the esophagus with stricture of the esophagus and pylorus. Permanent wave neutralizers may contain acetic acid. Vapors are capable of producing bronchial constriction with a clinical picture similar to that produced by other irritant gases and vapors (10).

Dichloroacetic Acid

Dichloroacetic acid does not possess the unusual metabolic actions of monochloroacetic acid, and it is a somewhat weaker acid than trichloroacetic acid. Like trichloroacetic and acetic acids its toxicity may be attributed largely to its corrosive action.

Trichloroacetic Acid (Sulfosalicylic Acid)

Trichloroacetic acid is a corrosive organic acid that rapidly penetrates and "fixes" tissues. Systemic effects are presumably secondary to gastrointestinal damage and to acidosis, not due to the trichloroacetate ion except after large doses.

Tannic Acid

Tannic acids are produced in plants from low-molecular-weight polyphenols as a result of tissue injury to the plant (14). They serve to protect the plant from potential infection by "tanning" an invading virus or fungus. Medicinal tannic acid is an extract containing various concentrations of polyphenol. This preparation had been used for years by radiologists to improve the contrast in barium sulfate diagnostic enemas. Various plant extracts containing tannins have been used for centuries in the treatment of diarrhea and as astringents, antiseptics, and styptics on the skin and mucous membranes.

Tannic acid is readily absorbed from the gastrointestinal tract (GIT), and blood concentrations reach their peak in approximately 3 hours (14). Tannic acid is a protoplasmic poison as well as a hepatotoxin (15), and its toxic effects are dose-related.

Formic Acid

Use

Formic acid is a caustic organic acid used in industry and agriculture capable of causing full-thickness skin injury and systemic toxicity. Formic acid, but not its sodium salt, produces prompt burns and local necrosis, like the strong mineral acids. Formic acid is present in readily available descaling agents and stain-removing fluids. It is also used extensively in agriculture as a hay preservative.

Complications

Accidental ingestions of formic acid usually have a good prognosis, as the pungent odor and corrosive characteristics prevent the intake of large volumes. Severe poisoning with formic acid is rare, but can lead to life-threatening systemic complications such as shock, extreme metabolic acidosis, and severe hemolysis, in addition to the local caustic effects (16). Systemic toxicity has been reported following cutaneous absorption. Hemolysis appears to be caused by the direct effect of formic acid on the red cells.

Treatment

Initial management consists of aggressive wound lavage. Acidosis, if present, should be treated with intravenous bicarbonate. Minor hemolysis needs no treatment. Mannitol may be used to expand plasma volume and promote osmotic diuresis in the event of significant hemolysis. Exchange transfusion and hemodialysis have been used in formic acid poisoning and may be required for patients in whom substantial cutaneous absorption has occurred (16).

DESICCANTS

The deleterious effects of these agents are caused both by excessive heat production and by tissue dehydration (6,17).

Sulfuric Acid (Oil of Vitriol, Battery Acid)

Sulfuric acid, when pure, is an odorless, colorless, oily liquid; but with slight impurities, it becomes yellow or brown and may have an unpleasant odor. It is used in the steel industry for casting iron and steel.

The caustic and chemical properties of concentrated sulfuric acid differ greatly from those of diluted acid. Concentrated sulfuric acid appears to attach to the tissues chemically in a different and a more destructive manner than can be explained simply on the basis of hydrogen ion concentration. When the acid is diluted, the caustic and chemical properties become similar to those of simpler acids, such as hydrochloric acid. Sulfuric acid is an exceedingly potent desiccant that produces a hard eschar, under which an indolent, deep ulcer forms. Destruction of all carbon-containing tissue occurs, and considerable heat is released during the reaction.

Mechanism of Toxicity of Acids

Acid agents produce primarily a coagulation-type necrosis (Table 24–5) (6,18). The leathery eschar formed by reducing substances and desiccants usually stops acid penetration and typically results in damage limited to the mucosa. Although burns to the oropharynx and esopha-

TABLE 24–5. *Differences in toxic properties between alkalis and acids*

Property	Alkalis	Acids
Type of injury	Liquefaction necrosis Saponification of fats Intense tissue destruction	Coagulation necrosis Eschar formation Limited tissue involvement
Typical location of injury	Mouth Pharynx Esophagus	Stomach
Long-term effects	Esophageal stricture	Pyloric stenosis Gastric scarring

gus do occur, acids tend to produce less damage to the upper airway or the esophagus than do alkalis because they pass rapidly through the esophagus (19). The esophagus is spared because of the relative resistance of the squamous epithelium to acid damage and the short duration of contact as a result of the rapid transit of the acid through the esophagus (7,18). There may be obvious burns to the mucosal surface of the lips, tongue, and mucosa of the oropharynx. The epiglottis may be involved, although the larynx is usually spared (5).

Acids usually produce necrotic gastric or proximal intestinal lesions with eschar formation (20). Usually, the lower two thirds of the stomach is involved (21). When the acid reaches the stomach, it progresses from the gastroesophageal junction along the lesser curvature to the pylorus (18). Pylorospasm usually develops immediately, resulting in pooling of the acid in the antrum, where the greatest injury occurs (17). The pooling of the agent caused by the pylorospasm may also cause acute gastric perforation, peritonitis, and death (11,20).

Most of the late complications are sequelae of severe toxic effects of acid to the gastric mucosa and muscular layers (11). The natural processes of wound repair result in fibroplasia and cicatrix formation. The end result of this process is pyloroantral stenosis as the most common late complication. Nutritional depletion secondary to gastric outlet obstruction, dysmotility, and a contracted intragastric volume may be exacerbated by a protein-losing gastroenteropathy (4).

METABOLIC COMPETITORS

Metabolic competitors produce their detrimental effects by binding or inhibiting calcium or other inorganic ions necessary for tissue viability and function. Metabolic competitors and inhibitors include oxalic acid, monochloroacetic acid (Table 24–6), and hydrofluoric acid (Chapter 28).

Oxalic Acid

Oxalic acid is used for removing ink stains and iron mold and for cleaning leather (Table 24–7). It is found in disinfectants, household bleach, antirust products, furniture polishes, and metal cleaners. Many plants contain oxalate, notably rhubarb leaves, dieffenbachia, beets, and spinach. Other potential metabolic sources of oxalate include ethylene glycol, glyoxylic acid, and glycolic acid.

TABLE 24–6. *Metabolic competitors*

Oxalic acid
Monochloroacetic acid
Hydrofluoric acid

TABLE 24–7. *Uses, sources, and toxic effects of oxalic acid*

Uses
Removal of ink stains
Leather cleaning
Antirust agent
Metal polish
Cleaning agents
Sources
Plants
Rhubarb leaves
Dieffenbachia
Beets
Spinach
Marigold
Other sources
Ethylene glycol
Glyoxylic acid
Glycolic acid
Furniture polish
Toxic effects
Burns
Muscular tremors
Hypocalcemia
Seizures
Vascular collapse

In dilute solution oxalic acid and its salts act by binding ionizable calcium from blood and tissues, thereby inactivating or poisoning protoplasm, preventing muscle contraction, and at times causing symptomatic hypocalcemia. Strong solutions of the acid are corrosive to the alimentary tract mucosa.

In acute poisoning from ingestion, there is local irritation and corrosion of the mouth, esophagus, and stomach; pain and vomiting are followed quickly by muscular tremors, convulsions, and collapse. Death may occur within a few minutes. If the victim does not die quickly from the local gastrointestinal injury, absorption and consequent systemic intoxication may become manifest. With dilute oxalate solutions, it is possible that gastrointestinal symptoms may be entirely absent; symptoms are then delayed, and the first evidence of poisoning may be muscle twitching, cramps, or central nervous system (CNS) depression. The neuromuscular effects can be explained largely by the calcium-complexing actions of oxalate, which depress the level of ionized calcium in body fluids. Treatment consists of establishing an intravenous line and placing the patient on a cardiac monitor. A 12-lead electrocardiogram (EKG) should be obtained, and serum calcium should be measured. Symptomatic hypocalcemia should be treated with calcium chloride (10 mL of 10% solution in adults).

Monochloroacetic Acid (Chloroacetic Acid, MCA)

Monochloroacetic acid is corrosive and is stronger than acetic acid. It is readily absorbed after ingestion and

TABLE 24–8. *Monochloroacetic acid*

Uses
Production of
carboxymethyl cellulose
phenoxyacetates
pigments
drugs
Effects
Enters tricarboxylic acid cycle (TCA cycle)
Converted to chlorocitrate
Inhibits TCA cycle

also after skin contact. Monochloroacetic acid is used in the production of carboxymethyl cellulose, phenoxy acetates, pigments, and drugs. Monochloroacetic acid is transported as an 80% solution, as flakes, or as its sodium salt by road, rail, and sea (Table 24–8).

Monochloroacetic acid enters the tricarboxylic acid cycle like any two-carbon atom acetate. It is converted by primary enzymes to chlorocitrate. These enzymes cannot metabolize the chlorocitrate further and the body is then left with the poison, which blocks the tricarboxylic acid cycle by inhibiting the aconitase system and thus, acetate oxidation. Monochloroacetic acid probably also reacts with sulfhydryl groups in enzymes and other substances. These two effects cause severe tissue damage in energy-rich organs such as the heart, CNS, and skeletal muscles (22).

Clinical Features

The features of monochloroacetic acid poisoning may be summarized as follows. Vomiting and diarrhea are common early signs of systemic poisoning. CNS features may be seen and include CNS excitability with disorientation (which is an early sign of systemic poisoning), delirium, convulsions followed by CNS depression and coma; cerebral edema is also seen. Severe myocardial depression with shock and EKG changes or nonspecific myocardial damage may also be observed. Progressive renal failure may be expected as well as hypokalemia and severe metabolic acidosis. Hypocalcemia may be delayed for 1–2 days. High activities of creatine kinase, aspartate aminotransferase, and alanine aminotransferase are signs of extensive tissue damage (skeletal muscles, heart, brain). Myoglobulinuria due to rhabdomyolysis may be seen (Table 24–9).

TABLE 24–9. *Toxicity of monochloroacetic acid*

Gastrointestinal
Nausea
Vomiting
Diarrhea
Central nervous system
Excitability
Disorientation
Delirium
Seizures
CNS depression
Coma
Cerebral edema
Laboratory abnormalities
Creatine kinase
Aspartate
Aminotransferase
Alanine aminotransferase
Myoglobinuria

Treatment

After exposure to liquid monochloroacetic acid, urgent decontamination and removal of contaminated clothing are the most important measures. After ingestion, emesis should be induced at the accident site, despite the risk of corrosive damage, as systemic poisoning of monochloroacetic acid is so severe. If more than 1% of the body surface is exposed to liquid monochloroacetic acid, the patient should be hospitalized. Thereafter, supportive therapy should be employed in all cases. This includes adequate fluid therapy, correction of acid-base and electrolyte disturbances, alkalinization of the urine to prevent myoglobin deposition in the tubuli, inotropic support in case of myocardial insufficiency, and controlled hyperventilation to prevent and treat cerebral edema (22).

BORIC ACID

Boric acid has been used extensively in irrigating solutions, talcum and baby powders, and dermatologic products. Although the medicinal use of boric acid has diminished as a result of its potential toxicity, boric acid is currently available in ophthalmic solutions, topical disinfectants, and roach powders and tablets. Borates are present in vegetables, fruits, orange juice, breads, and cereals (23).

Boric acid is well absorbed from the GIT, mucous membranes, and abraded skin but not from intact or unbroken skin. Greater than 90% of an oral dose is excreted unchanged by the kidneys within 96 hours. Half-lives varying from 5 to 10 hours up to 21 hours have been reported.

Clinical Findings

Acute poisonings have followed ingestion, parenteral injection, enemas, lavage of serous cavities, irrigation of the bladder, and application of powders and ointments to burned and abraded skin (23). Borate poisoning produces gastrointestinal, CNS, skin, renal, and hepatic toxicity (Table 24–10).

TABLE 24–10. *Toxicity of boric acid*

Gastrointestinal disturbances
Hemorrhagic gastroenteritis
CNS changes
Restlessness
Irritability
Headache
Delirium
Seizures
Coma
Dermatologic
Desquamating skin lesion ("boiled lobster")
Miscellaneous
Acute tubular necrosis
Liver damage

Clinical findings commonly consist of gastrointestinal disturbances, including hemorrhagic gastroenteritis, erythematous skin eruptions, and signs of CNS stimulation followed by depression. CNS effects include restlessness, irritability, headache, delirium, seizures, and coma. Death is due to vascular collapse in the early stages or to CNS depression later in the course of poisoning (24).

A classic erythematous rash that starts in the axillary, inguinal, and facial regions and then becomes more generalized to cover the entire body within 1 to 2 days of exposure has been described. The rash desquamates 2 to 3 days later, resulting in a "boiled lobster" appearance.

Acute tubular necrosis with oliguria or anuria has been reported. Mild liver damage is less common. Death results from circulatory collapse or renal failure.

Boric acid levels are obtained to document that boric acid was ingested in sufficient quantities to result in elevated levels but are not used to determine initial treatment (23).

Treatment

For patients weighing less than 30 kg, observation only is recommended for ingestions of less than 200 mg/kg, ipecac syrup in the home for ingestions of 200 to 400 mg/kg, if that can be verified, and lavage in an emergency department with a boric acid level obtained at 2 to 3 hours postingestion for ingestions of more than 400 mg/kg. Activated charcoal poorly adsorbs boric acid and therefore can be withheld unless there was suspicion of a mixed ingestion (24).

For patients weighing 30 kg or more, observation only is recommended for ingestions of less than 6.0 g, ipecac syrup for ingestions of 6.0 to 12.0 g, and lavage in an emergency department with a boric acid level obtained at 2 to 3 hours postingestion for ingestions of greater than 12 g.

Chronic toxicity or toxicity in the newborn is of greater consequence; therefore, more rigorous therapeutic intervention is required for newborns or those chronically exposed to boric acid.

REFERENCES

1. Pense SC, Wood WJ, Stempel TK, Zwemer FL, Wachtel TL: Tracheosophageal fistula secondary to muriatic acid ingestion. *Burns Incl Them Inj* 1988; 14:35–38.
2. Wason S, Karkal S: Coping swiftly and effectively with caustic ingestions. *Emerg Med Rep* 1989;10:25–32.
3. Sugawa C, Lucas C: Caustic injury of the upper gastrointestinal tract in adults: a clinical and endoscopic study. *Surgery* 1989;106:802–807.
4. Levine D, Surawicz C: Severe intestinal damage following acid ingestion with minimal findings on early endoscopy. *Gastrointest Endosc* 1984;30:247–249.
5. Jena G, Lazarus C: Acid corrosive gastritis. *S Afr Med J* 1985;67: 473–474.
6. Jelenko C: Chemicals that "burn." *J Trauma* 1974;14:65–72.
7. Nelson R, Walson P, Kelley M: Caustic ingestion. *Ann Emerg Med* 1983;12:559–562.
8. Klein M: Addressing the controversies of caustic ingestions. *Emerg Med Rep* 1983;4:155–160.
9. Ulin L: Caustic ingestions. *Curr Top Emerg Med* 1981;3:1–5.
10. Horvath O, Olah T, Zentai G: Emergency esophagogastrectomy for treatment of hydrochloric acid injury. *Ann Thorac Surg* 1991;52:98–101.
11. Zargar S, Kochhar R, Nagi B, et al: Ingestion of corrosive acids: spectrum of injury to upper gastrointestinal tract and natural history. *Gastroenterology* 1989;97:702–707.
12. Scott J, Jones B, Eisele D, et al: Caustic ingestion injuries of the upper aerodigestive tract. *Laryngoscope* 1992;102:1–8.
13. Stewart C: Chemical skin burns. *Am Fam Physician* 1985;31:149–157.
14. Boyd E, Bereczky K, Godi I: The acute toxicity of tannic acid administered intragastrically. *Can Med Assoc J* 1965;92:1292–1297.
15. Eschar J, Friedman G: Acute hepatotoxicity of tannic acid added to barium enemas. *Dig Dis* 1974;19:825–829.
16. Verstraete A, Vogelaers K, Van Den Bogaerde J, et al: Formic acid poisoning. *Am J Emerg Med* 1989;7:286–290.
17. Friedman E, Lovejoy F: The emergency management of caustic ingestions. *Emerg Med Clin North Am* 1984;2:77–86.
18. Penner G: Acid ingestion: toxicology and treatment. *Ann Emerg Med* 1980;9:374–379.
19. Knapp M, Bunn W, Stave G: Adult respiratory distress syndrome from sulfuric acid fume inhalation. *South Med J* 1991;84:1031–1033.
20. McAuley C, Steed D, Webster M: Late sequelae of gastric acid injury. *Am J Surg* 1985;149:412–415.
21. Zamir O, Hod G. Lernau O, et al: Corrosive injury to the stomach due to acid ingestion. *Am Surg* 1985;51:170–173.
22. Kulling P, Andersson H, Bostrom K, et al: Fatal systemic poisoning after skin exposure to monochloroacetic acid. *J Toxicol Clin Toxicol* 1992;30:643–652.
23. Ishii Y, Fujizuka N, Takahashi T, et al: A fatal case of acute boric acid poisoning. *J Toxicol Clin Toxicol* 1993;31:345–352.
24. Litovitz T, Klein-Schwartz W, Oderda G, et al: Clinical manifestations of toxicity in a series of 784 boric acid ingestions. *Am J Emerg Med* 1988.6:209–213.

ADDITIONAL SELECTED REFERENCES

Davis L, Raffensperger J, Novak G: Necrosis of the stomach secondary to ingestion of corrosive agents. *Chest* 1972;62:48–51.

Ellis E, Brouhard B, Lynch R, et al: Effects of hemodialysis and dimercaprol in acute dichromate poisoning. *J Toxicol Clin Toxicol* 1982;19:249–258.

Fitzpatrick K, Moylan J: Emergency care of chemical burns. *Postgrad Med J* 1985;78:189–194.

Hardin J: Caustic burns of the esophagus. *Am J Surg* 1956;91:742–748.

Michel L, Grillo H, Malt R: Esophageal perforation. *Ann Thorac Surg* 1982;33:202–210.

Oakes D, Sherck J, Mark J: Lye ingestion. *J Thorac Cardiovasc Surg* 1982; 83:194–204.

Okonek S, Bierbach H, Atzpodien W: Unexpected metabolic acidosis in severe lye poisoning. *Clin Toxicol* 1981;18:225–230.

CHAPTER 25

Work-Up of Patient with Gastrointestinal Burns

This chapter discusses the clinical manifestations of acid and alkali burns, the acute and chronic complications of burns, laboratory determinations including discussion of esophagoscopy, as well as treatment of the patient with a gastrointestinal burn.

INFORMATION FOR BURN HISTORY

History should include the type of substance ingested, the time since ingestion, the quantity taken, and whether or not vomiting has occurred; the pH of the emesis should also be determined (Table 25–1). In addition, the presence of pain and its location, any difficulty in swallowing or breathing, and whether or not hematemesis has occurred should be ascertained (1). Nevertheless, it is not possible on the basis of history or physical examination to predict the degree of esophageal involvement in many patients who have ingested a caustic or corrosive substance (2–4).

CLINICAL MANIFESTATIONS OF ACID AND ALKALI BURNS

Clinical manifestations may include dysphagia, hypersalivation with drooling, pain, and edema of the tongue, oral mucosa, lips, or palate (5). Drooling and the inability to clear secretions are indicative of significant posterior pharyngeal or upper esophageal injury (6). Drooling may cause the solid caustic to drain over the chin so that circumoral burns develop (5,7). Examination of the mouth may reveal soapy, white mucous membranes that might later become edematous (8).

Acute respiratory distress may occur as a result of posterior pharyngeal edema or spillage of the caustic agent into the upper airway. The patient may also complain of burning substernal, back, and abdominal pain and may vomit copious amounts of bloody material. There are patients, however, who are asymptomatic and have no oral burns but who are subsequently shown to have esophageal injuries (3,5,6). As many as 8%–20% of patients without lip or oropharyngeal burns show damage to the esophageal wall on endoscopy (9). The absence of oral burns therefore does not rule out the possibility of significant esophageal burns (2,10,11). Symptoms that suggest severe injury include dyspnea, dysphagia, chest pain, and hematemesis (12,13).

TABLE 25–1. *Information for burn history and clinical manifestations of burns*

History
Type of substance ingested
Estimated quantity of substance ingested
Time since ingestion
? Emesis
Determination of emesis pH
Clinical manifestations
Ingestion
Dysphagia
Hypersalivation
Drooling
White or black mucous membranes
Acute respiratory distress
Pain
Tongue
Lips
Palate
Substernum
Abdomen
Back
Edema
Tongue
Lips
Palate
Oral mucosa
Dyspnea
Hematemesis
Inhalation
Dyspnea
Cyanosis
Pulmonary edema
Hemoptysis
Ocular contact
Conjunctivitis
Pain
Lacrimation
Photophobia
Corneal abrasion

ACUTE AND LONG-TERM COMPLICATIONS OF ORALLY INGESTED CAUSTIC AGENTS

Esophageal burns characteristically evolve through three stages: acute, latent, and chronic, each characterized by distinct pathologic features.

The acute phase of caustic ingestion, the immediate inflammatory period, lasts 1 or 2 weeks. Usually, the patient who survives this phase of injury without complications enters a latent phase or postinflammatory period lasting 2 to 6 weeks. In the latent phase, which may occur 5 to 15 days after the acute injury, necrosis occurs, cellular debris sloughs off, and neovascularization and fibroblast proliferation occur. During this time, in the natural course of healing, cicatricial stenosis may occur. When this manifests itself as an obstructive problem, one is said to have entered the chronic phase of the disease process.

Acute Phase

Intraorally, chemical agents can cause serious damage to the oral mucous membranes, lips, and tongue. Deep burns of the lips and mouth can lead to scar contracture of the circumoral tissues with a marked reduction in the size of the oral aperture and vestibular depth, and a limited range of tongue movement. The mouth tends to become an inelastic and unyielding structure that impairs mastication and communication (14).

Acute complications of orally ingested caustic agents also include airway obstruction, esophageal ulcers, and esophageal, gastric, or intestinal perforation leading to mediastinitis or peritonitis (Table 25–2). Other complications include aspiration pneumonia, burns of the epiglottis and vocal cords, and laryngeal obstruction, tracheoesophageal fistula, peritonitis, pneumonia, sepsis, and death. Gastric ulcerations may occur, but they are less common in alkali ingestion than in acid ingestion. Mediastinitis may occur without frank perforation owing to bacterial invasion through the damaged mucosa (15).

TABLE 25–2. *Acute and long-term complications of significant caustic burns*

Local
Airway obstruction
Asphyxia
Laryngeal edema
Glottic edema
Esophageal (alkalis > acids)
Ulceration
Perforation
Stricture
Carcinoma (late sequelae)
Gastric (acids > alkalis)
Perforation
Ulceration
Achlorhydria
Systemic
Mediastinitis
Peritonitis
Circulatory failure
Shock
Infection
Pulmonary complications
Disseminated intravascular coagulation

Clinicians are most likely to encounter esophageal burns in the acute phase, which encompasses the first 4 to 5 days after injury. This phase is characterized by local thrombosis and inflammation, with or without secondary bacterial invasion, which may rarely produce an intramural abscess (9).

Latent Phase

Following the acute phase of the injury, a latent period begins, during which time stricture formation may occur. The process may proceed as rapidly as 1 month or during a period of years (16).

Chronic Phase

The hallmark of the subsequent chronic phase, the third week onward, is cicatrization, which may go on to produce an esophageal stricture (9,17).

Esophagorespiratory fistula may arise as a late complication of corrosive injury to the esophagus associated with a stricture (4,12). This is a rare lesion (18). Those with stricture at the mid-esophagus are at a higher risk of the development of fistula to one of the main bronchi. The lesion may be attributed to persisting inflammation within the esophageal wall, concomitant involvement of carinal and peribronchial lymph nodes, and finally, erosion of the adjacent membranous bronchial wall (19).

Patients who have sustained moderate to severe esophageal injury and survive the acute phase usually have severe damage. Stricture formation with possibly long segments of involvement as well as esophageal atony may result. Strictures may be mild and cause only slight alterations of diet or may be severely debilitating. Long-term management involves repeated hospitalizations for dilations with difficulties maintaining adequate nutritional status and chronic anemia. These sequelae can be debilitating. Late stricture formation is related to the agent ingested. Some substances such as household ammonia and bleaches may produce marked mucosal edema but rarely penetrate deeply enough to injure the submucosa or muscularis propria. There are isolated reports, however, of household-strength (3% to 10%) ammonia causing severe mucosal burns (1).

Other complications include circulatory failure and shock, asphyxia from glottic or laryngeal edema (20), intercurrent infection, inanition, and pulmonary complications. There is approximately a 1,000-fold increase in the incidence of cancer of the esophagus in patients who have sustained caustic burns of the esophagus over that of normal individuals. Squamous cell carcinoma of the esophagus has been reported and may develop more than 10 to 20 years after ingestion; this sequela occurs most commonly in patients who have sustained esophageal damage from lye. The incidence of this varies from 2% to 5% (14).

Late achlorhydria has been noted with acid burns and may be due to antral destruction, effectively producing a physiologic antrectomy. The achlorhydria is usually but not always permanent (21). Achlorhydria results from replacement of gastrin-producing mucosa by a thin, friable mucosa in which squamous metaplasia occasionally develops (22). Squamous cell carcinoma and adenocarcinomas have been reported in patients years after corrosive gastric injuries (23).

Disseminated intravascular coagulation has been described in patients who have ingested acid. The major tissue damage to the stomach and hemorrhage from the damaged gastrointestinal tract may be contributing factors to this condition.

PHYSICAL EXAMINATION

The oropharynx should be examined first by direct visualization. This should be followed by laryngoscopy. A supraglottic–epiglottic burn with erythema and edema heralds further edema formation, which will lead to airway obstruction and is thus an indication for early endotracheal intubation or tracheostomy (14).

The prognostic significance of clinical signs and symptoms and laboratory tests is not consistently predictive of the gastroesophageal involvement. Certain symptoms, however, do indicate severe esophageal injuries including dysphagia, retrosternal pain, or abdominal pain. Hoarseness or stridor suggests laryngeal or tracheal injury. Hamman's sign is an auscultatory crunching sound indicating air in the mediastinum secondary to esophageal rupture (8).

LABORATORY EXAMINATION IN CAUSTIC INGESTIONS

Chest and abdominal roentgenograms, including upright films, are usually indicated to check for signs of pulmonary injury or aspiration, evidence of free intra-abdominal air secondary to gastric perforation (7), or pneumomediastinum secondary to esophageal perforation or to locate an ingested disk battery (Table 25–3) (15,24). A barium esophagogram is not recommended in the acute phase because it provides little reliable information about the damage, it may cause perforation and mediastinitis, and it may also obscure the endoscopic picture. An esophagogram is of value in the recovery stage, when evaluation of stricture formation is important (15).

TABLE 25–3. *Laboratory work-up in caustic ingestion*

Upright chest roentgenogram
Upright abdominal roentgenogram
Complete blood count
Serum electrolytes
Blood urea nitrogen
Serum glucose
Blood type and cross-match
Toxicologic screen
Heavy metal concentrations

Routine baseline studies such as a complete blood count and measurement of electrolytes, blood urea nitrogen, and glucose should be obtained in the symptomatic individual. If necessary, blood should be typed and cross-matched, and a drug screen should be obtained (1). Heavy metal concentrations should be obtained in blood and urine in those patients who have ingested a disk battery if it is not passing quickly through the gastrointestinal tract.

TREATMENT OF ALKALI AND ACID BURNS

Much of the difficulty in managing patients who have ingested a caustic substance is related to the rapid onset of tissue damage. Although many other forms of poisoning can be treated effectively after an initial delay, measures instituted at the hospital for caustic ingestion may have little or no effect on the extent of tissue damage or outcome. Treatment, therefore, must be administered as soon as possible after ingestion to have the best chance of lessening the destructive potential of caustic agents (5,9).

Initial treatment for ingestion of all caustic agents is directed at minimizing the extent of tissue damage and then preventing and treating both short- and long-term complications (Table 25–4). In general, this consists of

TABLE 25–4. *Treatment of gastrointestinal burns*

Adequate ventilation
Intravenous infusion of crystalloid solution
Nothing by mouth (except for dilution)
Medication for relief of pain
Emesis or lavage (contraindicated)
Charcoal and cathartic (contraindicated)
Blood type and cross-match (for hematemesis)
Dilution with water or milk
Neutralization (contraindicated)
Esophagoscopy (within 24 hours)
Prophylactic antibiotics (withhold)
Tetanus prophylaxis
Steroids (withhold)
Parenteral nutrition

immediate dilution and subsequent direct examination of involved tissue, usually by endoscopy (7).

The first step in treating gastrointestinal burns is to rinse the mouth with water or milk, which is then expectorated. This may prevent swallowing of crystals that adhere to the oral cavity (5,24).

As with any acute intoxication, the first issue in management is to ensure that the patient has the ability to maintain adequate ventilation and that the cardiovascular status is acceptable (25). Because respiratory tract involvement suggests significant injury, control of the airway may be necessary (24). Blind nasotracheal intubation is contraindicated because of the risk of inducing tracheal or pharyngeal perforation. Oral endotracheal intubation under direct visualization is the preferred procedure, but cricothyrotomy may be performed in the patient requiring airway control who cannot be intubated. Although airway obstruction is not common, laryngeal edema or edema of the base of the tongue may produce significant airway obstruction that requires careful intubation.

Intravenous access should be initiated immediately, and hypotension should be treated initially with crystalloid solution through multiple large-bore intravenous lines. If the clinical picture suggests impending perforation, blood should be typed and cross-matched in preparation for emergency surgical intervention. Once the diagnosis is confirmed, a narcotic analgesic should be given in adequate doses to control pain (5).

The importance of adequate nutrition cannot be overemphasized. Patients with significant esophageal injury should receive parenteral nutrition early in their course. In a child, the clinician should look for other injuries, such as cigarette burns, scars, and other signs of body and head trauma, to exclude the possibility of child abuse.

Emesis, Lavage, or Charcoal and Cathartic

Gastric lavage and emesis are contraindicated in caustic ingestions because they may lead to iatrogenic esophageal perforation, cause an aspiration, or cause another burn as the material is passed back through the esophagus (15). Oral fluids, therefore, should never be forced to the point of emesis, and patients with a caustic injury should not receive oral fluids until they are able to swallow their own saliva (24). The primary focus of initial management should be to prevent vomiting.

Activated charcoal and cathartics are contraindicated for caustic ingestions for a number of reasons. The instantaneous nature of the injury negates any benefit from the use of these substances, and in addition charcoal is a poor adsorbent of caustic agents. Charcoal may also interfere with the subsequent use of the endoscope, and, most important, the administration of activated charcoal may cause an emesis. This emesis may reintroduce the corrosive material on the epiglottis, vocal cords, and larynx, leading to more severe injury, edema, and acute airway obstruction. Additionally, regurgitated materials may be aspirated, leading to potentially severe chemical pneumonitis.

TABLE 25–5. *Dilution of caustic agents*

Agents of choice
Water
Milk
Contraindications
Emesis
Acute airway obstruction
Perforation of esophagus, stomach, or intestine

Dilution

Although water is widely recommended as a diluent in patients who have ingested caustic substances, there are no data to support its efficacy. Despite this, water is relatively benign if aspirated and may be effective in diluting residual alkali or acid (Table 25–5) (26). Accordingly, it is not unreasonable to consider its use in small quantities immediately after a caustic substance has been ingested (25,27). If diluents are to be used, the clinician must recognize the inherent dangers of the induction of vomiting and the potential for aspiration and must weigh these factors against the lack of demonstrated efficacy (12). Dilution is contraindicated in patients with acute airway swelling and obstruction or in those who have clinical evidence of esophageal, gastric, or intestinal perforation.

Neutralization

Many product labels inappropriately suggest neutralization of the caustic (27). Neutralizing a chemical burn often produces an exothermic reaction, in which a thermal burn is added to the chemical burn (28). Mild acids or alkalis that are administered to neutralize ingested caustics should therefore not be used because they may aggravate the chemical burn by the further production of heat (15,25,27).

Esophagoscopy

Direct examination of the esophagus is essential in determining the medical management of each case. The role of endoscopy in caustic ingestion has changed considerably. This is mainly due to a change from the rigid endoscope, which may cause a perforation as it passes damaged mucosa, to the use of the flexible fiberoptic endoscope, which allows for the safe visualization of the esophagus and stomach. Unless the patient is unstable or pharyngeal injury precludes the study, esophagoscopy with a flexible endoscope should be performed within the first 12 to 24 hours (2,7,12). Delaying beyond 48 hours will cause the procedure to coincide with the period when the injured wall is at its weakest (19). All adult patients, especially those who have attempted suicide, and children with a reliable history of significant ingestion should be evaluated by esophagoscopy. Although many have insisted that the esophagus be visualized only as far as the first evidence of esophageal injury, this may underestimate the severity of esophageal injury if judged solely on the appearance of the most proximal injury (25,29). Although endoscopic perforation of a friable esophagus has been reported, this risk is minimized when a small fiberoptic endoscope is passed carefully into the esophagus with minimum air insufflation. The high incidence of actual ingestion in patients who have no supporting clinical history or physical findings on initial examination urges esophageal examination in most patients (16).

Endoscopic findings may be classified as superficial, transmucosal, or transmural and are classified in the same manner as burns of the skin (Figure 25–1; Table 25–6) (2). Superficial lesions are mild and show nonulcerative esophagitis and hyperemia of the mucosa but no loss of tissue. A superficial lesion is analogous to a first-degree burn with hyperemia, superficial sloughing of the mucosa, and mucosal edema (7). A transmucosal or second-degree burn demonstrates mild to moderate transmucosal involvement with shallow ulcers or deep craters and involvement of the muscle layer. Blistering, exudate, and loss of mucosa may also be noted (30). Grading of esophageal burns has been modified by some authorities. Grade 2 burns have been separated into those patients with transmucosal lesions but with no circumferential burns (grade 2a) and patients with circumferential lesions (grade 2b) (30). This separation is based on the fact that grade 2b burns may develop stenosis in contrast with

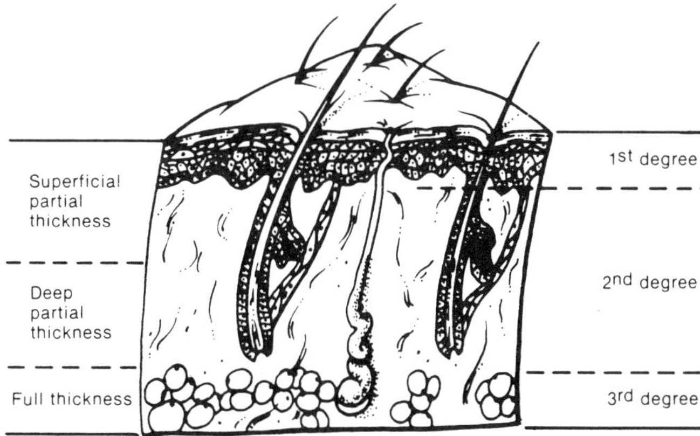

FIG. 25-1. Depth of burns. Adapted with permission from Marion Laboratories, Inc.

TABLE 25–6. *Esophagoscopy in the evaluation of a chemical burn*

Examination
First 24 hours after ingestion
Flexible esophagoscope
Findings
Superficial (first-degree burn)
Mild, nonulcerative lesions
Hyperemia of mucosa
Transmucosal (second-degree burn)
Shallow ulcers with involvement of muscular layer
Transmural (third-degree burn)
Ulcerative lesions
Severe, widespread tissue destruction
Possible mediastinitis and abscess formation
Contraindications
Significant posterior pharyngeal burns
Laryngeal burns
Respiratory distress

those with superficial ulceration. A transmural or third-degree burn is described as ulcerative and severe with widespread tissue destruction. Erosion through the esophagus into the periesophageal tissues may ensue, leading to mediastinitis (7), abscess formation, and peritonitis (12). If peritoneal signs, severe hemorrhage, or documented perforation are found, emergency laparotomy is mandatory (23).

The findings at endoscopy enable appropriate management to be determined (10). If no burns are noted, the patient may be saved an expensive and unnecessary hospitalization. First-degree injuries do not progress to stricture (2), but some second-degree burns may stenose (grade 2b), although this is rare. A great majority of third-degree injuries produce a clinically significant esophageal stricture, especially when they are of the circumferential type (2). In addition, if perforation is found surgical management is mandatory. In severe cases, this may involve total resection of the esophagus. In those patients with severe esophageal or gastric injury, close follow-up by a medical team is essential. Patients are hospitalized in an intensive care environment with frequent daily observations. In those patients with mild esophagitis or gastritis, less intensive observation and early hospital discharge are usually appropriate. Endoscopic reevaluation of all second- and third-degree burns should be performed 2 to 3 weeks after the initial injury (14).

The presence of significant posterior pharyngeal burns with edema is a contraindication to early esophagoscopy because of the risk of airway obstruction. Other contraindications include burns involving the larynx and evidence of respiratory distress, frank shock, or mediastinitis.

If there is evidence of inhalation or aspiration of a caustic agent such as subglottic edema noted on intubation, abnormal blood gases, or patchy infiltrates on the chest x-ray, bronchoscopy should be done with careful inspection of the entire tracheobronchial tree, realizing that an endotracheal tube may obscure the proximal tracheal or subglottic injury and should be removed briefly for inspection of this area and repositioned over the bronchoscope (31). If significant tracheal mucosal injury is seen, early tracheostomy should be performed and intubation done with a low-pressure or foam cuff, which should be closely monitored.

Antibiotics

Use of antibiotics is controversial. Because of the low risk of infection in uncomplicated esophageal burns, prophylactic antibiotics should generally be avoided but certainly instituted at the first sign of infection. Prophylactic antibiotics have not been shown to diminish the infection rate or to improve overall patient survival rate (3). Nevertheless, two widely accepted indications for antibiotics are the presence of a perforation and the need for prophylaxis against infection when steroids are to be used (2,5,15).

Steroids

The goal of the use of steroids is to decrease stricture formation without hindering the healing process of the esophageal mucosa (32). Nonetheless, the lack of adequately controlled clinical trials of steroids prevents any conclusion about their efficacy (5,24,33). Studies have shown that steroids given in pharmacologic doses impair wound healing, depress the body's immune defense, and mask important physical findings of infection and visceral perforation (3). In addition, superficial esophageal burns rarely proceed to stricture formation even in the absence of medical intervention. Transmural esophageal burns with concomitant tissue necrosis are likely to proceed to perforation, and steroid therapy may aggravate an already serious situation (34). Transmucosal injuries may benefit from steroid therapy, but this has yet to be shown conclusively (24).

The use of steroids in patients with circumferential esophageal burns from potent liquid alkali remains controversial (2). Methylprednisolone 54 (2 mg/kg/day) has been considered the intravenous steroid of choice once esophagoscopy is completed (12). The recommended dosage is 40 mg every 8 hours in patients older than 2 years and half that dose for younger patients (5).

Steroids may be useful in those patients with dyspnea stridor, hoarseness, or other evidence of respiratory compromise. In such cases, steroids decrease tracheal and laryngeal edema and ameliorate respiratory dysfunction (9).

Steroids are associated with serious side effects, especially an increased vulnerability to infection, and many have questioned their efficacy in the prevention of strictures after severe esophageal injury (32,35).

Steroids are of dubious value in those who have ingested acids, because steroids can obscure the diagnosis of peritonitis as well as enhance the likelihood of gastric ulceration and hemorrhage (9).

REFERENCES

1. Klein M: Addressing the controversies of caustic ingestions. *Emerg Med Rep* 1983;4:155–160.
2. Buntain W, Cain W: Caustic injuries to the esophagus: a pediatric overview. *South Med J* 1981;74:590–593.
3. Cello J, Fogel R, Boland R: Liquid caustic ingestion. *Arch Intern Med* 1980;140:501–504.
4. Gaudreault P, Parent M, McGuigan M, et al: Predictability of esophageal injury from signs and symptoms: a study of caustic ingestion in 378 children. *Pediatrics* 1983;71:767–770.
5. Ulin L: Caustic ingestions. *Curr Top Emerg Med* 1981;3:1–5.
6. Wason S: The emergency management of caustic ingestions. *J Emerg Med* 1985;2:175–182.
7. Kirsh M, Ritter F: Caustic ingestion and subsequent damage to the oropharyngeal and digestive passages. *Ann Thorac Surg* 1976;21: 74–82.
8. Scott J, Jones B, Eisele D, et al: Caustic ingestion injuries of the upper aerodigestive tract. *Laryngoscope* 1992;102:1–8.
9. Wason S, Karkal S: Coping swiftly and effectively with caustic ingestions. *Emerg Med Rep* 1989;10:25–32.
10. Adam J, Birck H: Pediatric caustic ingestion. *Ann Otol Rhinol Laryngol* 1982;91:656–658.
11. Crain E, Gershel J, Mezey A: Caustic ingestions. *Am J Dis Child* 1984;138:863–865.
12. Howell J: Alkaline ingestions. *Ann Emerg Med* 1986;15:820–825.
13. Gorman R, Gyi M, Klein-Schwartz W, et al: Initial symptoms as predictors of esophageal injury in alkaline corrosive ingestions. *Am J Emerg Med* 1992;10:189–194.
14. Rubin M, Jui V, Cozzi G: Treatment of caustic ingestion. *J Oral Maxillofac Surg* 1989;47:286–290.
15. Friedman E, Lovejoy F: The emergency management of caustic ingestions. *Emerg Med Clin North Am* 1984;2:77–86.
16. Friedman E: Caustic ingestions and foreign bodies in the aerodigestive tract of children. *Pediatr Clin North Am* 1989;36:1403–1409.
17. Kochhar R, Mehta S, Nagi B, et al: Corrosive acid-induced esophageal intramural pseudodiverticulosis: a study of 14 patients. *Clin Gastroenterol* 1991;13:371–375.
18. Rakic, S, Gerzic Z: Esophagobronchial fistula associated with corrosive stricture of the esophagus. *Ann Thorac Surg* 1992:53:142–143.
19. Nargar S, Kochhar R, Mehta S, et al: The role of fiberoptic endoscopy in the management of corrosive ingestion and modified endoscopic classification of burns. *Gastrointest Endosc* 1991;37:165–169.
20. Williams D: Acute respiratory obstruction caused by ingestion of a caustic substance. *Br Med J* 1985;291:313–314.
21. McAuley C, Steed D, Webster M: Late sequelae of gastric acid injury. *Am J Surg* 1985;149:412–415.
22. Zargar S, Kochhar R, Nagi B, et al: Ingestion of corrosive acids: spectrum of injury to upper gastrointestinal tract and natural history. *Gastroenterology* 1989;97:702–707.
23. Pense SC, Wood WJ, Stempel TK, Zwemer FL, Wachtel TL. Tracheoesophageal fistula secondary to muriatic acid ingestion. *Burns Incl Therm Inj* 1988;14:35–38.
24. Nelson R, Walson P, Kelley M: Caustic ingestion. *Ann Emerg Med* 1983;12:559–562.
25. Wasserman R, Ginsburg C: Caustic substance injuries. *J Pediatr* 1985;107:169–174.
26. Homan C, Maitra S, Lane B, et al: Therapeutic effects of water and milk for acute alkali injury of the esophagus. *Ann Emerg Med* 1994; 24:14–20.
27. Rumack B, Burrington J: Caustic ingestions: a rational look at diluents. *Clin Toxicol* 1977;11:27–34.
28. Rodenheaver G, Hiebert J, Edlich R: Initial treatment of chemical skin and eye burns. *Compr Ther* 1982;8:37–43.
29. Meredith W, Kon N, Thompson J: Management of injuries from liquid lye ingestion. *J Trauma* 1988;28:1173–1180.

30. Sugawa C, Lucas C: Caustic injury of the upper gastrointestinal tract in adults: a clinical and endoscopic study. *Surgery* 1989;106:802–807.
31. Chen Y, Ott D, Thompson J, et al: Progressive roentgenographic appearance of caustic esophagitis. *South Med J* 1988;81:724–728.
32. Anderson K, Rouse T, Randolph J: A controlled trial of corticosteroids in children with corrosive injury of the esophagus. *N Engl J Med* 1990;323:637–640.
33. Levine D, Surawicz C: Severe intestinal damage following acid ingestion with minimal findings on early endoscopy. *Gastrointest Endosc* 1984;30:247–249.
34. Sarfati E, Jacob L, Servant J, et al: Tracheobronchial necrosis after caustic ingestion. *J Thorac Cardiovasc Surg* 1992;103:412–413.
35. Lovejoy F: Corrosive injury of the esophagus in children. Failure of corticosteroid treatment reemphasizes prevention. *N Engl J Med* 1990;323:668–669.

ADDITIONAL SELECTED REFERENCES

Davis L, Raffensperger J, Novak G: Necrosis of the stomach secondary to ingestion of corrosive agents. *Chest* 1972;62:48–51.

Ellis E, Brouhard B, Lynch R, et al: Effects of hemodialysis and dimercaprol in acute dichromate poisoning. *J Toxicol Clin Toxicol* 1982;19:249–258.

Fitzpatrick K, Moylan J: Emergency care of chemical burns. *Postgrad Med J* 1985;78:189–194.

Hardin J: Caustic burns of the esophagus. *Am J Surg* 1956;91:742–748.

Michel L, Grillo H, Malt R: Esophageal perforation. *Ann Thorac Surg* 1982;33:202–210.

Oakes D, Sherck J, Mark J: Lye ingestion. *J Thorac Cardiovasc Surg* 1982; 83:194–204.

Okonek S, Bierbach H, Atzpodien W: Unexpected metabolic acidosis in severe lye poisoning. *Clin Toxicol* 1981;18:225–230.

CHAPTER 26

Burns of the Skin

Patients with chemical skin injuries compose a small percentage of the patients treated in emergency departments, yet these patients require prompt initial treatment, and the potential for systemic toxicity due to cutaneous absorption must be recognized. Because therapy is dependent upon recognition of the caustic agent, treatment begins with a good history (1).

The severity of a chemical burn, unlike that of a thermal burn, is determined not only by the duration of exposure but also by the amount, concentration, penetrating ability, and mechanism of action of the offending agent (2). By knowing the percent concentration or the pH of the alkaline products, one can estimate the degree of pain and injury secondary to exposure. Alkaline substances with more than 1% concentration or pH greater than 11.5 produce irreversible damage. Concentrated sodium hydroxide solutions of 25% to 50% cause skin irritation within 3 minutes (3). In contrast, a 4% solution creates subjective irritation only after hours because of an initial anesthetic effect on intact skin. Thus, exposure to lower concentrations of sodium hydroxide can lead to serious injury requiring skin grafting despite the lack of early warning signs or symptoms (4).

This chapter discusses burns from elemental metals, white phosphorus, phenol and cresol, hydrocarbons, cantharides, dimethyl sulfoxide (DMSO), nitrogen mustard, and lewisite. A general discussion of the treatment of skin burns follows.

ELEMENTAL METALS

Sodium and Potassium

The primary use of elemental metals occurs in industry where metallic potassium is used as a condensation, polymerization, and reduction catalyst and as a heat transfer medium in a sodium–potassium alloy and where metallic sodium is used in photoelectric cells as a coolant in nuclear reactors, as a polymerization catalyst, and in the manufacture of tetraethyl lead (2). Both metallic sodium and potassium react vigorously upon exposure to water, with the liberation of heat and the generation of hydrogen gas and hydroxide (5).

The evolved heat from this reaction is sufficient both to ignite the evolved hydrogen gas and to cause significant thermal burns in and of itself. Additionally, the formation of the hydroxide compound in reaction may result in significant chemical injury to exposed tissue. Elemental metal exposures may therefore be particularly severe in that burns occur secondary to both thermal and chemical injury. The reaction occurs more readily and tends to be more severe with elemental potassium than with sodium (6). This effect has been attributed to the trace amount of potassium superoxide that forms when elemental potassium is exposed to room air. The superoxide is extremely reactive and may hydrolyze in moist air to form both oxygen and hydrogen peroxide with the liberation of heat (2).

Treatment

The standard treatment for chemical burns has traditionally consisted of prompt, prolonged, and copious lavage with water, followed by standard burn treatment appropriate for the nature and severity of the lesion. In the case of elemental metal exposures, however, the initial treatment plan is modified. At the accident site, clothing should be removed rapidly and any obvious metallic particles extracted from the skin. Water lavage is contraindicated. The burn should be covered with oil to insulate any unreacted metal from water. The patient should then be transported to the nearest emergency department, where the wound should be debrided and any metallic fragments removed. Deeply embedded fragments may require surgical extraction.

WHITE PHOSPHORUS

White phosphorus is commonly used as an incendiary in the manufacture of munitions. The military population is at increased risk of sustaining white phosphorus injuries. The use of white phosphorus in the manufacture of certain fertilizers and fireworks also puts a select civilian population similarly at risk.

In the presence of air, white phosphorus is rapidly oxidized to phosphorus pentoxide. This exothermic reaction causes the phosphorous to burst into a yellow flame and give off dense white smoke with a characteristic garlic-like odor. The oxidation of phosphorous can be interrupted by eliminating the presence of oxygen; this is done by quenching the fire with water. When munitions containing white phosphorus explode, multiple particles may be embedded in skin and soft tissue. These retained particles continue to smolder, and even if doused with water initially, can reignite once the white phosphorus dries. Clothing often ignites, producing larger burns than those due solely to embedded white phosphorus particles.

Absorption of phosphorous from the burn may occur and produce systemic toxicity. Though systemic toxicity from cutaneous phosphorous absorption is not well defined, the potential for its occurrence exists. In patients with extensive white phosphorus burns, serum electrolyte concentrations should be measured serially and the electrocardiogram (EKG) monitored to detect potential systemic toxicity from phosphorous absorption (1).

Treatment

The initial treatment of white phosphorus burns consists of removal of all clothing. This is particularly important in hot climates or after an explosion, as the melting point of white phosphorus is 44°C; and at room temperatures greater than this, the liquid phase of white phosphorus may be present in clothing and difficult to identify. The skin must be irrigated with water to halt the ongoing oxidation, remove particles from the skin surface, and prevent reignition. The patient should be transported in saline or water-soaked dressings to prevent reignition of retained particles, and the dressing must be kept moist until adequate debridement is accomplished.

The ingestion of phosphorus as a rodenticide is discussed in Chapter 79.

PHENOL (CARBOLIC ACID, PHENIC ACID, PHENYLIC ACID)

Phenol, an aromatic hydrocarbon also known as carbolic acid or monohydroxybenzene, is extremely caustic in high concentrations. Toxic exposure to phenol has the potential to be widespread. Phenol and cresols are marketed in many forms and sold widely for their antiseptic activity. They are often used in homes and on farms as disinfectants, barn deodorants, and sanitizers.

Phenols are commercially available as disinfectants, deodorants, and sanitizers. In dilute aqueous solution, phenol has been used as an antiseptic and a topical anesthetic. The phenols are used in industry as bases for plastics and organic polymers. In addition, they are used widely in a variety of industrial manufacturing processes, such as the production of resin, industrial coating, agricultural products, dyes, perfumes, fungicides, lubrication oils, textiles, and chemicals. Today, phenol is used in podiatric and dermatalogic procedures and to establish permanent nerve blocks. The concentration stored on the office shelf, before dilution, usually is 89%. Phenol also remains an active part of cosmetic surgery for chemical face peeling, and is still occasionally used in preparations for treatment of localized skin disorders, as well as a local anesthetic.

Phenol is derived from coal tar, which is a highly reactive, corrosive contact poison in high concentrations. It is also a general protoplasmic poison and is toxic to all cells (7). It can be obtained as pure crystals or in a solution. Concentrations before processing often are between 40% and 100%. Ten percent solutions of phenol regularly produce corrosion, and occasionally skin necrosis is seen with solutions as dilute as 1%. Phenol is found in concentrations of 2% to 5% in some disinfectants and insecticides and in some over-the-counter preparations, such as Campho-Phenique and Chloraseptic. Self-administration of abortifacients, such as oral cotton root bark or Lysol douches, also can result in toxic phenol exposure (8).

Phenols in strong concentrations rapidly produce a brown or whitish stain that turns to a greenish-black or copper-colored eschar. Concentrated solutions of phenol cause second- and third-degree burns of the skin unless very promptly removed (Table 26–1). Formation of a coagulation necrosis of the dermis delays absorption, but this delay is only temporary. If skin absorption is significant, it may result in toxic effects on the central nervous system (CNS) and the cardiovascular system. Coagulation necrosis occurs quickly, and penetration into tissues continues secondary to phenol's high lipid solubility. Dilution of phenol with water may increase tissue penetration by allowing the water-solubilized phenol to penetrate the thick avascular eschar produced by contact with the more concentrated agent. Water irrigation is therefore not uniformly recommended unless a high-density shower is available (8).

Phenol is more soluble in polyethylene glycol, and a polyethylene glycol wash will more effectively remove the phenol from the skin. Propylene glycol, glycerol, vegetable oil, and soap and water have also been employed, but are less effective than polyethylene glycol

TABLE 26–1. *Toxic effects of phenols and cresols*

Caustic burn
CNS depression
Hypotension
Intravascular hemolysis
Pulmonary edema
Central lobular necrosis of liver
Shock
Death

(9). A 50% solution of polyethylene glycol in water should be used because higher concentrations produce a significant exothermic reaction when the skin moisture further dilutes the glycol. If polyethylene glycol is not immediately available, intense water irrigation should be done followed by polyethylene glycol used as a second wash once it is obtained. Polyethylene glycol should also be removed from the skin surface by copious water irrigation because it too has been reported to produce systemic toxicity when absorbed through the burn wound.

Phenol is extremely toxic and may produce multisystem effects. With substantial absorption, CNS depression, hypothermia, hypotension, intravascular hemolysis, pulmonary edema, shock, and death will result. Supportive measures are not specific and may include mechanical ventilation, invasive hemodynamic monitoring, and exchange transfusion. Obviating systemic absorption is most important in phenol burns and is done by washing the phenol from the skin as soon as possible (9).

CRESOLS (TRICRESOL, CRESYLIC ACID)

Like phenol, cresol is a derivative of coal tar. The cresols are the most important alkyl derivatives of phenol, and they occur as three isomers, orthocresol, metacresol, and paracresol; there are other cresol-like compounds as well (Table 26–2). The ortho and para isomers are even more toxic than phenol. The bactericidal potency of the cresols is about three times that of phenol; consequently, cresol solutions are used widely as disinfectants. Other commonly used compounds that are closely related are creosote, which is a distillate of coal and wood tars and is used as a wood preservative and as an expectorant; resorcinol, which is often used in bactericidal and fungicidal ointments; hexylresorcinol, which is used as an antiseptic (10); thymol, which is used as a fungicide; and hexachlorophene, which is used as an antiseptic.

The corrosive action of cresols is slightly greater than that of the phenols, whereas the systemic effects appear to be a little milder because of cresol's slower absorption. The extent of the burn and necrosis that may follow an ingestion or exposure depends on the concentration of cresol in the agent. The systemic effects depend on the amount absorbed, which is dependent on the area of contact and the duration of contact. There may be prominent CNS effects with depression of consciousness (Table 26–1) (11). There may also be central lobular necrosis of the liver with jaundice, kidney damage, and Heinz-body anemias (12).

TABLE 26–2. *Uses of cresol and cresol-like compounds*

Compound	Use
Cresol (orthocresol, metacresol, paracresol)	Bacteriocide
Creosote	Wood preservative, expectorant
Resorcinol	Bacteriocide, fungicide
Hexylresorcinol	Antiseptic
Thymol	Fungicide
Hexachlorophene	Antiseptic

HYDROCARBONS

Gasoline is either distilled from crude oil or is manufactured synthetically, and combined with additives such as tetraethyl lead, antioxidant, and preignition additives, rust inhibitors, lubricants, and anti-icing substances. Cutaneous injury from immersion in gasoline and other hydrocarbons does occur, and is often overlooked in victims of motor vehicle accidents who sustain prolonged exposure during extraction (1).

Hydrocarbons' solvent properties promote cell membrane injury and dissolution of lipids, resulting in skin necrosis. The high lipid solubility of hydrocarbons leads to penetration of cell membranes and dissolution of fatty elements (13). The degree of cutaneous injury is related to hydrocarbon concentration and time of exposure (13). Fortunately, most injuries are partial-thickness in character, although full-thickness injuries can occur. Epidermal necrolysis has been reported after prolonged contact with kerosene (1).

Systemic toxicity, which often occurs after ingestion or inhalation, has been described from cutaneous absorption (14). The well-documented systemic manifestations of gasoline absorption include CNS impairment ranging from intoxication to coma, pulmonary hemorrhage, pulmonary edema, pneumonitis, severe cardiac dysrhythmias, hepatic enzyme elevation, and renal dysfunction (13). Hydrocarbons are excreted through the lungs and absorption by any route may produce chemical pneumonitis and bronchitis (1), direct cellular damage, and surfactant inhibition. Despite its rarity, respiratory failure may therefore be the most significant systemic injury resulting from a gasoline contact burn (13).

Tetraethyl lead, an additive of gasoline, is absorbed through the skin, and lead poisoning due to this has been described. Blood and urine lead levels should be monitored.

The treatment of hydrocarbon exposure consists of removal of all clothing and water irrigation as soon as possible. In addition, lead poisoning from cutaneous absorption may require treatment with a chelating agent.

Gasoline ingestion is discussed in Chapter 53.

ALKYL MERCURIC AGENTS

The many actions of the alkyl mercuric agents include skin irritation. This can progress to severe skin lesions and burns, which have been reported with both ethyl and methyl mercuric compounds. The metallic mercury within the blister fluid can also be absorbed. These compounds are discussed further in Chapter 61.

VESICANTS

The vesicant agents produce their damage through a series of physiologic changes that results in blistering and edema. Frequently they liberate histamine or serotonin at the site of contact, and the net result is local production of ischemia and anoxic necrosis. Among the important vesicants are the cantharides (Spanish fly), dimethyl sulfoxide (DMSO), mustard gas (dichlorodiethyl sulfide), and lewisite [dichloro(2-chlorovinyl)arsine].

Cantharides (Spanish Fly, Blister Beetle)

Cantharides can be obtained from dried *Cantharis vesicatoria*, the blister beetle, and contain cantharidin, which is an irritant and vesicant to the skin. A dose of 1 mg, or contact with a single insect, can produce distressing symptoms that may commence immediately or be delayed for as long as 12 hours.

Preparations of cantharides have been used externally as rubefacients, counterirritants, and vesicants. Two preparations containing cantharidin are Cantharone and Verr-Canth. Cantharone liquid is a preparation for the treatment of warts and contains 0.7% cantharidin in a vehicle of acetone and colloidin. More concentrated cantharides produce severe, partial-thickness lesions. Cantharides are frequently used by farmers as veterinary aphrodisiacs and occasionally human contact occurs as a result of the mistaken belief that the material has aphrodisiac effects in humans. On skin contact, because of a severe histaminic response, papular lesions may occur that may then result in the burns previously described.

After ingestion of a cantharide, there may be burning pain in the throat and stomach with difficulty in swallowing and there may be nausea, vomiting, colic, bloody diarrhea, tenesmus, renal pain, frequent urination, hematuria, syncope, and circulatory failure. Treatment is nonspecific and supportive.

Dimethyl Sulfoxide

Dimethyl sulfoxide (DMSO) is a colorless, highly polar, organic liquid that was discovered in 1866 (15,16). DMSO is an inexpensive by-product of paper manufacturing. It has a high dielectric constant and therefore exhibits exceptional solvent properties for both organic and inorganic chemicals; it is widely used as an industrial solvent for resins, fungicides, dyes, and pigments (Table 26–3). It is also used as a reaction medium to accelerate rates of chemical combination and as antifreeze, hydraulic fluid, paint remover, a cryopreservative for platelets, and as a transport medium to facilitate transcutaneous drug absorption (16).

TABLE 26–3. *Uses of dimethyl sulfoxide (DMSO)*

Nonmedicinal
Industrial solvent for resins, fungicides, dyes, pigments
Reactant for chemical synthesis
Antifreeze
Hydraulic fluid
Paint remover
Medicinal
Anti-inflammatory agent (not FDA-approved)
Treatment of cerebral edema (not FDA-approved)
Cryopreservative for platelets
Treatment of interstitial cystitis (FDA-approved)
Treatment of scleroderma (approved for use in Canada)
Transport medium for drug absorption (not FDA-approved)

DMSO is reported to have various pharmacologic actions, including membrane penetration, anti-inflammatory effects, local analgesia, weak bacteriostasis, diuresis, vasodilation, and dissolution of collagen (7). Its one approved use in the United States is for interstitial cystitis, a urologic condition of unknown etiology that causes irritative voiding symptoms and suprapubic pain that usually improves after urination (7,11). Three preparations—Demasorb, Rimso-50, and Rimso-100—are available for use for this condition for intravesicular instillation; the last two of these are 50% and 100% sterile, pyrogen-free preparations. DMSO is also a potent osmotic agent and is gaining increasing acceptance as adjunctive therapy for severe cerebral edema secondary to massive stroke or head trauma (12).

Nonapproved medical applications for DMSO include use as an analgesic and anti-inflammatory agent in musculoskeletal disorders by application to the skin (12), but its value in specific diseases has not been shown. Topical DMSO has been used to treat arthritis, sports injuries, scleroderma, and keloids. A 90% solution is also approved as a veterinary medication for topical use. In Canada, DMSO is approved as a 70% solution for cutaneous use in patients with scleroderma.

Properties

DMSO is readily absorbed through the body surface and readily crosses most membranes without apparently destroying their integrity (17). This is a result of reversible configurational changes of protein molecules due to temporary water substitution by DMSO. In other words, it is the movement of DMSO through the skin that influences the movement of other molecules through the skin. It is also readily absorbed by injection and by mouth (18).

DMSO has come into use as a penetrating solvent to aid absorption of drugs through the skin, such as testosterone, corticosteroids, and salicylates. Impurities in DMSO preparations are also distributed systemically (it should be noted that the manufacturer makes no claim regarding the absence of contaminants). If the skin is contaminated with dirt or chemicals, DMSO may carry these compounds through the skin and into the circulation. Rubber gloves do not necessarily provide adequate protection from absorption of DMSO.

DMSO permeates body water, and serum concentrations reach their peak 4 hours after administration by mouth and 4 to 8 hours after percutaneous administration (18). Most of a dose is converted to an odorless compound, but about 3% to 6% is converted to a malodorous dimethyl sulfide and is excreted through the lungs. This gives a characteristic garlic odor to the breath (7).

Toxicity

The rate of absorption of DMSO is directly related to the relative concentration. Large amounts of high concentrations applied to the skin may cause burning, discomfort, itching, erythema (19), occasional vesiculation, hemoglobinuria, hemolysis, and profound release of histamine and serotonin in the immediate area (18). Severe tissue edema and ischemia may also result (11,19).

Long-term eye toxicity has included lens opacification in animals; this has not been documented in humans. A reddish discoloration of the urine may be secondary to the transient systemic hemolysis. Despite the hemoglobinuria, no long-term renal damage has been demonstrated (12). DMSO may also increase serum osmolality (20). Treatment for DMSO consists of decontamination and supportive care.

Nitrogen Mustard Gas

In military history, several chemical substances with different compositions have been used in chemical warfare. In accordance with their pathogenic effects these chemical war agents have been classified into those that cause suffocation, sneezing, tears, poisoning of the nervous system, or blisters. The nitrogen mustard gas is an example of a vesicant or blister agent (17).

Mustard gas is of scientific historic interest because it is the first substance observed to act by an alkylation reaction, or by binding to tissue proteins. During World War I, mustard gas was used as a vesicant and for chemical warfare. In an aqueous medium, it rearranges into a form that is highly reactive with sulfhydryl acid, carboxyl acid, amino acids, proteins, and the hydroxyl ions of water (21). This rearrangement is very stable and alters the functional and physicochemical properties of enzymes and other proteins so that they are denatured or inactivated.

Nitrogen mustard is an oily, colorless, or pale yellow liquid, sparingly soluble in water but freely soluble in organic solvents. It smells like garlic. The chemical composition of this substance is bis-2-chlorethyl-sulfide, and it is easily vaporized by heat and then quickly spread by the wind. In chemical war, the vesicant agents usually have been used as aerial bombs or artillery shells (22).

Topical nitrogen mustard has been used as a therapeutic measure in the management of patients with eczematous premycotic phase and plaque stage of mycosis fungoides. This topical application produces an allergic contact sensitization in approximately 50% of patients, and eventually a contact urticaria or even anaphylactoid reaction has been reported.

Clinical Manifestations

Although mustard gas reacts very quickly with tissues, delayed symptoms are characteristic (Table 26–4). Mustard gas penetrates the skin for 20 to 30 minutes without causing any warning signals, such as itching, burning, or sensations of wetness or cold. This latent period varies between several hours and several days. Nevertheless, decontamination must be carried out within seconds of exposure to be effective in preventing injury.

Patients exposed to nitrogen mustard may show extensive involvement of the skin characterized by widespread erythema and detachment of epidermis resembling scalding or toxic epidermal necrolysis. Confluence of vesicles leads to large flaccid bullae of irregular shape. These features in addition to the positivity of Nikolsky's sign and the mucous membranes involved closely resemble toxic epidermal necrolysis (21).

Residual hyperpigmentation may follow nearly any inflammatory eruption, particularly in more pigmented

TABLE 26–4. *Nitrogen mustard*

Delay in onset of symptoms
Lesions resemble toxic epidermal necrolysis
Residual pigmentation develops
Increased vulnerability in
Pubic area
Underarms
Neck
Intertrigineous areas
Periorbital areas
Signs and symptoms
Ophthalmic
Sand in eyes
Pain
Tearing
Blepharospasm
Conjunctivitis
Respiratory
Shortness of breath
Dryness in throat
Purulent diphtheroid bronchitis
Pneumonia
Formation of pseudomembrane

patients. This pigmentation starts as a small brown or black macule in the perifollicular location, closely resembling the initial events of the vitiligo repigmentation.

Certain regions of the body are particularly susceptible to skin damage because of their higher temperature, humidity level, sebaceous and sweat gland density, and relative thinness of the stratum corneum. Therefore, the vulnerable regions include the pubic area, the underarms, the neck, the skin between the fingers and toes, and the area around the eyes.

The eyes are one of the most frequently damaged organs. As early as 2 hours after contact, the effects begin with a feeling as if sand grains were in one's eyes. A painful burning sensation follows, which leads to tearing. The eyelids swell to the point of closure. At the same time, the conjunctivae also swell. The consequences include hypersensitivity to light and a lid cramp, resulting in a practical loss of vision.

The most dangerous effects of mustard gas are manifested in the respiratory tract. The substance can be inhaled in droplet or vapor form. The latent period for respiratory tract damage is approximately 2 to 3 hours.

Symptoms begin with a lump sensation in the throat, followed by tickling and dryness, an urge to cough, difficulty in swallowing, and shortness of breath. At the same time the mucous membranes swell and develop an inflamed redness.

After massive inhalation a serious, purulent diphtheroid bronchitis develops, followed by pneumonia. This pneumonia may be localized, lobular, or gangrenous, and is often hemorrhagic. In these serious cases, death often results when the pseudomembranes completely block the bronchial or tracheal passages, leading to suffocation.

Lewisite

Lewisite is an extremely toxic member of a group of arsenic compounds that produce lesions of the epithelium of the skin and respiratory system as a result of their vesicant action. It received considerable attention in World War I and World War II as a potential agent in chemical warfare. Lewisite reacts with thiol groups of tissue proteins, and an effective antidote known as British antilewisite (BAL) or dimercaprol was produced specifically for its actions (17).

TREATMENT OF SKIN BURNS

If the material is on the skin, removal by irrigating the area with copious amounts of water under low pressure for long periods of time is indicated (Table 26–5). Particulate matter should be debrided from the wound before or during irrigation. Prompt removal of clothing and copious irrigation with water should occur as soon as possible after contact with any caustic agent. Shoes must be removed because they may trap the agent against the skin, causing prolonged contact. The severity of the burn and the duration of hospital stay have both been shown to decrease when water lavage is initiated in the field (1).

TABLE 26–5. *Treatment of cutaneous burns*

Copious irrigation with water
Removal of particulate matter
Topical antibiotic
Tetanus prophylaxis
Careful follow-up

Lavage effectively dilutes the chemical in contact with the skin and washes off unreacted reagents not yet at the skin–chemical interface. No role exists for neutralizing acid and alkali injuries, as time is wasted searching for specific reagents, and the exothermic reaction produced by neutralization may extend the depth of the burn by increasing the temperature at the chemical–skin interface.

Severe alkaline burns can result if no dilution of the affected skin is immediately initiated and maintained for at least 1 hour. Treatment delays of more than 1 hour have been shown to damage skin to such a degree that subsequent continuous irrigation or hydrotherapy will have little or no effect on subcutaneous pH and the outcome (4). Cutaneous burns are like thermal injuries in that they require cleansing with soap, the application of a topical antibiotic such as silver sulfadiazine (Silvadene), and tetanus prophylaxis.

Steroids have no demonstrated role in cutaneous alkaline burn management. In most cases of full-thickness alkaline burns, a burn center should be consulted, and the need for a grafting procedure should be considered (4).

REFERENCES

1. Mozingo D, Smith A, McManus W, et al: Chemical burns. *J Trauma* 1988;28:642–647.
2. Clare R, Krenzelok E: Chemical burns secondary to elemental metal exposure: two case reports. *Am J Emerg Med* 1988;6:355–357.
3. Wason S, Karkal S: Coping swiftly and effectively with caustic ingestions. *Emerg Med Rep* 1989;10:25–32.
4. Lorette J, Wilkinson J: Alkaline chemical burn to the face requiring full-thickness skin grafting. *Ann Emerg Med* 1988;17:739–741.
5. Meredith W, Kon N, Thompson J: Management of injuries from liquid lye ingestion. *J Trauma* 1988;28:1173–1180.
6. Rubin M, Jui V, Cozzi G: Treatment of caustic ingestion. *J Oral Maxillofac Surg* 1989;47:286–290.
7. Bowman C, Muhleman M, Walters E: A fatal case of creosote poisoning. *Postgrad Med J* 1984;60:499–500.
8. Spiller H, Quandrani-Kushner D, Cleveland P: A five year evalua-

tion of acute exposures to phenol disinfectant (26%). *J Toxicol Clin Toxicol* 1993;31:307–313.
9. Hunter D, Timerding B, Leonard R, et al: Effects of isopropyl alcohol, ethanol, and polyethylene glycol/industrial methylated spirits in the treatment of acute phenol burns. *Ann Emerg Med* 1992;21:1301–1307.
10. Stewart C: Chemical skin burns. *Am Fam Physician* 1985;31:149–157.
11. Pegg S, Campbell D: Children's burns due to cresol. *Burns* 1985;11: 294–296.
12. Cote M, Lyonnais J, Leblond P: Acute Heinz-body anemia due to severe cresol poisoning: successful treatment with erythrocytapheresis. *Can Med Assoc J* 1984;130:1319–1322.
13. Schneider M, Mani M, Masters F: Gasoline-induced contact burns. *J Burn Care Rehabil* 1991;12:140–143.
14. Williams J, Ahrenholz D, Solem L, et al: Gasoline burns: the preventable cause of thermal injury. *J Burn Care Rehabil* 1990;11:446–450.
15. Litovitz T, Butterfield A, Holloway R, et al: Button battery ingestion: assessment of therapeutic modalities and battery discharge state. *J Pediatr* 1984;105:868–873.
16. Rumack B, Rumack C: Disc battery ingestion. *JAMA* 1983;249: 2509–2511.
17. Klein M: Addressing the controversies of caustic ingestions. *Emerg Med Rep* 1983;4:155–160.
18. Early S, Simpson R: Caustic burns from contact with wet cement. *JAMA* 1985;254:528–529.
19. Buntain W, Cain W: Caustic injuries to the esophagus: a pediatric overview. *South Med J* 1981;74:590–593.
20. Friedman E, Lovejoy F: The emergency management of caustic ingestions. *Emerg Med Clin North Am* 1984;2:77–86.
21. Requena L, Requena C, Sanchez M, et al: Chemical warfare. *J Am Acad Dermatol* 1988;19:529–536.
22. Eisenmenger W, Drasch G, von Clarmann M, et al: Clinical and morphological findings on mustard gas [Bis(2-chloroethyl)sulfide] poisoning. *J Forensic Sci* 1991;36:1688–1698.

ADDITIONAL SELECTED REFERENCES

Davis L, Raffensperger J, Novak G: Necrosis of the stomach secondary to ingestion of corrosive agents. *Chest* 1972;62:48–51.

Ellis E, Brouhard B, Lynch R, et al: Effects of hemodialysis and dimercaprol in acute dichromate poisoning. *J Toxicol Clin Toxicol* 1982;19: 249–258.

Fitzpatrick K, Moylan J: Emergency care of chemical burns. *Postgrad Med J* 1985;78:189–194.

Hardin J: Caustic burns of the esophagus. *Am J Surg* 1956;91:742–748.

Michel L, Grillo H, Malt R: Esophageal perforation. *Ann Thorac Surg* 1982;33:202–210.

Oakes D, Sherck J, Mark J: Lye ingestion. *J Thorac Cardiovasc Surg* 1982; 83:194–204.

Okonek S, Bierbach H, Atzpodien W: Unexpected metabolic acidosis in severe lye poisoning. *Clin Toxicol* 1981;18:225–230.

CHAPTER 27

Burns of the Eye

Occasionally, strong alkalis and acids are used or purposefully poured on the face or in the eye. The immediate management may be the single most important factor in determining the outcome (1).

Chemical burns to the cornea can be the most visually threatening ocular insult. Alkali and acid burns are true ocular emergencies (2). Their immediate treatment is essential to preservation of sight. Their prognosis is variable and progressively worsens as the time between exposure to and removal of the chemical lengthens. Less caustic agents generally produce only superficial injury with good prognosis but likewise must be treated as emergencies (3).

This chapter will discuss alkali and acid injuries to the eye, with specific reference to azides, detergents, super glue, and mace (or tear gas). This will be followed by a discussion of the general management of ocular chemical injuries.

ALKALI

Alkali damages the eye by increasing the hydroxyl ion concentration beyond the limits of protein stability. This results in the formation of alkaline proteinates that react with the lipid cellular membranes, causing them to saponify and lyse. By this process, the alkali rapidly penetrates the ocular tissue. A strong corrosive spilled into the eye may produce immediate whitening of the cornea and sclera (4). The anterior chamber pH rises within 2 to 3 minutes, causing damage to the iris, lens, and ciliary body. This may lead to irreversible loss of vision within minutes. If the burn is mild, only the epithelium will be lost; this is equivalent to a corneal abrasion and can be seen on fluorescein staining (5).

Large volumes or higher concentrations of alkali readily penetrate the corneal stroma, causing injury of the endothelium with resultant corneal edema. Initially, there is intense pain generated from the stimulation of free nerve endings, especially in the epithelium (6). The pain is enhanced by a sudden rise of the intraocular pressure induced by the direct effect of the alkali. This rise in intraocular pressure is prolonged as a result of prostaglandin release within the eye.

ACIDS

As a rule, acids produce less severe ocular injury than alkalis, yet acids do have the potential to cause ocular devastation equal to that of alkalis. Acids cause tissue protein precipitation which limits penetration through the cornea and into the eye. The sequelae of acid injury can be prolonged and difficult to manage but on the whole have a better visual prognosis than those of alkali burns (3). Hydrofluoric, sulfuric, sulfurous, and chromic acids are exceptions to this rule (7). Concentrated mineral acids cause extensive necrosis of the conjunctiva and corneal epithelium. They penetrate and injure the stroma of the cornea, with resulting perforation or with permanent opaque scar formation. Only rarely is the lens or iris injured.

Dilute acids, including 4% to 6% acetic acid as present in ordinary vinegar, may cause immediate pain, conjunctival hyperemia, and sometimes injury of the corneal epithelium, but the latter regenerates promptly and corneal opacities are uncommon.

Long-term sequelae secondary to significant chemical eye burns include corneal perforation or ulceration, iritis, lens damage, cataracts, and possible atrophy of the globe (2).

AZIDES

Azides are found in automobile airbags that have become an accepted part of motor vehicle safety systems and are now widely available on most new cars (8).

The idea of an airbag is that if the velocity of change exceeds 12 mph, the velocity sensors detect a sufficiently severe crash and an electrical signal ignites a primer in the airbag canister. This triggers ignition of about 70 g of sodium azide, which converts to inert nitrogen gas. Byproducts of this combustion include sodium hydroxide, sodium carbonate, and other metallic oxides, which create a fine alkaline aerosol. The specific reaction varies with the oxidizing agents used by various manufacturers.

Alkaline keratitis has been reported as a result of release of these sodium compounds from deployed automobile airbags. Alkaline keratitis is a potentially serious threat to vision that requires specific treatment. In this setting, its recognition is dependent on obtaining the history of eye pain after motor vehicle trauma in which an airbag has deployed. The diagnosis is confirmed when pH paper is used to show that ocular secretions have a pH of 8 or more, most conveniently determined by placing the paper in the inferior fornix (9). Fluorescein is used in conjunction with a Wood's light or slit-lamp to detect either an associated corneal abrasion or abnormal corneal epithelium caused by chemical burn (10). In many cases, fluorescein uptake is not punctate, and it will not be possible to determine if the abnormal corneal epithelium is from physical abrasion or is purely chemical keratitis. Differentiating between these two is not clinically relevant when the pH is shown to be alkaline (8).

ORGANIC SOLVENTS

Organic solvents and detergents, from industrial and home accidents, usually cause only superficial, self-limited injury to the cornea. Solvents denude epithelium in a geographic or punctate pattern without damaging underlying stroma.

DETERGENTS

Detergents cause conjunctival irritation and variable corneal epithelial compromise. Both can cause iritis, which is easily treated with cycloplegic agents (3).

In contrast to oral and dermal exposures, in which a minority of patients exposed to liquid automatic dishwashing detergent develop toxic symptoms, a majority of patients with an ocular exposure developed either mild or moderate symptoms (11). Conjunctivitis and corneal abrasions are most commonly noted. Liquid automatic dishwashing detergents are not solutions but appear to be aqueous slurries of solute (12). Therefore, it is difficult to discern if the ocular irritation is secondary to mechanical injury from particulate matter or to the highly alkaline nature of the products or to both. Usually patients do not develop permanent sequelae resulting from their ocular exposure.

SUPER GLUE

Cyanoacrylate adhesive was introduced in 1959. This adhesive has the unique property of being rapidly converted from a liquid to a solid state by anionic polymerization that occurs at room temperature without the need for catalysts, solvents, or application of pressure (13). Although cyanoacrylates are colorless, clear liquids as monomers, they become chalky white solids within 10 to 20 seconds upon polymerization. The cyanoacrylates have, for many years, been used in medicine and surgery. Many bottles used for nail glue appear identical to those used for ophthalmic solutions. The use of artificial nails has attained increased popularity in the last few years. Poorly sighted individuals, careless persons, and children run the greatest risk of mistaking these dispensers for eye medication (14).

Type of Injury

Rapid setting "super" glues are often inadvertently placed in the eyes and harden quickly on contact with moisture. Following instillation, there may be an intense burning or stinging pain. As the glue hardens within the conjunctival sac and the lids adhere to each other there is contact between this foreign body and the corneal surface. This results in corneal and conjunctival epithelial abrasion and punctate epithelial keratopathy (15).

Treatment

If the eyelids are glued together, they can be separated with gentle traction and/or by dissolving the glue with acetone. Acetone, however, must not be allowed to contact the eye itself as it dissolves corneal epithelium. Removal of glue adhered to the cornea will result in an epithelial defect that can be successfully treated as a simple corneal abrasion (16).

MACE (TEAR GAS)

Mace is the prototype of the nonexplosive, pressurized, solvent tear gas weapons. Tear gas is actually a common term for a family of chemical compounds that have been otherwise referred to as "harassing agents" because of their ability to cause temporary disablement. These agents have been used by law enforcement agencies for riot control, although private use of these agents has also become prevalent.

Some 15 chemicals have been used worldwide as tear gas agents. Four of these—chloroacetophenone (CN), chlorobenzylidenemalonitrile (CS), chlorodihydrophenarsazine, and bromotolunitrile—have been used extensively (Table 27–1) (10,17). Of these agents, only CN and CS have been widely employed in the United States, and all but one of the over-the-counter products contain CN.

TABLE 27–1. *Lacrimatory agents*

CS—Chlorobenzylidenemalonitrile
CN—Chloroacetophenone
DM—Diphenylaminechlorarsine
BBC—Bromobenzyl cyanide

These agents are primarily intended to incapacitate an individual without causing illness or permanent bodily harm (18).

Both CN and CS are alkylating agents that react with sulfhydryl groups (10). They were first synthesized during World War I for use as lacrimatory agents. CS is approximately 10 times more potent than CN as an irritant and at the same time is less systemically toxic (18). CN is generally acknowledged to be of greater toxicity than CS, being more likely to cause permanent corneal damage on contact with the eye and primary and allergic contact dermatitis. Since its introduction, CS has virtually replaced CN as the riot control agent of choice in the United States.

Chemical mace consists of a potent lacrimator (usually CN) dissolved in a mixture of hydrocarbons resembling kerosene. The mixture is maintained in a metal container and released as a spray of small liquid droplets directed in a stream that may travel 6 to 10 feet. Most of the active ingredient is dispersed before it reaches the target. The droplets of oily spray very effectively wet and spread on the skin.

Symptoms

The acute transient clinical effects of both CN and CS are similar (Table 27–2). In very low concentrations in air, CN gas has an odor resembling apple blossoms. Major symptoms involve the eyes and respiratory tract. Instantaneous conjunctivitis is characteristic and is accompanied by stinging and burning sensations in the eyes that induces outpouring of tears and involuntary closure of the lids. The burning and pain persists for 2 to 5 minutes and usually disappears abruptly. Conjunctivitis remains intense for 25 to 30 minutes. Erythema of the eyelids occurs and may persist for 1 hour. The profuse lacrimation that invariably occurs usually continues for 12 to 15 minutes.

TABLE 27–2. *Symptoms of exposure to lacrimating agents*

Eyes
- Conjunctivitis
- Lacrimation
- Blepharospasm
- Chemosis

Nose
- Rhinorrhea
- Pain

Mouth and throat
- Salivation
- Irritation

Skin
- Contact dermatitis

Respiratory system
- Cough
- Dyspnea
- Pulmonary edema (rare)

The nose may be painful, and there may be an associated rhinorrhea. Excessive salivation and irritation in the throat are common. A burning sensation in the chest associated with tightness, coughing, and occasionally dyspnea also may be noted. If the material is swallowed, some epigastric discomfort and eructation may develop later. Most symptoms usually clear within 20 minutes, although some may persist.

Respiratory symptoms include a stinging sensation in the nose and mouth and breath holding. High concentrations may lead to the development of acute pulmonary edema after latencies of 8 hours to several days, and death after exposure to high concentrations of CN gas has been reported. These effects may be delayed, and a symptom-free interval after exposure may be observed.

Permanent eye injury has been reported with these agents, although most have been associated with exposure to explosive-type devices discharged close to the face. CN has been known to cause chemical injury to the cornea as well as chemosis. These effects are more likely to occur when the agent is in powder or liquid form.

Fatalities have been reported to occur from 4 hours up to 4 days after exposure to CN. Common causes have been pulmonary edema, focal intra-alveolar hemorrhage, and early bronchopneumonia.

In addition to the irritant effects of these agents, repeated exposure may result in a contact dermatitis consisting of erythema, edema, and pruritus within 48 hours after exposure (19). Contact dermatitis is most common with CN. An allergic blepharitis has also been reported. First- and second-degree burns of the skin may occur, particularly if in contact with abraded areas.

Injury by these agents should prompt a search for projectiles that may have accompanied an aerosol spray or explosive canister (3).

Treatment

Other than prompt withdrawal from the area in which the aerosol is present, specific treatment is not required and recovery is usually prompt. In the management of the conjunctivitis, topical anesthetics are not recommended. Cutaneous reactions should be managed by decontamination with copious amounts of water. Prevention of secondary exposure of medical personnel through contact with residual aerosols on skin or clothing must also be considered, which means that rubber gloves should be worn and contaminated clothing should be placed in plastic bags.

Because of the delayed pulmonary symptoms with the inhalation of large amounts of these chemicals, all patients who have been exposed to high concentrations of tear gas should be carefully observed for several days (9).

GENERAL TREATMENT OF EYE BURNS

Chemical burns to the eye are serious ophthalmologic emergencies and must be treated immediately and appropriately. The single most important treatment of ocular chemical burns is the immediate and complete removal of the offending agent from the eye (10). This is most effectively done with copious irrigation that is started at the time and place of injury with any available source of water (3). The importance of time so outweighs other considerations that the first water, or innocuous watery solution at hand, should be used (5). Time should not be wasted in looking for some special irrigation fluid. A lid speculum may be necessary to open the eyes before irrigation. Irrigation can continue in the emergency department through a small-bore catheter fixed in the palpebral sulcus until the pH of the cul-de-sac returns to neutrality (10). Generally, 1 to 2 L during one half hour to 1 hour is administered through a Morgan lens. The pH should return to normal (7.3 to 7.7) immediately and should remain normal one-half hour after irrigation. The fornices of the lids should be swabbed to eliminate any particulate material that might be lodged there. When irrigation is complete, examination of the eye should be performed (20). Tetanus prophylaxis is also indicated.

For the patient's comfort, a drop of local anesthetic and slightly warmed water can be applied to the injured eye. The duration of irrigation depends on the nature of the chemical and on the concentration and quantity involved.

The rise of intraocular pressure that occurs after the burn frequently responds to the oral administration of carbonic anhydrase inhibitors such as acetazolamide (Diamox, 125 mg four times a day). Soft contact lenses may facilitate re-epithelialization by covering and protecting fresh epithelium from exposure to the air and by reducing the shearing stress of blinking.

Immediate ophthalmic consultation should be sought if there is a corneal opacification, conjunctival blanching, or additional ocular injury. Such severe chemical burns often necessitate anterior chamber paracentesis to lower intraocular pressure and remove alkali or hydrogen ions from the eye. This procedure carries considerable risk and should be performed only by those familiar with the technique. After emergency treatment, patients having sustained severe chemical burns are admitted to the hospital for observation and treatment of complications, glaucoma, corneal perforation, corneal ulceration, adhesions of the eyelid to the globe, cataract, and retinal detachment (21).

REFERENCES

1. Herr R, White G, Bernhisel K, et al: Clinical comparison of ocular irrigation fluids following chemical injury. *Am J Emerg Med* 1991;9: 228–231.
2. Jelenko C: Chemicals that "burn." *J Trauma* 1974;14:65–72.
3. Lubeck D, Greene J: Corneal injuries. *Emerg Med Clin North Am* 1988;6:73–94.
4. Rodenheaver G, Hiebert J, Edlich R: Initial treatment of chemical skin and eye burns. *Compr Ther* 1982;8:37–43.
5. Pfister R, Koski J: Alkali burns of the eye: pathophysiology and treatment. *South Med J* 1982;75:417–422.
6. Leape L, Ashcraft K, Scalpelli D, et al: Hazard to health—liquid lye. *N Engl J Med* 1971;284:578–581.
7. Stewart C: Chemical skin burns. *Am Fam Physician* 1985;31:149–157.
8. Smally A, Binzer A, Dolin S, et al: Alkaline chemical keratitis: eye injury from airbags. *Ann Emerg Med* 1992;21:1400–1402.
9. Wasserman R, Ginsburg C: Caustic substance injuries. *J Pediatr* 1985;107:169–174.
10. Vancura E, Clinton J, Ruiz E, et al: Toxicity of alkaline solutions. *Ann Emerg Med* 1980;9:118–122.
11. Krenzelok E: Liquid automatic dishwashing detergents: a profile of toxicity. *Ann Emerg Med* 1989;18:60–63.
12. Scharph L, Hill I, Kelly R: Relative eye-injury potential of heavy-duty phosphate and non-phosphate laundry detergents. *Food Cosmet Toxicol* 1972;10:829–837.
13. Cavanaugh T, Cottsch J: Infectious keratitis and cyanoacrylate adhesive. *Am J Ophthalmol* 1991;111:466–472.
14. Toriumi D, Raslan W, Friedman M, et al: Histotoxicity of cyanoacrylate tissue adhesives. *Arch Otolaryngol Head Neck Surg* 1990; 116:546–550.
15. DeRespinis P: Cyanoacrylate nail glue mistaken for eye drops. *JAMA* 1990;263:2301.
16. Lyons C, Stevens J, Block J: Superglue inadvertently used as eyedrops. *Br Med J* 1990;300:328.
17. Hu H, Fine J, Epstein P, et al: Tear gas—harassing agent or toxic chemical weapon? *JAMA* 1989;262:660–663.
18. Cello J, Fogel R, Boland R: Liquid caustic ingestion. *Arch Intern Med* 1980;140:501–504.
19. Tucker J, Yarington C: The treatment of caustic ingestion. *Otolaryngol Clin North Am* 1979;12:343–351.
20. Williams J, Ahrenholz D, Solem L, et al: Gasoline burns: the preventable cause of thermal injury. *J Burn Care Rehabil* 1990;11:446–450.
21. Burkhart K, Brent J, Kirk M, et al: Comparison of topical magnesium and calcium treatment for dermal hydrofluoric acid burns. *Ann Emerg Med* 1994;24:9–13.

ADDITIONAL SELECTED REFERENCES

Davis L, Raffensperger J, Novak G: Necrosis of the stomach secondary to ingestion of corrosive agents. *Chest* 1972;62:48–51.

Ellis E, Brouhard B, Lynch R, et al: Effects of hemodialysis and dimercaprol in acute dichromate poisoning. *J Toxicol Clin Toxicol* 1982;19: 249–258.

Fitzpatrick K, Moylan J: Emergency care of chemical burns. *Postgrad Med J* 1985;78:189–194.

Hardin J: Caustic burns of the esophagus. *Am J Surg* 1956;91:742–748.

Michel L, Grillo H, Malt R: Esophageal perforation. *Ann Thorac Surg* 1982;33:202–210.

Oakes D, Sherck J, Mark J: Lye ingestion. *J Thorac Cardiovasc Surg* 1982; 83:194–204.

Okonek S, Bierbach H, Atzpodien W: Unexpected metabolic acidosis in severe lye poisoning. *Clin Toxicol* 1981;18:225–230.

CHAPTER 28

Hydrofluoric Acid

GENERAL INFORMATION

Hydrofluoric acid, one of the strongest inorganic acids known (1), has been in industrial use since its ability to dissolve silica was recognized in the late 17th century. Hydrofluoric acid has a number of chemical and industrial applications. In 1976, the National Institute of Occupational Safety and Health listed 57 occupations with an estimated 22,000 workers who had potential exposure to hydrofluoric acid on a daily basis (Table 28–1) (2–4).

The use of hydrofluoric acid in the semiconductor industry has radically increased the number of workers exposed. It is used as a cleaning agent, in the production of high octane fuels, refrigerants, propellants, Teflon, and semiconductors, as well as in glass frosting and stone engraving (5). Products containing hydrofluoric acid are also available for consumer use. These include rust-removal agents in solution or as gels (6% to 8% hydrofluoride) and aluminum and chrome cleaning solutions (2% to 8% hydrofluoride) (6). Hydrofluoric acid is also used as a catalyst in alkylation units in the petroleum industry (7,8) as well as in dental laboratories to clean and etch castings that are fused with porcelain (9–11). This acid is also used in the pesticide and fertilizer industries and in the production of fire extinguishers, aluminum germicides, and tanning agents.

TABLE 28–1. *Uses of hydrofluoric acid*

Glass etching
Petroleum refining
Dental work
Rust removal
Fertilizers
Manufacturing of
fire extinguishers
dyes
tanning agents
refrigerants
aerosol propellants
plastics
semiconductors
Cleaning agent
Aluminum
Chrome

PHYSICAL PROPERTIES

Hydrogen fluoride is a colorless liquid or gas manufactured by the reaction of sulfuric acid with high-grade fluorospar (97% calcium fluoride) to produce the gas, which is then cooled and liquefied (12). Aqueous solutions fume above concentrations of 40% to 48%. Chemically, concentrated solutions are strong protonic acids, and the more common dilute solutions are weak acids because of the strong hydrogen bonding of all forms of hydrogen fluoride (5). Although hydrofluoric acid is referred to as a very strong acid, this only applies to the anhydrous hydrogen fluoride, and its concentrated aqueous solutions. Its weaker solutions are relatively weak acids. Hydrogen fluoride is 1,000 times less dissociated than hydrochloric acid, and it is the undissociated fluoride moiety that causes tissue damage (13).

Hydrofluoric acid is therefore the inorganic acid of elemental fluorine. The fluoride ion has a strong affinity with apatite crystals, which are present in all calcified tissue. Thus, on direct contact hydrofluoric acid causes liquefaction necrosis by disrupting the horny layer of the skin and immediately destroys the subcutaneous tissue (1).

Hydrogen fluoride solutions are more damaging than the stronger halogen acids (hydroiodic, hydrobromic, and hydrochloric acids) (4). It is available as a liquid in various concentrations, from dilute solutions in erusticators (<10%) to highly concentrated solutions (70%). This exceedingly corrosive material is lethal in small quantities, even at low concentrations (2,10,14).

EFFECTS OF HYDROFLUORIC ACID

Hydrofluoric acid is unique among corrosives in the acute toxicity that results from dermal, ocular, inhalation, and oral exposures (15). Most acids produce immediate pain on contact due to the chemical burn caused by dissociated H^+ ions (14,16). However, because of the affinity of the F^- ion, hydrofluoric acid is a relatively weak acid in dilute solutions, and few free H^+ ions exist. Because there may be little or no initial pain with exposure to weaker solutions, the burn may go undiscovered for a period of time. This time lag between exposure and decontamination allows time for deeper penetration of the fluoride in the undissociated hydrofluoric acid form and a more severe burn (17).

Although hydrofluoric acid is a corrosive agent, its hydrogen ion plays a relatively insignificant role in the pathophysiology of burns. The acid does produce caustic injury to the skin, but it causes less surface damage that equimolar solutions of stronger acids such as hydrochloric and sulfuric acids (18). Hydrofluoric acid has two stages of biologic effects in contrast to the more commonly used hydrochloric or sulfuric acids (2). It acts first as a corrosive to the superficial tissues, as any other inorganic acid. Second, owing to the highly permeable fluoride ions, it causes liquefaction necrosis, bone decalcification, and intense, delayed pain in deep tissues (5). As the fluoride ions penetrate deeper tissues, they complex with calcium and magnesium to form insoluble fluoride salts (Table 28–2) (1,7). This destruction continues until the hydrogen fluoride is precipitated as calcium or magnesium fluoride by natural tissue magnesium or calcium compounds or by compounds administered medically (4). This process can produce hypocalcemia and hypomagnesemia.

Fluoride ion also acts as a general enzyme inhibitor and inhibits cellular metabolism and the glycolytic enzymes, interferes with electrical membrane function, and decalcifies bone (2). It appears that the fluoride ion binds the calcium on the cell membrane, leading to increased permeability of the membrane to potassium and thus to altered membrane potential and spontaneous depolarization; this produces pain and necrosis (14). Severe hydrofluoric acid burns have been associated with systemic fluoride poisoning sometimes resulting in death (19). One hydrofluoric acid death was caused by the electrolyte abnormalities described above from a burn involving 2.5% of the body surface (20).

As little as 7 cc of anhydrous hydrogen fluoride will bind all the free calcium in a normal-sized person. It has been suggested that the lethal oral dose of hydrogen fluoride is 1.5 g (13). Household preparations, which generally contain very weak concentrations of hydrofluoric acid are particularly dangerous. With delays of as much as 24 hours before symptoms appear, these exposures can result in considerable tissue loss (18).

TABLE 28–2. *Effects of hydrofluoric acid*

Corrosive-type burn (onset may be delayed)
Complexion with cations (may result in hypocalcemia or hypomagnesemia)
Bone decalcification
Increased cellular permeability to potassium
- Altered membrane potential
- Increased spontaneous depolarization

Interference with
- Glycolytic enzymes
- Cellular metabolism
- Electrical membrane function

Systemic fluoride poisoning

NATIONAL INSTITUTES OF HEALTH CLASSIFICATION

The National Institutes of Health has classified hydrofluoric acid burns only according to the concentration of the acid to which the victim is exposed. No reference is made of the duration of exposure.

Solutions of up to 20% may not produce erythema and pain until 24 hours after exposure; burns from 20% to 25% solutions usually manifest themselves in 1 to 8 hours; and solutions greater than 50% produce immediate pain and rapid tissue destruction (15).

Patients believed to be at greatest risk for hypocalcemia are those with a wound of 1% of the body surface area or greater caused by exposure to a 50% or greater hydrofluoric acid concentration, or a wound of 5% body surface area caused by exposure to any hydrofluoric acid concentration, or inhalation of fumes from hydrofluoric acid concentration of 69% or greater. These patients do not show the usual signs of hypocalcemia such as tetany or carpopedal spasm. These patients must be closely monitored and have frequent serum calcium levels checked (13).

DERMAL EXPOSURE

The most common hydrofluoric acid exposure is dermal. Skin burns are characterized by (a) an intense, deep pain that may be delayed in onset (4), (b) development of thick, coagulated skin at the site of initial burn, (c) progressive tissue destruction with the absence of treatment, even into bony erosions, and (d) a predilection for subungual involvement (Table 28–3) (5).

Initial presentation may vary from mild skin erythema to severe third-degree burns. Untreated, the lesions progress to indurated, whitish, and blistered vesicles and bullae that contain caseous necrotic tissue (16). Severe burns can progress to ulceration, full-thickness tissue loss, and even loss of digits (1). Scarring and permanent disability may result.

The onset of signs and symptoms may be delayed for up to several hours after dermal exposure to compounds containing less than 20% hydrofluoric acid. Dermal injuries secondary to hydrofluoric acid exposure consist of two distinct phases. The immediate damage is caused by the high tissue hydrogen ion concentration. The second phase can produce more severe injury and may result in continued tissue necrosis over a period of several days (21).

TABLE 28–3. *Exposure to hydrofluoric acid*

Dermal	
	Deep intense pain
	Binding of fluoride ion to Ca, Mg
	Release of intracellular K
	Liquefaction necrosis
	Progressive tissue destruction
	Subungual involvement
Systemic	
	Hypocalcemia
	Abnormal EKG
	Cardiac dysrhythmias
Inhalation	
	Systemic toxicity
	Hemorrhagic pulmonary edema
	Atelectasis
	Tracheobronchial hemorrhage
Ocular	
	Pain
	Tearing
	Conjunctival injection
	Corneal opacification

The deep and intense pain is thought to be due to the binding of the fluoride ions to intracellular calcium and magnesium to form insoluble salts that interfere with the cellular functions and cause cellular death. This releases intracellular potassium, which, when combined with an increase of extracellular potassium due to binding of ionic calcium, causes nerve irritation. As the fluoride penetrates through the skin and subcutaneous tissue, it causes a liquefaction necrosis, with decalcification of underlying bone. The fluoride penetration seems to be facilitated by the initial corrosive effect of its weak acid (5).

Burns of the fingers also require special attention because they often involve the subungual areas that lack the protection of the stratum corneum and thus are particularly vulnerable. Moreover, the nail acts as a barrier to effective therapy, resulting in rapid progression to significant injury (18). Exposure of nail beds may produce permanent nail disfigurement and onycholysis (1). After a latent period, painful, deep ulcers may be noted beneath an exceedingly tough coagulum. If allowed to progress, it may destroy bone of the distal phalanx (15).

SYSTEMIC TOXICITY

Systemic manifestations of hydrofluoric acid burns stem primarily from hypocalcemia. Surprisingly, small exposures to concentrated hydrofluoric acid can lead to systemic effects. If left untreated, a burn with as little as 7 mL of 99% hydrofluoric acid can theoretically bind all of the available calcium in a 70-kg person. The hypocalcemia is silent, because it does not typically produce tetany; only the serum calcium level and the EKG are reliable indicators (19). In addition, the hypocalcemia of hydrofluoric acid burns induces cardiac arrhythmias that are particularly resistant to treatment (18).

Patients thought to be at high risk for systemic hypocalcemia and who require monitoring are those with (a) > 1% total body surface area exposure to a 50% or greater solution, (b) > 5% exposure to any solution, and (c) inhalation of a > 60% solution (5).

INHALATIONAL EXPOSURE

Serious injury from inhalation of hydrogen fluoride (HF) fumes is rare. It usually involves explosions that produce high concentrations of fumes or exposure of the skin and clothing of the upper body to high concentrations of hydrofluoric acid. Inhalation of HF not only can cause local adverse effects but also leads to rapid absorption of fluoride into the blood stream and may cause significant systemic toxicity. This absorption should not be surprising because fluoride ion is known to equilibrate rapidly across biologic membranes.

The vapor of hydrofluoric acid is also intensely irritating to the lungs and conjunctivae and may itself produce skin burns. In addition, inhalation has produced oropharyngeal, airway, and lower respiratory tract damage with respiratory distress and pulmonary edema (22). Several cases of inhalation exposure in humans have been reported that resulted in rapid hemorrhagic pulmonary edema (22), atelectasis, frank tracheobronchial hemorrhage, and death 30 to 150 minutes after exposure. In addition, delayed pulmonary effects have also been described (15). Respiratory symptoms may persist for months to years following inhalation injury. Deaths have been reported from inhalation of hydrofluoric acid vapors (10,11,20).

OCULAR EXPOSURE

Ocular exposures are of particular concern. The rapid penetration of the fluoride ion may cause substantial injury to the deep tissues of the eye, with devastating results (18). Exposure of the eye to hydrofluoric acid solution or vapors produces more extensive damage than that of other acids in similar concentrations. Hydrochloric acid produces damage only to the superficial structures of the eye. Its penetration is limited by a precipitated protein barrier. The fluoride ion's ability to penetrate deep into tissue make hydrofluoric acid more destructive to ocular tissue.

Signs and symptoms of eye exposure include the rapid onset of pain, tearing, conjunctival injection, and corneal opacification. Complications include decreased visual acuity, globe perforation, uveitis, glaucoma, conjunctival scarring, lid deformities, and keratitis sicca.

TABLE 28–4. *Laboratory determinations in hydrofluoric acid exposure*

Complete blood cell count
Liver function studies
Blood urea nitrogen
Serum creatinine concentration
Serum electrolytes
Serum calcium concentration
Serum magnesium concentration
Serum fluoride concentration
Electrocardiogram

LABORATORY DETERMINATIONS

Blood should be obtained for stat determination of serum calcium, magnesium, and potassium levels. Because of the rapid development of hypocalcemia and hypomagnesemia, empiric IV administration of calcium and magnesium should begin. Patients also may require immediate treatment of hyperkalemia.

Early administration of calcium can antagonize the abnormal cardiac effects of hyperkalemia. Frequent assessment of serum calcium, magnesium, and potassium levels as well as continued cardiac monitoring are necessary for optimal management of electrolyte abnormalities (6).

After a significant exposure to hydrofluoric acid, blood should be drawn immediately for a complete blood cell count, to determine liver function, and to measure blood urea nitrogen, electrolytes, and serum creatinine, calcium, magnesium, and fluoride concentrations. The electrocardiogram should be monitored continuously for prolongation of the QT interval (Table 28–4).

TREATMENT

Nonspecific

Despite the differences described between hydrofluoric acid and other inorganic acids, the initial care of such burns is the same. This includes complete disrobing of the patient, immediate copious irrigation of the area with tepid water, an attempt to identify the offending agent, and treatment of systemic toxicity when present (17).

The treatment of hydrofluoric acid burns of the skin consists of two phases. The first is decontamination of the skin by immediate and copious irrigation with the nearest available nontoxic liquid, usually water (Table 28–5). The speed with which irrigation is undertaken is of utmost importance because hydrofluoric acid rapidly penetrates the skin. Limiting the duration of exposure decreases the severity of toxicity. The danger of exposure to dilute hydrofluoric acid is that it is often not detected by the victim until hours later, when penetration and tissue destruction have already taken place. Irrigation, preferably under a shower or faucet, should be continued for at least 15 to 30 minutes. After irrigation is complete, appropriate wound care, such as cleansing and debridement, is undertaken.

TABLE 28–5. *Treatment of hydrofluoric acid exposure*

Nonspecific
Decontamination
Maintenance of electrolyte balance
Monitoring for renal and hepatic toxicity
Intravenous therapy
Electrocardiographic monitoring
Ingestion
Lavage
Endoscopy
Hemodialysis
Antiarrhythmic agents
Ophthalmic
Prolonged irrigation
Ophthalmic anesthetic drops
Delayed visual acuity check
Skin
Copious water lavage
Calcium gluconate gel (2.5%)
Local calcium gluconate infiltration
Intra-arterial calcium gluconate infusion
Systemic
Treat
Hypocalcemia
Systemic fluorosis
Cardiac dysrhythmias
Hyperkalemia
Hypotension
Dialysis
Fluorosis
Hyperkalemia

All blisters should be deroofed at the time of initial presentation to remove any necrotic tissue potentially harboring fluoride ion. The blister base is then treated with gel (18).

Most brief exposures to dilute concentrations of hydrofluoric acid will do well with this initial burn care and close follow-up obviating the need for invasive therapy.

Burns to the fingers must be examined closely to rule out subungal involvement. If definite injury exists or subungual injury is strongly suspected, all or part of the fingernail should be removed under local anesthesia. The nail bed must be thoroughly irrigated with water and given routine care with gel or injection. If the burn is extensive and the removal of more than one nail is necessary, intra-arterial therapy should be considered as a less morbid alternative.

The second phase of treatment is aimed at detoxifying the fluoride ion, usually by promoting formation of an insoluble calcium salt (15).

Treatment of Ingestion

As a first-aid measure in the home, milk should be administered immediately to dilute the acid and perhaps bind some of the fluoride ion. Because of hydrogen fluoride's propensity to cause significant systemic fluoride toxicity, gastric emptying after ingestion of a significant amount would seem desirable. If spontaneous vomiting has not occurred and the time between ingestion is brief (<90 minutes), then gastric lavage should be considered. The addition of 1% calcium gluconate to the lavage fluid may have an advantage over plain tap water or saline because of the availability of free calcium to bind the fluoride. The risk of perforating the stomach secondary to the procedure is small compared with the high morbidity and mortality associated with absorption of fluoride and systemic poisoning. The induction of emesis with syrup of ipecac is not advised. There is no data or guidelines for the amount of lavage fluid required for decontamination of the stomach in this setting. However, it should require substantially less volume than that required for removal of tablets or pill fragments.

Stabilization of an airway is of primary importance if there is clinical evidence of upper airway burns or obstruction. Other life-threatening symptoms that require immediate stabilization include hypovolemic shock from gastrointestinal bleeding and cardiac dysrhythmias. Endoscopy should follow after patient stabilization (6).

Hemodialysis may be used after excessive fluoride absorption to remove fluoride anion and correct serum chemistries. Serum fluoride levels (normal 0.01 mmol/L), although not as readily available as serum calcium, magnesium, or potassium levels, also can be useful in determining therapy.

Antiarrhythmic agents and/or cardioversion–defibrillation may be necessary should dysrhythmias develop.

Inhalational Injury and Treatment

Inhalation of the vapors of hydrofluoric acid can lead to life-threatening complications. Hydrofluoric acid vapor produces caustic burns with severe swelling of the oropharynx and tracheobronchial tree, occasionally necessitating tracheostomy. Inhalation injuries are also associated with a characteristic late-onset pulmonary edema (18). The management of inhalation exposure and injury consists of removing the victim from the source and into fresh air, accompanied by decontamination of clothes and skin. If respiratory symptoms are present, humidified oxygen should be administered and the patient transported to a health care facility where monitoring for laryngeal edema, pneumonitis, pulmonary edema, pulmonary hemorrhage, and systemic toxicity can be undertaken (15).

Inhalational injuries require initial management with 100% oxygen. Intubation is indicated if localized edema with airway compromise develops. Although some have suggested administering 2.5 to 3.0% calcium gluconate solution via a nebulizer, there is no experimental evidence to support its use (15). A constant vigilance for delayed pulmonary edema must be maintained. Steroid administration has been reported to be helpful in treating pulmonary edema, but no control studies exist (18).

Ocular Exposure and Treatment

All burns of the eye are considered ophthalmic emergencies. Immediate and copious irrigation of the exposed eye is the mainstay of treatment and is more important than transport to a hospital. Irrigation should be continued for at least 30 minutes after exposure, including during transport to a health care facility where an ophthalmic examination can be performed promptly.

Local ophthalmic anesthetic drops will increase patient comfort and compliance with prolonged irrigation. The pH of the eye fluid should be checked periodically with litmus paper, and irrigation continued until it is normal. A Morgan lens can facilitate irrigation (18). Assessment of visual acuity should be delayed until eye irrigation is completed.

Subsequent therapy is aimed at binding dissociated fluoride ion and preventing complications. Attempts to extrapolate dermal therapy to the eye are attractive but fraught with hazard, and magnesium oxide, magnesium sulfate, Hyamine, and benzalkonium chloride, as well as subconjunctival infiltration with 10% calcium gluconate have produced marked injury to eyes. Irrigation with water or isotonic saline are the only treatments that have been found to be nontoxic and of therapeutic benefit (15).

Specific Treatment

Authorities differ about the most effective specific treatment for hydrofluoric acid burns. Some suggest magnesium oxide ointment, topical or systemic calcium gluconate, and topical quaternary ammonium compounds (14). The first two treatments depend on the precipitation of the fluoride ion into insoluble magnesium and calcium salts, respectively. The action mechanism of the quaternary ammonium compounds is unknown, but it is postulated that ionized chloride is exchanged for the fluoride ion to produce a nonionized fluoride complex. It appears that calcium gluconate is more effective than other methods. The optimal therapy for hydrofluoric acid dermal burns has yet to be determined (21).

Calcium Gluconate Gel

Liberal and frequent application of 2.5% calcium gluconate gel to hydrofluoric acid burns has been recommended and is probably the early topical therapy of choice (14,23). Experimentally, it has been shown to be more effective than water or magnesium ointment in limiting burn severity when applied to burns. The main limitation of topical therapy is the impermeability of the skin to the calcium. Percutaneous penetration of calcium ion into subcutaneous tissue may be enhanced by formulating the gel with dimethyl sulfoxide (DMSO).

Calcium gluconate gel can be a useful first aid technique and in some cases may be all that is necessary (14, 23). Calcium gluconate gel (2.5%) made for this purpose can be gently massaged into the contaminated areas until the pain is relieved. Commercial preparations of calcium gluconate gel for the topical therapy of hydrofluoric acid burns are available in the United Kingdom, Canada, France, Germany, Italy, and the Netherlands (21) but not in the U.S. A calcium gel is not stocked in most hospital pharmacies, yet a 2.5% calcium gluconate gel may be formulated by mixing 3.5 g of calcium gluconate powder USP to 150 mL (5 oz) of a water-soluble lubricant. A dressing soaked with a calcium salt solution and applied to the burn is a suitable alternative. The gel or dressing may be secured with an occlusive barrier (e.g., latex glove or plastic wrap) if prolonged topical therapy is desired.

Topical therapy offers many advantages. The gel is painless and easy to apply. The mixture is stable over time and can be kept at the worksite. Therefore, therapy can be readily continued on an outpatient basis after the initial evaluation (18).

Calcium Gluconate Infiltration

Calcium gluconate infiltration is thought of as the more definitive treatment of choice for hydrofluoric acid skin burns (10,14). If used appropriately, local calcium gluconate infiltration may provide excellent symptomatic relief and prevent serious tissue destruction (2).

After vigorous flooding of the involved area with water, ampules of 10% calcium gluconate should be diluted with physiologic saline solution to obtain a 5% concentration of calcium gluconate. This solution may be injected into the burned areas with a 25- or 27-gauge needle to bind the fluoride ions. The usual recommendation is that injections be limited to 0.5 mL per square centimeter of involved tissue (1,16,24). The administration of calcium gluconate in concentrations greater than 5% tends to produce severe irritation of the tissues, which may cause keloid development and scarring.

Because pain is an excellent indicator of the extent of tissue involvement, use of local anesthesia should be delayed until the calcium infiltrations are complete. When pain recurs after injection of calcium gluconate, it indicates that free fluoride ions are again present.

Despite the acceptance of local infiltration with calcium gluconate, several disadvantages have been noted with this technique, especially when treating the digits: (a) the injections may be very painful, requiring block anesthesia; (b) vascular compromise may result from infiltration of too much fluid and may promote tissue necrosis; (c) local hyperosmolarity and inherent toxicity of calcium to skin cell may promote more tissue damage; (d) limited amounts of calcium can be delivered to the tissue—0.5 mL of 10% calcium gluconate contains 4.2 mg of elemental calcium which can neutralize only 0.025 mL of 20% hydrofluoric acid; and (e) removal of the nail is often required when subungual tissue is involved (15).

The overwhelming clinical experience to date has been with calcium gluconate, and it is the agent of choice. The infiltration of calcium chloride may cause tissue necrosis, and its use is not recommended.

Intra-arterial Infusion of Calcium Gluconate

Combined therapy with topical and subcutaneous calcium gluconate is generally effective. However, intra-arterial therapy may be of value in certain circumstances, particularly severe digital burns, which may be inadequately treated with gel and injections because of limited penetration and volume restrictions (18).

The intra-arterial technique varies among reports but it generally consists of identifying the arterial supply to the injured area and placing an intra-arterial catheter in the appropriate vascular supply in close proximity to the lesion (e.g., radial, ulnar, or brachial artery); Dilute solution of calcium salts may then be infused over 4 hours. The solutions used have been either 10 mL solution of 10% calcium gluconate or calcium chloride mixed in 40 to 50 mL of 5% dextrose and repeated if pain returned within 4 hours, or 10 mL of 20% calcium gluconate in 40 mL of normal saline for radial or ulnar artery infusion, and 20 mL of 20% calcium gluconate in 80 mL of normal saline for brachial artery infusion and repeated at 12-hour intervals if needed. The sooner the therapy is begun, the better the response obtained.

If the burn is of suitable size, such as to a limb, hand, or foot, then an intra-arterial infusion of calcium gluconate should be considered (25). If the burn is to the hand, the infusion can be performed through the radial artery with the aid of digital subtraction if the patient is able to cooperate (16). This has been shown to be of considerable benefit in significant exposures in that much greater amounts of calcium gluconate can be administered, which may then offset local calcium deficits and bind remaining fluoride ion (26). The efficacy of this method is difficult to determine because adequate controls have not been present. In general, however, pain relief is achieved and most patients require more than one treatment to maintain relief.

Intra-arterial therapy appears to be quite effective and may be most suitable for digital burns because it provides the best calcium ion delivery and avoids the prolonged morbidity associated with fingernail removal. It also allows delivery of higher doses of calcium in a more uniform manner to the tissues. However, the invasive nature and high cost of intra-arterial infusion, as well as the necessity for specialized equipment and personnel, warrant its use only in certain circumstances when more conventional therapy has failed. It requires more time, resources, and expense, such as monitoring of serum calcium, an infusion pump, and probable hospital admission for repeated infusions. Precise guidelines do not exist, but consideration should be given to the use of intra-arterial therapy if no improvement is noted after several hours of topical and subcutaneous treatment (18). This technique has not been proved to be superior to local infiltration, and it should be reserved for use on severe distal extremity burns and by those who are comfortable with the technique and have considerable experience in the evaluation and treatment of these burns.

Systemic Treatment

Systemic therapy for the severely burned patient is generally supportive and includes maintenance of electrolyte balance, careful monitoring for signs of renal or hepatic toxicity, and maintenance of respiratory and cardiac function. Intravenous therapy should be initiated as soon as possible, and the electrocardiogram should be monitored continuously for evidence of hypocalcemia. The results of frequent electrolyte monitoring or clinical signs of hypocalcemia may indicate the need for intravenous calcium or magnesium (or both). Profound hypocalcemia may occur in the absence of clinical tetany. Observation should be continued for 24 to 48 hours.

Hypocalcemia should be anticipated in significant exposures, whether by skin, ingestion, or inhalation, and corrected with 10% intravenous calcium gluconate. Serial serum calcium measurements should be obtained for the duration of the intoxication. Systemic fluorosis can be a concern with any significant exposure. EKG changes, such as Q-T prolongation, may provide valuable evidence of hypocalcemia (17).

Correcting systemic acidosis with sodium bicarbonate to near normal seems logical and should be guided by arterial blood gas measurements. Mild alkalosis may be beneficial in acute fluoride toxicity.

Cardiac arrhythmias may occur secondary to electrolyte imbalance, acidosis, or hypoxia, and the underlying cause should be identified and corrected. Fluoride-induced hyperkalemia may play a significant role in producing arrhythmias. Dialysis may be required to remove the excess serum potassium and fluoride. Hypotension should be managed with volume expansion and vasopressors, if needed.

REFERENCES

1. Adam J, Birck H: Pediatric caustic ingestion. *Ann Otol Rhinol Laryngol* 1982;91:656–658.
2. Ashcraft K, Padula R: The effect of dilute corrosives on the esophagus. *Pediatrics* 1974;53:226–232.
3. Edmonson M: Caustic alkali ingestions by farm children. *Pediatrics* 1987;79:413–416.
4. Skiendzielewski J: Cement burns. *Ann Emerg Med* 1980;9:316–318.
5. Chick L, Borah G: Calcium carbonate gel therapy for hydrofluoric acid burns of the hand. *Plast Reconstruct Surg* 1990;86:935–940.
6. Stremski E, Grande G, Ling L: Survival following hydrofluoric acid ingestion. *Ann Emerg Med* 1992;21:1396–1399.
7. Early S, Simpson R: Caustic burns from contact with wet cement. *JAMA* 1985;254:528–529.
8. Mercurius-Taylor L, Jayaraj A, Clark C: Is chronic detergent ingestion harmful to the gut? *Br J Indust Med* 1984;40:279–281.
9. Scharph L, Hill I, Kelly R: Relative eye-injury potential of heavy-duty phosphate and non-phosphate laundry detergents. *Food Cosmet Toxicol* 1972;10:829–837.
10. Kirchner S, Buckspan G, O'Neill J, et al: Detergent enema: a cause of caustic colitis. *Pediatr Radiol* 1977;6:141–146.
11. Burrington J: Clinitest burns of the esophagus. *Ann Thorac Surg* 1975;20:401–404.
12. Mofenson H, Greensher H, Caraccio T, et al: Ingestion of small Rat disc batteries. *Ann Emerg Med* 1983;12:88–90.
13. Conway E, Sockolow R: Hydrofluoric acid burn in a child. *Pediatr Emerg Care* 1991;7:345–347.
14. Lacouture P, Gaudreault P, Lovejoy F: Clinitest tablet ingestion: an in vitro investigation concerned with initial emergency management. *Ann Emerg Med* 1986;15:143–146.
15. Caravati E: Acute hydrofluoric acid exposure. *Am J Emerg Med* 1988;6:143–150.
16. O'Conner H, Grant A, Axon A, et al: Fatal accidental ingestion of Clinitest in an adult. *J R Soc Med* 1984;77:963–965.
17. Bertolini J: Hydrofluoric acid: a review of toxicity. *J Emerg Med* 1992;10:163–168.
18. Mistry D, Wainwright D: Hydrofluoric acid burns. *Am Fam Physician* 1992;45:1748–1754.
19. Kulig K, Rumack C, Rumack B, et al: Disc battery ingestion. *JAMA* 1983;249:2502–2504.
20. Temple D, McNeese M: Hazards of battery ingestion. *Pediatrics* 1983;71:100–103.
21. Saadi M, Hall A, Hall P, et al: Hydrofluoric acid dermal exposure. *Vet Hum Toxicol* 1989;31:243–246.
22. Levine D, Surawicz C: Severe intestinal damage following acid ingestion with minimal findings on early endoscopy. *Gastrointest Endosc* 1984;30:247–249.
23. Levine M, Jacob H, Rubin M: Battery ingestion: a potential form of alkaline injury to the gastrointestinal tract. *Ann Emerg Med* 1984;13:143–145.
24. Yasui T: Hazardous effects due to alkaline button battery ingestion: an experimental study. *Ann Emerg Med* 1986;15:910–916.
25. Litovitz T: Button battery ingestions. *JAMA* 1983;249:2495–2500.
26. Litovitz T: Battery ingestions: product accessibility and clinical course. *Pediatrics* 1985;75:469–476.

ADDITIONAL SELECTED REFERENCES

Davis L, Raffensperger J, Novak G: Necrosis of the stomach secondary to ingestion of corrosive agents. *Chest* 1972;62:48–51.

Ellis E, Brouhard B, Lynch R, et al: Effects of hemodialysis and dimercaprol in acute dichromate poisoning. *J Toxicol Clin Toxicol* 1982;19:249–258.

Fitzpatrick K, Moylan J: Emergency care of chemical burns. *Postgrad Med J* 1985;78:189–194.

Hardin J: Caustic burns of the esophagus. *Am J Surg* 1956;91:742–748.

Michel L, Grillo H, Malt R: Esophageal perforation. *Ann Thorac Surg* 1982;33:202–210.

Oakes D, Sherck J, Mark J: Lye ingestion. *J Thorac Cardiovasc Surg* 1982;83:194–204.

Okonek S, Bierbach H, Atzpodien W: Unexpected metabolic acidosis in severe lye poisoning. *Clin Toxicol* 1981;18:225–230.

CHAPTER 29

Alkaline Batteries

Alkaline disk batteries are used to power watches, cameras, games, computers, calculators, and hearing aids. Although ingestion of small batteries was seldom reported in the late 1970s, with the trend toward electronic miniaturization, ingestion of miniature or "button batteries" is now frequent (1,2). Easy access to the button batteries in these electronic devices and careless disposal of used batteries in the home have led to a rising incidence of their ingestion in children. Hearing aid batteries are ingested to a great extent, apparently due to the large supply in the homes of hearing aid users, due to the limited life span of the hearing aid battery (1,3). People have intentionally ingested button batteries to harm themselves and accidentally while attempting to "test" the battery under the tongue. However, the vast majority of button battery ingestions occur when curious children explore their environment. Although the age distribution of battery ingestors is predominantly pediatric, no age group appears to be exempt from accidental battery ingestion (4).

Button batteries are formed by compacting metals and metal oxides on either side of an electrolyte-soaked separator (Fig. 29–1) (5). The metal undergoes oxidation on one side of the electrolyte-soaked separator while the metal oxide is reduced to the metal on the other side (6–8). This reaction produces a current when a conductive path is provided. In an ingestion, a small percentage of batteries may spontaneously leak electrolyte solution. In addition to causing the production of NaOH, this local current also allows the button battery to contribute to its own dissolution (9). In any battery, the maximum current density occurs at the point where the anode and cathode come closest together. This occurs at the seal in button batteries. When the battery is in an acid environment, electrochemical reactions occur that lead to dissolution of the cathode, primarily in the crimp area, or the area of the seal. This tends to promote disassembly of the button battery with the subsequent release of the contents. In a neutral or alkaline environment, the reactions proceed at a much slower pace and act to deposit oxides in the crimp area.

It has become increasingly clear that it is not necessary for the battery to "leak" alkali to cause mucosal damage. It has been demonstrated that button batteries enclosed in a double capsule to prevent leakage of alkali produce the same degree of necrosis as regular unenclosed button batteries. This is because when a battery encounters any type of liquid in the gastrointestinal tract (GIT), it generates an electrical current and electrolysis is produced. The hydrogen ion produced escapes as gas, and progressive loss of hydrogen ions results in local alkalosis. The hydroxyl ion combines with dissolved sodium ion to form sodium hydroxide, which accumulates at the anode region of the battery to produce liquefaction necrosis identical in appearance to that produced by leakage of alkali from a disrupted battery (10).

In addition to electrolysis, pressure necrosis may occur if the battery is lodged in the GIT. Fatalities have resulted when the battery was wedged in the esophagus at the thoracic inlet with resulting esophageal perforation (11).

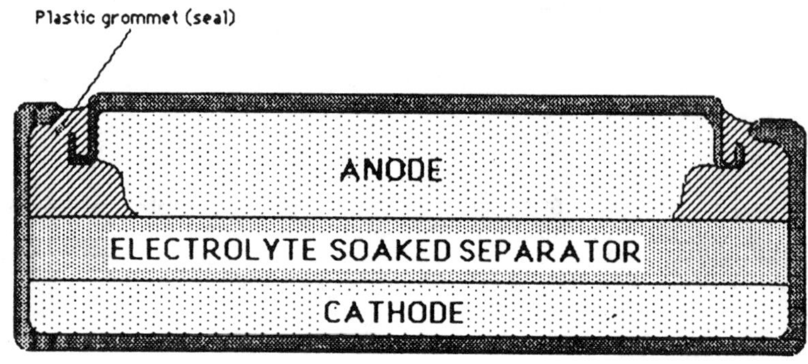

FIG. 29-1. This drawing represents a cross-section of a typical button battery. The metal casing serves to hold the battery together while allowing for a flow of electrons. The plastic grommet acts to seal the contents of the battery inside, anchors the cathode and anode together, and electrically insulates the anode from the cathode.

There are three mechanisms by which a button battery can cause injury. The first is the liquefaction necrosis that results directly from the leakage of the battery in the GIT. The second mechanism of injury is an electrochemical burn that may result from a direct current of the battery during the process called electrolysis. A third mechanism by which button batteries can be harmful is toxicity from absorption of the heavy metal itself.

There are many chemicals in alkaline batteries. Their major ingredients are alkalis such as sodium or potassium hydroxide, and their ingestion results in delivery of caustic material to the gastrointestinal tract without obvious accompanying oropharyngeal lesions. Toxicity of the battery depends on leakage from its casing, duration of contact with the mucosa, location in the gastrointestinal tract, and inherent toxicity of the chemicals.

HEAVY METAL TOXICITY AND BUTTON BATTERIES

The batteries currently available consist of various substances including a heavy metal salt and an alkali. The major forms of mercury in these batteries are mercuric oxide and elemental mercury (Table 29–1). Silver oxide, manganese dioxide, zinc oxide, or lithium hydroxide are among the other metallic salts commonly present. These metals may be systemically absorbed. A typical button battery may contain from 15% to 50% mercuric oxide leading to a possible ingestion of up to 5 g mercury, an amount known to be lethal (5).

The possibility of heavy metal poisoning, especially from mercury has been the subject of speculation. However, this theoretical threat of toxicity from mercury poisoning has not been borne out by clinical experience (5). The majority of ingested mercuric oxide batteries do not cause elevation of mercury levels or signs of mercury toxicity. This may be because mercuric oxide is reduced to insoluble metallic mercury in a discharged battery and because mercuric oxide is converted into elemental mercury in the presence of gastric acid and iron from the battery casing.

TABLE 29–1. *Heavy metals and batteries*

Item	Heavy metal
Calculator battery	Silver Mercury
Camera battery	Manganese Mercury
Computer game battery	Mercury Silver
Hearing aid battery	Mercury Silver Zinc
Watch battery	Lithium Mercury Silver

Other materials found in button batteries have not been well studied. Lithium is present in button batteries in the form of lithium hydroxide. There are no data on the amount and bioavailability of this form of lithium. Cadmium exerts its toxicity mainly by inhalation and is probably not a cause for concern in button battery ingestions. The small amount of zinc present in a button battery is unlikely to cause problems

SYMPTOMS

Button batteries do not cause problems unless they become lodged in the GIT. The likelihood that a button battery will lodge in the esophagus is a function of the size of the battery as well as of the age of the patient. A button battery that traverses the esophagus is very unlikely to lodge at any other location.

Button batteries range in size from 6 to 23 mm in diameter. Almost all of the batteries (96%) are small (7.9–11.6 mm in diameter). Larger batteries, greater than 15 mm in diameter, account for less than 3% of reported cases. Batteries larger than 18 mm in diameter are likely to be caught in the esophagus (12) yet large battery size does not necessarily lead to lodgment. There have been reports of 23-mm batteries that have traversed the esophagus and passed into the stomach (5).

HISTORY AND PHYSICAL EXAM

History should include time of ingestion; the presence of dysphasia, abdominal pain, or drooling in children should be noted.

Physical exam should address the vital signs and the presence of drooling, black flecks in the saliva, or abdominal guarding or tenderness (5). Children with battery lodgment in the esophagus typically present with refusal to take fluids, increased salivation, dysphagia, vomiting, and sometimes hematemesis.

Button batteries have been found outside of the GIT as well. The ear canal and nares have been reported as a site of impaction of button batteries. These sites should not be forgotten, and can be confirmed by a radiograph (13).

RADIOGRAPHIC EVALUATION

When a foreign body ingestion is suspected or witnessed, posteroanterior and lateral roentgenograms of the nasopharynx, chest, and abdomen are promptly required (6–8). In children with tracheoesophageal foreign bodies, it is important to distinguish between a coin and a button battery. Button batteries have a distinctive appearance on radiography with a "double density" on a posteroanterior

(PA) view and a "step off" at the junction of the cathode and anode, on a lateral view. Often on a PA view, a button battery is mistaken for a coin or an EKG lead on the chest, and only a lateral view on a radiograph will help to make the distinction (14). Radiographic evaluation will yield one of four groups of patients (4):

Group I—those with no evidence of a button battery
Group II—those with the battery in the esophagus
Group III—those with the battery in the stomach
Group IV—those with the battery lodged beyond the pylorus and duodenum.

An attempt should be made to identify the battery diameter and chemical system by determining the imprint code of a duplicate battery, by measuring the battery compartment within the product or battery instructions and packaging (7).

TREATMENT OF ALKALINE BATTERY INGESTION

Clinical experience indicates that in most cases of battery ingestion the battery is eventually passed through the gastrointestinal tract without incident. The degree of medical intervention remains a matter of judgment (Table 29–2). Most ingestions result in subclinical tissue damage as the battery moves through the digestive tract. Detection of impediment to a normal transit through the gastrointestinal tract or lodging of the battery in the esophagus are indications for prophylactic, aggressive removal.

Ipecac-induced emesis is usually unsuccessful in removing an ingested battery and should not be attempted (2,12,15). In addition, a complication of ipecac administration may occur, with incomplete retrograde movement of a battery leading to esophageal lodgment requiring emergent endoscopic retrieval. Other complications of ipecac-induced emesis may occur. Ipecac or other emetics could lead to perforation of the stomach or esophagus if the battery has already produced a full-thickness burn. Therefore, ipecac and any other emetic should be avoided in cases of button battery ingestion. Activated charcoal, which has been advocated as a marker, should not be administered because it may obscure examination of the stool (16).

When mercuric oxide cells are ingested, blood and urine mercury levels are necessary only if the cell is observed to split in the GIT or radiopaque droplets are evident in the gut. Chelation therapy need not be initiated in asymptomatic patients until toxic mercury levels are documented.

No clear differentiation of blood or urine mercury levels that are nontoxic, abnormal, symptomatic, or require chelation has been determined, especially following acute mercury exposure. However, population surveys demonstrate that 90% of adults have blood levels less than 2 to 4 μg/L and urine levels less than 10 to 20 μg/L. Symptoms are usually not evident with urine mercury levels less than 300 μg/L (17).

TABLE 29–2. *Treatment of battery ingestion*

Chest roentgenogram
Emesis (ineffective)
Activated charcoal (withhold)
Locate by roentgenogram
Esophagus, remove
Stomach, remove after 24 hours or observe until 24 hours
Respiratory tract, remove
Serial roentgenogram
Examination of stool for passage
Operative indications
Mediastinitis
Bowel perforation
Leakage of battery contents

Batteries in the Esophagus

A battery less than 18 mm in diameter (less than the size of a penny) is unlikely to be lodged in the esophagus (14). If the battery is in the esophagus or respiratory tract, immediate removal by endoscopy is indicated because there is a high risk of burns and perforation associated with esophageal lodgment (2,3,6–8,12). Burns due to esophageal lodgment have occurred as early as 4 hours after ingestion, and perforation has occurred as soon as 6 hours after ingestion (17). Attempts at blind retrieval either with the use of a Foley catheter or magnetized tube techniques are not recommended due to the necessity of direct inspection of the esophagus to determine the extent of injury and presence or absence of esophageal perforation (18). Endoscopy is the procedure of choice because it is the most effective technique and allows viewing of the extent of damage at the time of removal. If there is no mucosal damage, the ingestion may be treated as any other foreign body removed by esophagoscopy. The patient may be discharged after recovery from anesthesia or sedation.

Severe damage noted on endoscopy should lead to further diagnostic studies to rule out perforation or need for ICU monitoring. Esophageal lodgment is further implicated by the rapid development of symptoms such as dysphagia, vomiting, anorexia, and fever. If signs or symptoms suggesting esophageal or bowel perforation develop, operative intervention is recommended.

Batteries in the Stomach

Button batteries in the acid environment of the stomach are expected to undergo corrosive reactions that result in dissolution of the steel can, especially along the crimp area, or battery seal. When the cell passes to regions with neutral or slightly alkaline pH, the corrosive reactions are predicted to be slower, resulting in the formation of iron oxides and hydroxides instead. Not only is the reaction expected to be slower in the alkaline medium, but the oxides are expected to precipitate along the crimp area, possibly reducing or preventing further can dissolution or disassembly.

Endoscopy may also be performed to remove a battery in the stomach, or it may be allowed to pass through the pylorus. If the battery remains in the stomach for more than 24 hours, it should be removed (3). If a large button battery were ingested > 15 mm, x-rays may be obtained every 48 to 72 hours. If the battery appears to lodge in a diverticulum (2,7,19), surgical removal is also indicated. Spontaneous passage without morbidity may take as long as 7 days (12).

In theory, administration of cimetidine (Tagamet), antacids, or metoclopramide (Reglan) to minimize corrosion of the battery case by gastric acid may be of some additional value. Neither metoclopramide nor cimetidine lead to a significant slowing in battery dissolution in animals, although this has not been fully tested in humans. In addition, neither steroids nor antibiotics have a role in the treatment of button battery ingestions, including esophageal lodgment.

If the battery has passed beyond the esophagus, if the patient is asymptomatic, and if there is no radiologic evidence of leakage, the patient may be discharged with serial roentgenographic follow-up and with instructions to return to the hospital if fever, abdominal pain, vomiting, tarried or bloody stools, or decreased appetite ensue. Stools should also be checked for evidence of the battery.

REFERENCES

1. Wason S: The emergency management of caustic ingestions. *J Emerg Med* 1985;2:175–182.
2. Howell J: Alkaline ingestions. *Ann Emerg Med* 1986;15:820–825.
3. Mofenson H, Greensher H, Caraccio T, et al: Ingestion of small Rat disc batteries. *Ann Emerg Med* 1983;12:88–90.
4. Sarghouty N: Management of disc battery ingestion in children. *Br J Surg* 1991;78:247.
5. Kuhns D, Dire D: Button battery ingestions. *Ann Emerg Med* 1989; 18:293–300.
6. Litovitz T: Button battery ingestions. *JAMA* 1983;249:2495–2500.
7. Litovitz T: Battery ingestions: product accessibility and clinical course. *Pediatrics* 1985;75:469–476.
8. Litovitz T, Butterfield A, Holloway R, et al: Button battery ingestion: assessment of therapeutic modalities and battery discharge state. *J Pediatr* 1984;105:868–873.
9. Levine D, Surawicz C: Severe intestinal damage following acid ingestion with minimal findings on early endoscopy. *Gastrointest Endosc* 1984;30:247–249.
10. Friedman E: Caustic ingestions and foreign bodies in the aerodigestive tract of children. *Pediatr Clin North Am* 1989;36:1403–1409.
11. Levine M, Jacob H, Rubin M: Battery ingestion: a potential form of alkaline injury to the gastrointestinal tract. *Ann Emerg Med* 1984;13: 143–145.
12. Rumack B, Rumack C: Disc battery ingestion. *JAMA* 1983;249: 2509–2511.
13. Fosarelli P, Feigelman S, Pearson E, et al: An unusual intranasal foreign body. *Pediatr Emerg Care* 1988;4:117–118.
14. Wason S, Karkal S: Coping swiftly and effectively with caustic ingestions. *Emerg Med Rep* 1989;10:25–32.
15. Adam J, Birck H: Pediatric caustic ingestion. *Ann Otol Rhinol Laryngol* 1982;91:656–658.
16. Sheikh A: Button battery ingestions in children. *Pediatr Emerg Care* 1993;9:224–229.
17. Litovitz T, Schmitz B: Ingestion of cylindrical and button batteries: an analysis of 2382 cases. *Pediatrics* 1992;89:747–757.
18. Votteler T, Nash I, Rutledge J: The hazard of ingested alkaline disc batteries in children. *JAMA* 1983;249:2504–2506.
19. Lacouture P, Gaudreault P, Lovejoy F: Clinitest tablet ingestion: an in vitro investigation concerned with initial emergency management. *Ann Emerg Med* 1986;15:143–146.

ADDITIONAL SELECTED REFERENCES

Davis L, Raffensperger J, Novak G: Necrosis of the stomach secondary to ingestion of corrosive agents. *Chest* 1972;62:48–51.

Ellis E, Brouhard B, Lynch R, et al: Effects of hemodialysis and dimercaprol in acute dichromate poisoning. *J Toxicol Clin Toxicol* 1982;19:249–258.

Fitzpatrick K, Moylan J: Emergency care of chemical burns. *Postgrad Med J* 1985;78:189–194.

Hardin J: Caustic burns of the esophagus. *Am J Surg* 1956;91:742–748.

Michel L, Grillo H, Malt R: Esophageal perforation. *Ann Thorac Surg* 1982;33:202–210.

Oakes D, Sherck J, Mark J: Lye ingestion. *J Thorac Cardiovasc Surg* 1982; 83:194–204.

Okonek S, Bierbach H, Atzpodien W: Unexpected metabolic acidosis in severe lye poisoning. *Clin Toxicol* 1981;18: 225–230.

CHAPTER 30

Oxidizing Agents

The agents discussed in this chapter have in common their ability to cause local effects resembling a chemical burn as well as additional systemic effects. These agents consist of oxidizing agents such as the dichromates, hypochlorites and bleach, potassium permanganate, and hydrogen peroxide (Table 30–1). These agents produce damage because they become oxidized when in contact with body tissue, which often releases a toxic moiety.

DICHROMATES

Dichromate salts of sodium, potassium, and ammonium are water-soluble, crystalline substances that are highly corrosive to skin and mucosa (1). Accidental poisoning with dichromates is not uncommon, particularly in industrial settings (2).

Dichromates are derived from chromite ($FeCr_2O_4$), a chromium-containing ore (3). Potassium and sodium dichromate are strong oxidizing agents that exist in the hexavalent form but are highly reactive and spontaneously convert to the trivalent form in vivo (1,3). Although aqueous suspensions of dichromic acid salts are generally of intermediate pH, solutions containing dichromate may range in pH from 0.5 (chromic acid) to 13 (ammonium dichromate). Thus, the toxicity of dichromate-containing compounds may be attributed in part to their caustic potential as well as to the powerful oxidizing action of the hexavalent molecule (4).

TABLE 30–1. *Oxidizing agents*

Chlorinated lime
Chlorinated trisodium phosphate
Dichromates
Hydrogen peroxide
Hypochlorites
Calcium
Magnesium
Potassium
Sodium (bleach)
Javel water
Labarraque's solution
Potassium permanganate

Chromium is required in glucose and lipid metabolism, and the total body burden of chromium in a 70-kg person is less than 6 mg. In the trivalent state, chromium is strongly bound to plasma proteins. The metabolic effects of toxic amounts of chromium are not fully understood (3). Toxic tissue accumulation of chromium has been reported in kidney, liver, brain, spleen, lung, bone marrow, and muscle. The major excretory route for chromium is through the kidney (3), and approximately 60% is excreted through the kidneys within 8 hours after ingestion; elimination through the intestine and in breast milk may also occur.

Potassium dichromate (also called chromic acid, dichromic acid, potassium bichromate, chromium trioxide, and chromic oxide) is a common industrial and laboratory reagent. It is used in electroplating, aircraft building, ship building, dye casting, metal cleaning, and tanning (3). A pungent yellow liquid, it is a powerful oxidizing agent and is explosive when it comes in contact with small quantities of alcohol, ether, glycerin, and other organic substances (5). Potassium dichromate is dangerous because of its oxidizing potency, not its acidity. As little as 0.5 to 1 g is considered a lethal dose.

Sodium dichromate is also extremely toxic, with an estimated oral lethal dose between 1 to 10 g in an adult. Fatalities often result from poisonings with this compound as well as with potassium dichromate despite various therapies (3).

Ammonium dichromate is used in pyrotechnics, photography, and dyeing, in the glass-making and tanning industries, and in photoengraving (6). Ammonium dichromate is a powerful irritant when it comes in contact with the skin. When the skin is broken and frequent contact is established, chronic chromic sores or ulcers develop. Deaths from ammonium dichromate are unusual; reports of fatalities primarily involve sodium and potassium dichromate.

Manifestations of Dichromate Exposure

Manifestations of oral dichromate poisoning are immediate and include oral burns, nausea, vomiting, diarrhea,

TABLE 30–2. *Toxic effects of dichromates*

Gastrointestinal
Caustic burns
Nausea
Vomiting
Diarrhea
Gastrointestinal hemorrhage
Esophageal necrosis
Hematologic
Thrombocytopenia
Intravascular hemolysis
Hemorrhage
Neurologic
Vertigo
Coma
Myalgia
Inhalation
Rhinitis
Nasal septum perforation
Bronchitis
Miscellaneous
Methemoglobinemia
Liver damage
Renal damage
Peripheral vascular collapse

gastrointestinal hemorrhage, esophageal and gastric necrosis, and shock (Table 30–2) (5). Renal failure due to tubular damage, with glycosuria and gross and microscopic hematuria, may also be noted. In addition, thrombocytopenia, intravascular hemolysis, and hemorrhagic diathesis have been seen as well as toxic hepatitis and encephalopathy.

Contact with chromium and its salts may cause diffuse dermatitis in hypersensitive individuals and can also cause deep perforating ulcers known as "chrome holes." Protein coagulation with ulcer and blister formation occurs after cutaneous contact. If inhaled, chromic dusts cause rhinitis and ulcers of the nasal septum and may also cause bronchitis, gastritis, and other inflammatory conditions. Peripheral vascular collapse, vertigo, muscle cramps, coma, and liver damage have also been reported. The dichromates may cause methemoglobinemia because they oxidize hemoglobin to methemoglobin (2).

Morbidity and mortality rates in dichromate poisoning appear to be biphasic, with early multisystem involvement leading to shock and death. If the patient survives the initial phase, hepatic and renal failure may occur 8 to 10 days after ingestion (3).

Treatment

Treatment for dichromate poisoning should center on early supportive measures. Dialysis may be warranted when renal failure occurs, but because it does not remove large quantities of chromium it is ineffective in the treatment of systemic dichromate toxicity (3). Various agents have been suggested for the treatment of dichromate poisoning (1), including dimercaprol and other chelating agents, but their efficacy has not been shown.

HYPOCHLORITES

Hypochlorite salts (sodium, potassium, calcium, and magnesium) serve as bleaches, disinfectants, deodorizers, and water purifiers (7). Dilute hypochlorites are found in almost every home in the form of laundry bleach (such as Clorox), which is usually about 5% sodium hypochlorite. Ingestion of household bleach may include mild mucosal burns and edema, but extensive necrosis and stricture formation do not usually occur, although rare cases have been reported. Products intended for industrial use may have much higher hypochlorite concentrations, but in these products the active ingredient is usually calcium hypochlorite.

Hypochlorite toxicity arises from the material's corrosive activity on skin and mucous membranes (8). This corrosiveness stems from the oxidizing potency of the hypochlorite ion, which is measured in terms of available chlorine (5). The effects of ingested hypochlorite are related to concentration rather than dose. Solutions with 4% to 6% available chlorine, such as Clorox, are not usually seriously toxic. Higher concentrations, as found in commercially available solutions of hypochlorite, are more dangerous because the free chlorine that is released coagulates cutaneous proteins as well as the protein of mucous membranes. Ingestion of these stronger compounds often leads to esophageal stricture as a late complication.

Other available hypochlorite solutions may be more dangerous because of other toxic ingredients. Some of these more dangerous hypochlorite solutions are Labarraque's solution, which in addition to sodium hypochlorite, also contains sodium hydroxide or carbonate; chlorinated trisodium phosphate, which is best described as phosphate-buffered sodium hypochlorite; Javel Water, which, in addition to potassium hypochlorite, contains an unspecified amount of potassium hydroxide; calcium hypochlorite; chlorinated lime; and chloramine T.

HOUSEHOLD BLEACH

The risk of significant esophageal injury after ingestion of household bleach is low. Typically, erythema is the only problem. Immediate dilution is therefore the only therapy required in most cases (9). Because of the extremely low incidence of stricture formation, the decision to perform endoscopy after a bleach ingestion should be made on clinical grounds (10). Symptomatic patients with pain on swallowing, shortness of breath, significant oropharyngeal burns, or chest pain should undergo endoscopy (11,12).

TABLE 30–3. *Symptoms of potassium permanganate intoxication*

Burning of the throat
Nausea and vomiting
Dysphagia
Hematochezia
Hepatic dysfunction
Renal impairment
Circulatory collapse

There are many drug users in the U.S. who share needles and syringes with others, which is a known risk behavior for human immunodeficiency virus (HIV) infection. Many advocate the use of household bleach to clean the injection equipment of this group. Thus, there probably will be increasing instances of intravenous injections of hypochlorites (13).

POTASSIUM PERMANGANATE

Poisoning by ingestion of potassium permanganate is rare and generally occurs mainly in infants or as a result of a suicide attempt (14). Potassium permanganate is a powerful oxidizing agent that is used as an abortifacient, a topical astringent, and an antiseptic agent in aqueous solution. Deaths have resulted from the use of solutions as douches in attempted abortions. As an astringent, it is diluted 1:500 to 1:10,000. Dilute solutions (1% to 3%) may be only mildly irritating, and the patient may experience burning in the throat, nausea, vomiting, moderate gastroenteritis, and some difficulty in swallowing (Table 30–3) (14,15). Concentrated solutions or the dry crystals are highly corrosive. In addition, concentrated solutions (8%) may result in some renal toxicity, hematochezia, hepatic dysfunction, and circulatory collapse. Because the material is poorly absorbed, systemic effects are typically not of great concern (5). If absorption does occur, delayed neurologic and gastrointestinal effects may be noted. Treatment consists of careful observation and supportive care.

HYDROGEN PEROXIDE

Hydrogen peroxide is a colorless, odorless, clear liquid that is acidic to taste and to litmus paper. The pH of a 1% solution is 5–6. It is soluble in water and alcohol. The primary toxicity of hydrogen peroxide results from its interaction with catalase, which liberates water and oxygen on contact with organic tissue, some metals, and alkaline solutions. It acts as an oxidizing agent that produces its antimicrobial effect.

Use

Hydrogen peroxide is a medicinal primarily used for its antimicrobial effects and is a fairly common household product. A 3% solution is available over the counter and is used as a disinfectant and deodorant. Other common household and medicinal applications include its use for ear wax removal, as a gargle for stomatitis, vaginal douches, enemas for fecal impaction, and hair bleaching. Highly concentrated technical grades (27% to 90%) are used commercially to bleach, cleanse, or deodorize textiles, wool, fur, and paper. Hydrogen peroxide in the concentrated form is also used in the production of rocket fuel and foam rubber and also in the electroplating industry. Concentrated hydrogen peroxide also is promoted as a health aide to be used in "hyperoxygen" therapy. Industrial strength hydrogen peroxide has been promoted illegally to treat AIDS, cancer, and more than 60 other conditions. It is sold as "35% Food Grade HP" for use in "Hyper-oxygenation Therapy" (9). Distributors purchase the liquid in bulk form from chemical plants in Texas and Mexico; they then repackage it into pint, quart, and gallon containers. The product, sometimes called Biowater and H_2O_2, can be purchased by mail order distributors (16).

A 35% solution contains 35% hydrogen peroxide in an aqueous solution with a stabilizing agent. One milliliter of hydrogen peroxide solution can release about 115 mL of oxygen. High concentrations of hydrogen peroxide are caustic to the skin and mucous membranes and can result in a white eschar (17).

Toxicity

The more common route of exposure is by ingestion, followed by dermal and ocular exposures. The rare routes of exposure include inhalation, parenteral, and rectal, and many times these routes of exposure involve patients with psychiatric problems (9). There have been reports of fatal ingestion with high concentrations of hydrogen peroxide in children (18). In these cases, death usually was caused by respiratory complications. Ingestion of high-concentration hydrogen peroxide in adults usually is not fatal but often requires hospitalization.

Ingestions of household strength peroxides (3% to 9%) cause no significant effects. It is mildly irritating to the mucous membranes resulting in spontaneous emesis or mild abdominal bloating, yet this concentration (3%) of hydrogen peroxide has caused gas embolism to the portal venous system. Small bowel perforation, coma, and respiratory distress have been attributed to gas embolism after irrigation of wound with hydrogen peroxide (19). Ingestions of industrial strength (>10), on the other hand, can result in severe burns of the oropharynx and gastrointestinal tract. There is also the potential for rupture of the hollow viscus secondary to the liberation of oxygen, and cases of rupture of the colon, proctitis, and ulcerative colitis have been reported following hydrogen peroxide enemas (20).

REFERENCES

1. Behari J, Tandon S: Chelation in metal intoxication: part VIII: removal of chromium from organs of potassium chromate-administered rats. *Clin Toxicol* 1980;16:33–40.
2. Iserson K. Banner W, Froede R, et al: Failure of dialysis therapy in potassium dichromate poisoning. *J Emerg Med* 1983;1:143–149.
3. Ellis E, Brouhard B, Lynch R, et al: Effects of hemodialysis and dimercaprol in acute dichromate poisoning. *J Toxicol Clin Toxicol* 1982;19:249–258.
4. Kaufman D, Dinicola W, McIntosh R: Acute potassium dichromate poisoning. *Am J Dis Child* 1970;119:374–376.
5. Jelenko C: Chemicals that "burn." *J Trauma* 1974;14:65–72.
6. Reichelderfer T: Accidental death of an infant caused by ingestion of ammonium dichromate. *South Med J* 1968;61:96–97.
7. Hoy R: Accidental systemic exposure to sodium hypochlorite during hemodialysis. *Am J Hosp Pharmacol* 1981;38:1512–1514.
8. Hostynek J, Wilhelm K, Cua A, et al: Irritation factors of sodium hypochlorite solutions in human skin. *Contact Dermatitis* 1990;23: 316–324.
9. Hostynek J, Wilhelm K, Maibach C: Irritation factors of sodium hypochlorite solutions on human skin. *Contact Dermatitis* 1990;23: 316–324.
10. Landau G, Saunders W: The effect of chlorine bleach on the esophagus. *Arch Otolaryngol* 1964;80:174–176.
11. French R, Tabb H, Rutledge L: Esophageal stenosis produced by ingestion of bleach. *South Med J* 1970;63:1140–1144.
12. Howell J: Alkaline ingestions. *Ann Emerg Med* 1986;15:820–825.
13. Morgan D: Intravenous injection of household bleach. *Ann Emerg Med* 1992;21:1394–1395.
14. Holzgraefe M, Poser W, Kijewski H, et al: Chronic enteral poisoning caused by potassium permanganate. *Clin Toxicol* 1986;24:235–244.
15. Huntly A: Oral ingestion of potassium permanganate or aluminum acetate in two patients. *Arch Dermatol* 1984;120:1363–1365.
16. Luu T, Kelley M, Strauch J, et al: Portal vein gas embolism from hydrogen peroxide ingestion. *Ann Emerg Med* 1992;21:1391–1393.
17. Humberston C, Bean B, Krenzelok E: Ingestion of 35% hydrogen peroxide. *J Toxicol Clin Toxicol* 1990;28:95–100.
18. Giberson T, Kern J, Pettigrew D, et al: Near-fatal hydrogen peroxide ingestion. *Ann Emerg Med* 1989;18:778–779.
19. Christensen D, Faught W, Black R, et al: Fatal oxygen embolization after hydrogen peroxide ingestion. *Crit Care Med* 1992;20:543–544.
20. Bilotta J, Waye J: Hydrogen peroxide enteritis: the "snow white" sign. *Gastrointest Endosc* 1989;35:428–430.

ADDITIONAL SELECTED REFERENCES

Engberg A, Frodin L, Jonsson G: The use of dimethylsulfoxide in the treatment of interstitial cystitis. *Scand J Urol Nephrol* 1978;12:129–131.

Goodfellow R: Hydrofluoric acid burns. *Br Med J* 1985;290:937

Iverson R, Laub D, Madison M: Hydrofluoric acid burns. *Plast Reconstruct Surg* 1971;48:107–112.

Pike D. Peabody J, Davis E, et al: A re-evaluation of the dangers of Clorox ingestion. *J Pediatr* 1963;63:303–305.

Sperling S, Larsen I: Toxicity of dimethylsulfoxide (DMSO) to human corneal endothelium in vitro. *Acta Ophthalmol* 1979;57:891–898.

PART VI

GASES AND ABNORMAL HEMOGLOBIN FORMATION

CHAPTER 31

Inhalational Injuries

Innumerable chemicals are now present throughout the environment, and the potential exposure to a toxic agent occurs on a daily basis in today's society. The inhalation of various toxins can lead to a wide spectrum of illness, often with vague and inconsistent presentations. Although the acute exposure is frequently obvious, it can also be obscure, with little to suggest the occurrence of an inhalation exposure or the toxin involved. To further complicate the picture, an exposure need not involve just a single agent. For example, in an exposure to a fire there are various products of combustion, which often results in multiple hazards being encountered. Assorted combustibles, such as those containing synthetic polymers, can considerably increase the variety of toxins found in smoke, including hydrogen cyanide, hydrogen chloride, nitrogen dioxide, sulfur dioxide, ammonia, acrolein, and phosgene (1).

Health care personnel are typically inexperienced in the evaluation and treatment of inhalation exposures, with the exception of a few common toxic inhalations. Fortunately, the treatment of a toxic inhalation is only supportive in most cases. However, in others the quick administration of a specific antidote is essential for patient survival (2).

This chapter will discuss smoke inhalation, respiratory irritants, such as aldehydes, acrolein, formaldehyde, oxides of nitrogen, chlorine gas, chloramine gas, ammonia, phosgene, sulfur dioxide, and the treatment of an inhalational injury.

Mechanism of Injury

Despite the variable characteristics of these inhalational toxins and their varied presentations, injuries occur by two basic mechanisms: through regionalized pulmonary damage or by systemic absorption (3).

The pulmonary damage, which includes direct pulmonary injury and pulmonary sensitization, occurs most commonly after the inhalation of respiratory irritants and those agents that commonly induce immunologic reactions. Systemic toxicity occurs most commonly after the inhalation and absorption of asphyxiants, organophosphates, volatile hydrocarbons, and metal fumes.

Some inhalational exposures can result in both direct pulmonary and systemic injuries. Smoke inhalation, which refers to the inhalation of the products of combustion, typically includes both mechanisms of toxicity. The pulmonary injury also can be multifaceted, as there often are thermal lung injuries associated with the direct pulmonary irritant and chemical effects of the inhaled pathogens (4).

General Signs and Symptoms of Exposure

The signs and symptoms of exposure to respiratory irritants depend in large part on the specific agent's aqueous solubility.

Effect of Water Solubility

Highly water-soluble agents, such as ammonia, produce immediate irritation of eyes, nose, mouth, and upper airway. This property allows a good warning potential and, when possible, an avoidance of long exposures. When long exposures are unavoidable, the highly soluble agents can cause lower airway and alveolar effects, leading to more severe injury and even death.

Moderately water-soluble agents, such as chlorine, produce their main injuries on the lower airways, and generally have less warning properties when used in low concentrations. The lower-solubility agents, such as phosgene, produce their main injury at the alveolar level, often with a latent stage.

SMOKE INHALATION

Smoke inhalation is that injury to the airway and lungs resulting from the inhalation of combustion products that emanate from an active fire. Smoke is defined as the airborne products released by the thermal decomposition of material. Smoke consists of gases, volatilized organic molecules, free radicals, aerosols, and particles (3).

Smoke inhalation is now recognized as a major cause of increased morbidity and mortality in burn victims who incur it as an associated injury along with their skin burn. At the present time, smoke inhalation is the leading cause of death in burn victims, with a reported mortality ranging from 20%–80% (5).

TABLE 31–1. *Toxic products of smoke inhalation*

Acrolein
Wood
Cotton
Newspaper
Petroleum products
Aldehydes
Wood
Cotton
Newspaper
Ammonia
Melamine resins
Nylon
Silk
Wool
Benzene
Carbon dioxide
Carbon monoxide
Fires
Incomplete combustion of any fuel
Methylene chloride
Formaldehyde
Insulating material
Paper
Particleboard
Photochemical smog
Plastics
Plywood
Rubber
Textiles
Formic acid
Nitrocellulose film
Wood
Cotton
Newspaper
Petroleum products
Polyurethane
Melamine resins
Hydrogen chloride
Polyvinyl chloride
Polyester resins
Hydrogen cyanide
Polyurethane
Melamine resins
Plastics
Natural fibers
Nitrogen dioxide
Acetylene
Electric arc welding
Fabrics
Glass blowing
Nitrocellulose film
Phosgene
Polyvinyl chloride
Sulfur dioxide

Almost all materials when burned will generate toxic gases, the most common being carbon monoxide and carbon dioxide. Although carbon monoxide remains the most common toxic gas present in smoke from fires there are more than 25 toxic products of combustion that have been identified. Other gases may also be produced in toxicologically significant quantities, depending on the chemical structure of the burning material and the conditions present in the fire. Toxic compounds may include acrolein, benzene, hydrogen chloride, nitrogen dioxide, sulfur dioxide, and ammonia (Table 31–1) (6).

Most of the toxic compounds in smoke are rarely produced in concentrations that would be lethal by themselves. Rather than being primary causes of acute fire deaths, these combustion products could contribute to mortality by synergistic potentiation of the asphyxiant effects of the main smoke toxins, carbon monoxide and hydrogen cyanide (7).

Pathogenesis of Smoke Inhalation

Smoke inhalation injuries can be divided into three types. Asphyxia or obtundation syndrome is due to high levels of carbon monoxide and hydrogen cyanide or acute hypoxemia (6). In addition, upper airway injury may lead to airway obstruction. This is reliably diagnosed endoscopically and can be managed with early tracheal intubation. Finally, primary pulmonary parenchymal injury may occur due to smoke inhalation. This often leads to acute respiratory insufficiency, which is a major cause of morbidity and mortality in burn patients (8).

Smoke inhalation significantly alters normal respiratory physiology, resulting in a broad pattern of upper and lower airway injury. Respiratory epithelia may be damaged to the extent of complete necrosis, causing airway obstruction from shed epithelial cells forming pseudomembraneous casts. Smoke poisons cilia that line the trachea and small bronchioles. It induces bronchospasm and can cause hemorrhagic tracheal bronchitis in its severe form. It destroys alveolar macrophages, allowing bacteria to proliferate. Fibrin casts pose a significant threat to survival, as they may cause partial or complete respiratory obstruction.

Toxicity and Free Oxygen Radicals

Inhaled products of combustion are known to activate neutrophils, in part through the alternate pathway of the complement system, subsequently damaging pulmonary tissues through release of proteases and free oxygen radicals. Similarly, stimulation of pulmonary macrophages following respiratory tract injury produces prostanoids and cytokines that further contribute to the pathophysiology of inhalation injury and the morbidity and mortality of the host.

Some of the lung lesions result from the action of oxygen free radicals released from polymorphonuclear leukocytes marginating in the pulmonary microcirculation and tracheobronchial region. Peroxide and the hydroxyl ion have been implicated as mediators in the increased microvascular permeability, and consequently, pulmonary edema seen in inhalational injury.

Smoke destroys not only whatever surfactant is present in the lung, but also the alveolocyte that makes the surfactant. It is evident that smoke induces a capillary leak by causing changes in microvascular permeability. Such damage to the respiratory anatomy results in multiple complications, including upper airway edema, loss of compliance, atelectasis, interstitial edema, laryngotracheal bronchitis, pneumonia, and ultimately, respiratory failure (5).

Determinants of Toxicity

Many factors affect the inherent toxicity of an inhaled substance. Most important are the individual agent's underlying chemical activity, physiologic properties, such as particle size, and solubility. These physical properties help determine the level in the respiratory tract where the inhaled toxin will be deposited and its degree of systemic absorption.

Components of Smoke Inhalation

The different smoke components can be divided, with some overlap, into four categories: heat and thermal injury, particulate materials, systemic toxins, and respiratory irritants.

The water/lipid solubility ratio of the gases is a major determinant of their deleterious effects. Water-soluble gases, such as ammonia and hydrogen chloride, react with the water of the mucous membranes to produce strong acids and alkalis, resulting in an intense inflammatory reaction. Their most marked effect is at the earliest point of contact with the mucous membranes. On the other hand, oxides of nitrogen, aldehydes, and phosgene are toxic because of their solubility in the cellular membrane lipid fraction, and these agents exert their effects more slowly.

THERMAL INJURY

The damage to lung tissues following smoke inhalation is unlikely to be the result of thermal damage because the heat-carrying capacity of dry air is very low and the heat-dissipating capacity of the upper airways is very efficient. Although burns of the nasal and oropharyngeal mucosa are common in fire victims, thermal injury below the vocal cords is rarely seen because of the very efficient heat exchange in the upper air passages. Because of this, the temperature of inhaled heated dry air rapidly drops before the lower respiratory tract is reached.

PARTICULATE MATTER

In general, agents primarily causing upper airway injuries tend to be more irritating, more water soluble, and of a larger (>5 μm) particle size. Substances of a smaller (<5 μm) size and of lower water solubility are more likely to cause alveolar or parenchymal injury after inhalation (2).

Smoke particles consist mostly of carbon, which is chemically inert. However, inhalation of charcoal dust has been demonstrated to increase airway resistance in humans. More important, particles may be coated with irritating chemical substances, such as aldehydes and hydrogen chloride, and thus carry these irritants as far as the alveoli.

RESPIRATORY IRRITANTS

Combustion of commonly used structural materials or home furnishings produces a large number of respiratory irritants, such as aldehydes, halogen acids, phosgene, oxides of nitrogen, sulfur compounds, and ammonia.

Aldehydes and Acrolein

Aldehydes are among the most important of the lipid-soluble substances. They are produced in significant quantities when cellulose materials, such as wood, cotton, and paper, are burned.

The highly reactive aldehydes irritate mucous membranes. Accordingly, aldehyde gases have been incriminated as one of the causes of pulmonary edema in wood smoke inhalation. Aldehydes that reach the alveolar areas either in a gaseous form or bound to the surface of small particles may also affect the permeability of the alveolar capillary membrane.

Acrolein, a three-carbon aldehyde that is related to formaldehyde, is much more irritating than formaldehyde and has been shown to cause pulmonary edema and death. Acrolein is used in the manufacture of plastics, pharmaceuticals, synthetic fibers, resins, textiles, and herbicides. It is used in sewer treatment, and is a combustion product of cellulose products, including wood, paper, and cotton. Acrolein is a major contributor to the irritancy of cigarettes and photochemical smog. Acrolein is a clear yellow liquid with a pungent odor. It is a direct upper respiratory tract irritant with strong mucous membrane involvement, giving it excellent warning properties. Exposure is both by inhalation of vapors and by skin absorption.

Clinical manifestations include severe pulmonary irritation and intense lacrimation. High concentrations of the vapor can lead to pulmonary edema.

Formaldehyde

Formaldehyde, also known as formalin, methyl aldehyde, and methylene oxide, is a colorless gas that has a pungent irritating odor. It is ubiquitous in nature and presents widespread possibilities for exposure through its numerous commercial, medical, and industrial applications.

Formaldehyde-based resins are used in plywood, particleboard, insulating material, paper, plastics, textiles, and rubber products. It is used medically as an antiseptic, tissue fixative, embalming agent, and deodorant. It is used in agricultural products, pharmaceuticals, fumigants, and disinfectant production. Formaldehyde is also a combustion product of gas stoves and heaters and a contaminant of cigarette smoke and photochemical smog.

The potential for exposure in the home is primarily related to its use in urea-formaldehyde insulation and particleboard made with urea-formaldehyde resins. Chronic home exposure to such toxins should be considered in patients presenting with recurrent or unexplained respiratory symptoms.

Oxides of Nitrogen

Nitrogen dioxide is a reddish-brown gas that is heavier than air and has a pungent odor. The nitrogen oxides, including nitrogen dioxide and nitrogen tetroxide, are produced in the manufacture of dyes, fertilizers, and lacquer. They are formed in acetylene and electric arc welding and glass blowing. Oxides of nitrogen are produced in small quantities during thermal decomposition of fabrics and in larger quantities from cellulose nitrate and celluloid. Patients and fire fighters are at risk in chemical plant, nitrocellulose, and mattress fires. Farmers are at risk of "silo fillers' disease" when nitrogen oxides form from the oxidation of nitrogen-rich fertilizer that can adhere to crops within the first few hours to days of storage.

Apart from being a weak irritant of the upper airways, nitrogen dioxide is capable of reaching the bronchioles and alveoli. Nitrogen dioxide is a powerful oxidant. Traces of nitrogen dioxide have been reported to induce peroxidation of lung lipids with formation of highly destructive free radicals.

In addition, nitrogen dioxide hydrolyzes to nitrous and nitric acids. The nitrates and nitrites formed from the dissociation of these acids cause tissue damage in a dose-dependent fashion. Depending on the nitrogen dioxide concentration either a slight increase in lung capillary permeability or a profound chemical pneumonitis with frank alveolar edema ensues.

TABLE 31–2. *Toxicity of oxides of nitrogen*

Pulmonary
Acute bronchiolitis
Mucosal irritation
Bronchospasm
Dyspnea
Noncardiogenic pulmonary edema
Bronchiolitis obliterans
Chronic interstitial lung disease
Systemic
Hypotension
Methemoglobinemia
Cardiovascular depression

Toxicity of Oxides of Nitrogen

Pulmonary Toxicity

The pattern of toxicity from nitrogen dioxide has been described as triphasic. In the initial phase of acute bronchiolitis, mucosal irritation leads to symptoms of bronchospasm, dyspnea, vomiting, nausea, headache, and chest pain (Table 31–2). Symptoms can dissipate after a few hours but may persist for weeks, even when exposure was mild. This is followed by the delayed phase of noncardiac pulmonary edema occurring within a few to 36 hours. Although pulmonary edema may occur acutely, with lesser degrees of exposure it characteristically develops after a latent period of between several hours and one day. The third phase may develop weeks later and is characterized by bronchiolitis obliterans, a chronic interstitial lung disease.

Systemic Toxicity

In addition to the local pulmonary damage, the dissolution of nitrogen dioxide in body fluids may contribute to hypoxia, acidosis, and cardiovascular depression in smoke inhalation. Nitrous and nitric acids enhance acidosis. Methemoglobin is formed when nitrite ions react with hemoglobin. Additionally, nitric and nitrate ions induce systemic hypotension by direct action on the vascular smooth muscle.

HALOGEN ACIDS

Many formulations of the synthetic materials presently in use contain one of the halogens, which can react during combustion to form the corresponding halogen acid gases, hydrogen fluoride and hydrogen chloride.

Hydrogen Chloride

Hydrogen chloride is a typical example of a respiratory irritant whose action is usually confined to the upper airways but which is capable of producing pulmonary damage at the alveolar level with the formation of pulmonary edema if sufficient airway concentrations are present.

Chlorine Gas

Chlorine is a highly reactive greenish-yellowish gas, 2.5 times denser than air, with a distinctive, irritating odor. It is the most frequent cause of direct respiratory irritant injury. Chlorine gas was used as a chemical agent in World War I. Exposure now occurs both in industrial and nonindustrial settings and frequently involves more than one individual.

Chlorine gas inhalation injury is often the result of an industrial accident, which may lead to numerous simultaneous casualties. Small numbers of patients are injured from inhalation of chlorine used in the treatment of swimming pools or when household bleach containing hypochlorite is mixed with strong acids, releasing chlorine gas. Water dissolves approximately two times its volume of chlorine gas, forming a mixture of hydrochloric and hypochlorous acids.

Clinical Symptoms and Physical Examination

The duration and severity of symptoms varies directly with the concentration of chlorine gas and the duration of exposure. The threshold limit of exposure to chlorine gas is 1 ppm, and this can usually be tolerated for up to 8 hours.

Short exposures at 3–5 ppm are well tolerated. However, prolonged exposure at this level will produce symptoms. Major exposure may lead to a severe pneumonitis, pulmonary edema, and respiratory compromise.

Mechanism of Toxicity

Chlorine is corrosive because of its acidity and its oxidizing potential. The primary mechanism of injury is through the release of nascent oxygen when chlorine gas comes in contact with water on the mucous membranes of the patient. The oxygen free radicals as well as hydrochloric acid are all directly toxic to respiratory mucosa (9).

Clinical Manifestations

Chlorine gas acts as an irritant to mucous membranes, causing rhinorrhea and lacrimation (Table 31–3). In less severe exposure the patient may present with cough, chest pain, muscle weakness, headache, and a feeling of oropharyngeal dryness. Other clinical manifestations in mild exposure include conjunctival irritation, sore throat, chest burning, dyspnea, and nausea. Severe exposure can lead to severe tracheobronchitis, pulmonary edema, respiratory failure, severe cough, nausea, vomiting, dyspnea, and a burning sensation in the throat and substernal region (10).

TABLE 31–3. *Clinical manifestations of chlorine gas*

Pulmonary
Chest pain
Cough
Dyspnea
Pulmonary edema
Substernal burning
Tracheobronchitis
Miscellaneous
Conjunctival irritation
Lacrimation
Nausea
Rhinorrhea
Sore throat
Vomiting

Physical Examination and Laboratory Studies

Physical examination is usually normal, with decreased breath sounds being the most frequent finding. Bronchospasm is often present, but may be detectable only with early pulmonary function studies. Arterial blood gases may be normal, or may reveal hypoxia or metabolic acidosis in severe cases. Initial chest x-ray may demonstrate signs of pulmonary edema in severe exposure but is usually normal (11).

Pulmonary function studies have indicated both obstructive and restrictive disease following chlorine gas exposure. There is no conclusive evidence that these effects are long-term. Patients may complain of exercise intolerance for several days following exposure, even if they are asymptomatic at rest.

Pathologic changes include bronchial epithelium sloughing, ulcerative tracheobronchitis, purulent intraluminal exudate, hyaline membranes in the alveolar space, and interstitial and alveolar pulmonary edema (12).

Chloramine Gas

Mixing ammonia with household bleach preparations containing hypochlorite leads to the formation of chloramines. Monochloramine and dichloramine are soluble in water, and decompose to ammonia and hypochlorous acid. Chloramines are sometimes used as disinfectants in water purification. Exposure to the acrid fumes of chloramines produces lacrimation, irritation of membranes of the respiratory passages, and nausea (4).

Ammonia and Ammonium Hydroxide

Gaseous ammonia in its pure form was first isolated in 1790. Ammonia is produced as a by-product in the distillation of coal, by the action of steam on cyanamide, and by the catalytic combination of nitrogen and hydrogen gases at high temperature and pressure. It also results from the decomposition of nitrogenous materials, and is released in fires from the combustion of wool, silk, and nylon, but its concentration is low in most ordinary building fires. Because anhydrous ammonia is 82% nitrogen, it is a good fertilizer and thus is used extensively in agriculture. It is also used in the manufacturing of synthetic fibers, such as nylon and rayon, and in the dyeing and scouring of natural fibers. Oxidation of ammonia produces nitric acid, used in the production of trinitrotoluene, nitroglycerin, and other substances. Inhalation exposures are often the result of industrial or transportation accidents, as it is in widespread use as an industrial chemical. The ingestion of commercial strength ammonia solutions produces effects similar to ingestions of other corrosive alkalis. In addition, respiratory signs and symptoms should be anticipated after ingestion as a consequence of aspiration of the solution or inhalation of the vapors (8).

Ammonia is a colorless gas that is readily liquefied and is highly soluble in water, with which it combines to form ammonium hydroxide. Ammonium hydroxide in various concentrations is used in a number of products, such as cleaning agents, liniments, and aromatic spirits. It is also used extensively in refrigeration, petroleum refining, and the manufacturing of fertilizers, nitric acid, explosives, dyes, plastics, and other chemicals (Table 31–4). The strongest solution of ammonium hydroxide commonly available contains 28% ammonia. A 10% solution is also in common use, and so-called household ammonia ranges in concentration from 5% to 10% ammonia (13).

TABLE 31–4. Sources and uses of ammonia

Sources
Antirust agents
Aromatic spirits
Hair dyes
Jewelry cleaners
Metal cleaners
Toilet bowl cleaners
Window cleaners
Uses
Cleaning agents
Refrigeration
Petroleum refining
Manufacture of
Dyes
Explosives
Fertilizers
Nitric acid
Plastics

Pathophysiology of Injury

The pathophysiology of injury from ammonia gas exposure is secondary to the irritant and caustic effects of ammonium hydroxide, which is formed from the combination of the gas with water in the moisture of the mucosal membranes. Due to the high water solubility of ammonia gas this primarily occurs in the upper respiratory tract.

Ammonium hydroxide differs from other alkalis in its volatility. Because of this, the vapor, even in low concentrations, is extremely irritating to skin, eyes, and respiratory passages. Inhalation of ammonia in high concentrations has caused pulmonary edema. This is the most frequent cause of death after exposure to ammonia.

The severity of symptoms and tissue damage produced is related directly to the concentration of hydroxyl ions present. Three anatomic areas are most commonly involved: the skin, the respiratory system, and ocular structures (8).

Relationship Between Concentration and Clinical Effect

When long-term exposure to low concentrations occurs, the lungs efficiently absorb ammonia because of its high solubility in water. However, acute contact with high concentrations can produce rapid and severe changes in the pulmonary parenchyma. There is considerable degradation of collagen after inhalation of concentrated ammonia vapors, as evidenced by elevated urinary metabolites of hydroxylysine. This degradation is most likely that of respiratory structures.

A concentration of 100 ppm is usually tolerable for several hours; minor irritation of the eyes and mucosal surfaces may occur at 400–450 ppm; eye injuries are seen at 700 ppm; coughing and laryngospasm are noted at 1700 ppm, with edema of the glottic region seen within a few hours (Table 31–5). Concentrations of 2500–4500 ppm can be fatal in approximately 30 minutes; concentrations above 5000 ppm usually produce rapid respiratory arrest. Because of its lipophilic and hydrophobic properties, the epidermis is usually a good barrier to water-soluble substances. However, highly alkaline sub-

TABLE 31–5. *Relationship between ammonia concentration and clinical effect*

Parts per million	Clinical effect
100	Tolerable
400–450	Minor eye and mucosal irritation
700	Eye injury
1700	Cough, laryngospasm
2500–4500	Fatal in 30 min
5000	Rapid respiratory arrest

TABLE 31–6. *Effects of ammonia*

Respiratory
Cough
Hemoptysis
Pharyngitis
Laryngitis
Tracheobronchitis
Pulmonary edema
Bronchiectasis
Chronic bronchitis
Subatropic pharyngolaryngitis
Ocular—short-term
Lacrimation
Conjunctivitis
Palpebral edema
Blepharospasm
Photophobia
Corneal ulceration
Ocular—long-term
Iritis
Corneal opacification
Cataracts
Glaucoma
Retinal atrophy
Dermal
Partial-thickness burn

stances, such as ammonia, quickly saponify epidermal fats and breach the barrier to enter the more hydrophilic dermis.

Respiratory Effects

A mild insult to the respiratory system can produce cough and hemoptysis, as well as pharyngitis, laryngitis, and tracheobronchitis (Table 31–6). Severe injuries demonstrate fulminant pulmonary edema and bronchiectasis; 7–10 days after injury ulceration of the tracheobronchial mucosa and subsequent bronchospasm are often seen. In survivors of such exposures, late sequelae can include chronic bronchitis and subatropic pharyngolaryngitis.

As expected, pulmonary complications and sequelae are not uncommon. Although prolonged exposures to low concentrations may produce no acute problems, long-term sequelae are common. Some sequelae are often seen, even in patients who improved within the first few days after exposure. Late pulmonary sequelae may include hyperreactive bronchoconstriction and obstruction of residual central and peripheral airways. Fibrous obliteration of small airways has also been described. As with any chemical pneumonitis, bacterial infection is a great danger, and appropriate preventive measures should be taken (14).

Ocular Effects

Ocular injuries are also common in acute exposures, with permanent damage as a result of tissue destruction and large elevations in intraocular pressure. Mild ocular injuries can include increased lacrimation, conjunctivitis, palpebral edema, blepharospasm, and photophobia. More severe insults result in corneal ulceration and destruction.

Ocular sequelae reported include iritis, anterior and posterior synechiae, corneal opacification, cataracts, glaucoma, and retinal atrophy. Coagulopathy has been reported shortly after exposure.

Dermal Effects

Skin injuries can range from superficial to partial-thickness tissue loss. Lesser skin injuries appear as gray-yellow soft regions. Severe exposures result in black and leathery tissue. Anhydrous ammonia is usually stored at approximately –28°C, and exposure to such extreme temperatures produces thrombosis of surface vessels with subsequent ischemia and necrosis.

Examination

The initial physical examination of the chest may provide the best prognostic indicator; patients who are found to have a normal chest examination are often discharged within 24 hours (15).

Treatment

The most important stage of treatment of injuries from anhydrous ammonia is immediately after exposure and in the succeeding 24 hours. All clothing should be removed quickly, and prompt and vigorous irrigation with water should be started at the scene and continued for 15–20 minutes. This should be continued at regular intervals for the first 24 hours. Standard resuscitative measures should be taken if the total body surface involved is greater than 20%. The use of salves and greasy ointments should be discouraged because these seem to increase the depth of penetration of the chemicals. Nonviable tissue should be debrided early. Small full-thickness injuries may be excised and either closed primarily or skin grafted.

If the patient has significant facial or pharyngeal burns, early orotracheal or nasotracheal intubation should be considered because severe laryngeal edema will develop within 24 hours. Tracheostomy, despite its description in the management of this problem, should be avoided (14).

Phosgene

Phosgene is a pulmonary irritant that was once used as a war gas. It is a poorly soluble colorless gas that is slightly heavier than air, and has the odor of freshly mown hay or green corn at low concentrations and a pungent, mildly irritating odor at higher concentrations.

TABLE 31–7. *Sources of phosgene*

Fires and decomposition of
Arc welding
Carbon tetrachloride
Dry cleaning fluids
Methylene chloride
Organochlorine compounds
Paint removers
Solvents
Trichloroethylene

Phosgene, while not naturally occurring, has many industrial sources. Under special circumstances of intense heat, such as in a fire, some halogenated hydrocarbons, such as carbon tetrachloride, trichloroethylene, and methylene chloride, are able to decompose to phosgene (Table 31–7). These agents have produced serious toxicity and death. Phosgene is used in the manufacture of dyestuffs, insecticides, pharmaceuticals, and plastics. It is a decomposition product of arc welding and organochloride compounds and can be produced when common household substances, such as solvents, paint removers, or dry cleaning fluids are exposed to heat or fire.

Clinical Manifestations

Phosgene is poorly water soluble, so warning properties are poor and toxic levels may be reached prior to detection since phosgene is only mildly irritating to upper airway tissues. When inhaled it passes through to the deeper structures, hydrolyzing in mucosal water to form hydrochloric acid and carbon dioxide. This reaction occurs slowly, producing primarily alveolar injury. The pathologic action is multifactorial. The alveolar injury is through direct epithelial damage and necrosis of the small airways and capillary membranes. Even in potentially lethal exposures, the initial symptoms are mild and transient. The danger period is usually 6–24 hours after exposure with the development of peribronchial edema, pulmonary congestion, and alveolar edema, all leading to death from anoxia (8).

Phosgene also causes a sympathetic paralysis, inducing a vasoconstriction of pulmonary venules. This action causes an exacerbation of the alveolar injury and increased permeability, leading to hypovolemia, hemoconcentration, worsening pulmonary edema, and adult respiratory distress syndrome (15).

Sulfur Dioxide and Sulfuric Acid

Sulfur dioxide is a colorless irritating gas twice as heavy as air that has a characteristic pungent odor. Along with the nitrogen oxides it is a primary air pollutant and is a principal source of acid rain and photochemical smog. Sulfur dioxide, by virtue of its high water solubility, is primarily an upper respiratory tract irritant that produces sulfurous acid on contact with water. Sulfuric acid is also formed when inhaled sulfur dioxide is hydrated on the bronchial mucosa. Sulfuric acid is encountered in the manufacture of lead-acid batteries, fertilizers, acid pickling of steel products, and even in smog as the result of the combustion of fossil fuels (16).

Clinical manifestations include cough, sneezing, lacrimation, headache, vomiting, diarrhea, conjunctival erythema, and upper airway edema. Severe exposure can lead to upper airway obstruction, cyanosis, and pulmonary edema (17).

DIAGNOSIS OF INHALATIONAL INJURY

The majority of patients with inhalation injury after smoke inhalation do not show overt symptoms of wheezing or the production of copious amounts of carbonaceous sputum at the time of admission. In fact, these symptoms do not become apparent until 24–48 hours after injury (12).

History

The diagnosis of smoke inhalation is made essentially on history. The clinical history surrounding the events of the fire, obtained from patient and first responders is important (Table 31–8). As an example, one should ascertain whether the fire was in an enclosed space, whether there was the potential inhalation of noxious gases or smoke, the length of time the victim was in the structure prior to rescue, and whether the patient was unconscious or had cardiopulmonary resuscitation at the scene. Any patient with a history of being burned in a closed space should be assumed to have smoke inhalation injury until proven otherwise. In addition, any patient with flame burns or the acrid smell of smoke on the clothes should be suspected of having inhaled smoke.

TABLE 31–8. *History and physical for smoke inhalation*

History
Was fire in enclosed space?
Potential inhalation of smoke?
Length of exposure
History of loss of consciousness, seizure, decerebrate or decorticate?
Physical
Facial burns
Singed nasal hairs
Carbonaceous sputum
Wheezing
Rales
Intercostal retractions

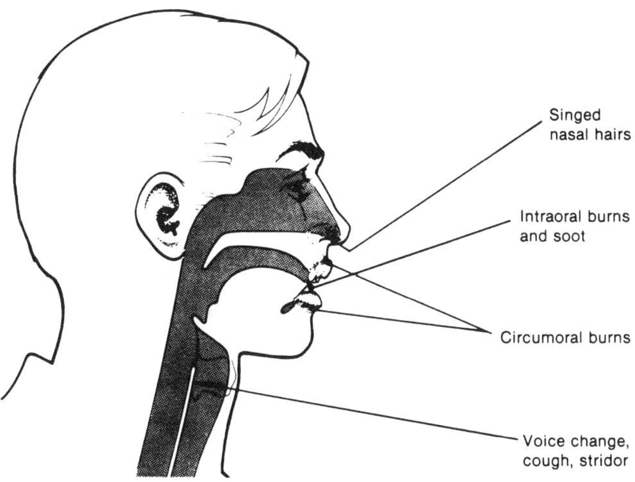

FIG 31–1. Physical findings suggestive of inhalation injury. Adapted with permission from Marion Laboratories, Inc.

Physical Examination

Physical findings may include burns of the face, lips, mouth, neck, and head; singed nasal hair and eyebrows; erythema; edema; ulceration in the mouth or pharynx; and carbonaceous sputum. Wheezing, hoarseness, rales, burned nasal mucosa, and sooty sputum are not of themselves reliable as early signs but are signs of serious involvement when present (Fig 31–1) (18,19). The location of the carbon in the tracheobronchial tree is important. When it is present above and below the vocal cords, the likelihood of small airway injury is greater than if carbon is found only in the pharynx. Less common physical signs are bronchorrhea, wheezing, hoarseness, and intercostal retractions. The admission chest film is usually normal (12).

A diagnosis of pulmonary parenchymal injury may be suspected with closed space injury, carbonaceous sputum, an elevated carboxyhemoglobin level, or in patients who lost consciousness at the scene of a fire. A normal carboxyhemoglobin level may not reliably suggest the degree of inhalation injury since most patients have inspired 100% oxygen for varying periods of time during transport to the hospital.

LABORATORY

Chest radiographs in the inhalation patient are usually initially clear since radiographic evidence lags behind the patient's condition and so is not a reliable indicator of the patient's status.

The insensitivity of chest roentgenograms and the unreliability of the clinical signs of inhalation injury necessitate use of other diagnostic techniques. The most easily performed reliable diagnostic modality is fiberoptic bronchoscopic examination of both the supra- and infraglottic airway to identify inflammatory changes and damage of the airway mucosa.

Fiberoptic bronchoscopy is considered the standard diagnostic technique used to diagnose smoke inhalation and pulmonary injury. It readily identifies airway edema and inflammation, mucosal necrosis, and the presence of soot and charring in the airway. It is helpful in determining the likelihood of upper airway obstruction due to tracheal edema and, therefore, the need for prophylactic intubation.

Due to progressive swelling in the upper airways, serial fiberoptic bronchoscopic examinations are recommended in the first 18–24 hours, and are useful for diagnosis of inhalation injury when used with other criteria (20). Bronchoscopy must be performed within the first 24 hours of injury to be helpful diagnostically because tracheal suction causes similar mucosal changes. The use of serial bronchoscopic findings identifies approximately twice as many patients with inhalation injury as compared to diagnosis based on clinical criteria alone (12).

Fiberoptic bronchoscopy can be performed in the emergency department to rule out upper airway injury. If no injury is noted, the patient can be admitted to a nonintensive care environment. There have been no complications associated with bronchoscopy, and it is considered a safe and useful diagnostic tool. Bronchoscopic evidence of inhalation injury includes mucosal edema, erythema, ulceration, and carbonaceous material.

Bronchoscopic examination may also fail to detect injury caused by the inhalation of a finely particulate aerosol since the site of airway deposition of particles with a mass median diameter of less than 5 μm is principally in the terminal bronchioles and pulmonary parenchyma. While only the upper airways can be evaluated by fiberoptic bronchoscopy, air trapping from small airway obstruction can be identified by xenon-133 scanning. This technique, however, has not become widely available.

Although xenon perfusion and ventilation tests have been used, they are expensive, they involve moving a sick patient to the nuclear medicine department, and they may give false positive results in patients with previous pulmonary pathology.

The arterial blood gases should be drawn early, although they may not deteriorate for 12–24 hours after exposure. Serial arterial blood gases can be monitored to maintain adequate oxygenation and to correct acid-base problems.

TABLE 31–9. *Laboratory determinations in smoke inhalation*

Chest roentgenography
Arterial blood gas test
Fiberoptic bronchoscopy
Xenon ventilation/perfusion scan

Although fiberoptic bronchoscopy and xenon scanning have improved diagnostic accuracy of inhalation injuries, emergency department diagnosis depends on a high index of suspicion, a suggestive history, careful examination of the upper airway, the presence of clinical symptoms, and suggestive arterial blood gases (Table 31–9).

TREATMENT OF INHALATIONAL INJURY

The early management of inhalation injury must begin before confirmation of the diagnosis. Regardless of the agent of exposure, withdrawal from exposure and removal of contaminated clothing should be coincident with institution of the basic ABCs of resuscitation.

The treatment of inhalation injury is guided by the severity of the resulting pulmonary insufficiency. In patients with minimal disease, the administration of warm humidified oxygen may be the only treatment needed. In patients with more severe airway injury, frequent suctioning may be necessary to remove secretions and debris. Cylindrical casts of the airway composed of necrotic endobronchial mucous, inspissated exudate, and inflammatory cells may cause acute obstruction of the airway, necessitating emergency bronchoscopy using a rigid bronchoscope to extract the occluding debris (5).

Of paramount importance is the maintenance of a patent airway. Early endotracheal intubation may be required because of imminent oropharyngeal or laryngeal edema. Oxygen administration of inspired oxygen concentrations of 100% should be administered at the accident site or as soon as possible thereafter. Warm humidified oxygen by face mask may help soothe bronchial irritation. In the case of severe exposure or inhalation of lower airway or alveolar irritants, continuous positive airway pressure or intubation with positive end-expiratory pressure may be necessary. It is very important to adequately but carefully fluid-resuscitate burn victims with inhalation injury. Fluid must be given to optimize resuscitation without overloading the patient with pulmonary damage. If there are signs of impending airway obstruction, endotracheal intubation should be considered.

Patients with inhalation injuries accompanied by coma or respiratory depression, posterior pharyngeal swelling, nasolabial full thickness burns, or circumferential neck burns are candidates for early intubation as well. Once intubated, these patients can receive aggressive pulmonary toilet and humidified oxygen and be placed on a ventilator to receive continuous positive airway pressure if needed. Tracheostomy plays an important part in the management of patients with pulmonary complications secondary to an inhalation injury (2).

Prophylactic use of antibiotics has been shown to be of little or no benefit and can lead to resistant strains (8). Antibiotic intervention, however, is clearly indicated when infections are documented. This requires surveillance of sputum for bacterial colonization. Steroids have little usefulness in treating inhalation injuries. Bronchodilators are effective if bronchospasm occurs. Bronchoconstriction may be treated with inhaled β agonists, subcutaneous epinephrine, or intravenous aminophylline (10). Symptomatic relief of the cough may be accomplished with an antitussive containing codeine.

With a history of significant toxic inhalation, patients should be admitted to the hospital for inpatient observation because of the well-documented latent toxicity of many compounds (21).

REFERENCES

1. Heimbach D, Waeckerle J: Inhalation injuries. *Ann Emerg Med* 1988; 17:1316–1320.
2. Tredget E, Shankowsky H, Taernum T, et al: The role of inhalation injury in burn trauma. *Ann Surg* 1990;212:720–727.
3. Purdue G, Hunt J: Inhalation injuries and burns in the inner city. *Surg Clin N Am* 1991;71:385–397.
4. Prien T: Toxic smoke compounds and inhalation injury—a review. *Burns* 1988;14:451–460.
5. Traber L, Linares A, Herndon D: The pathophysiology of inhalation injury—a review. *Burns* 1988;14:357–364.
6. Noguchi T, Eng J, Klatt E: Significance of cyanide in medicolegal investigations involving fires. *Am J Forensic Med* 1988;9:304–309.
7. Blinn D, Slater H, Golfarb W: Inhalation injury with burns: a lethal combination. *J Emerg Med* 1988;6:471–473.
8. Rorison D, McPherson S: Acute toxic inhalations. *Emerg Clin N Am* 1992;10:409–435.
9. Bosse G: Nebulized sodium bicarbonate in the treatment of chlorine gas inhalation. *J Toxicol Clin Toxicol* 1994;32:233–242.
10. Clark W, Nieman G: Smoke inhalation. *Burns* 1988;14:473–494.
11. Vinsel P: Treatment of acute chlorine gas inhalation with nebulized sodium bicarbonate. *J Emerg Med* 1990;8:327–329.
12. Herndon N, Barrow R, Linares H, et al: Inhalation injury in burned patients: effects and treatment. *Burns* 1988:5:349–356.
13. Morenson H, Caraccio T, Brody G: Carbon monoxide poisoning. *Am J Emerg Med* 1984;2:254–261.
14. Cox R, Osgood K: Evaluation of intravenous magnesium sulfate for the treatment of hydrofluoric acid burns. *J Toxicol Clin Toxicol* 1994; 32:123–136.
15. Pruitt B, Cioffi W, Shimazu T, et al: Evaluation and management of patients with inhalation injury. *J Trauma* 1990;30:S63–S69.
16. Hanley Q, Koenig J, Larson T, et al: Response of young asthmatic patients to inhaled sulfuric acid. *Am Rev Respir Dis* 1992:145:326–331.
17. Knapp M, Bunn W, Stave G: Adult respiratory distress syndrome from sulfuric acid fume inhalation. *South Med J* 1991;84:1031–1033.
18. Dolan M: Carbon monoxide poisoning. *Can Med Assoc J* 1985;133: 392–399.
19. Kravis TC, et al: *Emergency Medicine: A Comprehensive Review*, 3rd ed. New York: Raven Press, 1993.
20. Nargar S, Kochhar R, Mehta S, et al: The role of fiberoptic endoscopy in the management of corrosive ingestion and modified endoscopic classification of burns. *Gastrointest Endosc* 1991;37:165–169.
21. Pietzman A, Shires G, Teixidor H, et al: Smoke inhalation injury: evaluation of radiographic manifestations and pulmonary dysfunction. *J Trauma* 1989;29:1232–1239.

CHAPTER 32

Carbon Monoxide

Carbon monoxide (CO) contamination and poisoning dates back to the roots of civilization and industrialization (1). It was mentioned as early as the ancient Roman era, and early Greek physicians stated that carbon monoxide was harmful to the human body. Carbon monoxide was used by both the Greeks and Romans to execute criminals (2). In 1895, Haldane first demonstrated that carbon monoxide combined with hemoglobin to form carboxyhemoglobin (COHb), which blocks oxygen binding and thereby decreases the amount of hemoglobin available for oxygen transport (3–5).

In the United States, CO poisoning accounts for more than 3,800 accidental and suicidal deaths each year, making it the leading cause of death by poisoning in this country today (6,7).

Many deaths are accidental because as little as 0.1% [1000 parts per million (ppm)] of the gas in inspired air can be lethal (3–5). Carbon monoxide is normally present in the atmosphere at a concentration of less than 0.001% (10 ppm) (8–10). Even low-level exposure is associated with severe toxicity. Breathing air with CO concentrations of as little as 0.1% for only minutes may result in COHb levels of greater than 50% (6,8–10).

TABLE 32–1. *Sources of carbon monoxide*

Exogenous
Automobile exhaust
Cigarette smoke
Coal gas
Fireplace with faulty flue
Fires
Charcoal-burning grills
Incomplete combustion of any fuel
Methylene chloride
Natural gases
Sea plants
Sterno
Volcanic activity
Water gas
Endogenous
Hemolytic anemia

PHYSICAL PROPERTIES

Carbon monoxide is a combustible, colorless, tasteless, and odorless gas that is nonirritating to the respiratory tract. It readily mixes with air without stratification because it has about the same density as air. Because of these physical properties, carbon monoxide may give no warning of its presence.

Carbon monoxide binds to hemoglobin and the resultant compound, carboxyhemoglobin, and it is a completely reversible complex that appears and disappears from the body only through the lungs and only in the course of respiration. Less than 1% of carbon monoxide is oxidized within the body to carbon dioxide (11,12).

SOURCES OF CARBON MONOXIDE

Carbon monoxide is ubiquitous in the environment and is formed exogenously as a by-product of the incomplete combustion of any carbonaceous solid, liquid, or gaseous material (Table 32–1). Internal combustion engines account for 75% of the CO generated by human activities, with automobile engines being the most prolific (7).

Fatalities associated with suicide are most likely to be linked to exposure to automobile exhaust. Most cases of sublethal exposure can be traced to automobile engines, the use of solid fuels in home heating or cooking, tobacco smoke, or industrial plant exposure (6).

Fires

The most obvious source of carbon monoxide intoxication is smoke from any type of fire; and since the beginning of the use of fires for heat, carbon monoxide accumulation has been a problem. Smoke from fires may contain from 0.1%–10% carbon monoxide (11). Cyanide and other toxic inhalants may also be liberated (9,13). Fireplaces with faulty flues may be sources of carbon monoxide (14).

Fuels

Environmental pollution probably constitutes the most common source of carbon monoxide (9). The exhaust from gasoline engines may contain 6%–10% carbon monoxide and diesel engines up to 7% or 70,000 ppm (10,11,15–18). Not only does the automobile contribute to the sublethal concentrations of carbon monoxide in the atmosphere, but it can also be a source of high-level exposure to its occupants when exhaust fumes enter the passenger compartment and build to lethal concentrations (7). It has been shown that automobile exhaust can saturate a car's interior or the interior of a small garage with lethal amounts of carbon monoxide in less than 20 minutes (19,20). The use of gas-powered ice-surfacing machines at skating rinks has led to carbon monoxide intoxication in those enclosed areas (11,21).

Virtually any inadequately vented indoor appliance that relies on combustion of fuels can give rise to toxic levels of CO. Even though natural gas burns quite cleanly, proper oxygenation is required to avoid incomplete combustion. However, what makes natural gas particularly dangerous is that potentially lethal levels of CO may be reached without the warning of indicator fumes.

Older household fuels, such as coal gas and water gas, are made from coke, and contain up to 40% carbon monoxide, hydrogen, methane, and other hydrocarbons. Natural gas does not contain carbon monoxide, but if it is improperly or incompletely combusted the by-product may be carbon monoxide (5,10,22,23). Ironically, there is now an increased potential for carbon monoxide poisoning resulting from improved home insulation and increased use of space heaters because both space heaters and kerosene heaters produce variable amounts of carbon monoxide (15). Water heaters are also a common source of carbon monoxide, as CO is formed when a flame touches a surface cooler than the ignition temperature of the gaseous portion of the flame (24). If these heaters are not properly vented, the room atmosphere readily becomes contaminated. Sterno, a canned fuel used to heat food, contains ethyl alcohol, methanol, and acetone and has also been shown to elevate carbon monoxide concentrations in the surrounding air (5,25).

Cigarette Smoke

The inhaled smoke of most tobacco cigarettes contains approximately 400 ppm carbon monoxide (16,26). The smoking of tobacco products can produce carboxyhemoglobin concentrations in the smoker from 5%–18%, depending on the number of cigarettes smoked (27). A moderate smoker may have a carboxyhemoglobin concentration of 5%–8%, and a heavy smoker (2–3 packs/day) may have concentrations as high as 18% (5). Because normal values for smokers may range from 10%–15% immediately after smoking a cigarette to chronic values ranging from 3%–8%, a smoking history is significant in a patient with suspected CO exposure (6). These individuals are usually asymptomatic. Significant increases in carbon monoxide (concentrations higher than those observed with conventional cigarettes) have been noted with the smoking of nontobacco cigarettes, such as clove cigarettes. In smoke-filled environments, nonsmoking individuals or "passive smokers" are exposed to elevated carbon monoxide concentrations. In addition, "sidestream" smoke, which is emitted by the burning tip of a cigarette, contains two and a half times more carbon monoxide than "mainstream" inhaled smoke (11).

Charcoal-Burning Grills

Deaths have occurred from the use of charcoal-burning grills because the incomplete combustion of charcoal briquettes can produce high concentrations of carbon monoxide in poorly ventilated spaces (11,16,28).

Methylene Chloride

Methylene chloride (dichloromethane) is usually considered one of the safest of the chlorinated hydrocarbons (17,29). It has numerous industrial applications, such as a degreaser, an aerosol propellant, and a solvent for plastic films and cement (30). Domestically, it is used in furniture and paint stripping (31).

Using methylene chloride paint remover in an enclosed room may lead to absorption of a large amount of the solvent through the lungs (11,17,32). The chemical is then released slowly from body tissues and is metabolized to carbon monoxide endogenously, which may result in significant poisoning (5,16). The biologic half-life of carbon monoxide formed from methylene chloride is 2–2.5 times longer than that of carbon monoxide exposure taken into the body from the environment. This is because of the slow release of methylene chloride from endogenous tissue stores even after contact with the compound has terminated (31). Methylene chloride is therefore particularly hazardous because the carboxyhemoglobin concentration continues to increase after cessation of exposure (32). The amount of carbon monoxide formed in the body is directly related to the amount of methylene chloride absorbed; the greater the minute respiratory volume or the poorer the room ventilation, the greater the absorption of methylene chloride and the higher the elevation of carboxyhemoglobin concentration (33).

Natural Sources

Natural sources of carbon monoxide include forest fires, volcanic activity, natural gases, certain sea plants, and photochemical degradation of organic compounds. These and other natural sources are large producers of carbon monoxide and are estimated to produce greater amounts of carbon monoxide than all automobile and industrial sources combined.

Catabolism of hemoglobin and other heme-containing protoporphyrins to bilirubin and carbon monoxide accounts for a baseline carboxyhemoglobin level of 0.3%–3.0% in nonsmokers (10,11). In patients with hemolytic anemias, the concentration may rise to 4%–6% (15,16,26).

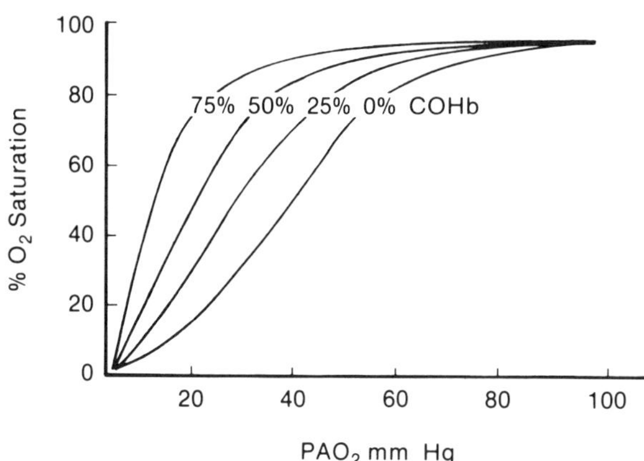

FIG 32–1. Oxyhemoglobin dissociation curve in the presence of carbon monoxide.

MECHANISM OF TOXICITY

Carbon monoxide causes toxicity in three ways: (a) by the formation of carboxyhemoglobin; (b) by shifting the oxyhemoglobin dissociation curve to the left; and (c) by binding to other heme-containing proteins including the cytochrome system and myoglobin.

The degree of carbon monoxide uptake depends on ventilatory rate, the duration of exposure, and the relative concentrations of carbon monoxide and oxygen.

Formation of Carboxyhemoglobin

Each molecule of hemoglobin has four heme groups and can reversibly bind up to four oxygen or carbon monoxide molecules in any combination. Carbon monoxide competes with oxygen for these binding sites on the hemoglobin molecule, and its affinity for hemoglobin is approximately 240 times greater than that of oxygen (5, 11,34–36). Thus, extremely low concentrations of carbon monoxide in the air may produce poisoning (16). Carbon monoxide is incapable of binding oxygen and because the oxygen-carrying capacity of blood is solely limited by the amount of hemoglobin not bound by carbon monoxide this results in tissue hypoxia. Bonding one or more of the four hemes of the hemoglobin molecule to carbon monoxide also appears to increase the bond strength between the remaining hemes and oxygen in the same molecule. In other words, the presence of some carboxyhemoglobin in an erythrocyte causes the remaining hemoglobin in the same erythrocyte to hold oxygen much more tightly than normal (see discussion of oxyhemoglobin dissociation below) (5). Because this binding is reversible, carbon monoxide can be competitively removed from hemoglobin by high concentrations of oxygen (14).

The reduction in oxygen-carrying capacity of blood is proportional to the amount of carboxyhemoglobin formed. Because the affinity for carbon monoxide is so many times that of oxygen, a small concentration of carbon monoxide in inspired air can tie up a large proportion of circulating hemoglobin. For example, carboxyhemoglobin concentrations of 0.01%, 0.02%, 0.1%, and 1% eventually saturate 11%, 19%, 54%, and 92% of the hemoglobin, respectively.

Shift in Oxyhemoglobin Dissociation Curve

The formation of carboxyhemoglobin inhibits oxyhemoglobin dissociation by shifting the oxyhemoglobin saturation curve to the left and by altering the shape of the curve toward a more hyperbolic form (Fig. 32–1) (5,37,38).

The leftward shift results in the availability of even less oxygen to the tissues than the carboxyhemoglobin saturation would suggest because of decreased unloading of oxygen at the tissues (12,39). In other words, tissue oxygen tensions must become extremely low before the remaining oxyhemoglobin can give up its oxygen (11). This effect is especially marked at carboxyhemoglobin concentrations greater than 45% (15). Thus, carbon monoxide results in a lower tissue end-capillary or venous oxygen tension (40). In pathophysiologic terms, this means that carbon monoxide causes a hypoxemia that is similar to but more severe than anemic hypoxia. Carbon monoxide-induced hypoxemia, in contrast to hypoxic hypoxia, does not reduce arterial oxygen partial pressure and, in contrast to anemic hypoxia, does not lower blood viscosity.

Binding to Other Heme-Containing Proteins

Although most of the body stores of CO in humans are chemically bound to hemoglobin, 10%–15% of total body CO is in extravascular tissues bound to other heme proteins, such as myoglobin, cytochromes, including cytochrome P-450, catalase, and peroxidase (14). Carbon monoxide in these locations can interfere with oxygen transport (5,41–44). Among the reactions with these proteins, the most significant are the reactions with cytochrome (a3) oxidase, cytochrome P-450, and myoglobin.

Cytochromes

The cytochromes are located in the mitochondria and are the seat of cellular respiration. The inhibitory effect of carbon monoxide on cytochrome oxidase therefore inhibits cellular respiration by competing with oxygen receptors in the cytochrome system. It is thought that the direct toxic effects on these cellular enzymes account for the often noted disparity between carboxyhemoglobin concentration and the patient's clinical condition, although this has not been shown. The affinity of the cytochrome system for oxygen is nine times that of carbon monoxide, so that, in adequately oxygenated individuals, carbon monoxide does not compete effectively for cytochrome oxidase (11). This may be altered, however, during carbon monoxide exposure when tissue oxygen content may be severely reduced (45).

Although the affinity of carbon monoxide for cytochrome oxidase is relatively low because the rate of dissociation is slow, it is conceivable that the interaction may result in a relatively prolonged impairment of oxidative metabolism. This may cause the electron transport chain to become fully reduced, and electrons may leak from mitochondrial oxidoreductase sites proximal to cytochrome oxidase. Mitochondria appears to be a source of oxygen-based free radicals within the first several hours after carbon monoxide poisoning.

Myoglobin

Except for hemoglobin, myoglobin is the most plentiful hemoprotein in the body and appears to act as a short-term oxygen store. Myoglobin also probably facilitates oxygen transport and diffusion across the cytoplasm from cell membrane to mitochondria. Carbon monoxide combines with myoglobin and interferes with this process (46). It binds to cardiac and skeletal muscle myoglobin, with cardiac muscle taking up about three times as much as skeletal muscle (11). This indicates that in individuals with a carboxyhemoglobin concentration of 10% approximately 30% of cardiac myoglobin is saturated with carbon monoxide. This significantly decreases the oxygen reserve available to the myocardium (47–49).

Carboxymyoglobin dissociation is slower than carboxyhemoglobin dissociation because of the increased affinity of CO for myoglobin. A "rebound effect" with delayed return of symptoms has occasionally been observed, corresponding to a recurrence of carboxyhemoglobin elevation. Presumably, this effect is caused by late release of CO from myoglobin and subsequent binding to hemoglobin (45).

Under hypoxic conditions, CO binding to proteins should increase, which may profoundly alter CO metabolic effects. In the case of myoglobin, when PaO_2 drops below 40 torr, 20%–40% of intravascular CO may be shifted into muscle. Hypoxia will increase CO binding to cytochrome oxidase, which may adversely affect oxidative metabolism (46). Because the rate of dissociation of CO from cytochrome oxidase is slow, concern has been raised that CO may cause a relatively prolonged adverse effect despite only transient hypoxia (50).

As COHb levels rise, cerebral vessels dilate and both coronary blood flow and capillary perfusion increase. Acutely, these compensatory reactions are accompanied by tachypnea and alveolar hyperventilation. As CO exposure continues, central respiratory depression occurs possibly secondary to cerebral hypoxia.

Acute mortality from CO may be mediated through cerebral hypoxia, either from respiratory depression or from a decreased PaO_2 caused by pulmonary shunting or ventilation/perfusion mismatch (50).

Absorption/Excretion

Carbon monoxide is readily absorbed into the bloodstream through the alveolar capillary network. As with uptake, the main route of excretion is also pulmonary and depends on many factors, one of the most important of which is minute ventilation (6).

MEASUREMENT OF CARBOXYHEMOGLOBIN CONCENTRATION

Carboxyhemoglobin concentrations obtained from venous or arterial blood (16), although the pH is better assessed with arterial samples and acidosis that may be profound, is more adequately monitored by means of arterial blood gases (51).

Blood carboxyhemoglobin is usually expressed as percent saturation. The terms percent saturation and carboxyhemoglobin concentration are used interchangeably, and both imply the percentage of hemoglobin combined with carbon monoxide (51). Both are calculated with the following formula:

Carboxyhemoglobin Concentration = (blood CO content/(blood CO capacity) × 100

The percentage of carboxyhemoglobin is the ratio of carboxyhemoglobin to hemoglobin. As an example, a carboxyhemoglobin concentration of 50% means that in a patient with 16 g of hemoglobin 8 g is carboxyhemoglobin. The percentage may be misleading, especially in the presence of anemia (50).

THE AIR AND CO (PPM)

Even very low concentrations of CO in the air will combine with large amounts of hemoglobin when equilibrium is reached. At a concentration of 0.01% of CO in the inspired air (100 ppm), the equilibrium concentration of carboxyhemoglobin in the blood is 14%. When higher concentrations of CO, such as 0.05% (500 ppm) are inspired, the equilibrium concentration of COHb increases to the highly toxic level of 45%. The rate at which the equilibrium concentration is reached on exposure to CO in the air depends on the minute ventilation of the subject. An increase in minute ventilation, such as that associated with exercise, shortens the length of time necessary for CO to reach the equilibrium concentration (41).

SIGNS AND SYMPTOMS OF CARBON MONOXIDE INTOXICATION

Carbon monoxide intoxication has symptoms referable to those tissues or organs that are most sensitive to the disruption of aerobic metabolism (Table 32–2) (34,52). These tissues or organs are also those with the highest metabolic rates. Therefore the brain and heart are the organs most susceptible to the effects of carbon monoxide poisoning (11,39,53,54). Children, because of their increased respiratory exchange requirements, may be more susceptible than adults to carbon monoxide intoxication (15). Patients with coronary artery disease also are at high risk of developing cardiac symptoms after carbon monoxide exposure (47,55). Sudden, acute exposure to a high atmospheric concentration of carbon monoxide may result in symptoms without elevated carboxyhemoglobin concentrations. Likewise, chronic exposure to carbon monoxide may result in elevated carboxyhemoglobin concentrations without symptoms (55).

All factors that increase respiration and circulation accelerate this process and shorten the latent period before toxic signs and symptoms appear. Exercise, fever, and anemia increase the hazard from carbon monoxide. Symptoms of poisoning are therefore related to the blood carboxyhemoglobin concentration, which may be affected by (a) the amount of inspired carbon monoxide or the amount in the environment; (b) the degree of physical activity; (c) the duration of exposure or contact with the gas; (d) the degree of alveolar COHbilation; (e) the level of cardiac output; and (f) the presence of cardiovascular or cerebrovascular disease (Table 32–3) (53,55).

Correlation Between Symptoms and Carboxyhemoglobin Concentration

Although there are rough guidelines concerning carboxyhemoglobin concentrations and symptomatology, often the correlation between these two factors is poor. In addition, unless exposure to carbon monoxide is suspected, carboxyhemoglobin concentrations may not be measured because there are no pathognomic symptoms, so that the presentation may easily imitate other illnesses (56). This may cause a dangerous delay in diagnosis. The possibility of carbon monoxide poisoning must therefore be considered when headache, nausea, dizziness, extreme fatigue, confusion, or collapse occur in an environment in which carbon monoxide could be present.

Only a few symptoms of carbon monoxide poisoning occur at carboxyhemoglobin concentrations of less than 10% to 13% (Table 32–4), although even low concentrations of carboxyhemoglobin significantly impair the delivery of oxygen to tissues. As an example, with blood carboxyhemoglobin concentrations of 1% to 4%, myocardial blood flow increases but no adverse effects are clearly demonstrable. At 5% to 9%, patients with coro-

TABLE 32–2. *Effects of carbon monoxide poisoning*

Effects
Respiratory
Dyspnea on exertion
Hyperpnea
Respiratory failure
Neurologic
Headache
Giddiness
Irritability
Dizziness
Vomiting
Excitement
Hallucinations
Seizures
Stupor
Syncope
Coma
Cardiac
Angina pectoris
Myocardial infarction
Palpitations
Tachycardia
Bradycardia
Cutaneous
Dermatographia
Papules
Tropic erythema
Vesicles
Blistering
Visual
Blurred vision
Blindness
Flame-shaped hemorrhages
Paracentral scotoma
Papilledema
Visual field defects
Musculoskeletal
Rhabdomyolysis
Myoglobinemia
Myoglobinuria

TABLE 32–3. *Conditions affecting the degree of carbon monoxide intoxication*

Concentration of inspired carbon monoxide
Degree of physical activity
Duration of exposure or contact with gas
Alveolar ventilation
Cardiac output
Pre-existing cardiovascular disease
Pre-existing cerebrovascular disease

nary artery disease demonstrate a decreased threshold for exercise-induced angina (48).

Typically, with carboxyhemoglobin concentrations between 10% to 20%, which corresponds to 70–120 ppm carbon monoxide in the air, the earliest symptom noted with carbon monoxide is a slight headache or tightness across the forehead (43). With concentrations between 20%–30%, the headache may become more pronounced and be experienced as a throbbing pain (1). Headache is presumed to be secondary to reflex cerebral vasodilation and increased cerebral blood flow resulting from relative tissue hypoxia. With carboxyhemoglobin concentrations of 30%–40%, muscular weakness, palpitations, dizziness, dimness of vision, nausea, vomiting, and mental confusion may occur. Excitement and reckless behavior may also follow. These symptoms may progress to tachycardia and cardiovascular collapse when the carboxyhemoglobin concentration is in the range of 40%–50% (1). At concentrations greater than 50%, coma and intermittent seizures may appear. Concentrations greater than 60% may lead to death (15). This corresponds to carbon monoxide concentrations as low as 0.1% inhaled for several minutes (50).

In addition, a particular carbon monoxide concentration can have a more profound effect on tissue oxygenation at high altitudes than at sea level because of the reduced oxygen partial pressures at high altitudes. The risk of carbon monoxide is also greater above 7,000 feet than at sea level because the reduced amount of oxygen at high altitudes results in poor combustion of motor fuels, causing vehicles to emit much more carbon monoxide.

Carboxyhemoglobin concentrations may be within the normal range and not reflect the true insult (51–59). This may be particularly true when there is a significant delay between cessation of exposure and drawing of the blood sample or if supplemental oxygen has been administered. Some patients may have a circulating carboxyhemoglobin concentration of 25% and be severely acidotic and unconscious, whereas others with concentrations of 40% or more may be awake and alert and only manifest a headache (55). A carboxyhemoglobin concentration that is within normal limits therefore does not rule out a significant case of carbon monoxide poisoning (5,15,57,60). This is because the tissue concentration may more accurately reflect the degree of insult, a measurement that may have to be inferred from the clinical state and examination. The carboxyhemoglobin concentration is in such a case only one of many factors.

Respiratory Effects

The principal chemoreceptors that sense a reduction in oxygen and initiate cardiovascular and respiratory reflex responses are located in the carotid artery and the aortic bodies. With carbon monoxide intoxication, the partial pressure of oxygen in the blood is normal because blood is still in tension equilibrium with alveolar gas. The actual oxygen saturation is low, however. Because the carotid artery and aortic body chemoreceptors are sensitive to oxygen tension and not to the oxygen content of the arterial blood, no respiratory compensation for the tissue hypoxia occurs in most patients until very high blood concentrations of carbon monoxide are attained. Acute pulmonary edema has also been reported secondary to carbon monoxide intoxication (61).

TABLE 32–4. *Carboxyhemoglobin concentration and symptomatology*

Carboxyhemoglobin concentration (%)	Carbon monoxide in air (%)	Clinical effect
0–10		None
10–20	0.007–0.012	Mild headache, fatigue
20–30	0.012–0.022	Throbbing headache, giddiness, blurred vision, dyspnea on exertion, irritability, impaired motor dexterity
30–40	0.022–0.035	Weakness, dizziness, nausea, voiding, blurred vision, confusion, excitement, palpitations
40–50	0.035–0.052	Weakness, ataxia, tachypnea, syncope, tachycardia, confusion, hallucinations
50–60	0.052–0.080	Syncope, stupor, seizures, coma, hyperpnea
60–70	0.080–0.122	Coma, bradycardia, bradypnea, seizures, incontinence
>70	0.195	Respiratory failure, death

TABLE 32–5. *Neurologic effects secondary to carbon monoxide intoxication*

Change in mental status
Coma
Decerebrate rigidity
Decreased comprehension
Decreased coordination
Decreased spatial reasoning
Decreased visual acuity
Extensor plantar responses
Short-term memory loss
Spatial disorientation
Transient cortical blindness

Neurologic Effects

Neurologic symptoms may include throbbing headache, excitability, confusion, visual complaints, seizures, and dizziness. Subtle neuropsychiatric symptoms may also be present after carbon monoxide poisoning (Table 32–5) (52). Physicians should be aware that signs of cortical dysfunction, particularly of the frontal and parietal lobes, may mimic psychiatric symptoms. In many cases, the earliest and most common neurological accompaniment to the comatose state is a tonic disorder or decerebrate rigidity associated with increased deep tendon reflexes and extensor plantar responses. Cortical blindness is usually transitory and characterized by visual loss but intact pupillary reactions to light. Carbon monoxide poisoning may also result in cerebral edema secondary to hypoxia and interference with cellular respiration (11).

Cardiac Effects

Carbon monoxide intoxication causes coronary artery vasodilation and an increase in coronary blood flow that is linearly related to the reduction in arterial oxygen content (58,62,63). The heart may be unduly compromised with carbon monoxide poisoning because it must increase its output if peripheral oxygen transport is to be maintained, yet at the same time its own oxygen supply is compromised (64). Therefore, in patients with ischemic heart disease, whose oxygen transport systems are marginal, very small increments in carboxyhemoglobin concentration can exacerbate symptoms (41).

Most tissues respond to CO-induced hypoxia by increasing oxygen extraction from the blood. If oxygen demands are still not met, cardiac output increases (56). This increases cardiac workload and thus the oxygen requirement of the heart, which is also operating in a hypoxic environment. Under normal circumstances, the heart operates at near maximal oxygen extraction (41). To make up for the decreased oxygen delivery and the increased consumption, the coronary arteries vasodilate to increase blood flow. In patients with coronary artery disease, increases in coronary blood flow may be impaired because of fixed proximal stenotic lesions, which put them at risk for infarction (65). Exacerbation of angina pectoris with or without myocardial infarction is a well-established complication of carbon monoxide poisoning (48,54). Electrocardiographic changes may include ST segment and T wave abnormalities suggestive of myocardial ischemia, or infarction, extrasystoles, and other dysrhythmias. Such abnormalities are sensitive indicators of myocardial damage (10).

An electrocardiogram should be ordered for all patients, and if it is abnormal, serial creatine kinase and lactate dehydrogenase levels should be determined and the patient should be closely observed (45).

Cutaneous Effects

Cutaneous manifestations of carbon monoxide poisoning include dermatographia, papules, vesicles, blisters, and bullae (66), which are often mistaken for burns or trauma in the unconscious patient (11). The most common skin manifestation is tropic erythema, which may appear on the face and extremities and is not necessarily related to pressure areas (67).

Because the formation of carboxyhemoglobin imparts a bright red color to the skin, patients may be profoundly hypoxic without manifesting cyanosis. Nevertheless, the cherry-red appearance of the skin is relatively uncommon, occurring only in a minority of severe cases, and should therefore never be relied on for making the diagnosis (5,68,69).

Visual Effects

Visual effects of carbon monoxide poisoning include temporary or permanent loss of vision, visual field defects, paracentral scotomas, decreased light sensitivity, and decreased dark adaptation (16). Flame-shaped superficial retinal hemorrhages have been reported in long-term, subacute carbon monoxide poisoning (11,70). Papilledema may also be seen on funduscopic examination. These visual changes may be permanent, even in the acute carbon monoxide exposure.

Musculoskeletal Effects

Although myonecrosis complicating carbon monoxide poisoning is uncommon, it has been recognized for many years (68,71,72). In the comatose patient, the crushing effect of the patient's body on certain muscle groups leads to their injury; this has occurred both with and without coma. The resulting myoglobinuria may lead to acute renal failure with terminal hyperkalemia (12,73). Al-

TABLE 32–6. *Late complications of carbon monoxide intoxication*

Adult respiratory distress syndrome
Aspiration pneumonitis
Myocardial damage
Neurologic abnormalities (see Table 32–7)
Ocular abnormalities
Renal insufficiency
Rhabdomyonecrosis

though rhabdomyolysis can occur secondary to pressure necrosis, it may also be a result of a direct cellular toxic effect in patients with long-term exposure (5).

Late Complications

Late complications of carbon monoxide poisoning are often not considered during initial management but can be more devastating than the effects of the original insult (Table 32–6) (38,68,74). Late complications include aspiration pneumonitis, myocardial damage, renal insufficiency, adult respiratory distress syndrome (67), and, most important, neuropsychiatric disturbances (Table 32–7) (4,52,68,75). These complications may occur days to weeks after exposure, be varied and unpredictable, and occur after an initial period of recovery (5).

Central nervous system damage resulting from carbon monoxide poisoning is similar to that from other severe hypoxic insults (76–78). Postanoxic encephalopathy may begin 7–21 days after the initial insult and has been described only after episodes of severe CNS hypoxia (52). Occasionally, a victim may appear to recover but suffer a relapse of neurologic manifestations.

TABLE 32–7. *Late neurologic sequelae of carbon monoxide intoxication*

Cerebral demyelination
Cortical blindness
Deafness
Dementia
Memory impairment
Mental retardation
Necrosis of globus pallidus
Necrosis of substantia nigra
Parietal lobe dysfunction
Visual agnosia
Temporospatial disorientation
Constructional apraxia
Dysnomia
Parkinsonism
Peripheral neuritis
Personality changes
Psychosis
Wernicke–Korsakoff syndrome

Delayed neurologic sequelae include a triad of gait disturbances, incontinence of urine, and mental deterioration. Long-term neuropsychologic sequelae have included almost every type and degree of neurologic deficit, such as memory impairment, mental retardation, cortical blindness (79), transient deafness, diabetes insipidus (80), and Korsakoff's psychosis (75). Personality alterations include irritability, impulsiveness, mood changes, violence, and verbal aggressiveness. Occasional frank psychosis has ensued (59). Specific signs of parietal lobe dysfunction, such as visual agnosia, temporospatial disorientation, constructional apraxia, dysnomia, and dysgraphia may be noted. Parkinsonism (81,82), chorea, spasticity, hyperreflexia, and polyneuritis have also been seen (62). Demyelination with widespread foci of cellular degeneration in the cerebrum, cerebellum, and basal ganglia may be noted.

There are no clear clinical signs that accurately predict which patients presenting with carbon monoxide poisoning will have delayed neurologic effects. Mild cases may at times go on to delayed relapse (63). Although these delayed neurologic sequelae may spontaneously resolve, improvement may require a convalescent period of two years (50). The highest cerebral function is recovered last (52). Neurologic symptoms may also worsen over time (5).

Death

The major cause of death associated with acute carbon monoxide poisoning is cardiac dysrhythmias (54,74,83). Carbon monoxide poisoning may also result in lethal cerebral edema as a consequence of cell death caused by hypoxia and interference with cellular respiration (75).

Carbon Monoxide in Pregnancy

Fetal COHb concentration depends on maternal COHb concentration, placental diffusing capacity of CO, endogenous fetal CO production, and the relative affinities of maternal and fetal hemoglobin for CO and O_2 (84). Carbon monoxide crosses the placental barrier, either by simple diffusion or mediated by a carrier, and enters the fetal blood supply (2,85). Chronic exposure in pregnancy is usually a result of cigarette smoking by the mother, and there is a well-established, direct relationship between the number of cigarettes smoked per day and the decrease in birth weight (86). In addition, there is a reported increase in the rate of fetal wastage independent of birth weight as well as an increase in the rate of placenta previa, abruptio placentae, and premature rupture of membranes (15,87,88). The fetus is more susceptible to carbon monoxide poisoning than the mother for two reasons: (a) during normal steady-state production, the human fetal-maternal COHb concentration is

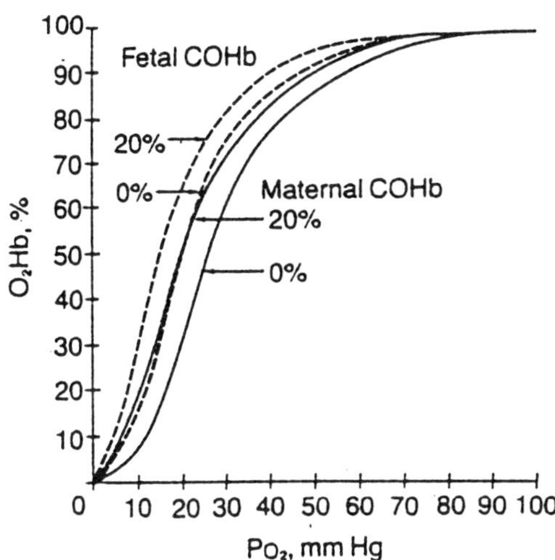

FIG 32–2. Fetal (*dashed lines*) and maternal (*solid lines*) oxyhemoglobin (O_2Hb) saturation curves demonstrating effect of carbon monoxide. Fetal curve normally lies to left of maternal curve. In presence of carbon monoxide, both curves are further shifted to left. COHb, carboxyhemoblobin; pO_2, partial oxygen pressure. Adapted from data of Longo (2).

1.1 to 1. Hence, fetal COHb levels are 10%–15% higher at steady state than maternal COHb levels (2,84) and the normal shift to the left of the fetal oxyhemoglobin dissociation curve accentuates the hemoglobin-binding properties of carbon monoxide (Fig. 32–2) (2,84). In addition, normal fetal arterial PaO_2 is low, at about 20 mm Hg, with an O_2 content of 12 mL/dL (89). The fetal system normally operates on the steep part of the oxyhemoglobin dissociation curve; thus, a small drop in O_2 tension can dangerously lower the fetal arterial O_2 concentration (84).

Carbon monoxide absorption and elimination occur more slowly in the fetal circulation. Following maternal exposure to CO, the fetal COHb rises more slowly than the maternal COHb but will continue to rise for several hours after acute exposure until it eventually reaches an equilibrium (89). Therefore, maternal levels may be greatly reduced while the fetus is encountering high COHb levels. Fetal hemoglobin binds CO more avidly than does hemoglobin A, and with slow transplacental transport, fetal levels decrease much more slowly than do levels in the mother (90). This accounts for the occasional occurrence of fetal death in nonfatal maternal exposure (45).

The fetal COHb concentration cannot be estimated only on the basis of a maternal blood sample. The fetal COHb level depends on the exposure pattern and equilibrium with maternal COHb (86). The maternal COHb level measured in the emergency department may be considerably lower than the patient's peak COHb level if a significant time has elapsed since exposure or if O_2 has been administered during transport (84).

When hyperbaric oxygen (HBO) therapy is not available to the pregnant female, normobaric oxygen therapy should be continued for approximately five times longer than normal due to the persistence of COHb in the fetus.

DIAGNOSIS OF CARBON MONOXIDE POISONING

History

The protean symptoms associated with carbon monoxide intoxication probably lead to a gross underestimation of its true incidence (91). The most common misdiagnosis is a flu-like viral illness because of symptoms of headache, dizziness, nausea, vomiting, and shortness of breath (11,92–95). Carbon monoxide poisoning should be considered in the differential diagnosis of an acute encephalopathic state. Appropriate settings for pathogenesis include a long automobile trip, smoke inhalation, and exposure to incompletely combusted domestic fuel; a history of suicidal thoughts or attempts is also grounds for suspecting carbon monoxide poisoning (96). Patients seen during winter months with severe headache, nausea, vomiting, unusual weakness, decreased cognitive function, new-onset angina pectoris, or exacerbation of chronic cardiopulmonary disorders should be questioned concerning similarly affected cohabitants of the home, faulty ventilation, defective heating, or the use of space heaters. Group exposures to carbon monoxide may be misdiagnosed as food poisoning, especially if vomiting is present (11).

Physical Examination

Unless there is a diligent search for pathognomonic signs, findings on physical examination are of little specific help in the diagnosis. A thorough neurologic examination should be performed so as not to miss the subtle signs that may be the only manifestation of poisoning (96). A funduscopic examination may reveal flame-shaped retinal hemorrhages, but this is a nonspecific indicator of subacute exposure to carbon monoxide (92,97).

Psychometric Testing

Psychometric assessments have shown that a patient's overall performance on a battery of tests decreases with increased carboxyhemoglobin levels. These tests involve comprehension, short-term memory, spatial orientation, visual motor speed, coordination, visual acuity, spatial reasoning, attentional ability, and fine motor control, and are measures of cerebral functioning (Table 32–8). The mental status examination may also be a sensitive diagnostic indicator of carbon monoxide intoxication.

TABLE 32–8. *Psychometric testing*

Comprehension
Short-term memory
Spatial orientation
Visual motor speed
Coordination
Visual acuity
Spatial reasoning
Attentional ability
Fine motor control

Neuropsychiatric testing is controversial in that some groups have shown that patients evaluated immediately after poisoning, who have abnormal test results, have not been shown to have a higher risk of morbidity (14). More data are needed to clarify this area.

Groups at Increased Risk

An interesting practical point is that animals with high basal metabolic rates are particularly susceptible to carbon monoxide and frequently succumb before the development of symptoms in humans (2,15,16). Infants, the elderly, and patients with cardiovascular disease, anemia, lung disease, and an increased metabolic rate are at greater risk (98).

Laboratory Analysis

Several factors need to be considered when examining a patient for CO poisoning. The possibility of thermal injury or other gas inhalation should be investigated. If poisoning is the result of a suicide attempt, a drug screen should be ordered, and acetaminophen, salicylate, and ethanol levels should be obtained (45). Routine laboratory studies (Table 32–9) may also offer no specific clues to the diagnosis (96).

Arterial Blood Gas

Arterial blood gases should be determined, but the values may be normal because the partial pressure of oxygen is a measure of the oxygen dissolved in plasma and is not affected by changes in hemoglobin saturation (99). Arterial oxygen tension may also be low, depending on the magnitude of the carboxyhemoglobin level, the fraction of inspired oxygen, and the nature and partial pressures of other inhaled gases, which are sometimes quite abnormal in cases of smoke inhalation. An anion gap metabolic acidosis due to lactic acidosis may be seen in severely poisoned patients (98).

TABLE 32–9. *Laboratory studies suggested in carbon monoxide poisoning*

Arterial blood gas determination
Carboxyhemoglobin concentration monitoring
Chest roentgenography
Electrocardiography
Spirometry
Urinalysis

Arterial Oxygen Saturation Gap

Many hospital laboratories calculate the oxygen saturation from the oxygen partial pressure by means of a slide rule nomogram (100). With carbon monoxide present the arterial oxygen partial pressure is normal if the patient is breathing normally, and calculated oxygen saturation may then be grossly incorrect (101). It is therefore mandatory to have a direct measurement of the oxygen saturation and to compare the calculated with the measured saturation (5,57,92). A difference of more than 5% is considered significant, and carbon monoxide poisoning should be considered (102).

Pulse Oximetry

Pulse oximetry is used widely in emergency situations. The technique relies on the different absorption of light by oxyhemoglobin and reduced hemoglobin. Adult blood usually contains four species of hemoglobin: oxyhemoglobin, reduced hemoglobin, methemoglobin, and carboxyhemoglobin. Being two-wavelength devices, pulse oximeters can differentiate only two species of hemoglobin. At 940 nm, carboxyhemoglobin absorbs very little light, but at 660 nm it absorbs as much light as oxyhemoglobin. Carboxyhemoglobin is therefore registered by the pulse oximeter as oxyhemoglobin. Pulse oximetry, therefore, may be misleading during CO poisoning as the pulse oximeter does not differentiate between oxyhemoglobin and carboxyhemoglobin (103,104).

An electrocardiogram may be abnormal, showing nonspecific ST-T wave changes. Atrial dysrhythmias and various conduction disturbances and occasionally evidence of myocardial infarction may also be noted (10,48, 54). Serial electrocardiograms and cardiac enzyme measurements may be necessary to screen for immediate and delayed evidence of myocardial toxicity (101).

Spirometry can be a sensitive indicator of smoke inhalation. This may be indicated in cases where the diagnosis is unclear. Both the forced expiratory volume and the forced vital capacity may be abnormal.

A chest roentgenogram of acutely intoxicated patients may show a ground-glass appearance, perihilar haze, peribronchial and perivascular cuffing, and intra-alveolar edema. The ground-glass appearance can be considered parenchymal interstitial edema caused by tissue hypoxia or the toxic effects of carbon monoxide on alveolar membranes. Pulmonary edema may also be noted.

There are currently four spot tests for carboxyhemoglobin, but the presence of carboxyhemoglobin cannot be determined accurately by any of these tests; they should therefore be abandoned (97). A urinalysis may be helpful in identifying myoglobinuria. Glycosuria and proteinuria may be seen secondary to renal tubular hypoxia.

There are relatively accurate portable breath analyzers for carbon monoxide that indicate immediately whether or not a patient has been exposed (105–107). Other poisonous compounds do not appear to interfere with accurate carboxyhemoglobin readings from these instruments, which operate on the basis of an electrochemical principle. Estimates based on measurement of expired air, in parts per million, are less accurate than directly measuring carboxyhemoglobin concentrations.

The definitive diagnosis is made by measuring blood carboxyhemoglobin concentration; this measurement should therefore be taken as early as possible. This can be done spectrophotometrically with a co-oximeter, which provides a rapid and accurate determination. This study is mandatory in all symptomatic patients to establish the diagnosis, to aid in determining the degree of intoxication, and to help plan the treatment needed (108).

Carbon monoxide is not produced by decomposition, nor is it absorbed in significant amounts by a body when exposed to an environment rich in CO. COHb persists for weeks in the human body and may be accurately quantified even after embalming and burial (89).

It must again be emphasized that the carboxyhemoglobin concentration may not adequately reflect the diagnosis if supplemental oxygen therapy has been instituted or if there is a long period of time between exposure and drawing of a blood sample (5,16). Consequently, patients can remain in a depressed clinical state even after the apparent elimination of carbon monoxide from the body. This situation may be the result of either an undetectable amount of carbon monoxide still bound in the tissues or a residual hypoxia (109).

Computed tomographic scans and magnetic resonance imaging have shown white matter to be particularly sensitive to cerebral hypoxia brought about by CO intoxication. Although gray matter has greater metabolic oxygen needs, the more restricted vascular supply of the white matter limits its tolerance for reduced oxygen tensions and thus increases its susceptibility to damage during hypoxic events (50).

Computed tomographic brain scanning of patients exposed to carbon monoxide has demonstrated symmetrical bilateral necrosis of the basal ganglia, most often the globus pallidus (36,110,111), and of the red zone of the substantia nigra, many times with abnormal contrast enhancement of the pallidum (52,76,112). This lesion is a pathologic but nonspecific hallmark of carbon monoxide intoxication; barbiturate intoxication, cyanide poisoning, hydrogen sulfide poisoning, and hypoglycemia have a similar appearance (113). Early evidence of low-density areas in the globus pallidus in comatose patients correlates with a high risk of death or poor neurologic outcome (11,16,63). Patients exposed to carbon monoxide who have normal tomographic scans have shown good recovery. An electroencephalogram may reveal diffuse frontal slow-wave activity consistent with a metabolic encephalopathy (93).

Although computed tomography-observed abnormalities are reflective of moderate to severe poisoning, patients with changes in the gray matter (e.g., hypodensity in the region of the basal ganglia) may still have good clinical recoveries. The presence of lesions in the white matter, however, more often reflects a poor prognosis (50).

TREATMENT

General

The management of carbon monoxide poisoning involves reversing the pathophysiologic process as quickly as possible. The first priority of treatment is removal of the patient from the poisoned environment and the administration of as much oxygen as possible (11,48). Resuscitation of patients who have evidence of stupor, coma, or severe motor neurologic impairment may require intubation with sedation or curarization and fluid restriction. In addition, treatment should include ruling out other causes of symptomatology (114). If the patient presents with an altered mental state, dextrose in water, thiamine, and naloxone should be administered. Cardiac rhythm should be monitored during transport and in the emergency department (11). There is no specific treatment for the patient presenting with delayed neurologic sequelae secondary to carbon monoxide poisoning (15,16).

Fluid and Electrolyte Balance

Fluid and electrolyte balance should be carefully maintained to guard against overhydration and further pulmonary complications. Positive end expiratory pressure may be helpful in raising the functional residual capacity. Although some authorities suggest not treating a mild acidosis (5,10) because of the shift of the oxyhemoglobin dissociation curve to the right, care should be taken in the patient with myonecrosis because this condition decreases excretion of the toxin (115,116). If ventilatory assistance is required, the use of a volume respirator is recommended because of increased airway resistance and decreased patient compliance (45).

Steroids

Steroids have been recommended by some investigators to combat cerebral edema. To date, there is no convincing evidence that steroids improve the prognosis for patients with diffuse cerebral edema. This is still an area of controversy. If steroids are used, they should be administered early in the course of treatment as a single, large intravenous bolus.

Oxygen

Oxygen therapy is the mainstay of treatment for carbon monoxide poisoning, and should be instituted as quickly as possible with the greatest concentration available. In addition to providing for one third of the body's total oxygen requirement by simple dissolution in plasma, 100% oxygen also reduces the half-life of CO in the body to approximately 80–90 minutes from the 240-minute half-life of CO when breathing normal room air (6). Hyperbaric oxygen may be indicated, but when there are no hyperbaric oxygen facilities available or when there is no clinical indication for hyperbaric oxygen and the patient is cooperative, a tightly fitting face mask should be used to administer 100% oxygen. The plastic "rebreather" mask typically used in emergency departments may not deliver 100% oxygen, even at a flow rate of 10 L/min (117). Furthermore, the unconscious or uncooperative patient may require intubation and mechanical ventilation to receive 100% oxygen. Supplementation with 5% carbon dioxide has been suggested because carbon dioxide shifts the oxyhemoglobin dissociation curve to the right, which tends to negate the carbon monoxide-induced shift (15). This therapy is not recommended, however (5,10).

Comparison of Oxygen Therapies

Carbon monoxide is eliminated from the body with different half-lives, depending on the percentage of inspired oxygen and atmospheric pressure. There are conflicting reports on the actual half-life of carbon monoxide in different environmental atmospheres. The half-life of carbon monoxide in the blood of healthy volunteers breathing room air is approximately 320 minutes, with a range of 120–400 minutes (Table 32–10). It is decreased to approximately 80–90 minutes with a tight-fitting mask and the patient breathing 100% oxygen. Hyperbaric oxygen at 3 atm decreases the half-life of carbon monoxide to less than 30 minutes (5). Although these times may be different in the symptomatic patient in a clinical setting, there is no question that carboxyhemoglobin concentrations decrease dramatically when oxygen is administered (68).

TABLE 32–10. *Half-life of carbon monoxide in blood*

Source	Half-life (min)
Room air	240–320
100% oxygen	80–100
Hyperbaric oxygen (three atmospheres)	20–30

Hyperbaric Oxygen Therapy

Hyperbaric oxygen (HBO) therapy has been suggested as the optimal treatment for cases of significant carbon monoxide poisoning (3,4,75). There are no prospective trials that document superiority of HBO over sea-level oxygen in CO poisoning. Nevertheless, the rationale for the use of HBO is sound, and the risks of therapy are minimal (118). Availability of hyperbaric oxygen chambers, although still limited, has improved with the use of helicopter and other air transport (117). It is important that personnel establish liaison with the hyperbaric treatment facilities in their communities so that referral can be expeditiously accomplished when needed (49).

TYPES OF CHAMBERS FOR HYPERBARIC OXYGEN THERAPY

There are two types of HBO chambers, a multiplace chamber and a monoplace chamber.

Multiplace Chambers

Multiplace chambers are large tanks accommodating 2 to 14 people. The are usually built to achieve pressures up to 6 atm and have a chamber lock-entry system that allows personnel to pass through without altering the pressure of the inner chamber. The chamber is filled with compressed air; patients breathe 100% oxygen through a face mask, head hood, or endotracheal tube. Although fire hazards restrict the use of certain electronic equipment, some monitors and ventilators with solid-state circuitry can be used within the chamber, allowing intensive care of critically ill patients (119).

Monoplace Chambers

Monoplace chambers are far less costly than their larger counterparts and have allowed hospitals to institute HBO programs without prohibitive capital outlays. Most chambers are sized to allow a single patient to lie supine under a transparent acrylic dome or viewing port. The internal environment of the monoplace chamber is maintained at 100% oxygen; thus, the patient does not wear a mask. Specially adapted ventilators and monitoring systems do allow treatment of critically ill patients (120).

Mechanism of Action of Hyperbaric Oxygen

At sea level in room air, hemoglobin is approximately 97% saturated with oxygen. An increase in pO_2 has a negligible impact on total hemoglobin oxygen content; however, it does result in an increase in the amount of oxygen dissolved directly into plasma. With 100% inspired oxygen the amount of plasma oxygen increases to 2.09 vol %. At 3 atmospheric pressure absolute (ATA) plasma contains 6.8 vol % oxygen, a level equivalent to the average tissue requirements for oxygen. Thus, HBO treatment could and has sustained life without hemoglobin (120). Increasing pressure in HBO therapy is often expressed in multiples of atmospheric pressure absolute (ATA). One ATA equals 735.5 mm Hg. Most HBO treatments are performed at 2–3 ATA (121).

Hyperbaric oxygen therapy provides a patient with breathing oxygen at pressures greater than one atmosphere so that high alveolar partial pressures of oxygen are attained. It is considered that 3 atm (66 feet below sea level) of oxygen is the maximum safe pressure to which humans may be exposed for any considerable length of time (122).

The mode of action of hyperbaric oxygen treatment follows the laws of mass action: high concentrations of oxygen drive carbon monoxide from hemoglobin, the cytochromes, and myoglobin. With increased amounts of oxygen available the ratio of oxygen to carbon monoxide is increased, and the carbon monoxide is driven off more quickly (3,4). In addition, tissue oxygenation is improved as a result of the increased amount of dissolved oxygen in plasma because hyperbaric oxygen provides oxygen independent of hemoglobin (98).

Beneficial Effects of Hyperbaric Oxygen

Among the beneficial effects of hyperbaric oxygen are (a) a greatly diminished carboxyhemoglobin half-life; (b) enhanced tissue clearance of residual carbon monoxide; (c) reduced cerebral edema; and (d) reversal of cytochrome oxidase inhibition (36). Carbon monoxide is considered a category-one indication for hyperbaric oxygen, which essentially means that research and clinical experience have left little doubt about the efficacy of this therapy (117). Hyperbaric oxygen decreases the period of symptoms and may also reduce the incidence of long-term sequelae (53,123,124). Although the results of animal studies appear to confirm this latter effect (125), no controlled clinical studies with humans have done so (59). It has not been ascertained whether 100% oxygen or hyperbaric oxygen treatment can alter the long-term sequelae of carbon monoxide poisoning (8).

Although HBO significantly shortens the time needed to remove CO from hemoglobin, this is not the most pronounced effect of HBO (84). The increased amount of oxygen carried in the plasma provides oxygen for the local tissues and reverses the effects of CO on the cytochrome oxidase A3 system at the local tissue level (119). This effect is much more important than the clearing of CO from hemoglobin (126).

Another beneficial effect of hyperbaric oxygen is the reduction in intracranial pressure that occurs in a few minutes after the patient begins to breathe oxygen at pressure. This is due to the vasoconstrictive effect of oxygen and its consequent contraction of the intracranial vascular space (3,4).

Criteria for Hyperbaric Oxygen Therapy

The criteria for selection of patients for hyperbaric oxygen therapy should take into account the availability of a hyperbaric facility (15,16). Some investigators recommend that where a hyperbaric oxygen chamber facility exists, all patients with carboxyhemoglobin saturation of 25% or more should be treated by hyperbaric oxygen regardless of symptoms. The rationale for this is partly because at this level electrocardiographic signs of myocardial ischemia begin to appear (68). Others consider carboxyhemoglobin concentrations greater than 30% or 40% as the cut-off point for hyperbaric oxygen therapy, regardless of the patient's symptoms. In addition, any level of carboxyhemoglobin is an indication for hyperbaric oxygen therapy if the patient is comatose, irrespective of whether he or she is conscious on admission to the hospital (3,4).

Other evidence of neurologic sequelae, such as a clouded sensorium, posturing, or the inability to perform serial sevens or threes are also indications for hyperbaric oxygen (Table 32–11) (53). Mild headache and nausea by themselves are not indications for therapy. The pregnant patient should be considered for hyperbaric oxygen therapy for the reasons stated earlier. Finally, if there is evidence of acute electrocardiographic changes, symptoms of angina, or evidence of a metabolic acidosis (15), hyperbaric oxygen therapy is indicated.

TABLE 32–11. *Criteria for hyperbaric oxygen therapy in carbon monoxide poisoning*

Criteria
Availability of hyperbaric oxygen chamber
Carboxyhemoglobin concentration greater than 25%, 35%, or 40%
Any carboxyhemoglobin concentration with neurologic sequelae (coma, posturing, clouded sensorium)
Acute electrocardiographic changes
Symptoms of angina
Metabolic acidosis
Pregnancy

Although there is legitimate concern regarding the transfer of a critically ill, unstable patient from the initial receiving hospital to a facility providing hyperbaric oxygen therapy, complications associated with this practice are rare (50). With regard to interhospital transfer, if a patient has not experienced cardiac or respiratory arrest before or during the initial emergency department resuscitation, the likelihood of an arrest for the first time during transfer or HBO therapy is small. Therefore, therapy should not be withheld for fear of these potential complications during transfer (119).

Procedure for Hyperbaric Oxygen Therapy

The general procedure for hyperbaric oxygen therapy is to administer 100% oxygen at 2.5 to 3.0 atm for 40–45 minutes (127,128). Depending on the patient's response, this period may be extended but interspersed with breaks. Patients who remain unconscious are given a second hyperbaric oxygen treatment 6–7 hours later (3,75). The goal of hyperbaric oxygen is to reduce the carboxyhemoglobin concentration to less than 5%–10% in addition to providing complete symptomatic relief as quickly as possible (121).

Complications of Hyperbaric Oxygen Therapy

Complications of HBO therapy are usually the result of either barometric pressure changes or oxygen toxicity. The most common complications involve cavity trauma due to change in pressure. Any air-filled cavity that cannot equilibrate with ambient pressure, such as the middle ear when the eustachian tube is blocked, is subject to deformity and barotrauma during pressure changes in HBO therapy (120). (Table 32–12) (15). Occasionally, a myringotomy may be necessary, but it should not delay definitive treatment (3). Other complications include decompression sickness due to intravascular and intracellular expansion of dissolved nitrogen with formation of bubbles, oxygen toxicity with resultant seizures, cerebral gas embolism, and the potential to increase the size of a small pneumothorax (16). Patients who are severely poisoned with CO frequently require intubation, positive pressure ventilation, chest compressions, or central venous catheterization during resuscitation, interventions that are all associated with the risk of iatrogenic pneumothorax infection (126).

TABLE 32–12. *Complications of hyperbaric oxygen therapy*

Cerebral gas embolism
Decompression sickness
Emesis
Explosion
Fire
Increasing size of pneumothorax
Oxygen toxicity
Retrolental fibroplasia (fetal)
Rupture of tympanic membrane

If air becomes trapped in the intrapleural space or alveoli distal to an outflow obstruction during hyperbaric compression (descent) or at depth, it will expand during decompression (ascent), according to Boyle's Law (126). Because small pneumothoraces can develop at any time, attentive pulmonary examination and chest radiography immediately before and following HBO therapy should be instituted for those patients with prior chest compressions, intubation, central venous catheterization, or a history of asthma or chronic obstructive airway disease. These high-risk patients must be assumed to have a tension pneumothorax if hypotension, respiratory distress, or cardiac arrest occur while in the HBO chamber or following decompression. The anticipation of a tension pneumothorax mandates that a large-bore needle be available for needle thoracostomy both during and after HBO therapy (119). Air embolism may also occur from holding the breath during the decompression phase.

When treating a CO-toxic patient with HBO therapy, continued consideration of the potential for emesis, agitation, seizures, arterial hypotension, and cardiac dysrhythmia is warranted because of the frequency and timing of these complications relative to HBO (119).

The risk of fire or explosion in the oxygen-rich atmosphere can be diminished by keeping the humidity high, and vomiting, especially during decompression, can best be avoided by routine emptying of the patient's stomach before treatment. Although a concern in premature newborns, retrolental fibroplasia has not been noted in infants, children, or adults undergoing HBO therapy (120). HBO given at pressures and durations that correspond to treatment schedules routinely used for CO intoxication appear to be well-tolerated by the fetus in early or late pregnancy (84). Major complications of hyperbaric oxygen are rare.

The risks of hyperbaric oxygen therapy should be carefully weighed against the possible benefits, particularly in cases of chronic sinusitis, history of spontaneous pneumothorax, upper respiratory infection, epilepsy, emphysema with carbon dioxide retention, and history of ear surgery. Untreated pneumothorax is an absolute contraindication (126).

Exchange Transfusion

Although some reports suggest treatment of carbon monoxide poisoning by exchange transfusion (16,58), the cornerstone of treatment remains immediate therapy with as high a level of inspired oxygen as is available. Because of the ability of 100% inspired oxygen to decrease the half-life of carboxyhemoglobin, oxygen therapy must be viewed as a more rapid and effective treatment than attempting exchange transfusion for any patient with clinically significant carbon monoxide poisoning.

REFERENCES

1. Somogyi E, Balogh I, Rubanyi G, et al: New findings concerning the pathogenesis of acute carbon monoxide (CO) poisoning. *Am J Forensic Med Pathol* 1981;2:21–39.
2. Longo L: The biological effects of carbon monoxide on the pregnant woman, fetus, and newborn infant. *Am J Obstet Gynecol* 1977;129: 69–102.
3. Myers R: Carbon monoxide poisoning. *J Emerg Med* 1984;1:245–248.
4. Myers R, Messier L, Jones D, et al: New directions in the research and treatment of carbon monoxide exposure. *Am J Emerg Med* 1983; 2:226–230.
5. Morenson H, Caraccio T, Brody G: Carbon monoxide poisoning. *Am J Emerg Med* 1984;2:254–261.
6. Llano A, Raffin T: Management of carbon monoxide poisoning. *Chest* 1990;97:165–169.
7. Hampson N, Norkool D: Carbon monoxide poisoning in children riding in the back of pickup trucks. *JAMA* 1992;267:538–540.
8. Olson K: Carbon monoxide poisoning: mechanisms, presentation, and controversies in management. *J Emerg Med* 1984;1:233–243.
9. Olson K, Becker C: Hyperbaric oxygen for carbon monoxide poisoning. *JAMA* 1982;248:172–173.
10. Zimmerman S, Truxal B: Carbon monoxide poisoning. *Pediatrics* 1981;68:215–224.
11. Dolan M: Carbon monoxide poisoning. *Can Med Assoc J* 1985;133: 392–399.
12. Bessoudo R, Gray J: Carbon monoxide poisoning and nonoliguric acute renal failure. *Can Med Assoc J* 1978;119:41–44.
13. Clark C. Campbell D, Reid W: Blood carboxyhemoglobin and cyanide levels in fire survivors. *Lancet* 1981;1:1332–1335.
14. Hardy K, Thom S: Pathophysiology and treatment of carbon monoxide poisoning. *J Toxicol Clin Toxicol* 1994;32:613–630.
15. Crocker P, Walker J: Pediatric carbon monoxide toxicity. *J Emerg Med* 1985;3:443–448.
16. Crocker P: Carbon monoxide poisoning, the clinical entity and its treatment: a review. *Mil Med* 1984;149: 257–259.
17. Stewart R: The effect of carbon monoxide on humans. *J Occup Med* 1976;18:304–309.
18. Stewart R, Hake C: Paint-remover hazard. *JAMA* 1976;235:398–401.
19. Landers D: Unsuccessful suicide by carbon monoxide: a secondary benefit of emissions control. *West J Med* 1981;135:360–363.
20. Landa J, Avery W, Sackner M: Some physiologic observations in smoke inhalation. *Chest* 1972;61:62–63.
21. Levesque B, Dewailly E, Lavoie R, et al: Carbon monoxide in indoor ice skating rinks: evaluation of absorption by adult hockey players. *Am J Public Health* 1990;80:594–598.
22. Heckerling P, Leikin J, Maturen A, et al: Predictors of occult carbon monoxide poisoning in patients with headache and dizziness. *Ann Intern Med* 1987;107:174–176.
23. Heckerling P: Occult carbon monoxide poisoning. *Am J Emerg Med* 1987;5:201–214.
24. Murray T: Carbon monoxide in the modern society. *Can Med Assoc J* 1978;118:758–760.
25. Murray T: Carbon monoxide poisoning from Sterno. *Can Med Assoc J* 1978;118:800–802.
26. Jackson D, Menges H: Accidental carbon monoxide poisoning. *JAMA* 1980;243 :772–774.
27. Heckerling P, Leikin J, Terzian C, et al: Occult carbon monoxide poisoning in patients with neurologic illness. *J Toxicol Clin Toxicol* 1990;28:29–44.
28. Wilson E, Rich T, Messman H: The hazardous hibachi. *JAMA* 1972; 221:405–406.
29. Stewart R, Fisher T, Hosko M, et al: Experimental human exposure to methylene chloride. *Arch Environ Health* 1972:25:342–348.
30. Ratney R, Wegman D, Elkins H: In vivo conversion of methylene chloride to carbon monoxide. *Arch Environ Health* 1974;28:223–226.
31. Rioux J, Myers R: Methylene chloride poisoning: a paradigmatic review. *J Emerg Med* 1988;6:227–238.
32. Fagin J, Bradley J, Williams D: Carbon monoxide poisoning secondary to inhaling methylene chloride. *Br Med J* 1980;281:1461.
33. Stewart R, Stewart S, Stamm W, et al: Rapid estimation of carboxyhemoglobin level in fire fighters. *JAMA* 1976;235:390–392.
34. Burney R, Wu S, Nemiroff M: Mass carbon monoxide poisoning: clinical effects and results of treatment in 184 victims. *Ann Emerg Med* 1982;11:394–399.
35. Leikin J, Vogel S: Carbon monoxide levels in cardiac patients in an urban emergency department. *Am J Emerg Med* 1986;4:126–128.
36. Garland H, Pearce J: Neurological complications of carbon monoxide poisoning. *Q J Med* 1967;34:445–454.
37. Gossel TA, Bricker JD: *Principles of Clinical Toxicology, 3rd ed.* New York: Raven Press, p. 111, 1994.
38. Anderson E, Andelman R, Strauch J, et al: Effect of low level carbon monoxide exposure on onset and duration of angina pectoris. *Ann Intern Med* 1973;79:46–50.
39. Winter P, Miller J: Carbon monoxide poisoning. *JAMA* 1976;236: 1502–1504.
40. Larkin J, Brahos G, Moylan J: Treatment of carbon monoxide poisoning: prognostic factors. *J Trauma* 1976;16:111–114.
41. Marius-Nunez A: Myocardial infarction with normal coronary arteries after acute exposure to carbon monoxide. *Chest* 1990;97:491–494.
42. Goldbaum L, Orellano T, Dergal E: Mechanism of the toxic action of carbon monoxide. *Ann Clin Lab Sci* 1976;6:372–376.
43. Goldbaum L, Orellano T, Dergal E: Studies on the relation between carboxyhemoglobin concentration and toxicity. *Aviat Space Environ Med* 1977;48:969–970.
44. Goldbaum L, Ramirez R, Absalon K: What is the mechanism of carbon monoxide toxicity? *Aviat Space Environ Med* 1975;46:1289–1291.
45. Sadovnikoff N, Varon J, Sternbach G: Carbon monoxide poisoning: an occult epidemic. *Postgrad Med J* 1992;92:86–96.
46. Florkowski C, Rossi M, Carey M, et al: Rhabdomyolysis and acute renal failure following carbon monoxide poisoning: two case reports with muscle histopathology and enzyme activities. *J Toxicol Clin Toxicol* 1992;30:443–454.
47. Aronow W: Effect of cigarette smoking and of carbon monoxide on coronary heart disease. *Chest* 1976;71: 514–518.
48. Aronow W, Isbell M: Carbon monoxide effect on exercise-induced angina pectoris. *Ann Intern Med* 1973;79:392–395.
49. Zeller W, Miele A, Suarez C: Accidental carbon monoxide poisoning. *Clin Pediatr* 1984;23:694–695.
50. Thom S, Keim L: Carbon monoxide poisoning: a review epidemiology, pathophysiology, clinical findings, and treatment options including hyperbaric oxygen therapy. *J Toxicol Clin Toxicol* 1989;27:141–156.
51. Chung S: Formulas predicting carboxyhemoglobin resulting from carbon monoxide exposure. *Vet Hum Toxicol* 1988;30:528–532.
52. Choi I: Delayed neurologic sequelae in carbon monoxide intoxication. *Arch Neurol* 1983;40:433–435.
53. Norkool D, Kirkpatrick J: Treatment of acute carbon monoxide poisoning with hyperbaric oxygen: a review of 115 cases. *Ann Emerg Med* 1985;14:1168–1171.
54. Scharf S, Thames M, Sargent R: Transmural myocardial infarction after exposure to carbon monoxide in coronary-artery disease. *N Engl J Med* 1974;291:85–87.
55. Davis S, Levy R: High carboxyhemoglobin level without acute or chronic findings. *J Emerg Med* 1984;1:539–542.
56. Allred E, Bleecker E, Chaitman B, et al: Short-term effects of carbon monoxide exposure on the exercise performance of subjects with coronary artery disease. *N Engl J Med* 1989;321;1426–1432.
57. Crapo R: Smoke-inhalation injuries. *JAMA* 1981;246:1694–1696.
58. Yee L, Brandon G: Successful reversal of presumed carbon monoxide-induced semicoma. *Aviat Space Environ Med* 1983;54:641–643.
59. Huber J: Do awake patients with high carboxyhemoglobin levels need hyperbaric oxygen? *J Emerg Med* 1984;1:555–556.
60. Fisher J: Occult carbon monoxide poisoning. *Arch Intern Med* 1982; 142:1270–1271.
61. Naeije R, Peretz A, Cornil A: Acute pulmonary edema following carbon monoxide poisoning. *Intensive Care Med* 1980;6:189–191.
62. Ginsburg R, Romano J: Carbon monoxide encephalopathy: need for appropriate treatment. *Am J Psychiatr* 1976;133:317–320.

63. Ginsberg M: Carbon monoxide intoxication: clinical features, neuropathology and mechanism of injury. *Clin Toxicol* 1985;23:281–288.
64. Moar J: Early acute fatal carbon monoxide poisoning: assessment of the survival period. *S Afr Med J* 1984;68:650–652.
65. Williams J, Lewis R, Kealey G: Carbon monoxide poisoning and myocardial ischemia in patients with burns. *J Burn Care Rehabil* 1992;13:210–213.
66. Myers R, Snyder S, Majerus T: Cutaneous blisters and carbon monoxide poisoning. *Ann Emerg Med* 1985;14:603–606.
67. Nagy R, Greer K, Harman L: Cutaneous manifestations of acute carbon monoxide poisoning. *Cutis* 1979;24:381–383.
68. Anderson G: Treatment of carbon monoxide poisoning with hyperbaric oxygen. *Mil Med* 1978;143:538–541.
69. Anderson R, Allensworth D, deGroot W: Myocardial toxicity from carbon monoxide poisoning. *Ann Intern Med* 1967;67:1172–1182.
70. Kelley J, Sophocleus G: Retinal hemorrhages in subacute carbon monoxide poisoning. *JAMA* 1978;239: 1515–1517.
71. Linton A, Adams J, Lawson D: Muscle necrosis and acute renal failure in carbon monoxide poisoning. *Postgrad Med J* 1968;44:338–341.
72. Loughridge L, Leader L, Bowen D: Acute renal failure due to muscle necrosis in carbon monoxide poisoning. *Lancet* 1958;2:349–351.
73. Howse A, Seddon H: Ischemic contracture of muscle associated with carbon monoxide and barbiturate poisoning. *Br Med J* 1966;1:192–195.
74. Myers R, Snyder S, Emhoff T: Subacute sequelae of carbon monoxide poisoning. *Ann Emerg Med* 1985;14:1163–1167.
75. Myers R, Snyder S, Lindberg S, et al: Value of hyperbaric oxygen in suspected carbon monoxide poisoning. *JAMA* 1981;246:2478–2480.
76. Lacey D: Neurologic sequelae of acute carbon monoxide intoxication. *Am J Dis Child* 1981;135:145–147.
77. Siesjo B: Oxygen deficiency and brain damage: localization, evolution in time, and mechanisms of damage. *Clin Toxicol* 1985;23:267–280.
78. Siesjo B: Carbon monoxide poisoning: mechanism of damage, late sequelae and therapy. *Clin Toxicol* 1985;23:247–248.
79. Werner B, Back W, Akerblom H, et al: Two cases of acute carbon monoxide poisoning with delayed neurological sequelae after a "free" interval. *Clin Toxicol* 1985;23: 249–265.
80. Halebian P, Yurt R, Petito C, et al: Diabetes insipidus after carbon monoxide poisoning and smoke inhalation. *J Trauma* 1985;25:662–663.
81. Klawans H, Stein R, Tanner C, et al: A pure parkinsonian syndrome following acute carbon monoxide intoxication. *Arch Neurol* 1982;39: 302–304.
82. Davous P, Rondol P, Marion M, et al: Severe chorea after acute carbon monoxide poisoning. *J Neurol Neurosurg Psychiatr* 1986;49: 206–208.
83. Myers R, Linberg S, Cowley R, et al: Carbon monoxide poisoning: the injury and its treatment. *JACEP* 1979;8:479–484.
84. Van Hoesen J, Camporesi E, Moon R, et al: Should hyperbaric oxygen be used to treat the pregnant patient for acute carbon monoxide poisoning? *JAMA* 1989;261:1039–1043.
85. Goldstein DL: Carbon monoxide poisoning in pregnancy. *Am J Obstet Gynecol* 1965;92:526–528.
86. Woody R, Brewster M: Telencephalic dysgenesis associated with presumptive maternal carbon monoxide intoxication in the first trimester of pregnancy. *J Toxicol Clin Toxicol* 1990;28:467–475.
87. Copel J, Bowen F, Bolognese R: Carbon monoxide intoxication in early pregnancy. *Obstet Gynecol* 1982;59:26s–28s.
88. Venning H, Roberton D, Milner A: Carbon monoxide poisoning in an infant. *Br Med J* 1981;284:651.
89. Farrow J, Davis G, Roy T, et al: Fetal death due to nonlethal maternal carbon monoxide poisoning. *J Foren Sci* 1990;35:1448–1452.
90. Caravati E, Adams C, Joyce S, et al: Fetal toxicity associated with maternal carbon monoxide poisoning. *Ann Emerg Med* 1988;17:714–717.
91. Binder J, Roberts R: Carbon monoxide intoxication in children. *Clin Toxicol* 1980;16:287–295.
92. Grace T, Platt F: Subacute carbon monoxide poisoning. *JAMA* 1981; 246:1698–1700.
93. Barret L, Danel V, Faure J: Carbon monoxide poisoning, a diagnosis frequently overlooked. *Clin Toxicol* 1985;23:309–313.
94. Castle S, Lapham S, Troutman W, et al: Carbon monoxide intoxication: diagnostic considerations. *JAMA* 1984;251:2350.
95. Gemelli F, Cattani R: Carbon monoxide poisoning in childhood. *Br Med J* 1985;291:1197.
96. Turnbull T, Hart R, Strange G, et al: Emergency department screening for unsuspected carbon monoxide exposure. *Ann Emerg Med* 1988;17:478–483.
97. Otten E, Rosenberg J, Tasset J: An evaluation of carboxyhemoglobin spot tests. *Ann Emerg Med* 1985;14:850–852.
98. Meredith T, Vale A: Carbon monoxide poisoning. *Br Med J* 1988; 296:77–79.
99. Myers R, Britten J: Are arterial blood gases of value in treatment decisions for carbon monoxide poisoning? *Crit Care Med* 1989;17: 139–142.
100. Lebby T, Zalenski R, Hyrhorczuk D, et al: The usefulness of the arterial blood gas in pure carbon monoxide poisoning. *Vet Hum Toxicol* 1989;31:138–139.
101. Heckerling P, Leikin J, Matuiren A, et al: Screening hospital admissions from the emergency department for occult carbon monoxide poisoning. *Am J Emerg Med* 1990;8:301–304.
102. Hall A, Linden C, Kulig K, et al: Cyanide poisoning from Laetrile ingestion: Role of nitrite therapy. *Pediatrics* 1986;78:269–272.
103. Vegfors M, Lennmarken C: Carboxyhaemoglobinaemia and pulse oximetry. *Brit M Anaes* 1991;66:625–626.
104. Buckley R, Aks S, Esham J, et al: The pulse oximetry gap in carbon monoxide intoxication. *Ann Emerg Med* 1994;24:252–255.
105. Wald N, Idle M, Boreham J, et al: Carbon monoxide in breath in relation to smoking and carboxyhemoglobin levels. *Thorax* 1981;36:366–369.
106. Wald N, Idle M, Boreham J, et al: Inhaling habits among smokers of different types of cigarettes. *Thorax* 1980;35:925–928.
107. Vogt T, Selven S, Widdowson G, et al: Expired air carbon monoxide and serum thiocyanate as objective measures of cigarette exposure. *Am J Public Health* 1977;67:545–549.
108. Hampson N: Arterial oxygenation in carbon monoxide poisoning. *Chest* 1990;948:1538–1539.
109. Cramer C: Fetal death due to accidental maternal carbon monoxide poisoning. *J Toxicol Clin Toxicol* 1982;19:297–301.
110. Smith J, Brandon S: Acute carbon monoxide poisoning: 3 years' experience in a defined population. *Postgrad Med J* 1970;46:65–70.
111. Smith J, Brandon S: Morbidity from acute carbon monoxide poisoning at three-year follow-up. *Br Med J* 1973;1:318–321.
112. Nardizzi L: Computerized tomographic correlate of carbon monoxide poisoning. *Arch Neurol* 1979;36:38–39.
113. Destee A, Courteville V, Devos P, et al: Computed tomography and acute carbon monoxide poisoning. *J Neurol Neurosurg Psychiatr* 1985;48:281–291.
114. Rioux J, Myers R: Hybaric oxygen for methylene chloride poisoning: report on two cases. *Ann Emerg Med* 1989;18:691–695.
115. Mendelsohn D, Hertzanu Y: Carbon monoxide poisoning. *S Afr Med J* 1983;64:751–752.
116. Finley J, VanBeek A, Glover J: Myonecrosis complicating carbon monoxide poisoning. *J Trauma* 1977;17:536–540.
117. Kindwall E: Hyperbaric treatment of carbon monoxide poisoning. *Ann Emerg Med* 1985;14:1233–1234.
118. Deger D, Welch L: Carbon monoxide controversies: Neuropsychiatric testing, mechanism of toxicity, and hyperbaric oxygen. *Ann Emerg Med* 1994;24:242–251.
119. Sloan E, Murphy D, Hart R, et al: Compilations and protocol considerations in carbon monoxide-poisoned patients who require hyperbaric oxygen therapy: report from a ten-year experience. *Ann Emerg Med* 1989;18:629–634.
120. Grim P, Gottlieb L, Boddie A, et al: Hyperbaric oxygen therapy. *JAMA* 1990;263:2216–2220.
121. Tibbles P, Perrotta PL: Treatment of carbon monoxide poisoning: a critical review of human outcome studies comparing normobaric oxygen with hyperbaric oxygen. *Ann Emerg Med* 1994;24:269–282.
122. Van Meter K, Weiss L, Harch P: Should the pressure be off or on in the use of oxygen in the treatment of carbon monoxide-poisoned patients? *Ann Emerg Med* 1994;24:283–288.
123. Ziser A, Shupak A, Halpern P, et al: Delayed hyperbaric oxygen treatment for acute carbon monoxide poisoning. *Br Med J* 1984;289: 960.
124. Mathieu D, Nolf M, Durocher A, et al: Acute carbon monoxide poi-

soning: risk of late sequelae and treatment by hyperbaric oxygen. *Clin Toxicol* 1985;23:315–324.

125. Goulon M, Barois A, Rapin M, et al: Carbon monoxide poisoning and acute anoxia due to breathing coal gas and hydrocarbons. *J Hyperbaric Med* 1986;1:23–41.
126. Murphy D, Sloan E, Hart R, et al: Tension pneumothorax associated with hyperbaric oxygen therapy. *Am J Emerg Med* 1991;9:176–179.
127. Vorosmarti J: Hyperbaric oxygen therapy. *Am Fam Physician* 1981; 23:169–173.
128. Hart G, Strauss M, Lennon P, et al: Treatment of smoke inhalation by hyperbaric oxygen. *J Emerg Med* 1985;3:211–215.

ADDITIONAL SELECTED REFERENCES

Benowitz N, Jacob P, Yu L, et al: Reduced tar, nicotine, and carbon monoxide exposure while smoking ultralow- but not low-yield cigarettes. *JAMA* 1986;256:241–246.

Buehler J, Berns A, Webster J, et al: Lactic acidosis from carboxyhemoglobinemia after smoke inhalation. *Ann Intern Med* 1975;82:803–805.

Castleden C, Cole P: Variations in carboxyhemoglobin levels in smokers. *Br Med J* 1974;4:736–738.

Cohen M, Guzzardi L: Inhalation of products of combustion. *Ann Emerg Med* 1983;12:628–632.

Cordasco E, Van Ordstrand H: Air pollution and COPD. *Postgrad Med J* 1977;62:124–127.

Dinman B: The management of acute carbon monoxide intoxication. *J Occup Med* 1974;16:662–664.

Flanagan N, Wootton D, Smith G, et al: An unusual case of carbon monoxide poisoning. *Med Sci Law* 1978;18: 117–119.

Gold A, Burgess A, Clougherty E: Exposure of firefighters to toxic air contaminants. *Am Ind Hyg Assoc J* 1978;39: 534–539.

Gozal D, Ziser A, Shupak A, et al: Accidental carbon monoxide poisoning. *Clin Pediatrics* 1985;24:132–135.

Hauck H, Neuberger M: Carbon monoxide uptake and the resulting carboxyhemoglobin in man. *Eur J Appl Physiol* 1984;53:186–190.

Jett G: Red retinal vein (Jett) sign. *Ann Emerg Med* 1984;13:2802–2803.

Kachulis C: Secondhand cigarette smoke. *Postgrad Med J* 1981;70:77–79.

Kizer K: Toxic inhalations. *Emerg Med Clin North Am* 1984;2:649–666.

Manning R: The serial sevens test. *Arch Intern Med* 1982;142:1192.

Neubauer R: Carbon monoxide and hyperbaric oxygen. *Arch Intern Med* 1979;139:829.

Pulst S, Walshe T, Romero J: Carbon monoxide poisoning with features of Gilles de la Tourette's syndrome. *Arch Neurol* 1983;40:443–444.

Remick R, Miles J: Carbon monoxide poisoning: neurologic and psychiatric sequelae. *Can Med Assoc J* 1977;17:651–657.

Spiller D: Carbon monoxide exposure in the home: source and epidemiology. *Vet Hum Toxicol* 1987;29:383–386.

Stevenson M, Cooper G, Chenoweth M: Effect on carboxyhemoglobin of exposure to aerosol spray paints with methylene chloride. *Clin Toxicol* 1978;12:551–561.

Stewart R, Peterson J, Fisher R, et al: Experimental human exposure to high concentrations of carbon monoxide. *Arch Environ Health* 1973;26:1–7.

Takahashi M, Maemura K, Sawada Y, et al: Hyperamylasemia in acute carbon monoxide poisoning. *J Trauma* 1982;22:311–314.

Terrill J, Montgomery R, Reinhardt C: Toxic gases from fires. *Science* 1978;200:1343–1347.

Utidjian H: The criteria for a recommended standard. I. Recommendations for a carbon monoxide standard: occupation exposure to carbon monoxide. *J Occup Med* 1973;15:446–451.

Webster J, McCabe M, Karp M: Recognition and management of smoke inhalation. *JAMA* 1967;201:71–74.

Williams R: Vehicular carbon monoxide screening: identification in a cross-cultural setting of a substantial public health risk factor. *Am J Public Health* 1985;75:85–86.

Zarem H, Rattenborg C, Harmel M: Carbon monoxide toxicity in human fire victims. *Arch Surg* 1973;107:851–853.

Zikria B, Weston G, Chodoff A, et al: Smoke and carbon monoxide poisoning in fire victims. *J Trauma* 1972;12:641–645.

CHAPTER 33

Cyanide

Cyanide is one of the oldest toxins known (1). In ancient Egyptian documents, administering cyanogenic peach kernel preparations is mentioned as a form of execution. Ancient Greeks and Romans used a cherry laurel distillate for suicides, murders, and judicial executions (2). In 1782, hydrogen cyanide liquid was isolated by the chemist Karl Wilhelm Scheele through the action of sulfuric acid on Prussian blue, from which the name prussic acid for hydrocyanic acid derives. Scheele died 4 years after his discovery from inhaling hydrogen cyanide gas when he accidentally broke a beaker of the deadly acid (3).

Although cyanide poisoning is very rarely encountered by clinicians, few poisons are more rapidly lethal. Furthermore, cyanide is one of the few poisons for which specific antidotes exist (4). The inhalation of hydrogen cyanide commonly produces reactions within a few seconds and death within minutes, although patients may survive at sublethal doses with symptoms lasting several hours (5). Chronic cyanide poisoning also occurs throughout the world secondary to intake of cyanogenic glycosides as part of normal diets. An increasing number of nonindustrial cases of cyanide poisoning are being reported; these are probably related to the increasing availability of Laetrile and the release of cyanide gas from burning synthetic materials.

SOURCES AND USES OF CYANIDE

Cyanide poisoning is most often due to cyanide ingestion, immersion in solutions of cyanide salts, ingestion of cyanogenic substances, inhalation of hydrogen cyanide gas in industrial accidents, smoke inhalation, or inhalation or dermal exposure to cyanogenic nitrile compounds.

Cyanide is a fairly widespread potential hazard of industrial and nonindustrial environments (Tables 33–1 and 33–2). Hydrocyanic acid and sodium and potassium cyanide are found in vermicidal fumigants, insecticides, rodenticides, metal polishes (especially silver polish), and electroplating solutions (6). Cyanide is used in metallurgy for the extraction of gold and silver metals from their ores, in chemicals used to remove hair from hides, in processing photographic film, and in chemical synthesis and research.

Hydrocyanic acid is an effective agent in the fumigation of ships, army posts, navy stations, large buildings, flour mills, private dwellings, freight cars, and airplanes that have become infested with rodents and insects. As a fumigant it is applied directly as a solution, or the gas is generated from one of the cyanide salts by the action of dilute mineral acid. Cyanide has also been used as an insecticide and in the process of soil sterilization. Potassium cyanide crystals may be used in coyote "gitter" traps: when an animal bites into the meat in the trap, a shell explodes and releases cyanide (6). Human intoxica-

TABLE 33–1. *Sources and uses of cyanide*

Cigarette smoke
False nail (glue) remover
Fires
Horsehair
Wool
Silk
Polyurethanes
Polyacrylonitriles
Industrial uses
Metal polish
Electroplating
Extracting silver and gold from ore
Removing hair from hides
Photography
Chemical synthesis
Plastics
Phencyclidine
Synthetic rubber
Judicial executions
Laboratories
Pest control
Vermicidal fumigant
Insecticide
Rodenticide
Soil sterilization
Coyote "gitter" traps
Plants and fruits
Cassava
Amygdalin (Laetrile)
Pits and seeds
Product tampering
Sodium nitroprusside

TABLE 33–2. *Compounds containing cyanide*

Calcium cyanide
Cyanamide
Cyanates
Cyanogen
Cyanogenic glycosides
Hydrogen cyanide
Isobornyl thiocyanoacetate
Nitriles
Acetonitrile
Acrylonitrile
Butyronitrile
Malononitrile
Succinonitrile
Nitroprusside
Potassium cyanide
Potassium ferricyanide
Prussic acid
Sodium cyanide

tion may occur if the unwary were to step on the cyanide or somehow to allow the cyanide to be released.

Cyanide is used in the production of nitriles and cyanohydrins, which are chemicals used in the manufacture of many plastics (7).

Fires

Incomplete combustion of products containing carbon and nitrogen may liberate cyanide. Fires where there is combustion of organic nitrogen-containing polymers, both natural (wool and silk) and synthetic (polyurethanes and polyacrylonitriles), which are used extensively in domestic furnishings, may therefore yield significant amounts of hydrogen cyanide (Table 33–3) (4,7,8). Plastics of any type, such as the plastics in electrical wires, can also yield cyanide when heated (8). The massive growth of the polymer industry makes it likely that cyanide will be encountered with increasing frequency in fires (9). This may have practical medical significance in the treatment of severe smoke inhalation (10). Firefighters involved in nonfatal fires have been found to have elevated cyanide concentrations in their blood (11). In addition, propionitrile (ethyl cyanide), which is used in organic synthesis and as a solvent, is toxic if ingested, inhaled, or absorbed through the skin (12).

TABLE 33–3. *Household materials that yield cyanide when burned*

Material	Location
Wool	Clothing, fabric, blankets
Silk	Clothing, fabric, blankets
Polyurethane	Insulation, upholstery material
Polyacrylonitrile	Appliances, plastics
Polyamide (nylon)	Carpeting, clothing
Melamine resins	Household goods
Plastics	Wiring

Microorganisms

Some microorganisms, notably *Pseudomonas aeruginosa*, have the ability to produce cyanide. These organisms may become a source of abnormally high cyanide concentrations in patients with an overwhelming infection, which can be a consequence of burns and sepsis (13). These cyanide concentrations, however, may be forensically misleading (14).

Sodium Nitroprusside

Nitroprusside is a ferrocyanide compound that contains 44% cyanide. Sodium nitroprusside at therapeutic doses has been shown to release cyanide in vivo by reaction with hemoglobin to form cyanomethemoglobin. Because each nitroprusside molecule contains five cyanide groups, and because nitroprusside is metabolized to cyanide (15), if a patient requires prolonged nitroprusside treatment the need for higher and higher doses to achieve the same effect (tachyphylaxis) may lead to cyanide intoxication (4,15–18). The cyanide concentration obtained from therapeutic doses does not typically lead to cyanide intoxication because of the rapid uptake of cyanide by erythrocytes, incorporation of cyanide into hydroxycobalamin (vitamin B_{12a}) to produce cyanocobalamin (vitamin B_{12}), and adequate hepatic metabolism of cyanide by mitochondrial sulfurtransferase (rhodanase) to thiocyanate, which is less toxic (19).

Prolonged administration of nitroprusside or administration in large dosages (greater than 10 μg/kg/min) may result in cyanide intoxication (15,20,21). Cyanide is released when the drug interacts with sulfhydryl groups found in body fluids and tissues. The toxicity of nitroprusside is dose related, and 3–10 hours of nitroprusside infusion at a dose of 5–10 μg/kg/min could cause lethal cyanide intoxication. In clinical practice, these infusion rates are never reached, although lesser quantities coupled with longer therapy could lead to toxicity in selected patient groups. Although an adult with normal renal function can easily handle 1 μg/kg/min for short periods of time, smaller amounts may be lethal in children or in patients with chronic renal failure (15,22,23). Deaths attributable to cyanide have been reported from the purposeful ingestion of nitroprusside (18).

Cigarette Smokers

Cigarette smokers have been found to have mean whole blood cyanide concentrations that are more than

2.5 times the mean for nonsmokers because of the natural cyanide found in tobacco (6). In addition, smokers have increased whole blood thiocyanate concentrations.

Phencyclidine Manufacturing

Potassium cyanide is necessary in the most commonly employed method of illicit synthesis of phencyclidine. In addition, improperly synthesized phencyclidine may be contaminated by an intermediary containing cyanide (cyclohexanecarbonitrile).

Mass Extermination

Cyanide was also used in the extermination centers operated by the Hitler regime during World War II, and the use of cyanide in judicial executions has been reinstituted as a form of capital punishment in some areas of the United States. Potassium cyanide was implicated in the deaths of more than 900 individuals in Jonestown, Guyana (24).

Product Tampering

In 1982, seven persons died in metropolitan Chicago after ingesting acetaminophen capsules that contained cyanide. In 1986, two persons died in Seattle after ingesting cyanide-containing analgesic capsules. In 1991, three persons in western Washington state were poisoned with cyanide-containing Sudafed 12-hour capsules. As a consequence of these incidents, many over-the-counter medications were repackaged to make them "tamper-resistant."

Acetonitrile

Acetonitrile (methyl cyanide, ethanenitrile, cyanomethane, ethyl nitrile, methane carbonitrile) is an organic solvent widely used for industrial and laboratory applications (25). Other nitriles include propionitrile, malononitrile, butyronitrile, acrylonitrile, and succinonitrile (26). Although the acute toxicity of unchanged acetonitrile is relatively low, major toxicity is exhibited due to the in vivo formation of cyanide as a metabolite (27). Acetonitrile liberates cyanide during oxidative metabolism through the cytochrome P-450 dependent hepatic microsomal enzyme system (28). Initial oxidation to a cyanohydrin intermediate is followed by spontaneous degradation to hydrogen cyanide and an aldehyde (29)

One use of acetonitrile is as a solvent remover of acrylic sculptured nails that are bonded to the natural nail with glues (26). These products come in a variety of containers in volumes ranging from 30–180 mL (27). Most of them are sold without child-resistant caps and without specific warnings (30). It may not always be clear whether nail glue remover (acetonitrile) or nail polish remover (acetone) is involved. The initial symptoms of both ingestions are similar (25).

The failure of the product label to clearly identify the potential generation of a lethal cyanide metabolite contributes to the confusion in diagnosis. Sufficient acetonitrile is contained in a typical 2-ounce sculpted nail remover bottle for several fatal doses even in a child's single swallow.

Signs and Symptoms of Acetonitrile Toxicity

Because the parent compound is believed to have little toxicity but is metabolized in vivo to hydrogen cyanide, delayed toxic effects may be anticipated (31). After a latent period of several hours and sometimes as much as 13 hours during which metabolism occurs and cyanide is slowly released, symptoms develop (27). This can obscure the seriousness of the poisoning and lead to a false sense of security.

Vomiting is not usually a major sign or important clue in inorganic cyanide poisoning, but delayed vomiting has immediately preceded major toxicity in virtually all case reports of acetonitrile poisoning.

The osmolal gap has been a traditional test for ingestion of low molecular weight water-miscible solvents, such as the alcohols. Ingestion of acetonitrile should produce an increase in osmolality slightly greater than that produced by a similar amount of ethanol (25). This is predicted from its slightly lower molecular weight and an expectation of similar volumes of distribution. Acetonitrile should now be included in the differential diagnosis of a systemic acidosis with both anion and osmolar gaps (27).

Cyanide in Plants

The natural environment contains various cyanogenic glycosides that can release hydrogen cyanide when exposed to acid or appropriate enzymes (Table 33–4).

TABLE 33–4. *Plants containing cyanogenic glycosides*

Rosaceae family
Amygdalin
Prunin
Linamarin
Lima bean
Cassava
Bamboo sprout
Flax
Hydrangea
Johnson grass
Macadamia nuts
Sorghum

(See Table 33–5).

Certain plants produce free hydrocyanic acid or cyanogenic glycosides because they lack the ability to convert all the available amino acids into proteins. For these species the production of cyanogenic glycosides is a side reaction in protein metabolism.

There are at least 360 varieties of fruits and vegetables in 41 families that can yield hydrocyanic acid. Members of the family Rosaceae, including the plum, peach, pear, apple, apricot, cherry, and almond, contain various quantities of amygdalin (mandelonitrile-ß-glucosido-6-ß-glucoside), a glycoside of gentiobiose, hydrocyanide, and benzaldehyde (32–34). Other species of this family, notably the cherry laurel, contain a related cyanogenic glycoside termed prunin, which has also been responsible for a number of cyanide poisonings (35). The bitter almond is not to be confused with the somewhat larger sweet almond, which is nontoxic. Another glycoside of this group, linamarin, has been responsible for a federal restriction on the importation of some varieties of lima bean into the United States (15).

Amygdalin

Natural sources of cyanide include amygdalin and other cyanogenic glycosides. The glycosides are found in apricot and peach pits, as well as in the seeds of apples, pears, plums, and cherries. Bamboo sprouts, cassava, lima beans, almonds, and macadamia nuts also contain cyanide, as do hydrangeas, Johnson grass, sorghum, and flax. Although human consumption of cyanogenic plants or nuts is common, fatalities are rare (22). Death has occurred after the ingestion of large quantities of almonds, apricot pits, or choke cherries. Ingestion of lesser quantities by small children or pets may be fatal.

Pits and seeds that contain amygdalin (Table 33–5) usually also contain a group of enzymes, the emulsin complex, which breaks the linkages of the amygdalin to yield hydrogen cyanide (15,36). These enzymes are activated when the plant tissue is crushed or otherwise disrupted, such as in chewing. The cyanide content of amygdalin is approximately 6%, and it has been estimated that 15 to 60 varieties of seeds containing amygdalin can, when ingested, result in severe intoxication or death (37). For example, the cyanide content of moist apricot pits varies from 8.9–409 mg/100 g (38); peach pits contain 88 mg/100 g; and bitter almonds contain 469 mg/100 g (15). Amygdalin is only toxic by the oral route; when administered intravenously the parent compound is almost completely excreted in the urine (39).

TABLE 33–5. *Pits and seeds of fruits containing amygdalin (*Prunus *species)*

Apple
Apricot
Bitter almond
Cherry
Cherry laurel
Peach
Pear
Pin cherry
Plum
Western choke cherry
Wild black cherry

A neurotoxicologic role for cyanide has been suggested in tobacco-associated amblyopia and in a report of amygdalin-associated peripheral neuropathy.

Laetrile

Amygdalin was first used as an antineoplastic agent in the 1890s in Germany but was discarded after excessive toxicity and a lack of antineoplastic properties were found. Amygdalin was reintroduced in the 1950s under the trade name Laetrile as an anticancer agent that is still not approved by the Food and Drug Administration (FDA); this agent contains various cyanogenic glycosides, not a single chemical entity (40). Laetrile as originally developed was a natural substance derived from apricot pits. In recent years, pure amygdalin isolated from apricot kernels is used, although peach kernels have also been reported as a source (39,41).

According to proponents of the use of Laetrile, malignant cells convert the drug into hydrocyanic acid in greater concentrations than normal cells, which kills the malignant cells (42). It has also been stated that tumor tissue is deficient in rhodanase, the enzyme that detoxifies cyanide; therefore, tumor tissue is selectively attacked by cyanide because normal cells contain a high concentration of rhodanase (43). Although there are no studies showing beneficial effects of Laetrile in this setting, (44–47) the drug has had great popularity with the public and lay practitioners, and its use is now rather widespread (45).

The use of Laetrile is legal in many states and is legal for use nationwide with a Federal court order (47). A dose of Laetrile contains from 30–150 mg of cyanide per tablet. Orally administered Laetrile is marketed only in 500-mg tablets and is approximately 6% cyanide by weight (15). Laetrile and seeds are two of the most commonly reported sources of cyanide poisoning in the medical literature (4,36,48,49). The toxic effects of oral ingestion of Laetrile are presumably due to the action of gastric acids on the amygdalin, releasing hydrogen cyanide (39). Although Laetrile is a toxic drug, its toxicity is limited to oral ingestion because by intravenous administration there is no liberation of cyanide. The drug is rapidly cleared from the blood and is largely excreted unchanged in the urine (39).

The mechanism of toxic action of Laetrile is similar to that of seeds and pits. The amygdalin in Laetrile is broken down by the enzymes in vegetables (celery, lettuce, green peppers, carrots, mushrooms, and bean sprouts), nuts (almonds), and fruits (peaches and plums), so that cyanide can be released with the co-ingestion of the drug and these foods (31). Also, hydrolysis by β-glucosidase can occur in the alkaline medium of the intestine and cause the same effect. Acute cyanide poisoning has also followed the administration of Laetrile enemas (4,50).

Miscellaneous Products

The cyanide ion may originate in vivo from hydrocyanic acid; salts and complexes of cyanide; biotransformations of cyanohydrins, aliphatic nitriles, thiocyanate, and nitrile glycosides; and even the interaction in the stomach of ingested chlorinogenic water purifiers (such as halazone tablets) and the amino acids of some foods.

CHRONIC CYANIDE INTOXICATION

Cassava (*Manihot esculenta*) is a carbohydrate staple in many sub-Saharan tropical countries. This food provides more than 70% of the caloric intake in some diets in these regions. Cassava contains large amounts of linamarin in its outer layers, which acts as a pesticide. Processing disrupts the root tissue, liberating an endogenous glucosidase that hydrolyzes linamarin to yield hydrogen cyanide (51). Incorrect preparation of cassava has resulted in chronic cyanide intoxication in humans. With continued ingestion over a period of time, individuals may develop neuropathy manifesting as optic atrophy, nerve deafness, and ataxia (Nigerian ataxic neuropathy) due to sensory spinal nerve involvement (14,39,52,53).

Another condition secondary to chronic cyanide ingestion is Konzo. This was first described in Africa in 1938. It is characterized by abrupt onset of varying degrees of symmetrical, isolated, and permanent, but not progressive, spastic paraparesis. Epidemics in East Africa have been attributed to the combined effect of high cyanide and low sulfur intake from exclusive consumption of insufficiently processed bitter cassava roots (51).

MECHANISM OF ACTION OF CYANIDE

Cyanide binds avidly to iron in the ferric (trivalent) state but not in the ferrous (divalent) state (54). Cyanide, therefore, does not react with the iron in hemoglobin, which is ferrous. Any iron-containing enzymes that cycle between the ferric and ferrous states during reduction-oxidation reactions are particularly susceptible to inactivation by cyanide because the cyanoferric complex is relatively stable and the enzyme remains trapped in this form.

Cyanide produces a cellular hypoxia by inhibiting the reoxidation of cytochrome oxidase; this hemoprotein has iron in the ferric state. Essentially, cyanide combines reversibly with cytochrome oxidase (cytochrome aa3), inhibiting the final step of oxidative phosphorylation and the transfer of electrons to oxygen, thereby inhibiting cellular respiration and preventing the formation of adenosine triphosphate (48,54,55). Because the ATP–ADP cycle is the fundamental mechanism in which energy is exchanged intracellularly, cyanide causes severe disruption of the energy state of the cell. This results in anaerobic metabolism (4). Pyruvate, which can no longer be incorporated into the tricarboxylic acid cycle, is reduced to lactate ion, which accumulates rapidly. Elevated lactate levels produce a severe metabolic acidosis; as serum bicarbonate buffers the excess acid, the anion gap increases. Therefore, the mechanism of cyanide toxicity is to block aerobic metabolism, the major pathway of high-energy phosphate production (48). The patient essentially suffocates, not from the inability to obtain or transport oxygen, but from the inability to use it (4). Venous blood may retain the bright red color of oxyhemoglobin, and the patient will not usually appear to be cyanotic. This differs from carbon monoxide intoxication, in which hypoxia is due to decreased oxygen transport. The cytochrome oxidase–cyanide complex is dissociable, and if death does not intervene the mitochondrial enzyme sulfur transferase (rhodanase) mediates the transfer of sulfur from thiosulfate to the cyanide ion. Thus thiocyanate is formed, the respiratory enzyme is released, and cell respiration is restored (54).

Although cyanide preferentially binds to ferric iron, some cyanide binds to the ferrous iron of normal hemoglobin. This cyanohemoglobin cannot transport oxygen.

Cyanide can also form complexes with other hematin compounds, such as catalase, peroxidase, cytochrome peroxidase, and methemoglobin, as well as with nonhematin metal-bearing compounds, such as tyrosinase, ascorbic acid oxidase, xanthine oxidase, amino acid oxidase, succinic, lactic, and formic dehydrogenase, phosphatase, and hydroxycobalamin (a precursor of vitamin B_{12}). The acute pathophysiologic effects of cyanide, however, are attributable to its action on cytochrome oxidase alone. In contrast to higher mammals, bacteria are not harmed by cyanide and are able to use the nitrogen of the poison to make their proteins (56).

In addition to multiple enzymes being affected by cyanide, there are differences in cytochrome oxidase in various organs. The predominant site of lethal effects of cyanide is the centtral nervous system because the cytochrome oxidase in the brain is the most susceptible to the toxic effects of cyanide (1).

Absorption

Cell membranes are highly permeable to cyanide, and the compound is rapidly absorbed through any body surface, such as the alveolar membranes, intestinal mucosa, or skin. Neither the liquid nor the vapor is irritating to the skin or membranes of the respiratory tract. A maximal effect is seen with either intravenous administration or inhalation of hydrocyanic acid vapors (57). Gas masks usually provide inadequate protection from poisoning (4,8). The oral route is less rapid because of a slower rate of entry of cyanide into the circulation; it gains entry through the hepatic portal system and passes through the liver, which is the main site of the body's detoxification system.

Metabolism

There are five routes through which cyanide is metabolized, two of which have clinical import. Absorbed cyanide is excreted in small amounts unchanged by the lungs. In addition, a small amount is excreted in the urine. Cyanide is also oxidized to formate ion and carbon dioxide and is incorporated into methyl groups to produce choline and methionine. Approximately 15% of cyanide reacts with cystine and is excreted. These routes of excretion are not of clinical import in intoxication.

A minor route of detoxification, but one with clinical importance, is the incorporation of cyanide into hydroxycobalamin to form cyanocobalamin (vitamin B_{12}). This minor route is under investigation as therapy for the cyanide-poisoned patient.

The major mechanism of detoxification, accounting for 80% of cyanide metabolism, is the conversion of cyanide to the relatively harmless thiocyanate ion by an enzymatic reaction mediated by the mitrochondrial enzyme rhodanase with thiosulfate as substrate. This enzyme is widely distributed in tissues, but the greatest amounts occur in the liver (1). Rhodanase has a large capacity to combine with cyanide but is relatively slow with respect to elimination of a toxic overdose, so that the reaction may be limited by the endogenous supply of thiosulfate (54). The resulting thiocyanate formed has some inherent toxicity but is rapidly excreted by the kidneys (57).

Toxicity

Clinical Features

Cyanide is a fast-acting poison and is capable of causing death in a matter of minutes. The manifestations of cyanide toxicity depend on the degree of tissue hypoxia: the more rapidly the individual acquires cyanide, the more acute are the signs and symptoms of poisoning and the smaller is the total absorbed dose required to produce toxicity. Short-term inhalation of 50 ppm of hydrogen cyanide causes acute symptoms of central nervous system, gastric, and respiratory tract disturbances, and inhalation of 130 ppm can be fatal (52). The lethal dose of sodium or potassium cyanide is approximately 200–300 mg, and the lethal dose of hydrogen cyanide is 50 mg (1,48,58).

Onset of symptoms depends on the form of cyanide ingested, the route of ingestion, and the amount ingested. In actual practice, the most rapidly acquired form of poisoning occurs from the inhalation of hydrogen cyanide vapor, with little difference noted between this and the intravenous route.

As with other chemical asphyxiants, the critical organs are those that are most sensitive to oxygen deprivation, notably the brain and the heart. In low concentrations, the cyanide ion stimulates respiration. The sites of action are the chemoreceptors of the carotid and aortic bodies, which respond to a decreased partial pressure of oxygen in the blood. Upon hyperventilating, more hydrogen cyanide is inhaled and, as a result, there is a positive feedback situation in which cyanide intake increases even more. In prolonged hyperventilation, carbon dioxide is blown off with a decrease in pCO_2, which has a depressive effect upon the central nervous system, particularly the respiratory center. The decrease in arterial pCO_2 causes cerebral arterial constriction and severe circulatory collapse, drastically reducing cerebral blood supply. This respiratory response may also be related to early, low-level lactic acid accumulation from cyanide inhibition of cellular respiration (15). This stimulation of ventilation may actually worsen the effects of cyanide inhalation (59). The transient central nervous system stimulation is followed by central nervous system depression and finally hypoxic convulsions, with death due to respiratory arrest. Although the heart shows toxic effects, it usually continues to function for some minutes after respirations have ceased.

Recovery from cyanide poisoning may be complete or may be followed by sequelae due to hypoxic and hemodynamic brain damage similar to that seen after other hypoxic insults.

Inhaled and Intravenous Cyanide

Hydrogen cyanide gas, when produced, is rapidly diffused in air and is quickly absorbed upon inhalation. It has a dramatic and immediate incapacitative effect consisting of a rapid loss of consciousness accompanied by severe disruptive changes in respiration, cardiac rhythm, and central nervous system function, as detected clinically by the respiratory rate and electrocardiogram changes (57).

Symptoms of intoxication from inhaled or intravenous cyanide in large amounts include a very brief sensation of dryness and burning in the throat from local irritation, a suffusing warmth, and air hunger. The first breath is followed immediately by hyperpnea, which is due to stimu-

TABLE 33–6. *Symptoms of cyanide overdose by inhalation*

Dryness of mouth
Air hunger
Hyperpnea
Apnea
Coma
Seizures

lation of the chemoreceptors in the carotid and aortic bodies. Apnea, coma, and seizures may occur in less than 1 minute and are often accompanied by cardiovascular failure. As stated above, the heart may continue to beat with various irregularities and blocks for as long as 3–4 minutes after the last breath (Table 33–6) (8).

Ingested Cyanide

The most common mode of suicide involving cyanide is ingestion of salts of cyanide. The salts cause a less acute syndrome because they are absorbed slowly and variably from the gastrointestinal tract and because their toxicity is attenuated by passage through the liver (4).

Central nervous system effects predominate from oral ingestion of cyanide. Within 1–5 minutes hyperpnea develops from chemoreceptor stimulation (Table 33–7). Vomiting occurs secondary to central hypoxic stimulation. Vomiting is due to the sodium and potassium salts of cyanide being strongly alkaline and therefore irritative to the gastric mucosa. Neurologic symptoms, such as anxiety, confusion, vertigo, giddiness, headache, and generalized seizures and trismus, often occur (15,59). In addition, within 5–20 minutes the patient may exhibit flushed, hot, and dry skin, a rapid, irregular pulse that may lead to bradycardia, and gasping respiratory efforts. This is followed by hypoxic dilatation of the pupils and vascular collapse.

TABLE 33–7. *Symptoms of cyanide overdose by ingestion*

Gastrointestinal
Nausea
Vomiting
Neurologic
Confusion
Vertigo
Giddiness
Seizures
Cardiac
Tachycardia
Bradycardia
Respiratory
Hyperpnea
Respiratory depression
Pulmonary edema

Although Laetrile may cause cyanide intoxication, after a toxic dose has been ingested there may be a delay in the development of symptoms because the enzyme emulsin does not normally hydrolyze amygdalin until it is transported into the alkaline environment of the small intestine (60,61). This delay of symptomatology may last from 90–120 minutes after ingestion of the drug (15,25).

Pulmonary edema has also been reported in oral cyanide intoxication (3,4,15,62). This may be the result of the direct toxic effect of cyanide on capillary endothelia or an indirect neurogenic effect leading to increased pulmonary capillary permeability.

DIAGNOSIS

Diagnosis of cyanide poisoning may be difficult because of a lack of a positive history (Table 33–8) (15). Exposure to cyanide may not be considered even when clinical and laboratory evidence are highly suggestive. The key to making a correct diagnosis of cyanide poisoning is having a high index of suspicion in patients with an altered level of consciousness and an otherwise unexplained metabolic acidosis (4,63). High-risk groups, such as laboratory technicians, chemists, pharmacists, physicians, and others with easy access to cyanide and its compounds, should be suspected of having ingested cyanide (4,15). Industrial accidents and fires may suggest cyanide as the causative factor of symptoms of toxicity (64).

The odor of hydrocyanic acid released into the air from solutions of sodium or potassium cyanide can be detected by most individuals, even in small concentrations, but it is estimated that 20%–40% of the population is unable to detect cyanide by odor (4,6,15,48,65). The odor and the taste of hydrocyanic acid have a characteristic musty quality that resembles that of bitter almonds or macaroons (66).

Because of poor oxygen use, venous blood may retain the bright red color of arterial blood; for example, retinal veins and arteries have been reported to be equally red when examined on funduscopic examination (6), yet this examination may be impractical in the emergency department.

Although the diagnosis of the comatose, hypotensive, apneic patient with dilated pupils presents a difficult

TABLE 33–8. *Diagnostic clues for cyanide poisoning*

High index of suspicion
Appropriate clinical setting
Unexplained cardiac arrest
Odor of bitter almonds
Abolition of difference between arterial and venous oxygen saturation
Anion-gap metabolic acidosis
Absence of cyanotic appearance

problem, the associated features of bradycardia and the absence of cyanosis resulting from cellular inability to use oxygen could lead to a consideration of cyanide poisoning. Although poisoning by carbon monoxide may present a similar picture, including bradycardia and pink mucous membranes, the patient's history may reveal circumstances that might better suggest the diagnosis of cyanide poisoning.

LABORATORY ANALYSIS

Routine toxicologic screens do not check for cyanide, so that the screen will be negative even in cases of pure cyanide ingestion. There are no readily available cyanide assays that confirm the poisoning within the time needed to treat an acutely poisoned patient. Confirmatory laboratory analysis specific for cyanide in the acute situation is seldom useful in prognosis or treatment and is also time-consuming. Specimens should be saved, however, in case a chemical analysis is needed for legal purposes (67). Because the toxicity of cyanide is due to the intracellular concentration of cyanide, the actual blood concentration finally reported may be misleading (68). As a result of the tight binding of cyanide to cytochrome oxidase, serious poisoning has occurred with only modest blood concentrations, especially several hours after ingestion (69).

Cyanide concentration may be measured in whole blood, gastric contents, tissues, and urine. The usual technique is a colorimetric diffusion method, although measurement by a specific electrode can be performed (Table 33–9) (1,6,6,70). Normal cyanide levels are higher in smokers than in nonsmokers and in whole blood as compared to plasma (13). Whole blood cyanide concentration in nonsmokers is approximately 0.02 μg/mL and in smokers is 0.04 μg/mL 1; this is measured from the cyanide found predominately in vitamin B_{12} or intermediaries of 1-carbon metabolism (3). Although difficult to measure and correlate with symptoms, the approximate toxic range is 0.1–0.2 μg/mL, and the fatal range is usually considered greater than 1–3 μg/mL in whole blood (1,4,71). Thiocyanate concentrations normally range from 1–4 μg/mL in nonsmokers and from 3–12 μg/mL in smokers (72).

Spectrophotometric and colorimetric methods for the estimation of blood cyanide concentration have adequate sensitivity but lack specificity because they react with thiocyanate as well as with cyanide and are also subject to interference with thiosulfate. These substances may be present in blood samples obtained after cyanide intoxication if nitrite-thiosulfate therapy was administered.

TABLE 33–9. *Blood cyanide concentrations and associated symptoms*

Concentration (μg/mL)	Symptoms
0.2–0.5	None
0.5–1.0	Tachycardia flushing
1.0–2.5	Depressed level of consciousness
2.5–3.0	Coma
>3.0	Death

Adapted with permission from Hall A, Rumack B: Clinical toxicology of cyanide. *Ann Emerg Med* 1986:15:1070. © 1986 American College of Emergency Physicians.

Lee-Jones Test

Because sophisticated laboratory confirmation of cyanide is time-consuming, a simple chemical test is available to measure cyanide concentration in gastric aspirate (Lee-Jones test) (6,73). This test is reported to detect as little as 50 mg of ingested cyanide. The test is based on the Prussian blue reaction and uses reagents that are stable and can be kept in the emergency department or an adjacent laboratory. A few small crystals of ferrous sulfate are added to 5 mL of gastric aspirate, and 4–5 drops of 20% sodium hydroxide solution are added to precipitate the iron. The mixture is boiled, cooled, and acidified with 8–10 drops of 10% hydrochloric acid. A greenish-blue precipitate, the color of which intensifies on standing, indicates the presence of cyanide. The reaction is not obtained with barbiturates, phenothiazines, benzodiazepines, or tricyclics, nor is the color reaction changed appreciably by the presence of these drugs in addition to cyanide. A color change does occur with salicylate, so that confusion with this substance could be a problem (3,60,73). Although this test could be used as an adjunct in making the diagnosis of cyanide intoxication, it should not be relied on for making or excluding the diagnosis.

Role of Saturation Gap

An arterial percent oxygen "saturation gap," which is the difference between the calculated and the measured values, may be of value in carbon monoxide poisoning (74). This saturation gap would not be expected, though, in cyanide intoxication because cyanide attaches to ferric iron, (Fe^{3+}), rather than to ferrous iron (Fe^{2+}). Since there is negligible cyanohemoglobin formed, there would be no reason to expect a saturation gap (74).

An anion-gap metabolic acidosis has been associated with cyanide intoxication. This is caused by lactic acidosis (63). It is postulated that, because oxidative phosphorylation is blocked by cyanide, the rate of glycolysis is markedly increased, leading to lactic acidosis (6). There is decreased tissue perfusion associated with the circulatory effects of cyanide, which also contributes to a lactic acidosis (75). Because of the possibility of lactic acidosis, arterial blood gas and blood lactate determinations

TABLE 33–10. *Laboratory determinations for cyanide overdose*

Arterial blood gas
Serum lactate concentration
Lee-Jones test
Cyanide concentration
Thiocyanate concentration

should be obtained, if possible, in the cyanide-intoxicated patient; these measurements may provide both therapeutic and prognostic information (Table 33–10) (3).

TREATMENT

Initial treatment of cyanide poisoning should include airway support, oxygen therapy, cardiac monitoring, decontamination of the skin and clothing, gastric lavage if necessary, and sodium bicarbonate as indicated for severe acidosis (Table 33–11) (76). Rescuers entering a contaminated area to remove an individual should first protect themselves with rubber boots and gloves. If a gas mask is used, the canister must be appropriate for hydrogen cyanide because the usual canister does not protect against cyanide (4,8).

Even if cyanide has been ingested, gastric lavage should follow, not precede, the initiation of more specific treatment for the symptomatic individual (77). Patients have survived even when cardiac asystole has occurred, so that vigorous treatment should be instituted immediately. In mild cases of cyanide poisoning, in which the individual may present with weakness, vertigo, headache, nausea, and vomiting, it may be only necessary to remove the individual from exposure and administer supportive care (78). In severe cases, specific antidotal therapy may be indicated. In some cases, patients who have ingested a potentially lethal dose of cyanide may survive with only nonspecific supportive measures (4,6). One survivor of cyanide intoxication, who had a blood concentration of 2.9 μg/mL, was treated with supportive measures alone; this was the largest overdose of cyanide successfully treated in this way. Survival with antidotal therapy has been reported with cyanide concentrations of 3.2–16.3 μg/mL (6,39.54).

Survival following acute cyanide poisoning with the development of life-threatening symptomatology has been reported when only supportive treatment was administered, but the highest reported whole blood cyanide level in such a survivor was 2.3 μg/mL. In contrast, patients receiving various specific antidotes as well as supportive therapy have survived with whole blood cyanide levels ranging from 3.2–40 μg/mL (79).

TABLE 33–11. *Treatment of cyanide poisoning*

Airway support
Oxygen
Cardiac monitoring
Decontamination
Amyl nitrite
Sodium nitrite
Adult: 300 mg
Child: 10 mg/kg
Sodium thiosulfate
Adult: 12.5 g
Child: 1.5 mL/kg
Methods not approved by the FDA
Dicobalt edetate
Hydroxycobalamin
Aminophenol
Rhodanase
Stroma-free methemoglobin

Oxygen

The effect of oxygen therapy cannot be overemphasized; oxygen therapy has been shown experimentally to abolish the inspiratory gasp and improve the electroencephalographic and electrocardiographic abnormalities associated with cyanide poisoning (4,48,80,81). Its low toxicity and ease of administration recommend it for use in any cyanide-intoxicated patient. The proposed salutory effect of oxygen is unexpected, and may be based on a cyanide-oxygen interaction at the cytochrome level (1,2). Cyanide may combine with reduced rather than oxidized cytochrome oxidase, thus allowing the possibility of oxygen competition with cyanide.

Dextrose, Thiamine, and Naloxone

Dextrose, thiamine, and naloxone should also be administered to any cyanide-intoxicated patient with an altered mental status. Naloxone should also be administered, both as a nonspecific agent when the diagnosis is unknown as well as when the diagnosis of cyanide poisoning has been made. This is because of the potential for naloxone to reverse the endorphin-induced respiratory depression that may also occur with cyanide intoxication (82).

Antidotal Therapy

The decision to treat a potentially lethal ingestion of cyanide with a toxic treatment regimen many times rests on nonspecific circumstantial evidence. Yet it may be this quick recognition and treatment that is lifesaving.

The rational therapeutic approach to cyanide toxicity is to prevent the cyanide ion from binding to cytochrome oxidase or to reverse the binding once it has occurred. In the United States, treatment of cyanide intoxication consists of two separate antidotes that, when used jointly, can potentiate each other's beneficial effect. One of these antidotes produces methemoglobin, an oxidation product of the normal blood pigment hemoglobin (83). Production of methemoglobin causes the ferric ion to act as an alternative site to cytochrome oxidase for cyanide binding (4,84–87). Although the cyanomethemoglobin complex is less tightly bound than the cyanide-cytochrome oxidase complex, the relatively greater amounts of methemoglobin generated in this procedure favor the formation of cyanomethemoglobin (24). The methemoglobin is capable of binding any cyanide in the plasma, but, more important, it can effectively compete for cyanide already bound to cytochrome oxidase. Recent evidence casts doubt on the traditionally proposed mechanism (1,6).

At one time, methylene blue was used for cyanide poisoning because of its ability to form methemoglobin (4,88). It was determined, however, that methylene blue is not an efficient antidote because it forms methemoglobin poorly. Methylene blue more efficiently reverses the reaction and is an effective antidote in the treatment of methemoglobinemia.

Nitrite Therapy

The formation of methemoglobin is accomplished with the administration of nitrites (84–87). The first nitrite used to antagonize cyanide was amyl nitrite; sodium nitrite was used subsequently.

The suggested regimen for nitrite therapy in the United States consists of the application of amyl nitrite pearls over the patient's nose or through positive-pressure breathing apparatus for 30 seconds of each minute (so that the patient can also be adequately oxygenated). Amyl nitrite is recommended because of the speed with which it can be administered. Amyl nitrite inhalation produces a relatively low concentration of methemoglobin, and must be followed by intravenous sodium nitrite. If sodium nitrite is immediately available, amyl nitrite can be omitted.

The goal of nitrite therapy is to attain a methemoglobin concentration that is approximately 10%–40% of the patient's total hemoglobin (6,89).

The recommended dose of sodium nitrite for adults is 300 mg or 10 mL of a 3% solution; for children the dose is 10 mg/kg or 0.2 mL/kg and not to exceed 10 mL (15). The nitrite solution should be administered at a rate not greater than 2.5–5 mL/min (90).

Normal methemoglobin is approximately 1% of the total hemoglobin. The initial amyl nitrite inhalation may raise the methemoglobin concentration to approximately 5% (4,15). The first dose of sodium nitrite should continue to raise the methemoglobin concentration to approximately 25% (4). The resulting compound, cyanomethemoglobin, has relatively low toxicity. The methemoglobin thus produced is spontaneously reconverted to oxyhemoglobin by intraerythrocyte enzymes. The co-oximeter does not detect cyanomethemoglobin, and there is no readily available assay for this compound (6). The methemoglobin concentration may not be accurately measured as a consequence.

Sodium Thiosulfate Therapy

Sodium thiosulfate produces the relatively nontoxic thiocyanate, which is then excreted by the kidneys. Sodium thiosulfate acts as a sulfur donor and provides a substrate for the liver enzyme rhodanase to convert cyanide released from methemoglobin to thiocyanate (6, 39). It is believed that three times more thiosulfate than cyanide must be present for successful detoxification. Administration of sodium thiosulfate has no significant toxic effects (3,60).

The dose of sodium thiosulfate for adults is 50 mL of a 25% solution (12.5 g) administered intravenously; for children the dose is 1.5 mL/kg (15). A continuous intravenous infusion has also been suggested, but this is not yet widely accepted (20).

The Lilly Kit

Although nitrite and thiosulfate have approximately equal antidotal activity, when they are used together there is a potentiation of effect; the combination of nitrite and thiosulfate is therefore suggested. A kit is marketed for this purpose (Eli Lilly & Co., Indianapolis, IN).

A temporary improvement in the patient's condition after the initial medication may occur but does not ensure complete recovery. The patient should be closely monitored, and if symptoms recur both the nitrite and the thiosulfate should be administered at one-half the original dose (91).

Precautions

Care should be taken to administer the correct dose of sodium nitrite to children because a fatal methemoglobinemia may result if too much is administered (4). Although the pediatric dose of nitrite should ideally be based on the amount of hemoglobin, generally it is not feasible to wait until this is determined. An initial dose of 10 mg/kg is safe, and blood should be drawn immediately to measure both hemoglobin and methemoglobin concentrations. Subsequent nitrite doses can be calculated on the basis of these values (92–94).

Sodium nitrite should be administered slowly to lessen the chance of developing hypotension; nitrite can significantly decrease mean blood pressure when injected as a bolus. The toxicity of sodium thiosulfate is low, and doses of 12.5–50 g by intravenous injection are well tolerated.

Evaluation of Nitrite-Thiosulfate Combination

Nitrite and thiosulfate are two distinct antidotes that are used for two distinct effects. The nitrite-thiosulfate kit is used to cause methemoglobin to form, to which the cyanide ion attaches. Although this is not ideal, it may be lifesaving (54). Recent studies suggest that methemoglobin formation by sodium nitrite may be only a partial explanation for the therapeutic benefit of nitrites in cyanide poisoning. Nitrites may act through effects on the cardiovascular system or changes in blood flow to organs (1). Certainly, it seems that the mechanism of action of the nitrites is more complex than previously believed (6,54).

The effect of thiosulfate is a stimulation of what naturally takes place in the body, that is, the rhodanase system, which normally detoxifies cyanide. Because this detoxification is a relatively slow process, and because the rate-limiting factor is usually a limited supply of sulfur ions, sodium thiosulfate is administered so that more rhodanase may form and detoxify the cyanomethemoglobin. The thiocyanate thus formed is excreted through the kidneys (93).

Methemoglobin Levels and Symptomatology

A concentration of 30% methemoglobin does not usually produce significant symptoms; a concentration of 40% is considered to cause mild symptoms and 70% is considered lethal (4). Because 30% methemoglobin does not usually produce symptoms and because the lethal dose of sodium nitrite for an adult is about 2 g, a dose of 300–600 mg of sodium nitrite is well within safe limits.

Adjunctive Therapy to Nitrite-Thiosulfate

Although the mechanism of action is not clear, oxygen is often recommended as a therapeutic adjunct in cyanide poisoning, as previously mentioned. In one study, oxygen alone, even at hyperbaric pressures, had only a slight protective effect against cyanide in mice, but it dramatically potentiated the protective effects of thiosulfate alone or in combination with nitrite (79).

Hemodialysis has been shown to remove thiocyanate but not cyanide. It may therefore be indicated in the patient with renal failure after antidotal treatment is instituted.

Limitations of Nitrite-Thiosulfate Therapy.

There are several disadvantages to the nitrite-thiosulfate combination. For example, the production of methemoglobin by nitrites is relatively slow. It has been reported that peak methemoglobin concentrations are attained in approximately 30 minutes (89). In addition, the higher percentage of methemoglobin decreases the oxygen-carrying capacity of the blood, so that a profound hypotension can result from the rapid administration of nitrites (54). Most important, however, the cyanide is not removed quickly from the body by this method, but remains bound in the erythrocytes while awaiting conversion to thiocyanate.

Antidotes Not Approved by the FDA

Cobalt Salts

Although the cobalt salts were among the earliest antidotes used to antagonize the lethal effects of cyanide, they have not received widespread acceptance in the U.S. (95). Despite their apparent lack of use, many toxicologists believe that cobalt compounds either alone or in combination with sodium thiosulfate should be the primary antidote for cyanide poisoning.

Cobalt salts are believed to exert their detoxifying effect primarily by combining directly with cyanide ion as a chelate rather than indirectly by methemoglobin formation (96). The reason for the preferential use of cobalt compounds is that the cobalt ion has a higher affinity for cyanide than either methemoglobin or cytochrome oxidase, and can also bind cyanide more rapidly than nitrite can convert hemoglobin to methemoglobin for subsequent binding to cyanide. Furthermore, cobalt forms a stable, presumably nontoxic, complex with the cyanide ion that is excreted within 24 hours. The inherent toxicity of cobalt compounds is considered less than that of the nitrite-thiosulfate combination, and the large amount of methemoglobin generated by sodium nitrite can be dangerous and has resulted in the death of at least one child.

It has been shown that cobalt chloride in combination with sodium nitrite produces additive antidotal effects in experimental cyanide poisoning. More striking are the results that showed the combination of cobalt and sodium thiosulfate to be much more effective than the traditional nitrite-thiosulfate combination against the lethal effects of cyanide (46).

Hydroxycobalamin (Vitamin B_{12a})

Hydroxycobalamin is a cobalt antidote shown to be effective against cyanide (21,97,98). Hydroxycobalamin has been used for more than 15 years in France with very little associated toxicity (7). It has also been suggested for use in combination with thiosulfate (7,96).

Hydroxycobalamin contains a central cobalt atom in a porphyrin-like ring structure. It has one cyanide less than cyanocobalamin (vitamin B_{12}), and combines in equimolar amounts with cyanide to form cyanocobalamin (52), which is extremely stable and is excreted in the urine

(7,68). It does this by giving up one hydroxyl group and binding one cyanyl group. Hydroxycobalamin has the advantage of low toxicity, with no toxic effects seen in moderate doses (99). It has a greater affinity for cyanide than cytochrome oxidase and can free the respiratory enzyme to resume its normal activity (100).

Hydroxycobalamin is considered unsuitable for use in the U.S. because it is not manufactured in a sufficiently concentrated form. It is commercially available in a solution of 1 mg/mL (99). This concentration has been used experimentally to prevent cyanide accumulation during nitroprusside administration (100). The recommended dose for cyanide intoxication is approximately 50 mg/kg (4,6,15,100). Hydroxycobalamin is considered an orphan drug and is currently available in the U.S. under an investigational license as a powder in combination with sodium thiosulfate (4,100). A proposed dose is 4 g combined with 8 g of sodium thiosulfate (1,100).

As much as 50% of hydroxycobalamin is excreted unchanged in the urine (98), but it may still play an active role in cyanide detoxification by binding cyanide to form vitamin B_{12}. The cyanide is excreted in this form or is later given up to rhodanase for complexing with thiocyanate; hydroxycobalamin is thereby regenerated (99).

Problems associated with the use of hydroxycobalamin include limited solubility in a reasonable volume, scarcity of the preparation, expense, and stability of the solution. Proper storage of the powder is necessary to maintain potency; otherwise deterioration will occur, liberating cobalt ions (21). Minor side effects reported from hydroxycobalamin include urticaria, which may be related to the vehicle in which the material is suspended. It may also cause a transient reddish-brown discoloration of the urine, skin, and mucous membranes (1,100,101). There is currently no commercial production of antidotal hydroxycobalamin in the United States, although a research preparation has been produced for use in a Phase II clinical study.

Further clinical investigations are necessary to evaluate the place of cobalt compounds in the treatment of cyanide poisoning. Although these agents appear to be promising, sodium nitrite-thiosulfate therapy should still be considered the treatment of choice in the United States. Perhaps the main use of cobalt compounds in the future will be in combination with sodium thiosulfate because, as mentioned above, cobalt compounds rapidly bind cyanide and then can be detoxified with thiosulfate.

Dicobalt EDTA

Dicobalt edetate is an effective cobalt compound that has had clinical use in Europe. Dicobalt edetate is commercially available in Europe as Kelocyanor. The kit consists of ampules, each containing 300 mg of dicobalt edetate in 20% glucose (102). The manufacturer recommends injecting two ampules (40 mL) initially. If there is no response, two more doses are given (79). The product formed, presumably cobalticyanide, is considered stable and of low toxicity; the toxicity of dicobalt edetate is greater when it is not chelating cyanide (4). Symptoms of intoxication may include hypertension, hypotension, cardiac dysrhythmias, and cardiac insufficiency (6,39).

Stroma-Free Methemoglobin

Stroma-free methemoglobin solution is made by oxidizing stroma-free hemoglobin solution, which is produced by releasing hemoglobin from erythrocytes. Stroma-free hemoglobin and methemoglobin solutions are free of membrane lipids. In theory, stroma-free methemoglobin binds cyanide, as does intracellular methemoglobin, but does not cause a reduction in the patient's oxygen-carrying capacity. It can also be administered intravenously (58). This antidote has been tried experimentally and may offer advantages over the nitrite-thiosulfate combination (48,58).

Rhodanase

Recent applications of crystalline rhodanase have been promising. This antidote may be of value in the future management of cyanide poisoning.

Aminophenols

The aminophenols have been used in Europe as a cyanide antidote. They have a mechanism of action that is similar to that of the nitrates. (4)-Dimethylaminophenol (DMAP) is a more rapid producer of methemoglobin than the nitrites and has been successfully used in animal models. DMAP has also been shown to be effective in sulfide and mercaptan poisonings because the mechanism of toxicity is similar to that of cyanide (8). Some investigators have promoted the use of aminophenols over the nitrites because they form methemoglobin more rapidly than the nitrites (24).

Hyperbaric Oxygen Therapy

Hyperbaric oxygen therapy has been proposed as a treatment for cyanide poisoning, but evidence supporting the use of this modality is inconclusive (48). In addition, animal studies have not shown that hyperbaric oxygen is more efficacious than the administration of 100% oxygen at one atmosphere (6). Even in view of these studies, the Undersea Medical Society has classified cyanide as a category-one condition, essentially stating that hyperbaric oxygen is mandatory for cyanide intoxication. If hyperbaric oxygen is readily available, it may be appropriate to administer it to cyanide-intoxicated patients who do not respond to supportive measures and antidotal therapy (6,15). Because the accumulated evidence does not point to any clear-cut conclusions, however, hyperbaric oxygen should not be considered the standard of care for cyanide poisoning (6).

REFERENCES

1. Becker C: The role of cyanide in fires. *Vet Hum Toxicol* 1985;27: 487–490.
2. Peters C, Mundy J, Rayner P: Acute cyanide poisoning. *Anaesthesiology* 1982;37:582–586.
3. Graham D, Laman D, Theodore J, et al: Acute cyanide poisoning complicated by lactic acidosis and pulmonary edema. *Arch Intern Med* 1917;137:1051–1055.
4. Vogel S, Sultan T, Ten Eyck R: Cyanide poisoning. *Clin Toxicol* 1981;18:367–383.
5. Stewart R: Cyanide poisoning. *Clin Toxicol* 1974;7:561–564.
6. Hall A, Rumack B: Clinical toxicology of cyanide. *Ann Emerg Med* 1986;15:1067–1074.
7. Bismuth C, Baud F, Djeghout H, et al: Cyanide poisoning from propionitrile exposure. *J Emerg Med* 1987;5:191–195.
8. Weger N: Treatment of cyanide poisoning with 4-dimethylaminophenol (DMAP)—experimental and clinical overview. *Fundam Appl Toxicol* 1983;3:387–396
9. Noguchi T, Eng J, Klatt E: Significance of cyanide in medicolegal investigations involving fires. *Am J Forensic Med* 1988;9:304–309.
10. Bell R, Stemmer K, Barkley W, et al: Cyanide toxicity from the thermal degradation of rigid polyurethane foam. *Ann Ind Hyg Assoc J* 1979;40:757–762.
11. Symington I, Anderson R, Oliver J, et al: Cyanide exposures in fires. *Lancet* 1978;2:91–92.
12. Ballantyne B: Toxicology and hazard evaluation of cyanide fumigation powders. *J Toxicol Clin Toxicol* 1988;26:325–335.
13. Silverman S, Purdue G, Hunt J, et al: Cyanide toxicity in burned patients. *J Trauma* 1988;28:171–176.
14. Way J: Cyanide antidotes. *Drug Ther* 1977;7:99–100.
15. Litovitz T, Larkin R, Myers R: Cyanide poisoning treated with hyperbaric oxygen. *Am J Emerg Med* 1983;1:94–101.
16. Atkins D: Cyanide toxicity following nitroprusside induced hypotension. *Can Anaesth Soc J* 1977;24:651–660.
17. Perchau R, Modell J, Bright R, et al: Suspected sodium nitroprusside-induced cyanide intoxication. *Anesth Analg* 1977;56:533–537.
18. Smith R, Kruszyna H: Nitroprusside produces cyanide poisoning via a reaction with hemoglobin. *J Pharmacol Exp Ther* 1974;191:557–563.
19. Sales J, Kennedy K: Epiglottic dysfunction after isocyanate inhalation exposure. *Arch Otolaryngol Head Neck Surg* 1990;116:725–727.
20. Ivankovich A, Braverman B, Kanuru R, et al: Cyanide antidotes and methods of their administration in dogs: a comparative study. *Anesthesiology* 1980;52:210–216.
21. Posner M, Tobey R, McElroy H: Hydroxycobalamin therapy of cyanide intoxication in guinea pigs. *Anesthesiology* 1976;44:157–160.
22. Gonzales J, Sabatini S: Cyanide poisoning: pathophysiology and current approaches to therapy. *Int J Artif Organs* 1989;12:347–355.
23. Vesey C, Cole P, Simpson P: Cyanide and thiocyanate concentrations following sodium nitroprusside infusion in man. *Br J Anaesth* 1976; 48:651–660.
24. Wesson D, Foley R, Sabatini S, et al: Treatment of acute cyanide intoxication with hemodialysis. *Am J Nephrol* 1985;5:121–126.
25. Geller R, Ekins B, Iknoian R: Cyanide toxicity from acetonitrile-containing false nail remover. *J Emerg Med* 1991;9:268–270.
26. Moore S, Whitney S, Purser C, et al: The effect of activity state upon the production of lethalities due to the inhalation of the toxic pyrolysis products of polyacrylonitrile. *Vet Hum Toxicol* 1987;29:20–24.
27. Caravati E, Litovitz T: Pediatric cyanide intoxication and death from an acetonitrile-containing cosmetic. *JAMA* 1988;260:3470–3473.
28. Michaelis H, Clemens C, Kijewski H, et al: Acetonitrile serum concentrations and cyanide blood levels in a case of suicidal oral acetonitrile ingestion. *J Toxicol Clin Toxicol* 1991;29:447–458
29. Kurt T, Day L, Reed W, et al: Cyanide poisoning from glue-on nail remover. *Am J Emerg Med* 1991;9:271–272.
30. Losek J, Rock A, Boldt R: Cyanide poisoning from a cosmetic nail remover. *Pediatrics* 1991;88:337–340.
31. Rainey P, Roberts W: Diagnosis and misdiagnosis of poisoning with the cyanide precursor acetonitrile: nail polish remover or nail glue remover? *Am J Emerg Med* 1993;11:104–108.
32. Rubino M, Davidoff F: Cyanide poisoning from apricot seeds. *JAMA* 1979;241:359.
33. Sayre J, Kaymakcalan S: Cyanide poisoning from apricot seeds among children in central Turkey. *N Engl J Med* 1964;270:1113–1115.
34. Townsend W: Cyanide poisoning from ingestion of apricot kernels. *MMWR* 1975;24:8–10.
35. Pijoan M: Cyanide poisoning from chokecherry seeds. *Am J Med Sci* 1942;204:550–553.
36. Humbert J, Tress J, Braico K: Fatal cyanide poisoning: accidental ingestion of amygdalin. *JAMA* 1977;238:482.
37. Schwarting A: Poisonous seeds and fruits. *Prog Chem Toxicol* 1963; 1:385–401.
38. Grabois B: Exposure to hydrogen cyanide in the processing of apricot kernels. *NY State Dept Labor Mon Rev* 1974;33:33–36.
39. Hall A, Linden C, Kulig K, et al: Cyanide poisoning from laetrile ingestion: role of nitrite therapy. *Pediatrics* 1986;78:269–272.
40. Lewis J: Laetrile. *West J Med* 1977;127:55–62.
41. Greenberg D: The vitamin fraud in cancer quackery. *West J Med* 1975;122:345–348.
42. Cassileth B: Sounding boards: after laetrile, what? *N Engl J Med* 1982;306:1482–1484.
43. Levi L, French W, Bickis I, et al: Laetrile: a study of its physiochemical and biochemical properties. *Can Med Assoc J* 1965;92:1057–1061.
44. Baker J, Lokey J, Price N, et al: Against legalization of laetrile. *N Engl J Med* 1976;295:679.
45. Moss M, Khabl N, Gray J: Deliberate self-poisoning with laetrile. *Can Med Assoc J* 1981;125:1126–1127.
46. Moertel C, Fleming T, Rubin J, et al: A clinical trial of amygdalin (laetrile) in the treatment of human cancer. *N Engl J Med* 1982;306: 201–206.
47. Moertel C, Ames M, Kavach J, et al: A pharmacologic and toxicological study of amygdalin. *JAMA* 1981;245:591–594.
48. Krieg A, Saxena K: Cyanide poisoning from metal cleaning solutions. *Ann Intern Med* 1987;16:582–584.
49. Sadoff L, Fuchs K, Hollander J: Rapid death associated with laetrile ingestion. *JAMA* 1978;239:1532.
50. Ortega J, Creek J: Acute cyanide poisoning following administration of laetrile enemas. *J Pediatrics* 1978;93:1059.
51. Tylleskar T, Banea M, Bikangi N, et al: Cassava cyanogens and konzo, an upper motoneuron disease found in Africa. *Lancet* 1992; 339:208–211.
52. Blanc P, Hogan M, Mallin K, et al: Cyanide intoxication among silver-reclaiming workers. *JAMA* 1985;253:367–371.
53. Freeman A: Chronic cyanide intoxication. *Br Med J* 1981;282:1321.
54. Hall A, Doutre W, Ludden T, et al: Nitrite/thiosulfate-treated acute cyanide poisoning: estimated kinetics after antidote. *Clin Toxicol* 1987;25:121–133.
55. Burrows G, Liu D, Way J: Effect of oxygen on cyanide intoxication: physiologic effects. *J Pharmacol Exp Ther* 1973;184:739–748.
56. Ware G, Painter H: Bacterial utilization of cyanide. *Nature* 1955;175: 900–902.
57. DiNapoli J, Hall A, Drake R, et al: Cyanide and arsenic poisoning by intravenous injection. *Ann Emerg Med* 1989;18:308–311.
58. Ten Eyck R, Schaerdel A, Lynett J, et al: Stroma-free methemoglobin solution as an antidote for cyanide poisoning: A preliminary study. *Clin Toxicol* 1984;21:343–358.
59. Carella F, Grazzi M, Savoiardo M, et al: Dystonic-parkinsonian syndrome after cyanide poisoning: clinical and MRI findings. *J Neurol Neurosurg Psychiat* 1988;51:1345–1348.
60. Beamer W, Shealy R, Prough D: Acute cyanide poisoning from laetrile ingestion. *Ann Emerg Med* 1983;12:449–451.
61. Don R, Paxinos J: The current status of laetrile. *Ann Intern Med* 1978; 89:389–397.
62. Winek D: Cyanide poisoning as a mode of suicide. *Forensic Sci* 1978; 11:51–55.
63. Samo D: Cyanide poisoning and the anion gap. *Ann Emerg Med* 1988;17:298–299.

64. Nakatani T, Kosugi Y, Mori A, et al: Changes in the parameters of oxygen metabolism in a clinical course recovering from potassium cyanide. *Am J Emerg Med* 1993;11:213–217.
65. Kirk R, Stenhouse N: Ability to smell solutions of potassium cyanide. *Nature* 1953;171:698–699.
66. DeBusk R, Seidl L: Attempted suicide by cyanide: a report of two cases. *Calif Med* 1969;110:394–396.
67. Yagi K, Ikeda S, Schweiss J, et al: Measurement of blood cyanide with a microdiffusion method and an ion-specific electrode. *Anesthesiology* 1990;73:1028–1031.
68. Cottrell J, Casthely P, Brodie J, et al: Prevention of nitroprusside-induced cyanide toxicity with hydroxycobalamin. *N Engl J Med* 1978;298:809–811.
69. Soffer A: Chicken soup or laetrile—which would you prescribe? *Arch Intern Med* 1977;137:994–995.
70. Groff W, Stemler F, Kaminskis A, et al: Plasma-free cyanide and blood total cyanide: a rapid, completely automated microdistillation assay. *Clin Toxicol* 1985;23: 133–163.
71. Marbury T, Sheppard J, Gibbons K, et al: Combined antidotal and hemodialysis treatments for nitroprusside-induced cyanide toxicity. *Clin Toxicol* 1982;19:475–482.
72. Baud F, Barriot P, Toffis V, et al: Elevated blood cyanide concentrations in victims of smoke inhalation. *N Engl J Med* 1991;325:1761–1766.
73. Lee-Jones M, Bennett M, Sherwell J: Cyanide self-poisoning. *Br Med J* 1970;4:780–781.
74. Curry S, Patrick H: Lack of evidence for a percent saturation gap in cyanide poisoning. *Ann Emerg Med* 1991:20:523–528.
75. Johnson R, Mellors J: Arteriolization of venous blood gases: a clue to the diagnosis of cyanide poisoning. *J Emerg Med* 1988;6:401–404.
76. McKiernan M: Emergency treatment of cyanide poisoning. *Lancet* 1980;2:86.
77. Bain J, Knowles E: Successful treatment of cyanide poisoning. *Br Med J* 1967;2:763.
78. Lambert R, Kindler B, Schaeffer D: The efficacy of superactivated charcoal in treating rats exposed to a lethal oral dose of potassium cyanide. *Ann Emerg Med* 1988;17:595–598.
79. Johnson W, Hall A, Rumack B: Cyanide poisoning successfully treated without "therapeutic methemoglobin levels." *Am J Emerg Med* 1989;7:437–440.
80. Cope C: The importance of oxygen in the treatment of cyanide poisoning. *JAMA* 1961;175:1061–1064.
81. Isom G, Way J: Effects of oxygen on the antagonism of cyanide intoxication: cytochrome oxidase in vitro. *Toxicol Appl Pharmacol* 1984;74:57–62.
82. Leung P, Sylvenster D, Chiou F, et al: Stereospecific effect of naloxone hydrochloride on cyanide intoxication. *Toxicol Appl Pharmacol* 1986;83:525–530.
83. Kirk M, Gerace R, Kulig K: Cyanide and methemoglobin kinetics in smoke inhalation victims treated with the cyanide antidote kit. *Ann Emerg Med* 1993;22:1413–1418.
84. Chen K, Rose C, Clowes G: Amyl nitrite and cyanide poisoning. *JAMA* 1933;100:1920–1922.
85. Chen K, Rose C, Clowes G: Comparative vaiues of several antidotes in cyanide poisoning. *Am J Med Sci* 1934;188:767–781.
86. Chen K, Rose C: Nitrite and thiosulfate therapy in cyanide poisoning. *JAMA* 1952;149:113–119.
87. Chen K, Rose C: Treatment of acute cyanide poisoning. *JAMA* 1956; 162:1154–1155.
88. Geiger J: Cyanide poisoning in San Francisco. *JAMA* 1932;99:1944–1945.
89. Ten Eyck R, Schaerdel A, Ottinger W: Comparison of nitrite treatment and stroma-free methemoglobin solution as antidotes for cyanide poisoning in a rat model. *Clin Toxicol* 1986;23:477–487.
90. Wolfsie J, Shaffer C: Hydrogen cyanide: Hazards, toxicology, prevention and management of poisoning. *J Occup Med* 1959;1:281–288.
91. Andrews J, Sweeney E, Grey T, et al: The biohazard potential of cyanide poisoning during postmortem examination. *J Foren Sci* 1989; 34:1280–1284.
92. Berlin C. The treatment of cyanide poisoning in children. *Pediatrics* 1970;46:793–796.
93. Berlin C: Accidental childhood poisoning. *Pediatrics* 1971;47(6):1093.
94. Berlin C: Cyanide poisoning—a challenge. *Arch Intern Med* 1977; 137:993–994.
95. Rose C, Worth R, Kikuchi K, et al: Cobalt salts in acute cyanide poisoning. *Proc Soc Exp Biol Med* 1965;120:780–783.
96. Evans C: Cobalt compounds as antidotes for hydrocyanic acid. *Br J Pharmacol* 1964;23:455–475.
97. MacRae W, Owen M: Severe metabolic acidosis following hypotension induced with sodium nitroprusside: case report. *Br J Anesth* 1975;46:795.
98. Wilson J, Linnell J, Matthews D: Plasma-cobalamins in neuro-ophthalomological diseases. *Lancet* 1971;1:259.
99. Forsyth J, Mueller P, Becker C, et al: Hydroxycobalamin as a cyanide antidote: safety, efficacy and pharmacokinetics in heavily smoking normal volunteers. *J Toxicol Clin Toxicol* 1993:31:277–294.
100. Hall A, Rumack B: Hydroxycobalamin/sodium thiosulfate as a cyanide antidote. *J Emerg Med* 1987;5:115–121.
101. Curry S, Connor D, Raschke R: Effect of the cyanide antidote hydroxycobalamin on commonly ordered serum chemistry studies. *Ann Emerg Med* 1994;24:65–647.
102. Hillman B, Bardhan D, Bain J: The use of dicobalt edetate (kelocyanor) in cyanide poisoning. *Postgrad Med J* 1974;581:171–174.

CHAPTER 34

Sulfide Poisoning

Sulfide poisoning usually occurs after exposure to hydrogen sulfide, carbon disulfide, one of the mercaptans, or a soluble salt of sulfide. Hydrogen sulfide, a highly dangerous gas that occurs naturally and is a by-product of many industrial processes, and soluble salts of sulfides are potent poisons and have a toxicity comparable to that of cyanide (1,2). The common soluble salts and the sulfur acids all produce nearly identical toxic syndromes because sodium and other soluble sulfides are promptly and completely hydrolyzed in body fluids so that in terms of their systemic effects, no toxicological distinctions are recognized between them. In general, the route of administration is not a critical determinant of the toxic effects (3).

PROPERTIES OF SULFIDES

Hydrogen Sulfide

Hydrogen sulfide (H_2S) is a nonflammable, colorless, irritating gas whose odor is similar to that of rotten eggs (4–6). Hydrogen sulfide is heavier than air, and for this reason it accumulates in underground locations, such as sewers and wells. Hydrogen sulfide gas usually occurs in the setting of degrading protein waste. Although it has a strong and identifiable odor, it causes olfactory fatigue after short exposure and at relatively low concentrations (7). Hydrogen sulfide is poorly soluble in water. The proposed safe air concentration is 10 parts per million (ppm) (8).

Hydrogen sulfide is used or encountered in diverse industries such as farming, glue making, rubber vulcanizing, and rayon manufacturing (Tables 34–1 and 34–2) (1,9).

Farm workers may be exposed to fumes from liquid manure or from pouring hydrochloric acid into a farm well that has a high content of organic material. Large quantities of hydrogen sulfide are used in the production of elemental sulfur, sulfuric acid, and heavy water for nuclear reactors (9,10). It is a natural constituent of volcanic gases and occurs in some deposits of natural gas and petroleum (8). Hydrogen sulfide may also be encountered in mining and felt manufacturing (11). A mixture of sulfuric acid and bleach can release hydrogen sulfide, as

TABLE 34–1. *Sources of sulfides*

Hydrogen sulfide
Carbon disulfide
Mercaptans
Sulfides found or used in
Sulfur springs
Volcanic gases
Liquid manure
Insecticides
Soil fumigants
Petroleum industry
Farm industry
Jet fuels
Metal refining

TABLE 34–2. *Occupations at risk for hydrogen sulfide exposure*

Sulfides used in the manufacture of
Rubber vulcanizing
Synthetic fabrics
Heavy water
Leather
Plastics
Asphalt roofing
Carbon disulfide
Felt
Glue
Hydrogen sulfide
Natural gas
Phosphorus sequisfulfide production
Potential for workers to be exposed in
Caisson work
Chemical laboratory work
Industrial waste disposal
Industrial fishing
Liquid manure storage
Mining
Petroleum refining
Septic tank cleaning
Sulfur dye production
Sulfuric acid purification
Tannery work
Well digging

can an industrial cleaner with plaster of Paris in a cast room (8). Hydrogen sulfide is produced endogenously from sulfur-containing proteins in the alimentary canal of animals.

Occupational exposure to hydrogen sulfide is prevalent in the petrochemical, paper pulp, leather tanning, food processing, and sewage industries. The general public also faces the risk of H_2S exposure as a result of major industrial accidents emanating from these industries (12).

Sulfide Salts

Hydrogen sulfide is released in vivo from ingested or injected soluble inorganic sulfide salts. Sodium sulfide is therefore completely hydrolyzed in body fluids, and there is no toxicologic distinction between it and hydrogen sulfide. Mixing liquid sodium sulfide with an acid-containing agent, mixing acid and alkaline drain cleaners, and breathing fumes from sodium sulfide have been responsible for cases of poisoning (5). The leather industry uses substantial amounts of sodium sulfide in preparing hides for tanning. Sodium sulfide monohydrate, a common commercial form of sulfide salt, is highly hydroscopic and corrosive (13).

Carbon Disulfide

Carbon disulfide is a colorless liquid with a sweet odor that vaporizes at room temperature (14). Because of this, inhalation is the major route of entry. Hydrogen sulfide is necessary for the production of carbon disulfide (13). Carbon disulfide is used widely as an insecticide, soil fumigant, and solvent for rubber, sulfur, phosphorus, lipids, and waxes. The production of carbon disulfide is most prominent in oil and gas exploration and processing (15).

Mercaptans

The mercaptans are toxic, flammable gases. There are two mercaptans of note: ethyl and methyl mercaptan. These compounds are used in the production of pesticides, jet fuels, and plastics. They are extremely foul-smelling agents and are added in very small concentrations as warning agents for the release of natural gases and other gases because their odor can be detected well below the concentrations necessary to produce toxicity.

METABOLISM OF SULFIDES

Hydrogen sulfide and similar compounds may be detoxified spontaneously by various oxidative mechanisms with formation of nontoxic products, such as polysulfides, thiosulfate, and sulfate, all of which are excreted by the kidneys (2,6,16). These reactions are catalyzed by heavy metals, particularly in the presence of proteins, and occur with low concentrations of the sulfide (17). Other modes of sulfide elimination whose significance is unknown include urinary excretion of unoxidized sulfide and pulmonary excretion of the gas (18).

MECHANISM OF TOXICITY

The sulfides are intracellular toxins; their mechanism of poisoning is similar to that of cyanide (1,5,6). Like cyanide, hydrogen sulfide inhibits the cytochrome oxidase system. It binds to the cytochrome oxidase ferric (F3+3) moiety, inhibits the cytochrome oxidase ferric moiety, and inhibits oxidative phosphorylation (4). This inhibition blocks cellular respiration, leading to cellular anoxia. Anaerobic metabolism and lactic acid accumulation result (5,6). Both cyanide and sulfides also act as inhibitors of the ferric iron peroxidases and catalases. In addition, the sulfides inhibit succinic dehydrogenase, carbonic anhydrase, and other enzymes (17).

In body fluids, dissociated and undissociated hydrogen sulfide exist in approximately equal proportions. The undissociated acid penetrates biologic membranes more rapidly than the hydrosulfide anion. It is thought that the hydrosulfide anion inhibits the cytochrome oxidase system by interrupting electron transport. This is done by formation of a dissociable complex with ferric heme groups in cytochrome oxidase, producing sulfmethemoglobin. Sulfmethemoglobin is therefore analogous to cyanomethemoglobin. When the mitochondrial electron transport system is unable to function properly, cellular respiration continues anaerobically with production of organic acid by-products.

Two differences are recognized between cyanide binding to methemoglobin and sulfide binding to the same ferric heme sites. The first is that sulfmethemoglobin undergoes gradual auto-oxidation, reduction to ferrohemoglobin, and the second is that cyanide is bound more tenaciously than sulfide by a factor of 200 (13).

Sulfhemoglobin and Sulfmethemoglobin

There has been a great deal of confusion regarding the relationship between sulfhemoglobin and the toxicity associated with the sulfides (10). Sulfmethemoglobin is unrelated to sulfhemoglobin, and even though many investigators refer to sulfhemoglobinemia as a cause of death in sulfide poisoning, no abnormal pigments including sulfhemoglobin are found in significant concentrations in those fatally poisoned by sulfide (11,13).

Sulfhemoglobin is a bright green derivative of hemoglobin (19). This derivative has a sulfur atom incorporated into the porphyrin ring. It is ineffective for oxygen transport. Although it can be formed in vitro from oxyhemoglobin by various compounds that oxidize hemoglobin, it is rarely found in life (20). Sulfhemoglobin has not been generated in vivo; its formation requires exogenous sulfide or some other unknown form of sulfur, together with only distinctly unphysiologic chemicals and conditions. Such pigments have been generated in high yield, but only in vitro, or postmortem (18). Sulfhemoglobin, in contrast to sulfmethemoglobin, has rarely been encountered in those who survive sulfide poisoning, but its postmortem formation may be responsible for the various tissue discolorations noted (11,13). Unlike carbon monoxide, the sulfides do not combine with hemoglobin during life. The formation of sulfmethemoglobinemia occurs after death as a result of the decomposition of tissues. The many cases of sulfhemoglobin in published reports involve phenacetin, nitrites, nitrates, and sulfa drugs such as dapsone (21–23). These drugs also cause methemoglobinemia, and this may very well be the pigment that is read as sulfhemoglobin. It has also been associated with drug abuse and exposure to polluted air (20). This pigment may more precisely be called pseudosulfhemoglobin, and may be a mixture of oxidized and denatured hemoglobin that may have formed abnormal disulfide bridges with sulfhydryl compounds (11,13). Some investigators hold that sulfhemoglobinemia is probably a relatively nontoxic syndrome, if it truly exists (20).

TOXICITY

Clinical Effects

The most important route of absorption of hydrogen sulfide is through the lungs. Under appropriate circumstances hydrogen sulfide can penetrate the intact skin to produce signs of systemic intoxication. The intensity of exposure accounts for the highly diverse clinical patterns of hydrogen sulfide poisoning. At concentrations of 150 ppm, hydrogen sulfide is detectable by its rotten egg odor and is a local irritant to the conjunctival membranes and respiratory tract (Table 34–3). With levels of 150 ppm, slight systemic symptoms will occur after several hours (12). Low concentrations of approximately 0.01%–0.15% (100–150 ppm) cause paralysis of the olfactory nerve (6,8). At 0.02% (200 ppm), hydrogen sulfide depresses the central nervous system, and may cause acute pulmonary edema. In moderate concentrations it stimulates the nervous system and respiration. At concentrations greater than 500 ppm, cardiovascular collapse may ensue. In high concentrations of 0.1% (1000 ppm) or more it directly paralyzes the central nervous system, including the respiratory center. Because the body has an inherently large capacity for detoxifying sulfide, the toxicity of gas mixtures is more closely related to concentration than to length of exposure (5).

TABLE 34–3. *Sulfide concentration and symptomatology*

ppm	Percent	Symptoms
25	0.025	Detection of odor
100–150	0.01–0.15	Paralysis of olfactory nerve
150	0.15	Local irritation
200	0.02	Central nervous system depression
500	0.05	Cardiovascular collapse
1000	0.1	Central nervous system paralysis, death

Low Concentrations of Hydrogen Sulfide

At 25 ppm the odor of hydrogen sulfide may be detected (16). Odor is considered unreliable, however, because, as mentioned above, concentrations of approximately 150 ppm or greater cause rapid paralysis of the olfactory nerve (Table 34–4) (6). At these low concentrations (50–200 ppm), symptoms of sulfide intoxication are due chiefly to local tissue irritation of the eyes and respiratory tract rather than to systemic actions (6). The gas is relatively harmless at low concentrations except for its unpleasant odor and the irritation it causes to the eyes, respiratory tract, and gastrointestinal tract. The most characteristic effect is on the eyes, where superficial injury to the conjunctivae and corneas may be noted. This keratoconjunctivitis is known as "gas eye" and is manifested after several hours or days of exposure as a scratchy, irritated sensation with tearing and burning. Recovery is almost always complete and spontaneous unless secondary infection occurs (11).

Other local reactions may include pharyngitis, bronchitis, and pneumonia. Hydrogen sulfide may also pro-

TABLE 34–4. *Symptoms of hydrogen sulfide intoxication*

Low concentration
- Irritation
  - Eye ("gas eye")
  - Respiratory tract (pharyngitis, bronchitis)
  - Gastrointestinal tract
- Headache
- Nausea
- Vomiting
- Weakness

High concentration
- Neurologic
  - Agitation
  - Coma
  - Seizures
  - Respiratory paralysis
- Cardiac
  - Disorders of conduction
  - Various dysrhythmias
- Local
  - Caustic burn

duce significant hyperpnea by direct chemostimulation of the carotid body. Nonspecific effects in mild poisonings may include headache, nausea, vomiting, and generalized weakness. As stated earlier, at approximately 200 ppm (0.02%) hydrogen sulfide depresses the central nervous system.

High Concentrations of Hydrogen Sulfide

Serious consequences are the result of increasing exposures above 150 ppm, beginning with pulmonary irritation and edema after prolonged exposure at 200 ppm. Above 700 ppm, intoxication is often immediate and fatal, the result of respiratory failure from respiratory center paralysis and asphyxia followed by cardiac failure (7).

In high concentrations (1000 ppm), a single breath or a few breaths can lead to various neurological alterations ranging from agitation to abrupt loss of consciousness, coma, and death (10). It has been thought that the respiratory paralysis noted is due to central depression of the hypothalamic respiratory center (8). Apnea is often followed by hypoxic seizures, cardiovascular collapse, and death. Once apnea has developed, breathing generally does not begin again spontaneously. Pulmonary edema may be noted in a significant number of individuals poisoned with sulfide (5,9,11,13).

The direct toxic action of sulfide on the heart has been associated with various dysrhythmias, disorders of conduction, and disorders of ventricular repolarization. Carbon disulfide appears to have a greater affinity for the central nervous system and cardiovascular system than does hydrogen sulfide. Because soluble salts of sulfides are alkaline substances, they may cause a caustic burn.

Most deaths due to hydrogen sulfide intoxication occur at the site of exposure. Those patients arriving alive at a treatment facility generally experience complete recovery without sequelae.

Common neurological symptoms associated with acute hydrogen sulfide exposure include nervousness, fatigue, weakness of the extremities, headache, dizziness, lightheadedness, sleep disturbances, spasms, convulsions, disturbed equilibrium, agitation, and delirium (24).

Survivors of acute toxic episodes sometimes show other neurologic sequelae, such as amnesia, intention tremor, neurasthenia, disturbance of equilibrium, or more serious brain stem and cortical damage, but complete recovery is the general rule.

LABORATORY DETERMINATIONS

Patients exposed to compounds that can cause sulfmethemoglobin should undergo tests for arterial blood gases, serum electrolytes, and complete blood count.

TABLE 34–5. *Laboratory determinations in sulfide intoxication*

Determination
Arterial blood gas
Calculated arterial oxygen saturation
Measured arterial oxygen saturation
Carboxyhemoglobin concentration
Methemoglobin concentration
Serum electrolytes
Complete blood count

Additionally, arterial saturation should be both measured and calculated (Table 34–5). Sulfhemoglobin concentrations may be obtained, but their significance is unclear. They should not be used to determine or guide therapy in hydrogen sulfide poisoning (2). Sulfmethemoglobin concentrations may be more appropriate to obtain, but this assay is not widely available.

TREATMENT

Initial treatment for patients intoxicated with sulfides involves vigorous prehospital and hospital care. Rapid removal from the toxic environment to fresh air is necessary (Table 34–6). (8,11,13) Because sulfide is so rapidly detoxified in the body, any decrease in the exposure intensity may result in a rapid and spontaneous revival (4). Rescuers should be cautious and should wear protective clothing and face masks because ill-advised rescue attempts often lead to rescuers' exposure (12). Decontamination methods should be performed, especially if the sulfide was on the skin. Providing 100% supplemental oxygen with assisted ventilation if required is important. Although the use of 100% oxygen by itself is not life-saving, the use of oxygen may encourage noncytochrome oxidase-mediated aerobic cellular respiration (11,25,26). Support of the vital signs, including pulse and blood pressure, by standard means is also necessary. Seizures should be treated with diazepam or a short-acting barbiturate. Patients should be monitored closely for development of pulmonary edema (27).

TABLE 34–6. *Treatment of sulfide poisoning*

Comment	Treatment
Acute exposure	Rapid removal from environment
	Oxygen
	Supportive care
	Decontamination
Seizures	Diazepam
Antidotes	Amyl nitrite
	Sodium nitrite*

*Dosage: adult: 10 mL of 3% solution (300 mg); Child: 10 mg/kg of 3% solution.

Nitrite Therapy

Although advocated by many investigators, there is controversy surrounding the use of nitrites as sulfide antidotes (2,5). Because of the similarity between sulfide and cyanide toxicity, and because of the formation of sulfmethemoglobin, the chemical induction of methemoglobinemia has been suggested as an effective antidotal procedure in acute sulfide poisoning (2,8). Induction of methemoglobinemia with nitrites is thought to reverse the effects of sulfides by the competitive binding of methemoglobin with the hydrosulfide anion (8). The important role of methemoglobin may be the trapping of free sulfide because methemoglobin has a greater affinity for sulfide than does cytochrome oxidase (6). As sulfide is exchanged from cytochrome oxidase, aerobic metabolism returns. The nontoxic sulfmethemoglobin is then degraded to nontoxic oxidized forms of sulfur, which are excreted primarily by the kidneys (8,10,11). It may also be that nitrites act by mechanisms other than methemoglobin formation, such as vasodilation or a more direct effect on cytochrome oxidase (5).

Although amyl nitrite pearls may be used, if sodium nitrite is available amyl nitrite is not necessary. Ten milliliters of a 3% solution (300 mg) of sodium nitrite can be injected intravenously at a rate of 2.5–5 mL/min in an adult (8,11). In a child, 10 mg/kg should be administered. If signs and symptoms of systemic poisoning recur, administration of half these doses is indicated.

If nitrites are used, methemoglobin concentrations should be monitored in the critically ill patient so as to ensure that no compromise of oxygen delivery occurs (11,13). Even with all the controversial data concerning nitrite therapy, it is prudent to use this therapy when confronted with a comatose patient who is intoxicated with hydrogen sulfide (6). It should be remembered, however, that the efficacy of antidotal therapy is controversial and that there are serious side effects associated with the use of nitrites in this context.

Thiosulfate Therapy

Although thiosulfate appears to be an effective antidote for cyanide, it is not suggested in the case of sulfide poisoning. This is because rhodanase is necessary to convert cyanide to thiocyanate, but no comparable detoxification pathway is known to exist for sulfide (11,13).

Other Antidotal Therapy

The effectiveness of hydroxycobalamin and other agents such as *p*-aminopropiophenone for the treatment of sulfide poisoning remains to be shown (13).

Hyperbaric Oxygen Therapy

The use of hyperbaric oxygen in sulfide poisoning is another area of controversy, and its role has yet to be defined with certainty (2). Hydrogen sulfide intoxication is considered a category-two condition by the Undersea Medical Society, which means that there are insufficient data to assess the efficacy of hyperbaric oxygen for this condition (5). At this time it should be reserved for the patient who does not respond to maximal supportive care, 100% oxygen, and sodium nitrite.

REFERENCES

1. Beck J, Bradbury C, Connors A, et al: Nitrite as an antidote for acute hydrogen sulfide intoxication? *Am Ind Hyg Assoc J* 1981;42:805–809.
2. Smilkstein M, Bronstein A, Pickett H, et al: Hyperbaric oxygen therapy for severe hydrogen sulfide poisoning. *J Emerg Med* 1985;3:27–30.
3. Rabvinovitch S, Greyson N, Weiser W, et al: Clinical and laboratory features of acute sulfur dioxide inhalation poisoning: two-year follow-up. *Am Rev Respir Dis* 1989;139:556–558.
4. Burnett W, King E, Grace M, et al: Hydrogen sulfide poisoning: review of 5 years' experience. *Can Med Assoc J* 1977:117:1277–1280.
5. Hoidal C, Hall A, Robinson M, et al: Hydrogen sulfide poisoning from toxic inhalations of roofing asphalt fumes. *Ann Emerg Med* 1986;15:826–830.
6. Stine R, Slosberg B, Beacham B: Hydrogen sulfide intoxication. *Ann Intern Med* 1976;85:756–758.
7. Bhambhani Y, Singh M: Physiological effects of hydrogen sulfide inhalation during exercise in healthy men. *J Appl Physiol* 1991;71: 1872–1877.
8. Peters J: Hydrogen sulfide poisoning in a hospital setting. *JAMA* 1981;246:1588–1589.
9. Deng J, Chang S: Hydrogen sulfide poisonings in hot spring reservoir cleaning: two case reports. *Am J Ind Med* 1987;11:447–451.
10. Smith R, Gossellin R: Hydrogen sulfide poisoning. *J Occup Med* 1979;21:93–97.
11. Smith R: Hydrogen sulfide poisoning. *Can Med Assoc J* 1978;118: 775–776.
12. Wasch H, Estrin W, Yip P, et al: Prolongation of the P-300 latency associated with hydrogen sulfide exposure. *Arch Neurol* 1989;46: 902–904.
13. Smith R, Kruszyna R, Kruszyna H: Management of acute sulfide poisoning: effects of oxygen, thiosulfate and nitrite. *Arch Environ Health* 1976;31:166–169.
14. Peters H, Levine R, Matthews C, et al: Extrapyramidal and other neurologic manifestations associated with carbon disulfide fumigant exposure. *Arch Neurol* 1988;45:537–540.
15. Chapman L, Sauter S, Henning R, et al: Finger tremor after carbon disulfide-based pesticide exposures. *Arch Neurol* 1991;48:866–870.
16. Whitcraft D, Bailey T, Hart B: Hydrogen sulfide poisoning treated with hyperbaric oxygen. *J Emerg Med* 1985; 3:23–25.
17. Thompson D, Szarek J, Altiere R, et al: Nonadrenergic bronchodilation induced by high concentrations of sulfur dioxide. *J Appl Physiol* 1990;69:1786–1791.
18. Smith R: Chemicals reacting with various forms of hemoglobin: biological significance, mechanisms, and determination. *J Forensic Sci* 1990;31:662–672.
19. Nichol A, Hendry I, Morell D, et al: Mechanism of formation of sulphaemoglobin. *Biochem Biophys Acta* 1968;156:97–108.
20. Park C, Nagel R, Blumberg W, et al: Sulfhemoglobin. *J Biol Chem* 1986;261:8805–8810.
21. Lim T, Lower D: "Enterogenous" cyanosis. *Am Rev Respir Dis* 1970; 101:419–422.
22. Medeiros M, Bechara E, Naoum P: Oxygen toxicity and hemoglobin

in subjects from a highly polluted town. *Arch Environ Health* 1983; 38:11–16.
23. Lambert M, Sonnet J, Mathieu P, et al: Delayed sulfhemoglobinemia after acute dapsone intoxication. *J Toxicol Clin Toxicol* 1982;19:45–50.
24. Sheppard D: Sulfur dioxide and asthma—a double-edged sword. *J Allergy Clin Immunol* 1988;82:961–964.
25. Park C, Nagel R: Sulfhemoglobinemia. *N Engl J Med* 1984;310: 1579–1584.
26. Carrico R, Blumberg W, Peisach J: The reversible binding of oxygen to sulfhemoglobin. *J Biol Chem* 1978;253:7212–7215.
27. Thoman M: Sewer gas: Hydrogen sulfide intoxication. *Clin Toxicol* 1969;2:383–386.

CHAPTER 35

Drugs and Toxins Causing Methemoglobinemia

In biochemical terms, methemoglobin (MetHb), or ferrihemoglobin, is an oxidation product and chemical analog of the normal blood pigment hemoglobin (1). When iron is oxidized from the ferrous state in hemoglobin to the ferric state, methemoglobin is produced (2). Oxygen bound to methemoglobin is so firmly attached that it is not available to tissues; consequently, methemoglobin is not an oxygen-transporting pigment (3). Methemoglobin is normally present in a low concentration in red blood cells; total blood pigment is usually about 1%–2% methemoglobin and the remainder is hemoglobin, with iron in the normal reduced state (3–5). The percentage of methemoglobin is the ratio of methemoglobin to hemoglobin. For example, a methemoglobin concentration of 50% means that in a patient with 16 g of hemoglobin 8 g is methemoglobin. The percentage can therefore be misleading, especially in the presence of anemia (6).

MECHANISMS FOR OXIDIZING METHEMOGLOBIN

Physiologically, within the red blood cell hemoglobin shifts continually from the reduced, functional, ferrous form to the oxidized, nonfunctional, ferric form (Fig. 35–1) (7,8). An equilibrium exists between hemoglobin and methemoglobin, the latter being continuously reduced in the cell. The body has four mechanisms for maintaining methemoglobin levels at or below 1%; two are enzymatic, and the other two act directly.

Of the two enzyme systems that exist in the red blood cell to limit the accumulation of methemoglobin, the main mechanism is reduced nicotinamide adenine dinucleotide (NADH)-MetHb reductase, which accounts for about 95% of in vivo methemoglobin reduction (2). This reaction uses flavin-containing cytochrome b5 as an electron-carrying intermediate between NADH, derived from glycolysis, and methemoglobin.

The second enzyme system, using reduced nicotinamide adenine dinucleotide phosphate (NADPH) from the pentose phosphate shunt, is not essential under physiologic conditions. This enzyme requires an artificial electron carrier, such as methylene blue, to become active; there is no known physiologic substance in the erythrocyte that can function in place of methylene blue. In addition to these two enzymatic pathways, ascorbic acid and glutathione can reduce methemoglobin directly, but quantitatively they are not very important, accounting for a very small amount of the methemoglobin reduction (9).

Although the second enzymatic system is usually not an important mechanism because there is no endogenous electron acceptor, when the methemoglobin concentra-

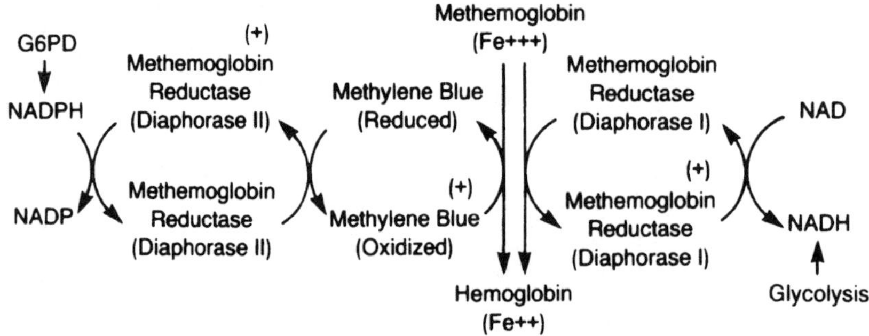

FIG. 35–1. Mechanisms of methemoglobin reduction. G6PD indicates glucose-6-phosphate dehydrogenase; NADP, nicotinamide adenine dinucleotide phosphate; NADPH, nicotinamide adenine dinucleotide phosphate, reduced; NAD, nicotinamide adenine dinucleotide. Reprinted with permission from Harris J, Rumack B, Peterson R, et al: Methemoglobinemia resulting from absorption of nitrates. *JAMA* 1979;242;2871. © 1979 American Medical Association.

tion in the cell rises to more than the physiologic 1%–2%, its activity can increase by up to a factor of 60. In addition, this mechanism may be activated by the presence of exogenously added electron carriers, such as methylene blue. Although this system plays no physiologic role, its therapeutic activation is an important procedure for the management of acute acquired methemoglobinemia. Under physiologic conditions, it is the NADH-dependent pathway that plays the major role in methemoglobin reduction.

MECHANISM OF TOXICITY

In methemoglobinemia the oxidized complexes do not bind oxygen, thus lowering hemoglobin's saturation without affecting arterial oxygen tension or arterial carbon dioxide pressure (10). Moreover, as with carbon monoxide, the remaining iron atoms in the hemoglobin tetramer bind oxygen more avidly in the presence of methemoglobin, causing a leftward shift in the oxyhemoglobin dissociation curve (2,4,11). Both phenomena decrease oxygen delivery to the tissues.

TYPES OF METHEMOGLOBINEMIAS

Methemoglobinemia may result from (a) exposure to drugs or chemicals that accelerate the oxidation of hemoglobin beyond the reductive and protective capabilities of the cell; (b) deficiency in the ability to reduce methemoglobin (hereditary deficiency of NADH-methemoglobin reductase); and (c) the presence of a structural abnormality in hemoglobin. This chapter deals only with exogenous substances that can cause an oxidation of hemoglobin (acquired methemoglobinemia) (1).

ACQUIRED METHEMOGLOBINEMIA

Acquired methemoglobinemia results when the rate of formation of methemoglobin exceeds the rate of reduction secondary to the action of certain chemicals. A number of substances are capable of oxidizing hemoglobin directly to methemoglobin. In general, the cause of methemoglobinemia relates to drugs, industrial exposure to certain chemicals, cultural dietary patterns, and recreational abuse of certain compounds. Compounds causing methemoglobinemia include the nitrites, chlorates, hydrogen peroxide, alloxan, the quinones, aniline dyes, local anesthetics, nitrobenzene, phenazopyridine, phenacetin, and others (Table 35–1) (1).

Nitrates and Nitrites

Nitrites are the chemicals that most frequently produce methemoglobinemia. They are present in medicinal agents, such as amyl nitrite, nitroglycerin (11), and spirits of nitrite (12), as well as many other compounds (13, 14). Some of the nitrites are so toxic that only a small amount can rapidly cause intoxication that, if not treated, can lead to death (15). Although the substances that contain nitrites are myriad, they may be divided into inorganic and organic compounds. The inorganic compounds are generally more toxic. These consist of sodium nitrite, potassium nitrite, bismuth subnitrate, and others. Organic nitrites include many drugs used in medicine (15,16).

Because of its similarity in appearance to table salt and its use as a meat preservative and curing agent (1), sodium nitrite is frequently the cause of methemoglobinemia associated with purposeful ingestion or with ingestion of contaminated food (17). Methemoglobinemia has been caused by nitrites added to sausage. Many times, nearly maximum amounts of nitrite are added to meats because enhanced color is a desirable marketing technique (18).

Methemoglobinemia has been reported in burn patients treated with silver nitrate (19,20). The apparent mechanism for development of methemoglobinemia in these patients is nitrate reduction by bacteria on areas of granulation tissue with subsequent absorption of nitrite (2,21).

TABLE 35–1. *Causes of acquired methemoglobinemia*

Nitrates and nitrites
Bismuth subnitrate (Pepto-Bismol)
Nitrate-rich foods
Nitrate-rich water
Nitroglycerin
Nitroprusside (Nipride)
Silver nitrate
Sodium nitrite
Volatile nitrites
Amyl nitrite
Butyl nitrite
Isobutyl nitrite (Bolt, Hardware, Satan's Scent, Locker Room, Quick Silver)
Local anesthetics
Benzocaine (Unguentine, Solarcaine)
Lidocaine (Xylocaine)
Prilocaine (Citanest)
Procaine (Novocain)
Aromatic amino and nitroso compounds
Aniline dyes (inks, shoe polishes)
Nitrobenzene
Nitrochlorobenzene
Paranitroaniline
Metachloroaniline
Dinitrotoluene
Phenazopyridine (Pyridium)
Sulfonamides
Dapsone
Miscellaneous
Acetanalid
Chlorates
Methylene blue (large doses)
Phenacetin
Primaquine

There are many reports of nitrite-induced methemoglobinemia in infants fed well water contaminated with high concentrations of nitrates (2,22–28). Nitrates are toxic only in amounts higher than those encountered in foods. The potential hazard of nitrates in water or food is their conversion to nitrite either before or after ingestion. Methemoglobinemia has also been reported in a home dialysis patient who was using well water high in nitrate concentrations (25).

Methemoglobinemia and Infants

Although persons of any age may be affected by methemoglobinemia, infants are particularly susceptible during the first 4 months of life (1,25). Newborn infants normally have a low concentration of erythrocyte cytochrome b5 reductase. Infants are also at risk from the ingestion of vegetables rich in nitrates, such as spinach, beets, carrots, turnips, and cabbage (20,29). Nitrates do not directly oxidize hemoglobin to methemoglobin, but nitrates can be converted by intestinal microflora to nitrites. It has been found that nitrates normally present in these vegetables are reduced by bacteria, especially *Escherichia coli*, that colonize the upper gastrointestinal tract of some infants; these are introduced during preparation or storage of purees, soups, and stews (2,15,20). Infants may be more susceptible to bacterial conversion because, during the first few months of life, they have a low gastric acidity, which can result in proliferation of bacterial species capable of reducing nitrates to nitrites.

Well water polluted by nitrate-containing fertilizers is an additional cause of methemoglobinemia that should be considered in neonates (28). The gastric pH of neonates is elevated, allowing for the growth of nitrite-producing bacteria. In addition, neonates have decreased amounts of methemoglobin reductase and a large percentage of fetal hemoglobin, which is more susceptible than normal hemoglobin to oxidation. In view of these facts, neonates are at risk of developing methemoglobinemia when such contaminated water is used in the preparation of formulas.

Volatile Alkyl Nitrites

Although the volatile organic nitrites may cause methemoglobinemia (30,31), they are primarily inhaled as drugs of abuse (9,32–37). For this reason, they are discussed with other chemical inhalants that are abused (see Chapter 53).

Miscellaneous Nitrite Compounds

Cases of methemoglobinemia that are due to nitrates have been reported after the use of bismuth subnitrate (Pepto-Bismol), ammonium or potassium nitrate, and amyl nitrite and from the inhalation of nitrous gases by arc welders (38). Various reports list sublingual, oral, and intravenous nitroglycerin as well as intravenous nitroprusside as causes of methemoglobinemia (39,40).

Local Anesthetics

Local anesthetics have induced methemoglobinemia (41). This has also been reported when benzocaine was applied as a gel to the gums of infants for the relief of teething pain (2,42,43). Although prilocaine has been implicated most frequently (44), topical procaine and lidocaine have also been noted to cause methemoglobinemia (45–46). The case reports involving lidocaine all occurred in patients with enzyme deficiencies or some other condition predisposing them to methemoglobinemia (47–48).

Aromatic Amino and Nitroso Compounds

Aniline Dyes and Nitrobenzene

In its pure form, aniline is a colorless, oily liquid most commonly found in the chemical and rubber industries. It is used in the manufacture of synthetic rubber, dyes, inks, varnishes, perfumes, shoe polish, paint remover, photographic chemicals, explosives, herbicides, and fungicides, as well as in other products (49).

Aniline, nitrobenzene, and their derivatives are found in many household products (Table 35–2). Aniline does not produce methemoglobinemia, but it is metabolized to active compounds in the body that are capable of forming methemoglobin (50). Among these are the aminophenols, the phenylhydroxylamines, and the phenylenediamines (29). The most potent methemoglobin-generating metabolite is phenylhydroxylamine. This compound is unstable and is readily oxidized to nitrosobenzene, which is the form that predominates in the circulation (15).

Because aniline is a volatile liquid, it can gain access to the body by inhalation as well as by skin penetration (51). When aniline dyes were in common use as laundry markers, dermal absorption from diaper markings caused

TABLE 35–2. *Aniline compounds*

Coloring agents
Dyes
Inks
Laundry markers
Paints
Shoe polishes
Aniline converted to
Aminophenol
Phenylenediamine
Phenylhydroxylamine

numerous cases of methemoglobinemia (2,12). In addition to methemoglobinemia, aniline has long been known to produce a Heinz-body hemolytic anemia (29,52).

Phenazopyridine (Pyridium)

Toxic reactions to phenazopyridine, an azo dye, appear to be exceedingly rare (53). Both methemoglobinemia and hemolytic anemia have been reported after an overdose of phenazopyridine as well as in patients with renal disease who were receiving the drug in therapeutic doses (3,54). Patients with glucose-6-phosphate dehydrogenase deficiency have also been reported to develop methemoglobinemia after therapeutic doses of phenazopyridine (55). Metabolism of phenazopyridine results in the formation of large quantities of aniline, and the production of methemoglobinemia by phenazopyridine is probably due to the aniline metabolites (56).

Because the azo dye is deposited in the skin, a yellow skin pigmentation has been noted in cases of azo dye intoxication (53,57).

The hemolysis secondary to the ingestion of phenazopyridine and other oxidizing agents may result in the appearance of bizarre red cell forms in the peripheral blood smear (58). One such form has been named the "bite cell" or degmacyte because these red cells appear as though a bite has been taken out of them (52).

Sulfonamides: Dapsone

Dapsone, a sulfonamide derivative, has been used in the treatment of malaria, leprosy, and dermatitis herpetiformis, and most recently in the prophylactic treatment of *Pneumocystis carinii* pneumonia in patients infected with the human immunodeficiency virus. The predominant toxic effect of Dapsone is oxidation of the ferrous iron in heme to ferric iron, with the resultant production of methemoglobinemia (59). Common side effects include a dose-dependent hemolytic anemia and methemoglobinemia in normal individuals (60,61).

Miscellaneous Compounds: Chlorates

The chlorates (sodium and potassium) have occasionally been used therapeutically in mouthwashes and gargles; they are also used in furniture polishes (62). They are widely used in industry and as a nonselective weed killer. Because they have strong oxidizing properties, they have also been used commercially in the manufacture of explosives, matches, dyestuffs, tanning chemicals, and leather-finishing chemicals (1). One of the characteristic features of chlorate poisoning is the great variability in toxic effects.

The chlorates have three main actions: (a) a local action that causes nausea, vomiting, and abdominal pain; (b) the production of methemoglobinemia; and (c) a late production of acute tubular necrosis (62–64). The gastrointestinal symptoms are secondary to a direct action of the chlorates on the gastrointestinal tract. Because of their potent oxidizing action, methemoglobinemia may ensue. The direct toxic effect on the red cell membrane may cause intense hemolysis (65). The renal impairment appears to be due to a direct toxic effect on the proximal tubule with resultant anuria. This blocks the main route of elimination of the drug and prolongs the exposure time of the red blood cells to the oxidant effects.

SIGNS AND SYMPTOMS OF METHEMOGLOBINEMIA

Methemoglobinemia is manifested clinically by cyanosis. Because methemoglobin is incapable of binding with oxygen, the symptoms of methemoglobinemia are attributable to the hypoxia produced by the lowered oxygen-carrying capacity of the blood. As mentioned before, the oxygen-hemoglobin dissociation curve is also shifted to the left (2,4), which makes the remaining oxyhemoglobin bind more tenaciously to the available oxygen. The severity of the symptoms is related to the quantity of methemoglobin present, the rapidity with which the methemoglobinemia develops, and the capacity of the patient's cardiorespiratory and hematopoietic system to adjust to hypoxia (66).

Methemoglobin is darker than unoxygenated hemoglobin and can produce a marked cyanosis even when present at concentrations that do not threaten life (Table 35–3). Symptoms of methemoglobinemia may vary from anxiety to headaches, fatigue, coma, and death. In patients without anemia, cyanosis first appears at methemoglobin

TABLE 35–3. *Methemoglobin concentrations and symptomatology*

Methemoglobin concentration (%)	Symptoms
10–15	Cyanosis "Chocolate cyanosis"
20–40	Headache Fatigue Weakness Dizziness
40–60	Lethargy Dyspnea Bradycardia Respiratory depression Stupor
60–80	Seizures Coma Death

concentrations of about 15% (2). As the cyanosis increases, the lips, ears, and mucous membranes develop a violet cast that is unlike the bluish discoloration seen in oxygen desaturation (2). This "chocolate cyanosis" is the hallmark of methemoglobinemia. In addition, methemoglobinemia-induced cyanosis improves little when even high concentrations of oxygen are administered. This cyanosis may be difficult to appreciate in dark-skinned individuals although the nailbeds and mucous membranes will be discolored.

In general, patients with acquired methemoglobinemia tolerate concentrations of methemoglobin up to 20% without ill effects (67). At concentrations of 20%–25%, symptoms such as headache, fatigue, tachycardia, weakness, and dizziness may appear. When methemoglobin concentrations reach 55%–60%, oxygenation of tissues becomes inadequate; this may result in dyspnea, lethargy, metabolic acidosis, and sinus bradycardia and other dysrhythmias. Neurologic manifestations, such as paralysis, coma, and seizures, may also occur. Death occurs with concentrations greater than 70% and is due to heart failure from hypoxia (1,2). The urine may be brown to black as a result of the presence of methemoglobin (68).

The toxic signs of acquired methemoglobinemia have been noted to be more severe than those produced by a corresponding degree of anemia. This is because methemoglobin, like carboxyhemoglobin, not only decreases the available oxygen-carrying pigment but also increases the affinity of the unaltered hemoglobin for oxygen, thus further impairing oxygen delivery (1).

TOXIC EFFECTS UNRELATED TO METHEMOGLOBINEMIA

An acute toxic methemoglobinemia causes more pronounced symptoms than chronic methemoglobinemia. Methemoglobin concentrations that are relatively benign when caused by congenital defects are likely to produce more severe signs if induced by a chemical for two reasons. First, otherwise normal subjects do not have the compensatory mechanisms that develop over a lifetime, and second, a strong possibility always exists of additional toxic effects or side effects of the chemical agent. Any chemical agent used to generate methemoglobin may have additional toxic effects, which may make profound contributions to the toxic syndrome. Some aromatic amino and nitro compounds, such as aniline and nitrobenzene, have central and prominent cardiac effects. Chlorate salts produce intravascular hemolysis, gastroenteritis, and nephritis (2). Inorganic salts of nitrite and organic nitrates and nitrites also act directly as peripheral vasodilators. It is doubtful that any chemical agent produces an otherwise uncomplicated methemoglobinemia. Therefore, it is inappropriate and misleading to suggest that there is a lethal concentration of methemoglobin without taking into account the particular agent involved.

The effects of methemoglobin may be additive or even synergistic with those of carbon monoxide poisoning as both the inhibition of oxygen binding and delivery are shared between them. Poisoning with carboxyhemoglobin and methemoglobin might result in significant symptoms at individual levels that would be expected to be well tolerated.

DIAGNOSIS

An arterial blood gas that is "chocolate brown" with a normal PaO_2 suggests this diagnosis (69). Standard blood gas determinations do not measure arterial blood oxygen saturation (SaO_2), but, rather, report a derived value based on pHa and PaO_2. Co-oximetry of arterial blood accurately identifies this condition, because SaO_2 is measured rather than calculated (70). The co-oximeter measures the absorbance of seven specific wavelengths through a film of the sample, thereby analyzing the specific hemoglobin derivatives oxyhemoglobin, deoxyhemoglobin, methemoglobin, and carboxyhemoglobin (2,71).

The diagnosis of methemoglobinemia, therefore, is based largely on history of exposure to an offending agent, the characteristic central cyanosis that is unresponsive to oxygen administration, a normal pO_2, and a normal calculated oxygen saturation, but a decreased measured (direct) saturation (70). The diagnosis of methemoglobinemia is not difficult to make if it is considered in the differential diagnosis of the cyanotic patient, particularly in the absence of cardiac or pulmonary disease and if the cyanosis is not promptly alleviated by oxygen therapy (2). Direct measurements of methemoglobin will confirm the diagnosis.

About 5 g of deoxyhemoglobin per 100 mL of blood are required to produce visible cyanosis, but a comparable discoloration is produced by 1.5–2 g of methemoglobin per 100 mL (1,21,54). The greater visible effects of this abnormal pigment are due to alterations in the absorption spectra (7,8). A confirmation of the diagnosis can therefore be made by means of a spectrophotometric method, which measures the amount of methemoglobin present. Although methemoglobin concentrations expressed as a percentage of total hemoglobin in the methemoglobin form are reported, the total hemoglobin must always be taken into consideration (2).

LABORATORY

Normally, less than 1%–2% of hemoglobin circulates in the oxidized state. When concentrations greater than this occur, methemoglobinemia is said to exist.

Pulse oximetry is a major advance in the noninvasive monitoring of oxygen saturation. It has been quickly accepted in clinical practice because it is easy to perform, painless, rapid in response, and accurate when arterial saturations are greater than 65%. However, pulse oximetry gives an inaccurate estimate of arterial oxygen saturation in the presence of dyes, abnormal types of hemoglobin, or when saturation is below 65%.

The pulse oximetry findings in methemoglobinemia are notable. Methemoglobin has an absorption characteristic similar to that of deoxygenated hemoglobin and therefore lowers the saturation as read on the pulse oximeter (72). In contrast, the saturation as reported on the arterial blood gas test is a calculated value based on the partial pressure of dissolved oxygen and assumes no abnormal hemoglobin present. Therefore, the reported oxygen saturation from the laboratory is generally higher than that measured with the pulse oximeter. Because all pulse oximeters now available function at essentially the same wavelengths, all should be equally affected by similar amounts of methemoglobin (69). Normal pO_2 in the presence of a decreased oxygen saturation, measured directly, is highly suspicious of methemoglobinemia or carbon monoxide poisoning.

TREATMENT

Profound methemoglobinemia shares with narcotic overdose, hypoglycemia, organophosphate poisoning, and cyanide poisoning the need for treatment before a definitive diagnosis is made. Many times a decision must be made on the basis of strong clinical suspicion (73). Survival is possible with methemoglobinemia concentrations of 75% if immediate treatment with antidotal therapy is instituted (Table 35–4).

Acute overdose should be treated with gastric lavage followed by the administration of oral charcoal and a cathartic. Because some of the agents that cause methemoglobinemia can be percutaneously absorbed, a patient's contaminated clothing should be removed and the skin decontaminated by a thorough washing with soap and water. Supplemental oxygen, even in the presence of normal oxygen partial pressure, is recommended, the aim being to saturate the remaining functional hemoglobin with oxygen.

In cases where the methemoglobin concentration is less than 45%, supportive care will usually suffice. In the absence of serious signs of hypoxia, removal of the offending chemical agent is the only therapy required because normal reducing mechanisms within the erythrocyte will usually convert methemoglobin to hemoglobin within 48–72 hours. Usually, no specific therapy is required unless stupor or coma is present.

TABLE 35–4. *Treatment of acquired methemoglobinemia*

Condition	Modality
Acute ingestion	Lavage Charcoal and cathartic Naloxone or glucose
Dermal exposure	Decontamination Supplemental oxygen
Stupor or coma	Methylene blue (1–2 mg/kg of 1% sterile solution)

Methylene Blue

When the degree of methemoglobinemia is so pronounced that semistupor or unconsciousness is present, an emergency exists and treatment must be prompt (7). The chief feature of antidotal treatment consists of the intravenous injection of methylene blue (tetramethylthionine chloride).

Methylene blue acts as a cofactor in the transfer of an electron from NADPH to ferric iron in a reaction catalyzed by methemoglobin-NAPDH reductase. In this reaction methylene blue is first reduced to leukomethylene blue, which then reduces methemoglobin to normal hemoglobin (74). There is no endogenous cofactor to act as an electron acceptor for NADPH, so that the reaction catalyzed by NADPH methemoglobin reductase is normally responsible for, at most, 5% of the reduction of methemoglobin. However, with the addition of methylene blue, methemoglobinemia should be resolved within 1 hour.

It may seem to be paradoxical that methylene blue, which is a methemoglobin former, is effective in decreasing methemoglobinemia. Actually, methylene blue is not a good methemoglobin former in vivo in humans. Doses much smaller than those that produce methemoglobin are capable of reducing methemoglobin because, in low concentrations, methylene blue forms a reversible oxidation-reduction system that can enhance erythrocyte reduction of methemoglobin. In high concentrations, however, it can oxidize hemoglobin to methemoglobin and thus increase methemoglobinemia (6,7). When methylene blue is administered in its oxidized form, it is reduced to a colorless, reduced form called leukomethylene blue. Leukomethylene blue acts as an electron donor and nonenzymatically reduces methemoglobin to hemoglobin (2,7,12,75).

Methylene blue, when indicated, should be administered in a dose of 1–2 mg/kg intravenously as a 1% sterile aqueous or saline solution. It can be administered from a 10 mL syringe over 5 minutes; this is repeated in 1–2 hours if necessary (3,4,7,15). The total dose should not exceed 7 mg/kg (2,7,15).

Maximal response to methylene blue usually occurs within 30–60 minutes; therefore, methemoglobin concentrations should be monitored for approximately 1 hour after administration (74). If the patient does not respond to methylene blue treatment within 30–60 minutes, other possibilities for the diagnosis should be considered. For example, there may be an associated glucose-6-phosphate dehydrogenase deficiency that could lead to hemolysis, there may be a subclinical deficiency

TABLE 35–5. *Side effects of methylene blue*

Precordial pain
Dyspnea
Restlessness
Apprehension
Tremors
Blue urine
Dysuria
Urinary frequency
Hemolytic anemia (with large doses in glucose-6-phosphate dehydrogenase deficiency)
Methemoglobinemia (with large doses)

in methemoglobin reductase, or the diagnosis may be incorrect (76).

Methylene blue has been implicated as a cause of hemolytic anemia but only in very large doses (usually greater than 7 mg/kg) or in the presence of glucose-6-phosphate dehydrogenase deficiency (Table 35–5). Nonspecific side effects of methylene blue seen with high doses include apprehension, precordial pain, dyspnea, restlessness, and tremors. Often, the urine appears dark blue because some of the dye is present in the blue or oxidized form. Because of the irritating effect of this compound in the excreted form, dysuria may occur. Finally, as mentioned above, high concentrations of methylene blue may cause methemoglobinemia by directly oxidizing hemoglobin to methemoglobin (77).

Ascorbic Acid

Although ascorbic acid can also reduce methemoglobin and has been used to treat hereditary methemoglobinemia, it has no place in the management of acquired methemoglobinemia because the rate at which it reduces methemoglobin is too slow to be of any benefit for severe poisoning (45,78). In addition, it may produce a large number of Heinz bodies.

Exchange Transfusion

There has been only limited experience with exchange transfusion in methemoglobinemia. As a treatment, it has the advantage of reducing blood concentrations of the offending chemical as well as restoring functional blood pigment. This advantage, however, must be weighed against the attendant risks of multiple blood transfusions (29).

Hyperbaric Oxygen

Hyperbaric oxygen has been recommended for the treatment of chemically induced methemoglobinemia, but there is no evidence that it is effective and there is little experience with its use (79).

REFERENCES

1. Rodansky O: Methemoglobinemia and methemoglobin-producing compounds. *Pharmacol Rev* 1951;3:144–196.
2. Curry S: Methemoglobinemia. *Ann Emerg Med* 1982;11:214–221.
3. Cohen B, Bovasso G: Acquired methemoglobinemia and hemolytic anemia following excessive pyridium (phenazopyridine hydrochloride) ingestion. *Clin Pediatr* 1971;10:537–540.
4. Fibuch E, Cecil W, Reed W: Methemoglobinemia associated with organic nitrate therapy. *Anesth Analg* 1979;58:521–523.
5. Smith R, Olson M: Drug-induced methemoglobinemia. *Semin Hematol* 1973;10:253–268.
6. White C, Weiss L: Varying presentations of methemoglobinemia: two cases. *J Emerg Med* 1991;9:45–49.
7. Cohen R, Sachs J, Wicker D, et al: Methemoglobinemia provoked by malarial chemoprophylaxis in Vietnam. *N Engl J Med* 1968;279: 1127–1131.
8. Cohen S: The volatile nitrites. *JAMA* 1979; 241:2077–2078.
9. Metz E, Balcerzak S, Sagone A: Mechanisms of methylene blue stimulation of the hexose monophosphate shunt in erythrocytes. *J Clin Invest* 1976;58:797–802.
10. Avner J, Henretig F, McAneney C: Acquired methemoglobinemia. *Am J Dis Child* 1990;144:1229–1230.
11. Gibson G, Hunter J, Raabe D, et al: Methemoglobinemia produced by high-dose intravenous nitroglycerin. *Ann Intern Med* 1982:96:615–616.
12. Chilcote R, Williams B, Wolff L, et al: Sudden death in an infant from methemoglobinemia after administration of "Sweet spirits of nitre." *Pediatrics* 1977;59:280–282.
13. Smith M, Stair T, Rolnick M: Butyl nitrite and a suicide attempt. *Ann Intern Med* 1980;92:719–720.
14. Smith R: The nitrite methemoglobin complex—its significance in methemoglobin analyses and its possible role in methemoglobinemia. *Biochem Pharmacol* 1967;16:1655–1664.
15. Schimelman M, Soler J, Muller H: Methemoglobinemia: nitrobenzene ingestion. *JACEP* 1978;7:406–408.
16. Buenger J, Mauro V: Organic nitrate-induced methemoglobinemia. *DICP* 1989;23:283–288.
17. Ten-Brink W, Wiezer J, Luijpen A, et al: Nitrate poisoning caused by food contaminated with cooling fluid. *J Toxicol Clin Toxicol* 1982; 19:139–147.
18. Bakshi S, Fahey J, Pierce L: Sausage cyanosis—acquired methemoglobinemic nitrite poisoning. *N Engl J Med* 1967;277:1082.
19. Cushing A, Smith S: Methemoglobinemia with silver nitrate therapy of a burn: report of a case. *J Pediatr* 1967;74:613–615.
20. Geffner M, Powars D, Choctaw W: Acquired methemoglobinemia. *West J Med* 1981;134:7–10.
21. Strauch B, Buch W, Grey W: Successful treatment of methemoglobinemia secondary to silver nitrate therapy. *N Engl J Med* 1969;281: 257–258.
22. Comly H: Cyanosis in infants caused by nitrates in well water. *JAMA* 1987;257:2788–2792.
23. Grant R: Well water nitrate poisoning review: a survey in Nebraska, 1973 to 1978. *Nebr Med J* 1981;66:197–200.
24. Johnson C, Bonrud P, Dosch T, et al: Fatal outcome of methemoglobinemia in an infant. *JAMA* 1987; 257:2796–2797.
25. Miller L: Methemoglobinemia associated with well water. *JAMA* 1971;216:1642–1643.
26. Shearer L, Goldsmith J, Young C, et al: Methemoglobin levels in infants in an area with high nitrate water supply. *Am J Public Health* 1972;62:1174–1180.
27. Vigil J, Warburton S, Haynes W, et al: Nitrates in municipal water supply cause methemoglobinemia in an infant. *Public Health Rep* 1965;80:1119–1121.
28. Bradberry S, Gazzard B, Vale J: Methemoglobinemia caused by the accidental contamination of drinking water with sodium nitrite. *J Toxicol Clin Toxicol* 1994;32:173–178.
29. Kearney T, Manoguerra A, Dunford J: Chemically induced methe-

moglobinemia from aniline poisoning. *West J Med* 1984;140:282–286.
30. Wason S, Detsky A, Platt O, et al: Isobutyl nitrite toxicity by ingestion. *Ann Intern Med* 1990;92:637–638.
31. Elkayam U: Tolerance to organic nitrates: Evidence, mechanisms, clinical relevance, and strategies for prevention. *Ann Intern Med* 1991;114:667–677.
32. Dixon D, Reisch R, Santinga P: Fatal methemoglobinemia resulting from ingestion of isobutyl nitrite, a "room odorizer" widely used for recreational purposes. *J Forensic Sci* 1981;26:587–593.
33. Horne M, Waterman M, Simon L, et al: Methemoglobinemia from sniffing butyl nitrite. *Ann Intern Med* 1979;91:417–418.
34. Lowry T: Amyl nitrite and the EEG: a pilot study. *J Psychedelic Drugs* 1979;11:239–241.
35. Munjack D: Sex and drugs. *Clin Toxicol* 1979;15:75–89.
36. Shesser R, Mitchell J, Edelstein S: Methemoglobinemia from isobutyl nitrite preparations. *Ann Emerg Med* 1981;10:262–264.
37. Bradberry S, Whittington R, Parry D, et al: Fatal methemoglobinemia due to inhalation of isobutyl nitrite. *J Toxicol Clin Toxicol* 1994;32: 179–184.
38. Kearns G, Fiser D: Metoclopramide-induced methemoglobinemia. *Pediatrics* 1988;82:364–366.
39. Marshall J, Ecklund R: Methemoglobinemia from overdose on nitroglycerin. *JAMA* 1980;244–330.
40. Challoner K, McCarron M: Ammonium nitrate cold pack ingestion. *J Emerg Med* 1988;6:289–293.
41. Anderson S, Hajduczek J, Barker S: Benzocaine-induced methemoglobinemia in an adult: Accuracy of pulse oximetry with methemoglobinemia. *Anesth Analg* 1988;67:1099–1101.
42. McGuigan M: Benzocaine-induced methemoglobinemia. *Can Med Assoc J* 1981;125:816.
43. O'Donohue W, Moss L, Angelillo V: Acute methemoglobinemia induced by topical benzocaine and lidocaine. *Arch Intern Med* 1980; 140:1508–1509.
44. Ludwig S: Acute toxic methemoglobinemia following dental analgesia. *Ann Emerg Med* 1981;10:265–266.
45. Potter J, Hillman J: Benzocaine-induced methemoglobinemia. *JACEP* 1979;8:26–27.
46. Ferraro L, Zeichner S, Greenblott G, et al: Cetacaine-induced acute methemoglobinemia. *Anesthesiology* 1988;69:614–615.
47. Weiss L, Generalovich T, Heller M, et al: Methemoglobin levels following intravenous lidocaine administration. *Ann Emerg Med* 1987; 16:323–325.
48. Collins J: Methemoglobinemia as a complication of 20% benzocaine spray for endoscopy. *Gastroenterology* 1990;98:211–213.
49. Phillips D, Gradisek R, Heiselman D: Methemoglobinemia secondary to aniline exposure. *Ann Emerg Med* 1990;19:425–429.
50. Potter J, Krill C, Neal D, et al: Methemoglobinemia due to ingestion of *N,N*-dimethyl-*p*-toluidine, a component used in the fabrication of artificial fingernails. *Ann Emerg Med* 1988;17:1098–1100.
51. Harrison M: Toxic methemoglobinemia. *Anaesthesia* 1977;32:270–272.
52. Greenberg M: Heinz-body hemolytic anemia. *Arch Intern Med* 1976; 136:153–155.
53. Alano F, Webster G: Acute renal failure and pigmentation due to phenazopyridine (Pyridium®). *Ann Intern Med* 1970;72:89–91.
54. Zimmerman R, Green E, Ghurabi W, et al: Methemoglobinemia from overdose of phenazopyridine hydrochloride. *Ann Emerg Med* 1980;9: 147–149.
55. Jeffery W, Zelicoff A, Hardy W: Acquired methemoglobinemia and hemolytic anemia after usual doses of phenazopyridine. *Drug Intell Clin Pharmacol* 1982;16: 157–159.
56. Fincher M, Campbell H: Methemoglobinemia and hemolytic anemia after phenazopyridine hydrochloride (Pyridium) administration in end-stage renal disease. *South Med J* 1989;82:372–373.
57. Eybel C, Armbruster K, Ing T: Skin pigmentation and acute renal failure in a patient receiving phenazopyridine therapy. *JAMA* 1974;228: 1027–1028.
58. Nathan D, Siegel A, Bunn F: Acute methemoglobinemia and hemolytic anemia with phenazopyridine. *Arch Intern Med* 1977;137:1636–1638.
59. Linakis J, Shannon M, Woolf A, et al: Recurrent methemoglobinemia after acute dapsone intoxication in a child. *J Emerg Med* 1989;7:477–480.
60. Cooke T: Dapsone poisoning. *Med J Aust* 1970;1:1158–1159.
61. Iserson K: Methemoglobinemia from dapsone therapy for a suspected brown spider bite. *J Emerg Med* 1985;3: 285–288.
62. Steffen C, Seitz R: Severe chlorate poisoning: report of a case. *Arch Toxicol* 1981;48:281–288.
63. Jackson R, Elder W, McDonnell H: Sodium chlorate poisoning. *Lancet* 1961;2:1381–1383.
64. Timperman J, Maes R: Suicidal poisoning by sodium chlorate. *J Forensic Med* 1966;13:123–129.
65. Stoodley B, Rowe D: Hematological complications of chlorate poisoning. *Br Med J* 1970;2:31–32.
66. Hoffman R, Sauter D: Methemoglobinemia resulting from smoke inhalation. *Vet Hum Toxicol* 1989;31:168–170.
67. Hall A, Kulig K, Rumack B: Drug and chemical induced methemoglobinemia. *Med Toxicol* 1986;1: 253–260.
68. Schott A, Vial T, Gozzo I, et al: Flutamide-induced methemoglobinemia. *DICP Ann Pharmacother* 1991:25:600–601.
69. Barker S, Tremper K, Hyatt J: Effects of methemoglobinemia on pulse oximetry and mixed venous oximetry. *Anesthesiology* 1989;70: 112–117.
70. Eisenkraft J: Pulse oximeter desaturation due to methemoglobinemia. *Anesthesiology* 1988;68:279–281.
71. Watcha M, Connor M, Hing A: Pulse oximetry in methemoglobinemia. *Am J Dis Child* 1989;143:845–847.
72. Delwood L, O'Flaherty D, Prejean E, et al: Methemoglobinemia and its effect on pulse oximetry. *Crit Care Med* 1991;19:988.
73. Caudill L, Walbridge J, Kuhn G: Methemoglobinemia as a cause of coma. *Ann Emerg Med* 1990;19:677–679.
74. Sheehy M, Way J: Nitrite intoxication: Protection with methylene blue and oxygen. *Toxicol Appl Pharmacol* 1974;30:221–226.
75. Lukens J: The legacy of well-water methemoglobinemia. *JAMA* 1987;257:2793–2795.
76. Harris J, Rumack B, Peterson R, et al: Methemoglobinemia resulting from absorption of nitrates. *JAMA* 1979;242:2869–2871.
77. Whitman J, Taylor A, White J: Potential hazard of methylene blue. *Anaesthesia* 1979;34:181–182.
78. Bolyai J, Smith R, Gray C: Ascorbic acid and chemically induced methemoglobinemia. *Toxicol Appl Pharmacol* 1972;21:176–185.
79. Goldstein G, Doull J: Treatment of nitrite-induced methemoglobinemia with hyperbaric oxygen. *Proc Soc Exp Biol Med* 1971;138:137–139.

PART VII

THE ALCOHOLS

CHAPTER 36

Ethyl Alcohol

Probably the most frequent cause of a patient presenting to an emergency department with an altered mental status involves the acute ingestion of ethyl alcohol (1,2). Ethanol is the most widely abused "drug" and is a component of overdose in up to 70% of cases (3–6). In addition, physicians frequently encounter sequelae from the multisystem dysfunction caused by the chronic ingestion of ethanol (7). Therefore, the physician must be aware of the effects expected from both the acute and chronic ingestion of ethyl alcohol or its substitutes (2,4). Substitutes consist of methanol, ethylene glycol, and isopropyl alcohol (Table 36–1) (1).

Ethanol has great impact on the practice of emergency medicine. It taxes resources as well as physician and nursing personnel and patience. Many patients who present to the emergency department have been drinking recently and may have illnesses or injuries related to alcohol ingestion or intoxication. The clinician must be able to identify and treat acute and chronic alcohol intoxication and acute ingestion of ethylene glycol and methanol, and to use serum osmolality and anion gap measurements in rendering a diagnosis of a toxic or medical disorder. Although commonly encountered in emergency practice, acute intoxication with ethanol or the more dangerous alcohols may be mismanaged or misdiagnosed.

The chapters in this section are devoted to a discussion of each of these alcohols and of the manner in which to evaluate the patient who may have ingested an alcohol substitute, an act that can lead to permanent organ damage. The alcohols of concern are ethyl alcohol, isopropyl alcohol (Chapter 37), and methyl alcohol and ethylene glycol (Chapter 38). All are low-molecular-weight, water-soluble substances with prominent multiorgan toxicity. Although they are related, each one has a separate toxicity (8).

TABLE 36–1. *The alcohols*

Ethyl alcohol (ethanol)
Ethylene glycol
Isopropyl alcohol (isopropanol)
Methyl alcohol (methanol)
Propylene glycol
Diethylene glycol

ETHYL ALCOHOL (ETHANOL): SOURCES AND USES

Intoxication from ethanol beverages is the most common cause of acute intoxication encountered in clinical practice. However, other products, such as alcohol-containing medications, colognes, mouthwash, aftershave, hair tonics, solvents, and other household products, may also contain ethanol. These in particular may be sources of ethanol ingestion in the pediatric population (Table 36–2).

Ethanol as a Medicinal Agent

Ethanol is used as a solvent in many medicinal and nonmedicinal preparations, including antiseptics (2,9–11). Applied locally, ethanol acts as an astringent and antimicrobial. It also acts as an irritant. Ethyl alcohol is used externally as a solvent of many drugs as well as a skin disinfectant (12). Ethanol is injected as a nerve block in the management of certain types of intractable pain, as with trigeminal neuralgia, inoperable cancer, and sciatica. Intravenous ethanol is also used for the treatment of methanol and ethylene glycol poisoning because of its ability to be preferentially metabolized by the common enzyme alcohol dehydrogenase.

Ethanol in Other Pharmaceuticals

Other easily available substances may contain ethanol, although the presence or the amount of ethanol may be unknown to the user. Household ethanol sources include

TABLE 36–2. *Uses of ethanol*

Solvent
Antiseptic (local)
Astringent (local)
Antimicrobial (local)
Nerve block
Treatment of methanol overdose
Treatment of ethylene glycol overdose

TABLE 36–3. *Usual concentration of ethyl alcohol in common products*

Product	Concentration (%)
Aftershave	15–80
Cements	7–30
Cough preparations	25
Elixirs	2–10
Extracts	40–90
Gasohol	10
Glass cleaners	10
Hair tonics	25–65
Liquid hand-washing detergent	1–10
Mouthwash	15–25
Paint stripper	25
Perfumes	25–95
Rubbing alcohol	70–90

perfumes, colognes, aftershaves, mouthwashes, antiseptics, elixirs, and food extracts (Table 36–3) (13). As an example, in the five most popular mouthwashes the concentration of ethanol ranges from 14%–27%. Because mouthwashes are classified as cosmetics, they are not well regulated, are thought to be innocuous, and are often kept within easy reach of children. In addition, mouthwashes are frequently sold in containers large enough to supply a fatal dose of ethanol to a child (14). Colognes and perfumes are more than 60% ethanol, and lemon extract is as much as 80% ethanol (2,15). Most liquid-based oral medications contain some ethanol in widely variable concentrations. Liquid medications commonly prescribed for coughs, colds, congestion, and asthma usually contain ethanol in the range of 15%–20% (16).

Ethanol in Beverages

The use of ethanol-containing beverages goes back almost to the beginning of recorded history. Wine is produced from the fermentation of grapes and other fruits, which causes the alcohol content of the fermentation liquid to rise to 12%–18% (2). Wines may be distilled to produce brandies with higher ethyl alcohol content or be fortified with added ethanol (Table 36–4) (17). Another source for ethanol-containing beverages is cereal grains. Corn produces bourbon, barley produces scotch, potatoes produce vodka, and molasses produces rum. Typically, beer and ale, which are produced from the fermentation of cereals, contain 3%–6% ethanol; wine is 10%–18% ethanol; brandy is approximately 40% ethanol; and hard liquors contain 40%–50% ethanol (2). The characteristic taste and odor of ethanol are augmented by impurities, such as aldehydes and other alcohols (18).

The strength of ethanol is usually stated in volume-percent, which indicates the volume of ethanol in 100 volumes of fluid. The term proof indicates twice the concentration in volume-percent, so that 100 proof equals 50 volume-percent or 50% ethanol (2).

Thirty milliliters (1 oz) of 80-proof whiskey can be expected to raise the serum ethanol concentration by approximately 25–30 mg/dL in a 70-kg individual (1). A 12-oz can of beer and 4-oz glass of wine raise the ethanol as much as 1 oz of liquor (2,13). Conversions of ethanol to SI units are found in Table 36–5.

TABLE 36–4. *Sources of ethanol for use as a beverage*

Beverage	Source	Alcohol content (%)
Wine	Grape	12–18
Brandy	Wine	40–50
Bourbon	Corn	40–50
Scotch	Barley	40–50
Vodka	Potatoes	40–50
Rum	Molasses	40–50
Beer	Cereals	3–6
Ale	Cereals	3–6

TABLE 36–5. *Blood ethanol conversions*

mg/dL	mmol/L
10	2.17
20	4.34
30	6.50
40	8.69
50	10.84
60	13.02
70	15.19
80	18.38
90	19.52
100	21.7
150	32.55
200	43.4
300	65.1
400	86.8
500	108.5

Example: To convert an ethanol of 160 mg/dL to SI units: 160/4.6 = 34.78 mmol/L

PHARMACOKINETICS

Blood ethanol concentrations after an ingestion of ethanol are affected by the rate of absorption from the gastrointestinal tract, the space of distribution in the body, and the rate of elimination (19).

The rate of ethanol absorption is affected by several factors. The presence of food, especially fat-containing foods in the stomach, delays absorption considerably and reduces the peak blood alcohol concentration achieved. The amount of ethanol consumed, the time period of consumption, as well as metabolic differences, also influence the shape of the blood alcohol concentration versus time curve. Following the ingestion of ethanol into an empty stomach, peak blood ethanol levels may occur in 30–75 minutes. Ethyl alcohol is absorbed rapidly by diffusion mainly from the small intestine and to a lesser extent from the stomach and large intestine (20,21). A large amount of food may delay absorption so that the peak may not be achieved until 3 hours after ingestion. Carbonation appears to increase the rate of absorption of ethanol (22). The volume of distribution of ethanol is 0.6 L/kg, which is approximately equal to that of total body water, so that ethanol diffuses freely in body tissues. It is neither accumulated to any extent by specific organs nor preferentially bound to cellular components. No binding of ethanol to plasma proteins occurs (11). Ethanol is a water-soluble compound with a molecular weight of 46 and specific gravity of 0.79 g/mL (8).

METABOLISM

The metabolism of ethanol occurs principally through oxidative metabolism in the liver (Fig. 36–1) (19). Consequently, after an initial equilibrium phase, the primary determinant of the duration and extent of ethanol's pharmacologic actions is the rate of its oxidative metabolism by alcohol dehydrogenase to form acetaldehyde; this process requires nicotinamide adenine dinucleotide (NAD) (22). Acetaldehyde is then oxidized to acetate by the enzyme aldehyde dehydrogenase. Acetate (acetic acid) is then oxidized through the Krebs cycle, with the eventual production of carbon dioxide and water, mostly in the peripheral tissues (2,21). This first reaction, in which the enzyme alcohol dehydrogenase is used, essentially occurs by zero-order kinetics, with the rate of decay being constant and independent of concentration (1,2). This is thought to be caused by early depletion of NAD, which is a cofactor for alcohol dehydrogenase. The action of alcohol dehydrogenase is the rate-limiting step of metabolism (23).

There may be three separate pathways for the metabolism of ethanol in the liver (22). The alcohol dehydrogenase pathway is the predominant system, and this system has been found to contain a number of isoenzymes that appear to account for the great variability in metabolism among individuals. The second pathway is the microsomal ethanol-oxidizing system located in the endoplasmic reticulum. There is considerable controversy concerning the role of this system, which may be associated with the cytochrome P-450 mixed-function oxidase system in the liver (24). The third system involves the catalases located in the perioxisomes. The alcohol dehydrogenase system metabolizes ethanol under most conditions, but the microsomal system functions importantly in ethanol oxidation in the chronic heavy user or abuser of alcohol. In most individuals, the rate of metabolism of ethanol is in the range of 15–25 mg/dL/hr regardless of the plasma concentration (2,25). This variation parallels the history of ethanol use: it is approximately 12 mg/dL/hr in nondrinkers, 15 mg/dL/hr in social drinkers, and up to 30 mg/dL/hr in alcoholics (20). In other words, it takes a 150-lb person approximately 1 hour to metabolize the amount of ethanol in 10 oz of beer.

Most authorities no longer hold that the rate of ethanol metabolism can be materially increased by the co-administration of other substances, such as fructose or other sugars, hormones, vitamins, or enzymatic cofactors (26–30).

Intoxication from ethanol ingestion largely depends on how quickly a blood ethanol concentration has been attained as well as on the length of time it has been maintained (31). Because ethyl alcohol is rapidly absorbed from the stomach, the blood concentration is usually at or near maximum on evaluation.

Ethanol	alcohol dehydrogenase →	acetaldehyde
Acetaldehyde	aldehyde dehydrogenase →	acetic acid
Acetic acid	Krebs cycle →	carbon dioxide + water

FIG. 36–1. Metabolism of ethanol.

ACUTE INTOXICATION

Because alcohol often induces euphoria, it is frequently mistakenly classified as a stimulant rather than as a depressant because inhibitory synapses in the brain are depressed slightly earlier than are excitatory synapses with low doses of ethanol (2). Ethanol, however, acts as a sedative-hypnotic throughout the entire central nervous system (32).

For the most part, the patient acutely poisoned by ethanol has intentionally ingested a large amount of ethanol. Occasionally, the central nervous system depression itself may cause the patient to be brought to an emergency department, but usually the physician finds ethanol ingestion an additional finding in evaluating a patient who has concomitant trauma or other medical problems (27).

The acute ingestion of ethanol may result in decreased inhibitions, visual impairment, diplopia, nystagmus, lack of muscular coordination, slurred speech, ataxia, slowing of reaction time, tachycardia, vasodilation, stupor, and depression of the deep tendon reflexes (21,34–37). In severe stages, hypothermia, hypoventilation, hypotension, and possibly cardiovascular collapse may be seen (38–40).

Ethanol and Hypoglycemia

Metabolic effects may include hypoglycemia, which is primarily due to impaired gluconeogenesis because of NAD depletion (41). This is especially seen in children. A number of factors including age, prior fasting state, and underlying medical conditions can affect individuals' susceptibility to ethanol-induced hypoglycemia. Normal euglycemic control is accomplished by a combination of intestinal absorption, glycogenolysis, and gluconeogenesis (41). Ethanol-induced hypoglycemia requires a significant fasting state to exhaust the first two mechanisms. The liver contains enough glycogen to maintain euglycemia for 8–10 hours without any contribution from gluconeogenesis (42). During the oxidation of ethanol to acetaldehyde and acetate, NAD is reduced to NADH. The rate of NAD reduction exceeds mitochondrial NADH oxidation, thus increasing the NADH/NAD ratio. This increased redox ratio provides an adverse environment for the oxidation of substrate, such as lactate and glutamate to pyruvate and α-ketoglutarate, respectively. Because the conversion of these substrates is necessary for gluconeogenesis, the process is halted (42).

Blood Concentrations of Ethanol

The intoxicating effects of ethanol correlate roughly with blood concentrations, which in turn reflect levels present in the brain. Blood concentrations can be expressed in units of milligrams per deciliter, as percent by volume (vol/vol), or in SI units as millimoles per liter. A level of 11 mmol/L in SI units corresponds to 50 mg/dL (8).

Blood concentrations greater than 50 mg/dL (0.05%) may be associated with some impairment, and concentrations greater than 100 mg/dL (0.1%) are generally used as evidence of driving while intoxicated. Interpretations of the physiologic effects of a particular blood alcohol concentration may be difficult because there is such wide variability among individuals. This is especially true in the individual who chronically ingests ethyl alcohol (20). Despite large individual variation, if a patient is comatose at a blood concentration of 50 or 100 mg/dL, it is likely that another problem coexists. Ethanol concentrations in the range of 100–250 mg/dL generally cause mental confusion, ataxia, nystagmus, exaggerated emotional states, and lack of coordination (43). Most fatal intoxications are associated with ethanol concentrations greater than 400 mg/dL, although the highest reported concentration in a survivor was 1510 mg/dL (44,45). The physiologic effects that may be expected in the occasional drinker are listed in Table 36–6.

Several factors can modify the relation between the blood ethanol concentration and neurologic impairment. For example, the severity of intoxication at a given ethanol concentration is typically greater when the concentration is rising than when it is falling—a phenomenon known as the Mellanby effect. This is due in part to pharmacokinetic factors, but it may also reflect the occurrence of acute tolerance to ethanol during a single episode of drinking (46).

TABLE 36–6. *Ethanol concentration and acute symptomatology*

Concentration		
(mg/dL)	mmol/L	Symptoms
50	11	Mild muscle incoordination
50–100	11–22	Incoordination Slow reaction time Decreased inhibitions Blurred vision
10–300	22–65	Visual impairment Ataxia Hypoglycemia Slurred speech Decreased motor skills
300–400	65–87	Marked incoordination Stupor Hypoglycemia Hypothermia Seizures
>400	>87	Coma Respiratory failure Death

Chronic tolerance, which develops as a consequence of prolonged, frequent, and excessive ethanol use, may permit alcoholic patients to remain sober in the face of blood ethanol concentrations that would normally be fatal and to survive despite concentrations exceeding 1000 mg/dL (217 mmol per liter) (46).

LABORATORY ANALYSIS

When ethyl alcohol use is combined with multiple drug overdose, head injury, coma, major trauma, seizures, or psychosis, it is particularly important to obtain an ethanol concentration (20,33,47). The most commonly used specimen for obtaining an ethanol level is the blood (25), although the breath and occasionally the urine may be used. The saliva is infrequently used. Capillary and arterial blood most accurately indicate the brain ethanol concentrations; venous blood lags slightly in ethanol content during the absorption-distribution phase. The determination of serum ethanol concentration can be done in most hospital laboratories in 30–60 minutes. Postmortem blood is subject to putrefaction and fermentation, whereby the destruction and neoformation of ethyl alcohol is possible.

Techniques for the determination of serum ethanol include diffusion or distillation, oxidation of the alcohol, and osmometric, enzymatic, and gas chromatographic procedures. Early techniques for blood ethanol determination used distillation, aeration, or diffusion to separate the alcohol from plasma (46). This was a colorimetric method that was nonspecific and gave a reaction with all volatiles, including ketones. Osmometry by freezing-point depression was also nonspecific because all alcohols cause an osmolal gap. Enzymatic methods employ alcohol dehydrogenase, which reacts primarily with ethanol but not with methanol or acetone. This is a spectrophotometric method that is specific for ethanol. Gas chromatographic methods by flame ionization separate the alcohols on a chromatographic column and are specific for most alcohols. Laboratory differentiation of the alcohols should be performed with gas chromatography whenever possible.

The breath alcohol analyzer has been studied extensively and shown to be sufficiently accurate for clinical use (20,48). The pocket-sized instrument measures the amount of ethyl alcohol in a sample of expired air by electrochemical oxidation and gives a digitally displayed reading of the equivalent blood ethanol. Breath is a reliable specimen for the measurement of ethanol because there is a fairly constant equilibrium of ethanol in blood and alveolar air. The breath analyzer should not be used within 15 minutes of the last drink because it gives a falsely high reading (22). Its use as legal evidence, however, has been questioned (8).

Although breath alcohol analyzers have been available for years, they have inherent limitations, especially in the uncooperative patient. In addition, breath analysis determinations require the use of a conversion factor, and may be inaccurately high and not truly reflective of blood alcohol concentration secondary to ethanol in the mouth, regurgitated stomach air or liquid contents, or ventilation-perfusion abnormalities. A saliva dipstick method of determining alcohol use is a new method that may correlate well with serum alcohol and breath alcohol levels (8,49).

Urine may be used as an alternative specimen, but the ethanol in a random urine specimen is not necessarily in equilibrium with that in the blood. This is because the bladder contents represent urine produced over a period of time, during which the blood ethanol concentration may have risen or fallen (48).

Serum osmolality is a useful adjunct laboratory test, particularly in centers where blood alcohol may be difficult to obtain (50). The presence of an "osmolal gap," which is the difference between the measured osmolality by freezing-point depression and the calculated osmolality, if greater than 10 suggests the presence of another osmotically active substance (ethanol, methanol, ethylene glycol, isopropanol, sorbitol, mannitol, ketones) (50). Ethanol is the most common cause of hyperosmolality, and if ethanol is the known ingestant, the elevation in the osmolal gap can be used to estimate the blood ethanol level (See Chapter 39). (51).

TREATMENT

Although acute ethyl alcohol coma may be a potentially life-threatening situation, the treatment of the acute ingestion is relatively straightforward (Table 36–7). Treatment of acute intoxication is largely supportive. Serial examinations to confirm primary ethanol intoxication and to rule out co-existing anatomic or metabolic abnormalities are essential (8). Prevention of aspiration and observation for development of respiratory depression are crucial. Placement of the patient in the lateral decubitus position with head forward may help prevent aspiration. Intravenous access should be obtained in any patient with seizures, hypovolemia, change in mental status, or complicating features, or in whom the diagnosis of acute intoxication alone is in doubt (52). If the patient presents with an altered mental status, 2 mg of naloxone, 25 g of glucose, and 50–100 mg of thiamine should be administered (21). If the patient responds to the dextrose, a continuous infusion of 10% dextrose should be administered. The administration of oxygen and electrocardiogram monitoring may be appropriate in certain patients, especially if co-existing pulmonary or myocardial disease is suspected. Unless concomitant ingestion of other drugs is suspected, gastric lavage is probably useful only if performed within 2 hours of ingestion of ethanol. There have been conflicting reports as to the adsorption of ethanol by charcoal. Some investigators have reported no significant adsorption, and others found moderate adsorption (53). Physical restraints may be used when required to prevent the patient from escaping. Care must be taken to avoid unnecessary trauma by their use.

If alveolar hypoventilation is present, a patent airway with supportive mechanical ventilation must be established. Correction of fluid deficits, acid-base disturbances, and hypothermia are important ancillary measures (16). Hypotension generally responds well to volume replacement (23). Further treatment consists of treating any associated medical conditions. Analeptic agents are not only useless but dangerous and are to be avoided.

TABLE 36–7. *Treatment of ethyl alcohol overdose*

Condition	Treatment
Altered mental status	Naloxone Glucose Thiamine
Hypoventilation	Mechanical ventilation
Ketoacidosis	Glucose Normal saline
Hypotension	Normal saline Trendelenburg's position Vasopressors

Repletion of electrolytes is often necessary, especially in the chronic alcoholic patient. It may be advisable to begin repletion of suspected deficiencies before the laboratory values become available if there is clinical evidence of deficiencies. Most alcoholic patients have a total body depletion of magnesium and thus will require supplementation. Calcium repletion is rarely needed; magnesium repletion will usually allow spontaneous correction of hypocalcemia, if present, to occur. The routine use of phosphorus is not encouraged but phosphorus levels should be followed closely.

Ketoacidosis can be treated with glucose and saline solution. Insulin is not indicated, and bicarbonate therapy is usually not necessary. In alcoholic ketoacidosis, regeneration of bicarbonate from the metabolism of lactate, ketoacids, and acetate occurs with conservative treatment.

There have been many claims concerning the beneficial effect of fructose on accelerating the metabolism of ethyl alcohol and leading to a shortened clinical course. In theory, because ethyl alcohol requires NAD for its metabolism and because fructose can enhance the production of NAD by enhancing oxidation of NADH (the reduced form of NAD), enhanced alcohol metabolism results from administration of fructose. Nevertheless, because the rate of oxidation of alcohol is limited by the enzyme alcohol dehydrogenase and not by the availability of NAD, it is not surprising that this theory has not been substantiated (26). Fructose, then, has not been shown to effectively accelerate the rate of ethanol metabolism or to decrease the amount of time of coma. In addition, the use of fructose has been associated with increased serum uric acid and lactate concentrations (28), leading to the increased likelihood of lactic acidosis.

Forced diuresis is ineffective in enhancing the removal of ethanol because most ethanol is eliminated by hepatic metabolism (21). Hemodialysis increases ethanol elimination but is rarely required clinically because most patients can be effectively managed conservatively. The development of an alcohol antagonist may be helpful in the future for diagnosis of the inebriated patient with a concomitant medical condition.

Thiamine repletion is routinely indicated both to increase pyruvate dehydrogenase activity and to provide prophylaxis against the development of Wernicke's encephalopathy.

Medicolegal Considerations

Medicolegal considerations in the setting of acute intoxication may be complex. When procedures requiring consent are being considered, the usual criteria for ability to sign consent must be met. If the patient is unable to sign for himself or herself, the chain of custody in the state must be followed. It is advisable to treat patients appropriately with their best interests in mind, rather than postponing medically necessary treatment.

One of the most common dilemmas involves the patient's request to sign out against medical advice. If the physician judges the patient to have an altered mental status, the patient must not be allowed to sign out against medical advice. Physicians may be held responsible for the consequences resulting from premature discharge of intoxicated patients.

REFERENCES

1. Becker C: The alcoholic patient as a toxic emergency. *Emerg Clin North Am* 1984;2:47–61.
2. Tong T: The alcohols. *Crit Care Q* 1982;4:75–85.
3. Barnsley J, Sellers E: An interview study of hospitalized drug overdose patients. *Can Fam Physician* 1978; 24:850–855.
4. Patel A, Roy M, Wilson G: Self-poisoning and alcohol. *Lancet* 1972; 2:1099–1102.
5. Rangno R, Dumont C, Sitar D: Effects of ethanol ingestion on outcome of drug overdose. *Crit Care Med* 1982;10:180–185.
6. Halpern J, Davis J: Use and abuse of alcohol: further perspectives. *J Emerg Nurs* 1983;9:49–52.
7. Bernstein L, Tong T: Alcoholism. *Calif Pharm* 1979;6:26–30.
8. Marco C, Kelen G: Acute intoxication. *Emerg Med Clin N Am* 1990; 8:731–748.
9. Cardoni A: The alcohol in liquid medicinals: information for the pharmacist. *Guidelines Prof Pharm* 1978;5:1–2.
10. Varma B, Cincotta J: Mouthwash-induced hypoglycemia, editorial. *Am J Dis Child* 1978;132:930–931.
11. Weller-Fahy E, Berger L, Troutman W: Mouthwash: a source of acute ethanol intoxication. *Pediatrics* 1980;66:302–305.
12. Goldfinger T, Schaber D: A comparison of blood alcohol concentration using non-alcohol and alcohol containing skin antiseptics. *Ann Emerg Med* 1982;11:665–667.
13. Rubinstein J: Beware of these drugs when you prescribe for a recovering alcoholic. *Resident Staff Physician* 1980;62–66.
14. Moore J, Christian P, Datz F, et al: Effect of wine on gastric emptying in humans. *Gastroenterology* 1981;81:1072–1075.
15. Scherger D, Wruk K, Kulig K, et al: Ethyl alcohol (ethanol)-containing cologne, perfume, and after-shave ingestions in children. *Am J Dis Child* 1988;142:630–632.
16. Gerson B: Alcohol. *Clin Lab Med* 1990;10:355–374.
17. Petroni N, Cardoni A: Alcohol content of liquid medicinals. *Drug Ther* 1978;8:72–93.
18. Lerman B, Bodony R: Ethanol sensitivity. *Ann Emerg Med* 1991;20: 1128–1130.
19. Li T, Bosron W: Genetic variability of enzymes of alcohol metabolism in human beings. *Ann Emerg Med* 1986;15:997–1004.
20. Gibb K: Serum alcohol levels, toxicology screens, and use of the breath alcohol analyzer. *Ann Emerg Med* 1986;15:349–353.
21. Litovitz T: The alcohols: ethanol, methanol, isopropanol, ethylene glycol. *Pediatr Toxicol* 1986; 33:311–323.
22. Lieber C: Metabolism and metabolic effects of alcohol. *Med Clin North Am* 1984;68:3–31.
23. Schelling J, Howard R, Winter S, et al: Increased osmolal gap in alcoholic ketoacidosis and lactic acidosis. *Ann Intern Med* 1990:113:580–582.
24. Holtzman J, Gebhard R, Eckfeldt J, et al: The effects of several weeks of ethanol consumption on ethanol kinetics in normal men and women. *Clin Pharmacol Ther* 1985;38:157–163.
25. Jatlow P: Acute toxicology of ethanol ingestion—role of the clinical laboratory. *Am J Clin Pathol* 1980;74: 721–724.
26. Crow K, Newland K, Batt R: The fructose effect. *N Z Med J* 1981;93: 232–234.
27. Iber F: The effect of fructose on alcohol metabolism. *Arch Intern Med* 1977;137:1121.
28. Levy R, Elo T, Hanenson I: Intravenous fructose treatment of acute alcohol intoxication. *Arch Intern Med* 1977;137:1175–1177.

29. Meyer R, Mueller F, Hundt H: The effect of fructose on blood alcohol levels in man. *S Afr Med J* 1982;62:719–721.
30. Sprandel U, Troger H, Liebhardt E, et al: Acceleration of ethanol elimination with fructose in man. *Nutr Metab* 1980;24:324–330.
31. Koch-Weser J, Sellers E, Kalant H: Alcohol intoxication and withdrawal. *N Engl J Med* 1976;294:757–762.
32. Deitrich R, Dunwiddie T, Harris A, Erwin V: Mechanism of action of ethanol: initial central nervous system actions. *Pharmacol Rev* 1989; 41:489–533.
33. Bailey D: Comprehensive toxicology screening: the frequency of finding other drugs in addition to ethanol. *Clin Toxicol* 1984;22:463–471.
34. Madison L: Ethanol-induced hypoglycemia. *Adv Metabol Disord* 1968;3:85–109.
35. MacLaren N, Valman H, Levin B: Alcohol-induced hypoglycaemia in childhood. *Br Med J* 1970;1:278–280.
36. Miquel C, Rubies-Prat J: Effects of ethanol-induced hypoglycemia. *Br Med J* 1977;2:027.
37. Rittencourt P. Wade P, Richens A, et al: Blood alcohol and eye movements. *Lancet* 1980;2:981.
38. Hoppe P: Alcohol and the heart. *Ann Intern Med* 1983;97:109–110.
39. Abelmann W: Effects of alcohol on the cardiovascular system. *Hosp Pract* 1981;16:80A–80X.
40. Knochel J: Cardiovascular effects of alcohol. *Ann Intern Med* 1983; 98:849–854.
41. Arky R: Hypoglycemia associated with liver disease and ethanol. *Endocrinol Metab Clin N Am* 1989;18:75–90.
42. Sporer K, Ernst A, Conte R, et al: The incidence of ethanol-induced hypoglycemia. *Am J Emerg Med* 1992;10:403–405.
43. Lopez G, Yealy D, Krenzelok E: Survival of a child despite unusually high blood ethanol levels. *Am J Emerg Med* 1989;7:283–285.
44. Johnson C, Jackson D: Alcohol and sex. *Heart Lung* 1983;12:93–97.
45. Johnson R, Noll E, Rodney W: Survival after a serum ethanol concentration of 1 1/2%. *Lancet* 1982;2:1394.
46. Charness M, Simon R, Greenberg D: Ethanol and the nervous system. *N Engl J Med* 1989;321:442–454.
47. Pierce R: Stuporous alcoholics: metabolic considerations. *South Med J* 1982;75:463–469.
48. Simpson G: Accuracy and precision of breath-alcohol measurements for a random subject in the postabsorptive state. *Clin Chem* 1987;33: 261–268.
49. Wax P, Hoffman R, Goldfrank L: Rapid quantitative determination of blood alcohol concentration in the emergency department using an electrochemical method. *Ann Emerg Med* 1992;21:254–259.
50. Snyder H, Williams D, Zink B, et al: Accuracy of blood ethanol determination using serum osmolality. *J Emerg Med* 1992;10:129–133.
51. Galvan L, Watts M: Generation of an osmolality gap-ethanol nomogram from routine laboratory data. *Ann Emerg Med* 1992;21:1343–1348.
52. Marx J: Alcohol and trauma. *Emerg Med Clin N Am* 1990;8:929–935.
53. Minocha A, Herold D, Barth J, et al: Activated charcoal in oral ethanol absorption: lack of effect in humans. *Clin Toxicol* 1986;24: 225–234.

CHAPTER 37

Isopropyl Alcohol

Isopropyl alcohol (isopropanol or 2-propanol) is a three-carbon alcohol used as an industrial solvent and that also has found many uses in medicine. It is an ingredient in rubbing alcohol; various cosmetics, such as aftershaves, perfumes, and colognes; skin disinfectants, aerosol products, de-icing and antifreeze preparations, and hair tonics (Table 37–1) (1). Rubbing alcohol may contain either ethanol or isopropanol in concentrations of 70%–90% (2). Isopropyl alcohol is also an ingredient in mouthwashes and solvent mixtures. This alcohol is a clear, colorless, volatile liquid that has an odor different from that of ethanol and a distinctly disagreeable bitter taste except when highly diluted (1,2).

Accidental and suicidal ingestions of isopropyl alcohol-containing products continue to be a common occurrence and are most often encountered in the alcoholic who has ingested rubbing alcohol or aftershave lotion as a substitute for ethanol or in an accidental ingestion by a child. It is estimated that one swallow of rubbing alcohol that contains 70% isopropyl alcohol may produce a toxic level in a small child (3). Secondary and tertiary alcohols are less toxic than their primary alcohols. The toxicity of isopropanol is between that of ethanol and *n*-propanol. *N*-Propyl alcohol (1-propanol) appears to be more toxic than isopropyl alcohol. In the past this compound was mistaken for isopropyl alcohol, which led to a greater concern over isopropyl alcohol than was warranted.

TABLE 37–1. *Sources and concentrations of isopropyl alcohol*

Source	Concentration (%)
Antifreeze	40–55
Cements	5–20
Glass cleaners	3–15
Liquid detergents	5–12
Mouthwash	15–25
Paint stripper	2–10
Paint thinner	5–10
Rubbing alcohol	70–90
Windshield de-icer	60–80

PHARMACOKINETICS

The volume of distribution of isopropyl alcohol is 0.6–0.8 L/kg, which is similar to that of ethanol (1). Although about 10% of isopropyl alcohol may be metabolized in the body to glucuronide, the major metabolic pathway is first-order kinetics with the enzyme alcohol dehydrogenase acting to convert isopropanol to acetone, carbon dioxide, and water (4). Eighty percent of ingested isopropyl alcohol is metabolized to acetone by hepatic alcohol dehydrogenase (5). Twenty percent is excreted unchanged by the kidneys or lungs with small amounts being resecreted into the stomach or saliva (6). This is a different metabolic process from that of ethanol, which saturates its metabolic mechanisms at low levels and usually is eliminated independent of concentration (zero-order elimination). Isopropyl alcohol has a half-life of 2.5–4.2 hours, yet longer half-lives of 7 hours have been noted in patients with chronic liver disease (6). Chronic ethanol abuse, hepatic enzyme induction, ethanol-induced hepatic damage, changes in respiratory rate, and the use of activated charcoal and cathartics in patient management may affect the observed isopropyl alcohol and acetone disposition (7). Concentrations of isopropyl alcohol in urine closely parallel those in the blood, which indicates that it is not substantially concentrated in the urine.

Acetone

Acetone has a much longer half-life, approximately 22 hours, compared to isopropyl alcohol (3). Once absorption is complete, there is an inverse relationship between the dissipation of isopropyl alcohol and rising levels of acetone. Eventually, acetone levels may actually exceed isopropyl alcohol blood levels and persist longer than isopropyl alcohol in both blood and urine due to the continuous generation of acetone from isopropyl alcohol and the slower elimination rate of acetone. The acetone formed is excreted predominantly by the kidneys and in small amounts by the lungs. The acetone metabolite contributes to the central nervous system depression produced by isopropanol. Because of its higher molecular weight, isopropanol produces a smaller osmolal gap than a corresponding quantity of ethanol. Serum acetone may be measurable as soon as 30 minutes postingestion, and by 3 hours postingestion, the urine may be positive for acetone (8).

ABSORPTION

Isopropanol is absorbed easily through the gastrointestinal tract and, if not delayed by food, may be completely absorbed in less than 30 minutes (1,2). Isopropanol is also absorbed by the lungs. It is not significantly absorbed through the skin (2,4,7,9,10). Large amounts of isopropyl alcohol applied topically have little effect (1,11). Although there are reports of deep coma from the local application of isopropanol to the skin of infants, this appears to have been caused by inhalation of the alcohol during sponging procedures in poorly ventilated areas (6,7,10,12,13). Concentrations greater than 120 mg/dL have been reported after sponging (2). Isopropyl alcohol may also be absorbed by rectal mucosa.

ACUTE TOXICITY

Isopropyl alcohol is a central nervous system depressant with twice the potency of ethanol (14,15). It has a longer duration of action (and thus intoxication) than ethanol because it is metabolized more slowly and because its major metabolite, acetone, is also a central nervous system depressant (1,14–16). The initial phase of exhilaration that is noted with the ingestion of ethanol and is the usual reason for ingesting the material is not noted with isopropanol ingestion (4).

Many of the same problems associated with ethanol overdose can be seen with isopropanol overdose (Table 37–2). It is much more irritating to the gastrointestinal tract and more likely to produce nausea, vomiting, and abdominal pain than ethanol (2,17). In addition, pancreatitis, dizziness, confusion, and ataxia may be noted. Hematemesis and melena may appear early, and they are related to ulceration of the gastric mucosa (1,18). Coma may occur with concentrations of approximately 120 mg/dL (19–21). Coma can be prolonged for several days. Acetone probably contributes to the prolonged central nervous system depression that follows ingestions of large amounts of isopropyl alcohol (22). The pupil size is variable. Hypothermia, hypoglycemia, and respiratory and renal failure are frequently reported with significant ingestions of isopropanol (14,18,23). Isopropanol-induced hypotension is thought to result from peripheral vasodilation and direct cardiac depression (24). In adults, hypotension associated with coma is considered the best prognostic indicator of a potentially fatal intoxication, and hemodialysis to accelerate elimination of isopropanol is recommended (6,17). In the event of hypotension secondary to isopropyl alcohol, causes of volume depletion, such as gastrointestinal bleeding, should also be investigated. Death may occur from respiratory arrest.

TABLE 37–2. *Features of isopropyl alcohol overdose*

Gastrointestinal
Nausea and vomiting
Abdominal pain
Gastritis
Gastrointestinal hemorrhage
Neurologic
Dizziness
Contusion
Ataxia
Coma
Hypothermia
Hypotension
Hypoglycemia
Respiratory failure

DIAGNOSIS AND LABORATORY ANALYSIS

It is often difficult to make the diagnosis of isopropyl alcohol intoxication, even when it is the sole toxin involved (1). A presumptive diagnosis of isopropanol ingestion can be made in the intoxicated-appearing patient who has acetonuria and acetonemia but no glycosuria, hyperglycemia, or acidemia (25). The presence of the odor of acetone on the breath may aid in the diagnosis (26). In addition, an osmolal gap may be noted. In other words, if no history is available for a patient who has a normal anion gap associated with strongly positive serum ketones and normal serum bicarbonate and blood sugar concentrations, the diagnosis of isopropyl alcohol intoxication should be strongly considered (27). If rapid urine testing is to be used to diagnose potential exposure to isopropyl alcohol, Acetest reagent tablets may be used. Although these tablets are not as sensitive to acetone as they are to acetoacetic acid, they may be sensitive enough to qualitatively identify acetone associated with subtoxic-dose isopropyl alcohol ingestion. Serum acetone may be measurable as soon as 30 minutes postingestion, and by 3 hours postingestion the urine may be positive for acetone (8). Acetone may be present in sufficient quantities in large exposures, even in the absence of isopropyl alcohol, for up to 24 hours (28). The persistence of the acetone marker enables the clinician to confirm the suspicion of an isopropyl alcohol overdose many hours after the ingestion. The lack of acetone in the blood within 30–60 minutes or in the urine within 3 hours effectively eliminates the possibility of an isopropyl alcohol exposure.

Isopropyl alcohol intoxication differs from that of the other alcohols because acidemia is not a part of the clinical picture. Although isopropanol ingestion is a cause of ketosis, unlike the other ketones acetone is not an acid and does not cause a decreased bicarbonate or an elevated anion gap (7,14,25,27). Where acidosis is noted, its etiology is probably lactic acid accumulation in the presence of isopropanol-induced hypotension. In addition, isopropanol is less toxic than both methanol and ethylene glycol, and causes no permanent retinal injury or renal damage. When isopropanol is ingested in preparations not intended for ingestion, other volatile aromatics such as methyl salicylate, menthol, naphthalene, and camphor may contribute to toxicity (1,2).

The diagnosis of isopropyl alcohol ingestion can be confirmed by gas chromatography. After a subtoxic dose of isopropyl alcohol, isopropyl alcohol serum concentrations may be undetectable while serum acetone concentrations remain elevated (29). Therefore, the presence of acetone in the serum without measurable isopropyl alcohol does not rule out exposure to isopropyl alcohol. As the concentration of isopropyl alcohol decreases, it can be expected that the serum acetone concentration will rise because of the continued production of this compound (15,16,30). Enzymatic methods involving alcohol dehydrogenase may underestimate the amount of isopropyl alcohol (8). A Breathalyzer test for isopropyl alcohol is also unreliable.

Although these guidelines are not absolute, toxic symptoms have been noted when isopropyl alcohol concentrations are approximately 50 mg/dL (29). Coma may be associated with concentrations of 120 mg/dL or more (14). Depending on the method used, there may be a cross-reaction with ethanol measurements.

TREATMENT

The treatment of isopropanol overdose is essentially the same as that of ethanol, and consists of naloxone, glucose, and thiamine, if the patient presents with an altered mental status, and, if appropriate, an attempt to prevent further absorption (Table 37–3). Although isopropyl alcohol has been demonstrated to be secreted into the stomach, it is not necessary to use continuous nasogastric suction. Supportive care should be instituted in much the same way as with ethanol intoxication. In the hypotensive patient, intravenous fluids should be administered. The patient should be placed in Trendelenburg's position. Vasoconstrictor agents such as dopamine or norepinephrine are usually not necessary. Usually with supportive care and artificial ventilation alone even large doses of isopropyl alcohol can be survived (3). Dialysis can be effective but is only indicated in the rare instances when hypotension is present and the patient is unresponsive to alternate medical management (1,7,17,19,20,31). Because hemodialysis will rapidly remove both isopropyl alcohol and acetone by increasing clearance more than 40-fold, it should be considered in patients with coma associated with hypotension (5).

TABLE 37–3. *Treatment of isopropyl alcohol overdose*

Condition	Treatment
Altered mental status	Glucose Thiamine Oxygen
Hypotension	Normal saline Trendelenburg's position Vasopressors Dialysis
Hypoventilation	Mechanical ventilation

REFERENCES

1. Lacouture P, Wason S, Abrams A, et al: Acute isopropyl alcohol intoxication. *Am J Med* 1983;75:680–686.
2. Litovitz T: The alcohols: ethanol, methanol, isopropanol, ethylene glycol. *Pediatr Clin North Am* 1986;33:311–323.
3. Burkhart K, Martinez M: The adsorption of isopropanol and acetone by activated charcoal. *J Toxicol Clin Toxicol* 1992;30:371–375.
4. Grant D: The pharmacology of isopropyl alcohol. *J Lub Clin Med* 1923;8:382–386.
5. Gaudet M, Fraser G: Isopropranol ingestion: case report with pharmacokinetic analysis. *Am J Emerg Med* 1989;7:297–299.
6. Vicas I, Beck R: Fatal inhalational isopropyl alcohol poisoning in a neonate. *J Toxicol Clin Toxicol* 1993;31:473–481.
7. Smith M: Solvent toxicity: isopropanol, methanol, and ethylene glycol. *Ear Nose Throat J* 1983;62:126–135.
8. Lacouture P, Heldreth D, Shannon M, et al: The generation of acetonemia/acetonuria following ingestion of a subtoxic dose of isopropyl alcohol. *Am J Emerg Med* 1989;7:38–40.
9. Tong T: The alcohols. *Crit Care Q* 1982;4:75–85.
10. Moss M: Alcohol-induced hypoglycemia and coma produced by alcohol sponging. *Pediatrics* 1970; 46:445–447.
11. McGrath R, Einterz R: Absorption of topical isopropyl alcohol in an adult. *Crit Care Med* 1989;1:1233.
12. McFadden S, Haddow J: Coma produced by topical application of isopropanol. *Pediatrics* 1969;43:632–633.
13. Senz E, Goldfarb D: Coma in a child following use of isopropyl alcohol in sponging. *J Pediatr* 1958;53:323–324.
14. Adams S, Mathews J, Flaherty J: Alcoholic ketoacidosis. *Ann Emerg Med* 1987;16:90–97.
15. Lehman A, Chase H: The acute and chronic toxicity of isopropyl alcohol. *J Lab Clin Med* 1944;29:561–571.
16. Lehman A, Schwerma H, Rickards E: Isopropyl alcohol: rate of disappearance from the bloodstream of dogs after intravenous and oral administration. *J Pharmacol Exp Ther* 1944;82:196–201.
17. Adelson L: Fatal intoxication with isopropyl alcohol. *Am J Clin Path* 1962;38:144–151.
18. Juncos L, Taguchi J: Isopropyl alcohol intoxication—report of a case associated with myopathy, renal failure, and hemolytic anemia. *JAMA* 1968;204:732–734.
19. Freireich A, Cinque T, Xanthaley G, et al: Hemodialysis for isopropanol poisoning. *N Engl J Med* 1967; 277:699–700.
20. Mecikalski M, Depner T: Peritoneal dialysis for isopropanol poisoning. *West J Med* 1982;137:322–325.
21. Visudhiphan P, Kaufman H: Increased cerebrospinal fluid protein following isopropyl alcohol intoxication. *N Y State J Med* 1971;71:887–888.
22. Burkhart K, Kulig K: The other alcohols: methanol, ethylene glycol, and isopropanol. *Emerg Med Clin North Am* 1990;8:913–927.

23. Hawley P, Falko J: "Pseudo" renal failure after isopropyl alcohol intoxication. *South Med J* 1982;75:630–631.
24. Mydler T, Wasserman G, Watson W: Two-week old infant with isopropanol intoxication. *Pediatr Emerg Care* 1993;9:146–148.
25. Kreisberg R, Wood B: Drug- and chemical-induced metabolic acidosis. *Clin Endocrinol Metab* 1983; 21:391–411.
26. Bailey D: Detection of isopropanol in acetonemic patients not exposed to isopropanol. *J Toxicol Clin Toxicol* 1990;28:459–466.
27. Emmett M, Narins R: Clinical use of the anion gap. *Medicine* 1977; 56:38–54.
28. Pappas A, Ackerman B, Olsen K, et al: Isopropanol ingestion: a report of six episodes with isopropanol and acetone serum concentration time data. *J Toxicol Clin Toxicol* 1991;29:11–21.
29. Jerrard D, Verdile V, Yealy D, et al: Serum determinations in toxic isopropanol ingestion. *Am J Emerg Med* 1992;10:200–202.
30. Kelner M: Isopropanol ingestion: interpretation of blood concentrations and clinical findings. *J Toxicol Clin Toxicol* 1983;20:497–507.
31. Rosansky S: Isopropyl alcohol poisoning treated with hemodialysis: kinetics of isopropyl alcohol and acetone removal. *J Toxicol Clin Toxicol* 1982;19(3):265–271.

CHAPTER 38

Ethylene Glycol/Methanol

THE GLYCOLS

Ethylene Glycol

Ethylene glycol (1,2-ethanediol), a bivalent aliphatic alcohol, is structurally similar to alcohol but contains a hydroxyl group on each carbon (1). It was synthesized about 100 years ago and was considered of little commercial value until World War I, when a shortage of glycerin led to a widespread search for a practical nontoxic substitute to be used as a solvent for drugs (2). Although it is now known that ethylene glycol is toxic, for many years it was believed to be nontoxic on the basis of two independent experiments 10 years apart, when two investigators drank small amounts of ethylene glycol without ill effects. For that reason, it has been included as a solvent in detergents, paints, lacquers, drugs, dyes, hydraulic brake fluid, polishes, cosmetics, and industrial solvents (3,4). It also has been used as a glycerine substitute in enemas, as a coolant in the lunar module, and, in the past, as a preservative in juices and an ingredient in various early medicinals (5). Its most familiar use as radiator antifreeze is based on its high boiling point and its ability to depress the freezing point of aqueous solutions (Table 38–1) (6).

Intoxication by ethylene glycol is usually due to accidental ingestion, a suicide attempt, or consumption as a substitute for ethanol (4,7–10). The alcoholic patient, in an attempt to maintain an altered mental status, may ingest ethanol substitutes containing methanol, ethylene glycol, or isopropanol (11). The compound's viscosity, warmth, sweet taste, and aromatic odor, which resemble the features of some liqueurs, in addition to its availability and low cost, contribute to its popularity as a suicide agent or as a substitute for alcohol (12,13).

TABLE 38–1. *Sources and concentrations of ethylene glycol*

Source	Concentration (%)
Antifreeze	95
Brake fluid	70–95
Coolant	95
Windshield de-icer	50

Other Glycols

Among the various low molecular weight ethylene glycol derivatives, the presence of an ether linkage appears to be the predisposing factor to intense renal damage. Glycols with an ether linkage include diethylene glycol, dipropylene glycol, dioxane, and the monomethyl, ethyl, and butyl ethers of diethylene glycol. In contrast, the toxicity of simple esters resembles that of the parent glycol, to which they are hydrolyzed in the body.

Diethylene glycol

Diethylene glycol, which consists of two ethylene glycol moieties connected through an ether linkage, produces central necrosis of liver lobules as well as vacuolization of renal tubular cells and more severe renal damage than that produced by ethylene glycol (1,14). Calcium oxalate crystals are not produced because oxalate is not an end-product of the metabolism of this compound as a result of the stable ether linkage (15). Severe acidosis is also not a prominent feature of the clinical course with diethylene glycol poisoning. Dioxane, another glycol, is also not associated with a severe metabolic acidosis (16).

Propylene glycol

Propylene glycol (1,2-propanediol), a liquid, is another polyalcohol of low molecular weight that is considered safe for pharmacologic purposes and for use in food and cosmetics (17). It has been widely used as a solvent in the preparation of oral and injectable drugs, lotions, and ointments (18). It is generally considered a stable, pharmacologically inert substance with low systemic toxicity because it enters the normal metabolic pathways of the body. It is approved by the Food and Drug Administration as a solvent for certain drugs, such as injectable phenytoin and diazepam (Table 38–2) (19–22). Studies

TABLE 38–2. *Commonly used drugs that contain propylene glycol*

Diazepam (injection)
Digoxin (injection)
Ergocalciferol (oral liquid)
Eucerin (cream)
Hydralazine (injection)
Multivitamin (injection)
Nembutal (injection)
Nystatin (ointment and cream)
Phenobarbital (injection)
Phenytoin (injection)
Sulfamethoxazole and trimethoprim (injection)

Adapted with permission from *Pediatrics* 1987;79:623.

have shown that propylene glycol is partly metabolized to lactic and pyruvic acids, which then enter the glycolytic pathway and are excreted as carbon dioxide and water (1). It is theoretically possible, however, for lactic acidosis to occur, but this would be an extremely rare occurrence and would be noted only in a patient with impaired renal clearance of propylene glycol (17,23).

Although propylene glycol is generally considered nontoxic, there are reports of toxic effects in humans (18). These are mostly secondary to intravenous administration, and include cardiac dysrhythmias and asystole, renal damage, hemolysis, seizures, hepatic damage, and an increased osmolal gap (20,22).

Pharmacokinetic Properties of Ethylene Glycol

Ethylene glycol is a colorless, odorless substance; it appears to have color because artificial coloring is added to the finished product (24). Fluorescein, a fluorescent dye, is added to many commercial preparations of antifreeze to a final concentration of approximately 20 µg/mL. The high boiling point and low vapor pressure of ethylene glycol eliminates the danger of poisoning by inhalation. Ethylene glycol has a volume of distribution of approximately 0.7 L/kg (25), a half-life of approximately 3 hours, and a molecular weight of 62 (3,26,27). Although the half-life of ethylene glycol has been reported to vary from 3–5 hours, it can be prolonged to 17 hours with adequate ethanol blocking therapy (28). Its rate of elimination is more rapid than that of methanol, which means that the latent period for metabolic accumulation to toxic concentrations is usually shorter (29).

Eighty percent of ethylene glycol is passively reabsorbed in the kidneys, with 20% being excreted unchanged

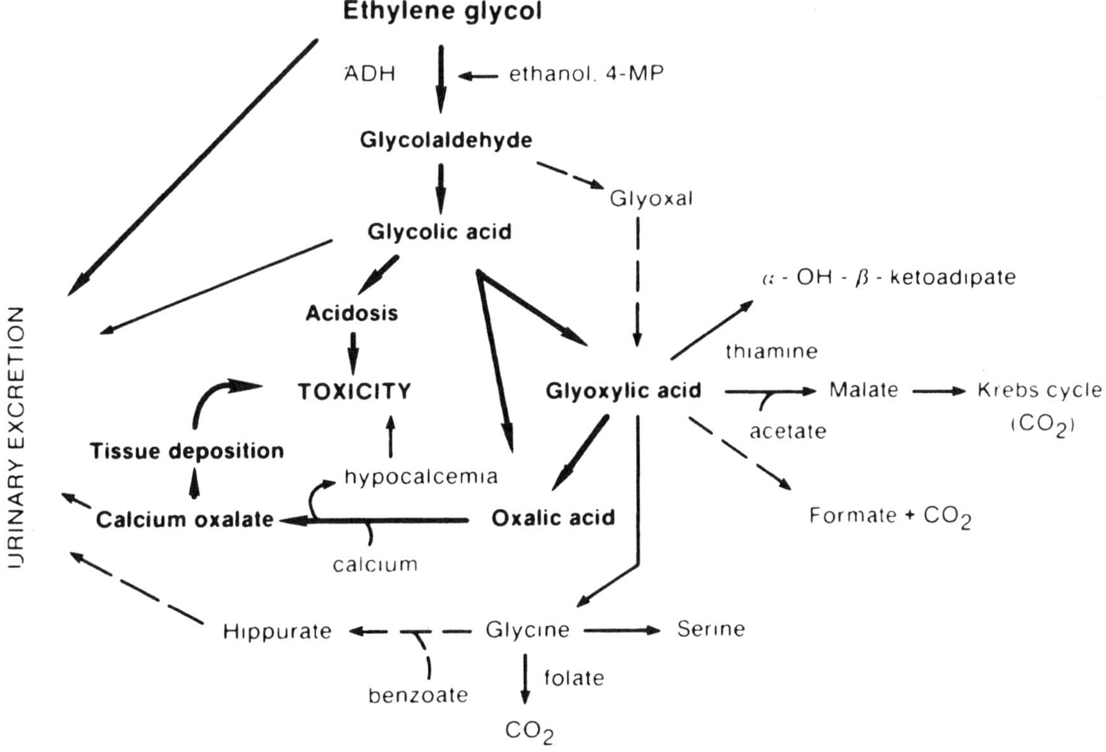

FIG 38–1. Pathways of ethylene glycol elimination. The thick solid arrows represent probable major pathways, the thin solid arrows less important pathways, and the broken arrows indicate theoretic pathways. Reprinted with permission from *Am J Med* 1988;84:146.

(28). The majority is converted to toxic metabolites, some of which have elimination half-lives of up to 12 hours (30).

Absorption

There is no toxicity associated with skin absorption of ethylene glycol, nor is there toxicity secondary to its inhalation. Toxicity is limited to the ingestion of the compound. The estimated lethal dose is considered approximately 100 mL, although a much smaller amount has been reported to cause death (5). Survival has been reported after ingestion of 400 mL.

Metabolism

Ethylene glycol intoxication may result in a profound, sometimes life-threatening, metabolic acidosis, but in its original form the substance is relatively nontoxic and has no effect on respiration, the citric acid cycle, or other biochemical pathways. It is the metabolites and intermediaries that are formed that contribute to the toxicity associated with ethylene glycol (13).

The major metabolites, in order of their appearance, are glycoaldehyde, glycolic acid, and glyoxylic acid (Fig. 38–1) (31). The initial step in the metabolism of ethylene glycol is oxidation of one of the hydroxyl moieties to an aldehyde, resulting in glycoaldehyde (29). This oxidation is catalyzed by the hepatic enzyme alcohol dehydrogenase. Glycoaldehyde is then further oxidized to glycolic acid. The second hydroxl group may then be oxidized, resulting in glyoxylic acid. Oxidation to formic acid and carbon dioxide occurs only to a small extent. A small fraction (3%–10%) of the glyoxylic acid is converted to oxalic acid. Glycoaldehyde, glycolic acid, and glyoxylic acid are more toxic than the parent compound.

Other compounds contributing to a metabolic acidosis include hippuric and lactic acids. These minor pathways are dependent on pyridoxal pyrophosphate and thiamine pyrophosphate (3,31,32) and occur primarily in the liver (33).

The Role of Oxalate

The role played by oxalate remains an unsolved problem in the etiology of ethylene glycol toxicity. It was once thought that oxalic acid was the major cause of the metabolic acidosis. Although oxalate is a minor metabolic product of ethylene glycol, oxalic acid may contribute to the organ damage noted in ethylene glycol intoxication (34,35). Oxalate crystalluria can be a striking feature of ethylene glycol intoxication (13). Oxalate rapidly precipitates as calcium oxalate (mainly in the monohydrate form), which is deposited in various tissues, such as the kidneys, myocardium, brain, and pancreas. The exact mechanism of the renal necrosis and failure is not known, and there appears to be a direct link between oxalate precipitation and the development of tubular necrosis (36).

The accumulation of oxalate has long been considered responsible for most of the clinical picture of ethylene glycol poisoning (37). Although oxalate is a highly toxic compound and can by itself produce extensive renal damage, acidosis, and death, it does not account for all the effects of ethylene glycol (3). Oxalic acid is an organic, dicarboxylic acid that is corrosive and has a marked affinity for calcium and magnesium. Although calcium oxalate crystals have been shown in some cases to physically block the renal tubules, this may be an incidental finding; it may be the oxalic acid itself, among other intermediaries, that is toxic to cells by chelating calcium or magnesium intracellularly, leading to acute tubular necrosis (38,39).

Crystalluria

Only up to 10% of ethylene glycol is excreted as calcium oxalate. The contribution of calcium oxalate crystal deposition to the toxicity of ethylene glycol is not known, but the crystals have been identified in renal, brain, and lung tissue. Two forms of urinary calcium oxalate crystals are now recognized (Fig. 38–2) (40). The less prevalent form is the octahedral dihydrate or "envelope" form. On microscopic examination these crystals resemble a square containing an "x" that connects the vertices (41). This form is present only at high concentrations of both calcium and oxalate (42). The monohydrate or needle-shaped crystal is seen more commonly because it is more thermodynamically stable under normal physiologic conditions (34). This form was previously thought to be composed of hippuric acid crystals. Hippuric acid crystals may be formed if patients consume antifreeze that contains benzoic acid as a preservative (13). Although calcium oxalate crystals are considered an important diagnostic marker for ethylene glycol poisoning, in some cases they may be absent (1,20). If the initial urine sample is free of crystals, repeated urine microscopy may be indicated (43).

Anion Gap Metabolic Acidosis

The anion gap in ethylene glycol intoxication is greater than that in any of the more common metabolic acidoses (13). It has been shown that glycolic acid is the metabolite that accumulates in the highest concentrations in the blood (4,34,35,44,45). This is because the rate of glycolic acid formation from ethylene glycol exceeds the rate of elimination (46,47). This acid therefore appears to be the major contributing factor to the acute toxicity of ethylene

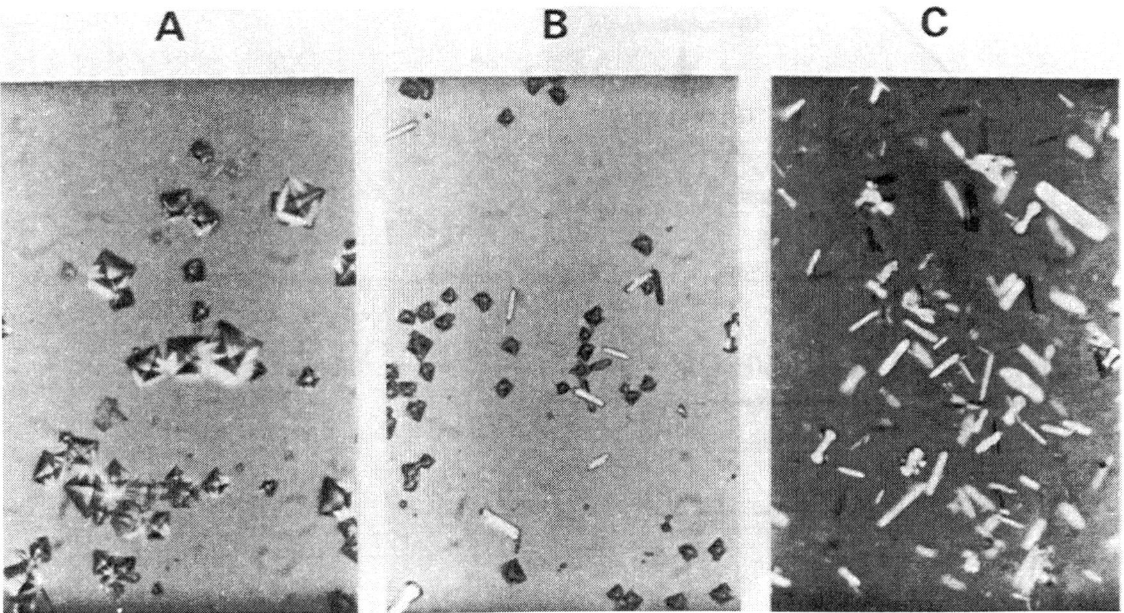

FIG 38–2. Crystalluria in ethylene glycol poisoning. Envelope-shaped crystals are the dihydrate, whereas needle-shaped crystals are the monohydrate. Reprinted with permission from *Am J Med* 1988;84:150. ©1988 Technical Publishing Company.

glycol as well as the major determinant of the metabolic acidosis (48). Serum and urine concentrations of glycolic acid have been found to correlate directly with clinical symptoms and mortality in poisoning cases, and glycolic acid may be found in the serum and urine longer than ethylene glycol (4). Lactic acidosis may also be present as a result of inhibition of the citric acid cycle by glyoxylic acid as well as the increased cellular reduction:oxidation ratio, which favors the buildup of lactate over pyruvate (13,34,35). The development of a concomitant lactic acidosis may be due to circulatory failure and poor tissue perfusion (13,46).

Acute Toxicity of Ethylene Glycol

Ethylene glycol has about the same central nervous system toxicity as ethanol, and is rapidly absorbed and evenly distributed throughout the body tissues (4). Blood concentrations reach their peak between 1 and 4 hours after ingestion (12). The toxicity of ethylene glycol is due to the breakdown products. Classically, descriptions of ethylene glycol toxicity include three stages. Clinically, however, patient presentations are rarely as well demarcated as the descriptions indicate (35). These stages may be confluent, and the different latent periods before each stage depend on the amount of ethylene glycol and ethyl alcohol ingested. These three stages are the initial central nervous system, gastrointestinal, and metabolic stages (stage 1), which are followed by the cardiopulmonary stage (stage 2) and then the renal stage (stage 3) (Table 38–3). Early diagnosis is essential because removal of the toxin by dialysis and reversal of the severe metabolic acidosis may be lifesaving.

Stage 1

During the first 12 hours after ingestion of ethylene glycol, central nervous system manifestations predomi-

TABLE 38–3. *Stages of ethylene glycol toxicity*

Stage 1 (30 minutes to 12 hours)
Intoxicated patient with no odor of alcohol
Nausea and vomiting
Metabolic acidosis
Crystalluria
Myoclonus
Seizures
Death
Stage 2 (12–24 hours)
Tachypnea
Tachycardia
Hypertension
Cyanosis
Pulmonary edema
Bronchopneumonia
Cardiac enlargement
Stage 3 (36–48 hours)
Crystalluria
Costovertebral angle tenderness
Acute tubular necrosis with oliguria
Renal failure

nate. These central nervous system manifestations are related to the aldehyde metabolites of ethylene glycol, which reach their maximal concentrations during this period (46). The aldehydes are toxic because they inhibit oxidative phosphorylation and glucose metabolism (28).

Clinically, the patient appears to be intoxicated with ethyl alcohol, but the typical odor of alcohol is absent. Nausea, vomiting, and ataxia are common. This stage of intoxication is associated with the profound metabolic acidosis being produced in the metabolic degradation of ethylene glycol.

Generalized or focal seizures are relatively frequent, as is myoclonus or tetany secondary to hypocalcemia. Hypocalcemia is believed to be due to chelation of the calcium ion by oxalate, forming relatively insoluble calcium oxalate crystals (35). Profuse calcium oxalate crystalluria, both before and after the period of anuria, is usually the hallmark of the renal sediment and may appear in the urine within 4–8 hours after ingestion (36).

Coma during this period is a frequent finding. Complete recovery from coma has occurred in a patient who was comatose for 17 days (47). Coma may be due to cerebral oxalosis and cytotoxic damage, with secondary cerebral edema developing (3).

Papilledema is seen and is usually due to cerebral edema, but occasionally it represents a toxic optic neuropathy with progressive loss of vision and optic atrophy similar to that seen in methanol ingestion (5). In rare circumstances, abnormal eye findings consisting of nystagmus, ophthalmoplegia, and papilledema with subsequent optic atrophy are noted (49,50). Although these eye findings have been reported on occasion, no methanol determinations were performed to rule out the possibility of methanol contamination of the liquid ingested (35).

Death, if it occurs during this stage, is accompanied by cerebral edema. Examination of the cerebrospinal fluid characteristically reveals features of a meningoencephalitis with leukocytosis, xanthochromia, elevated cerebrospinal fluid pressure, and increased cerebrospinal fluid protein. On postmortem examination, calcium oxalate crystals can be found in the brain, leptomeninges, and perivascular spaces (5). The aldehyde metabolite glycoaldehyde is thought to be responsible for much of the toxicity seen in this stage.

Stage 2

The second or cardiopulmonary stage occurs between 12 and 24 hours after ingestion and has less well-defined symptoms. These consist of tachypnea, tachycardia, mild hypertension, cyanosis, and congestive heart failure or pulmonary edema (46). Death, if it occurs, is associated with bronchopneumonia and cardiac enlargement. Fatalities in this stage are not as common as in the other stages.

The pathophysiology of the cardiopulmonary symptoms is not well known, but widespread capillary damage is assumed to be the primary lesion.

Stage 3

Stage 3, the renal stage, is noted 36–48 hours after ingestion. If the patient survives the initial 24–72 hours, renal failure usually becomes the predominant problem (51). The renal damage may vary from temporary azotemia to anuria lasting for many weeks. Other abnormalities associated with renal involvement may include destruction of epithelial cells, interstitial edema, focal hemorrhagic necrosis of the cortex, extensive hydropic degeneration, numerous cellular casts, and oxalate crystals in the convoluted tubules (46). Although oxaluria can occur during this stage, it can also be noted during stage 1. If the patient is alert, he or she may complain of flank pain, and costovertebral angle tenderness may be noted. Acute tubular necrosis with oliguria and hematuria may eventually lead to renal failure (52). Renal function may return to near normal if the patient survives (46).

Stage 4

A fourth stage has been postulated describing central nervous system effects different from those seen in stage 1. Cranial nerve palsies may manifest as bilateral facial paralysis. Other late neurologic findings that have been reported include anisocoria, blurred vision, dysphagia, hyperreflexia, and ataxia. The mechanism for these effects appears unclear (28). The cranial nerve dysfunction may be profound, slow to resolve, or even permanent (28).

Laboratory Diagnosis

Diagnosis of ethylene glycol intoxication involves measuring serum electrolytes and arterial blood gas, urinalysis, Wood's lamp examination, measuring serum cal-

TABLE 38–4. *Laboratory evaluation for ethylene glycol*

Serum electrolytes
Arterial blood gas
Blood urea nitrogen
Serum creatinine
Urinalysis
Wood's lamp examination
Serum calcium
Serum phosphorus
Measured serum osmolality
Calculated serum osmolality
Serum ethylene glycol
Serum glycolic acid
Electrocardiogram

cium and phosphorus concentrations, and measuring serum osmolality and calculating an osmolal gap (Table 38–4). The rise in the osmolal gap in ethylene glycol intoxication occurs only early in the poisoning, when unmetabolized ethylene glycol is present in the serum (4). Serum calcium concentration may be low because of the precipitation of calcium by oxalate (11). This may also be reflected in evidence of hypocalcemia on the electrocardiogram. The definitive diagnosis of ethylene glycol toxicity rests with the laboratory determination of the serum ethylene glycol concentration (53). A delay in diagnosis may exist because many hospital laboratories are not equipped to perform the assay and must transfer the specimen to an off-site reference laboratory.

Serum concentrations of ethylene glycol should also be measured in a known ethylene glycol ingestion. Most techniques presently available attempt to detect ethylene glycol in blood and urine. This approach can be unreliable in diagnosing the severity of the ingestion because of the rapid elimination of ethylene glycol by metabolic degradation or renal excretion (4). Techniques to measure toxic metabolites of ethylene glycol, including glycolic acid, glyoxylic acid, and oxalate are also available. Measurement of glycolic acid levels can be useful in diagnosis and monitoring clinical progress in ethylene glyco-poisoned patients (54). The detection of high concentrations of glycolic acid when there has been an extended period of time between ingestion and admission is valuable in the diagnosis and treatment. In these cases, the major portion of ethylene glycol has been metabolized and may be detected in small quantities or not at all. Because high-performance liquid chromatography can detect both ethylene glycol and glycolic acid, it is important to have both concentrations reported, especially when there has been an extended period of time between ingestion and admission (4).

False positive results may also be obtained. For example, in chronic alcoholics, 2,3-butanediol has been identified mistakenly as ethylene glycol; it may be formed as a novel metabolic product in alcoholism or can be produced enzymatically from the 2-butanone found in some denatured ethanol products. Propylene glycol, found in high concentrations in several parenteral medications, such as phenytoin and diazepam, may lead to falsely positive ethylene glycol measurements as well (28).

When interpreting blood ethylene glycol levels, carefully note the units reported by the laboratory. Levels reported in milligrams/liter rather than milligrams/deciliter have resulted in unnecessary hemodialysis treatment.

An anion gap metabolic acidosis may be noted early after measuring serum electrolytes. A measurement of arterial blood gas may confirm this finding. Although the osmolal gap may be useful, it may not be present late in the course of an intoxication. The rise in the osmolal gap occurs only early in the poisoning, when unmetabolized ethylene glycol is present in the serum. As ethylene glycol is metabolized and glycolic acid levels rise, there is an increase in the anion gap that corresponds to the amount of glycolic acid (55). The osmolal gap may not reflect this (4).

Fluorescence of Ethylene Glycol

Sodium fluorescein, a fluorescent dye, is added to some commercial antifreeze preparations to a final concentration of approximately 20 μg/mL. In a 30-mL volume of 100% antifreeze, which is potentially toxic to an adult, there can be 0.6 mg sodium fluorescein. Therefore, Wood's lamp examination of the urine or emesis may show fluorescence from the fluorescein coloring (56). If a urine sample is collected more than 4 hours after ingestion, fluorescence may not be seen, but a toxic serum concentration of ethylene glycol may be found. Because sodium fluorescein is not an additive to all commercially available antifreeze products, a negative test for fluorescence does not eliminate the possibility of a significant ingestion of ethylene glycol.

The pH of the sample specimen to be tested is important. At a pH of less than 4.5, the fluorescence of sodium fluorescein disappears. Therefore, the pH of the solution should be checked and appropriately adjusted to 4.5 or more before examination under ultraviolet light (56).

An approach to the workup of a patient potentially intoxicated with ethylene glycol is presented in greater detail in Chapter 39.

Treatment

The treatments for intoxication with ethylene glycol and methanol are similar enough that they can be discussed together (see below).

METHANOL

Methanol has been recognized as a serious toxic agent since the end of the 19th century. The classic method for producing methanol, or wood alcohol, relied on the distillation of hardwood, with fractionation yielding methanol, acetone, methylethylketone, and other products. With early distillation methods it produced such a vile odor and taste that it was not used as a substance of abuse. With the addition of deodorizing substances and the removal of many of the noxious impurities, the product became more palatable, and the number of poisonings increased substantially (57,58).

Uses

Methanol has been used as an adulterant or denaturant in other substances to discourage the oral use of that par-

TABLE 38–5. *Sources and concentrations of methanol*

Source	Concentration (%)
Sterno	4
Carburetor fluid	99
Cements	1
Glass cleaners	1–40
Denatured ethanol	2–5
Duplicator fluid	60–90
Gasohol	10
Gas line antifreeze	100
Model engine fuel	45–75
Paint stripper	2–25
Pipe sweetener	75
Windshield de-icer	4–90
Windshield-washing solution	17–100

ticular substance (59–61). During the early part of this century in the United States, it was legal to include methanol as a constituent of various spirits and whiskeys. In the past, it was not uncommon for "epidemics" of methanol poisoning to occur when methanol was ingested from a common contaminated source (34,35,57, 62,63). Methanol has also been used as an industrial solvent for shellac and paint thinners and in the manufacturing of rubber goods, synthetic textiles, antifreeze of the nonpermanent type, duplicating fluid, printing solutions, and cleaning solutions, and it is commonly used as a windshield-washing solution (Table 38–5) (64–69).

At present, many new uses of methyl alcohol are being proposed. These are primarily concerned with energy production or research on gasoline extenders, substitutes, and additives. Recently, methanol has been used as a synthetic fuel for automobiles because it has excellent combustion-mixing properties. Gasohol, the synthetic fuel, may contain 90% gasoline and 10% methanol or ethanol depending on local cost and availability. Sterno, which is 4% methanol, is marketed because of this combustion property (65). Methanol is also used in the production of formaldehyde and methylated compounds, such as methyl esters (35).

In industry, methanol is produced in large quantities by the catalytic reaction of carbon monoxide or carbon dioxide with hydrogen. Methanol is a normal constituent of saliva and expired air and can be detected in the blood. Dietary methanol arises in large part from fresh fruits and vegetables, where it occurs as free alcohol, methyl esters of fatty acids, or methoxy groups on polysaccharides, such as pectin.

Aspartame (Nutrasweet), a nutritive sweetener produced commercially from two amino acids (L-phenylalanine and L-aspartic acid), in theory has the ability to be converted to methanol. Studies have shown no increases in blood methanol with large doses (34 mg/kg), however, so that there is no concern of methanol intoxication from this artificial sweetener (67).

Pharmacokinetics

Methanol is a colorless substance with an odor distinctly different from that of ethanol and a bitter taste (57). This may often be difficult to recognize in the mixed liquids that cause poisonings (34). Methanol has a low molecular weight, distributes throughout total body water, and has a volume of distribution of 0.6 L/kg (71). Formate, the major metabolite that is responsible for toxicity, also has a low molecular weight and a volume of distribution of 0.5 L/kg.

Absorption

Absorption of methanol occurs by all routes. Methanol is rapidly absorbed from the gastrointestinal tract, with peak absorption occurring in 30–60 minutes. Blindness has been reported in a factory worker who accidentally spilled a gallon of methanol on a trouser leg (65,66,69), and an infant died as a result of being wrapped in methanol-soaked towels (70). Inhalation of vapors in excess of 200 ppm is associated with toxicity (65,71). Ingestion of as little as 4 mL has caused blindness (20,46, 57), and as little as 15 mL has caused death.

Metabolism (Fig. 38–3)

Although some methanol is eliminated by the lungs in expired air, the main route of metabolism is through successive oxidation by alcohol dehydrogenase. Whereas ethanol is metabolized to carbon dioxide and water by alcohol dehydrogenase, 40% of a dose of methanol is metabolized by the same enzyme undergoing zero-order kinetics to produce formic acid from formaldehyde (72). This is the rate-limiting step in the metabolism of methanol. The formaldehyde is then rapidly converted to formic acid, and further metabolized by a folate-dependent process to carbon dioxide and water. The half-life of formaldehyde is 1–2 minutes, so that no accumulation is detectable (34). The metabolism of methanol proceeds five times more slowly than that of ethanol, and approximately 30% of a dose of methanol remains unchanged in the body up to 48 hours after ingestion. Formic acid, which is six times more toxic than methanol, is responsi-

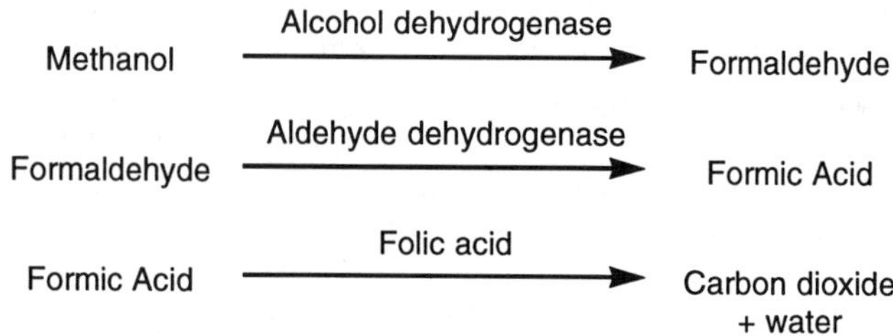

FIG 38–3. Metabolism of methanol.

TABLE 38–6. *Clinical manifestations of methanol intoxication*

General
Mild inebriation
Long latent period
Metabolic acidosis
Gastrointestinal
Nausea
Vomiting
Severe abdominal pain
Neurologic
Headache
Dizziness
Seizures
Stupor
Visual
Diminished sensation of light
Reduced central vision
Photophobia
Slurred vision
Retinal edema
Hyperemia of optic disks

ble for metabolic acidosis, an anion gap, and ocular toxicity (31,46,48,73–75).

Methanol is nontoxic, but its breakdown product, formic acid, may cause multisystem problems (76). Susceptibility to methanol poisoning is regulated by the functioning of the folate systems in each species. Only humans and monkeys develop methanol poisoning because of the absence of a pathway allowing large amounts of formate to be metabolized into carbon dioxide (35). The rate-limiting step for the production of formic acid, therefore, appears to be the availability of folic acid (65). This may have clinical importance in the management of methanol intoxication (47,77).

There is individual variation in the clinical presentation of the methanol-intoxicated patient, subject to such considerations as the amount of food in the patient's stomach, the quantity of methanol consumed, and the quantity of ethanol consumed. Individuals with folate deficiencies may be more susceptible to intoxication.

Acute Toxicity

Toxicity usually manifests itself in the visual, gastrointestinal, respiratory, and central nervous systems (Table 38–6) (78).

General Considerations

The initial period of inebriation is a disappointment to the intentional user because it is milder than expected, sometimes encouraging the user to ingest a greater quantity (32,35,79,80). This is in contrast to the later stage, when coma may occur as a result of the accumulation of metabolites. Early central nervous system depression after the ingestion of methanol may be due to the concomitant ingestion of ethanol (34). An important part of the natural course of methanol intoxication is the relatively long latent period between ingestion and significant toxic findings (79). A latent period of 6–72 hours, with an average of 24 hours between ingestion and toxic symptoms, is noted, and because the individual may be asymptomatic he or she may not seek medical attention until the toxic breakdown products have accumulated (35,65). This latent period can be explained as the time required for methanol to be converted to the toxic metabolites responsible for the characteristic syndrome (81,82). If ethanol is also ingested, the lag period before breakdown of methanol is even longer (35).

Visual Disorders

Visual disorders are very common (72). There may be complaints of a diminished sensation of light, reduced central vision, photophobia, blurred or indistinct vision with a perception of dancing spots over the eyes, the sensation of "skin over the eyes," flashes of gray, white, or yellow, or blindness (83). On funduscopic examination retinal edema may be observed, which develops over 2–4 days and may persist for up to 2 weeks (84). There may be dilated, sluggishly reactive pupils along with hyperemia of the optic disks (83). In patients with severe visual damage, optic atrophy may develop with cupping of the optic disk (85,86). The usual visual field defect is a central scotoma (87). The patient's subjective complaints and actual eye findings very seldom correlate (83).

Although in the past it was thought that formaldehyde caused optic toxicity, animal studies show unequivocally that visual impairment is caused by formic acid inhibiting cytochrome oxidase with resultant impairment of electron transport in the mitochondria (35,83,88). As a result formation of adenosine triphosphate is defective, and stasis of nerve flow occurs in the optic nerve head rather than the retinal ganglia (65). Axonal swelling develops because of the stasis, resulting in optic disk edema and leading to visual impairment (83). Optic atrophy, if it occurs, is a late finding. Although recovery from partial loss of vision may occur (57), the prognosis for recovery of vision from total blindness, if it occurs, is not favorable.

Metabolic Acidosis

In the early stages of methanol intoxication, formate accumulation is the main contributor to the metabolic acidosis. Lactic acidosis may appear at a late stage in severe methanol poisoning. This results mainly from formate inhibition of mitochondrial respiration, tissue hypoxia due to poor circulation, and altered lactate metabolism due to an increased ratio of reduced nicotinamide adenine dinucleotide (NADH) to nicotinamide adenine dinucleotide (NAD) (34,35,89).

Folate is a necessary co-factor for the conversion of formate to carbon dioxide. For this reason, nutritional folate deficiency predisposes the patient to more severe poisoning when methanol is ingested.

Neurologic Abnormalities

Headache and dizziness are frequently found with methanol intoxication; weakness and malaise are seen less commonly. In severely intoxicated patients, seizures, stupor, and coma may also be present (90). Prognosis is poor if the patient has these neurologic findings in conjunction with signs of increased intracranial pressure, such as bradycardia, hypertension, and dilated, nonreactive pupils. White blood cells in the cerebral spinal fluid and xanthochromia have also been reported (32). Survivors of serious methanol poisoning may be left with an extrapyramidal movement disorder due to permanent damage to the putamen (34,65,91).

Gastrointestinal Effects

The local effects on the gastrointestinal tract may cause the individual to seek medical attention before a large amount of the compound is metabolized. Fifty percent of patients experience nausea and vomiting, which is usually persistent and violent (92). Approximately two-thirds of patients experience abdominal pain, which may be violent and colicky and, at times, may simulate an acute abdomen or renal colic. An elevated serum amylase concentration is a relatively frequent finding associated with the severe abdominal pain caused by methanol (20,57,72).

Laboratory Analysis

Although there may be a poor correlation between blood methanol concentration and symptoms, a peak level greater than 50 mg/dL is considered toxic. Blood methanol concentrations are not as difficult to obtain as blood ethylene glycol concentrations; therefore, if the diagnosis of methanol poisoning is considered, serum concentrations should be measured.

Techniques are available for measuring blood formate concentrations (93). Elevated blood formate levels account for nearly all of the anion gap and diminished plasma bicarbonate observed in metabolic acidosis from methanol poisoning. Formate is also responsible for producing the ocular lesions, and formate levels of 50 mg/dL have been correlated with ophthalmologic injury (11,94).

When methanol poisoning is suspected, establish baseline visual acuity and obtain baseline laboratory studies, including serum electrolytes, measured serum osmolality by freezing-point depression, serum methanol and ethanol levels, arterial blood gases, serum calcium, serum amylase, complete blood count, liver and renal function tests, urinalysis, and serum formate levels, if available. Further work-up of the patient suspected of ingesting a methanol-containing compound is discussed more fully in Chapter 39.

TREATMENT FOR ETHYLENE GLYCOL AND METHANOL INTOXICATION

For the most part, the treatments of ethylene glycol overdose and methanol overdose are identical (Table 38–7). Treatment is directed first toward correcting the metabolic acidosis, then toward inhibiting the oxidation of the parent compound, and finally toward the removal of circulating amounts of the parent compound and its toxic metabolites (95). Because poisoning with these two alcohols causes such serious irreversible problems, treatment should be instituted as rapidly as possible, especially in patients who are symptomatic (29). Ethanol therapy may be offered while waiting for positive laboratory confirmation of a suspected ingestion. This is especially true in cases of suspected ethylene glycol poisoning (96).

Attempts to prevent further absorption using ipecac or lavage with subsequent administration of activated charcoal and a cathartic should be instituted (97). Skin decontamination should be performed in the methanol-exposed patient.

Alkali Therapy

If the patient is acidotic, intravenous alkali therapy should be started. It has been demonstrated that the mortality for methanol and ethylene glycol intoxication can be greatly influenced by prompt and generous sodium bicarbonate treatment, and it has been further shown that correction of metabolic acidosis alone significantly increases the patient's chance for survival (13). Because

TABLE 38–7. *Treatment of ethylene glycol and methanol overdose*

Prevent further absorption
Lavage
Charcoal
Cathartic
Alkalinization (2–3 mEq/kg)
Ethanol therapy (see Table 38–8)
Calcium (1 g $CaCl_2$)
Thiamine (50–100 mg)—for ethylene glycol
Pyridoxine (2–5 g intravenously)—for ethylene glycol
Folic acid (50–100 mg intravenously)—for methanol
Dialysis

methanol and ethylene glycol are responsible for the generation of organic acids, as opposed to conditions that block excretion (such as uremia), large amounts of bicarbonate may be required (98). In addition, unlike pure lactic acidosis or ketoacidosis, the anions generated in ethylene glycol and methanol intoxication are not metabolized to regenerate bicarbonate.

Bicarbonate therapy consists of continuous infusion of 5% sodium bicarbonate or administration of 2–3 mEq/kg of sodium bicarbonate, with frequent monitoring of electrolytes, arterial blood gases, and fluid status of the patient. Although large amounts of fluids may increase oxalate excretion, they may also increase the likelihood of pulmonary edema.

Ethyl Alcohol Therapy

Because it is the metabolic products of methanol and ethylene glycol that are toxic and not the parent compounds themselves, preventing the formation of these products will render these compounds nontoxic (99,100). Ethyl alcohol is suggested in the management of ethylene glycol and methanol ingestion because it competes with alcohol dehydrogenase, the enzyme responsible for the critical first step in the metabolism of methanol and ethylene glycol (101). Ethyl alcohol saturates this enzyme because its affinity for ethanol is 100 times greater than for either methanol or ethylene glycol (5,32,101). Ethanol increases the half-life of ethylene glycol from 3 hours to 17 hours (109,110). The administration of ethanol will therefore avoid a buildup of the toxic products of metabolism and allows for an increased excretion of unchanged parent compound through the kidneys. In theory, ethanol could be the only therapy for mild intoxication with these compounds. Severe intoxication requires more aggressive therapy (13). If clinical suspicion of methanol or ethylene glycol poisoning is high, treatment with ethanol should not be delayed for the report of blood concentrations.

The aim of ethanol therapy is to saturate the enzyme system. This can be accomplished at approximately 100 mg/dL (22 mmol/L) of ethanol (5,102). At an ethanol concentration of 100 mg/dL, more than 75% of the metabolites of ethylene glycol are blocked. At ethanol concentrations up to 200 mg/dL, more than 95% are blocked (5). To accomplish this goal, both a loading dose and a maintenance dose are necessary. Absolute ethanol or lesser concentrations of ethanol, administered either parenterally or orally, will produce the proper saturation of the enzyme. Advantages of oral administration of ethanol are the ease of administration and the ability to use a more concentrated solution than may comfortably be administered parenterally (26,27,102). Parenteral administration, however, produces the desired blood level more quickly and obviates concern about prior intestinal absorption. Parenteral administration of ethanol may also be required for the patient who is vomiting. In a comatose patient or a patient with variable ethanol absorption (as occurs after activated charcoal administration), the intravenous route is preferred (11).

With absolute ethanol (95%), a loading dose of 1 mL/kg in 5% dextrose in water over 10–15 minutes brings the blood concentration to approximately 100 mg/dL (5). A maintenance dosage consists of 0.1 mL/kg/hour, and therapy should be continued for 2–3 days (Table 38–8). Although absolute alcohol can be used, it should be diluted to approximately 10% for ease of parenteral administration because concentrations greater than 10% are associated with local irritation (95). The hospital pharmacy may be able to prepare this solution from absolute alcohol. A 5% ethanol solution is commercially available, but the volume of fluid that must be administered with this preparation is often excessive. Since intravenous ethanol is not pyrogen free, intravenous tubing with micropore filters should be used for its administration (102). Ethanol infusions may be uncomfortable for some patients because of their irritating nature, but postinfusion phlebitis is not common.

Because of the relatively short half-life of ethylene glycol, ethyl alcohol therapy should be started within 4–6 hours after ingestion. It should also be started as soon as possible for methanol, although the rate of breakdown of methanol is much slower than that of ethylene glycol. Close monitoring of levels is needed every 1–2 hours initially to adjust the maintenance infusion rate for the individual patient (104). Ethanol therapy should be continued until the levels of methanol or ethylene glycol fall to zero. If intravenous ethanol is not available at the institution, oral ethanol therapy may be given. A loading dose of ethanol for a 70-kg adult is approximately 4 ounces of 86-proof whiskey. One ounce per hour should serve as a

TABLE 38–8. *Ethyl alcohol management of ethylene glycol and methanol overdose*

Dose	95% Ethanol	40% Ethanol	10% Ethanol
Loading	1 mL/kg	2.5 mL/kg	10 mL/kg
Maintenance (without dialysis)	0.1 mL/kg/hour	0.3 mL/kg/hour	1 mL/kg/hour
Maintenance (with dialysis)	0.3 mL/kg/hour	1 mL/kg/hour	3 mL/kg/hour

Adapted with permission from Smith M: Solvent toxicity: isopropanol, methanol, and ethylene glycol. *Ear Nose Throat J* 1983;62:13. ©1983 Little, Brown, and Company.

maintenance dose until intravenous ethanol becomes available.

If dialysis is to be performed, increased amounts of maintenance ethanol should be administered because ethanol will also be eliminated in the dialysate. Alternatives to absolute ethanol therapy, as well as the suggested dose if dialysis is instituted, are suggested in Table 38–8. Treatment with ethyl alcohol should be continued for 24 hours after the ethylene glycol is removed from the plasma because various body tissues can act as reservoirs for the substance and release their contents even several days later.

Blood ethanol concentrations should also be routinely measured to assess whether dosage adjustments are needed to maintain the desired effect (5). With prolonged ethanol administration, hypoglycemia may result, especially in children (12).

Indications for intravenous ethanol therapy include a history of significant ingestion when blood levels cannot be obtained in a reasonable time period, the presence of symptoms following methanol ingestion, a history of ingesting 30 mL (0.4 mL/kg) or more, a blood methanol level of 20 mg/dL or greater, or the presence of an elevated anion gap metabolic acidosis following methanol ingestion. If there is a strong suspicion that either significant quantities of methanol or ethylene glycol have been ingested, empiric treatment with intravenous ethanol should begin, even while laboratory tests are pending (104).

Calcium

The suggested treatment for symptomatic hypocalcemic manifestations associated with ethylene glycol overdose is calcium chloride or calcium gluconate, although some investigators hold that the administration of calcium may increase the production of calcium oxalate crystals (51).

Pyridoxine and Thiamine

Two of the most rapidly used co-factors in the enzymatic metabolism of ethylene glycol are thiamine and pyridoxine. Pyridoxine is an important co-factor in converting glyoxylate to glycine rather than to oxalate. Thiamine assists in the metabolization of glyoxalate to γ-hydroxy-β-ketoadipate instead of to oxalate, although the importance of this pathway has recently been questioned (13). Thiamine (50–100 mg) and pyridoxine (2–5 g) should therefore be given prophylactically (3,12,105).

Folic Acid

Folic acid is suggested for the methanol-intoxicated individual because it enhances the oxidation of formic acid to carbon dioxide and water through a folate-dependent system (65). Folic acid (1 mg/kg or 50–100 mg) administered intravenously every 4 hours for a total of six doses is the suggested dosage regimen (106).

Pyrazole

Pyrazole compounds such as 4-methylpyrazole (4-MP) have been shown to be inhibitors of alcohol dehydrogenase and thus of the oxidation of methanol (107). It is an inhibitor of alcohol dehydrogenase rather than a competitive substrate like ethanol (35). 4-Methylpyrazole has been used experimentally in animals for modifying ethanol metabolism with few toxic effects (46,47, 73,107). It does not appear to exert central nervous system depression and has a longer duration of action than ethanol because it is metabolized and eliminated more slowly (108). Although pyrazoles are still experimental, they may offer another approach to the treatment of methanol and ethylene glycol overdose (65,106,109, 110).

A dose of 7 mg/kg of intravenous 4-MP decreases the rate of elimination of ethanol and suppresses the typical manifestations of alcohol ingestion in humans. Pyrazole, the parent compound of 4-MP, has well-documented toxic effects (111). In contrast, no side effects have been reported with the use of single doses of up to 20 mg/kg of 4-MP.

Dialysis

Dialysis is essential for the removal of both ethylene glycol and methanol (Table 38–9). Because these two alcohols have relatively small volumes of distribution and are freely water soluble, significant amounts can be removed by hemodialysis (5). Hemodialysis is superior to peritoneal dialysis (32,112–114), although either is effective for the removal of both the parent compounds as

TABLE 38–9. *Substances removed by dialysis in ethylene glycol and methanol intoxication*

Ethylene glycol
Ethylene glycol
Glycoaldehyde
Glycolic acid
Glyoxylic acid
Oxalic acid
Lactic acid
Methanol
Methanol
Formaldehyde
Formic acid
Lactic acid

TABLE 38–10. *Indications for dialysis in ethylene glycol and methanol intoxication*

Ethylene glycol
History of ingestion
Ethylene glycol concentration >50 mg/dL or
Symptomatic patient or
Acidotic patient
Methanol
History of ingestion
Methanol concentration >50 mg/dL or
Symptomatic patient or
Acidotic patient

well as the metabolic breakdown products (13,34,35,112, 115). Dialysis not only removes these toxins but also permits infusion of alkali without the danger of overloading the circulation and increasing the likelihood of pulmonary edema. If dialysis is necessary, ethyl alcohol can be added to the dialysate bath at a concentration of 100 mg/dL, thus lowering the amount required for parenteral or oral administration (4,96,101). In addition, hemodialysis aids in the correction of metabolic acidosis and other metabolic abnormalities while helping to maintain a therapeutic ethanol concentration.

Dialysis is indicated in ethylene glycol toxicity when a history of ingestion is obtained and the patient is symptomatic or when the patient is acidotic (95). If methanol is ingested, dialysis is indicated when the concentration exceeds 50 mg/dL or when the patient is symptomatic or has a metabolic acidosis (Table 38–10).

Frequently, there is a postdialysis rebound, probably due to a redistribution of ethylene glycol from fat stores. Consequently, intravenous ethanol should be continued until ethylene glycol levels are zero.

Hemoperfusion

Although coated activated charcoal hemoperfusion removes ethylene glycol and methanol and their metabolites, the column becomes saturated in about 2 hours, which renders the process ineffective.

SUMMARY

Both ethylene glycol and methanol are dangerous compounds that may cause permanent injury or death. There should be little delay in making the diagnosis of intoxication, with aggressive treatment undertaken once the diagnosis is made.

Ethylene Glycol

Patients who have ingested ethylene glycol and are symptomatic or acidemic, or have a serum concentration greater than 50 mg/dL should be given the full therapeutic regimen of alkali therapy, ethanol, and dialysis (24, 96). With ethylene glycol concentrations less than 50 mg/dL, completely asymptomatic patients (no anion gap, no osmolal gap) with normal renal function should be able to compensate and excrete the acids produced (5).

Methanol

Patients who have ingested methanol, have blood concentrations less than 50 mg/dL, are asymptomatic, and are not acidotic should be treated with ethanol only (115). For patients with concentrations greater than 50 mg/dL who are symptomatic with mental, visual, or funduscopic abnormalities or who have a metabolic acidosis should undergo alkali, alcohol, and dialysis therapy (Fig. 38–4) (20,32,72,96,112). A complete workup of the patient who may have ingested methanol or ethylene glycol is discussed in Chapter 39.

SUMMARY OF THE EFFECTS OF ALCOHOLS

Methanol typically produces eye findings usually late in the course of intoxication (Table 38–11). No characteristic odor of alcohol is noted on the breath. No urinary crystals or serum ketones are detected, and there is likely to be an osmolal gap.

Ethylene glycol typically produces no eye findings, and there is no characteristic ethyl alcohol odor on the

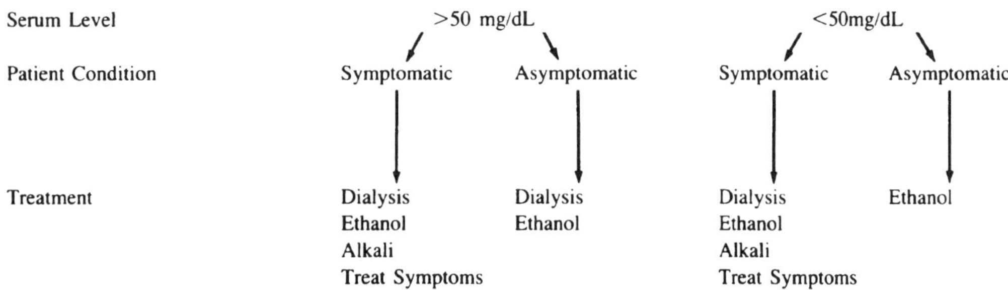

FIG 38–4. Summary of treatment for ethylene glycol and methanol intoxication.

TABLE 38–11. *Diagnostic clues to the presence of toxins commonly ingested by alcoholics*

Substance/condition	Eye findings	Anion gap metabolic acidosis	Distinct odor on breath	Urine crystals	Serum ketones	Osmolal gap
Ethanol	0	+	+	0	+	+
Methanol	+	+	0	0	0	++
Ethylene glycol	0	+	0	+	0	+
Isopropyl alcohol	0	0	+	0	+	+
Ketoacidosis	0	+	+	0	+	+/–

Adapted with permission from Emmett M, Narins R: Clinical use of the anion gap. *Medicine* 1977;56:46. ©1977 Williams & Wilkins Company.

patient's breath. Intoxication may exhibit one or both forms of calcium oxalate crystals in the urine. There are no serum ketones, and an osmolal gap occurs to a lesser extent than with methanol.

Isopropyl alcohol is not associated with eye findings or eye damage. There is a characteristic fruity odor from ketones on the breath. The urine contains no crystals but is positive for ketones. There may be an osmolal gap.

The molecular weights of ethylene glycol and isopropyl alcohol are similar, and both these compounds raise the gap approximately half as much as methanol.

REFERENCES

1. Turk J, Morrell J, Avioli L: Ethylene glycol intoxication. *Arch Intern Med* 1986;146:1601–1603.
2. Sangster B, Prenen J, De Groot G: Ethylene glycol poisoning. *N Engl J Med* 1980;302:465–466.
3. Parry M, Wallach R: Ethylene glycol poisoning. *Am J Med* 1974;57: 143–150.
4. Hewlett T, McMartin K. Lauro A, et al: Ethylene glycol poisoning: the value of glycolic acid determinations for diagnosis and treatment.*Clin Toxicol* 1986;24:389–402.
5. Bobbitt W, Williams R, Freed C: Severe ethylene glycol intoxication with multisystem failure. *West J Med* 1985;144:225–228.
6. Amstrup S, Gardner C, Myers K, et al: Ethylene glycol (antifreeze) poisoning in a free-ranging polar bear. *Vet Hum Toxicol* 1989;31: 317–319.
7. Bove K: Ethylene glycol toxicity. *Am J Clin Pathol* 1966;45:46–50.
8. Goldsher M, Better O: Antifreeze poisoning during the October 1973 war in the Middle-East: case reports. *Mil Med* 1979;144:314–315.
9. Gordon H, Hunter J: Ethylene glycol poisoning—a case report. *Anaesthesia* 1982;37:332–338.
10. Haggarty R: Toxic hazards: death from permanent antifreeze ingestion. *N Engl J Med* 1959;261:1296–1297.
11. Hall A: Ethylene glycol and methanol: poisons with toxic metabolic activation. *Emerg Med Rep* 1992;13:29–38.
12. Brown C, Trumbull D, Klein-Schwanz W, et al; Ethylene glycol poisoning. *Ann Emerg Med* 1983;12:501–506.
13. Gabow P, Clay K, Sullivan J, et al: Organic acids in ethylene glycol intoxication. *Ann Intern Med* 1986;105:16–20.
14. Cantarell M, Fort J, Camps J, et al: Acute intoxication due to topical application of diethylene glycol. *Ann Intern Med* 1987;106:478–479.
15. Winek C. Shingleton D, Shanor S: Ethylene and diethylene glycol toxicity. *Clin Toxicol* 1978;13:297–324.
16. Dean B, Krenzelok E: Clinical evaluation of pediatric ethylene glycol monobutyl ether poisonings. *J Toxicol Clin Toxicol* 1992;30:557–563.
17. Cate J, Hedreck R: Propylene glycol intoxication lactic acidosis. *N Engl J Med* 1980;303:1237.
18. Arulanantham K, Genel M: Central nervous system toxicity associated with ingestion of propylene glycol. *J Pediatr* 1978;93:515–516.
19. Gaunt I, Carpanini F, Grasso P, et al: Long-term toxicity of propylene glycol in rats. *Food Cosmet Toxicol* 1972;10:151–153.
20. Tong T: The alcohols. *Crit Care Q* 1982;4:75–85.
21. MacDonald M, Getson P, Glasgow A, et al: Propylene glycol: increased incidence of seizures in low birth weight infants. *Pediatrics* 1987;79:622–625.
22. Doenicke A, Nebauer A, Hoernecke R, et al: Osmolalities of propylene glycol-containing drug formulations for parenteral use. Should propylene glycol be used as a solvent? *Anesth Analg* 1992;75:431–435.
23. Bossaert L, Demey H: Propylene glycol intoxication. *Arch Intern Med* 1987;147:611–612.
24. Rothman A, Normann S, Manoguerra A, et al: Shortterm hemodialysis in childhood ethylene glycol poisoning. *J Pediatr* 1986;108:153–155.
25. Jacobsen D, Bredesen J, Eide I, et al: Anion and osmolal gaps in the diagnosis of methanol and ethylene glycol poisoning. *Acta Med Scand* 1982;212:17–20.
26. Peterson C, Collins A, Himes J, et al: Ethylene glycol poisoning: pharmacokinetics during therapy with ethanol and hemodialysis. *N Engl J Med* 1981;304:21–23.
27. Peterson P, Peterson J, Hardinge M, et al: Experimental treatment of ethylene glycol poisoning. *JAMA* 1963;186:955–957.
28. Saladino R, Shannon M: Accidental and intentional poisonings with ethylene glycol in infancy: diagnostic clues and management. *Pediatr Emerg Care* 1991;7:93–96.
29. Burkhart K, Kulig K: The other alcohols: methanol, ethylene glycol, and isopropanol. *Emerg Med Clin North Am* 1990;8:913–927.
30. Wrenn K: The delta gap: an approach to mixed acid-base disorders. *Ann Emerg Med* 1990;19:1310–1313.
31. Smith M: Solvent toxicity: isopropanol, methanol, and ethylene glycol. *Ear Nose Throat J* 1983;62:126–135.
32. Smith SR, Smith S, Buckley B: Lactate and formate in methanol poisoning. *Lancet* 1982;1:561–562.
33. Rowland J: Incidence of ethylene glycol intoxication in dogs and cats seen at Colorado State University Veterinary Teaching Hospital. *Vet Hum Toxicol* 1987;29:41–44.
34. Jacobsen D: Organic acids in ethylene glycol intoxication. *Ann Intern Med* 1986;105:799–800.
35. Jacobsen D, McMartin K: Methanol and ethylene glycol poisonings: mechanism of toxicity, clinical course, diagnosis and treatment. *Med Toxicol* 1986;1:309–334.
36. Jacobsen D, Hewlett T, Webb R, et al: Ethylene glycol intoxication: evaluation of kinetics and crystalluria. *Am J Med* 1988;84;145–152.
37. Friedman E, Greenberg J, Merrill J, et al: Consequences of ethylene glycol poisoning. *Am J Med* 1962;32:891–902.
38. Pons C, Custer R: Acute ethylene glycol poisoning: a clinico-pathologic report of eighteen fatal cases. *Am J Med Sci* 1946;211:544–552.
39. Underwood F, Bennett W: Ethylene glycol intoxication. *JAMA* 1973; 226:1453–1454.
40. Terlinsky A, Grochowski J, Geoly K, et al: Identification of atypical calcium oxalate crystalluria following ethylene glycol ingestion. *Am J Clin Pathol* 1981;76:223–226.
41. Linnanvuo-Laitinen M, Huttunen K: Ethylene glycol intoxication. *Clin Toxicol* 1986;24:167–174.
42. Steinke W, Arendt G, Mull M, et al: Good recovery after sublethal ethylene glycol intoxication: serial EEG and CT findings. *J Neurol* 1989;236:170–173.

43. Hewlett T, Jacobsen D, Collins T, et al: Ethylene glycol and glycolate kinetics in rats and dogs. *Vet Hum Toxicol* 1989;31:116–120.
44. Cadnapaphornchai P, Taher S, Bhathena D, et al: Ethylene glycol poisoning: diagnosis based on high osmolal and anion gaps and crystalluria. *Ann Emerg Med* 1981;10:94–97.
45. Cheng J, Beysolow T, Kaul B, et al: Clearance of ethylene glycol by kidneys and hemodialysis. *Clin Toxicol* 1987;25:95–108.
46. Kreisberg R, Wood B: Drug- and chemical-induced metabolic acidosis. *Clin Endocrinol Metab* 1983;12:391–411.
57. Clay K, Murphy R: On the metabolic acidosis of ethylene glycol intoxication. *Toxicol Appl Pharmacol* 1977;39:39–49.
48. Gabow P: Ethylene glycol intoxication. *Am J Kidney Dis* 1988;11: 277–279.
49. Ahmed M: Ocular effects of antifreeze poisoning. *Br J Ophthalmol* 1971;55:854–859.
50. Palmer B, Eigenbrodt E, Henrich W: Cranial nerve deficit: A clue to the diagnosis of ethylene glycol poisoning. *Am J Med* 1989;87: 91–92.
51. Levy R: Renal failure secondary to ethylene glycol intoxication. *JAMA* 1976;173:1210–1213.
52. Collins J, Hennes D, Holzgang C, et al: Recovery after prolonged oliguria due to ethylene glycol intoxication. *Arch Intern Med* 1970; 125:1059–1062.
53. Haupt M, Zull D, Adams S: Massive ethylene glycol poisoning without evidence of crystalluria: a case for early intervention. *J Emerg Med* 1988;6:295–300.
54. Karlson-Stiber C, Persson H: Ethylene glycol poisoning: experiences from an epidemic in Sweden. *J Toxicol Clin Toxicol* 1992;30:565–574.
55. Steinhart B: Case report: Severe ethylene glycol intoxication with normal osmolal gap—"A chilling thought." *J Emerg Med* 1990;8: 583–585.
56. Winter M, Ellis M, Snodgrass W: Urine fluorescence using a Wood's lamp to detect the antifreeze additive sodium fluorescein: a qualitative adjunctive test in suspected ethylene glycol ingestions. *Ann Emerg Med* 1990;19:663–667.
57. Bennett I, Cary F, Mitchell G, et al: Acute methyl poisoning: a review based on experiences in an outbreak of 323 cases. *Medicine* 1953;32: 431–463.
58. Bohn G, Nicolson I, Owens J: A report of a fatal accidental methanol self-poisoning. *Med Sci Law* 1974;14: 219–221.
59. Scrimgeour E, Dethlefs R, Kevau I: Delayed recovery of vision after blindness caused by methanol poisonings. *Med J Aust* 1982;2:481–483.
60. Scrimgeour E: Outbreak of methanol and isopropanol poisoning in New Britain, Papua New Guinea. *Med J Aust* 1980;1:36–38.
61. Scully R, Galdabini J, McNeely B: Case 38-1979: presentation of a case. *N Engl J Med* 1979;301:650–657.
62. Swartz R, Millman R, Billi J, et al: Epidemic methanol poisoning: clinical and biochemical analysis of a recent episode. *Medicine* 1981; 60:373–382.
63. Hashemy-Tonkabony S: Postmortem blood concentration of methanol in 17 cases of fatal poisoning from contraband vodka. *Forensic Sci* 1975;6:1–3.
64. Posner H: Biohazards of methanol in proposed new uses. *J Toxicol Environ Health* 1975;1:153–171.
65. Becker C: Methanol poisoning. *J Emerg Med* 1983;1:51–58.
66. Becker C: The alcoholic patient as a toxic emergency. *Emerg Med Clin North Am* 1984;2;47–60.
67. Stegink L, Brummel M, McMartin K, et al: Blood methanol concentrations in normal adult subjects administered abuse doses of aspartame. *J Toxicol Environ Health* 1981;7:281–290.
68. Chinard F, Frisell W: Methanol intoxication: biochemical and clinical aspects. *J Med Soc N J* 1976;73: 712–719.
69. Dutkiewicz B, Konezalik J, Karwacki W: Skin absorption of administration of methanol in man. *Int Arch Occup Environ Health* 1980; 48:81–88.
70. Kahn A, Blum D: Methyl alcohol poisoning in an 8-month-old boy: an unusual route of intoxication. *J Pediatr* 1979;94:841–843.
71. McCormick M, Mogabgab E, Adams S: Methanol poisoning as a result of inhalational solvent abuse. *Ann Emerg Med* 1990;19:639–642.
72. Grufferman S, Morris D, Alvarez J: Methanol poisoning complicated by myoglobinuric renal failure. *West J Med* 1985;3:24–26.
73. McMartin K, Makar A, Martin A, et al: Methanol poisoning: the role of formic acid in the development of metabolic acidosis in the monkey and the reversal by 4-methylpyrazole. *Biochem Med* 1975;13: 319–333.
74. McMartin K, Ambre J, Tephly T: Methanol poisoning in human subjects. *Am J Med* 1980;68:414–418.
75. Sejersted O, Jacobsen D, Ovrebo S, et al: Formate concentrations in plasma from patients poisoned with methanol. *Acta Med Scand* 1983; 213:105–110.
76. Emmett M, Narins R: Clinical use of the anion gap. *Medicine* 1977; 56:38–54.
77. Sharpe J, Hostovsky M, Bilbao J, et al: Methanol optic neuropathy: a histopathological study. *Neurology* 1982;32:1093–1100.
78. Martin D, Naughton J: Acute methanol poisoning: "the blind drunk." *West J Med* 1981;135:122–128.
79. Closs K, Solberg C: Methanol poisoning. *JAMA* 1970;211:497–499.
80. Fulop M: Methanol intoxication. *Lancet* 1982;1:338.
81. Heath A: Methanol poisoning. *Lancet* 1983;1:1139–1140.
82. Keeney A, Mellinkoff S: Methyl alcohol poisoning. *Ann Intern Med* 1951;34:331–338.
83. Hayreh M, Hayreh S, Baumbach G, et al: Methyl alcohol poisoning: ocular toxicity. *Arch Ophthalmol* 1977;95:1851–1858.
84. Dethlefs R, Naraqi S: Ocular manifestations and complications of acute methyl alcohol intoxication. *Med J Aust* 1978;2:483–485.
85. Jacobsen D, Jansen H, Wiik-Larsen E, et al: Studies on methanol poisoning. *Acta Med Scand* 1982;212:5–10.
86. Jacobsen D, Ostby N, Bredesen J: Studies on ethylene glycol poisoning. *Acta Med Scand* 1982;212:11–15.
87. Spillane L, Roberts J, Meyer A: Multiple cranial nerve deficits after ethylene glycol poisoning. *Ann Emerg Med* 1991;20:208–210.
88. Olson E, McEnrue J, Greenbaum D: Alcohols and miscellaneous agents. *Heart Lung J Crit Care* 1983;12:127–130.
89. Martens J, Verberckmoes R, Westhovens R, et al: Recovery without sequelae from severe methanol intoxication. *Postgrad Med J* 1982; 58:454–456.
90. Phang P, Passerini K, Mielke B, et al: Brain hemorrhage associated with methanol poisoning. *Crit Care Med* 1988;16:137–140.
91. McLean D, Jacobs H, Mielke B: Methanol poisoning: a clinical and pathological study. *Ann Neurol* 1980;8:161–167.
92. King L: Acute methanol poisoning: a case study. *Heart Lung J Crit Care* 1992;21:260–264.
93. Jacobsen D, Webb R, Collins T, et al: Methanol and formate kinetics in late diagnosed methanol intoxication. *Med Toxicol* 1988;3:418–423.
94. Galvan L, Watts M: Generation of an osmolality gap—ethanol nomogram from routine laboratory data. *Ann Emerg Med* 1992;21: 1342–1348.
95. Porter G: The treatment of ethylene glycol poisoning. *N Engl J Med* 1988;319:109–110.
96. Pappas S, Silverman M: Treatment of methanol poisoning with ethanol and hemodialysis. *Can Med Assoc J* 1992;126:1391–1394.
97. Garella S: Extracorporeal techniques in the treatment of exogenous intoxication. *Kidney Int* 1988;33:735–754.
98. Chew W, Berger E, Brines O, et al: Alkali treatment in methyl alcohol poisoning. *JAMA* 1946;130:61–64.
99. Bergeron R, Cardinal J, Geadah D: Prevention of methanol toxicity by ethanol therapy. *N Engl J Med* 1992; 307:1528.
100. Wacker W, Haynes H, Druyan R, et al: Treatment of ethylene glycol poisoning with ethyl alcohol. *JAMA* 1965;194:173–175.
101. Freed C, Bobbitt W, Williams R, et al: Ethanol for ethylene glycol poisoning. *N Engl J Med* 1981;304:976–977.
102. Peterson C: Oral ethanol doses in patients with methanol poisoning. *Am J Hosp Pharmacol* 1981;38:1024–1027.
103. Peterson C, Collins A, Keane W, et al: Reply to Dr. Freed et al (editorial). *N Engl J Med* 1981;304:977–978.
104. Curtin L, Kraner J, Wine H, et al: Complete recovery after massive ethylene glycol ingestion. *Arch Intern Med* 1992;152:1311–1313.
105. Robertson C, Sellers E: Alcohol intoxication and the alcohol withdrawal syndrome. *Postgrad Med J* 1978;64:133–138.
106. Noker P: Methanol toxicity: treatment with folic acid and 5-formyl tetrahydrofolic acid. *Alcohol Clin Exp Res* 1980;4:378–383.
107. Van Stee E, Harris A, Horton M, et al: The treatment of ethylene glycol toxicosis with pyrazole. *J Pharmacol Exp Ther* 1975;192:251–259.

108. McMartin K, Collins T: Distribution of oral 4-methylpyrazole in the rat: inhibition of elimination by ethanol. *J Toxicol Clin Toxicol* 1988; 26:451–466.
109. Narins R, Emmett M: Simple and mixed acid-base disorders: a practical approach. *Medicine* 1980;59:161–185.
110. Becker C: Acute methanol poisoning. *West J Med* 1981;135: 122–128.
111. Jacobsen D, Sebastian C, Barron S, et al: Effects of 4-methylpyrazole, methanol/ethylene glycol antidote, in healthy humans. *J Emerg Med* 1990;8:455–461.
112. Gonda A, Gaunt H, Churchill D, et al: Hemodialysis for methanol intoxication. *Am J Med* 1978;64:749–759.
113. Keyvan-Larijarni H, Tannenberg A: Methanol intoxication: comparison of peritoneal dialysis and hemodialysis treatment. *Arch Intern Med* 1974;134:293–296.
114. Vale J, Prior J, O'Hare J, et al: Treatment of ethylene glycol poisoning with peritoneal dialysis. *Br Med J* 1982;284:557.
115. Osterloh J, Pond S, Grady S, et al: Serum formate concentrations in methanol intoxication as a criterion for hemodialysis. *Ann Intern Med* 1986;104:200–203.

CHAPTER 39

Work-Up of the Patient with an Acid-Base Disorder

The preceding three chapters discussed the acute ingestion of ethanol and ethanol substitutes, many of which may offer the clinician a diagnostic challenge. Yet, physicians seldom entertain the possibility that an intoxicated patient may have ingested a toxic alcohol unless the presentation is complicated by coma, seizures, metabolic acidosis, or symptoms specific for such ingestions. This chapter discusses the work-up of a patient with an acid-base disorder that may involve some of the toxins previously discussed. A systematic plan for the work-up is presented.

The work-up of the alcoholic patient or a patient with suspected ethylene glycol or methanol ingestion presenting to the emergency department may consist of any or all of the following: electrolyte determinations, calculation of the anion gap, calculation of the osmolal gap, urinalysis, measurement of serum concentrations of potential toxic substances, electrocardiography (if available), and other studies (Table 39–1) (1).

SERUM ELECTROLYTES

Electrolytes should be measured because imbalances are relatively common in the alcoholic, usually as a result of nutritional deficiencies and dehydration (1). Serum electrolytes may also indicate an acid-base disorder (2).

TABLE 39–1. *Laboratory work-up of the alcohol-intoxicated patient*

Electrolytes
Anion gap
Arterial blood gas
Amylase
Ketones
Osmolal gap
Urinalysis
Serum concentrations of various agents
Electrocardiogram
Liver function tests
Complete blood cell count
Clotting studies

ANION GAP

The anion gap is an extremely useful aid in diagnosing disorders associated with both the alcoholic population and other groups with serious medical problems (3,4). Results of the serum electrolytes are necessary for this calculation, which is based on the measured cations (sodium) and anions (chloride and bicarbonate).

The formula for the calculation of the anion gap is

$$Na - (Cl + HCO_3)$$

This calculation of the anion gap is considered within normal limits if it is 8–12 mEq when potassium is not considered (2,3,5). Although potassium may be included in the formula, most experts do not recommend including K in the serum anion gap formula because its level is low in absolute terms and is not highly variable. The number obtained from this calculation can signify the type of acid-base disorder (6). Sodium is the only cation included in the formula for simplicity; the other cations are relatively stable and present in small concentrations (7). If the calcium or magnesium concentrations change greatly, however, the anion gap may be significantly altered (3). Even so, for all practical purposes laboratories do not routinely measure these cations because, in the normal state, sodium accounts for almost 90% of the extracellular cations (8).

Chloride and bicarbonate account for 85% of the extracellular anions (3,9). The unmeasured anions are albumin, which is an anion at physiologic pH, phosphate, sulfate, organic acids, and negatively charged proteins

TABLE 39–2. *Cations and anions not usually measured*

Anions
Proteins
Phosphate
Sulfate
Organic acids
Cations
Magnesium
Calcium

(Table 39–2). False elevations of serum chloride may result from the presence of other halide ions, as in patients intoxicated with bromide or iodide (10). These elevations occur because bromide and iodide interfere with both colorimetric and "ion-selective" techniques, resulting in reported values for chloride that exceed the sum of the true chloride concentration plus that of the other halide (8). Spurious hyperchloremia, with an equivalent apparent decrease in the anion gap, may also occur from the technical artifact caused by hypertriglyceridemia (3,11,12).

TABLE 39–3. *Causes of anion gap metabolic acidosis*

	Acronym: **A MUD PILE CAT**
A	Alcohol
M	Methyl alcohol
U	Uremia
D	Diabetic ketoacidosis
P	Paraldehyde
I	Iron, isoniazid
L	Lactic acidosis
E	Ethylene glycol
C	Carbon monoxide, cyanide
A	Aspirin
T	Toluene

Decreased Anion Gap

An anion gap of 7 mEq/L or less is unusual, but may be a clue to conditions such as multiple myeloma, halide poisoning, or an analytic artifact. The finding of a negative anion gap is helpful in that it indicates an analytic problem (13). Severe intoxication with lithium or magnesium reduces the anion gap by increasing unmeasured cations (14).

Severe hypoalbuminemia will reduce the anion gap by approximately 2.5–3.0 mEq/L for every gram/deciliter decline in the serum albumin level. Because albumin is also the principal component of so-called total weak acids, a decrease in plasma albumin concentration might result in so-called hypoproteinemic alkalosis (7).

Increased Anion Gap

For the most part, a significantly increased anion gap signifies a metabolic acidosis, although small increases in the anion gap (2–3 mEq/L) can be caused by dehydration or starvation ketosis (5), the administration of sodium salts, such as sodium sulfate for hypercalcemia, or the administration of certain antibiotics containing large amounts of sodium, such as disodium carbenicillin (in which the carbenicillin moiety acts as an anion and is not routinely measured) (4). In addition, respiratory alkalosis and hypocapnea may cause a slight increase in the anion gap.

An anion gap greater than 30 mEq/L usually indicates the presence of an organic acidosis. Values between 23 and 30 mEq/L are also suggestive of an organic acidosis, but the nature of the retained anion frequently cannot be established (6).

In a patient who is admitted with an acid-base disorder, the type of acid-base disturbance that has occurred must be determined. If the bicarbonate is low and there is an anion gap, it is necessary to know whether this reflects a respiratory alkalosis or a metabolic acidosis. Respiratory acidosis causes an increased gap because the primary defect is the enhanced pulmonary excretion of carbon dioxide, which lowers the serum bicarbonate concentration. If the disorder is due to an anion gap metabolic acidosis, further examination of the cause is appropriate. Both drug and nondrug causes should be considered (2,11). An acronym has been developed for causes of an anion gap metabolic acidosis (Table 39–3) (3,11).

Nondrug Causes of Anion Gap Metabolic Acidosis

Nondrug causes of an anion gap metabolic acidosis include lactic acidosis secondary to tissue hypoperfusion (as observed in hypotension and shock) or the body's inability to keep up with an increase in the metabolic demands (as seen in a grand mal seizure); diabetic ketoacidosis, in which the ketoacids contribute to the metabolic acidosis (15); alcoholic ketoacidosis in patients who are usually chronic alcoholics with a history of prolonged ethanol intake and a marked decrease in food intake before the development of the acidosis; and uremia due to the retention of sulfates, phosphates, urates, and unidentified acids (4,6,15,16). Not all ketones produce an acidosis; in fact, only β-hydroxybutyric acid and acetoacetic acid lead to acidosis. Acetone is a neutral ketone that does not change serum bicarbonate or affect the anion gap (3,16).

Drug Causes of Anion Gap Metabolic Acidosis

Drug causes of an anion gap metabolic acidosis include salicylates, which typically cause a respiratory alkalosis in adults (although a mixed acid-base picture can occur as well as an anion gap metabolic acidosis), iron, isoniazid, paraldehyde, toluene, Vacor, carbon monoxide, and cyanide (16).

Ethylene glycol can cause an anion gap metabolic acidosis because of the accumulation of glycolic acid (11). Methanol causes an anion gap metabolic acidosis because of the formation of formic acid. Both ethylene glycol and methanol can interfere with the Krebs cycle, resulting in lactic acidosis (4,16).

OSMOLAL GAP

In addition to the anion gap, the osmolal gap may also be helpful in making the diagnosis of an exogenous toxin (11,17). Osmolality is a reflection of the number of molecules of solute dissolved in a solvent or, in other words, of the total number of particles in a solution (18). In clinical practice, solute concentrations are measured per liter of solution (19). Usually sodium, urea, and glucose are the substances that primarily contribute to serum osmolality. In the normal state, the dependence of serum osmolality on electrolyte concentration is essentially a function of sodium alone (9).

Osmolality and Osmolarity

Osmolality differs from osmolarity only in that the number of particles are expressed per kilogram of solution rather than per liter, as in the case of osmolarity (20). Thus, osmolarity and osmolality are said to represent molar and molal concentrations of solutes, respectively (13).

For nonpolar solutes 1 mole of particles has an osmolarity defined as 1 Osm/L when dissolved in 1 L of solution. Polar solutes, such as sodium, contribute 2 Osm/L for each mole in solution because two osmotically active particles are obtained from each molecule. In general, osmolality is a measured parameter, whereas osmolarity is calculated (19).

The formula for the calculation of the serum osmolality is (2,3,9,11,18,19,21–24)

$$2(\text{Na}) + \text{glucose}/18 + \text{blood urea nitrogen}/2.8$$

The real osmotic coefficient for sodium chloride is 1.86, but the coefficient of 2 approximates the contribution that potassium, calcium, and magnesium would make (25). The units for glucose and blood urea nitrogen are milligrams per deciliter. The coefficients (or denominators) for glucose and urea are used to convert these values to millimolar concentrations (9). (When SI units are used, the formula is 2(Na) + glucose + blood urea nitrogen.) A normal serum osmolality is 280–295 mOsm/L of water (2,11). Normally, the calculated value is within 10 mOsm/L of the measured value (26). The calculated serum osmolality, however, does not take into account the possible presence of other osmotically active particles. When the measured value is greater than the calculated value by more than 10 mOsm, it is called an osmolal gap (16,21,27). This implies the presence of one or more exogenous, low-molecular-weight solutes in the blood (24). From a practical point of view the osmolal gap is normally less than 10 mOsm/L and consists mainly of calcium, lipids, proteins, and solutes not included in the formula (18).

An important reason for serum osmolality measurement is for detection of solute abnormalities when no primary disorder of sodium, glucose, or urea exists (21). Specifically, it is the detection of the hyperosmolal state caused by the presence of an osmotically active substance ordinarily absent from the blood (28). Typically, a substance contributes significantly to the osmolality of the serum only if it has a low molecular weight and achieves high blood concentrations (22).

Practically speaking, few drugs or intoxicants with the exception of the alcohols affect plasma osmolality (27). The alcohols that contribute in this regard are ethanol, methanol, ethylene glycol, and isopropanol (Table 39–4), with ethanol being the most commonly noted (21,29). Because the molecular weight of methanol is so low, it can produce a profound osmolal gap that can be 50% greater than that produced by ethanol (30). Although ethylene glycol has almost twice the molecular weight of methanol, the same amount of ethylene glycol produces only half the osmolal gap. An absence of an elevated osmolal gap with ethylene glycol, therefore, does not exclude the diagnosis of ethylene glycol intoxication, but detecting the presence of a gap can be crucial in making a rapid, accurate diagnosis (17). The osmolal gap is due to unchanged ethylene glycol itself; as it is metabolized, the osmolal gap decreases but the anion gap increases secondary to accumulation of glycolic acid. In addition to these alcohols, glycerol, mannitol (31), sorbitol, diatrizoate (a dye used in intravenous pyelography), and acetone can also contribute to an osmolal gap (19,28,32).

A lower than normal osmolal gap may be seen when water-insoluble substances are present in the blood; this is the case with hyperlipidemia or hyperproteinemia, in which the increase in plasma lipids or proteins in the serum causes an apparent reduction in the sodium and water concentration of the serum. Because globulins and lipids are not measured in osmolality, a low osmolal gap is reflected.

Two methods of osmolality measurement are freezing-point depression and vapor pressure. A vapor pressure osmometer is insensitive to the presence of volatile solutes in a sample, and the osmolality is not changed by these low-molecular-weight organic compounds. The

TABLE 39–4. *Substances that cause an osmolal gap*

Alcohols
Ethanol
Ethylene glycol
Isopropanol
Methanol
Propylene glycol
Sugars
Glycerol
Mannitol
Sorbitol
Diatrizoate
Acetone

TABLE 39–5. *Molecular weights of the alcohols*

Alcohol	Molecular weight
Ethanol	46
Ethylene glycol	62
Isopropanol	60
Methanol	32

TABLE 39–7. *Coefficients associated with the alcohols for use in osmolal gap calculations*

Alcohol	Coefficient
Ethanol	5
Methanol	3
Ethylene glycol	6
Isopropanol	6

advantage of vapor pressure osmometers is that they can measure grossly lipemic serum. Nevertheless, most laboratories use freezing-point depression rather than vapor pressure for measuring serum osmolality (11). A freezing-point depression osmometer responds with increased osmolality when volatile substances, such as alcohols, are present in high concentrations.

The osmolal gap is noted with all four alcohols. Its magnitude is proportional to the amount ingested and inversely proportional to the molecular weight (MW) of the alcohol (Table 39–5). Appropriate blood concentrations of each alcohol can be predicted from osmolality measurements by means of the following formula (2)

$$\text{Predicted serum concentration} = (\text{osmolal gap} - 10) \times \text{MW}/10$$

The osmolal gap can also be used in the formula because it has been shown that for every 100 mg of ethanol per deciliter the osmolal gap increases by approximately 20 (Table 39–6). The amount of ethanol (in milligrams per deciliter) can therefore be divided by 5 to give an approximation of the amount of ethanol in the body. The same is true for other alcohols and alcohol-like substances. A serum methanol concentration of 100 mg/dL, for example, adds approximately 31 mOsm/L to the osmolal gap (30).

Only molecules that are unable to pass through a semipermeable membrane exert osmotic pressure. Any molecule that can freely diffuse through cellular membranes does not exert osmotic pressure. Solutes such as urea, ethyl alcohol, methanol, and ethylene glycol pass through cells freely; therefore, although they raise the osmolality, they do not cause any fluid shifts (19). In contrast, accumulation of impermeable solutes, such as sodium or glucose, leads to water movement from cells, intracellular dehydration, and symptoms secondary to the fluid shifts.

TABLE 39–6. *Interpretation of osmolal gaps in the presence of alcohols*

Alcohol (100 mg/dL increment)	Increase in osmolal gap
Ethanol	22
Methanol	31
Ethylene glycol	16
Isopropanol	17

The simplicity of osmolal analysis of serum permits rapid identification of the presence of a toxin in advance of formal quantitative toxicologic assay. All patients in whom there is a suspicion of alcohol intoxication, especially those who are comatose or acidemic, merit osmolal screening. When present, the osmolal gap must be reconciled with measured ethanol concentrations to determine whether there are additional or alternate toxins.

It is possible to use the osmolal gap to estimate the concentration of an osmotically active molecule (9,11). For instance, if the measured serum osmolality is 380 mOsm/L and the calculated serum osmolality is 310 mOsm/L, the gap is 70. If the osmotically active substance is ethanol, the gap of 70 corresponds to a serum concentration of 300 mg/dL (70 – 10 = 60, 60 × 5 = 300 mg/dL) (33). The concentrations of methanol, isopropanol, and ethylene glycol can also be calculated from this formula (Table 39–7) (26).

There may be several causes of an elevated anion gap or osmolal gap, but there are few conditions, except the ingestion of methanol or ethylene glycol, that will concomitantly elevate both anion and osmolal gaps.

It should be remembered that significant levels of the toxic alcohols may be present despite a normal osmolal gap (34). An osmolal gap of 10 mOsm/kg water may represent an ethylene glycol level of 50 mg/dL if the patient's osmolal gap was initially zero. False negative results also have been reported by laboratories. Therefore, the suspicion of an ethanol substitute is supported by the presence of an osmolal gap, and may indicate the need for therapeutic interventions, but the absence of a gap does not rule out the presence of an ethanol substitute.

Very early or very late in the course of an intoxication with either ethylene glycol or methanol an osmolal gap may disappear. Although methanol and ethylene glycol are rapidly absorbed, if serum levels are drawn too soon after ingestion, significant blood levels will not be present, and hence, no osmolal gap will be found. In this circumstance, acidemia will not be present. Additionally, after the toxin has been completely metabolized, no osmolal gap will be present. However, acidemia may persist, reflecting the continued presence of the acidic metabolic products of the catabolized ethylene glycol or methanol.

TABLE 39–8. *Oxalate-rich plants and foods*

Diffenbachia
Rhubarb
Spinach
Cola drinks
Beets
Tea

URINALYSIS

A urinalysis may be useful in a patient suspected of being intoxicated with an alcohol-like substance; analysis should be directed toward evidence of crystalluria, ketonuria, proteinuria, microscopic hematuria, and myoglobinuria. Calcium oxalate crystals appear in the urinary sediment of an ethylene glycol–intoxicated patient in octahedral (dihydrate) (35) or envelope (36) form and, more commonly, in a monohydrate (dumbbell or rod) form. The monohydrate form has previously been misinterpreted as hippuric acid crystals (11,37,38). These findings must not be overinterpreted, however, because oxalate crystals can be a normal constituent of urine, especially when certain foods, such as rhubarb, spinach, tea, and cola drinks, are ingested (Table 39–8).

Because of the fluorescein-based coloring added to ethylene glycol preparations, if a 30-mL volume of antifreeze is ingested 0.6 mg of fluorescein is also ingested. This may be noted on Wood's lamp examination of the emesis, gastric aspirate, or urine if performed in a timely fashion. This could be an adjunctive diagnostic test while awaiting definitive quantitation analysis of serum ethylene glycol concentration (39).

SERUM CONCENTRATIONS OF VARIOUS AGENTS

It may be necessary to measure serum concentrations to make a diagnosis of ingested agents that can cause an anion gap metabolic acidosis. Salicylate, iron (and iron-binding capacity), methanol, ethylene glycol, isopropyl alcohol, and ethanol should be measured if there is a suspicion of ingestion of any of these substances. Other more sophisticated toxicologic analyses may also be required.

ELECTROCARDIOGRAM

An electrocardiogram should be performed if there is a suspicion of ingestion of an alcohol-like substance, as this test will find evidence of hypocalcemia (in ethylene glycol poisoning) or hypomagnesemia and hypokalemia (in ethanol poisoning) (27).

MISCELLANEOUS STUDIES

Liver function studies, a complete blood cell count, and clotting studies should also be performed for baseline values in the patient who has ingested an alcohol or alcohol-like substance.

REFERENCES

1. Goldfrank L, Starke C: Metabolic acidosis in the alcoholic. *Hosp Physician* 1979;15:34–38.
2. Becker C: The alcoholic patient as a toxic emergency. *Emerg Clin North Am* 1984;2:47–61.
3. Emmett M, Narins R: Clinical use of the anion gap. *Medicine* 1977; 56:38–54.
4. Gabow P, Kaehny W, Fennessey P, et al: Diagnostic importance of an increased serum anion gap. *N Engl J Med* 1980;303:854–858.
5. Scully R, Galdabini J, McNeely B: Case 38-1979: presentation of a case. *N Engl J Med* 1979;301:650–657.
6. Kreisberg R, Wood B: Drug- and chemical-induced metabolic acidosis. *Clin Endocrinol Metab* 1983;12:391–411.
7. Fenel V, Rossing T: Acid-base disorders in critical care medicine. *Ann Rev Med* 1989;40:17–29.
8. Oster J, Perez G, Materson B: Use of the anion gap in clinical medicine. *South Med J* 1988;81:229–237.
9. Dorwart W, Chalmers L: Comparison of methods for calculating serum osmolality from chemical concentrations, and the prognostic value of such calculations. *Clin Chem* 1975;21:190–194.
10. Sestoft L, Bartels P: Biochemistry and differential diagnosis of metabolic acidoses. *Clin Endocrinol Metab* 1983;12:287–302.
11. Epstein F: Osmolality. *Emerg Med Clin North Am* 1986;4:253–261.
12. Herr R, Swanson T: Psuedometabolic acidosis caused by underfill of vacutainer tubes. *Ann Emerg Med* 1992;21:177–180.
13. Wrenn K: Osmolality. *Ann Intern Med* 1991;114:337–338.
14. Winter S, Pearson R, Gabow P, et al: The fall of the serum anion gap. *Arch Intern Med* 1990;150:311–313.
15. Schelling J, Howard R, Winter S, et al: Increased osmolal gap in alcoholic ketoacidosis and lactic acidosis. *Ann Intern Med* 1990;113:580–582.
16. Adams S. Mathews J, Flaherty J: Alcoholic ketoacidosis. *Ann Emerg Med* 1987;16:90–97.
17. Turk J, Morell L: Ethylene glycol intoxication. *Arch Intern Med* 1986;146:1601–1603.
18. Lund M, Banner W, Finley P, et al: Effect of alcohols and selected solvents on serum osmolality measurements. *J Toxicol Clin Toxicol* 1983;20:115–132.
19. Gennari F: Serum osmolality: uses and limitations. *New Engl J Med* 1984;310:102–105.
20. Galvan L, Watts M: Generation of an osmolality gap-ethanol nomogram from routine laboratory data. *Ann Emerg Med* 1992;21:1343–1348.
21. Glasser L, Sternglanz P, Combie J. et al: Serum osmolality and its applicability to drug overdose. *Am J Clin Pathol* 1973;60:695–699.
22. Tintinalli J: Of anions, osmols and methanol poisoning. *JACEP* 1977; 6:417–421.
23. Felts P: Ketoacidosis. *Med Clin North Am* 1983;67:831–843.
24. Hoffman R, Smilkstein M, Howland M, et al: Osmolal gaps revisited: normal values and limitations. *J Toxicol Clin Toxicol* 1993:31: 81–93.
25. Doenicke A, Nebauer A, Hoernecke R, et al: Osmolalities of propylene glycol-containing drug formulations for parenteral use. Should propylene glycol be used as a solvent? *Anesth Analg* 1992;75:431–435.
26. Cadnapaphornchai P, Taher S, Bhathena D, et al: Ethylene glycol poisoning: diagnosis based on high osmolal and anion gaps and crystalluria. *Ann Emerg Med* 1981;10:94–97.
27. Tong T: The alcohols. *Crit Care Q* 1982;4:75–85.
28. Jacobsen D, Bredesen J, Eide J, et al: Anion and osmolal gaps in the diagnosis of methanol and ethylene glycol poisoning. *Acta Med Scand* 1982;212:17–20.
29. Robinson A, Loeb J: Ethanol ingestion—commonest cause of elevated plasma osmolality. *N Engl J Med* 1971;284:1253–1255.

30. Smith M: Solvent toxicity: Isopropanol, methanol, and ethylene glycol. *Ear Nose Throat J* 1983;62:126–135.
31. Huff J: Acute mannitol intoxication in a patient with normal renal function. *Am J Emerg Med* 1990:8:338–339.
32. Stem E: Serum osmolality in cases of poisoning. *N Engl J Med* 1974; 290:1026.
33. Snyder H, Williams D, Zink B, et al: Accuracy of blood ethanol determination using serum osmolality. *J Emerg Med* 1992;10:129–133.
34. Steinhart B: Case report: Severe ethylene glycol intoxication with normal osmolal gap—"A chilling thought." *J Emerg Med* 1990;8:583–585.
35. Madison L: Ethanol-induced hypoglycemia. *Adv Metab Disord* 1968; 3:85–109.
36. Williams H: Alcoholic hypoglycemia and ketoacidosis. *Med Clin North Am* 1984;68:33–38.
37. Godolphin W, Meagher E, Sanders H, et al: Unusual calcium oxalate crystals in ethylene glycol poisoning. *Clin Toxicol* 1980;16: 479–486.
38. Terlinsky A, Grochowski J, Geoly K, et al: Identification of atypical calcium oxalate crystalluria following ethylene glycol ingestion. *Am J Clin Pathol* 1981;76:223–226.
39. Winter M, Ellis M, Snodgrass W: Urine fluorescence using a Wood's lamp to detect the antifreeze additive sodium fluorescein: a qualitative adjunctive test in suspected ethylene glycol ingestions. *Ann Emerg Med* 1990;19:663–667.

CHAPTER 40

Associated Medical Conditions of the Alcoholic

It is important to know the associated medical conditions of the patient group that may be more likely to be poisoned by ethanol and ethanol substitutes. Knowing what disorders to expect will aid in understanding the rationale for the suggested workup of the patient.

The patient who chronically ingests an alcohol-like substance may present to the emergency department with an episode of ethanol intoxication, but there may be any number of associated medical conditions (Table 40–1). The chronic alcoholic may have evidence of alcoholic liver disease, cirrhosis, or neurologic abnormalities associated with alcohol intake (1). Mental deterioration, nystagmus, and ophthalmoplegias suggestive of Wernicke-Korsakoff syndrome may also occur (2,3). The alcoholic has many nutritional deficiencies that should be considered. Multiple vitamin deficiencies, including decreases in folate, thiamine, and vitamin B_{12}, are common (4,5). Complaints of abdominal pain may be secondary to liver disease, pancreatitis, gastritis, or Mallory-Weiss syndrome (6). Hematologic disturbances may consist of bleeding diathesis, thrombocytopenia, pancytopenia, or anemia (either macrocytic or microcytic). Hypothermia may be a problem secondary to exposure. Infection and the sequelae of trauma should always be considered in the alcoholic.

A concomitant ingestion of any drug should be considered in any patient with an altered mental status, but consideration should especially be given to the ingestion of ethylene glycol, methanol, and isopropyl alcohol because these are substances that are considered substitutes for ethyl alcohol (7,8).

The electrolyte disorders noted in this group can be varied and profound. Hypoglycemia may result from the depletion of glycogen stores and impairment of gluconeogenesis (9). Normally, blood glucose is maintained by liver glycogen stores, by gluconeogenesis, and by the amount of carbohydrate intake. The nutritionally deficient alcoholic also has decreased glycogen stores and is dependent on gluconeogenesis to maintain a normal blood glucose concentration. Because alcohol inhibits gluconeogenesis, hypoglycemia may result (10). This inhibitory effect appears to develop gradually, which accounts for the relatively slow decrease in serum glucose concentration and the late onset of symptoms of hypoglycemia after ingestion of alcohol (10). The ingestion of alcohol is the most common cause of profound, disabling, and lethal hypoglycemic coma in adults and children, although there does not appear to be a direct relationship between the blood alcohol concentration and hypoglycemia (11–13).

In normal adults, a fast of 42–72 hours is necessary to induce alcoholic hypoglycemia, whereas infants and children seem to be particularly susceptible to this condition.

TABLE 40–1. *Associated medical conditions in the alcoholic*

Alcoholic liver disease with cirrhosis
Polyneuritis
Mental deterioration (Wernicke–Korsakoff syndrome)
Cardiac toxicity
Nutritional deficiencies
Abdominal pain
Liver disease
Pancreatitis
Gastritis
Mallory–Weiss syndrome
Hematologic disturbances
Bleeding diathesis
Thrombocytopenia
Pancytopenia
Anemia
Macrocytic
Microcytic
Hypothermia
Infection
Trauma
Overdose
Ethylene glycol
Methanol
Isopropyl alcohol
Other toxins
Electrolyte disorder
Hypoglycemia
Hypomagnesemia
Hypophosphatemia
Hypokalemia
Acid-base disorder
Lactic acidosis
Ketoacidosis

Both the period of fasting and the latent period from time of ingestion of ethanol to hypoglycemic coma are shorter in children than in adults; an overnight fast has been sufficient to cause hypoglycemia in healthy infants and children (11,12,14). Although ethanol-induced hypoglycemia occurs most frequently in combination with malnutrition and chronic alcoholism, it also appears in both adult and adolescent "binge" drinkers (15).

Hypomagnesemia, hypophosphatemia, and hypokalemia may also be observed. These electrolyte disorders are thought to contribute to the dysrhythmias noted in the alcoholic population (16). Atrial fibrillation is the most frequent conduction abnormality noted and is followed by atrial flutter and isolated premature contractions (17). Alcoholic cardiomyopathy may also develop; this condition may have an insidious onset but may result in florid congestive failure.

Acid-base disturbances may be noted frequently, especially an anion gap metabolic acidosis secondary to lactic acidosis, ketoacidosis, or the concomitant ingestion of another drug causing an acidosis (18). Both lactic acidosis and ketoacidosis are related to the fact that alcohol depletes nicotinamide adenine dinucleotide (NAD) during its metabolism, which leads to a buildup of reduced NAD (NADH) (19,20). A functional block in NADH reoxidation also appears to exist, possibly because of the accumulation of acetaldehyde (Fig 40–1) (10,21). Lactic acidosis occurs because of inhibition of lactate transformation into pyruvate (22–24). Ketoacidosis is produced through the increased oxidation of fatty acids to acetoacetic acid, which is consequently reduced to β-hydroxybutyric acid and then cannot be reoxidized to acetoacetic acid (10,12).

Because β-hydroxybutyric acid is not measured by Acetest tablets or by a dipstick test (acetoacetate is the measured ketone), serum and urine ketones may be read as negative (24). Many times patients have no measurable blood alcohol concentration because they stopped their alcohol intake 24–72 hours before presentation and at the same time consumed few calories (9,10).

In addition to these disorders, alcoholic withdrawal and delirium tremens may present either as a life-threatening situation or a condition that requires medical intervention.

ALCOHOL WITHDRAWAL

Chronic consumption of alcoholic beverages can result in tolerance and physical dependence. Tolerance to ethanol occurs in alcoholism by three mechanisms. The metabolic rate may be increased significantly, largely because of increased metabolism by the microsomal ethanol oxidizing system. In addition, a cellular tolerance occurs as cell membranes make neurochemical adaptations. Behavioral tolerance is the third mechanism. It is postulated that addiction occurs after cellular adaptation, when ethanol is required for optimal neural function (25).

Because of the widespread abuse of ethyl alcohol, withdrawal from chronic ethanol consumption is the most common withdrawal syndrome encountered in the emergency department (26–30). Ethanol is a cellular depressant, so that with its abrupt cessation a rebound neuronal hyperexcitability occurs, the severity of which is directly related to the amount of ethyl alcohol that was regularly consumed (4,31).

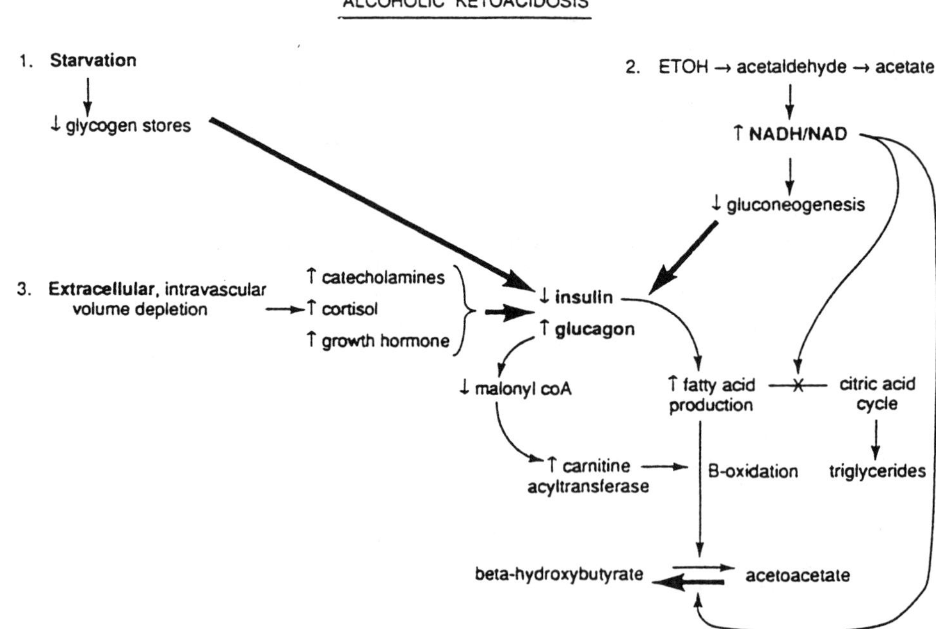

FIG 40–1. Simplified scheme of pathophysiology of alcoholic ketoacidosis. Reprinted with permission from the *American Journal of Medicine*.

Prolonged heavy alcohol intake causes a variety of changes in neurotransmission and neural functions (32). For example, adrenergic, cholinergic, serotonergic, tryptaminergic, and excitatory glutaminergic functions increase, while GABA-ergic, enkephalinergic, and, possibly, dopaminergic functions decrease during the acute withdrawal syndrome (1). The basic mechanisms behind these changes are multiple, including intramembrane effects of ethanol on receptor proteins embedded in the membrane, nonspecific changes in membrane properties, changes in neurotransmitter biosynthesis, or catabolism caused by ethanol's biotransformation.

The early stages of ethanol withdrawal are characterized by hyperactivity of the autonomic nervous system manifested by tachycardia and hypertension, diaphoresis, motor activity manifested by generalized tremulousness, and central nervous system hyperactivity manifested by insomnia and irritability (Table 40–2) (33,34). These withdrawal symptoms begin within 12–24 hours after the cessation of ethanol ingestion and may last for 48–72 hours.

The earliest and most common withdrawal syndrome is characterized by a generalized tremor, which may be accompanied by perceptual disturbances, autonomic hyperactivity, nausea, vomiting, insomnia, and a mild confusional state with agitation. The perceptual disorder may take the form of nightmares or of visual and auditory illusions or hallucinations. Symptoms begin within hours of the onset of withdrawal and are typically most pronounced at 24–36 hours. They can be suppressed by the resumption of drinking or by the administration of benzodiazepines, β-adrenergic receptor antagonists, or α_2-adrenergic receptor agonists. In severe reactions the early symptoms are followed by signs of increasing autonomic activity, disorientation, confusion, and auditory or visual hallucinations. Seizures may occur between 12 and 48 hours after drinking (35).

Acute ethanol withdrawal syndrome, with its inherent morbidity and mortality, can be complicated by its traditional pharmacologic management. Most patients experiencing acute alcohol withdrawal do not require pharmacologic intervention. A small percentage, however, may develop severe complications requiring pharmacologic intervention. Complications may include significant dysrhythmias or hypertension, seizures, hallucinations, and delirium tremens (36). In the past, sedative hypnotics, such as barbiturates, were used for withdrawal (5). These agents have their own inherent toxicity and their use has been discouraged, but they are still advocated by some authorities (37).

TABLE 40–2. *Signs and symptoms of ethanol withdrawal*

Mild to moderate
Tremor
Tachycardia
Hypertension
Diaphoresis
Insomnia
Irritability
Severe
Dysrhythmias
Hypertension
Seizures
Hallucinations
Delirium tremens

The benzodiazepines are now considered one of the safest classes of compounds for the treatment of alcohol withdrawal (38). They are prescribed to alcoholics more often than any other psychoactive drug (39). Not only are the benzodiazepines effective in suppressing the withdrawal symptoms and in treating or preventing seizures, but they also are of unequalled safety because they cause minimal respiratory and cardiac depression. These drugs may be abused by this group of patients, however.

Considerable evidence exists that a nonmedical setting without pharmacotherapy for detoxification can be safe, efficient, and effective in the uncomplicated patient undergoing mild to moderate withdrawal. However, patients with medical complications or with progressive or moderate to severe withdrawal should all be assessed medically, and pharmacotherapy on an outpatient or inpatient basis should be considered.

It has been shown that reassurance, reality orientation, frequent monitoring of signs and symptoms, and general supportive nursing care can be effective in decreasing the severity of selective alcohol withdrawal symptoms and signs (40). However, supportive care alone does not prevent the occurrence of seizures, hallucinations, or arrhythmias. Hence, pharmacotherapy is also required for all patients in moderate and severe alcohol withdrawal or with past histories or current evidence of complications.

In the last few years, clonidine has also been shown to be effective in reducing the adrenergic manifestations of both narcotic and alcohol withdrawal. The mechanism of action appears to be mediated through stimulation of centrally located α_2-adrenergic receptors. β-Blockers have also been used in alcohol withdrawal (41). Although they appear to be effective for the symptoms of withdrawal that are due to a hyperadrenergic state, they are of little value in preventing delirium or seizures. They may also be partially responsible for hallucinations (39).

Withdrawal Seizures

Seizures in withdrawal are typically single and generalized. If they occur, they most often develop between 6 and 48 hours after drinking has stopped. Electroencephalograph findings are usually normal or changes are nonspecific in nature. Management is required only if the seizures recur or are continuous or life threatening. Seizures usually respond to anticonvulsant therapy such as intravenous benzodiazepines (4,42). Many patients with alcohol withdrawal seizure disorder are also treated with phenytoin, which in this instance is of questionable efficacy (1,30,43). The development of status epilepticus has a high morbidity and mortality and should be aggressively treated. Patients who are having their first ethanol-related seizure should be hospitalized to undergo diagnostic studies and to be observed for the occurrence of additional seizures or delirium tremens (36).

Delirium Tremens

Disorientation and global confusion are the diagnostic criteria of delirium tremens, and typically appear 48–96 hours after drinking. In the early stages of alcohol withdrawal, patients may have a mild disorientation of their sense of time with some impairment of memory. Few patients go on to have true delirium tremens, which is a delayed and serious clinical manifestation of ethanol withdrawal (44,45). Delirium tremens is the most advanced stage of alcohol withdrawal and includes hallucinatory behavior associated with severe tremors and autonomic hyperactivity. The essential feature of delirium tremens is a delirium, with impaired attention and memory, disorganized thinking, disorientation, a reduced level of consciousness, perceptual disturbances, and agitation that develops after recent cessation of or reduction in alcohol consumption, usually within 1 week. It usually occurs 2–3 days after cessation of alcohol ingestion and may last 3–5 days. Most significant complications occur during this phase and may include seizures, dysrhythmias, and hyperthermia (38).

Neuroleptics may be required to control perceptual disturbances, thought disorders, or severe agitation in withdrawal. The butyrophenone class of antipsychotics is usually chosen because they cause less sedation and hypotension. Haloperidol may be used. Because haloperidol decreases seizure threshold, patients should also receive a benzodiazepine to offset any increased risk of seizures (43).

REFERENCES

1. Diehl A: Alcoholic liver disease. *Med Clin North Am* 1989;73:815–830.
2. DeKeyser J, Deleu D, Solheid C, et al: Coma as presenting manifestation of Wernicke's encephalopathy. *J Emerg Med* 1985;3:361–363.
3. Marx J: The varied faces of Wernicke's encephalopathy. *J Emerg Med* 1985;3:411–413.
4. Becker C: The alcoholic patient as a toxic emergency. *Emerg Clin North Am* 1984;2:47–61.
5. Scott R, Mitchell M: Aging, alcohol, and the liver. *J Am Geriatr Soc* 1988;36:255–265.
6. Tong T: The alcohols. *Crit Care Q* 1982;4:75–85.
7. Barnsley J, Sellers E: An interview study of hospitalized drug overdose patients. *Can Fam Physician* 1978; 24:850–855.
8. Patel A, Roy M, Wilson G: Self-poisoning and alcohol. *Lancet* 1972; 2:1099–1102.
9. Rangno R, Dumont C, Sitar D: Effects of ethanol ingestion on outcome of drug overdose. *Crit Care Med* 1982;10:180–185.
10. Halpern J, Davis J: Use and abuse of alcohol: further perspectives. *J Emerg Nurs* 1983;9:49–52.
11. Cardoni A: The alcohol in liquid medicinals: information for the pharmacist. *Guidelines Prof Pharm* 1978;5:1–2.
12. Varma B, Cincotta J: Mouthwash-induced hypoglycemia, editorial. *Am J Dis Child* 1978;132:930–931.
13. Sporer K, Ernst A, Conte R, et al: The incidence of ethanol-induced hypoglycemia. *Am J Emerg Med* 1992;10:403–405.
14. Weller-Fahy E, Berger L, Troutman W: Mouthwash: a source of acute ethanol intoxication. *Pediatrics* 1980;66:302–305.
15. Mizock B, Falk J: Lactic acidosis in critical illness. *Crit Care Med* 1992;20:80–93.
16. Goldfinger T, Schaber D: A comparison of blood alcohol concentration using non-alcohol and alcohol containing skin antiseptics. *Ann Emerg Med* 1982;11:665–667.
17. Petroni N, Cardoni A: Alcohol content of liquid medicinals. *Drug Ther* 1978;8:72–93.
18. Owen O, Caprio S, Reichard G, et al: Ketosis of starvation: a revisit and new perspectives. *Clin Endocrinol Metab* 1983;12:359–379.
19. Rubinstein J: Beware of these drugs when you prescribe for a recovering alcoholic. *Resident Staff Physician* 1980;62–66.
20. Wrenn K, Slovis C, Minion G: The syndrome of alcoholic ketoacidosis. *Am J Med* 1991;91:119–127.
21. Challoner K, McCarron M, Newton E: Pentazocine (Talwin®) intoxication: report of 57 cases. *J Emerg Med* 1990;8:67–74.
22. Moore J, Christian P, Datz F, et al: Effect of wine on gastric emptying in humans. *Gastroenterology* 1981;81:1072–1075.
23. Li T, Bosron W: Genetic variability of enzymes of alcohol metabolism in human beings. *Ann Emerg Med* 1986;15:997–1004.
24. Gibb K: Serum alcohol levels, toxicology screens, and use of the breath alcohol analyzer. *Ann Emerg Med* 1986;15:349–353.
25. Charness M, Simon R, Greenberg D: Ethanol and the nervous system. *N Engl J Med* 1989;321:442–454.
26. Koch-Weser J, Sellers E, Kalant H: Alcohol intoxication and withdrawal. *N Engl J Med* 1976;294:757–762.
27. Knott D, Lerner W, Davis-Knott T, et al: Decision for alcohol detoxication—a method to standardize patient evaluation. *Postgrad Med J* 1961;69:67–75.
28. Brown C: The alcohol withdrawal syndrome. *Ann Emerg Med* 1982; 11:276–280.
29. Brown C: Alcohol. *Ann Emerg Med* 1986;15:989–990.
30. Vance M: Drug withdrawal syndromes. *Top Emerg Med* 1985;7:63–68.
31. Rosenbloom A: Optimizing drug treatment of alcohol withdrawal. *Am J Med* 1986;81:900–904.
32. Wright C, Moore R: Disulfiram treatment of alcoholism. *Am J Med* 1990;88:647–655.
33. Baumgartner G, Rowen R: Clonidine vs chlordiazepoxide in the management of acute alcohol withdrawal syndrome. *Arch Intern Med* 1987;147;1223–1226.
34. Robertson C, Sellers E: Alcohol intoxication and the alcohol withdrawal syndrome. *Postgrad Med J* 1978;64:133–138.
35. Romach M, Sellers E: Management of the alcohol withdrawal syndrome. *Annu Rev Med* 1991;42:323–340.
36. Ng S, Hauser W, Brust J, et al: Alcohol consumption and withdrawal in new-onset seizures. *N Engl J Med* 1988;319:666–673.
37. Young G, Rores C, Murphy C, et al: Intravenous phenobarbital for alcohol withdrawal and convulsions. *Ann Emerg Med* 1987;16:847–850.
38. Liskow B, Goodwin G: Pharmacological treatment of alcohol intoxication, withdrawal and dependence: a critical review. *J Stud Alcohol* 1987;48:356–370.
39. Peachey J, Naranjo C: The role of drugs in the treatment of alcoholism. *Drugs* 1984;27:171–182.
40. Susick R, Zannoni V: Effect of ascorbic acid on the consequences of acute alcohol consumption in humans. *Clin Pharmacol Ther* 1987;41: 502–509.
41. Schelling J, Howard R, Winter S, et al: Increased osmolal gap in alcoholic ketoacidosis and lactic acidosis. *Ann Intern Med* 1990:113: 580–582.
42. Sellers E, Naranjo C, Giles H, et al: Intravenous diazepam and oral ethanol interaction. *Clin Pharmacol Ther* 1980;28:638–645.
43. Chance J: Emergency department treatment of alcohol withdrawal seizures with phenytoin. *Ann Emerg Med* 1991;20:520–522.
44. West L, Maxwell D, Noble E, et al: Alcoholism. *Ann Intern Med* 1984;100:405–416.
45. Merrin E: Withdrawal states and alcoholic hallucinosis. *Am J Psychiatr* 1980;137:1280–1281.

PART VIII

DRUGS OF ABUSE

CHAPTER 41

Drugs of Abuse: Overview

The use and misuse of mind-altering substances has existed since antiquity and the history of mankind is marked by the constant search for new substances and forms of previously used substances with mind-altering effects (1,2). Drug abuse is now one of the major health problems in the United States and is implicated in many deaths, both directly from overdose and indirectly as a result of injuries sustained while the individual is intoxicated. Further, the number of available pharmaceuticals has increased greatly during the last few decades, as has societal use and dependence on medicines. Americans take prescription medications at an astonishing rate (3,4). In addition, a large number of illicit drugs containing psychoactive substances are consumed each year (5). The problems resulting from substance use and abuse appear to be more extensive in our modern society than ever before because of this increased availability and the increase in the number of available substances (6). There seems to be no limit to the type of material used to carry or disguise the drug or drug combination. The United States seems to be at the forefront of the problem, but there are few countries whose youth are not involved (7,8).

The definition of drug or substance abuse varies, but is generally defined as the use of a chemical for a desired pharmacologic effect in a developmentally inappropriate way (9). It may be considered an excessive and persistent self-administration of a drug without regard for medically or culturally accepted patterns of use (10). The use of the drug may interfere with the health and social functioning of an individual. The terms use and abuse are used interchangeably in this section (11).

It is clear that, in discussing drugs of abuse, all sections of the community are involved—from the accidental ingestion of drugs by young children, to experimentation by youth, to the isolated individual for whom hallucinogens or hard drugs are part of a lifestyle, to the middle-aged "housewife" who is on the roller coaster of barbiturates or benzodiazepines and amphetamines, to the harried business executive who needs tranquilizers or alcohol to face the problems of his or her hectic world (12–14).

Drugs of abuse include any substance or chemical used to alter an individual's mood, sense of well-being, or psychologic conception of his or her relation to the environment (5). Sometimes, there is a fine line between where therapeutic use ends and abuse begins. Although there are major classes of drugs that are abused, such as stimulants, narcotics, sedative-hypnotics, and hallucinogens, there are also drugs that fit into no particular class. In this section, drugs of abuse are discussed in separate chapters according to pharmacologic class, and miscellaneous agents are also discussed separately.

Drug abusers may have a number of complaints referable to many systems because they frequently abuse more than one substance and often ingest a large proportion of unknown diluents that are added without the observance of proper sterile precautions (15). They may not know or may withhold valuable information. Usually, only the more severe and dramatic complications of drug misuse are seen in the emergency department (16). They may consist of toxic physiologic, psychologic, and behavioral manifestations, such as life-threatening reactions resulting from intentional and unintentional overdose and abstinence syndromes of varying intensity. The major drugs of misuse that bring patients to the clinician's attention are the opiates, sedative-hypnotics, alcohol, and central nervous system stimulants (17). This chapter serves as an overview of the problem of the misuse of drugs for recreational purposes.

Identification of the drugs used by an acutely intoxicated or overdosed patient usually depends on the clinical picture of the patient as well as a sound knowledge of various pharmacologic syndromes associated with drugs that are abused. It must be remembered that drugs of abuse may not be pharmacologically pure because of the adulterants or "cutting" substances used. Combinations meant to mimic or enhance a drug's effect may complicate and confuse diagnosis and treatment (15).

ROUTES OF ADMINISTRATION

A drug of abuse can be administered by any means, including orally, by insufflation ("snorting"), by smoking, and by injection subcutaneously ("skin popping"), intramuscularly, or intravenously ("mainlining") (Table

TABLE 41–1. *Routes of administration of drugs of abuse*

Oral
Insufflation ("snorting")
Smoking
Injection
Subcutaneous ("skin popping")
Intramuscular
Intravenous ("mainlining")
Intra-arterial ("pinkie")
Web spaces of fingers
Web spaces of toes
Dorsal vein of penis
Internal jugular vein ("pocket shot")
Subclavian vein ("pocket shot")
Sublingual
Mucosal membranes
Vagina
Penis

41–1) (18). Administration into the web spaces of the fingers and toes, into the sublingual area, as well as by the dangerous internal jugular or subclavian route, has been attempted. This last is referred to as the "pocket shot" and is an attempt to obtain venous access by injecting into one of the large veins in the neck (19,20). This is used by long-term addicts who no longer have peripheral venous access. The patients inject themselves while looking in the mirror or have someone else perform the procedure. Because of the proximity of the apical pleura to the internal jugular vein, this approach frequently causes a pneumothorax (21).

Drugs that are taken intravenously are usually heated in a spoon or bottle cap, drawn into a syringe or eye dropper through cotton or other homemade filters to remove large impurities, and then injected without cleaning the skin. Frequently the same syringe is used by several persons. Also, it should be remembered that street drugs are impure substances (15,22,22).

ADULTERANTS AND SUBSTITUTES—"CUTTING SUBSTANCES"

Although there are classic effects that can be expected from the drugs of abuse, the effects seen are often unpredictable because the purity of the drug is usually unknown. Drugs obtained on the street are always mixed with "cutting" substances in a ratio of 20:1 to 100:1, and it may be those substances that cause adverse reactions (24). Therefore, a dose may contain only 5%–20% of the desired substance and 80%–90% of "cutting" substances, many of which have significant actions of their own. Of all the drugs of abuse, heroin and cocaine represent two of the most extensively adulterated compounds on the street.

Diluents and adulterants are terms that refer to exogenous substances, either active or inactive, added to a specimen after its chemical synthesis or refinement, but before its retail sale. A diluent would be added to expand the size of a sample, such as the use of starches in the "cutting" of heroin. An adulterant is added to enhance or mimic the effect of the primary agent, e.g., the addition of phenylpropanolamine to cocaine preparations to augment cocaine's stimulatory effect.

Complications can arise from the pharmacologic effect of the drug itself, from intentional or unintentional overdosing, or from toxicity caused by other pharmacologically active agents present as impurities, diluents, adulterants, or substitutes for the abused substances (25).

In addition to the inherent toxic effects encountered with the abuse of licit and illicit drugs, the presence of adulterants superimposes another spectrum of possible complications for the drug abuser. A variety of contaminants and microorganisms in the injected solutions may invoke foreign body reactions and a wide variety of infectious disorders. Likewise, the substitution of active ingredients, the wide variations in potency after the "cutting" procedure, and the presence of these adulterant substances result in unpredictable clinical effects following their use (26).

A number of agents are used as cutting substances, among which quinine is the most favored. In addition to quinine, cutting substances for drugs of abuse include sugars, local anesthetics, baking soda, starch, stimulants (including caffeine), central nervous system depressants (including barbiturates), powdered milk, and easily obtainable narcotic-like substances, such as propoxyphene (Table 41–2) (27).

TABLE 41–2. *"Cutting" substances for drugs of abuse*

Quinine
Sugars
Lactose
Mannitol
Dextrose
Inositol
Sucrose
Local anesthetics
Procaine
Lidocaine
Benzocaine
Tetracaine
Strychnine
Stimulants
Pseudoephedrine
Phenylpropanolamine
Depressants
Barbiturates
Propoxyphene
Phencyclidine
Inert substances
Microcrystalline cellulose
Talc
Starches
Wheat
Flour
Cornstarch
Rice
Potato starch
Heavy metals

Quinine

Quinine is a bitter-tasting white powder that was first used as a heroin adulterant when there was an epidemic of malaria in New York. Its use has continued, and for many drug dealers it is the preferred adulterant for two reasons: its bitter taste prevents the buyer from being able to test the heroin content by tasting for bitterness, and, when injected intravenously, quinine produces a "flush" because of its vasodilator action, mimicking the effect of intravenously administered heroin. Quinine itself has gastrointestinal, auditory, neurologic, ophthalmic, and renal toxicity, and by itself it may be responsible for side effects and mortality (28).

Small doses can produce cinchonism, with tinnitus, headaches, visual disturbances, vertigo, nausea, vomiting, and diarrhea. Owing to the irritant nature of quinine, its use can lead to gastrointestinal manifestations if used orally; tissue irritation and lesions with intradermal, subcutaneous, or intramuscular use; or thrombosis and precipitous hypotension from rapid administration if used intravenously (24). When applied to the nasal mucosa, quinine is rapidly absorbed and causes marked local irritation. Large doses have produced tinnitus and facial flushing.

The most troublesome toxic effects arising from the use of quinine include visual disturbances and the appearance of cardiac conduction defects, arrhythmias, or hypotension. Severe poisoning has resulted in renal damage, acute hemolytic anemia, coma, and death by respiratory arrest. Quinine amblyopia has been observed in heroin addicts.

Sugars

The inert sugars lactose, mannitol, dextrose, inositol, and sucrose are commonly found in heroin and cocaine samples, probably because of the unrestricted availability of these sugars. These sugars are normally regarded as safe for human use, hence their appearance in many pharmaceutical and nutritional products. However, most safety data are based on oral consumption, not parenteral or intrapulmonary use.

Commonly found mixed with cocaine, inositol is a water-soluble vitamin that is metabolically converted to glucose and is involved in the biosynthesis of phospholipids. Aside from being very irritating to the nasal mucosa, inositol is not known to cause clinical toxic effects (24).

Local Anesthetics

This group of adulterants is commonly found in cocaine and heroin samples. During the 1970s, procaine was by far the most common anesthetic used, followed by lidocaine, benzocaine, and tetracaine. Procaine appears to be the least toxic of the group; lidocaine is considered two to three times as toxic, and tetracaine about seven times as toxic as procaine. Although considered quite safe when applied topically, benzocaine is extremely hazardous when injected, probably because of its relative insolubility.

It appears that intranasal cocaine users cannot distinguish lidocaine and procaine from cocaine. Likewise, smoking lidocaine apparently gives effects similar to that of free-base cocaine smoking.

Strychnine

Commonly available as a rodenticide, strychnine is also used as a cocaine adulterant. It is readily absorbed through mucous membranes and, by competitive antagonism with glycine in the central nervous system, produces central nervous system stimulation. The toxicologic effects noted with strychnine exposure include agitation, nausea, and vomiting, muscle twitching and spasm, opisthotonos, and seizures without a change in sensorium. Lactic acidosis, rhabdomyolysis, myoglobinuria, and acute renal failure may also complicate the clinical picture.

Stimulants

These agents are commonly found alone or in combination. Included in this class are ephedrine, pseudoephedrine, and phenylpropanolamine, all of which are direct adrenergic agonists, and which provoke the release of norepinephrine at adrenergic nerve endings. Although all are chemically similar to amphetamine, differences exist in the magnitude of the clinical effects produced.

Phenylpropanolamine, considered the most toxic of the group, has been associated with intracerebral hemorrhage, central nervous system depression, seizures, hypertension, and death. Significant cardiovascular effects have included cardiac conduction delays, arrhythmias, and myocardial infarction.

Phencyclidine

Phencyclidine is one of the most common pharmacologically active adulterants found in the street drug trade. It is absorbed well by oral, pulmonary, and nasal routes, and although it is considered a dissociative anesthetic, phencyclidine produces central nervous system stimulation or depression, hallucinations, and marked paranoid behavior. As the dosage escalates, catatonia, rhabdomyolysis, coma, respiratory depression, hyperthermia, and hypertension may ensue.

"Inert" Substances

Intravenous abusers who inject the contents of capsules or crushed tablets expose themselves to excipients normally employed as binders, fillers, and distintegrants in tablet and capsule manufacture. Some of these compounds are intentionally added to illicit drugs to increase bulk prior to sale. Although technically inert, these substances can cause extensive embolic damage to vessels of the lung, liver, kidneys, endocardium, and brain if injected intravenously.

Microcrystalline Cellulose

Inadvertent intra-arterial injection of microcrystalline cellulose obtained from crushed tablets has produced gangrene, and a variety of pulmonary vascular complications. It is proposed that the injection of this insoluble material induces foreign body granulomas and pulmonary angiothrombosis, resulting in pulmonary hypertension and vascular changes within the lungs.

Talc

Magnesium silicate is very common in heroin and cocaine street preparations. This insoluble powder is used pharmaceutically as a capsule lubricant, glidant, and anticaking agent. Although talc consists primarily of magnesium silicate, aluminum silicate is often present in the commercial grade product.

Because the addict often injects intravenous preparations intended for oral use, inert "fillers" are injected and may embolize to the lungs. The resultant angiothrombosis may eventually cause pulmonary hypertension and right ventricular failure. Pulmonary talcosis appears to be irreversible. Evidence indicates that it progresses in severity even after the abuser abstains. This is commonly seen in patients who crush pills for injection that contain talc particles. Although many pills contain talc, tripelennamine and methylphenidate are two of the major substances that have been implicated as the causative agent of granulomas.

Starches

Starch is produced from various plant sources and is used pharmaceutically to enhance tablet disintegration, to increase powder bulk, and to enhance dispersal of powders during tablet manufacture. Wheat, flour, corn, rice, and potato starch have been isolated in a variety of illicit drugs. The intravenous injection of cornstarch obtained from crushing oral tablets has been reported to induce foreign body granulomas, produce emboli in the retina, and result in neovascularization of the disc and retina. Cornstarch has not been associated with significant toxic effects when ingested or administered intranasally, but supposedly contributes to the adverse pulmonary effects when smoked with cocaine.

"Cotton Fever"

The term "cotton fever" was first used to describe this particular entity in 1975. Cotton has been implicated as the cause of cotton fever in addicts who experience febrile reactions after injecting drug suspensions that have been filtered through cotton balls. Heroin, as an example, is generally purchased in a powdered form and dissolved in water prior to injection. It is common practice to strain the suspended drug through cotton balls or cigarette filters to remove particulate material (29).

Cotton fever may be a reaction to pyrogens in the cotton, transient bacteremia, multiple pulmonary microemboli, a pyrogenic reaction to heroin, or some other occult mechanism. Current research favors endotoxin from Gram-negative rods as the causative agent, since all parts of the cotton plant are heavily colonized with Gram-negative rods, and hence contain endotoxin. In the context of intravenous drug use, cotton fever appears to be a benign, self-limiting condition that may present in a very dramatic fashion, closely mimicking serious sepsis.

The onset of symptoms is thought to be from 5–10 minutes after injection (Table 41–3). Symptoms include headache, malaise, chills, rigors, dyspnea, palpitations, nausea, emesis, abdominal pain, low back pain, myalgias, and arthralgias. Patients typically preset looking acutely ill. Temperatures of 38.5°C to 40.3°C develop within the first hours after injection. Patients frequently exhibit tachycardia and tachypnea despite otherwise normal cardiorespiratory examinations and chest radiographs. The abdomen is typically diffusely tender, with no rebound

TABLE 41–3. *Cotton fever*

Gastrointestinal
Abdominal pain
Nausea
Vomiting
Neurologic
Headache
Musculoskeletal
Low back pain
Myalgia
Arthralgia
Cardiorespiratory
Dyspnea
Palpitations
Sinus tachycardia
Miscellaneous
Fever
Malaise
Chills

tenderness. Guarding may be present and diffuse muscle and joint tenderness has been noted. The syndrome is self-limiting and resolves spontaneously in 12–24 hours in most cases (29).

LABORATORY ANALYSIS OF DRUGS OF ABUSE

Drug misuse is often incompatible with honesty. Deception, distortion, and denial are typical of drug abusers. Thus, the physician should be aware of techniques commonly used to adulterate the urine sample and of methods to overcome them. Supervision may reduce some deceptive techniques, such as substituting a urine specimen from a non–drug-using person (30). Adulterating or diluting the specimen is likewise common practice. Contaminants include sodium hypochlorite, salt, lemon juice, vinegar, ammonia water, soap solutions, or caustic compounds, all of which may interfere with certain immunoassay procedures (Table 41–4).

For forensic purposes, the urine specimen for drugs of abuse must be accounted for from its exit from the body during its transport in a labeled, sealed container over the course of laboratory analysis. If collection of the urine specimen is unsupervised, the urine pH, temperature, and specific gravity should be recorded immediately after voiding. The allegedly freshly voided urinary temperature should range between 33°C and 36°C and the urinary pH should range between 4.6 and 8.0 (30).

The urine toxicology screening procedures, usually involving various types of immunoassay, must be differentiated from the more familiar toxicology screen (coma or tox screen). Tests for drugs of abuse in urine can be divided into two types of analytic procedures: screening tests and confirmatory tests. Screening tests allow rapid and relatively inexpensive results. Confirmatory tests are necessary to reduce the number of false-positive results (31). The most widely available and least expensive test used to detect drug use is the enzyme immunoassay (EIA) test. Other screening tests include radioimmunoassay (RIA), fluorescence polarization immunoassay (FPIA), and thin layer chromatography TLC (32).

TABLE 41–4. *Drug of abuse testing*

Common adulterants
Bleach
Salt
Lemon juice
Vinegar
Ammonia
Soap solutions
Caustic compounds
Urine testing
pH (4.6–8.0)
Temperature (33°–36°C)
Specific gravity
Screening tests
Enzyme immunoassay (EIA)
Radioimmunoassay (RIA)
Fluorescence polarization immunoassay (FPIA)
Thin layer chromatography (TLC)
Confirmatory tests
Gas chromatography (GC)
High performance liquid chromatography (HPLC)
Mass spectrometry

Results of a patient's drug of abuse toxicology screen may depend largely on which analyzer the laboratory is using and what value the laboratory chooses to determine as its "cut-off" value for positive results. Although the "gold standards" in toxicology for the majority of drugs of abuse continue to be mass spectrometry, gas chromatography, or high performance liquid chromatography, many small laboratories are unable to purchase the instruments needed for these procedures.

CLASSIFICATION OF CONTROLLED SUBSTANCES

Although drugs of abuse can be classified in several ways, in this text they are classified according to their most prominent central nervous system effects. Classes include the narcotics and narcotic antagonists, sedative-hypnotics, stimulants, hallucinogens, phencyclidine, cannabinoids, volatile inhalants, and miscellaneous drugs (Table 41–5).

The Drug Enforcement Administration of the U.S. Department of Justice has categorized the controlled substances as narcotics, depressants, stimulants, hallucinogens, and cannabis; these categories reflect their medical utility and abuse potential. Many of the drugs of abuse fall under the Comprehensive Drug Abuse Prevention and Control Act of 1970, which is more familiarly known as the Controlled Substances Act. The Drug Enforcement Administration of the Department of Justice is responsible for enforcing the provisions of the Controlled Substances Act.

There are five categories or schedules that the government has compiled for many of the drugs of abuse. These schedules rank drugs from those with high potential of abuse to those with very little potential for abuse.

TABLE 41–5. *Classification of drugs of abuse*

Narcotics
Sedative-hypnotics
Central nervous system stimulants
Hallucinogens
Phencyclidine
Cannabinoids
Volatile inhalants
Miscellaneous agents

TABLE 41–6. *Schedule I drugs*

Heroin
Lysergic acid diethylamide (LSD)
Marijuana (tetrahydrocannabinol)
Hashish
Methylene dioxyamphetamine
Methylene dioxymethamphetamine
Mescaline
Peyote
Psilocybin

Schedule I

The drugs listed in Schedule I are believed to have the highest potential for abuse and have no recognized medical use except for experimental purposes. Substances in Schedule I include heroin, marijuana, and the hallucinogen lysergic acid diethylamide (LSD). Because Schedule I drugs are almost always used within research institutions, there are no specific prescription requirements (Table 41–6).

Schedule II

These drugs have legitimate medical uses but have a high potential for abuse. Most narcotics are listed in Schedule II, along with barbiturates, amphetamines, and cocaine (Table 41–7).

Schedule III

Drugs in Schedule III, with moderate potential for abuse, include nonbarbiturate sedatives, nonamphetamine stimulants, and some narcotic preparations (Table 41–8).

TABLE 41–7. *Schedule II drugs*

Amphetamine
Cocaine
Methylphenidate
Phenmetrazine
Amobarbital
Methaqualone
Pentobarbital
Secobarbital
Codeine
Fentanyl
Hydrocodone
Levorphanol
Meperidine
Methadone
Morphine
Opium
Oxycodone
Oxymorphone
Phencyclidine

TABLE 41–8. *Schedule III drugs*

Benzphetamine
Glutethimide
Methyprylon
Acetaminophen with codeine
Aspirin, phenacetin, and caffeine (APC) with codeine
Acetylsalicylic acid (aspirin) with codeine
Paregoric

TABLE 41–9. *Schedule IV drugs*

Diethylpropion
Phentermine
Chloral hydrate
Chlordiazepoxide
Clonazepam
Chlorazepam
Diazepam
Mephobarbital
Phenobarbital
Propoxyphene
Pentazocine
Meprobamate

Schedule IV

Drugs in Schedule IV have less abuse potential than those in Schedule III and have a limited likelihood of creating physical and psychological dependence. These include some sedatives and analgesics that do not contain narcotics (Table 41–9).

Schedule V

Drugs in Schedule V contain small amounts of narcotics and are used to control coughs and diarrhea. They have a low potential for abuse, may lead to limited physical and psychological dependence, and require the least amount of control and scrutiny.

"Designer Drugs"

The term "designer drug" was first coined in 1980 by a California pharmacologist to describe the private synthesis of drugs slightly different from parent compounds that, by design, render them temporarily immune from the control of the Drug Enforcement Agency (33). The loophole was that until a drug was isolated, studied, and scheduled, no laws could apply to it. Designer drugs are those created in illegal laboratories in attempts to circumvent the law by manufacturing substances that are not yet controlled (34). This is because the law currently requires that the chemical structure of a controlled substance be specified. Illegal laboratories create noncontrolled substances by altering the chemical structure of certain compounds (28). Drugs manufactured in this way are of the amphetamine type with psychomimetic properties, such as methylene dioxymethamphetamine, the fentanyl derivatives, and the meperidine derivatives (35).

In place of the reactive approach of placing new abused substances under restricted status as they appear, a more prospective method has been adopted in the form of an amendment to the Controlled Substances Act. This amendment places under Schedule I restriction those chemicals which: 1) have structures similar to those of existing Schedule I or II drugs, 2) are stimulants, depressants, or hallucinogens, or 3) are represented as such.

The concept of a designer drug specifically does not include new forms or new dosing routes of old drugs, such as cocaine used in the crystalline free-base form (crack). Nor does it include legal, although abused, alternatives to controlled substances: phenylpropanolamine, ephedrine, caffeine, and butyl nitrite, for example. The term "designer drug" also does not refer to such drug combinations as "T's and Blues" (Talwin [pentazocine] and tripelenamine), speedballs (cocaine or amphetamine and heroin), or star search (cocaine and phencyclidine) (28).

REFERENCES

1. Khantzian E, McKenna G: Acute toxic and withdrawal reactions associated with drug use and abuse. *Ann Intern Med* 1979;90:361–372.
2. McGuigan M: Toxicology of drug abuse. *Emerg Med Clin North Am* 1984:2:87–101.
3. Giannini A, Price W, Giannini M: Contemporary drugs of abuse. *Am Fam Phys* 1986;33:207–216.
4. Giannini A, DeFrance D: Metronidazole and alcohol—potential for combinative abuse. *J Toxicol Clin Toxicol* 1983;20:509–515.
5. Vogel S, Leikin J: What's up (and down) in drug abuse: street drugs. *Top Emerg Med* 1986;8:57–75.
6. Moriarty K, Alagna S, Lake C: Psychopharmacology. *Psychiatr Clin North Am* 1984;7:411–433.
7. Ficarra B: Toxicologic states treated in an emergency department. *Clin Toxicol* 1980;17:1–43.
8. Shulgin A: Drugs of abuse in the future. *Clin Toxicol* 1975; 8:405–456.
9. Kulberg A: Substance abuse: clinical identification and management. *Pediatr Clin North Am* 1986;33:325–361.
10. Chiang W, Goldfrank L: Substance withdrawal. *Emerg Med Clin North Am* 1990;8:613–631.
11. Montagne M: Drug-taking paraphernalia. *J Psychoact Drugs* 1983; 15:159–175.
12. Sanders J: Adolescents and substance abuse. *Pediatrics* 1985; 76:630–632.
13. Smith H, Talbott G, Morrison M: Chemical abuse and dependence: an occupational hazard for health professionals. *Top Emerg Med* 1985;7:69–78.
14. Pope H, Ionescu-Pioggia M, Cole J: Drug use and life-styles among college undergraduates. *Arch Gen Psychiatr* 1981;38:588–591.
15. Klatt E, Montgomery S, Namiki T, et al: Misrepresentation of stimulant street drugs: a decade of experience in an analysis program. *Clin Toxicol* 1986;24:441–450.
16. Taliaferro E, Rund D, Brown C, et al: Substance abuse education in residency training programs in emergency medicine. *Ann Emerg Med* 1989;18:1344–1347.
17. Goldfrank L, Bresnitz E: Opioids. *Hosp Physician* 1978;14:26–37.
18. Glassroth J, Adama G, Schnoll S: The impact of substance abuse on the respiratory system. *Chest* 1987;596–602.
19. Bell C, Borak J, Loeffler J: Pneumothorax in drug abusers: a complication of internal jugular venous injections. *Ann Emerg Med* 1983;12:167–170.
20. Lewis J, Groux N, Elliot J, et al: Complications of attempted central venous injections performed by drug abusers. *Chest* 1980; 78:613–617.
21. Wisdom K, Nowak R, Richardson H, et al: Alternate therapy for traumatic pneumothorax in "pocket shooters." *Ann Emerg Med* 1986; 15:428–432.
22. Brown J, Malone M: Status of drug quality in the street-drug market: an update. *Clin Toxicol* 1976;9:145–168.
23. Brown J, Malone M: Legal highs—Constituents, activity, toxicology, and herbal folklore. *Clin Toxicol* 1978;12:1–31.
24. Shesser R, Jotte R, Olshaker J: The contribution of impurities to the acute morbidity of illegal drug use. *Am J Emerg Med* 1991; 9:336–342.
25. Alldredge B, Lowenstein D, Simon R: Seizures associated with recreational drug abuse. *Neurology* 1989;39:1037–1039.
26. Schauben J: Adulterants and substitutes. *Emerg Med Clin North Am* 1990;8:595–611.
27. Sloan M, Kittner S, Rigamonti D, et al: Occurrence of stroke associated with use/abuse of drugs. *Neurology* 1991;41:1358–1364.
28. Beebe D, Walley E: Substance abuse: The designer drugs. *Am Fam Phys* 1991;43:1689–1698.
29. Harrison D, Walls R: "Cotton fever": a benign febrile syndrome in intravenous drug abusers. *J Emerg Med* 1990;8:135–139.
30. Schwartz J, Zollars P, Okorodudu A, et al: Accuracy of common drug screen tests. *Am J Emerg Med* 1991;9:166–170.
31. Schwartz R: Urine testing in the detection of drugs of abuse. *Arch Intern Med* 1988;148:2407–2412.
32. Osterloh J, Lee B: Urine drug screening in mothers and newborns. *Am J Dis Child* 1989;143:791–793.
33. Jerrard D: "Designer drugs"—a current perspective. *J Emerg Med* 1990;8:733–741.
34. Buchanan J, Brown C: "Designer drugs": a problem in clinical toxicology. *Med Toxicol* 1988;3:1–17.
35. Sternbach G, Varon J: "Designer drugs": recognizing and managing their toxic effects. *Postgrad Med* 1992;91:169–176.

CHAPTER 42

Associated Medical Conditions of the Drug User

In general, those individuals who misuse drugs, especially when parenterally administered, suffer medical complications that can be severe to life threatening. The clinician should always suspect a coexisting medical or psychological problem in patients abusing drugs. In this regard, the heroin abuser may share the same type of problem as that seen with the intravenous cocaine user, and for that reason some of the medical complications of parenteral drug abuse are discussed in this chapter (Table 42–1).

INFECTIONS SECONDARY TO CONTAMINATION

Intravenous drug abusers are subject to numerous infectious diseases, some of which may be life threatening (1–3). Because of the lack of sterile technique among users, in addition to their custom of sharing paraphernalia, it is not surprising that the complications of intravenous drug abuse are often the result of serious infections, including localized cellulitis or abscess, bacteremia with septic arthritis, osteomyelitis, bacterial or fungal endocarditis, pneumonia, hepatitis, tuberculosis, and malaria.

Bacteremia is the most common hematologic complication of parenteral drug abuse (4). This leads to "seeding" and infections in other organs. It has been shown that, in the febrile intravenous drug user, clinical data and clinical judgment on the part of the physician are not good predictors as to which patient may have a serious or life-threatening problem, such as endocarditis. For this reason, a policy of admitting all febrile intravenous drug users with a thorough work-up of the source of the fever is important. Symptoms of chest pain and shortness of breath are common in intravenous drug users. The differential diagnoses of these complaints include a pulmonary embolus or septic pulmonary emboli, pneumothorax, pericarditis, pneumonia, and endocarditis.

Malaria was first described as a complication of narcotic abuse more than 50 years ago (5). Any of the naturally occurring forms of malaria may be seen in the abuser, and "epidemics" have been reported in various

TABLE 42–1. *Complications of parenteral drug abuse*

Skin
Necrotizing fasciitis
Gangrene
Thrombophlebitis
Lymphedema
Hyperpigmentation
Cellulitis
Abscess
Systemic
Bacteremia
Endocarditis
"Cotton fever"
Osteomyelitis
Viral hepatitis
Malaria
Tetanus
Acquired immune deficiency syndrome (AIDS)
Pulmonary
Pneumonia
Pulmonary edema
Atelectasis
Pulmonary embolism
Tuberculosis
Pulmonary hypertension
Granuloma
Pneumothorax
Neurologic
Cerebral edema
Transverse myelitis
Homer's syndrome
Cerebral infarction
Intracerebral hemorrhage
Polyarteritis
Seizures
Renal
Nephropathy
Renal tubular acidosis
Rhabdomyolysis
Acute tubular necrosis
Eye
Endophthalmitis
Blindness
Metabolic
Hypokalemia
Metabolic acidosis
Hypophosphatemia

cities from shared needles. Recently this phenomenon has decreased, possibly owing to the quinine added as an adulterant. With the return of Vietnam war veterans, an increase in the incidence of malaria was noted and was confined to the West Coast, where quinine was not in great use. In general, the most common side effect of parenteral drug use and shared needles is both acute and chronic hepatitis (6).

PULMONARY SEQUELAE

Pulmonary abnormalities, such as pneumonia, pulmonary edema, atelectasis, fibrosis, granuloma formation, and pulmonary embolism are frequently found (7). Infarcts may progress to cavitation, abscess, or empyema formation. Pneumonia is usually the result of infection with pneumococcus, *Hemophilus* sp, or *Staphylococcus aureus* that is often unilateral and typically located in the right middle or lower lobe (7–9). These pulmonary infections have been ascribed to the septicemia that accompanies the skin infections and right-sided endocarditis that occurs in the abuser. The roentgenographic appearance in this instance may be that of pulmonary consolidation (5). In addition, the incidence of tuberculosis is increased in this population (3,8).

Pneumothorax can be a traumatic complication of parenteral drug abuse because a growing number of long-term drug abusers are resorting to the use of central veins, particularly the jugular or subclavian veins, as preferred sites for venipuncture; these abusers gradually obliterate peripheral veins by an infectious or sclerotic process (10,11).

Because marijuana may be contaminated with various fungi, various pulmonary fungal infections, such as *Aspergillus pneumonitis*, may be noted (7).

NONCARDIOGENIC PULMONARY EDEMA

Noncardiogenic pulmonary edema is a frequently associated medical finding in the drug abuser, and the clinician should be on the lookout for signs such as cyanosis, diffuse rales, tachypnea, tachycardia, and foamy sputum (12). Symptoms may occur after intoxication by any route of administration of most classes of illicitly used substances, including narcotics, cocaine, hydrocarbons, and sedative-hypnotics (7). Individuals who develop pulmonary edema may do so almost instantaneously after injecting the substance. More commonly, the onset may be delayed up to 24 hours after administration (7,13). Pulmonary edema is usually bilateral, although it may appear in one or only a part of one lung (14–16). The chest roentgenogram may display fluffy, ill-defined densities in an alveolar pattern, radiating centrally to peripherally, with a normal-appearing heart (17). Physical examination reveals rales and ronchi, but absence of peripheral signs, such as gallop heart sounds, increased jugular venous distension, or hepatomegaly. Swan-Ganz catheterization reveals a normal left ventricular end-diastolic pressure (18).

Despite the fact that noncardiogenic pulmonary edema has been recognized for many years, a well-accepted mechanism for this entity is lacking. The pulmonary capillary wedge pressure is normal. The best explanation appears to be an increase in the capillary permeability, causing leakage of fluid into the alveoli. Management is supportive, and if uncomplicated by aspiration the edema usually resolves over a period of hours (19).

CARDIAC SEQUELAE

The highest rates of morbidity and mortality associated with drug abuse involve the cardiopulmonary system (20). Endocarditis should be considered in any abuser presenting with fever of unknown etiology and especially in older addicts with heart murmurs, pulmonary infarction, splenomegaly, positive blood cultures, or systemic embolic phenomena (3,21). In many cases, fever is the only indication of endocarditis (22). Endocarditis, both right- and left-sided, may occur, although right-sided endocarditis is most common, sparing the pulmonic valve and attacking the previously normal tricuspid valve in almost all cases (5). This is unusual for endocarditis from other causes, which usually affects the left side of the heart. Because right-sided endocarditis is more common, this group of patients may not have the classic signs or symptoms, and there is usually no history of predisposing heart disease.

The causative organism in right-sided endocarditis is not usually fungal in nature but typically *S. aureus* (3,21). Usually, this is a "silent" problem, only seen by evidence of peripheral effects. The first clue to the presence of tricuspid regurgitation may be the existence of multiple or repeated septic pulmonary emboli that may simulate pneumonia (21). This is in contrast to left-sided endocarditis, where physical signs of valvular disease are invariably apparent. Although the valve attacked usually has been previously normal, a left-sided endocarditis may be superimposed on old syphilitic, atherosclerotic, or rheumatic damage or on a prosthesis (23).

S. aureus is the most common bacterial organism causing disease, although *Streptococcus* sp, *Esche-richia coli*, *Klebsiella* sp, and *Pseudomonas* sp are relatively common as well (6). Fungal endocarditis is always due to *Candida albicans* and is almost always fatal (3). Death from bacterial endocarditis is most frequently due to heart failure.

The abuser with bacterial endocarditis may present with peripheral embolization (24). Physical findings most well recognized are Janeway's lesions of the fingers, splinter hemorrhages under the nails, petechiae of the conjunctivae, and Roth's spots in the fundi. Organisms may be cultured from these sites (16).

SKIN LESIONS

Drug abusers are subject to several types of skin lesions, some of which are pathognomonic for drug abuse. Signs of venous injections vary from a subtle but definite hyperpigmentation over the injected area, usually antecubital, to the extreme "railroad tracks," (5,25) which are cutaneous scars due to the repeated puncture of the skin overlying the accessible veins (3). Because of the many adulterants in illicit opioids, the veins eventually become sclerotic and grey, forming these tracks (14). Tattoos may be imprinted over the course of veins in an attempt to hide the tracks. Hyperpigmentation or tattooing may also result from repeated carbon that is deposited by needles heated with a match before use.

Abscess formation at the site of injection is the most common skin infection encountered (2). Another set of skin lesions is related to the administration of drugs by "skin popping" or subcutaneous injection, possibly leading to bacterial or chemical abscesses. Lesions secondary to subcutaneous administration may be round macular depressions with sharp borders, giving a "punched-out" appearance (20). Another type of skin lesion is the rosette of a cigarette burn on the upper anterior chest wall, which is due to the addict "nodding out" with a lighted cigarette in the mouth (3).

Other dermatologic abnormalities include cellulitis, lymphangitis, and thrombophlebitis. The "puffy hand syndrome," seen in those with longstanding addiction, is the result of occlusive thrombophlebitis, lymphatic obstruction, and lymphedema (5,26). Necrotizing fasciitis has also been seen in the parenteral drug user (9). It may begin in a manner similar to that of cellulitis but quickly spreads to a central zone of necrosis with eventual ulceration. It is important to differentiate this disorder from cellulitis so as to institute more appropriate treatment with antibiotics as *Bacteroides* sp are frequent pathogens in necrotizing fasciitis (23). Gangrene, which is caused by intra-arterial injection, may be accompanied by intense pain distal to the injection site and is characterized by swelling, cyanosis, and coldness of the extremity.

The most common pathogens responsible for most of the soft tissue infections caused by a single bacterium are *Staphylococcus aureus* and β-hemolytic streptococci. Enteric Gram-negative bacilli as well as normal flora may occasionally be noted. Tetanus, which is an uncommon disease in the United States, has a much greater incidence in the population of drug users than in any other group and often results from "skin popping" with resultant subcutaneous abscess formation.

RENAL INVOLVEMENT

Renal abnormalities include nephropathy, glomerulonephropathy, and rhabdomyolysis with acute tubular necrosis.

ACQUIRED IMMUNE DEFICIENCY SYNDROME (AIDS)

The acquired immune deficiency syndrome (AIDS) is a severe disorder first described in male and female drug abusers, hemophiliacs, Haitians, and homosexual men (6). It is now known that it is not limited to any subgroup (27). In AIDS, the depression of the individual's cellular immune system results in subsequent development of multiple opportunistic infections, unusual neoplasms, and an inability to mount a delayed hypersensitivity response. Patients with AIDS may exhibit lymphopenia, cutaneous anergy, hypergammaglobulinemia, and a reversal of the ratio of helper to suppressor T cells. These patients most often present with *Pneumocystis carinii* pneumonia, other unusual community-acquired opportunistic infections, and Kaposi's sarcoma (9,27).

BONE AND JOINT INFECTIONS

Bone and joint infections, which are usually caused by *Pseudomonas aeruginosa*, may occur in the lumbar spine, sternoclavicular joint, and cervical spine. Low back pain may therefore be due to an infection of the disk space rather than to muscle strain. The ^{99m}Tc bone scan is most helpful in localizing the site of infection before changes are visible in plain radiographs.

NEUROLOGIC ABNORMALITIES

Neurologic abnormalities include cerebral edema and transverse myelitis. The mechanism for these is unclear. Horner's syndrome from injection into the neck has also been reported (28). One common abnormality is an atraumatic mononeuropathy, which appears as a painless weakness shortly after injection. Seizures may be secondary to the effect of the drug, the adulterants of the compound, or from withdrawal from a drug of abuse (29). Cerebral infarction has been a sequela of intravenous drug abuse, either immediately after injection or hours later (30). This can be a direct result of the injection or secondary to infective endocarditis, with the cerebrovascular complications of embolization and subarachnoid hemorrhage being due to rupture of a mycotic aneurysm. Vascular changes due to polyarteritis (necrotizing angiitis) have been reported in persons who use amphetamines intravenously (principally methamphetamine) (9). These changes frequently result in cerebrovascular occlusion and intracerebral hemorrhage. Central nervous system stimulants administered parenterally or orally may also cause intracerebral or subarachnoid hemorrhage (30).

METABOLIC ABNORMALITIES

Inhalation of paint and glue has been associated with severe metabolic abnormalities, such as metabolic acidosis, which is often accompanied by hypokalemia, hypophosphatemia, renal tubular acidosis, and, occasionally, renal failure (31). Liver necrosis has been reported as a complication of solvent abuse, whereas cardiac fibrillation has been associated with inhalation of the fluorinated hydrocarbons. Solvents, such as methylethyl ketone and hexane, can produce motor polyneuropathy.

Many abusers, because they know about the problems of associated infections, take nonprescribed antibiotics that are purchased on the street to prevent infections. This may lead to a delay in proper treatment, may suppress bacterial growth in cultures, and may be a major factor promoting the development and spread of resistant organisms (32).

OPHTHALMIC ABNORMALITIES

Endophthalmitis is a serious and increasingly common ocular complication of intravenous drug abuse (33). Endophthalmitis is an inflammation of the ocular tissues. Bacterial endophthalmitis, which consists of eye pain and redness, lid swelling, and decreased or blurred vision, may develop suddenly within 24–48 hours after drug use (34). This condition should be suspected if pain, chemosis, lid edema, and anterior chamber and vitreous inflammation are present. Mycotic endophthalmitis has also been recognized as a complication of intravenous drug abuse. Species of *Candida, Aspergillus, Torulopsis, Helminthosporium*, and *Penicillium* have been reported to cause endophthalmitis secondary to intravenous drug use. The mycotic endophthalmitis, unlike bacterial endophthalmitis, has a slow, indolent course. In addition to endogenous metastatic endophthalmitis, talc retinopathy and ophthalmic manifestations of endocarditis may be caused by intravenous drug abuse (34).

Blindness has been reported from quinine amblyopia. Although permanent blindness is rare, a permanent reduction of visual acuity is not uncommon.

REFERENCES

1. Orangio G, Latta P, Marino C, et al: Infections in parenteral drug abusers. *Am J Surg* 1983;146:738–740.
2. Orangio G, Pitlick S, Latta P: Soft tissue infections in parenteral drug abusers. *Ann Surg* 1984;199:97–100.
3. Sapira J: The narcotic addict as a medical patient. *Am J Med* 1968;45:555–588.
4. Kozel N, Adams E: Epidemiology of drug abuse: an overview. *Science* 1986;234:970–974.
5. Sternbach G, Moran J, Eliastam M: Heroin addiction: acute presentation of medical complications. *Ann Emerg Med* 1980;9:161–169.
6. Aston R: Drug abuse: its relationship to dental practice. *Dent Clin North Am* 1984;28:595–610.
7. Glassroth J, Adama G, Schnoll S: The impact of substance abuse on the respiratory system. *Chest* 1987;596–602.
8. Gottlieb L, Boylen T: Pulmonary complications of drug abuse. *West J Med* 1974;120:8–16.
9. Jacobson J, Huschman S: Necrotizing fasciitis complicating intravenous drug abuse. *Arch Emerg Med* 1982;142:634–635.
10. Bell C, Borak J, Loeffler J: Pneumothorax in drug abusers: a complication of internal jugular venous injections. *Ann Emerg Med* 1983;12:167–170.
11. Lewis J, Groux N, Elliot J, et al: Complications of attempted central venous injections performed by drug abusers. *Chest* 1980; 78:613–617.
12. Duberstein J, Kaufman D: A clinical study of an epidemic of heroin intoxication and heroin-induced pulmonary edema. *Am J Med* 1971;51:704–714.
13. Steinberg A, Karliner J: The clinical spectrum of heroin pulmonary edema. *Arch Intern Med* 1968;122: 122–127.
14. Kulberg A: Substance abuse: clinical identification and management. *Pediatr Clin North Am* 1986;33:325–361.
15. Kushner D, Szanto P: Heart failure, fever and splenomegaly in a morphine addict. *JAMA* 1958;166:2162–2165.
16. Jaffe R, Koschmann E: Intravenous drug abuse: Pulmonary, cardiac and vascular complications. *Am J Roentgenol* 1970;109:107–120.
17. Frand U, Shim C, Williams M: Heroin-induced pulmonary edema. *Ann Intern Med* 1972;77:29–35.
18. Karliner J: Noncardiogenic forms of pulmonary edema. *Circulation* 1972;46:212–215.
19. Carlet J, Francoual M, Lhoste F, et al: Pharmacological treatment of pulmonary edema. *Intensive Care Med* 1980;6:113–122.
20. Khantzian E, McKenna G: Acute toxic and withdrawal reactions associated with drug use and abuse. *Ann Intern Med* 1979;90:361–372.
21. Banks T, Fletcher R, Ali N: Infective endocarditis in heroin addicts. *Am J Med* 1973;55:444–451.
22. Nicholi A: The nontherapeutic use of psychoactive drugs. *N Engl J Med* 1983;308;925–933.
23. Shesser R, Jotte R, Olshaker J: The contribution of impurities to the acute morbidity of illegal drug use. *Am J Emerg Med* 1991; 9:336–342.
24. Ramsey R, Gunnar R, Tobin J: Endocarditis in the drug addict. *Am J Cardiol* 1970;25:608–618.
25. Westerhof W, Wolters E, Brookbakker J, et al: Pigmented lesions of the tongue in heroin addicts: fixed drug eruption. *Br J Dermatol* 1983;109:605–610.
26. Shuster M, Lewis M: Needle tracks in narcotic addicts. *NY State J Med* 1968;68:3129–3134.
27. Small C, Klein R, Friedland G: Community-acquired opportunistic infections and defective cellular immunity in heterosexual drug abusers and homosexual men. *Am J Med* 1983;74:433–441.
28. Hawkins K, Bruckstein A, Guthrie T: Percutaneous heroin injection causing Horner's syndrome. *JAMA* 1977;237:1963–1964.
29. Alldredge B, Lowenstein D, Simon R: Seizures associated with recreational drug abuse. *Neurology* 1989;39:1037–1039.
30. Sloan M, Kittner S, Rigamonti D, et al: Occurrence of stroke associated with use/abuse of drugs. *Neurology* 1991;41:1358–1364.
31. Voigts A, Kaufman C: Acidosis and other abnormalities associated with paint sniffing. *South Med J* 1983; 76:443–447.
32. Novick D, Ness G: Abuse of antibiotics by abusers of parenteral heroin or cocaine. *South Med J* 1984;77:302–303.
33. McLane N, Carroll D: Ocular manifestations of drug abuse. *Surv Ophthalmol* 1986;30:298–313.
34. Kreeger R, Pearson P, Bullock J, et al: Endophthalmitis associated with intravenous drug abuse. *Ann Emerg Med* 1987;16:585–587.

CHAPTER 43

Withdrawal from Drugs of Abuse

Continued administration of drugs of abuse may lead to physical dependence, which is closely related to tolerance. Often, the terms *drug dependence, drug abuse*, and *drug addiction* are used interchangeably. Dependence can either be physical, associated with intense physical discomfort upon the discontinuation of the drug, or psychological, associated with an uncontrolled pattern of use despite adverse consequences. All the narcotics and sedative-hypnotics produce both physical and psychological dependence. Physical dependence refers to an alteration of the normal functions of the body necessitating the continued presence of a drug to prevent the withdrawal or abstinence syndrome. The abstinence syndrome then is another facet of the drug abuser's problems that may be seen by emergency department personnel. Although the withdrawal syndrome from narcotics may be dramatic and temporarily disabling, it represents the least life-threatening or permanently disabling danger when compared with withdrawal from the sedative-hypnotics (1).

TOLERANCE

Tolerance is the phenomenon whereby frequent drug use necessitates an increased dosage to produce the same physiologic effects. Tolerance is closely associated with the phenomenon of physical dependence. It is largely due to compensatory responses that mitigate the drug's pharmacodynamic action.

Both the pharmacologic principles of pharmacokinetics and receptor adaptation can contribute to this phenomenon. Pharmacokinetic tolerance is based upon increased drug clearance associated with repeated exposure to an agent. Receptor tolerance is demonstrated by the fact that an increasing drug concentration is necessary to achieve the same physiologic effect when a drug is chronically used (2). Metabolic tolerance due to increased disposition of the drug after chronic use is occasionally reported. Behavioral tolerance, an ability to compensate for the drug's effects, is another possible mechanism of tolerance (3).

Tolerance is common with chronic use of opioids and sedative-hypnotics. The patient first notices a shorter duration of effect of the drugs. Tolerance can be delayed by giving nonopioid analgesics concurrently. Tolerance to most of the adverse effects of opioids, including respiratory and central nervous system depression, develops at least as rapidly as tolerance to the analgesic effect. Tolerance, therefore, can usually be surmounted and adequate analgesia restored by increasing the dose. Cross-tolerance exists among all of the full agonists, but it is not complete, and switching to another opioid, starting with half the equianalgesic dose, may be helpful.

DEPENDENCE AND ADDICTION

Dependence is marked by the onset of predictable signs and symptoms of withdrawal brought about by cessation of a drug. Administration of the drug during withdrawal will abort signs and symptoms of withdrawal. Drug use may be continued to offset the discomfort of withdrawal, particularly if the withdrawal is severe. Physical dependence is the altered physiologic state resulting from the continued administration of a drug. This continued administration is required to prevent the development of a predictable group of clinical, biochemical, and toxicologic manifestations, i.e., the withdrawal or abstinence syndrome. Physical dependence is invariably associated with a psychological dependence.

Patients who take strong opioids will develop physical dependence and abstinence symptoms if the drug is discontinued suddenly or an opioid antagonist is given. Physical dependence can be detected after a few days of therapy, but clinically significant dependence develops only after several weeks of chronic treatment with relatively large doses of morphine-like opioids. Patients who take opioids for acute pain or cancer pain rarely experience euphoria and even more rarely develop psychic dependence or addiction to the mood-altering effects of narcotics.

Addiction is the state of drug intoxication that is detrimental to the individual or to society. Although many of these individuals may develop physical dependence on these drugs, physical dependence is not a necessary feature of addiction.

Psychological Dependence

Psychological dependence is manifested by the often overwhelming drive to continue administration of a drug either to achieve pleasure or to avoid discomfort related or unrelated to a well-defined physical dependence.

Cross-Dependence

Cross-tolerance is the capacity of a tolerant individual to respond to a different chemical agent in a manner as though prior exposure had occurred and tolerance had been achieved. Cross-tolerance may be partial or complete, depending on the similarities of the pharmacologic effects of the two agents.

WITHDRAWAL SYNDROME

A withdrawal syndrome is a constellation of symptoms chronologically following the abstinence or decreasing use of the drug to which the patient has become dependent (4). These symptoms must not be present before the instillation of the drug, should evolve and resolve over a well-defined period of time, and can resolve with varying degrees of success upon reinstitution of the appropriate amount of the drug or a drug that renders cross-tolerance.

The clinical characteristics of these syndromes depend on the pharmacologic and toxicologic action of the drug, the patient, the rate of withdrawal from the agent, and the pharmacokinetics of the drug itself.

Frequently, there is a lack of predictability of who will manifest withdrawal under what circumstances, and when the clinical characteristics will be noted. However, once a withdrawal syndrome is noted in the individual, symptoms in future abstinence periods from the same drug are usually replicated (5).

Opioid Withdrawal

Individuals who are physically dependent on opiate agonists may remain relatively asymptomatic as long as they are able to maintain their daily opiate agonist requirement. Individuals who are morphine-dependent will usually continue to exhibit miosis while those who are dependent on methadone may develop some tolerance to miosis. The clinician needs to be alert to the high probability that the typical patient undergoing opiate withdrawal may also be undergoing withdrawal from other drugs, including alcohol, benzodiazepines, or barbiturates.

Tolerance and withdrawal are receptor phenomena. Because both enkephalins and opioid agonists decrease sodium permeability in opiate receptors, opioid administration decreases the baseline need for endogenous enkephalin production and secretion. As endogenous production and secretion decreases, more exogenous narcotic can be tolerated without excessive adverse reaction. Sudden cessation of opioid administration does not allow adequate time for resumption of enkephalin production. The increasing sodium permeability results in neuronal excitability and symptoms of withdrawal. The rate of metabolism of narcotics does not increase with prolonged usage, yet tolerance to the analgesic, sedative, and euphoric effects does. Tolerance does not develop to respiratory depression, which is the most common cause of death.

The mechanism of development of tolerance and physical dependence is not related to pharmacokinetic factors, but is a true cellular adaptive response that is associated with changes in second messenger systems related to Ca^{2+} flux, adenyl cyclase inhibition, or G protein synthesis. Chronic exposure and tolerance to opioids is associated with an elevation of intracellular Ca^{2+} content—unlike acute exposure, which often causes a decrease. The effect appears to be related to a change in the receptor's ability to associate with G coupling proteins, increased level of G proteins, and an up-regulated cAMP system. In addition, the number of receptors may be reduced by internalization and by reduced synthesis.

The onset and duration of opiate withdrawal symptoms are directly related to the pharmacologic and biologic half-life of the abused drug. Several weeks of continuous high-dose narcotic abuse are necessary before withdrawal symptoms may manifest. There may be times where street narcotics may not be concentrated enough to cause tolerance and dependency. In patients who have taken up to 80 mg of morphine sulfate daily for up to 1 month, withdrawal symptoms are usually slight and require little or no treatment. A severe abstinence syndrome occurs if the patient has received 240 mg or more of morphine sulfate for 30 days or longer (6).

If the abstinence syndrome is precipitated by the parenteral administration of naloxone, symptoms will be apparent within a few minutes and maximal within 30 minutes after administration. Effects will usually be more severe than those following withdrawal of the opiate agonist. Induction of methadone abstinence in this manner is especially severe. Because of naltrexone's long duration of antagonist effect, withdrawal precipitated by the drug may be prolonged. Until the antagonist has been eliminated, large doses of opiate agonists will only partially suppress these symptoms.

Some investigators consider opiate withdrawal a model for other conditions, such as naturally occurring anxiety or panic states in humans, and have suggested that it is mediated by a major noradrenergic nucleus in the locus coeruleus in the brain.

TABLE 43–1. *Signs and symptoms of narcotic withdrawal*

Abdominal cramps
Body aches
Diaphoresis
Diarrhea
Fever
Gooseflesh
Irritability
Loss of appetite
Nausea/vomiting
Nervousness
Rhinorrhea
Sneezing
Tachycardia
Yawning

Clinical Manifestations of Opioid Withdrawal

Narcotic withdrawal usually begins to appear close to the time when the individual would have been taking the next dose and gradually intensifies to peak severity at about 48 hours. It then diminishes until no overt signs remain 7–10 days after the last. The opioid withdrawal syndrome has both voluntary and involuntary characteristics. The voluntary manifestations are the patients' pleas, demands, manipulations, or even mimicking and exaggerating signs of withdrawal in an attempt to obtain their needed drugs. This voluntary behavior may occur before the development of any objective withdrawal symptoms.

Early signs and symptoms of narcotic withdrawal that are involuntary include yawning, lacrimation, rhinorrhea, and sweating about 8–10 hours after the last dose (Table 43–1). Thereafter, the addict may fall into a restless sleep. As the abstinence syndrome continues, symptoms may progress to piloerection ("gooseflesh"), restlessness, irritability, anorexia, flushing, diaphoresis, tachycardia, tremor, and mydriasis. The term "cold turkey" is derived from the gooseflesh that is part of narcotic withdrawal. Later in the course of withdrawal, the individual may experience fever, nausea, vomiting, and abdominal pain as well as diarrhea, spontaneous ejaculation (in males), and involuntary muscle spasms (from which the term "kicking the habit" derives) (7). The patient is weak and depressed, may be socially withdrawn, and at this point may become suicidal.

Withdrawal from Meperidine

In patients who are physically dependent on meperidine, abstinence symptoms usually occur 3–4 hours after the last dose of the drug, reaching maximal intensity within 8–12 hours. Although symptoms associated with meperidine withdrawal are generally milder than those of morphine withdrawal, during the period of maximal intensity, muscle twitching, restlessness, and nervousness may be worse than with morphine. Symptoms of meperidine withdrawal decline until few are apparent after 4–5 days.

Withdrawal from Methadone

Because of the cumulative effects of methadone, abstinence symptoms following its withdrawal are less intense and more prolonged than those following withdrawal of other opiate agonists and may not be manifested until 3 or 4 days after the last dose. Peak intensity of symptoms occurs on the sixth day and may include weakness, anxiety, anorexia, insomnia, abdominal discomfort, headache, sweating, and hot and cold flashes. Few symptoms are apparent after 10–14 days, although patients may exhibit lethargy and anorexia for longer periods.

Withdrawal from Other Opioids

Other opiate agonists produce abstinence syndromes similar to those described previously. In general, the shorter the onset and duration of action of the drug, the greater the intensity and rapidity of onset of withdrawal symptoms. Those drugs that are eliminated slowly produce a mild, prolonged abstinence syndrome.

In a medical sense, the withdrawal from narcotics generally is not life threatening. Because of the excessive loss of fluids through sweating, vomiting and diarrhea, there is usually marked weight loss, dehydration, ketosis, and disturbances in acid-base balance. Cardiovascular collapse may occur especially in aged or debilitated patients. Seizures do not occur as a part of opiate withdrawal unless the abuser was continually supplied with a sedative-hypnotic as part of the narcotic. In that case, the seizure is secondary to the withdrawal of the sedative-hypnotic.

If no treatment is given, most observable symptoms disappear in 5–14 days; however, there appears to be a phase of secondary or chronic abstinence that may last for 2–6 months after withdrawal of the drug. This phase is associated with gradually decreasing insomnia, irritability, and muscular aches. In addition, the patient may have miosis and a slight lowering of blood pressure, pulse rate, and body temperature; respiratory centers exhibit a decreased response to the stimulatory effects of carbon dioxide.

Treatment of Opioid Withdrawal

Not all cases of narcotic withdrawal require treatment, and without treatment the syndrome eventually runs its course. Although the signs and symptoms of narcotic withdrawal can be reversed by another narcotic, the administration of a narcotic for withdrawal is strictly proscribed by law (8). Although some patients prefer to detoxify without the use of medications, most are frightened of the withdrawal syndrome and prefer treatment and medication. If treatment is deemed necessary, it should be symptomatic and supportive and treat the acute physical discomfort experienced by the patient. A phenothiazine, such as promethazine, 25–50 mg every 4–6 hours as needed, may be administered for nausea and vomiting and a nonnarcotic pain medication, such as ibuprofen, 400 mg every 4 hours as needed, can be given for pain relief. A nonnarcotic antidiarrheal agent, such as loperamide, can also be administered (Table 43–2).

In the treatment of physical dependence, the patient may be detoxified by gradual reduction of daily opiate agonist dosage. Temporary administration of tranquilizers and sedatives may aid in reducing patient anxiety and opiate agonist craving. Symptoms involving gastrointestinal disturbance or dehydration should be treated accordingly. Supportive social, vocational, psychiatric, and educational services should be available to the patient.

Several approaches are available for opioid detoxification. Classically, methadone has been the agent of choice. Alternative therapeutic agents that have been used in the treatment of opiate dependency include α_2-agonists, such as clonidine, buprenorphine, L-α-acetyl methadol (LAAM), and naltrexone (4).

Methadone

Methadone is a synthetic opioid similar in structure to propoxyphene. It has been used for over two decades for the treatment of opiate detoxification and in methadone-maintenance programs for the management of physical dependence to opiates such as heroin. When methadone is used, heroin detoxification can be accomplished in a relatively short time, usually between 7 and 180 days. When detoxification lasts longer than 180 days it is considered maintenance therapy, but there are no official guidelines concerning the length of either maintenance or detoxification programs. Methadone maintenance programs must have both the Food and Drug Administration and the designated state authority approval. To receive methadone maintenance treatment the addict must have a 2 year history of opioid dependence and must be older than 16 years of age.

TABLE 43–2. *Treatment of opiate withdrawal*

Nonspecific treatment
Nausea/vomiting
Promethazine
Pain
Ibuprofen
Diarrhea
Loperamide
Specific treatment
Methadone
Heroin detoxification
Methadone maintenance
L-α-Acetylmethadol (LAMM)
Long acting cogener of methadone
α_2-Agonists
Eliminates subjective symptoms of withdrawal
Buprenorphine
Partial opioid agonist
Long duration of action
Does not cause physical dependence
Naltrexone
Oral opioid antagonist
Used in highly motivated individuals

Levo-α-acetylmethadol

Levo-α-acetylmethadol (LAAM) is a congener of methadone that has a longer duration of action than methadone. Abstinence from opiates is maintained for up to 72 hours, compared to about 24 hours with methadone, allowing LAAM administration three times a week.

Large clinical studies have shown that LAAM is safe, acceptable, and effective as an alternative maintenance treatment to methadone (5). It may require 2–4 weeks for the long acting LAAM metabolites to attain adequate concentrations to prevent withdrawal symptoms prior to the next dose (5).

LAAM is rapidly absorbed from the gastrointestinal tract. The onset of opioid effects is approximately 2–4 hours.

Common adverse effects of LAAM, similar to those found with methadone, have included excessive sweating, constipation, abdominal pain, decreased libido, and delayed or absent ejaculation.

Buprenorphine

Buprenorphine appears to be the most promising partial opioid agonist for use in the opioid-dependent population. It exhibits a long duration of activity and has affinity for both μ- and κ-receptors. Buprenorphine is unusual because it tightly binds and very slowly dissociates from the μ-receptors. This results in both a long-term analgesic effect and a blockade of morphine or heroin effects because their site of action is already occupied.

When given chronically, buprenorphine produces little physical dependence. Neither abrupt withdrawal nor challenge with naloxone results in a severe withdrawal syndrome, possibly due to the tight binding to the receptor such that it is not dislodged by the antagonist.

Because buprenorphine is a partial agonist, a withdrawal response should occur when a large dose is administered to a heroin addict. If withdrawal symptoms do occur, they might interfere with the initiation of buprenorphine treatment.

α_2-Agonists

α_2-Agonists effectively treat many of the symptoms of acute physical withdrawal. Although clonidine is most commonly used, other agents, such as lofexidine, guanfacine, or guanabenz may prove to be just as effective without causing unacceptable sedation or hypotension.

The administration of clonidine (Catapres) has been successfully used to eliminate objective and subjective symptoms of withdrawal. Clonidine's effects last for 4–6 hours after oral administration. It has been proposed that this drug works directly on the locus coeruleus in the brain to inhibit many of the symptoms of withdrawal. Although it may be used on an acute basis in the emergency setting, it is doubtful that it would be of great benefit to those who may require days or weeks of outpatient therapy. Clonidine should be used primarily in an inpatient setting because of its associated effects of dizziness, postural hypotension, dyscoordination, and sedation.

Clonidine is especially effective when it is combined with a benzodiazepine. Since the advent of a transdermal patches, benzodiazepines have been used with good success, in that they are thought to promote a smoother withdrawal. Because of the time required to reach a therapeutic blood level with transdermal administration, though, an initial oral dose should be given (1).

Narcotic Antagonists

Opioid antagonists block the euphoria, respiratory depression, and analgesia produced by the opioids and precipitate opioid withdrawal in individuals chronically using opioid agonists. A transient, explosive abstinence syndrome can therefore inadvertently be precipitated by the administration of naloxone or other antagonists. Within 5 minutes of injection of the antagonist, withdrawal signs and symptoms appear. They peak in 10–20 minutes and subside in about 1 hour (5).

Oral agents have been used in the highly motivated individual that has already withdrawn from an opioid and is now post-withdrawal. Naltrexone is a potent oral opioid antagonist that antagonizes opioid effects, produces no dysphoria or euphoria, and does not cause tolerance or physical dependence. Naltrexone has an elimination half-life of about 10 hours and can be given once daily or, in larger doses, three times weekly.

When used in the doses necessary to block opioid agonist effects, naltrexone is safe and well-tolerated. However, because it possesses no opioid-agonist properties, it has not been well accepted by the addict population. Consequently, the retention of addicts in naltrexone programs has generally been poor. Therapy with naltrexone may be a useful adjunct in the maintenance of opiate cessation in some individuals formerly physically dependent on opiates and who have successfully undergone detoxification. To avoid precipitation of a withdrawal reaction, initiation of naltrexone therapy should not begin until the patient has been opioid-free for 7–10 days.

Neonatal Opiate Withdrawal

Neonates born to mothers physically dependent on opiate agonists may also be opiate dependent and usually exhibit withdrawal symptoms from 1–4 days after birth. These symptoms include generalized tremors and hypertonicity with any form of tactile stimuli, hyperalertness, sleeplessness, excessive crying, vomiting, diarrhea, yawning, and, occasionally, fever. Neonates with severe withdrawal symptoms may be given diluted opium tincture or paregoric. After withdrawal symptoms are relieved, dosage should be decreased gradually and withdrawn completely over a 2- to 4-week period.

Sedative-Hypnotic Withdrawal

Many cases of sedative-hypnotic dependence are preceded by medically supervised administration for therapeutic purposes. The likelihood of serious withdrawal reactions depends on both the dose and the duration of use. The abrupt cessation or reduction of high doses of sedative-hypnotics may result in a characteristic withdrawal syndrome that closely resembles the alcohol withdrawal syndrome (9,10). It should be recognized as a medical emergency that may be more serious than that of most other drugs of abuse (Table 43–3). Long-term intoxication with the equivalent of 600–800 mg of pentobarbital or secobarbital is sufficient to produce clinically significant physical dependency, and the equivalent doses of any of the other sedative-hypnotics may also cause a severe abstinence syndrome, ranging from tremulousness and irritability to seizures, delirium, and death (10).

The short-acting barbiturates, such as pentobarbital and secobarbital, and the short-acting benzodiazepines, such as triazolam, produce an acute withdrawal syn-

TABLE 43–3. *Clinical features of sedative-hypnotic withdrawal*

Abdominal cramps
Diaphoresis
Hallucinations
Insomnia
Myoclonus
Orthostatic hypotension
Restlessness
Seizures
Status epilepticus
Tremors
Vomiting
Weakness

drome similar to that of ethanol. The long-acting barbiturates, as well as other benzodiazepines, have a delayed onset of withdrawal symptoms. Symptoms may begin 48–72 hours after the last dose, and the clinical course may be prolonged (9). As with barbiturates, dependence and withdrawal reactions are more likely after chronic use of the shorter acting agents, such as triazolam, temazepam, and alprazolam. Because these drugs are often prescribed for anxiety disorders, the withdrawal symptoms may be difficult to distinguish from the patient's underlying disorder.

Typically, withdrawal may manifest itself after 12–16 hours, with symptoms of apprehension and weakness, tremors, insomnia, diaphoresis, and restlessness. Vomiting and abdominal cramps may develop. Major withdrawal reactions include seizures and delirium. Although similar to alcohol withdrawal in many respects, some differences are noteworthy. Because the half-life of some barbiturates is longer, withdrawal symptoms may begin later, about 1–5 days after the last dose, usually peaking around 40 hours later. Symptoms usually decline over a period of about 2 weeks. Seizures are more severe and more likely to be multiple. Barbiturate withdrawal should thus be regarded as a life-threatening event requiring skilled medical management. With severe withdrawal, major symptoms and neurologic manifestations appear, as well as orthostatic hypotension and seizures. Symptoms usually peak during the second or third day of abstinence from the short-acting barbiturates or meprobamate, but this may be delayed until the seventh or eighth day of abstinence from the long-acting barbiturates or some of the benzodiazepines. It is during this peak period that the major withdrawal symptoms usually occur. Myoclonic muscular contractions, spasmodic jerking of the extremities, and grand mal seizures may develop, sometimes leading to status epilepticus. Often after the seizure, hallucinations and delirium may develop (11). The hallucinations are usually auditory and may be indistinguishable from those of delirium tremens associated with alcohol withdrawal.

Because of the serious nature of the withdrawal from sedative-hypnotics, patients should be under medical supervision. Specific treatment of the withdrawal consists of replacing the sedative-hypnotic with a short- or long-acting barbiturate and gradually tapering this dose over a period of time.

Ethchlorvynol Withdrawal

Ethchlorvynol produces psychological dependence, tolerance, and physical dependence. A daily dose of 1.5 g may produce physical dependence. This dose is easily reached as continued tolerance to the effects of ethchlorvynol occur (12). Withdrawal has been reported with the usual 500 mg dose after a 4–5 month exposure. As dependence continues, up to 4 g ethchlorvynol may be required to reach the desired effect.

Features of ethchlorvynol withdrawal include a schizophrenic state with affective blunting and tactile, visual, and auditory hallucinations. Approximately 9 days after disuse, delirium, schizoid reactions, and unusual anxiety with agitation may occur (12).

Stimulant Withdrawal

Long-term users of central nervous system stimulants such as cocaine and amphetamine may present to the emergency department in an attempt to abstain from the drug. These patients should be fully evaluated for associated signs of drug abuse and referred to an appropriate facility for detoxification and rehabilitation. There is a strong risk of psychologic dependency from cocaine, and there appears to be a pharmacologic basis for the withdrawal symptoms noted after abrupt cessation of cocaine. Consistent use of cocaine may result in depression when the drug is discontinued. Because the drug affects the dopaminergic neuronal systems, long-term use of cocaine depletes the nerve terminals of dopamine, which contributes to the dysphoria and depression that develops during withdrawal and the subsequent craving for more of the drug.

With long-term use of stimulants, serious depression and suicidal ideation may occur and can be quite prolonged. After long-term high-dose use, abusers exhibit a profound depression, apathy, and fatigue (Table 43–4). Many have a disturbed, restless, yet prolonged sleep, sometimes up to 20 hours a day (13). There may also be a lingering impairment of perception and thought processes. This incapacitating tenseness, anxiety, and suicidal tendency may persist for weeks or months. Precautions against suicide should be enacted for patients withdrawing from amphetamines.

Management of the central nervous system stimulant abstinence syndrome, for the most part, consists of reassurance that the symptoms will pass. Drug therapy is usually not required, yet, in recent years it has been thought that pharmacologic intervention might decrease the relapse rate following stimulant withdrawal. Dopamine precursors have been used in an attempt to raise dopamine concentrations in the brain. Dopamine agonists, such as amantadine (Symmetrel), which releases dopamine from storage sites, and bromocriptine

TABLE 43–4. *Clinical features of stimulant withdrawal*

Apathy
Disturbed sleep
Fatigue
Profound depression
Suicidal ideation

(Parlodel), a dopamine substitute, have been used to decrease craving. Tricyclic antidepressants have been used in an attempt to reduce depression and drug craving. Evidence that these measures are clinically effective is not sufficiently strong to recommend their routine use at this time.

Caffeine Withdrawal

Evidence suggests that habituation to caffeine may occur at relatively low dosages easily obtained by both children and adults. The withdrawal in some respects may resemble caffeine overdose and consist of headaches, irritation, nervousness, anxiety, nausea, rhinorrhea, dizziness, and mild depression. In addition, there may be an inability to work effectively. The headache is a clinically recognizable syndrome known as caffeine withdrawal headache, which responds to caffeine therapy. These symptoms begin within 12–24 hours after the last use, peak at 20–48 hours, and last approximately 1 week. Symptoms have been reported to occur after the cessation of doses of caffeine as low as 100 mg/day, the equivalent of about one cup of coffee, two cups of tea, or three cans of caffeinated soft drinks. Withdrawal may persist for up to 1 week but usually requires no specific treatment.

Phencyclidine (PCP) Withdrawal

Acute withdrawal symptoms following cessation of PCP use include nervousness, anxiety, and depression. These symptoms, when they occur, are mild. Pharmacologic detoxification is not required. However, the persistence of PCP's effects may require the use of haloperidol and a benzodiazepine for a period of time.

Cannabinoid Withdrawal

A mild abstinence syndrome consisting of irritability, restlessness, nervousness, decreased appetite, insomnia, mild tremor, slightly increased body temperature, and chills has been reported after chronic, high-dose use. In reality, acute cannabinoid abstinence syndrome is rarely seen. Most abusers have lethargy, apathy, and difficulty concentrating. Because of its mild nature, cannabinoid abstinence syndrome does not require pharmacologic treatment.

Hallucinogen Withdrawal

Hallucinogens are not associated with an abstinence syndrome; therefore, detoxification is not required.

Inhalant Withdrawal

An abstinence syndrome consisting of hallucinations, abdominal cramps, chills, and delirium tremens has been reported with heavy, chronic inhalation of solvents. However, this syndrome is rarely seen. Abstinence syndromes have not been reported with nitrites or nitrous oxide.

Detoxification is rarely required for the solvent and aerosol abstinence syndrome. Because of the lack of nitrite and nitrous oxide abstinence syndromes, detoxification from these agents is not required (14).

REFERENCES

1. Milhorn H: Pharmacologic management of acute abstinence syndromes. *Am Fam Phys* 1992;45:231–239.
2. Schauben J: Adulterants and substitutes. *Emerg Med Clin North Am* 1990;8:595–611.
3. Kulberg A: Substance abuse: clinical identification and management. *Pediatr Clin North Am* 1986;33:325–361.
4. Chiang W, Goldfrank L: Substance withdrawal. *Emerg Med Clin North Am* 1990;8:613–631.
5. Fraser A: Clinical toxicology of drugs used in the treatment of opiate dependency. *Clin Lab Med* 1990;10:375–386.
6. Guthrie S: Pharmacologic interventions for the treatment of opioid dependence and withdrawal. *DICP Ann Pharmacother* 1990; 24:721–734.
7. Klatt E, Montgomery S, Namiki T, et al: Misrepresentation of stimulant street drugs: a decade of experience in an analysis program. *Clin Toxicol* 1986;24:441–450.
8. Kreeger R, Pearson P, Bullock J, et al: Endophthalmitis associated with intravenous drug abuse. *Ann Emerg Med* 1987;16:585–587.
9. Vogel S, Leikin J: What's up (and down) in drug abuse: street drugs. *Top Emerg Med* 1986;8:57–75.
10. Sanders J: Adolescents and substance abuse. *Pediatrics* 1985; 76:630–632.
11. Wisdom K, Nowak R, Richardson H, et al: Alternate therapy for traumatic pneumothorax in "pocket shooters." *Ann Emerg Med* 1986; 15:428–432.
12. Yell R: Ethchlorvynol overdose. *Am J Emerg Med* 1990;8:246–250.
13. Kushner D, Szanto P: Heart failure, fever and splenomegaly in a morphine addict. *JAMA* 1958;166:2162–2165.
14. Skinner M, Thompson D: Pharmacologic considerations in the treatment of substance abuse. *South Med J* 1992;85:1207–1219.

CHAPTER 44

Narcotics

The term narcotic has a number of different meanings depending on the context in which it is used. Strictly speaking, narcotics are opiates, which are substances isolated from the opium poppy. Opioids are drugs, naturally occurring or synthetic, that have opium or morphine-like activity. Narcotics also include the semisynthetic opium derivatives, all of which produce tolerance and dependence and have the ability to suppress narcotic withdrawal (1). In the popular sense, narcotics include any drug that can be substituted for heroin or morphine in abuse potential. This definition includes the synthetic opium derivatives, some of which are incapable of suppressing narcotic withdrawal. All these drugs are considered opioids. Endogenous opioids are released in response to stress, electrical brain stimulation, acupuncture, and exogenous opioid analgesics. Unless otherwise noted, the terms opioid, opiate, and narcotic are used interchangeably.

Many times, emergency department personnel are approached by patients requesting drugs for symptoms, such as headache, migraine, toothache, or other subjective complaints. The sophisticated user may also claim an allergy to agents of low potency and may even suggest what drug to prescribe (2). Narcotics abusers may try to obtain meperidine, morphine, pentazocine, hydromorphone, oxycodone, and propoxyphene. This chapter is devoted to a discussion of the various legitimate narcotic agents that are available and yet may be abused as well as some of the "designer drugs" that have not found any accepted legitimate use.

CLINICAL USE OF OPIOIDS

A major use of the opioids is for relief of intense pain. Typically, there is a suppression of the perception of pain and a reduction in the response to pain without loss of consciousness. In addition to this major use, narcotics are also used as a cough suppressant, by their direct suppression of the cough centers in the medulla, for the treatment of diarrhea, and for the treatment of cardiogenic pulmonary edema. The opioids are also used preoperatively for sedation and as a supplement to anesthesia (Table 44–1).

TABLE 44–1. *Uses of narcotic agents*

Relief of intense pain
Antitussive agents
Antidiarrheal agents
Cardiogenic pulmonary edema
Preoperative sedation
Supplement to anesthesia

ENDORPHINS AND ENKEPHALINS

The discovery of the endorphins, which are endogenous analgesic polypeptides, has led to an enormous expansion of knowledge about opiate receptors in the brain and peripheral nervous system. These endogenous polypeptides act as specific neurotransmitters and, in the pituitary, as hormone modulators (3). Thus, they are involved in pain perception and analgesia, appetite regulation, respiration, temperature control, and the pathophysiology of shock (4). A number of other opiate peptides have been identified, including the enkephalins, dynorphin, and casomorphine (5–7). These peptides bind to several opiate receptors in the brain and peripheral nervous system to produce their physiologic actions, which affect virtually all functions of the body, including opiate drug addiction, epilepsy, regulation of pancreatic secretions, and non-insulin-dependent diabetes (Table 44–2) (8). The naturally occurring alkaloids morphine and codeine, their

TABLE 44–2. *Physiologic effects and functions of endogenous opiates*

Analgesia
Blood pressure regulation
Drinking regulation
Feeding behavior alteration
Hormone regulation
Mental function and memory alteration
Respiratory function alteration
Sexual function alteration
Temperature regulation

Adapted, with permission, from Atkinson R: Endocrine and metabolic effects of opiate antagonists. *J Clin Psychiatr* 1984;45:20. ©1984 Physicians Postgraduate Press Inc.

semisynthetic derivatives, and other synthetic agents all either contain or mimic a piperidine ring structure, which is the active component.

Tolerance develops to synthetic enkephalins and endorphins because they appear to mimic morphine in every respect (9). Enkephalin is rapidly destroyed in vivo, and endorphin is stable and has a long duration of action. The endorphins and enkephalins function as neurotransmitters by inhibition of sodium permeability in opiate receptors (10). This decreases sodium conductance and permeability, thus inhibiting neuronal activity. Opioid antagonists, on the other hand, increase sodium permeability and cell firing (9). In actuality, the mechanism may be much more complex and involve the calcium ion or cyclic AMP (11).

Opiate Receptors

Opiate receptors are present in the highest concentration in the limbic system, thalamus, striatum, hypothalamus, midbrain, and spinal cord. Five opioid receptor types have been identified in humans: μ, κ, σ, δ, and ϵ. At this time, only μ-, κ-, and σ-receptors have been associated with pharmacologic activity in humans (12,13). The μ-receptor is the classic morphine-like receptor, which mediates euphoria, physical dependence, respiratory depression, and supraspinal analgesia (3). These receptors are located mainly at supraspinal sites in the brain stem and limbic system (Table 44–3) (11). Recently two distinct μ-receptor subtypes designated μ_1 and μ_2 have been identified (14).

The μ-receptor is localized in pain modulating regions of the central nervous system; the κ-receptor is localized in the deep layers of the cerebral cortex; the δ-receptor is localized in the limbic regions of the central nervous system; and the σ-receptor is thought to mediate the dysphoric and psychotomimetic effects of some opiate partial agonists (e.g., pentazocine) (15). The κ-receptors, which mediate pentazocine-like analgesia, sedation, and miosis and perhaps respiratory depression, are located, with high density, in the spinal cord. The σ-receptor seems related to the dysphoric, hallucinogenic, and cardiac stimulant effects. Both the μ- and κ-agonists can produce tolerance and physical dependence, but the abstinence syndromes differ for different receptor agonists, and there is no cross-tolerance for the most part (Table 44–4) (5,16).

TABLE 44–3. *Location of opiate receptors*

Amygdala
Area postrema of the chemoreceptor trigger zone
Medial thalamus solitary nucleus
Periacqueductal gray matter of the brain stem
Substantia gelatinosa
Vagal nerve fibers

TABLE 44–4. *Opiate receptor system*

	μ-Receptor	κ-Receptor	δ-Receptor
Agonists	Morphine Morphine-like analgesics	Pentazocine Nalorphine Cyclazocine	Pentazocine Nalorphine Cyclazocine
Antagonists	Pentazocine Cyclazocine Nalorphine Naloxone Naltrexone	Naloxone Naltrexone	Naloxone Naltrexone
Clinical effects	Analgesia Euphoria Respiratory depression Miosis Physical dependence	Analgesia Sedation Miosis ?Respiratory depression	Dysphoria Delusions Hallucinations Respiratory stimulation Vasomotor stimulation

Adapted, with permission, from *Drug Intell Clin Pharmacol* 1981;15. ©1981 Harvey Whitney Books.

In addition to the μ-, κ-, and σ-receptors, δ-receptors for the enkephalins and epsilon receptors for the endorphins have been proposed (17). Since an opioid drug might function as an agonist, partial agonist, or antagonist at each of these multiple receptor types, it is not surprising that these agents are capable of diverse effects (3,9).

EXOGENOUS OPIOIDS

The exogenous opioids are substances that mimic the action of the endogenous opioids (18). These compounds bind to stereospecific receptors in the central nervous system and have at least some morphine-like activity (19). Exogenously administered opioids are analgesic by acting like endogenous opioid peptides at opioid receptors (18). Exogenously administered opioids also act in part by releasing endogenous opioid peptides (3).

Morphine, the prototype opiate agonist, has agonist activity at the μ- and κ-receptors, but has little, if any, activity at the σ-receptor. Morphine may also have some agonist activity at the δ-receptor. Agonist activity at the μ- or κ-receptor can result in analgesia, miosis, and decreased body temperature. Agonist activity at the μ-receptor can also result in suppression of opiate withdrawal, whereas antagonist activity can result in precipitation of withdrawal. Respiratory depression may be mediated by μ-receptors, possibly μ_2-receptors (which may be distinct from the μ_1-receptors involved in analgesia); κ- and δ-receptors may also be involved in respiratory depression. The agonist-antagonists are thought to bind to the μ-receptor and to compete with agonists, but either they exert no action (competitive antagonism) or they exert only limited action (partial agonism).

TABLE 44–5. *Summary of opioid agonist and antagonist effects*

Drug	Receptor μ	κ	σ
Butorphanol	Antagonist	Agonist	Agonist
Morphine	Agonist	Agonist	
Nalbuphine	Antagonist	Agonist	Agonist
Nalorphine	Antagonist	Partial agonist	Agonist
Naloxone	Antagonist	Antagonist	Antagonist
Pentazocine	Antagonist	Agonist	Agonist

Reprinted, with permission, from Zola E, McLeod D: Comparative effects and analgesic efficacy of the agonist-antagonist opioids. *Drug Intell Clin Pharmacol* 1983;17:411–417. ©1983, Harvey Whitney Books.

TABLE 44–6. *Opiate agonists, partial agonists, and antagonists*

Agonists	Partial agonists	Antagonists
Alphaprodine	Butorphanol	Naloxone
Codeine	Levallorphan	Naltrexone
Fentanyl	Nalbuphine	
Hydrocodone	Nalorphine	
Hydromorphone	Pentazocine	
Levorphanol		
Meperidine		
Methadone		
Morphine		
Opium		
Oxycodone		
Oxymorphone		
Propoxyphene		

Drugs can have activities at one or several of the receptors. They can also function as agonists, partial agonists, or competitive antagonists at one or more of these receptors (Tables 44–4 to 44–6) (12). Nalorphine, for example, appears to be a competitive antagonist at the μ-receptor, a partial agonist at the κ-receptor, and an agonist at the σ-receptor.

The mixed antagonists-agonists, such as pentazocine and cyclazocine, also produce analgesia, but act mainly at the κ-receptor in the spinal cord. Their addiction liability is low in comparison to the μ-activators because of their ability to block the agonistic tendency to develop tolerance.

TYPES OF NARCOTICS

Narcotic drugs can be divided into three groups: natural, semisynthetic, and synthetic (Table 44–7). Aspects of the medical use of the narcotic drugs follow a typical life cycle. Each new drug is initially hailed as a potent nonaddictive analgesic agent that can safely be made available to medical practice and may even be useful in the treatment of pre-existing opiate addiction; such was the history of morphine and heroin. It should be considered that all the opioids have the potential for abuse and dependence.

TABLE 44–7. *Partial list of natural, semisynthetic, and synthetic narcotics*

Natural	Semisynthetic	Synthetic
Opium	Heroin	Meperidine
Morphine	Hydromorphone	Methadone
Codeine	Oxymorphone	Levorphanol
Thebaine	Oxycodone	Butorphanol
		Pentazocine
		Paregoric
		Diphenoxylate
		Fentanyl
		Propoxyphene

Opioids can also be classified on the basis of function into three groups; morphine-like opioids, opioid antagonists, and agonist-antagonist/partial agonists. The morphine-like agonists act primarily on μ- and κ-receptors, with possible weak interaction with δ-receptors, in the nervous system to alter pain perception and various other physiologic functions. Antagonists occupy but do not activate receptor sites and therefore they competitively block receptor activation by other opioid drugs. Agonist-antagonist drugs produce varied effects depending on the predominance of agonistic or antagonistic activities on the different types of receptors.

Table 44–8 lists some of the commercially available narcotic preparations.

TABLE 44–8. *Trade names of selected commonly used narcotics*

Narcotic	Trade name
Meperidine	Demerol Mepergan Pethadol
Propoxyphene	Darvon Darvon-N Dolene Pargesic Profene
Methadone	Dolophine Methadose
Oxymorphone	Numorphan
Butorphanol	Stadol
Hydrocodone	Entuss Hycodan Ru-Tuss Vicodin
Hydromorphone	Dilaudid
Pentazocine	Talwin Talwin Nx
Nalbuphine	Nubain
Opium	Pantopon Parepectolin
Oxycodone	Percocet Percodan Tylox

Naturally Occurring Narcotics

The naturally occurring narcotics include opium, morphine, codeine, and thebaine.

Opium

The poppy *Papaver somniferum* is the primary source of the nonsynthetic narcotics. It was grown in the Mediterranean region as early as 300 BCE and is found in countries around the world, including Mexico, Hungary, Yugoslavia, Turkey, India, Burma, and China. The milky fluid that oozes from the unripe poppyseed pod is air dried to form raw opium. Clandestine laboratories then process the base drug to make morphine, codeine, or heroin in addition to the approximately 25 organic substances extractable from the parent compound.

Opium was an ingredient in old medicines, and there were no legal restrictions on the importation or use of opium until the early 1900s (20). At that time, patent medicines often contained opium without any warning label. Today, although a small amount of opium is used to make antidiarrheal preparations, such as paregoric, virtually all the opium imported into the United States is broken down into its alkaloid constituents, principally morphine and codeine. With the exception of concentrated opium alkaloids, hydrochlorides, and rectal suppositories containing powdered opium, opium preparations are rarely used for analgesia. Paregoric, which consists of a combination of opium, camphor, benzoic acid, and anise oil, is still prescribed for diarrhea in children. The anise oil is used to flavor the medication, and the benzoic acid acts as a preservative. Paregoric has been reported to cause toxicity, including pulmonary edema (21), so that there is little rationale for the use of this drug to treat gastrointestinal problems (21). Paregoric and opium tincture are used principally as antidiarrheal agents; paregoric and opium tincture have also been used to treat opiate withdrawal in neonates born to addicted mothers.

Morphine

Morphine was isolated as early as 1803 and was named for Morpheus, the Greek god of dreams and sleep (10). Morphine is a pure opiate agonist and is the principal constituent of opium, ranging from 4%–20%. Although morphine produces many diverse effects, such as drowsiness, changes in mood, respiratory depression, decreased gastrointestinal motility, nausea, vomiting, and alterations of the endocrine and autonomic nervous system, its most important effect is analgesia (22). It is considered the prototype of the opiate agonists (3). Morphine and some of its alkaloid surrogates act supraspinally at the μ-receptor to produce analgesia; the effects at this locus also account for the addiction liability of these compounds.

Parenteral morphine is widely used in medicine both as an analgesic as well as in the treatment of cardiogenic pulmonary edema. Orally administered morphine is about one-third to one-sixth as potent as parenteral morphine because of a large first-pass effect by the liver, whereby only a small percentage of an oral dose reaches the systemic circulation. The analgesic effects of morphine are usually maximal within 1 hour after administration, regardless of route. After subcutaneous or intramuscular injection of morphine, plasma concentrations reach their peak within 30 minutes.

The major metabolite, morphine glucuronide, is inactive as an analgesic. Although codeine is a metabolite of morphine, the amounts produced appear to be small. A large amount of morphine is used in the manufacturing of codeine and hydromorphone. Morphine is not a widely abused drug.

Codeine

Codeine is a pure opiate agonist and, although it is a naturally occurring ingredient of raw opium (1%–2%), most of the available codeine is produced from morphine. Codeine is approximately 20% as potent as morphine and is metabolized by enzymes in the liver to morphine, which then enters the brain and accounts for the pharmacological actions of the drug (6). Codeine has great use as an analgesic in the relief of mild to moderate pain that is not alleviated by nonopiate agonists, and it is extensively used as an antitussive. Some liquid antitussive codeine preparations include Robitussin A-C, Cheracol, and elixir of terpin hydrate with codeine. It is as an antitussive that codeine is most frequently abused. In addition, codeine has found abuse as a constituent of "loads," which is a combination of glutethimide and codeine. Because of its availability in a variety of oral forms with antipyretic analgesics, accidental ingestion and resultant overdose are not uncommon (15) (see Chapter 49).

Codeine and its salts are well absorbed from the gut, reaching a peak concentration 1–1.5 hours after the ingestion. The oral bioavailability of codeine is 70%, appreciably higher than that of morphine, making codeine an attractive oral narcotic. Codeine plasma elimination half-life 3–4 hours, and the drug is 25% protein bound (15).

With routine use the most frequent adverse effects of codeine are gastrointestinal, with reports of abdominal pain, cramping, constipation, and occasional nausea and vomiting. Fatal intoxications due solely to the ingestion of codeine are rare but have occurred (23). Deaths are more common when codeine is mixed with analgesics, antihistamines, or sedatives. Codeine is more stimulating to the spinal cord than other narcotics, and as a result delirium and seizures may occur during coma, although death occurs from respiratory depression (23,24).

Thebaine

Thebaine is a minor constituent of opium and is not a drug of abuse, but it can be converted to other abuseable drugs, including oxycodone, codeine, oxymorphone, and hydrocodone.

Semisynthetic Narcotics

The semisynthetic narcotics include heroin, hydromorphone, oxycodone, and oxymorphone and are produced through minor chemical alterations of the poppy plant.

Heroin

Heroin (3,6-diacetylmorphine) is one of the most popular narcotic drugs of abuse because of its intense euphoria and long-lasting effect (25). It may be administered by all routes and has a rapid onset of action. Its duration of effect is approximately 3–5 hours (19). Heroin has been reported to be about 2.5 times more potent than morphine. Heroin is faster in inducing pain relief and has a shorter duration of effect than morphine after parenteral administration (25). These differences are from the rapid and extensive brain uptake of the more lipid-soluble heroin compared with morphine (26). For this reason, it has the greatest addictive potential (25,27).

Heroin has no legitimate use in the United States. It is produced by heating morphine in the presence of acetic acid and is nearly 10 times as potent as morphine (28). Once in the body, heroin is converted back to 6-monoacetylmorphine in the liver, brain, kidney, and heart (29,30). The 6-monoacetylmorphine is then slowly converted to morphine (26). Morphine is then conjugated with glucuronic acid or excreted unchanged. Both the 6-monoacetylmorphine metabolite and morphine have metabolic activity.

Heroin, in its pure form, is a white powder with a bitter taste. Illicit heroin varies in color because of impurities left from the manufacturing process or from additives such as food coloring, cocoa, or brown sugar, which act as "fillers." A "bag" of heroin is a slang term for a single dosage unit, which may weigh approximately 100 mg and usually contains less than 10% pure heroin. Street heroin is usually 2%–5% heroin, the remainder being adulterants. In particular, quinine is a popular filler because it tastes bitter, like heroin.

Hydromorphone

Hydromorphone (Dilaudid), a pure narcotic agonist, is a strong analgesic used in the relief of moderate to severe pain. It has 2–8 times the potency of morphine. Hydromorphone has a more rapid onset and shorter duration of action than morphine and is more sedative and less euphorant than morphine. The onset of action of hydromorphone is usually 15–30 minutes and analgesia is maintained for 4–5 hours, depending on the route of administration. Because of its greater potency, hydromorphone is a highly abused drug that is much sought after by narcotic addicts.

Oxycodone

Oxycodone, which is synthesized from thebaine, is similar in effect to codeine but is more potent and thus has a higher dependence potential. It is available only in combination products. Oxycodone is used to relieve moderate to moderately severe pain. Addicts take this drug orally as Percodan or Tylox or dissolve the tablets in water, filter out the insoluble material, and "mainline" the active drug.

Following oral administration, the analgesic effect occurs within 10–15 minutes, reaches its maximum in 30–60 minutes, and persists for 3–6 hours.

Synthetic Narcotics

Although the synthetic narcotics are structurally unrelated to morphine, they have many of the same properties as the agonists. Synthetic narcotics include meperidine, methadone, propoxyphene, pentazocine, diphenoxylate, fentanyl, and butorphanol. These drugs are narcotic agonists or partial agonists, the latter of which may have dual effects.

Meperidine

Meperidine (Demerol) is a pure narcotic agonist and was the first synthetic narcotic. It was initially synthesized as a substitute for atropine because of its anticholinergic effects (31,32). It therefore has a different chemical structure from that of morphine. Because of a significant first-pass effect through the liver, it is less than one-half as effective when taken orally as when given parenterally (33,34).

Meperidine is metabolized by the liver through two primary pathways: hydrolysis to meperidinic acid, and hydroxylation to normeperidine. Normeperidine is the only active metabolite. The half-life of normeperidine is 24–48 hours; hence, with repeated use, normeperidine accumulates (34). Normeperidine has half the analgesic potency of meperidine yet has twice the neurotoxicity. Normeperidine accumulation is more likely to occur in patients with decreased hepatic or renal function, in whom the metabolite cannot be effectively conjugated or eliminated.

Manifestations of toxicity include seizures, myoclonus, central nervous system stimulation, jitteriness, and tremors (35). These signs generally appear after several days of meperidine use and are due either to the anticholinergic activity of the compound or to the accumulation of normeperidine (35). Meperidine differs from other narcotics in that it does not produce miosis and, in fact, may cause mydriasis or no pupillary changes secondary to its anticholinergic effect (4).

Meperidine as a "Designer Drug"

Meperidine is a Schedule II controlled substance. MPPP is a little-known derivative of meperidine that has been used in the manufacture of industrial chemicals. It has recently surfaced as a "designer drug" of abuse.

MPPP is most often sold as heroin (19). Street names include "synthetic heroin," "new heroin," and "synthetic Demerol." 1-Methyl-4-phenyl-1,2,5,6-tetrahydropyridine (MPTP) is a contaminant created during the faulty synthesis of MPPP as MPPP requires sophisticated laboratory procedures to ensure purity. The contaminant has produced destructive lesions of the substantia nigra and a clinical picture similar to that of Parkinsonism. MPTP is converted by monoamine oxidase-B to a positively charged compound MPP+. This is then actively transported via the dopaminergic uptake carriers to the nigrostriatal dopamine neurons, where it induces cellular death, possibly by inhibiting mitichondrial respiration.

Injection of MPTP causes an atypical burning sensation and a dysphoric state. Within 1 week of using the drug, patients report initial sudden jerking of the extremities followed by bradykinesia and near-total immobility—hence the term "frozen addict." Physical examination reveals signs and symptoms of Parkinsonism, difficulty moving and speaking, flexed posture, constant drooling, increased muscle tone, a positive glabellar tap test, and cogwheel rigidity in the upper extremities. Unlike patients with idiopathic Parkinsonism, these patients have a postural tremor affecting the proximal muscles of the extremities that is more pronounced than the typical resting tremor.

Parkinsonism does not usually appear until 80% of the cells in the substantia nigra have been destroyed. The neurologic damage of brain cells by MPTP is irreversible and worsens with time, especially if the user has repeated exposures. The drug-induced syndrome is permanent, but like idiopathic Parkinsonism, treatment with L-dopa, bromocriptine, and anticholinergic drugs may improve the clinical condition.

Methadone

Methadone (Dolophine) is a pure opiate agonist and was first synthesized by German scientists during World War II because of a shortage of morphine. It is structurally similar to propoxyphene. It is, along with heroin, one of the more frequently abused narcotics and may be made available to abusers by those enrolled in a methadone maintenance program (29). As an analgesic, methadone has many advantages over some of the other narcotics in that it may be orally administered for a reasonable cost and has a prolonged duration of action with a mild abstinence syndrome on long-term usage. Methadone is used mainly in the detoxification and maintenance of opiate addicts.

A single dose of methadone produces less sedation and euphoria than morphine and has an extended duration of action (4–6 hours). Because of this long duration of action, depressant effects after overdosage may continue for 36–48 hours (19). Such an extended action is possibly due to the drug's high degree of protein binding, which allows slow elimination. Because of this, methadone can be given once daily. As an analgesic, methadone may be used in the relief of severe pain but should not be used in narcotic withdrawal or maintenance unless the individual is enrolled in an approved withdrawal or maintenance program (36).

Accidental methadone poisoning in children has been reported in relation to methadone maintenance programs because the drug is dispensed as a fruit-flavored solution to some patients, who then take the substance home and store it in the refrigerator (37,38).

Propoxyphene

Propoxyphene is a pure opiate agonist that is structurally similar to methadone and contains the phenylpiperidine moiety found in all narcotic analgesics. It is a weaker analgesic than codeine or salicylate in single doses and is solely available as an oral preparation. Propoxyphene is a very dangerous drug, with the potential for inducing seizures and cardiac dysrhythmias in addition to its typical narcotic effects. Some of these toxic effects of propoxyphene are not explained by its opiate-like properties; it is believed that they are due to the local anesthetic action of propoxyphene and its metabolite norpropoxyphene (39).

Propoxyphene is commercially available as the hydrochloride or napsylate salt. Toxic effects may develop more slowly with the napsylate salt because of its slower absorption, but, despite claims to the contrary, there is no evidence that the napsylate is any safer than the hydrochloride. A 65-mg dose of the hydrochloride is equivalent to 100 mg of the napsylate. Propoxyphene has mild analgesic effects at the usual dosage and has no antipyretic action.

One reason why propoxyphene is considered a dangerous drug is that only 15–20 tablets or capsules are sufficient to cause death, and smaller amounts may be fatal in combination with ethanol or other central nervous system

TABLE 44–9. *Clinical effects of propoxyphene*

Miosis
Coma
Respiratory depression
Pulmonary edema
Circulatory depression
Grand mal seizures
First degree atrioventricular block
Bundle-branch block
Ventricular dysrhythmias
Ventricular fibrillation
Ventricular tachycardia

depressants. In addition, the metabolite norpropoxyphene has been shown to cause both cardiac and excitatory central nervous system effects because it has a local anesthetic effect similar to that of amitriptyline and other antidysrhythmic agents. Propoxyphene has been shown to be a more potent blocker of sodium channels than lidocaine, quinidine, and procainamide. Intracardiac conduction delays attributable to high concentrations of norpropoxyphene may be of relatively long duration. Cardiac conduction disturbances reported include first-degree atrioventricular block, right and left bundle branch block, ventricular bigeminy, and ventricular fibrillation (23). Grand mal seizures have also been attributable to the effects of norpropoxyphene.

In the past, propoxyphene has been abused by dissolving the hydrochloride pellets in water and injecting the solution intravenously. This practice has been discontinued because the manufacturer now disperses propoxyphene uniformly throughout the capsule.

Acute toxicity from propoxyphene overdosage results in symptoms similar to those of acute opiate intoxication; these may include miosis, coma, respiratory depression, circulatory collapse, and pulmonary edema (Table 44–9) (40). Seizures, dysrhythmias, and bundle branch block occur frequently with propoxyphene intoxication and can be life threatening shortly after ingestion (23). Cardiac failure is also responsible for many of the deaths (41). Because of the rapid onset of action of propoxyphene, death may occur within the first hour, and a small number of deaths have occurred within the first 15 minutes. Although naloxone is effective as an antidote, large doses may be necessary. In addition, the action of propoxyphene may outlast that of naloxone. A temporary transvenous cardiac pacemaker may be necessary in some patients (41).

Diphenoxylate

Diphenoxylate is an ingredient in the antidiarrheal preparation Lomotil, which, in the United States, contains 2.5 mg of diphenoxylate and 0.025 mg of atropine in each tablet or 5 mL of liquid preparation. Intoxication with this agent has been reported in children in both therapeutic administration and accidental ingestion (42). Adults do not appear to be as sensitive to the effects of overdose as young children (43). Because of the combination of drugs contained in Lomotil, effects can vary from narcotic-like to anticholinergic-like. Delayed effects of this drug have been noted with a lag of as long as 12 hours after ingestion (43,44).

Diphenoxylate acts on smooth muscle of the intestinal tract in a manner similar to that of morphine, inhibiting gastrointestinal motility and excessive gastrointestinal propulsion. The drug has little or no analgesic activity. Although single doses in the usual therapeutic range produce little or no opiate effect, high doses (40–60 mg) may produce euphoria, suppression of the opiate abstinence syndrome, and physical dependence after chronic administration. Administration of opiate antagonists may precipitate withdrawal symptoms in patients following chronic administration of high doses of diphenoxylate hydrochloride; however, evidence of physical dependence to diphenoxylate has not been reported with the recommended dosage.

Commercial preparations of diphenoxylate contain a subtherapeutic quantity of atropine sulfate to discourage misuse, yet overdosage of diphenoxylate preparations may produce atropinism in some patients (42).

Overdosage of the commercially available preparations containing diphenoxylate and atropine produces reactions similar to those of acute toxicity from opiate analgesics. In addition, symptoms of atropinism have occurred in approximately 50% of reported acute toxicity cases. Children are particularly susceptible to toxic effects of these drugs, and fatalities have resulted from accidental ingestion of relatively small amounts.

At least 12 hours of monitoring are required to detect initial symptoms, and an additional 12 hours are needed to detect late symptoms. Early symptoms are caused by the combination of diphenoxylate and atropine, while late symptoms are caused by the accumulation of the metabolite, difenoxime (42).

Since the Canadian preparation of Lomotil contains only diphenoxylate, symptoms are not mixed, and resemble that of a pure narcotic overdose.

Fentanyl

Fentanyl is an opiate agonist related to the phenylpiperidines and is an ingredient in Sublimaze. It was first introduced in 1968 as an intravenous analgesic anesthetic. After parenteral administration, fentanyl is more prompt and less prolonged in its action than morphine or meperidine. Fentanyl is estimated to be 50–100 times more potent as an analgesic than morphine. Large doses of fentanyl produce marked muscular rigidity and almost instantaneous respiratory arrest (6,28). Pharmacologic properties of fentanyl include high lipophilicity, rapid serum clearance, high potency, and minimal histamine release. Fentanyl rapidly crosses the blood-brain barrier, producing analgesia in as little as 1.5 minutes (45). Serum fentanyl levels rapidly decline from peak concentrations due to extensive tissue uptake, producing a duration of action of 30–40 minutes.

A single dose of fentanyl administered intravenously has a more rapid onset and shorter duration of action than morphine. The greater potency and more rapid onset of action reflects the greater lipid solubility of fentanyl compared with that of morphine, which facilitates its passage across the blood-brain barrier (46).

Transdermal Fentanyl

Fentanyl, has now been marketed in a controlled-release transdermal formulation (Duragesic) for use in patients with chronic pain severe enough to require opioid analgesia. Duragesic is supplied as a patch and is released from a reservoir containing fentanyl and a small amount of alcohol (47). The amount of fentanyl released per hour is proportional to the surface area of the patch.

The drug is not detectable in the blood until about 2 hours after application of the patch to the skin. Serum fentanyl concentrations increase gradually after application, generally leveling off between 12 and 24 hours, and then remaining relatively constant until 72 hours after application, when the patch should be removed and a new one applied at a different site. After the first patch is removed, a depot of fentanyl in the skin continues to release the drug while a new depot builds up from the next patch (47).

Fentanyl as a "Designer Drug"

A methyl analog of fentanyl produced in clandestine laboratories has been sold along the West Coast as a "super heroin." α-Methyl fentanyl, known as "China White," is a synthetic opioid that may be as much as 200 times more potent than heroin. It was the first of more than ten "designer drugs" to appear on the street (Table 44–10) (48). 3-Methyl fentanyl is approximately 3000 times stronger than morphine sulfate (45).

Other street names for fentanyl derivatives are "Synthetic Heroin," "Mexican Brown," and "Persian White." A pure white powder is sold as "Persian White." A light tan powder is sold as "China White" or "Synthetic Heroin." A light brown powder is sold as "Mexican Brown"; the brown color is acquired by carmelizing the lactose filler or using a dye. The fentanyl derivatives are normally diluted with large amounts of "cutting" substances. Because the active ingredient is present in small quantities, it is unrecognizable by color, odor, or taste (14).

TABLE 44–10. *Fentanyl analogs*

Analog	Year of appearance	Minimum lethal dose
α-Methyl fentanyl	1979	125 μg
Benzyl fentanyl	1982	Unknown
p-Fluoro fentanyl	1981	120 μg
α-Methyl acetyl fentanyl	1983	Unknown
α-Methyl acryl fentanyl	1983	Unknown
3-Methyl fentanyl	1984	A few micrograms (6000 × potency morphine)
3-Methyl thienyl fentanyl	1985	Unknown
Thienyl fentanyl	1985	Unknown
β-Hydroxy-thienyl fentanyl	1985	Unknown
β-Hydroxy-(3 methyl)-thienyl fentanyl	1985	Unknown

Adapted, with permission, from Henderson G: Designer drugs. *J Forensic Sci* 1988;32:569—572. ©ASTM.

Although the "designer" fentanyls have been sold in powder form, the most common route of administration is intravenous. Smoking and insufflation of fentanyl are growing in popularity because the compounds are highly lipid soluble. These drugs can cause very rapid onset of respiratory arrest or pulmonary edema. Large doses of naloxone may be necessary as an antidote for overdosage with any of the fentanyl narcotics.

Sufentanil is a thienyl analog of fentanyl. The analgesic potency of sufentanil is 5–10 times that of fentanyl, which parallels the greater affinity of sufentanil for opioid receptors compared with that of fentanyl.

Alfentanil is an analog of fentanyl that is less potent and has one-third the duration of action of the parent opioid. 3-Methylfentanyl, the most powerful analog to date, is 2000 times stronger than morphine. These illicit derivatives are cut with lactose or sucrose for street sale. Given the strength of some derivatives, a mistake in the mixture can have lethal results.

CLINICAL EFFECTS OF NARCOTICS

Opioids interact with specific receptors in the central nervous system to inhibit the activity of pain fibers, either by decreasing neurotransmitter release or by producing cellular membrane hyperpolarization due to the opening of potassium channels. The result is the alteration of the effective component of the pain rather than an elevation of the sensory threshold; the result is that the patient perceives the pain but remains indifferent to it.

Opioid effects on the level of consciousness can vary from euphoria to dysphoria, and from mild analgesia or sedation to coma, but patients presenting to emergency departments are usually stuporous or in a coma (49).

The clinical effects of opioids include euphoria, which is why this class of drugs is abused, as well as drowsiness, apathy, lethargy, and sedation. In addition, nausea and vomiting, constipation, miosis, sleep, and respiratory depression are seen (19). Large doses of some opiate agonists, on the other hand, may induce excitation and seizures (Table 44–11). Nausea and vomiting are caused by stimulation of the chemoreceptor trigger zone in the medulla oblongata. After this initial stimulation the opiate agonists then depress the vomiting center, and subsequent doses of the drugs are unlikely to produce vomiting.

The classic triad for acute opiate intoxication is symmetrical pinpoint pupils, depressed respiratory rate, and coma (19,32,50). Opioid-induced respiratory depression is primarily a response of binding at μ-receptors in the medullary respiratory center, although activity at κ-receptors may also depress respiration. As a result, all agents in clinical use have the potential to affect respiration.

In addition, there may be cardiovascular effects and pulmonary edema (19,51,52). The precise etiology of pulmonary edema remains unknown. The prevailing theory holds that hypoxia secondary to ventilatory compromise results in precapillary pulmonary hypertension with increased pulmonary capillary permeability and fluid leak. A hypersensitivity reaction to heroin, a direct toxic effect of heroin on the alveolar membrane, a central neurogenic response to increased intracranial pressure, and increased capillary permeability secondary to opioid-mediated release of leukotrienes and histamine have also been proposed as pathophysiologic mechanisms.

The onset of central nervous system depressant effects may occur immediately after intravenous administration of the substance. Absorption of the opiates by nasal insufflation or by the subcutaneous or oral route may be sufficiently slow that narcotic effects may not reach their peak for 2 or more hours (32).

Normally, opiate-induced miosis is presumed to be due to an excitatory effect of the drug on the autonomic segment of the oculomotor nerve (32). This effect may be antagonized by anticholinergic drugs such as atropine. Therefore, if a patient's pupils are dilated, opiate ingestion cannot be ruled out. This is because mydriasis can result if Lomotil was ingested (from the atropine) or can be a direct effect of concurrently ingested nonnarcotic drugs if the patient is postictal or agitated or if asphyxia has occurred. Mydriasis can also result from an overdose of meperidine, a narcotic that causes a paradoxical pupillary response.

TABLE 44–11. *Clinical features of narcotic overdose*

Apathy
Constipation
Drowsiness
Excitement
Lethargy
Miosis
Nausea
Pulmonary edema
Respiratory depression
Vomiting

Opioids can also cause spasms in the biliary tract that can prevent emptying of duct contents, resulting in increased biliary pressure. Clinical symptoms of this effect range from mild epigastric pain to biliary colic.

Bradycardia may also occur as a result of opioid therapy. Bradycardia appears to involve μ-receptor mediation resulting in central vagal stimulation and a reduction in sympathetic tone.

Dilatation of cutaneous blood vessels, possibly as the result of histamine release, can manifest as flushing of the face, neck, and upper torso, sweating, and urticaria at the site of injection in patients receiving opioids.

LABORATORY ANALYSIS

There is usually no indication for determining serum concentrations of opiates in the clinical setting. It may be useful to know whether a narcotic was present, as can be determined from a qualitative drug screen, but concentrations of the particular narcotic are not helpful.

TREATMENT

In the treatment of opiate agonist overdosage, especially in the presence of apnea, primary attention should be given to re-establishment of adequate respiratory exchange by maintaining an adequate, patent airway, using assisted or controlled respiration and oxygen as necessary (52). A patent intravenous line should also be established. Naloxone (2 mg) should be administered and repeated as necessary. This is of both diagnostic and therapeutic importance. Although the preferred route of administration is intravenous, naloxone can be administered intramuscularly or sublingually or placed down the endotracheal tube if an intravenous line cannot be established (10,53,54). It should be remembered that the duration of respiratory depression following overdosage of an opiate agonist may be longer than the duration of action of the opiate antagonist. It should also be considered that use of an opiate antagonist in patients physically dependent on opiate agonists may precipitate an acute withdrawal syndrome that cannot be readily suppressed while the action of the antagonist persists.

If the offending drug has been taken orally, attempts to retrieve the material should be performed with gastric lavage if the patient has no gag reflex and has been previously intubated. Gastric lavage may be effective even many hours after drug ingestion since pylorospasm produced by the opiate agonist may cause much of the drug to be retained in the stomach for an extended period of time.

Treatment of noncardiogenic pulmonary edema, if it occurs, includes support of respiration and oxygen. Positive end-expiratory pressure may be added if oxygenation cannot be maintained, but it is seldom required and its use has certain hazards. If it is necessary to use mechanical ventilation, a volume-cycled respirator is recommended. The use of furosemide has also been suggested for this condition but has not been shown to be of benefit. Intravenous fluid administration should be kept to a minimum. Other customary components of pulmonary therapy are neither effective nor necessary. Response is usually dramatic, and physical findings usually clear within 1 day, with radiologic changes reverting to normal within 72–96 hours.

Cardiac dysrhythmias and hypotension rarely require specific treatment when caused by a narcotic and usually respond to effective ventilation and naloxone. Dialysis, diuresis, and hemoperfusion also should not be attempted for narcotic overdose because there is no evidence that any of these methods are beneficial.

REFERENCES

1. Buck M, Blumer J: Opioids and other analgesics. *Crit Care Clinics* 1991;7:615–637.
2. Aston R: Drug abuse: Its relationship to dental practice. *Dent Clin North Am* 1984;28:595–610.
3. Adams M, Brase D, Welch S, et al: The role of endogenous peptides in the action of opoid analgesics. *Ann Emerg Med* 1986; 15:1030–1035.
4. Dipalma J: Opiate antagonists: Naloxone. *Am Fam Phys* 1984; 29:270–272.
5. Barsan W: Narcotic agents. *Ann Emerg Med* 1986;15:1019–1020.
6. Snyder D: Opiate receptors in the brain. *N Engl J Med* 1977;296:266–271.
7. Snyder S: The opiate receptor and morphine-like peptides in the brain. *Am J Psychiatr* 1978;135:645–652.
8. Atkinson R: Endocrine and metabolic effects of opiate antagonists. *J Clin Psychiatr* 1984;45:20–24.
9. Handal K, Schauben J, Salamone F: Naloxone. *Ann Emerg Med* 1983;12.438–445.
10. Wald P, Weisman R, Goldfrank L: Opioids. *Top Emerg Med* 1985;7:9–17.
11. Way E: Sites and mechanisms of basic narcotic receptor function based on current research. *Ann Emerg Med* 1986;15:1021–1025.
12. Zola E, McLeod D: Comparative effects and analgesic efficacy of the agonist-antagonist opioids. *Drug Intell Clin Pharmacol* 1983; 17:411–417.
13. Martin W: Clinical evidence for different narcotic receptors and relevance for the clinician. *Ann Emerg Med* 1986;15:1026–1029.
14. Ford M, Hoffman R, Goldfrank L: Opioids and designer drugs. *Emerg Clin North Am* 1990;8:495–511.
15. Koren G, Maurice L: Pediatric uses of opioids. *Pediatr Clin North Am* 1989;36:1141–1156.
16. *Drug Intell Clin Pharm* 1981:15.
17. Basbaum A, Levine J: Opiate analgesia: how central is a peripheral target? *N Engl J Med* 1991;325:1168–1169.
18. McLane N, Caroll D: Ocular manifestations of drug abuse. *Surv Ophthalmol* 1986;30:298–313.
19. Kulburg A: Substance abuse: clinical identification and management. *Pediatr Clin North Am* 1986;33:325–361.
20. Moriarty K, Alagna S, Lake C: Psychopharmacology. *Psychiatr Clin North Am* 1984;7:411–433.
21. Rice T: Paregoric intoxication with pulmonary edema in infancy. *Clin Pediatr* 1984;23:101–103.
22. Robieux I, Koren G, Vandenbergh H, et al: Morphine excretion in breast milk and resultant exposure of a nursing infant. *J Toxicol Clin Toxicol* 1990;28:365–370.
23. Heaney R: Left bundle branch block associated with propoxyphene hydrochloride poisoning. *Ann Emerg Med* 1983;12:780–782.
24. Pearson M, Poklis A, Morrison R: A fatality due to the ingestion of (methyl morphine) codeine. *Clin Toxicol* 1979;15:267–271.
25. Sternbach G, Moran J, Eliastam M: Heroin addiction: acute presentation of medical complications. *Ann Emerg Med* 1980;9:161–169.
26. Inturrisi C, Max M, Foley K: The pharmacokinetics of heroin in patients with chronic pain. *N Engl J Med* 1984;310:1213–1217.
27. Bozarth M, Wise R: Toxicity associated with long-term intravenous heroin and cocaine self-administration in the rat. *JAMA* 1985;254:81–83.
28. Gay G, Inaba D: Treating acute heroin and methadone toxicity. *Anesth Analg* 1976;55:607–610.
29. Goldfrank L, Bresnitz E: Opioids. *Hosp Physician* 1978;14:26–37.
30. Goldfrank L, Bresnitz E, Weisman R: Opioids and opiates. *Curr Top Emerg Med* 1983;3:1–7.
31. Batterman R, Himmelsbach C: Demerol—a new synthetic analgesic. *JAMA* 1943;122:222–226.
32. Cuddy P: Management of acute opioid intoxication. *Crit Care Q* 1982;4:65–74.
33. Brena S: Oral analgesics: use and misuse. *Emerg Med Rep* 1983; 4:139–146.
34. Goetting M, Thirman M: Neurotoxicity of meperidine. *Ann Emerg Med* 1985;14:1007–1009.
35. Szeto H, Inturrisi C, Houde R, et al: Accumulation of normeperidine, an active metabolite of meperidine in patients with renal failure or cancer. *Ann Intern Med* 1977;86:738–741.
36. Nanji A, Filipenko J: Rhabdomyolysis and acute myoglobinuric renal failure associated with methadone intoxication. *J Toxicol Clin Toxicol* 1983;20:353–356.
37. Roland E, Lockitch G, Dunn H, et al: Methadone poisoning due to accidental contamination of prescribed medication. *Can Med Assoc J* 1984;131 :1357–1358.
38. Carin I, Glass L, Parekh A, et al: Neonatal methadone withdrawal. *Am J Dis Child* 1983;137:1166–1169.
39. Krantz T, Thisted B, Strom J, et al: Severe, acute propoxyphene overdose treated with dopamine. *Clin Toxicol* 1985;23:347–352.
40. Whitcomb D, Gilliam F, Starmer C, et al: Marked QRS complex abnormalities and sodium channel blockade by propoxyphene reversed with lidocaine. *J Clin Invest* 1989;84:1629–1636.
41. Strom J, Haggmark S, Madsen P, et al: Cardiac pacing and central hemodynamics in experimental propoxyphene-induced shock. *Clin Toxicol* 1985;23:353–356.
42. McCarron M, Challoner K, Thompson G: Diphenoxylate-Atropine (Lomitil®) overdose in children: an update (report of eight cases and review of the literature). *Pediatrics* 1991;87:694–700.
43. Rumack B, Temple A: Lomotil poisoning. *Pediatrics* 1974;53:495–500.
44. McGuigan M, Lovejoy F: Overdose of Lomotil (editorial). *Br Med J* 1978;1:990.
45. Vogel S, Leikin J: What's up (and down) in drug abuse: street drugs. *Top Emerg Med* 1986;8:57–75.
46. Lind G, Marcus M, Mears S, et al: Oral transmucosal fentanyl citrate for analgesia and sedation in the emergency department. *Ann Emerg Med* 1991;20:1117–1120.
47. Marquardt K, Tharratt R: Inhalation abuse of fentanyl patch. *J Toxicol Clin Toxicol* 1994;32:75–78.
48. Taliaferro E, Rund D, Brown C, et al: Substance abuse education in residency training programs in emergency medicine. *Ann Emerg Med* 1989;18:1344–1347.
49. Smith D, Leake L, Loflin J, et al: Is admission after intravenous heroin overdose necessary? *Ann Emerg Med* 1992;21:1326–1330.
50. Khantzian E, McKeena G: Acute toxic and withdrawal reactions associated with drug use and abuse. *Ann Intern Med* 1979; 90:361–372.
51. Frand U: Methadone-induced pulmonary edema. *Ann Intern Med* 1972;76:975–979.
52. Light R, Dunham R: Severe slowly resolving heroin induced pulmonary edema. *Chest* 1975;67:61–64.
53. Maio R, Gaukel B, Freeman B: Intralingual naloxone injection for narcotic-induced respiratory depression. *Ann Emerg Med* 1987; 16:572–573.
54. Maio R, Griener J, Clark M, et al: Intralingual naloxone reversal of morphine-induced respiratory depression in dogs. *Ann Emerg Med* 1984;13:1087–1091.

CHAPTER 45

Narcotic Antagonists

Narcotic antagonists are drugs that tend to block and reverse the effects of narcotics. They can be pure antagonists or partial antagonists, also referred to as mixed agonist-antagonists. Opioid agonist/antagonists were developed partly to avoid problems of abuse, although some have themselves been abused (1).

The pure antagonists and the agonist-antagonists, when given to a subject who has received an agonist, will have very different effects. Agonist–antagonist drugs usually produce sedation in addition to analgesia when given in therapeutic doses. At higher doses, sweating, dizziness, and nausea are common, but severe respiratory depression may be less common than with pure agonists. When it does occur, respiratory depression may be reversed by naloxone but not reliably by other agonist–antagonists, such as nalorphine (2). Psychotomimetic effects, with hallucinations, nightmares, and anxiety, have been reported following the use of agonist-antagonist agents.

TABLE 45–1. *Agonists and partial agonists for which naloxone and naltrexone are effective*

Agonists	Partial agonists
Alphaprodine	Butorphanol
Anileridine	Cyclazocine
Codeine	Levallorphan
Diphenoxylate	Nalbuphine
Fentanyl	Nalorphine
Heroin	Pentazocine
Hydromorphine	
Levorphanol	
Meperidine	
Methadone	
Opium	
Oxymorphone	
Propoxyphene	

PURE ANTAGONISTS

The pure antagonists are naloxone, the oral preparation naltrexone, and nalmefene, an investigational narcotic antagonist (3–10). These exhibit antagonistic activities at all three receptors.

Naloxone (Narcan)

Naloxone is a synthetic compound of oxymorphone originally derived from thebaine. It has also been used in the treatment of narcotic addiction (11,12). Naloxone is used for the treatment of respiratory depression induced by natural and synthetic opiates (Table 45–1). Naloxone is believed to act by competing for opioid receptor sites and displacing the opiate agonists because it binds to the receptors with greater affinity than the agonist without causing their activation. Although naloxone antagonizes the μ-, κ-, and σ-receptors, it is bound less avidly by the latter two receptors. Because it has no agonist activity, naloxone does not cause respiratory depression even if given in excessive amounts or in the absence of narcotic overdose. When the nature of the depression is not known, naloxone is the drug of choice because it will not cause further respiratory depression (5,13,14). Naloxone, like other narcotic antagonists, is ineffective in the treatment of respiratory depression caused by other central nervous system depressants (11,15–17).

Naloxone may be used in neonates for the treatment of asphyxia resulting from administration of opiates to the mother during labor and delivery. Naloxone has been given to the mother shortly before delivery, but many clinicians believe it is preferable to administer an opiate antagonist directly to the neonate if needed after delivery.

Method of Administration

Although the intravenous route is the preferred method for administration of naloxone, the drug must be administered frequently to patients with a scarcity of peripheral veins. Difficulty in obtaining venous access sometimes precludes the use of the intravenous technique (18). This problem may be encountered in the long-term drug abuser, obese patients, neonates, and children. Under these conditions, naloxone can be administered by the intramuscular or subcutaneous route; however, these routes provide less rapid, less predictable, and more erratic systemic absorption and therapeutic response. The sublingual and endotracheal routes, on the other hand, provide quick access to the systemic circulation (19). The ventral lateral surface of the tongue is a highly vascular area with an abundance of capillary beds; even in situations of low cardiac output, the tongue maintains its ability to autoregulate blood flow and to absorb material quickly (5,20,21).

Dosage

In the past, it was believed that many patients were given an insufficient amount of naloxone (14). For that reason, large doses of naloxone are currently recommended. In any adult patient with an altered mental status with respiratory depression, 2 mg of naloxone should be administered. It has been suggested that for neonates and children 0.01 mg/kg be administered (14,22), but the administration of a larger dose should cause no harm. The pupils should not be relied on as an indicator of whether naloxone should be administered (23). If there is a partial response, the same dose can be administered up to a total of 10 mg (13). In addition to naloxone, patients with an altered mental status should receive 50 mL of 50% dextrose intravenously, along with thiamine and oxygen.

The manufacturer of naloxone now makes at least two preparations of different concentrations. The first product marketed contained naloxone in a concentration of 0.4 mg in 1 mL. To give 2 mg required the administration of five ampules. The same manufacturer now makes a concentration of 1 mg/mL in a 2-mL ampule. These two preparations should not be confused. In addition, there is a preparation for multiple use as well as a neonatal preparation.

Continuous Infusion

Naloxone can be administered by continuous intravenous infusion by a number of methods. One method consists of placing 4 mg of naloxone in 1 L of 5% dextrose in water at an infusion rate of approximately 100 mL/hour (13,24). Another method for continuous infusion is to administer the bolus dose necessary to reverse the respiratory depressant effects of the opioid overdose and to follow that with an infusion of two-thirds the initial bolus dose each hour (20). In this regimen, half the loading dose may be administered 15–20 minutes after the first dose because of the transient decrease in naloxone levels (13). If a continuous infusion is to be used, patients should be monitored closely in an intensive care setting (24).

Onset of Action

Naloxone has an onset of action of 1–2 minutes after intravenous administration and 5–10 minutes after intramuscular injection. The rapid onset of action is related to the drug's rapid entry into the brain as a result of its high degree of lipid solubility (13). Its duration of action after intravenous administration is 45–90 minutes in adults and about 3 hours in neonates (5,13,15,24,25). Because the duration of action of naloxone is generally shorter than that of the opiate, the effects of the opiate may recur as the effects of naloxone disappear (26). Oral administration is 2% as potent as parenteral administration because of a prominent first-pass effect by the liver (5). Although oral administration of naloxone can be effective, large amounts are required (27).

TABLE 45–2. *Narcotic effects that naloxone acts to reverse*

Respiratory depression
Cardiovascular depression
Gastrointestinal effects
Central nervous system depression
Miosis
Analgesia
Psychomimetic effects of partial agonists

A positive response from naloxone typically consists of increased respirations, increased alertness, and reversal of miosis (Table 45–2). In addition, naloxone reverses the cardiovascular, gastrointestinal, analgesic, and emetic effects of the narcotics (28). Naloxone is the drug of choice when the nature of the depressant drug is not known because it will not cause further respiratory depression. If naloxone is used for long-term treatment of opiate dependence, an abstinence syndrome does not develop (29). The main drawback to the use of naloxone remains its relatively short duration of action and poor absorption when administered orally.

Naloxone and Withdrawal

Although 0.4 mg of naloxone hydrochloride administered subcutaneously will precipitate potentially severe withdrawal symptoms in patients physically dependent on opiates or pentazocine, oral administration of naloxone generally does not precipitate these symptoms unless the dose exceeds 10 mg. Even a 30-mg oral dose of naloxone usually induces only very mild abstinence symptoms (29).

Partial Response to Naloxone

A patient may have only a partial response to naloxone for a number of reasons (Table 45–3).The patient may have had a seizure with a subsequent postictal period or may have a mixed overdose of narcotic and nonnarcotic agents. In addition, there may be a concurrent head injury, hypoglycemia, or hypoxia that require

TABLE 45–3. *Reasons for partial response to naloxone*

Postictal period
Mixed overdose
Concurrent head injury
Hypoglycemia
Hypoxia

treatment before the patient can regain a normal level of consciousness.

Toxicity of Naloxone

The toxicity of naloxone is minimal. In those patients who are physically dependent on opiates, naloxone may cause an acute withdrawal (Table 45–4) (28). This may include the newborns of mothers who are physically dependent on opioids. Nausea and vomiting have been reported in postoperative patients who received a dose greater than the recommended dose, but such reports are rare. Up to 20 mg have been given to children without adverse effect (5). Several investigators have reported naloxone-induced hypertension that is possibly due to catecholamine release (30). Although a casual relationship to the drug has not been established, hypotension, coagulation disturbances, ventricular irritability, and pulmonary edema have been described after postoperative administration of naloxone, but these reports are also uncommon (28–32).

Other Uses of Naloxone

Although naloxone has been used on an investigational basis for detection of chronic opiate abuse, chemical methods used to detect the presence of opiates in the urine are preferable because naloxone may precipitate abstinence symptoms in patients who are physically dependent on opiates (28). Naloxone does not produce tolerance or physical or psychological dependence (29).

In addition to reversal of narcotic withdrawal, naloxone has been used investigationally in intoxicated patients to reverse alcohol-, diazepam-, and clonidine-induced coma and respiratory depression (5,11,16,17). Even though alcohol may in part act by releasing endogenous endorphins, there has never been satisfactory evidence that naloxone reliably reverses alcohol-induced coma (22,33,36). It has also been used investigationally in the management of high-altitude pulmonary edema, acute respiratory failure, senile dementia, ischemic neurologic deficits, and septic and cardiogenic shock (35). The efficacy of naloxone under these conditions has not been established (22,33,36).

TABLE 45–4. *Potential toxicity of naloxone (all uncommon)*

Acute withdrawal from opiates
Nausea
Vomiting
Hypertension
Coagulation disturbances
Ventricular irritability

Nalmefene

Nalmefene is a pure narcotic antagonist that has been recently released under the trade name Revex. It has a potential advantage over naloxone because of its 4–8 hour half-life (37). It is similar in effect to naloxone. Its safety profile is excellent, characterized by only mild and transient side effects (38).

Naltrexone (Trexan)

Naltrexone is a long-lasting orally administered synthetic narcotic antagonist. It is a structural analog of naloxone and is derived from thebaine (39). Naltrexone is almost ideal as an opiate antagonist in that it is long acting, active orally, does not cause physical dependence, antagonizes the euphoric effects of opiates, is not associated with tolerance, and has no serious side effects or toxicities (Table 45–5) (3).

Naltrexone is a pure opioid antagonist that markedly attenuates or completely and reversibly blocks the subjective effects of opioids, including those with agonist and antagonist activity (Table 45–1) (40). It appears to block the effects of opioids by competitive binding at the three opioid receptors. The major action, like that of naloxone, is on the μ-receptor. This makes the blockade potentially surmountable. Naltrexone appears to have a narcotic antagonist activity 2–9 times greater than that of naloxone (3).

Pharmacokinetics

Naltrexone is rapidly and nearly completely absorbed from the gastrointestinal tract. Concentrations reach their peak 1 hour after oral administration (3). Approximately 25% of naltrexone is bound to plasma proteins. It is rapidly and extensively metabolized by the liver. Naltrexone, like naloxone, undergoes extensive first-pass

TABLE 45–5. *Properties of naltrexone*

Pure opiate antagonist
No agonist effects
Long-acting oral agent
No tolerance noted
No serious side effects

hepatic metabolism, but its major metabolite, 6-β-naltrexol, is also a pure antagonist and contributes to opioid receptor blockade. The half-lives of naltrexone and 6-β-naltrexol are 4 hours and 13 hours, respectively (39). Urinary excretion is the most important route of elimination of naltrexone and its metabolite.

Naltrexone (50 mg) will block the pharmacologic effects of 25 mg of heroin for as long as 24 hours. Doubling the dose of naltrexone provides blockade for 48 hours, and tripling the dose provides blockade for about 72 hours (3).

The onset of opiate antagonism following oral administration of naltrexone has been reported to be 15–30 minutes. Administration of a single 15-mg oral dose of naltrexone immediately following a single 30-mg subcutaneous dose of morphine has been reported to produce opiate antagonism that is prominent within 6 hours, maximal within 12 hours, and persists for at least 24 hours. The extent and duration of the antagonist activity of naltrexone appear to be directly related to plasma and tissue concentrations of the drug.

Uses

Naltrexone has been approved for the long-term treatment of addiction to heroin and other opioids and can be used in those individuals who are highly motivated to stop taking a narcotic agent (3). For such patients the antagonist offers excellent protection against the temptation to use narcotics (39). Although naltrexone is an effective narcotic blocking agent, it does not block any other class of psychoactive substances (41). Patients may elect to accept naltrexone therapy and still abuse other psychoactive substances. Unlike patients who stop taking methadone and have withdrawal symptoms, patients who stop taking naltrexone experience no withdrawal (42). Patient compliance is then a major factor (3). In addition, although naltrexone blocks the effects of opioids it does not abolish the craving for narcotics (43). It appears to be most useful in discouraging impulsive use of narcotics, which is an important cause of relapse (44). Self-administration of large doses of heroin or other narcotics can overcome the blockade and may cause serious injury, including coma and death (45).

Narcotic antagonists precipitate withdrawal in opiate-dependent individuals. Therefore, a drug-free interval is necessary before induction. Typically, the treatment should not be attempted until the patient has remained opioid-free for 7–10 days (41). Before the first dose of naltrexone, 2 mg of naloxone may be administered intravenously to determine the presence of residual dependence and to avoid precipitating a more prolonged and severe withdrawal with naltrexone (46). Clonidine has also been used before naltrexone for narcotic abstinence. Tolerance does not appear to develop to the opioid antagonistic properties of naltrexone for up to 2 years of treatment (47).

Dosage

Approximately 50 mg of naltrexone blocks the opiate receptor for 24 hours, and 100–150 mg provides a block for several days (8). The usual dosage of naltrexone is 50 mg once daily or 350 mg/week in three divided doses. Sustained-release delivery systems for naltrexone to enhance compliance are currently under investigation.

Plasma Levels

Opiate antagonism correlates well with naltrexone plasma concentrations, and effective blockade of opiate effects can be expected at plasma concentrations of 2 ng/mL. The lack of readily available commercial assays that are reliably sensitive to 2 ng/mL with a suitable margin of error makes routine assessments of naltrexone plasma concentrations difficult (42).

Side Effects

Naltrexone causes few side effects that, when present, tend to be mild (3). In opiate-dependent individuals, naltrexone may precipitate acute opiate withdrawal. In the nonopiate-dependent individual, gastrointestinal irritation and clinically insignificant increases in blood pressure have been reported (48). Dosages of up to 800 mg/day have been administered with no untoward effects (3). Doses of about 5 times the usual dose for the opioid addict have caused increases in serum aminotransferase activity in some patients. These patients were clinically asymptomatic, and their enzyme abnormalities returned to normal in a few weeks. Naltrexone, therefore, should not be used in patients with acute hepatitis or hepatic failure.

PARTIAL ANTAGONISTS

The development of drugs for clinical use that antagonize the effects of morphine-like drugs began more than 40 years ago with the preparation of nalorphine, a partial antagonist-agonist (3–5,49). This was the prototypical agonist-antagonist. Agonists-antagonists in use today include buprenorphine, butorphanol, nalbuphine, and pentazocine (Table 45–6). Nalorphine and levallorphan act antagonistically at the μ-receptor while exhibiting agonistic properties at the two remaining opiate receptor sites (6,22). The major problems limiting the use of these drugs are the physical dependence noted after sustained use, an increase in respiratory depression and coma if a non-narcotic was taken, and intense dysphoria.

TABLE 45–6. *Partial opioid agonists*

Buprenorphine (Buprenex)
Butorphanol (Stadol)
Nalbuphine (Nubain)
Pentazocine (Talwin)
Nalorphine (Nalline)
Levallorphan
Dezocine (Dalgan)

The partial agonist buprenorphine is similar to the mixed agonist-antagonists pentazocine, butorphanol, nalbuphine, and dezocine. All of these drugs can precipitate withdrawal symptoms in patients physically dependent on full agonists. All are less likely to cause dependence than full agonists, but none is completely free of dependence liability. Only pentazocine is available for oral use and only in combination products.

Each opioid that is a mixed agonist-antagonist may act as an agonist, a partial agonist, or an antagonist at each receptor. Nalorphine, pentazocine, butorphanol, and nalbuphine are thought to produce their analgesic and sedative effects by interacting with κ-receptors. Each of them has affinity, but no efficacy, at μ-receptors and therefore acts as a morphine antagonist. Dysphoria and hallucinations are thought to be mediated by σ-receptors.

Buprenorphine, and dezocine also have agonist and antagonist effects, but they are thought to be partial agonists at μ-receptors. Buprenorphine has been shown to have extremely high affinity and relatively low efficacy at μ-receptors. When given alone, it produces effects which appear similar to morphine. When given after morphine, it displaces the full agonist and causes a reduction in opioid effect (1).

Nalorphine (Nalline)

Nalorphine is a partial narcotic agonist whose use has been supplanted by the pure narcotic antagonist naloxone. It is thought that nalorphine is antagonistic at the μ-receptor and agonistic at the two remaining receptor sites. When administered to a patient who has ingested a narcotic, nalorphine reverses the narcotic effect, thereby acting as an antagonist. If no narcotic has been ingested, however, the agonist action of nalorphine is noted, with further central nervous system and respiratory depression. This makes the use of nalorphine potentially dangerous because it may induce respiratory depression and apnea.

Buprenorphine

Buprenorphine (Buprenex) is a partial opiate agonist with behavioral and psychic effects similar to morphine, and, unlike pentazocine, it rarely causes psychotomimetic effects. Buprenorphine is a derivative of the morphine alkaloid thebaine and is a partial μ-agonist that also blocks the action of morphine. Its efficacy is 25 to 50 times greater than that of morphine when given in low doses parenterally, yet it is comparable to naloxone as an antagonist (50).

Buprenorphine has been used as a methadone substitute in pharmacotherapy for heroin addiction, but it may also elicit dependence, with withdrawal symptoms beginning 1 to 2 days after the last dose and peaking at 2 weeks (50).

Effect on Opioid Receptors

Buprenorphine exerts its analgesic effect due to a high degree of binding to μ-receptors in the central nervous system. Although buprenorphine may be classified as a partial agonist it behaves very much like classical μ-agonists, such as morphine. Buprenorphine binds slowly with and dissociates slowly from the μ-receptor (40). It is thought that the high affinity of buprenorphine for the μ-receptor and its slow binding to and dissociation from the receptor may account for the prolonged duration of analgesia and possibly in part for the limited physical dependence potential observed with the drug.

The opiate agonist and antagonist activities of buprenorphine appear to be dose related. At doses of up to 1 mg subcutaneously, buprenorphine has a potent analgesic effect; at doses greater than 1 mg subcutaneously, the opiate agonist activity of the drug decreases and the opiate antagonist activity predominates. The drug may antagonize its own opiate agonist activity when administered at doses within the opiate antagonist range. Buprenorphine does not antagonize respiratory depression produced by nonopiate analgesics and other drugs (1).

Buprenorphine and Dependence

Buprenorphine may produce psychological dependence and, infrequently, may also produce limited physical dependence. Signs and symptoms of mild withdrawal may appear following discontinuance of prolonged therapy with the drug alone (45). Because buprenorphine binds slowly with and dissociates slowly from the μ-receptor, elimination of the drug from the central nervous system is prolonged following abrupt discontinuance. Consequently, signs and symptoms of acute withdrawal are less intense than those produced by morphine and delayed in appearance (1).

In patients physically dependent on opiates, buprenorphine produces many of the subjective and objective effects of opiates. However, the drug may not be a satisfactory substitute for opiate agonists in all patients physically dependent on opiates. Tolerance to the drug's opiate agonist activity reportedly develops rarely, if at all.

Buprenorphine and Naloxone

Intravenous naloxone hydrochloride has been used to reverse signs of buprenorphine-induced respiratory depression. However, in the usual doses, naloxone is substantially less effective in reversing buprenorphine-induced respiratory depression than in reversing morphine-induced respiratory depression. Occasionally, naloxone is only partially effective or, more rarely, completely ineffective in reversing buprenorphine-induced respiratory depression. Larger than usual doses may be necessary when naloxone is used to reverse signs of respiratory depression in patients receiving buprenorphine.

Clinical Use

Buprenorphine has been used to reduce opiate consumption in individuals physically dependent on opiates. Like naltrexone, buprenorphine has also been used on a limited basis for its opiate antagonist effects in the initiation and short-term maintenance of opiate cessation in individuals physically dependent on opiates.

Because of buprenorphine's antagonist activity, the drug may precipitate mild-to-moderate signs and symptoms of withdrawal in some patients physically dependent on opiates. Signs and symptoms of mild withdrawal may also appear following discontinuance of prolonged therapy with buprenorphine alone. Although buprenorphine appears to have a low physical dependence liability, the drug should be used cautiously in patients who have a history of opiate abuse or who were formerly physically dependent on opiates. Because of buprenorphine's opiate antagonist activity, it occasionally may precipitate mild to moderate withdrawal in patients physically dependent on opiates. The drug may not be a satisfactory substitute for opiate agonists in all patients physically dependent on opiates.

Butorphanol (Stadol)

Butorphanol is a partial agonist that is structurally related to morphine but pharmacologically similar to pentazocine. The analgesic effect is believed to result from a stimulation of κ- and σ-receptors in the central nervous system, and the antagonistic effect appears to result from competitive inhibition at the μ-receptor. The analgesic activity is 4–7 times that of morphine. Although orally administered butorphanol is easily absorbed, because of significant first-pass metabolism only 17% of a dose reaches the circulation unchanged. Because the drug does not suppress the abstinence syndrome and may actually induce withdrawal in opiate-dependent patients, it cannot be substituted for opiate agonists after physical dependence has been established without prior detoxification.

Butorphanol is probably not an effective antidote in the treatment of cardiovascular, respiratory, or behavioral depression induced by opiate agonists because of its relatively weak antagonistic effects (51).

Tolerance and Dependence

Tolerance and psychological and physical dependence may occur in patients receiving butorphanol. Unnecessary increases in dosage or frequency of administration should be avoided. Although cases of butorphanol abuse or dependence have been reported, the relative dependence liability and abuse potential of butorphanol currently appears to be low to moderate.

Withdrawal

Following abrupt discontinuance after prolonged use of butorphanol, withdrawal symptoms similar to but more intense than those produced by pentazocine, have occurred and may include nausea, vomiting, abdominal cramping, diarrhea, increased temperature, diaphoresis, mydriasis, weight loss, restlessness, malaise, myalgia, rhinorrhea, increased blood pressure, itching, tachycardia, and "electric shocks" usually associated with a feeling of faintness. Acute withdrawal has been reported to develop within 4 to 24 hours after discontinuance of the drug in individuals who are dependent. Clonidine hydrochloride has been used in the management of acute butorphanol withdrawal.

Misuse of Butorphanol

Butorphanol has been misused in combination with diphenhydramine by drug abusers in a manner similar to the parenteral use of pentazocine and tripelennamine (known as "T's and blues"), since the combination's effects are purported to be similar to those of intravenous heroin.

Butorphanol Nasal Spray

Butorphanol is now being marketed as a nasal spray (Stadol-NS). The spray was approved by the Food and Drug Administration for any type of pain for which an opioid analgesic is appropriate. Butorphanol has not been scheduled as a controlled substance, but "possible abuse" has been reported with the intranasal formulation.

Dexocine (Dalgan)

Dezocine is a new synthetic opioid agonist/antagonist structurally related to pentazocine. Dezocine is a strong opioid analgesic that has analgesic potency. It has its highest affinity for μ-receptors and less interaction with κ-receptors. Its opioid antagonist activity is less than that of nalorphine but greater than that of pentazocine when measured by antagonism of morphine-induced narcosis. Although it is said to be equivalent in efficacy to morphine, its use is associated with the same problems observed with all agonist-antagonists.

Adverse Effects

Nausea, vomiting, and sedation occur with dezocine about as often as with other opioid analgesics. Dizziness, anxiety, disorientation, hallucinations, sweating, tachycardia, and skin reactions at the injection site have also been reported. Acute respiratory depression, which can be reversed with naloxone, can occur after intravenous dezocine. Fatal respiratory depression has not been reported, but dezocine could be dangerous in patients with diminished respiratory reserve.

Dezocine is not currently a controlled substance but, like buprenorphine, it causes subjective effects in nondependent drug abusers similar to those of morphine and different from those of nalbuphine or pentazocine.

Overdosage and Treatment

Although there have been no incidents of overdosage with dezocine during clinical trials, and thus no human experience with the drug, overdosage with dezocine is possible. Based on the pharmacology of dezocine, overdosage will produce acute respiratory depression, cardiovascular compromise, and delirium.

The pharmacologic treatment of suspected dezocine overdosage is intravenously administered naloxone. The respiratory and cardiac status of the patient should be evaluated constantly and appropriate supportive measures instituted, such as oxygen, intravenous fluids, vasopressors, and assisted or controlled respiration.

Nalbuphine (Nubain)

Nalbuphine is a strong κ-receptor agonist and μ-receptor antagonist that is given parenterally. Like opiate agonists, nalbuphine produces respiratory depression, sedation, and miosis (52). At higher doses there seems to be a definite ceiling—not noted with morphine—to the respiratory depressant effect. Unfortunately, when respiratory depression does occur, it may be relatively resistant to naloxone reversal. Naloxone reverses the analgesic and sedative effects of nalbuphine, however. The narcotic antagonist activity of nalbuphine is one-fourth as potent as nalorphine and 10 times that of pentazocine (52).

Because it does not suppress the abstinence syndrome and may induce withdrawal in opiate-dependent patients, nalbuphine cannot be substituted for opiate agonists after physical dependence has been established without prior detoxification. Because the drug's antagonist activity appears to be selective for the μ-receptor and relatively weak compared with nalorphine, nalbuphine is probably not an effective antidote in the treatment of many effects induced by opiate agonists. However, nalbuphine has effectively reversed or prevented postoperative respiratory depression induced by opiate agonists, without reversing analgesia, in many but not all patients.

Nalbuphine should be used with caution in patients who have been chronically receiving opiate agonists because nalbuphine does not suppress the abstinence syndrome in these patients, and high doses may precipitate withdrawal symptoms as a result of opiate antagonist effect.

The effects of nalbuphine are additive with those of other central nervous system depressants, such as general anesthetics, phenothiazines or other tranquilizers, sedatives, hypnotics, or alcohol. When nalbuphine is used concomitantly with other depressant drugs, the dose of one or both drugs should be decreased.

Tolerance and Dependence

Tolerance and psychological and physical dependence may occur in patients receiving nalbuphine, and unnecessary increases in dosage or frequency of administration should be avoided. Nalbuphine has been shown to have a low abuse potential. When compared with drugs which are mixed agonist-antagonists, it has been reported that nalbuphine's potential for abuse would be less than that of codeine and propoxyphene. Following abrupt discontinuance after prolonged use of nalbuphine, withdrawal symptoms, which are similar to but more intense than those produced by pentazocine, have occurred and may include abdominal cramps, nausea, vomiting, rhinorrhea, lacrimation, restlessness, anxiety, increased temperature, and piloerection.

Pentazocine (Talwin)

Pentazocine is a synthetic opiate agonist similar to butorphanol and nalbuphine with very weak antagonist effects. The analgesic and respiratory depressant activity of the drug apparently result mainly from the *l*-isomer. Pentazocine differs from other opioids in its action at μ-, κ-, and σ-receptors (36). It acts as both an agonist and an antagonist at μ-receptors, a partial agonist at κ-receptors, and unlike other opioids, an agonist at σ-receptors. Pentazocine has about 1/50 the antagonistic activity of nalorphine (53). Initially, pentazocine was developed with the intention of producing an analgesic with the potency of an opiate but with less potential for addiction because of its mixed agonist–antagonist properties. This was not the case, however.

Pentazocine does not antagonize morphine-induced respiratory depression, but it may precipitate opiate withdrawal symptoms in patients who have been receiving opiates regularly. In patients not tolerant to opiates, the analgesic effect of pentazocine and morphine may be additive; but, in patients tolerant to opiates, pentazocine may produce a dose-related reduction in the analgesic effect of morphine. Pentazocine produces respiratory depression, sedation, miosis, and antitussive effects.

In therapeutic dosages, pentazocine's agonist action at σ-receptors produces psychotomimetic effects, such as dysphoria, uncontrollable or unusual thoughts, anxiety, nightmares, and hallucinations. Orally administered pentazocine undergoes first-pass metabolism in the liver, and less than 20% of a dose reaches the systemic circulation unchanged.

The most common side effect of pentazocine is sedation with subsequent diaphoresis and dizziness. Psychologic side effects include hallucinations, depression, and psychosis. Pentazocine in large doses produces respiratory depression that may be reversed by naloxone. Because the affinity of naloxone for κ- and σ-receptors is less than that for μ-receptors, large doses are frequently required to produce antidotal effects (53).

"T's and Blues"

Pentazocine is often combined with tripelennamine, an antihistamine, to form a relatively common drug of abuse known as "T's and Blues" (11,41,43,46). T's and Blues, used intravenously, was first seen in the Chicago area in 1976 as an alternative to heroin, which was then in low supply there, and quickly spread to other major cities in the Midwest (47). "T's" refers to the pentazocine trade name Talwin and "Blues" is slang derived from the light blue color of the 50-mg tripelennamine tablet, an antihistamine of the ethylenediamine class that is marketed under the trade name Pyribenzamine.

Combinations of opioids and antihistamines have long been used as a "lytic cocktail," although there is no known mechanism to explain why this drug combination produces euphoric or heroin-like effects greater than those of pentazocine alone (41). It is said that tripelennamine prolongs and heightens the duration of the euphoria of the pentazocine (41). The reported injection of solutions of tripelennamine with or without narcotics dates back 20 years, when it was reported as a combination with heroin or paregoric known as "blue velvet." (41) As an antihistamine, tripelennamine can depress or stimulate the central nervous system. In patients with focal neurologic lesions, even small doses can precipitate seizures (43,46). In an overdose of T's and Blues, there is usually a phase of central nervous system depression that is followed by central nervous system excitement and culminates in seizures. The simultaneous injection of tripelennamine with pentazocine greatly increases the frequency of this complication, although seizures have been reported with pentazocine alone.

The constituents of T's and Blues are sold in their legitimate commercial solid dosage forms, and various ratios of the two drugs are used (46). The tablets are crushed and placed in a vial and allowed to dissolve in a small quantity of tap water. The resultant mixture is then filtered through cotton or a cigarette filter and then drawn into a syringe and injected intravenously.

The effect of injection of a "dose," which is typically two or three tablets of pentazocine and one tablet of tripelennamine, may be coma, after which the patient awakens and experiences a euphoric effect. Alternatively, the reaction may be an immediate "rush," which reportedly is indistinguishable from the heroin rush and lasts 5–10 minutes. For most users the rush is followed by dysphoria, so that the injection may be repeated (46). The brief rush may be followed by a feeling of well-being lasting up to 2 hours, which then subsides over the next few hours (46). Because of the purported intense feeling, alcohol or sometimes diazepam is frequently used as an additional drug. Tolerance develops to the repeated injections of the drug, and larger doses need to be injected for the same effect (53).

The oral dosage form of pentazocine was reformulated in 1983 to contain 0.5 mg of naloxone (Talwin Nx). The reformulation to a yellow, oblong caplet, rather than the round peach-colored pill, was intended to eliminate the drug's misuse in T's and Blues. Theoretically, because naloxone is inactive when administered orally in the amount present in this formulation, its presence does not affect the efficacy of oral pentazocine; however, if it is ground up, solubilized, and administered parenterally, the naloxone antagonizes the effects of pentazocine and precipitates withdrawal symptoms in the drug abuser. Despite the theoretical validity of this formulation, Talwin Nx in combination with tripelennamine continues to be abused. This may be due to the following effects. Pentazocine exerts its agonist effects at the κ- and σ-receptors; the euphoria attributed to the drug may derive from its σ-receptor activity. Naloxone predominantly affects μ-receptors and, at a dose of 0.5 mg, may have little or no effect on the κ- and σ-sites. In addition, tripelennamine may also exert some euphoric qualities that would not be blocked by naloxone. It may also be that the dose of naloxone in the preparation is inadequate to block the combined effects of pentazocine and tripelennamine. If the dose were effective, signs of neurologic toxicity after the administration of naloxone as an antidote in overdose

TABLE 45–7. *Clinical effects of "T's and Blues"*

Gastrointestinal
Nausea
Vomiting
Neurologic
Headache
Coma
Muscle tremors
Myoclonus
Seizures
Pulmonary
Shortness of breath
Bronchoconstriction
Congestive heart failure
Psychiatric
Dysphoria
Depression
Confusion
Hallucinations

would be secondary to the anticholinergic effects of the antihistamine.

The adverse effects of T's and Blues that are most often reported include nausea, vomiting, and headache (Table 45–7). More serious early effects of T's and Blues that are frequently reported are muscle tremors, myoclonus, and tonic–clonic seizures, which are possibly due to central excitation from tripelennamine (43). The most frequent and serious reported complication involves the pulmonary system: symptoms may include shortness of breath and wheezing, sometimes leading to pulmonary hypertension and right-sided heart failure (41). These symptoms are similar to those characteristic of intoxication with blue velvet. Evidence suggests that these respiratory symptoms result from intravenous administration of insoluble particulates, such as magnesium silicate (talc), which is found in tripelennamine preparations, or microcrystalline cellulose, which is used as a binder for pentazocine preparations. These may cause a granulomatous reaction that obliterates the smaller vessels in the lung, liver, kidneys, endocardium, and brain and leads to increased pulmonary artery resistance and pulmonary hypertension (41). Other complications of embolization include angiothrombosis of pulmonary arterioles leading to pulmonary infiltrates. Psychiatric disturbances associated with the abuse of pentazocine in T's and Blues include dysphoria, depression, confusion, and hallucinations.

REFERENCES

1. Rosow C: Agonist-antagonist opioids: theory and clinical practice. *Can J Anaesth* 1989;36:S5–S8.
2. Buck M, Blumer J: Opioids and other analgesics. *Crit Care Clin* 1991;7:615–637.
3. Crabtree B: Review of naltrexone, a long-acting opiate antagonist. *Clin Pharmacol* 1984;3:273–280.
4. Foldes F, Lunn J, Moore J, et al: *N*-Allylnoroxymorphone: a new potent narcotic antagonist. *Am J Med Sci* 1963;245:57–64.
5. Handal K, Schauben J, Salamone F: Naloxone. *Ann Emerg Med* 1983;12:438–445.
6. Martin W: Naloxone. *Ann Intern Med* 1976;85:765–768.
7. Foldes F, Duncalf D, Kuwabara S: The respiratory, circulatory, and narcotic antagonistic effects of nalorphine, levallorphan, and naloxone in anaesthetized subjects. *Can Anaesth Soc J* 1969;16:151–161.
8. Greenstein R, Arndt I, McLellan T, et al: Naltrexone: a clinical perspective. *J Clin Psychiatry* 1984;45:25–28.
9. Greenstein R, Resnick R, Resnick E: Methadone and naltrexone in the treatment of heroin dependence. *Psychiatr Clin North Am* 1984;7:671–679.
10. Atkinson R: Endocrine and metabolic effects of opiate antagonists. *J Clin Psychiatry* 1984;45:20–24.
11. Bell E: The use of naloxone in the treatment of diazepam poisoning. *J Pediatr* 1975;87:803–804.
12. Evans L, Swainson C, Roscoe P, et al: Treatment of drug overdosage with naloxone, a specific narcotic antagonist. *Lancet* 1973; 1:452–455.
13. Goldfrank L, Weisman R, Errick J, et al: A dosing nomogram for continuous infusion of intravenous naloxone. *Ann Emerg Med* 1986; 15:566–570.
14. Moore R, Rumack B, Conner C, et al: Naloxone. *Am J Dis Child* 1980;134:156–158.
15. Berkowitz B: The relationship of, pharmacokinetics to pharmacological activity: morphine, methadone and naloxone. *Clin Pharmacol* 1976;1:219–230.
16. Barros S, Rodriguez G: Naloxone as an antagonist in alcohol intoxication. *Anesthesiology* 1981;54:174.
17. Lyon L, Antony J: Reversal of alcoholic coma by naloxone. *Ann Intern Med* 1982;96:464 465.
18. Schneider S, Michelson E, Boucek C, et al: Dextromethorphan poisoning reversed by naloxone. *Am J Emerg Med* 1991;9:237–238.
19. Tandberg U, Abercrombie D: Treatment of heroin overdose with endotracheal naloxone. *Ann Emerg Med* 1982;11:443–445.
20. Wald P, Weisman R, Goldfrand L: Opioids. *Top Emerg Med* 1985;7:9–17.
21. Maio R, Griener J, Clark M, et al: Intralingual naloxone reversal of morphine-induced respiratory depression in dogs. *Ann Emerg Med* 1984;13:1087–1091.
22. Dipalma J: Opiate antagonists: Naloxone. *Am Fam Phys* 1984; 29:270–272.
23. Lovejoy F: Indications for naloxone in Lomotil poisoning. *Pediatrics* 1974;53:658.
24. Kulberg A: Substance abuse: Clinical identification and management. *Pediatr Clin North Am* 1986;33:325–361.
25. Fossel M, Rosen P: Naloxone treatment for codeine induced gastrointestinal symptoms. *J Emerg Med* 1984;2:107–110.
26. Khantzian E, McKenna C: Acute toxic and withdrawal reactions associated with drug use and abuse. *Ann Intern Med* 1979; 90:361–372.
27. Frand U: Methadone-induced pulmonary edema. *Ann Intern Med* 1972;76:975–979.
28. Schwartz J, Koenigsberg M: Naloxone-induced pulmonary edema. *Ann Emerg Med* 1987;16:1294–1296.
29. Zaks A, Jones T, Fink M, et al: Naloxone treatment of opiate dependence. *JAMA* 1971;215:2108–2110.
30. Tanaka G: Hypertensive reaction to naloxone. *JAMA* 1974; 228:25–26.
31. Michaelis L, Hickey P, Clark T, et al: Ventricular irritability associated with the use of naloxone hydrochloride. *Ann Thorac Surg* 1974;18:608–614.
32. Andree R: Sudden death following naloxone administration. *Anaesth Analg* 1980;59:782–784.
33. Banner W, Lund M, Clawson L: Failure of naloxone to reverse clonidine toxic effect. *Am J Dis Child* 1983;137:1170–1171.
34. Jeffcoate W, Hastings A, Cullen M, et al: Naloxone and ethanol antagonism. *Lancet* 1981;1:1052.
35. McNicolas L, Martin W: New and experimental therapeutic roles for naloxone and related opioid antagonists. *Drugs* 1984;27:81–93.
36. Mattila M, Neotto E, Seppala T: Naloxone is not an effective antagonist of ethanol. *Lancet* 1981;1:775–776.
37. Fudala P, Heishman S, Henningfield J, et al: Human pharmacology and abuse potential of nalmefene. *Clin Pharmacol Ther* 1991; 49:300–306.

38. Kaplan J, Marx J: Effectiveness and safety of intravenous nalmefene for emergency department patients with suspected narcotic overose: a pilot study. *Ann Emerg Med* 1993;22:187–190.
39. Volpicelli J, Alterman A, Hayashida M, et al: Naltrexone in the treatment of alcohol dependence. *Arch Gen Psychiatry* 1992;49:876–880.
40. Milhorn H: Pharmacologic management of acute abstinence syndromes. *Am Fam Phys* 1992;45:231–239.
41. O'Brien C, Childress A, McLellan A, et al: Use of naloxone to extinguish opioid-conditioned responses. *J Clin Psychiatry* 1984;45: 53–56.
42. O'Malley S, Jaffe A, Chang G, et al: Naltrexone and coping skills therapy for alcohol dependence. *Arch Gen Psychiatry* 1992;49:881–887.
43. Judson B, Goldstein A: Naltrexone treatment of heroin addiction: One year follow-up. *Drug Alcohol Depend* 1984;13:357–365.
44. Skinner M, Thompson D: Pharmacologic considerations in the treatment of substance abuse. *South Med J* 1992;85:1207–1219.
45. Guthrie S: Pharmacologic interventions for the treatment of opioid dependence and withdrawal. *DICP Ann Pharmacother* 1990;24: 721–734,
46. Ginzburg H, MacDonald M: The role of naltrexone in the management of drug abuse. *Med Toxicol* 1987;2:83–92.
47. Kleber H, Kosten T, Gaspari J, et al: Nontolerance to the opioid antagonism of naltrexone. *Biol Psychiatry* 1985;20:66–72.
48. Myer E, Morris D, Brase D, et al: Naltrexone therapy of apnea in children with elevated cerebrospinal fluid B-endorphin. *Ann Neurol* 1000;27:75–80.
49. Zola E, McLeod D: Comparative effects and analgesic efficacy of the agonist-antagonist opioids. *Drug Intell Clin Pharmacol* 1983;17: 411–417.
50. Ford M, Hoffman R, Goldfrank L: Opioids and designer drugs. *Emerg Clin North Am* 1990;8:495–511.
51. Fraser A: Clinical toxicology of drugs used in the treatment of opiate dependency. *Clin Lab Med* 1990;10:375–386.
52. Preston K, Bigelow G, Liebson I: Antagonist effects of nalbuphine in opioid-dependent human volunteers. *J Pharmacol Exp Ther* 1989; 248:929–937.
53. Challoner K, McCarron M, Newton E: Pentazocine (Talwin®) intoxication: report of 57 cases. *J Emerg Med* 1990;8:67–74.

CHAPTER 46

Sedative-Hypnotics

HISTORY

The use of depressant compounds is as old as the use of alcohol, which is the oldest of the depressant agents. In earlier days, alcohol was held to be a remedy for practically all diseases and problems. Since then, many compounds other than alcohol have been manufactured for many of the same effects.

Sedative-hypnotics are the drugs most frequently involved in deliberate overdosage situations, in part because of their general availability as the most commonly prescribed pharmacologic agents (1,2). The benzodiazepines are generally considered to be "safer" drugs in this respect. Yet, since most serious cases of drug overdosage, intentional or accidental, involve polypharmacy, when combinations of agents are taken, the practical "safety" of benzodiazepines may be less than the foregoing would imply (3).

The lethal dose of any sedative-hypnotic is variable. If discovery of the ingestion is made early and a conservative treatment regimen is started, the outcome is rarely fatal, even following very high doses. On the other hand, for most sedative-hypnotics, with the exception of benzodiazepines, a dose as low as ten times what is required for hypnosis may be fatal if the patient is not discovered or does not seek help in time. With severe toxicity, the respiratory depression from central actions of the drug may be complicated by aspiration of gastric contents in the unattended patient—an even more likely occurrence if ethanol is present. Loss of brain stem vasomotor control, together with direct myocardial depression, further complicates successful resuscitation. In such patients, treatment consists of mechanical respiration; maintenance of plasma volume, renal output, and cardiac function; and perhaps use of a positive inotropic drug, such as dopamine, that preserves renal blood flow. Hemodialysis or hemoperfusion may be used to hasten elimination of some of the sedative-hypnotics.

TYPES OF ACTIONS

The sedative-hypnotic compounds are drugs that have diverse chemical structures but have in common their ability to induce various degrees of behavioral depression (1,2). The method of classification arose primarily as an attempt to categorize the drugs according to the subjective and behavioral effects produced by them, that is, sedation and hypnosis (4). Hypnotics are used to produce sleep, and sedatives are used to relieve anxiety, restlessness, irritability, and tension (5). Often, there is no sharp distinction between the two effects, and the same drug may have both actions, depending on the method of use and the dose employed. Other terms that describe these drugs include minor tranquilizers, anxiolytic drugs, and antianxiety agents. These terms are often used interchangeably because there is no clear distinction among many of the drugs and their effects. In large amounts, these drugs produce a state of intoxication similar to that induced by ethanol and can, in addition, produce sedation, tranquilization, hypnosis, and anesthesia (2).

TYPES OF SEDATIVE-HYPNOTICS

Sedative-hypnotics are generally categorized as one of three main types: the barbiturates, the nonbarbiturate-nonbenzodiazepines, and the benzodiazepines (Table 46–1). Drugs in the first two classes have a greater potential for serious systemic sequelae of misuse than those in the last group (6). Although there are other drugs that have sedation as a property, such as the antihistamines, sedation is usually seen as a side effect in other drugs. Such drugs are therefore not included in this discussion.

Early agents, such as bromides and chloral hydrate, were replaced in great part by the barbiturates in the early 1900s (7). Currently, benzodiazepines, introduced in 1960, have supplanted most of the other agents and are among the most commonly prescribed drugs in the Western world (8).

Many of the effects from the sedative-hypnotics are similar, and much of the treatment after an overdose is symptomatic. As with the narcotics, there are two areas of concern: the management of the overdosed patient and the management of the withdrawal state, which is recog-

TABLE 46–1. *Sedative-hypnotic agents*

Barbiturates
Ultrashort-acting
Thiopental
Methohexital
Buthabital
Hexobarbital
Thiamylal
Short- and intermediate-acting
Amobarbital
Aprobarbital
Butabarbital
Butalbital
Pentobarbital
Secobarbital
Talbutal
Long-acting
Phenobarbital
Mephobarbital
Metharbital
Nonbarbiturate-nonbenzodiazepine
Buspirone
Carisoprodol (Soma)
Chloral hydrate
Chlormezanone (Trancopal)
Ethchlorvynol (Placidyl)
Glutethimide (Doriden)
Mebrobamate (Equanil)
Methaqualone (Quaalude)
Methyprylon (Noludar)
Paraldehyde
Zolpidem (Ambien)
Benzodiazepines
Antianxiety agents
Alprazolam (Xanax)
Chlordiazepoxide (Librium, Libritabs, Murcel, Reposans, Tenax, Zetran)
Clorazepate (Tranxene)
Diazepam (Valium)
Halazepam (Paxipam)
Lorazepam (Ativan)
Oxazepam (Serax)
Prazepam (Centrax)
Anticonvulsants
Clonazepam (Clonopin)
Clorazepate
Diazepam
Hypnotic agents
Flurazepam (Dalmane)
Midazolam (Versed)
Temazepam (Restoril)
Triazolam (Halcion)

nized as a medical emergency more serious than that of any other drug of abuse.

GENERAL CLINICAL EFFECTS

The members of the sedative-hypnotic class depress the activity of all excitable tissue, particularly nerve cells. This depressant effect is reversible and its action is transient on acute administration. The central nervous system is exquisitely sensitive to sedative-hypnotics in doses that produce little effect on skeletal, cardiac, or smooth muscle. Low doses of the sedative-hypnotics produce mild sedation (5). In larger doses, as in acute intoxication, the drugs can suppress function in cardiovascular activity and in other peripheral organs.

In high doses, the main cause of morbidity and mortality is the resulting coma and apnea. Tolerance to the intoxicating effects develops rapidly and may lead to a progressive narrowing of the margin of safety between an intoxicating and lethal dose of the drug. Drug abusers may be able to increase their daily dose up to 10–20 times the recommended therapeutic dose (5).

Toxic reactions from the sedative-hypnotics involve a general slowing of mental functions, slurred speech, ataxia, and impairment in thinking, including poor comprehension, memory disturbance, increased reaction time, poor judgment, limited attention span, labile mood, and a release of aggressive impulses. In large doses, sleep, stupor, coma, and death from respiratory and circulatory depression are possible (Table 46–2).

TABLE 46–2. *Toxic effects of sedative-hypnotics*

Slowing of mental function
Slurred speech
Ataxia
Memory disturbance
Increased reaction time
Poor judgement
Limited attention span
Release of aggressive impulses
Stupor
Coma
Respiratory depression
Circulatory depression

Alcoholics often take sedative-hypnotics, as do opiate and cocaine addicts. Short-acting barbiturates, such as pentobarbital ("yellow jackets") or secobarbital ("red devils"), are preferred by these users to long-acting agents, such as phenobarbital. Other sedative-hypnotics commonly used by alcoholics are meprobamate, glutethimide, methyprylon, methaqualone, and the benzodiazepines. Paraldehyde and chloral hydrate are still available but have been replaced by other drugs that do not have such noxious side effects (7).

LONG-TERM EFFECTS OF SEDATIVE-HYPNOTICS

Many of the sedative-hypnotics have actions and toxicities that are similar to those of the barbiturates. Barbiturates stimulate the hepatic microsomal enzyme system in the liver; meprobamate, chloral hydrate,

TABLE 46–3. *Sedative-hypnotics that stimulate the liver microsomal enzyme system*

Barbiturates
Chloral hydrate
Glutethimide
Methaqualone
Meprobamate

glutethimide, and methaqualone also stimulate this enzyme system (Table 46–3). The consequence is that an individual who has been taking any of these drugs chronically may need to increase the amount to achieve the same therapeutic effect. At the same time tolerance to the lethal dose does not change much, which causes greater morbidity and mortality than the safer alternatives, the benzodiazepines (8).

ROLE OF GAMMA AMINO BUTYRIC ACID (GABA)

GABA is thought to be the major inhibitory transmitter in the human central nervous system, being used by as many as 40% of neurons. GABA is synthesized from L-glutamate by the enzyme glutamic acid decarboxylase. GABA exerts it physiological actions at two classes of receptors, designated GABA-A and GABA-B. These receptors can be distinguished pharmacologically and physiologically. GABA-B receptors represent the minority of GABA sites and are insensitive to benzodiazepines or barbiturates.

At type A receptors, GABA promotes the direct opening of chloride-selective ion channels. In most neurons, electrochemical gradients drive an influx of chloride into neurons, thus hyperpolarizing the membrane and inhibiting cell firing. Agents that inhibit GABA-A function act as convulsants, presumably by mediating a decrement in GABA-A mediated inhibition.

In addition to having sites for agonists and inhibitors, the GABA-A complex is also a site of action for potentiating compounds, such as barbiturates, benzodiazepines, steroid anesthetics, and ethanol. These agents, acting through several distinct mechanisms, augment chloride currents that flow through the GABA-A ion channel. Because many sedative-hypnotic agents modulate GABA, this theory explains the similar effects of sedative-hypnotic agents and the cross-tolerance that exists among these agents (7).

GABA and Barbiturates

Barbiturates increase GABA responses by prolonging the length of time that chloride channels remain open. After treatment with barbiturates, the mean channel open time increases 4–5 times, without change in the single channel current amplitude. As a result, chloride flows through the GABA channel for a substantially longer time after the channel is exposed to barbiturates (9).

GABA and Benzodiazepines

Although the GABA-benzodiazepine receptor complex has not been fully characterized, research supports the concept of a neuronal cell surface protein complex containing a benzodiazepine receptor, a GABA receptor, and a chloride channel (10,11). These three sites are believed to be anatomically distinct but closely related functionally. Activation of the benzodiazepine receptor appears to increase the sensitivity of the GABA receptor complex to stimulation by GABA. Binding of GABA to postsynaptic sites causes an increase in the chloride conductance, with resultant membrane hyperpolarization. Benzodiazepines cause no change in their conductance or any alteration in the synthesis, release, reuptake, or degradation of GABA. There is also no competitive binding at GABA receptors. Some evidence suggests that benzodiazepine receptor sites are heterogeneous, with at least two central nervous system subtypes of benzodiazepine receptors being described to date [type 1 (BZ1) and type 2 (BZ2)] (12,13). This suggests that different benzodiazepine receptors, coupled to GABA-A receptors, may be responsible for anxiolytic and sedative effects (14).

Benzodiazepines act on the GABA-A receptor at sites distinct from those of barbiturates to alter GABA-mediated responses. It has become apparent that benzodiazepine receptors exhibit a complex pharmacology; these sites bind molecules that augment, inhibit, or have no effect on GABA responses (9).

A benzodiazepine binding site pharmacologically distinct from that associated with the GABA-A receptor has also been described. This protein is found in the brain and peripheral tissues and is associated with the mitochondria. The function of these peripheral-type receptors is unclear. These peripheral receptors may play a role in adaptive metabolic responses (15).

REFERENCES

1. Matthew H, Lawson A: Acute barbiturate poisoning: a review of two years' experience. *Q J Med* 1966;35:539–550.
2. Gault F: A review of recent literature on barbiturate addiction and withdrawal. *Bol Estud Med Biol* 1976;29:75–83.
3. Gillin J: The long and short of sleeping pills. *N Engl J Med* 1991;324:1735–1736.
4. Truog RT, Bewrde C, Mitchell C, et al: Barbiturates in the care of the terminally ill. *N Engl J Med* 1992;327:1678–1682.

5. Matthew H: Barbiturates. *Clin Toxicol* 1975;8:495–513.
6. Bertino J, Reed M: Barbiturate and nonbarbiturate sedative-hypnotic intoxication in children. *Pediatr Clin North Am* 1986;33:703–722.
7. Miller N, Gold M: Sedative-hypnotics: pharmacology and use. *J Fam Pract* 1989;29:665–670.
8. Dire D: Benzodiazepine toxicity: dealing with too much of a good thing. *Emerg Med Rep* 1992;13:73–80.
9. Zorumski C, Isenberg K: Insights into the structure and function of GABA-benzodiazepine receptors: ion channels and psychiatry. *Am J Psychiatry* 1991;148:162–173.
10. Haefely W: The biological basis of benzodiazepine actions. *J Psychoactive Drugs* 1983;15:19–39.
11. Tallman J: Benzodiazepines: from receptor to function in sleep. *Sleep* 1982;5:812–817.
12. Aarseth H, Bredesen J, Grynne B, et al: Benzodiazepine-receptor antagonist, a clinical double blind study. *J Toxicol Clin Toxicol* 1988;26:283–292.
13. Verma A, Snyder S: Peripheral type benzodiazepine receptors. *Annu Rev Pharmacol Toxicol* 1989;2(9):307–322.
14. Mullen K: Benzodiazepine compounds and hepatic encephalopathy. *N Engl J Med* 1991;325:509–511.
15. Bansky G, Meier P, Riederer E, et al: Effects of the benzodiazepine receptor antagonist flumazenil in hepatic encephalopathy in humans. *Gastroenterology* 1989;97:744–750.

CHAPTER 47

Barbiturates

Barbiturates are among the drugs still very commonly prescribed to induce sedation and sleep. Barbiturates are derivatives of barbituric acid and are formed from the condensation of urea and malonic acid (1). They acquire an alkyl or aryl group, which confers their sedative-hypnotic properties. The first barbiturates were prepared in 1864; since that time about 2,500 derivatives of barbituric acid have been synthesized, but only about 15 remain in medical use (2). Barbiturates are capable of producing all levels of central nervous system depression, from mild sedation to hypnosis to deep coma and death. The degree of depression depends on dose, route of administration, and pharmacokinetics of the particular barbiturate (3).

PATTERNS OF ABUSE

Patterns of abuse of the barbiturates vary from intermittent recreational use to compulsive daily use with chronic intoxication. Most barbiturate poisonings in adults are suicide attempts.

Some people abuse barbiturates to produce sleep, but more probably abuse them for the euphoria they cause. It is not uncommon for barbiturates and amphetamines to be abused at the same time. Abusers claim that this combination produces more elation than either class of drugs alone (2).

Many of the barbiturates have street names related to their colors. Phenobarbital pills are called "purple hearts." Secobarbital is red, so that the terms "reds," "red devils," and "red birds" are used. Amobarbital is blue and goes by the terms "blues" and "blue devils." A combination of reds and blues, or amobarbital and secobarbital, is Tuinal or "Christmas trees." Pentobarbital is yellow, so that the names "yellows" or "yellow jackets" are used.

MECHANISM OF ACTION

The mechanism of action of the barbiturates is not completely known. In the central nervous system, barbiturates facilitate inhibitory neurotransmission by inhibiting chemical neurotransmission across neuronal and neuroeffector junctions (1,4). Barbiturates increase GABA responses by prolonging the length of time that chloride channels remain open. After treatment with barbiturates, the mean channel open time increases 4–5 times, without change in the single channel current amplitude (5). As a result, chloride flows through the GABA channel for a substantially longer time after the channel is exposed to barbiturates. Barbiturates thus facilitate inhibitory neurotransmission in the central nervous system with a subsequent decrease in the activity of postsynaptic cyclic guanosine monophosphate and cyclic AMP (6). Although the drugs act throughout the central nervous system, a site of particular sensitivity is the polysynaptic midbrain reticular formation, which is concerned with the arousal mechanism (7). Barbiturates induce an imbalance in central inhibitory and facilitatory mechanisms influencing the cerebral cortex and the reticular formation (3). Although the drugs decrease the excitability of both presynaptic and postsynaptic membranes, it has not been determined which of the various actions of barbiturates at cellular and synaptic levels are responsible for their sedative and hypnotic effects (8).

PHARMACOKINETICS

The lipid solubility of the barbiturates is the dominant factor in their distribution through the body (1). Barbiturates suitable for clinical use as anesthetics are those that are the most lipid soluble and can most rapidly penetrate all tissues. In general, the more lipid soluble the barbiturate, the more rapid the onset of its action, the shorter the duration of its effects, and the greater the degree of its hypnotic activity. The highly lipid-soluble drugs penetrate the blood-brain barrier rapidly. Less lipid-soluble drugs, such as phenobarbital, penetrate and leave the brain more slowly and thus have a slower onset and longer duration of action. Termination of action with these barbiturates depends more on redistribution than metabolism (7).

CLASSIFICATION OF BARBITURATES

The duration of action of the barbiturates is multifactorial and depends on the rates of drug absorption, whether

TABLE 47–1. *Classification of barbiturates by duration of action*

Ultrashort-acting
Thiopental
Methohexital
Buthabital
Hexobarbital
Thiamylal
Short- and intermediate-acting
Amobarbital
Aprobarbital
Butabarbital
Butalbital
Pentobarbital
Secobarbital
Talbutal
Long-acting
Phenobarbital
Mephobarbital
Metharbital

elimination is primarily by metabolic degradation or excretion, and the rate of removal of the active drug from the central nervous system. On the basis of these differences in the duration of action, barbiturates are classified into three categories: ultrashort-acting, short- and intermediate-acting, and long-acting (Table 47–1) (1). The anticonvulsant primidone (Mysoline) is metabolized to phenobarbital and thus should be considered a barbiturate (4).

Following oral administration, the onset of action varies from 10–30 minutes for amobarbital, aprobarbital, butabarbital, pentobarbital, and secobarbital and from 20–60 minutes for metharbital, mephobarbital, and phenobarbital. There appears to be little difference in duration of the hypnotic action among barbiturates used orally as hypnotics (9). For this reason, barbiturates have recently been grouped according to their intended pharmacologic action, sedative-hypnotic or anesthetic, rather than according to the duration of their action, since classification problems also arose when it was found that the length of time that the drug action persisted did not parallel the time it took to eliminate half the dose of the drug, the elimination half-life. Although the old classification is not used, nothing has been devised to replace it. However, because of the convenience of categorizing barbiturates as to their duration of action, this method is used in this chapter.

The fatal dose of barbiturates with intermediate or short half-lives is usually lower than the fatal dose of drugs with longer half-lives. For example, to induce severe poisoning, it takes less pentobarbital than phenobarbital when they are compared on a milligram-to-milligram basis (3).

Ultrashort-Acting Barbiturates

The ultrashort-acting barbiturates are thiopental, methohexital, buthabital, hexobarbital, and thiamylal (10). These drugs are not a source of abuse, and there should be no occasion to see an overdose with these drugs in an emergency department setting.

Short- and Intermediate-Acting Barbiturates

The short-acting and intermediate-acting barbiturates, such as secobarbital and pentobarbital, are used for induction of general anesthesia. Their relatively swift onset and short duration of action allow for general anesthesia that is rapid and easily reversible. Ease of titration and low acute toxicity in usual doses add to their usefulness (2).

The short- and intermediate-acting barbiturates have an onset of action of 15–40 minutes and a duration of 6 hours. These drugs are the most widely used and abused barbiturates, both separately and in combination. They include, among others, pentobarbital, secobarbital, amobarbital, and butalbital (Table 47–2). Tuinal is a combination of amobarbital and secobarbital and is a favored drug for abuse. Overdoses of the short acting barbiturates have the highest mortality rate (4,11).

Long-Acting Barbiturates

The long-acting barbiturates have an onset of action of approximately 1 hour and a duration of action of up to 16

TABLE 47–2. *Selected trade names of commonly abused barbiturates*

Amobarbital
Amytal
Aprobarbital
Alurate
Butabarbital
Butal
Butalan
Butapan
Butazem
Buticaps
Butisol
Soduben
Butalbital
Fiorinal
Metharbital
Bemonil
Pentobarbital
Nembutal
PBR/12
Phenobarbital
Luminal
Phen-Squar
Sedadrops
Secobarbital
Seconal
Talbutal
Lotusate

hours. They are used as sedative-hypnotics, anticonvulsants, in treating gastrointestinal disorders, and as preanesthetic agents. Some of the drugs in this group (Table 47–2) are phenobarbital and drugs that act as or are converted to phenobarbital in the body, such as methylphenobarbital (12,13). These drugs are also abused but not to the same extent as the short-acting barbiturates (4).

METABOLISM

To some degree, all barbiturates undergo metabolic degradation by the liver (14,15). After ingestion, the short-acting barbiturates are initially and rapidly sequestered in the tissues so that their effects on the central nervous system are terminated rapidly. These agents are then mobilized slowly and immediately degraded by the liver, and their inactive products are excreted in urine. Long-acting drugs are metabolized by the slower process of urinary excretion. For example, 25%–50% of a dose of phenobarbital is excreted unchanged in the urine.

The barbiturates compete with other substrates that are metabolized by the cytochrome P-450. The barbiturates and other sedative-hypnotics combine with the cytochrome P-450 system to inhibit the biotransformation of those drugs that also combine with that system. More often, however, the barbiturates cause a marked increase in the microsomal enzyme system to accelerate the metabolism of other drugs, including the sedative-hypnotics themselves (Table 47–3). This drug-induced biotransformation of itself and other drugs is another source of tolerance and cross-tolerance. Various anesthetics, ethanol, and the sedative-hypnotic drugs are metabolized by and induce the microsomal enzyme systems, thus producing multidirectional cross-tolerance.

TOXICITY

Overdosage of barbiturates occurs through attempts to commit suicide, miscalculations by drug abusers, and accidents, such as might occur in children.

Clinical Features

Low doses of the barbiturates depress the sensory cortex, decrease motor activity, and produce sedation and drowsiness. In some patients, drowsiness may be preceded by a period of transient elation, confusion, euphoria, or excitement. This may be particularly true for children and the elderly (16). Barbiturates do not reduce pain. They may actually increase sensitivity to pain. If the patient is in pain when the barbiturate is taken, excitement instead of sedation may occur.

TABLE 47–3. *Sedative-hypnotics that stimulate the liver microsomal enzyme system*

Barbiturates
Chloral hydrate
Glutethimide
Methaqualone
Meprobamate

Mild to Moderate Overdose

Mild to moderate barbiturate intoxication may mimic the clinical picture of alcohol intoxication. The neurologic examination may reveal general incoordination with nystagmus, slurred speech, and dysmetria. On examination, one may observe nystagmus, finger-to-nose and heel-to-shin ataxia, and uncoordinated rapid alternating movements of the hands and tandem walking.

Severe Toxicity

The toxic dose of barbiturates varies considerably, but in general a severe reaction is likely to occur when the amount ingested is more than 10 times the usual oral hypnotic dose (9). Overdosage produces central nervous system depression ranging from sleep to coma and death (1). Respiratory depression may progress to Cheyne–Stokes respiration and central hypoventilation. Also noted are cyanosis, cold clammy skin, areflexia, tachycardia, hypotension, anuria, and hypothermia. Hypothermia results from depression of the temperature-regulating mechanism in the pons. It is usually seen in fairly deeply unconscious patients who have been exposed for several hours. Patients with severe overdosage often experience typical shock syndrome such as apnea along with circulatory collapse. Barbiturates may have a direct toxic effect on the myocardium, but large doses are required to achieve this effect (14,15). In addition, there may be a reduction in vasomotor tone of the smaller peripheral blood vessels with escape of fluid into the extravascular space, leading to hypotension and shock (Table 47–4). Because of the central and peripheral effects of the barbiturates, which often lead to hypoxia, hypotension, and shock, a lactic acidosis may ensue.

Short-acting barbiturates may cause respiratory depression as quickly as they produce unconsciousness. These agents are considered dangerous because many patients die before rescue efforts can be initiated (13).

Serious Complications of Overdose

The serious complications from barbiturate overdose include pulmonary complications, such as aspiration, pneumonia, and pulmonary edema (17). In addition, acute tubular necrosis subsequent to hypotension, hypo-

TABLE 47–4. *Clinical features of severe barbiturate overdose*

Neurologic
Areflexia
Cerebral edema
Coma
Hypothermia
Sleep
Respiratory
Apnea
Cyanosis
Respiratory depression
Cardiovascular
Circulatory collapse
Hypotension
Pulmonary edema
Tachycardia
Miscellaneous
Blisters
Acute tubular necrosis

volemia, and cerebral edema has also been reported. A severe overdose of barbiturates can also cause hypotension, profound shock, ventilatory depression, coma, and death as a result of cardioventilatory failure from depression of the vital medullary centers (17).

"Barbiturate Blisters"

Barbiturate blisters were first described about 50 years ago, and although blisters do not affect the outcome of a barbiturate-intoxicated patient they can be of considerable diagnostic importance (16). They can appear as early as 4 hours after ingestion and do not necessarily occur over areas of maximum pressure; rather, they most often occur where skin surfaces have been in contact with each other (18). These lesions are usually multiple and consist of erythematous, indurated, irregular patches progressing to bullous lesions. Their presence is not dependent on depth of coma or associated complications, such as hypotension and respiratory insufficiency. These bullous cutaneous lesions may heal slowly. Although the precise mechanism of development of these lesions is unknown, a local toxic effect has been postulated (19). These blisters are important in that, although barbiturates are just one of the drugs that can cause them, their presence may give a clue as to what was ingested (see Chapter 1) (20,21).

LABORATORY ANALYSIS

The serum barbiturate concentration is not regarded as an important indicator of the severity of poisoning because it is not necessarily closely related to the clinical state. It also has little prognostic value in determining depth or duration of coma (22). This is particularly so in epileptic patients and others habituated to these drugs (23). Serum barbiturate determinations may be of benefit, however, in discerning the etiology of coma and can distinguish short from long-acting agents. In assessing a patient with barbiturate poisoning, the serum concentration should always be considered in relation to the patient's history and clinical condition and should never take precedence over the latter (24).

TREATMENT

Supportive Therapy

The treatment of the barbiturate overdose (Table 47–5) consists mainly of supportive therapy. Because most deaths are due to respiratory causes, attention to the airway is the immediate priority. Maintenance of an adequate airway, administration of oxygen, and assisted respiration, if necessary, are extremely important (2). Measures to remove the remaining material from the gastrointestinal tract by lavage and by administering activated charcoal and a cathartic should be instituted. Fluids should be administered for blood pressure support and for diuresis if necessary (1). Often, the blood pressure may return to normal after dehydration has been corrected and adequate ventilation has been restored. Vasoconstrictors are usually not necessary for blood pressure support, and fluid administration is usually adequate to correct even severe hypotension.

Role of Analeptic Agents

Analeptic drugs should not be administered because they may produce paroxysmal cerebral activity, which may result in generalized seizures. In addition, it has been demonstrated that analeptics are incapable of stimulating respiration and exerting an arousal effect in patients with severe barbiturate poisoning and profound central nervous system depression.

Multiple-Dose Activated Charcoal

Recently, it has been shown that multiple-dose activated charcoal is of some benefit for phenobarbital over-

TABLE 47–5. *Treatment of barbiturate overdose*

Gastric lavage
Activated charcoal and cathartic
Maintenance of patent airway
Fluid administration for blood pressure support
Forced alkaline diuresis (for long-acting barbiturate over dose)
Hemodialysis (for long-acting barbiturate overdose)
Hemoperfusion (for long-acting barbiturate overdose)
Multiple-dose activated charcoal (for long-acting barbiturate overdose)

dose by decreasing the half-life of the drug, enhancing the elimination, and shortening the duration of coma (1,25–27). The charcoal can be administered either orally (if the patient is cooperative) or through a nasogastric tube every 2–6 hours (28). Activated charcoal, by adsorbing phenobarbital in the gastrointestinal tract, sets up a gradient differential that allows more phenobarbital to diffuse from blood into the bowel, where it is subsequently adsorbed by the charcoal (25). This is considered "intestinal dialysis." (29) In addition to its direct adsorptive properties, activated charcoal significantly shortens the elimination half-life and increases total body nonrenal clearance of the drug (30). The effectiveness of this procedure is comparable to forced alkaline diuresis or dialysis, and it can be promptly and easily initiated (28,29).

Urinary Alkalinization

Urinary alkalinization promotes ionization of barbiturates, which prevents tubular reabsorption and thus traps the drug in the kidney for excretion. An alkaline diuresis may only be useful in enhancing the excretion of the long-acting barbiturates (phenobarbital) or drugs that are converted to phenobarbital in the body (primidone and mephobarbital). It is ineffective for the short or intermediate-acting barbiturates (31). Although an alkaline diuresis removes reasonable amounts of the long-acting barbiturates, it should be reserved for the severely poisoned patient because there are risks associated with this procedure (32).

Extracorporeal Methods

Hemodialysis and, to a lesser extent, peritoneal dialysis also remove long-acting barbiturates in significant amounts in a severely poisoned patient (33). Hemoperfusion has also been shown to decrease the duration of coma caused by the long-acting barbiturates (33). The amounts of intermediate and short-acting barbiturates retrieved are not substantial, and dialysis should not be attempted in these situations. Extracorporeal measures should only be used if other measures are unsuccessful or in patients with impaired drug elimination due to renal failure. These methods should be necessary only in rare cases (31).

REFERENCES

1. Bertino J, Reed M: Barbiturate and nonbarbiturate sedative-hypnotic intoxication in children. *Pediatr Clin North Am* 1986;33:703–722.
2. Miller N, Gold M: Sedative-hypnotics: pharmacology and use. *J Fam Prac* 1989;29:665–670.
3. Gillin J: The long and short of sleeping pills. *N Engl J Med* 1991; 324:1735–1736.
4. Baltarowich L: Barbiturates. *Top Emerg Med* 1985;7:46–54.
5. Zorumski C, Isenberg K: Insights into the structure and function of GABA-benzodiazepine receptors: ion channels and psychiatry. *Am J Psychiatry* 1001;148:162–173.
6. Robinson R, Gunnells J, Clapp J: Treatment of acute barbiturate intoxication. *Mod Treat* 1971;8:561–579.
7. Truog RT, Bewrde C, Mitchell C, et al: Barbiturates in the care of the terminally ill. *N Engl J Med* 1992;327:1678–1682.
8. Johnson W, Hall A, Rumack B: Cyanide poisoning successfully treated without "therapeutic methemoglobin levels." *Am J Emerg Med* 1989;7:437–440.
9. Gary N, Tresznewsky O: Barbiturates and a potpourri of other sedatives, hypnotics, and tranquilizers. *Heart Lung* 1983;12:122–127.
10. Zink B, Darfler K, Saliuzzo R, et al: The efficacy and safety of methohexital in the emergency department. *Ann Emerg Med* 1991;20;1293–1298.
11. Goldfrank L, Osborn H: The barbiturate overdose. *Hosp Physician* 1977;13:30–33.
12. Hooper W, Kunze H, Eadie M: Qualitative and quantitative studies of methylphenobarbital metabolism in man. *Drug Metab Dispos* 1981;9:381–385.
13. Hooper W, Kunze H, Eadie M: Pharmacokinetics and bioavailability of methylphenobarbital in man. *Ther Drug Monit* 1981;3:39–44.
14. Matthew H, Lawson A: Acute barbiturate poisoning: a review of two years' experience. *Q J Med* 1966;35:539–550.
15. Gault F: A review of recent literature on barbiturate addiction and withdrawal. *Bol Estud Med Biol* 1976;29:75–83.
16. Khantzian E, McKeena G: Acute toxic and withdrawal reactions associated with drug use and abuse. *Ann Intern Med* 1979;90:361–372.
17. Shubin H, Weil M: Shock associated with barbiturate intoxication. *JAMA* 1971;215:263–268.
18. Beveridge G, Lawson A: Occurrence of bullous lesions in acute barbiturate intoxication. *Br Med J* 1965;1:835–837.
19. Groeschel D, Gerstein A, Rosenbaum J: Skin lesions as a diagnostic aid in barbiturate poisoning. *N Engl J Med* 1970;283:409–410.
20. Boyce M, Mason P: Blisters in unconscious patients. *Lancet* 1972;2:874.
21. Burdon J: "Barbiturate burns" caused by glutethimide. *Med J Aust* 1979;1:101–102.
22. Parker K, Elliott H, Wright J, et al: Blood and urine concentrations of subjects receiving barbiturates, meprobamate, glutethimide or diphenylhydanloin. *Clin Toxicol* 1970;3:131–145.
23. Rodichok L: A case of barbiturate poisoning with a readily-accessible laboratory reagent. *J Toxicol Clin Toxicol* 1992;30:455–458.
24. Drost R, Plomp T, Maes R: EMIT-ST drug detection system for screening of barbiturates and benzodiazepines in serum. *J Toxicol Clin Toxicol* 1982;19:303–312.
25. Goldberg M, Berlinger W: Treatment of phenobarbital overdose with activated charcoal. *JAMA* 1982;247:2400–2401.
26. Preskorn S, Denner L: Benzodiazepines and withdrawal psychosis. *JAMA* 1977;237:36–38.
27. Veerman M, Espejo M, Christopher M, et al: Use of activated charcoal to reduce elevated serum phenobarbital concentration in a neonate. *J Toxicol Clin Toxicol* 1991;29:53–58.
28. Berg M, Berlinger W, Goldberg M, et al: Acceleration of the body clearance of phenobarbital by oral activated charcoal. *N Engl J Med* 1982;307:642–644.
29. Pond S, Olson K, Osterloh H, et al: Randomized study of the treatment of phenobarbital overdose with repeated doses of activated charcoal. *JAMA* 1984;251:3104–3108.
30. Amitai Y, Degani Y: Treatment of phenobarbital poisoning with multiple dose activated charcoal in an infant. *J Emerg Med* 1990; 8:449–450.
31. Setter J, Maher J, Schreiner G: Barbiturate intoxication: evaluation of therapy including dialysis in a large series selectively referred because of severity. *Arch Intern Med* 1966;117:224–236.
32. Bloomer H: A critical evaluation of diuresis in the treatment of barbiturate intoxication. *J Lab Clin Med* 1966;67:898–905.
33. Yatzidis H; The use of ion-exchange resins and charcoal in acute barbiturate poisoning, in Matthew H (ed): Acute Barbiturate Poisoning. Amsterdam, Excerpta Medica, 1971;223–232.

CHAPTER 48

Benzodiazepines

The first benzodiazepine, chlordiazepoxide, was introduced in 1960 (1). They are currently the drugs of choice for the pharmacologic treatment of anxiety because of their low lethality, even when taken in massive amounts, and the fact that they do not activate the liver microsomal enzymes, so that their rate of metabolism and that of other drugs that may be in concurrent use is unchanged (2). When alcohol or other central nervous system (CNS) depressants are not used concomitantly, the benzodiazepines are the safest of all currently available antianxiety and hypnotic agents. They also have a wide margin of safety in cases of overdosage (3). Although they appear to have a low potential for abuse, these drugs are used by more Americans than any other single prescription item. Benzodiazepines are frequently prescribed in large quantities and are easily available (4). They are, therefore, prime agents for use in suicide attempts.

CLINICAL USES

Benzodiazepines are among the most widely used drugs in the world. In anesthesia and in the intensive care unit they have proved safe and effective agents for the induction of sedation for a variety of therapeutic goals: in the induction and maintenance of general anesthesia, for conscious sedation in shorter diagnostic and therapeutic procedures, for sedation of patients requiring mechanical ventilation, for the treatment of status epilepticus, and for the sedation of critically ill patients in anxiety-provoking situations. Although the benzodiazepines may be effective for musculoskeletal disorders, the required dose is higher than that currently used (5).

PHARMACOKINETICS

The determinant for onset of action of orally administered benzodiazepines is the rate of gastrointestinal absorption, which is proportional to the lipophilicity of the drug (6). Highly lipophilic benzodiazepines are rapidly absorbed and attain relatively high peak concentrations shortly after administration, causing rapid and intense single-dose effects. Diazepam and clorazepate are two of the most rapidly absorbed benzodiazepines; oxazepam and prazepam are the least rapidly absorbed (7).

Most of the benzodiazepines are metabolized in the liver by oxidation. This pathway has important clinical implications if the drug's metabolite is active, especially if the active metabolite has a long elimination half-life, in which case both the parent compound and the active metabolite accumulate with multiple dosing (Table 48–1). The elimination half-life of the benzodiazepines is prolonged in the elderly because of the age-related decrease in the hepatic transformation for the compounds (8). Chlordiazepoxide, clorazepate, diazepam, halazepam, flurazepam, and prazepam are transformed to active metabolites that have longer half-lives than the parent drug (Table 48–2) (9,10).

The elimination half-life of benzodiazepines is prolonged in elderly patients. Hepatic *N*-desmethylation declines with age secondary to decreased concentration of necessary enzymes. Also the increased proportion of fat to total body weight in the elderly increases the volume of distribution of lipid-soluble drugs. Benzodiazepines, therefore, that have long half-lives, or have active metabolites, should be used with great caution in geriatric patients.

TABLE 48–1. *Classification of benzodiazepines by length of half-life*

Short half-life
Midazolam
Triazolam
Intermediate half-life
Alprazolam
Clonazepam
Lorazepam
Oxazepam
Temazepam
Long half-life
Clorazepate
Chlordiazepoxide
Diazepam
Flurazepam
Halazepam
Prazepam

TABLE 48–2. *Benzodiazepine parent compounds that have active metabolites*

Chlordiazepoxide
Clorazepate
Diazepam
Halazepam
Flurazepam
Prazepam

MECHANISM OF ACTION

A feature of benzodiazepines is their selective action on the CNS. In pharmacologic doses, no direct effect on peripheral organs and tissues has been found; all changes induced by these drugs on peripheral functions are the result of their action on the CNS.

It has been found that the benzodiazepine drugs, as well as other minor tranquilizers, anticonvulsant and convulsant drugs, produce at least part of their pharmacologic effects by affecting one or more regulatory sites on a benzodiazepine receptor complex. This complex is thought to consist of a benzodiazepine receptor that is functionally coupled to a GABA receptor and an associated chloride channel.

The benzodiazepines augment GABA-mediated inhibition by increasing the affinity of GABA for its receptor. Benzodiazepines do not directly alter the properties of the chloride channel but, rather, enhance the ability of GABA to open the channel. As a result, the degree of effect of a benzodiazepine on a GABA response depends on the concentration of GABA. At low GABA concentrations, benzodiazepines produce a marked effect. At saturating agonist concentrations, benzodiazepines have no enhancing effect (11).

Peripheral receptors in the kidney, lung, liver, and heart are known to exist, but benzodiazepine binding to these receptors is fundamentally different from that in the CNS (12). The peripheral cardiac benzodiazepine receptors are believed to be of minimal clinical importance (13). The decrease in left ventricular stroke work and cardiac output that results from benzodiazepine intoxication is thought to arise from the CNS benzodiazepine-GABA receptor system which adversely affects cardiovascular regulation. Although the designation of peripheral-type receptors originally resulted from their relative absence from the brain, use of the specific, high-affinity ligands later demonstrated these sites in the CNS as well (14).

The GABA-enhancing effects of benzodiazepine agonists can be blocked by antagonists such as flumazenil (13). These antagonists do not alter GABA responses themselves but block the actions of benzodiazepine agonists and inverse agonists. The inverse agonists have the opposite effect of agonists, decreasing GABA-mediated chloride responses (11).

TABLE 48–3. *Selected list of benzodiazepines*

Antianxiety agents
Alprazolam (Xanax)
Chlordiazepoxide (Librium, Libritabs, Murcel, Reposans, Tenax, Zetran)
Clorazepate (Tranxene)
Diazepam (Valium)
Halazepam (Paxipam)
Lorazepam (Ativan)
Oxazepam (Serax)
Prazepam (Centrax)
Anticonvulsants
Clonazepam (Clonopin)
Clorazepate
Diazepam
Hypnotic agents
Flurazepam (Dalmane)
Midazolam (Versed)
Temazepam (Restoril)
Triazolam (Halcion)

ACTIONS

The benzodiazepines are capable of producing all levels of CNS depression, from mild sedation to hypnosis and coma (15). In addition, the benzodiazepines suppress the spread of seizure activity but do not abolish the abnormal discharge from a focus in epilepsy.

In therapeutic amounts, the benzodiazepines produce sedation and relief of anxiety and, at higher doses, muscle relaxation (16). Thus, the benzodiazepines are marketed variously as anticonvulsants, antianxiety drugs, and hypnotics, although all the benzodiazepines share these actions and no benzodiazepine has been shown to be superior to chlordiazepoxide or diazepam for the treatment of acute and chronic anxiety or insomnia (17,18). The wide margin of safety of benzodiazepines permits their use in various clinical situations (Table 48–3) (18). The clinical uses of the benzodiazepines are listed in Table 48–4 (19).

TOXICITY

As mentioned above, there are many factors involved in the onset and duration of clinical effects of the benzodiazepines, including metabolism, distribution, degree of protein binding, lipid solubility, and half-life (16). When taken alone, massive quantities of benzodiazepines can be ingested with little or no hazard of prolonged or serious CNS depression, and an overdose of benzodiazepines alone is rarely fatal. The combination of benzodiazepines and alcohol has been lethal, however (2,7,18,20).

Symptoms of overdose of the benzodiazepines include drowsiness, ataxia, dizziness, delirium, somnolence, confusion, and occasionally aggression (21,22). Hypotension and respiratory depression rarely occur (Table 48–5) (16). If deep coma with marked hypotension or cardio-

TABLE 48–4. *Clinical uses of benzodiazepines available in the United States*

Drug	Anxiety	Insomnia	Seizure	Muscle relaxant	IV anesthesia	Alcohol withdrawal
Alprazolam	+	–	–	–	–	+
Chlordiazepoxide	+	–	+	–	–	+
Clonozepam	–	–	+	–	–	–
Clorazepate	+	–	–	–	–	+
Diazepam	+	+	+	+	+	+
Estazolam	–	+	–	–	–	–
Flurazepam	–	+	–	–	–	–
Halazepam	+	–	–	–	–	–
Lorazepam	+	+	+	–	+	+
Midazolam	–	–	–	+	+	–
Oxazepam	+	–	–	–	–	+
Prazepam	+	–	–	–	–	–
Temazepam	–	+	–	–	–	–
Triazolam	–	+	–	–	–	–
Quazepam	–	+	–	–	–	–

+, Currently an indication used for; –, not currently an indication used for.

vascular collapse is clinically present, the clinician should suspect ingestion of another CNS depressant.

LABORATORY ANALYSIS

Single values of the plasma concentration of many of the benzodiazepines are not closely related to their therapeutic or toxic effects because of the presence of metabolites as well as other factors (23,24). Qualitative laboratory analysis may be useful, but quantitation is rarely of benefit (18,24).

TREATMENT

Treatment for benzodiazepine overdose is supportive. Even after a significant overdose of benzodiazepines, mechanical ventilation is not usually required, although, rarely, coma may persist for up to 3 days. Diuresis, dialysis, and hemoperfusion are not indicated (7,15,18).

FLUMAZENIL

It is often desirable to be able to terminate or interrupt sedation without waiting for the effect of the benzodiazepine to become dissipated by normal metabolism and excretion. This constitutes the basic rationale for the application of benzodiazepine antagonism in clinical practice. Flumazenil competitively blocks the effects of benzodiazepines on GABAergic pathway-mediated inhibition in the CNS (17). The drug appears to act at CNS but not peripheral benzodiazepine receptor binding sites. Flumazenil has a high therapeutic index and a wide margin of safety (Table 48–6) (25).

Before the introduction of flumazenil, various substances including naloxone, methylxanthines, and cholinergic agents were investigated as possible benzodiazepine antagonists, with disappointing results. Flumazenil is a ligand of the benzodiazepine receptor that has a high affinity and great specificity for the benzodiazepine receptor. It acts by displacing other centrally acting benzodiazepine agonists by competitive inhibition at receptor sites and reverses all effects of benzodiazepine receptor agonists. Flumazenil is available outside the United States as Anexate, and in the U.S. under the brand name Romazicon (17,25,26).

Pharmacokinetics

Oral doses are rapidly and completely absorbed, with peak levels reached after 20 to 90 minutes; however,

TABLE 48–5. *Clinical features of benzodiazepine overdose*

Aggression
Ataxia
Confusion
Dizziness
Drowsiness
Hypotension (rare)
Respiratory depression (rare)

TABLE 48–6. *Flumazenil*

High affinity for benzodiazepine receptor
Acts by competitive antagonism
Side effects
Nausea
Dizziness
Headache
Blurred vision
Diaphoresis
Anxiety
Panic attacks
Seizures

bioavailability is low by this route due to a hepatic first-pass effect with only 16% of the active drug reaching the general circulation in its original form (19). Flumazenil has a volume of distribution of 1.50 L/kg and a half-life of approximately 1 hour (27). The protein binding of flumazenil is approximately 40%. Any decrease in hepatic blood flow or any impairment of hepatic function prolongs the half-life of flumazenil and its effect.

Flumazenil has a shorter duration of action than most benzodiazepines (19,28). Benzodiazepine antagonism begins within 1 to 2 minutes after IV injection, reaches a peak in 6 to 10 minutes, and lasts for about 1 hour, when the residual effect of the agonist may return, depending on the doses of the agonist and antagonist (27).

Use

Flumazenil has been used to antagonize the effect of benzodiazepines used in general anesthesia and for sedation in conjunction with regional and local anesthesia. In the setting of isolated benzodiazepine overdose, flumazenil is capable of completely reversing coma within 1 to 2 minutes, with this effect lasting between 1 and 5 hours. Repeat doses can be given safely to reverse recurrent effects of longer-acting benzodiazepines. In multiple drug overdose and in coma of uncertain etiology, flumazenil administration has been noted to "unmask" the benzodiazepine component of coma. The need for additional diagnostic evaluations or invasive procedures may then be obviated (28).

Flumazenil may not be effective in treating benzodiazepine-induced respiratory depression. In patients with serious pulmonary disease who experience serious benzodiazepine-induced respiratory depression, primary therapy should be appropriate ventilatory support rather than flumazenil therapy. Flumazenil is an adjunct to, not a substitute for, appropriate supportive and symptomatic measures in the management of benzodiazepine overdosage (29).

Side Effects

When flumazenil is used in pure benzodiazepine overdose, side effects are mild and can usually be avoided by slow administration and with close observation of the patient's reactions (30). However, adverse events, possibly related to flumazenil administration, have been reported to be more frequent in mixed drug overdoses than in pure benzodiazepine intoxication, particularly when tricyclic antidepressants (TCAs) have been ingested. Seizures have been attributed to the unmasking of the proconvulsant effect of antidepressants (31).

Flumazenil can cause nausea, dizziness, headache, blurred vision, increased sweating, and anxiety, and may provoke panic attack in some patients (32,33). Anxiety, which has been reported inconsistently, has been the only significant adverse effect of flumazenil after benzodiazepine-induced general anesthesia. This adverse effect appears to be partially but not entirely dose-related.

The drug can cause convulsions in patients physically dependent on benzodiazepines or taking them to control epilepsy. Flumazenil is not recommended for use in patients with serious concurrent cyclic antidepressant overdosage; in such patients the drug should be withheld and the patient managed with ventilatory and circulatory supportive measures as needed until the signs of antidepressant toxicity have subsided (29).

Flumazenil has no known benefit other than reversal of benzodiazepine-induced sedation in patients with multiple-drug overdosage, and the antagonist should not be used in cases in which seizures from any cause are likely (12).

Because flumazenil has an elimination half-life of only about 1 hour, the effects of the antagonized benzodiazepines may recur. Residual benzodiazepine or metabolites remain after the effects of flumazenil have dissipated (31).

Dosage

For reversal of conscious sedation, an initial dose of 0.2 mg, injected intravenously over 15 seconds, should be given; it can be repeated at 1-minute intervals, if necessary, up to a maximum cumulative dose of 1 mg (32).

For treatment of benzodiazepine overdosage, the same initial dose should be given over 30 seconds, and subsequent doses of 0.3 and then 0.5 mg can be given at 1-minute intervals up to a cumulative dose of 3 mg. A few patients have received a total of 5 mg. However, some patients who exhibit a partial response after a 3-mg cumulative dose rarely may require additional doses up to a total of 5 mg. If no response is observed within 5 minutes after administration of an initial 5-mg cumulative dose of flumazenil, the major cause of sedation may not be a benzodiazepine and additional flumazenil doses likely will provide little if any beneficial effect (31). For recurrent sedation, the initial dose of flumazenil can be repeated at 30 minutes and possibly also at 60 minutes (32). Most patients respond to cumulative flumazenil doses of 0.6–1 mg, but individual requirements may vary considerably depending on the dose and duration of effect of the benzodiazepine administered and patient characteristics (30). In clinical situations where resedation is not yet apparent but must be prevented, the initial dosing regimen can be repeated at 30 and 60 minutes despite the current absence of manifestations of recurrence.

REFERENCES

1. Boyer R: Anticonvulsant properties of benzodiazepines: a review. *Dis Nerv Syst* 1966;27:35–42.
2. Greenblatt D, Allen M, Noel B, et al: Acute overdosage with benzodiazepine derivatives. *Clin Pharmacol Ther* 1977;21:497–500.
3. Greenblatt D, Shader R, Abernethy D: Current status of benzodiazepines: part I. *N Engl J Med* 1983;309:354–358.
4. Miller N, Gold M: Sedative-hypnotics: pharmacology and use. *J Fam Pract* 1989;29:665–670.
5. Greenblatt D, Shader R, Abernethy D: Current status of benzodiazepines: part II. *N Engl J Med* 1983;309:410–416.
6. Greenblatt D. Shader R, Koch-Weser J: Slow absorption of intramuscular chlordiazepoxide.*N Engl J Med* 1974;291:1116–1118.
7. Greenblatt D, Shader R, Koch-Weser J: Flurazepam hydrochloride. *Clin Pharmacol Ther* 1975;17:1–14.
8. Ramoska E, Linkenheimer R, Glasgow C: Midazolam use in the emergency department. *J Emerg Med* 1991;9:247–251.
9. Bertino J, Reed M: Barbiturate and nonbarbiturate sedative-hypnotic intoxication in children. *Pediatr Clin North Am* 1986; 33:703–722.
10. Gamble J, Dundee J, Assaf R: Plasma diazepam levels after single-dose oral and intramuscular administration. *Anaesthesia* 1975; 30:164–169.
11. Zorumski C, Isenberg K: Insights into the structure and function of GABA-benzodiazepine receptors: ion channels and psychiatry. *Am J Psychiatry* 1001;148:162–173.
12. Coates W, Evans T, Jehle D, et al: Flumazenil for the reversal of refractory benzodiazepine-induced shock. *J Toxicol Clin Toxicol* 1991;29:537–542.
13. Aarseth H, Bredesen J, Grynne B, et al: Benzodiazepine-receptor antagonist, a clinical double blind study. *J Toxicol Clin Toxicol* 1988;26:283–292.
14. Verma A, Snyder S: Peripheral type benzodiazepine receptors. *Annu Rev Pharmacol Toxicol* 1989;2(9):307–322.
15. Greenblatt D, Shader R, Koch-Weser J: Flurazepam hydrochloride, a benzodiazepine hypnotic. *Ann Intern Med* 1975;83:237–241.
16. Schauben J: Benzodiazepines. *Top Emerg Med* 1985;7:39–45.
17. Haefely W: The biological basis of benzodiazepine actions. *J Psychoactive Drugs* 1983;15:19–39.
18. Greenblatt D, Woo E, Allen M, et al: Rapid recovery from massive diazepam overdose. *JAMA* 1978;240:1872–1874.
19. Dire D: Benzodiazepine toxicity: dealing with too much of a good thing. *Emerg Med Rep* 1992;13:73–80.
20. Tallman J: Benzodiazepines: from receptor to function in sleep. *Sleep* 1982;5:812–817.
21. Mullen K: Benzodiazepine compounds and hepatic encephalopathy. *N Engl J Med* 1991;325:509–511.
22. Hooker E, Danzl D: Acute dystonic reaction due to diazepam. *J Emerg Med* 1988;6:491–493.
23. Drost R, Plomp T, Maes R: EMIT-ST drug detection system for screening of barbiturates and benzodiazepines in serum. *J Toxicol Clin Toxicol* 1982;19:303–312.
24. Lister R, File S, Greenblatt D: The behavioral effects of lorazepam are poorly related to its concentration in the brain. *Life Sci* 1983;32:2033–2040.
25. Hofer P, Scollo-Lavizzari G: Benzodiazepine antagonist Ro 15-1788 in self-poisoning. *Arch Intern Med* 1985;145:663–664.
26. O'Sullivan G, Wade D: Flumazenil in the management of acute drug overdosage with benzodiazepines and other agents. *Clin Pharmacol Ther* 1987;42:254–259.
27. Votey S, Bosse G, Bayer M, et al: Flumazenil: a new benzodiazepine antagonist. *Ann Emerg Med* 1991;20:181–188.
28. Martens F, Koppel C, Ibe K, et al: Clinical experience with the benzodiazepine antagonist flumazenil in suspected benzodiazepine or ethanol poisoning. *J Toxicol Clin Toxicol* 1990;28:341–356.
29. Chern T, -Hu S, Lee C, et al: Diagnostic and therapeutic utility of flumazenil in comatose patients with drug overdose. *Am J Emerg Med* 1993;11:122–124.
30. Amrein R, Leishman B, Bentzinger C, et al: Flumazenil in benzodiazepine antagonism. *Med Toxicol* 1987;2:411–429.
31. Lhjeureux P, Vranckx M, Leduc D, et al: Flumazenil in mixed benzodiazepine/tricyclic antidepressant overdose: a placebo-controlled study in the dog. *Am J Emerg Med* 1992;10:184–188.
32. Bansky G, Meier P, Riederer E, et al: Effects of the benzodiazepine receptor antagonist flumazenil in hepatic encephalopathy in humans. *Gastroenterology* 1989;97:744–750.
33. Derlet R, Albertson T: Flumazenil induces seizures and death in mixed cocaine-diazepam intoxications. *Ann Emerg Med* 1994; 23:494–498.

ADDITIONAL SELECTED REFERENCES

Costello J, Poklis A. Treatment of massive phenobarbital overdose with dopamine diuresis. *Arch Intern Med* 1981;141:938–940.

Faulkner T. Hayden J, Mehta C, et al: Dose-response studies on tolerance to multiple doses of secobarbital and methaqualone in a polydrug abuse population. *Clin Toxicol* 1979;15:23–37.

Hall S: Apnea after intravenous diazepam therapy. *JAMA* 1977;238:1052.

Hancock B: Acute barbiturate poisoning in young epileptics. *Postgrad Med J* 1974;50:242–244.

Kaplan S, Jack M, Alexander K, et al: Pharmacokinetic profile of diazepam in man following single intravenous and oral and chronic oral administrations. *J Pharmacol Sci* 1973;62:1789–1796.

Korttila K, Linnoila M: Absorption and sedative effects of diazepam after oral administration and intramuscular administration into the vastus lateralis muscle and the deltoid muscle. *Br J Anaesth* 1975;47:857–862.

Lightman S: Phenobarbital dyskinesia. *Postgrad Med J* 1978;54: 114–115.

Maes V, Huyghens L, Dekeyser J, et al: Acute and chronic intoxication with carbromal preparations. *Clin Toxicol* 1985;23:341–346.

McGuigan M, Lovejoy F: Overdose of Lomotil [editorial]. *Br Med J* 1978;1:990.

Murphy J, Sawasky F, Marquardt K, et al: Deaths in young children receiving nitrazepam. *J Pediatr* 1987;111:145–147.

Roytblat L, Bear R, Gesztes T: Seizures after pentazocine overdose. *Isr J Med Sci* 1986;22:385–386.

Sato S, Baud F, Bismuth C, et al: Arterial-venous plasma concentration differences of meprobamate in acute human poisonings. *Hum Toxicol* 1986;5:243–248.

CHAPTER 49

Nonbarbiturates-Nonbenzodiazepines

The barbiturates have been regarded as prototypes of the class because of their extensive use since their introduction approximately 80 years ago. The motivation to develop other sedative-hypnotics can be attributed to efforts to avoid certain undesirable features of the barbiturates, including their potential for addiction and physical dependence. Unfortunately, such efforts have not always been successful. For example, the piperidinediones such as glutethimide, introduced as "nonbarbiturates," are in fact chemically related and virtually indistinguishable from barbiturates in their pharmacologic properties (1). Because of the huge market for sedative-hypnotics, such "failed attempts" have often been commercially successful. The propanediol carbamates such as meprobamate are of distinctive chemical structure but are practically equivalent to barbiturates in their pharmacologic effects, and their clinical use is rapidly declining. The sedative-hypnotic class also includes compounds of simple chemical structure, including alcohols and the cyclic ethers. Chloral hydrate and its congeners, such as trichloroethanol, together with paraldehyde, continue to be used, particularly in institutionalized patients. Several newer drugs that appear to be more successful in avoiding some of the adverse effects of the barbiturates have been introduced recently. Buspirone is the first of these drugs to be approved for prescription use.

Many classes of compounds can produce sedation, many times as a side effect. Compounds of the antihistaminic type are an example of this, and these compounds are present in a number of over-the-counter sleep preparations, in which their autonomic properties as well as their long duration of action can result in unwanted side effects of sedation. These agents are discussed in Chapters 10 and 11.

This chapter will discuss sedative-hypnotics such as buspirone, carisoprodol chloral hydrate, glutethimide, methaqualone, ethchlorvynol, meprobamate, methyprylon, paraldehyde, and others (Table 49–1). The pharmacologic properties of these drugs are more alike than distinct. The abuse potential and addiction to these drugs develop readily and significantly (2).

TABLE 49–1. *Miscellaneous sedative-hypnotics*

Buspirone
Carisoprodol (Soma)
Chloral hydrate (Noctec)
Chlormezanone (Trancopal)
Ethchlorvynol (Placidyl)
Glutethimide (Doriden)
Meprobamate (Equanil)
Methaqualone (Quaalude)
Methyprylon (Noludar)
Paraldehyde
Zolpidem (Ambien)

Buspirone

Buspirone has been described as an anxioselective drug because, unlike benzodiazepines, it has no anticonvulsant or muscle relaxant activity, does not substantially impair psychomotor function, and has little sedative effect. This drug may cause less potentiation of the depressant actions of ethanol than conventional sedative-hypnotics (3).

Buspirone is "anxioselective," but this action may take more than a week to become established and makes the drug suitable mainly for chronic anxiety states. Though not strongly sedative, buspirone can cause drowsiness and confusion, and caution is advisable when it is used together with other central nervous system (CNS) depressant drugs, including alcohol.

Mechanism of Action

The precise mechanism of buspirone's anxiolytic action is not known but appears to be distinct from benzodiazepines, and probably involves several central neurotransmitter systems. A variety of sites in the CNS have been postulated as contributing to the anxiolytic action of the drug. Buspirone does not interact with GABAergic systems and may exert its anxiolytic action through interaction with 5-HT1A receptors. It is not effective in blocking the withdrawal syndrome resulting from cessation of use of benzodiazepines or other sedative-hypnotics. Because of the variety and location of the drug's effects on central neurotransmitter systems, including serotonergic, dopaminergic, cholinergic, and noradrenergic systems, buspirone has been described as a midbrain modulator.

Overdosage and Treatment

In general, overdosage of buspirone may be expected to produce effects that are mainly extensions of pharmacologic and adverse effects.

There is no specific antidote for buspirone intoxication, and treatment of overdosage with the drug generally involves symptomatic and supportive care. Following acute ingestion of buspirone, the stomach should be emptied immediately by gastric lavage. Pulse, blood pressure, and respiration should be monitored.

Carisoprodol (Soma)

Carisoprodol, first introduced in the late 1950s, is a nonscheduled skeletal muscle relaxant that is widely prescribed in the U.S. Carisoprodol is used by veterinarians and can be obtained without a prescription through mail-order veterinary catalogs (3).

Carisoprodol is a meprobamate precursor. It is a CNS depressant with sedative and skeletal muscle relaxant effects. Its exact mechanism of action is unknown but is thought to result from sedation rather than direct skeletal muscle relaxation. The drug does not directly relax skeletal muscle and, unlike neuromuscular blocking agents, does not depress muscle excitability. Carisoprodol produces muscle relaxation in animals by blocking interneuronal activity in the descending reticular formation and spinal cord. The onset of action is rapid and effects last 4 to 6 hours (4).

Carisoprodol is commonly prescribed as an adjunctive agent in the treatment of chronic back pain or headaches. Although it should only be used for a short period of time, many patients with chronic pain form a group at risk for the development of substance abuse and dependence. Carisoprodol may have a particularly reinforcing effect because it is a precursor to meprobamate.

Acute Toxicity

Overdosage of carisoprodol has produced symptoms which are similar to those of meprobamate overdosage; stupor, coma. shock, respiratory depression, and, very rarely, death (Table 49–2). In these patients, drowsiness, dizziness, headache, diplopia, and nystagmus on lateral gaze have occurred. The effects of an overdosage of carisoprodol and alcohol or other CNS depressants or psychotropic agents can be additive even when one of the drugs has been taken in the usual recommended dosage.

TABLE 49–2. *Signs and symptoms of carisoprodol overdose*

Mild
Drowsiness
Dizziness
Headache
Diplopia
Nystagmus
Moderate-severe
Stupor
Coma
Shock
Respiratory depression
First-dose effect
Agitation
Ataxia
Confusion
Diplopia
Disorientation
Dizziness
Dysarthria
Euphoria
Mydriasis
Quadriplegia (transient)
Weakness

On very rare occasions, the first dose of carisoprodol has been followed by idiosyncratic symptoms appearing within minutes or hours. Symptoms reported include extreme weakness, transient quadriplegia, dizziness, ataxia, temporary loss of vision, diplopia, mydriasis, dysarthria, agitation, euphoria, confusion, and disorientation. Symptoms usually subside over the course of the next several hours. Supportive and symptomatic therapy, including hospitalization, may be necessary.

Carisoprodol can be measured in biologic fluids by gas chromatography.

Treatment

Although limited information is available on the treatment of carisoprodol intoxication, treatment of meprobamate intoxication consists of general supportive therapy including maintenance of adequate airway, assisted respiration, and cautious administration of pressor agents, if necessary. Any drug remaining in the stomach should be removed and symptomatic therapy be given. If the patient is comatose, gastric lavage may be done if an endotracheal tube with cuff inflated is in place to prevent aspiration of gastric contents. Activated charcoal may be instilled after gastric lavage to adsorb any remaining drug, since relapse and death attributable to incomplete gastric emptying and delayed absorption may occur. Urinary output should be monitored and overhydration avoided.

Chloral Hydrate

Actions

Chloral hydrate (Cohidrate, H-S Need, Noctec, Oradrate, SK-Chloral Hydrate, Aquachloral) is one of the oldest of the sedative-hypnotics and was once a popular drug for inducing sedation and sleep. It was the source of "knockout drops," also known as the "Mickey Finn," the effect of which was due to the additive effects of chloral hydrate and alcohol and was never as rapid as depicted in movies.

Chloral hydrate has CNS depressant effects similar to those of barbiturates and was mainly used for children and the elderly, who tolerate barbiturates poorly, because it was thought that chloral hydrate produced less paradoxical excitement in these age groups (5). Chloral hydrate has little analgesic activity, and patients who ingest the drug may respond to pain with delirium or excitement.

Chloral hydrate is converted by liver alcohol dehydrogenase through a large first-pass hepatic effect to an active metabolite, trichloroethanol, which has a longer duration of action than the parent compound. Chloral hydrate is not a street drug of choice, and its main misuse is by the elderly (6).

Trichloroethanol is the pharmacologically active metabolite of chloral hydrate and has a half-life of 6–10 hours. However, its toxic metabolite, trichloroacetic acid, is cleared very slowly and can accumulate with the nightly administration of chloral hydrate. Furthermore, recurrent concerns regarding the possible carcinogenicity of chloral hydrate itself—or its metabolites—suggest that this drug should not be used until more data are available.

Toxicity

Clinical features of intoxication with chloral hydrate are similar to those for barbiturates and alcohol and may include drowsiness, lethargy, stupor, hypotension, hypothermia, and respiratory depression, the last of which sometimes can occur shortly after ingestion (6) (Table 49–3). These may be the direct results of the parent compound, whereas a prolonged coma appears to be the result of the active metabolite. Chloral hydrate is irritating to the gastric mucosa, and gastric necrosis has occurred after intoxicating doses (7). In addition, hepatotoxicity, renal failure, and cardiac dysrhythmias may occur (7). The dysrhythmias are generally atrial fibrillation, occasionally with aberrant conduction or premature ventricular contractions. Rare cases of ventricular tachycardia have been observed. Torsade de pointes has also been reported. Death may occur from respiratory failure or refractory hypotension or secondary to a dysrhythmia. The lethal oral dose of chloral hydrate in adults is about 10 g; however, ingestion of 4 g has caused death, and some patients have survived ingestion of as much as 30 g (6).

TABLE 49–3. *Clinical features of chloral hydrate overdose*

Central nervous system
Drowsiness
Hypotension
Hypothermia
Lethargy
Respiratory depression
Stupor
Cardiac dysrhythmias
Atrial fibrillation
Premature ventricular contractions
Torsade de pointes
Ventricular tachycardia
Miscellaneous
Gastric necrosis
Hepatotoxicity
Renal failure
Respiratory failure

As with all sedative-hypnotics, clinical assessment of the patient's condition is more important and reliable than a plasma concentration because of the various degrees of tolerance to the drug among individuals.

Treatment

Treatment for chloral hydrate ingestion is supportive and includes maintenance of an adequate airway, assisted respiration if necessary, oxygen administration, and maintenance of body temperature and circulation. Lidocaine or propranolol may be used for ventricular tachydysrhythmias. If torsade de pointes is present, overdrive pacing, isoproterenol, or atropine may be effective. Methods to enhance drug removal such as dialysis, diuresis, and hemoperfusion should not be attempted.

Chlormezanone (Trancopal)

Chlormezanone has CNS depressant actions similar to those of meprobamate. Although there is some evidence that chlormezanone has skeletal muscle relaxant effects, these effects are probably due to its sedative property.

Adverse Reactions

Adverse effects reported to occur with chlormezanone include drowsiness, drug rash, dizziness, flushing, nausea, depression, edema, inability to void, weakness, excitement, tremor, confusion, and headache. Rare instances of erythema multiforme, Stevens-Johnson syndrome, and toxic epidermal necrolysis have been reported. Jaundice, apparently of the cholestatic type, has been reported as occurring rarely during the use of chlormezanone, but is reversible on discontinuance of therapy.

Toxicity

Limited information is available on the acute toxicity of chlormezanone. Overdosage has resulted in mild sedation, confusion, flushing, vertigo, nausea, weakness, and drowsiness. In addition, coma, hypotension, absence of reflexes, and flaccidity have occurred in patients ingesting as little as 7 g of the drug; ingestion of higher doses reportedly may result in alternating periods of coma and excitement.

Ethchlorvynol

Ethchlorvynol (Placidyl) is a tertiary acetylenic alcohol that was introduced in the mid-1950s as a sedative-hypnotic (8). It has anticonvulsant and muscle relaxant properties as well as sedative-hypnotic activity. Ethchlorvynol has a pungent, aromatic odor that is often detectable on the breath and in gastric fluid (9). Known on the street as "Mr. Green Jeans," "Pickles," and "Jelly Beans," ethchlorvynol is a frequently abused drug with only a small margin of safety (3).

Pharmacokinetics

The clinical effect of ethchlorvynol is within 15 to 30 minutes with clinical effectiveness lasting about 3 hours (5). Blood concentrations reach their peak 60 to 90 minutes after ingestion (10). Only 10% of ethchlorvynol is excreted unchanged via the urine, feces, or as the volatile alcohol through the lungs. The remaining 90% of ethchlorvynol is hepatically altered by glucuronide conjugation or hydroxylation. Blood ethchlorvynol levels greater than 3.8 mg/dL are associated with coma, hypotension, areflexia, and respiratory depression. The usual hypnotic dose is 500 mg, producing a peak serum level of 0.65 mg/dL. A lethal dose of ethchlorvynol is about 10 to 15 g, which corresponds to lethal serum levels of 13 to 15 mg/dL (11).

Ethchlorvynol is considered very dangerous. Its half-life is long, between 10 and 25 hours, and can increase to more than 100 hours if the patient ingests large amounts of the drug. Ethchlorvynol is highly lipid-soluble and has a large volume of distribution, approximately 4 L/kg, with extensive distribution in adipose and brain tissue.

The half-life of ethchlorvynol can only be explained on a two-compartment kinetic basis. One to 3 hours after administration, about one-half of the dose will disappear from the bloodstream. The drug then is moved into the fat-soluble areas of the body, and 10 to 25 hours are required to eliminate half of this dose. For this reason, overdoses may result in a slow elimination of the drug, and the length of coma from excessive doses may depend on how much drug was taken.

Although the drug is available only in a soft capsule form, to be taken orally, intravenous abuse of the contents of the capsule has been reported. This is achieved by withdrawing the semiliquid contents of the capsule with a needle and syringe and injecting its contents.

Toxicity

Mild toxicity manifests itself in difficulty responding to verbal stimuli and sluggishly reacting pupils. Urinary retention, cholestatic jaundice, and positional nystagmus have been reported (9).

Major toxic reactions to ethchlorvynol include pancytopenia, dizziness, weakness, gastrointestinal upset, and thrombocytopenia. Apneic episodes, hemolysis, and bradycardia with hypotension are associated with severe ethchlorvynol overdose (10). Other manifestations include areflexia, hypothermia, severe respiratory depression, and prolonged deep coma which may last up to 300 hours (Table 49–4). Flat electroencephalogram readings have been reported (11).

Ocular symptoms include overshoot nystagmus, diplopia, macular degeneration, and chiasmal optic neuritis with toxic amblyopia. Ethchlorvynol intoxication can produce sudden painless bilateral blindness, disorientation, and muscle twitching. Ethchlorvynol may cause noncardiogenic pulmonary edema after illicit intravenous administration but also after oral administration (8,12). Experimentally it has been shown that ethchlorvynol exerts a direct toxic action on the alveolar capillary mem-

TABLE 49–4. *Clinical features of ethchlorvynol overdose*

CNS depression
Coma
Hypothermia
Hypotension
Bradycardia
Weakness
Respiratory depression
Death
Hematologic effects
Hemolysis
Pancytopenia
Thrombocytopenia
Ocular
Nystagmus
Diplopia
Macular degeneration
Blindness
Miscellaneous
Pulmonary edema
Peripheral neuropathy
Gastrointestinal disturbance

brane (12). This apparently is produced through nontoxic endothelial cell retraction involving arachidonic acid metabolites that are implicated in the vascular permeability. Death may result from respiratory failure or hypotension or as a complication of prolonged coma. A mint-like taste is usually reported after oral and intravenous use.

Treatment

Treatment for ethchlorvynol overdosage is supportive and includes maintenance of an adequate airway, assisted respiration, and oxygen administration. Hypotension should be treated with intravenous fluids. Because of the drug's large volume of distribution, dialysis, diuresis, and hemoperfusion are believed to be ineffective in its removal. There are reports of effective yields from resin hemoperfusion with Amberlite XAD-4, which is a styrene–divinylbenzene copolymer that acts as an uncharged exchange resin. Although this procedure may rid the body of the drug (13), it has not been reported to alter the clinical course of the overdose. In addition, some of the complications of hemoperfusion include anemia, thrombocytopenia, hypocalcemia, and pancreatitis. Care should be taken not to overtreat this type of patient with fluids because this may increase the likelihood of pulmonary edema.

Glutethimide

Actions

Glutethimide (Doriden, Dormtabs, Rolathimide) was introduced in 1954 as one of the earliest of the "new" sedative-hypnotics (5). The structure is virtually identical to that of the barbiturates except for one slight modification of the molecule. It is also similar structurally and in therapeutic activity to methyprylon, a nonbarbiturate sedative-hypnotic. It produces hypnosis and has no analgesic, antitussive, or anticonvulsant activity (1).

Since its introduction, glutethimide has been shown to have a mortality consistently greater than that of other sedative-hypnotics. Two of the reasons for this are its long duration of action and the fact that it is metabolized to another active compound, 4-hydroxy-2-ethyl-2-phenylglutarimide (8,14). This metabolite has twice the activity and potency of glutethimide and also a duration of action that is more than twice that of glutethimide (15). About half the parent compound is metabolized to the active metabolite. Although early studies suggested an important role for 4-hydroxyglutethimide in acute glutethimide poisoning, the role this metabolite plays appears to have been overemphasized. In human studies, no pharmacologic effects of 4-hydroxyglutethimide have been demonstrated when glutethimide has been administered.

Pharmacokinetics

Glutethimide stimulates the hepatic microsomal enzyme system and has pronounced antimuscarinic activity (15). The drug appears to be slowly and erratically absorbed from the gastrointestinal tract (16). Co-administration with ethanol appears to increase the oral absorption of glutethimide dramatically. Because of its high lipid solubility, once absorbed there is extensive tissue localization, with high concentrations found in the brain and adipose tissue. Glutethimide has a volume of distribution of approximately 3 L/kg (16). Peak plasma concentrations ranging from 2.9 to 7.1 mg/L are seen 1 to 6 hours after a therapeutic oral dose of 500 mg (16).

Ingestion of 5 g of glutethimide usually produces severe intoxication in adults, and the ingestion of 10–20 g of the drug is frequently lethal. Although glutethimide blood concentrations greater than 10 μg/mL are generally associated with intoxication, there is a poor correlation between glutethimide plasma concentration and the clinical course of the patient, possibly because of the formation and accumulation of an active metabolite, 4-hydroxy-2-ethyl-2-phenylglutarimide (4-HG).

Toxicity

An overdose of glutethimide produces symptoms similar to those of other sedative-hypnotics and may include profound and prolonged coma, hypotension, respiratory depression, shock, and hypothermia (8). There may be cyclic fluctuations in the depth of coma. There appears to be a poor correlation between the plasma concentration of glutethimide and its metabolite and the clinical course of the patient (16,17–19). In addition, because of the antimuscarinic activity, patients overdosed on this drug may exhibit mydriasis, urinary retention, tachycardia, and hypertension (Table 49–5).

A prominent feature of glutethimide poisoning is a characteristic fluctuation in the level of consciousness. This may be due to the formation of the metabolite, but alternative explanations for this phenomenon include further absorption of the parent compound from the gas-

TABLE 49–5. *Clinical features of glutethimide overdose*

Sedative-hypnotic effects
Coma
Hypotension
Hypothermia
Respiratory depression
Shock
Antimuscarinic effects
Hypertension
Tachycardia
Urinary retention
Mydriasis

trointestinal tract after recovery from an ileus, enterohepatic circulation of glutethimide and its metabolite, and release of the drug from body fat. Most of the drug that is absorbed is deposited rapidly in body tissues, leaving only a small fraction to circulate freely in the bloodstream.

Glutethimide and Codeine

In recent years glutethimide has become increasingly popular among drug users when it is mixed with codeine (16,18). The two drugs together have been termed "loads," "4's and Dors," or "setups" (19). This combination was reported more than a decade ago and is purported to produce a euphoria equal to that of heroin. It is also relatively inexpensive, is more readily available than heroin and can be taken orally. Also, because of the potent enzyme-inducing properties of glutethimide, more codeine may be converted to morphine than occurs with codeine alone. The effects may last for 3 to 12 hours (depending on the individual's degree of tolerance) without the side effects of intravenous administration. Although the typical intravenous "rush" is absent, it can be approximated when loads are taken on an empty stomach (20,21). One "load" may consist of two 500-mg glutethimide tablets combined with four 60-mg codeine tablets, and abusers may take from 3 to 12 "loads" per day. Intoxication is achieved within 20 minutes after ingestion, with the peak effect occurring after 40 minutes (20).

Clinical features of loads overdose may be the same as those expected from a combination of a sedative-hypnotic and a narcotic agent and are characterized by alternating states of dreamlike euphoria and "nodding," sometimes associated with prolonged sensorimotor disturbances in the extremities (1).

The finding of glutethimide by history or on a drug screen should prompt a search for codeine and vice versa, particularly when the presence of either drug by itself does not explain the clinical condition of the patient (18).

There are many problems associated with the use of glutethimide and codeine. First, this combination is highly addicting. Tolerance may develop quickly, requiring more frequent administration and increased doses. In addition, a high mortality is seen with acute toxicity due to the profound depressant effects on the CNS and respiration (1). Finally, withdrawal complications have been reported to be more severe than for heroin alone.

Treatment

Treatment for overdose of glutethimide or loads is directed toward supporting the patient and consists of attempts at removal of the drug by lavage, even many hours after ingestion, because it can remain in the gastrointestinal tract. Concretions may also form from a large amount of glutethimide. If a combination drug was ingested or if the patient exhibits an altered mental status, then naloxone should be administered. Dialysis, although initially thought to be of benefit, has been shown not to be clinically useful. This is due to the large volume of distribution of glutethimide and its high concentration in body fat (19). Hemoperfusion and diuresis are also ineffective.

The question of effectiveness of multiple-dose activated charcoal remains unanswered, but the known enterohepatic circulation of some of the metabolites of glutethimide suggests that continued administration of charcoal may be of benefit (18).

Meprobamate

Actions

Meprobamate (Bamate, Equanil, Mepripam, Meprotabs, Miltown, Neuromate, SK-Bamate, Suronil), which was first synthesized in 1950, is only one of a large number of carbamate derivatives currently on the market (22–24). It is a drug that still may be used by the elderly and is usually not a drug of abuse chosen by the younger population. Meprobamate acts as an intermediate barbiturate except that it also has muscle relaxant properties. Meprobamate does not produce sleep at therapeutic doses (8).

Pharmacokinetics

Oral administration of 400 mg of meprobamate produces peak plasma concentrations of 5–30 μg/mL within 1–3 hours. Plasma concentrations of 30–100 μg/mL are usually reached following mild overdosage and are associated with stupor or light coma. Plasma concentrations of 100–200 μg/mL are associated with deep coma and are potentially lethal; fatalities frequently occur when plasma concentrations exceed 200 μg/mL. The onset of sedative action is usually less than 1 hour following oral administration of meprobamate (25,26).

Toxicity

Overdosage of meprobamate produces symptoms similar to those of barbiturate overdosage; these may include drowsiness, stupor, ataxia, lethargy, coma, hypotension, shock, and respiratory depression. Hypotension may be marked, and pulmonary edema has been reported in a number of patients (Table 49–6). Large amounts of meprobamate may cause concretions. Because of this, clinical effects may be prolonged until the gastrointestinal tract is adequately emptied.

TABLE 49–6. *Clinical features of meprobamate overdose*

Ataxia
Coma
Drowsiness
Stupor
Hypotension
Lethargy
Pulmonary edema
Respiratory depression
Shock

Treatment

Treatment of meprobamate overdose consists of supportive care. Emesis or lavage should be followed by administration of activated charcoal and a cathartic. Hypotension should be treated with fluids. Dialysis, diuresis, and hemoperfusion do not enhance excretion and should not be used.

Methaqualone

Actions

Methaqualone (Quaalude, Sopor, Parest, Mequin) was originally marketed in the early 1970s as a safe, effective, nonaddicting substitute for barbiturates, but it was soon realized that the drug by itself or in combination could cause serious poisoning (8). Mandrax is a European trade name for methaqualone in combination with an antihistamine, diphenhydramine; in Great Britain, the first death from this compound was reported within a few months of its commercial availability (27,28). Of the nonbarbiturate drugs used clinically as hypnotics, methaqualone is probably the most widely abused member of the group.

In addition to sedative-hypnotic properties, methaqualone has anticonvulsant, antispasmodic, local anesthetic, and weak antihistaminic properties. The drug has antitussive properties comparable to those of codeine. In toxic doses, methaqualone may lead to a defect in platelet function and, because of this, to spontaneous bleeding (25,26).

Popular notions of the qualities of methaqualone have made it a widespread drug of abuse for more than a decade. Methaqualone was thought to have aphrodisiac qualities and has been referred to as the "love drug" (8,28). It is a low-potency sedative-hypnotic agent that appears to have an inordinate capacity to produce a dissociative "high" without sedation (29). Users describe a loss of the perception of physical and mental "self." At certain doses, a state of disinhibition or euphoria results. During such disinhibition an individual may feel euphoric about sexual experiences, but, as with all other sedatives, sensation may be increased but performance may be impaired (30). These effects may also be due to the drug's muscle relaxant qualities. Methaqualone also causes physiologic dependence and withdrawal (29).

Sometimes, the act of taking methaqualone, either singly or in combination with alcohol, is called "luding out." Methaqualone is available on the street from clandestine sales as well as by diversion from legal manufacturers or pharmacies. Although most manufacturers have voluntarily suspended production of the drug because of its widespread abuse, street forms are still available. Counterfeit "quaalude" tablets sold on the street do not necessarily contain methaqualone. They are prevalent on the illicit market and are similar in appearance to the well-known commercial product. Some patients have experienced necrotizing cystitis manifested by painful hematuria after ingestion of methaqualone purchased on the street. This reaction is believed to be due to orthotoluidine, which is a contaminant of the street drug.

Toxicity

Symptoms of overdosage with methaqualone include lethargy, coma, respiratory depression, and death (Table 49–7). In contrast to the coma of barbiturate overdose, the coma of severe methaqualone overdosage may be accompanied by pyramidal signs such as restlessness, excitement, muscle hypertonicity, myoclonus, and seizures (30). In addition, the methaqualone–diphenhydramine combination has been reported to cause delirium, signs of extrapyramidal stimulation, and grand mal seizures. Bullous lesions, seen with barbiturates, have also been reported with methaqualone.

Treatment

Treatment for overdose is similar to that for overdoses of intermediate-acting barbiturates and includes adequate emptying of the gastrointestinal tract with subsequent administration of activated charcoal and a cathartic as well as support for blood pressure and respiration. Dialysis and hemoperfusion are not effective, and forced diuresis may increase the risk of pulmonary edema.

TABLE 49–7. *Clinical features of methaqualone overdose*

CNS depression
Respiratory depression
Coma
Death
CNS stimulation
Muscle hypertonicity
Myoclonus
Seizures
Hyperreflexia
Restlessness
Miscellaneous effects
Bleeding
Blisters

Methyprylon

Methyprylon (Noludar) is a general CNS depressant introduced in 1955 for use as a hypnotic. The drug is similar in chemical structure to glutethimide.

After oral administration, the drug is metabolized by the microsomal enzyme system of the liver. Although the plasma half-life is 4 hours, higher dosages, as may be seen in acute overdosage, result in much longer half-lives. Overdosage may result in a coma lasting up to 5 days. Acute overdosage symptoms resemble those of barbiturate poisoning.

As with glutethimide and barbiturates, physical dependence on and tolerance to methyprylon do occur. Withdrawal symptoms, including seizures, are similar to those of barbiturate withdrawal.

Paraldehyde

Paraldehyde is a general CNS depressant, available only as a liquid. It is usually administered orally, but it can be given in an oil retention enema. Due to the extreme irritability of the drug on intramuscular or intravenous administration, these routes of administration have been discontinued.

Although the precise mechanism of action of paraldehyde is not known, it is believed to depress many levels of the CNS including the ascending reticular activating system to cause an imbalance between inhibitory and facilitatory mechanisms. Paraldehyde exhibits anticonvulsant activity in subhypnotic doses; however, the margin between the anticonvulsant and hypnotic dose is small. It is not an effective analgesic in subanesthetic doses, and it may produce excitement or delirium in the presence of pain. Therapeutic doses of the drug have little effect on respiration or blood pressure; however, high doses of paraldehyde produce respiratory depression and hypotension, and death may result from respiratory failure.

Pharmacokinetics

The usual hypnotic dose of paraldehyde is 4 mL to 8 mL although higher doses may be required in the treatment of alcohol withdrawal. Paraldehyde is rapidly absorbed from the gastrointestinal tract and from intramuscular injection sites. Paraldehyde's sedative effects begin about 20 minutes after oral ingestion. Maximum serum concentrations, which may range from 34 to 150 μg/mL, are reached within 20–60 minutes following oral administration of 10 mL of the drug or IM administration of 0.25 mL/kg. The half-life of paraldehyde is approximately 7.5 hours.

Paraldehyde is chemically unstable and after paraldehyde has been exposed to air, it rapidly decomposes to acetic acid. Paraldehyde is incompatible with plastic and must be measured and administered in glass containers.

Approximately 80–90% of a dose of paraldehyde is metabolized by the liver. In some patients with hepatic disease, the drug is metabolized slowly and the hypnotic effects are prolonged. Although the metabolic fate of paraldehyde has not been definitely established, it appears that the drug is depolymerized to acetaldehyde, which is oxidized by aldehyde dehydrogenase to acetic acid and then further metabolized via the tricarboxylic acid cycle to carbon dioxide and water.

The most impressive quality of paraldehyde is its putrid odor and taste. Once smelled or tasted, it will not be soon forgotten by staff or patients. The odor of paraldehyde makes the patient who has taken the drug readily identifiable. A substantial amount of the drug is excreted unchanged through the lungs, giving the breath a characteristic odor. It appears that paraldehyde is excreted across alveolar membranes in much the same manner as carbon dioxide. Only trace amounts of paraldehyde are excreted unchanged in urine.

Paraldehyde gained some of its use in the treatment of alcohol withdrawal because it had the reputation of being excreted by the lungs. This statement is misleading because 70% to 80% of the drug is metabolized in the liver, leaving less than 30% of the drug to be excreted through the lungs.

Overdosage

Paraldehyde overdosage produces symptoms similar to those of chloral hydrate overdosage which may include coma, severe hypotension, respiratory depression, pulmonary edema, and cardiac failure. Paraldehyde-induced coma may last for several hours because the rate of metabolism of the drug is slow. Diagnosis of paraldehyde overdosage is facilitated by the characteristic odor of the drug on the breath. Metabolic acidosis may also occur. Renal function may be impaired and may result in azotemia, oliguria, and albuminuria. Fatty changes in the kidneys, nephrosis, fatty changes in the liver, and/or toxic hepatitis may also occur.

Although fatalities are rare, administration of 25 mL of paraldehyde orally or 12 mL rectally has caused death. Death is usually caused by respiratory failure. A few fatalities have been attributed to pulmonary edema and right-sided heart failure or metabolic acidosis.

Zolpidem (Ambien)

Zolpidem is an imidazopyridine-derivative sedative and hypnotic. Although zolpidem is structurally unrelated to the benzodiazepines, it shares some of the pharmacologic properties of benzodiazepines. Subunit modulation of the GABA-A receptor chloride channel macromolecular complex is hypothesized to be responsible for sedative, anticonvulsant, anxiolytic, and myorelaxant drug properties. The major modulatory site of the GABA-A receptor complex is located on its alpha subunit and is referred to as the benzodiazepine (BZ) or omega (omega) receptor. At least three subtypes of the omega receptor have been identified.

Unlike some benzodiazepines, which nonselectively activate central type 1 (BZ1) and 2 (BZ2) receptors, as well as peripheral type 3 (BZ3) receptors, resulting in nonspecific pharmacologic actions, zolpidem reportedly may bind preferentially to BZ1 receptors.

Published reports of large case series with zolpidem have noted that the acute overdose of zolpidem is generally benign and requires no specific therapeutic measures (31).

REFERENCES

1. Bender F, Cooper J, Dreyfus R: Fatalities associated with an acute overdose of glutethimide (Doriden) and codeine. *Vet Hum Toxicol* 1988;30;332–333.
2. Gillin J: The long and short of sleeping pills. *N Engl J Med* 1991; 324:1735–1736.
3. Miller N, Gold M: Sedative-hypnotics: pharmacology and use. *J Fam Pract* 1989;29:665–670.
4. Littrell R, Hayes L, Stillner V: Carisoprodol (Soma): a new and cautious perspective on an old agent. *South Med J* 1993;86:753–756.
5. Gary N, Tresznewsky O: Barbiturates and a potpourri of other sedatives, hypnotics, and tranquilizers. *Heart Lung* 1983;12:122–127.
6. Young J, Vanedermolen L, Pratt C, et al: Torsade de pointes: an unusual manifestation of chloral hydrate poisoning. *Am Heart J* 1986;112:181–184.
7. Stalker N, Gambertoglio J, Fukumitso C, et al: Acute massive chloral hydrate intoxication treated with hemodialysis: a clinical pharmacokinetic analysis. *J Clin Pharmacol* 1978;18:136.
8. Bertino J, Reed M: Barbiturate and nonbarbiturate sedative-hypnotic intoxication in children. *Pediatr Clin North Am* 1986;33:703–722.
9. Teehan B, et al: Acute ethchlorvynol intoxication. *Ann Intern Med* 1970;72:875–882.
10. Westervelt F: Ethchlorvynol (Placidyl) intoxication. *Ann Intern Med* 1966;64:1229–1236.
11. Yell R: Ethchlorvynol overdose. *Am J Emerg Med* 1990;8:246–250.
12. Glauser F, Smith W, Caldwell A, et al: Ethchlorvynol-induced pulmonary edema. *Ann Intern Med* 1976;84:46–48.
13. Lynn R, Honig C, Jatlow P, et al: Resin hemoperfusion for treatment of ethchlorvynol overdose. *Ann Intern Med* 1979;91:549–553.
14. Crow J, Lain P, Bochner F, et al: Glutethimide and 4-OH glutethimide: pharmacokinetics and effect on performance in man. *Clin Pharmacol Ther* 1977;22:458–464.
15. Hansen A, Kennedy K, Ambre J, et al: Glutethimide poisoning: a metabolite contributes to morbidity and mortality. *N Engl J Med* 1975;292:250–252.
16. Curry S, Hubbard J, Gerkin R, et al: Lack of correlation between plasma 4-hydroxyglutethimide and severity of coma in acute glutethimide poisoning. A case report and brief review of the literature. *Med Toxicol* 1987;2:309–316.
17. Parker K, Elliott H, Wright J, et al: Blood and urine concentrations of subjects receiving barbiturates, meprobamate, glutethimide or diphenylhydantoin. *Clin Toxicol* 1970;3:131–145.
18. Chazan J, Cohen J: Clinical spectrum of glutethimide intoxication: hemodialysis re-evaluated. *JAMA* 1969;208:837–839.
19. Chazan J, Garella S: Glutethimide intoxication: a prospective study of 70 patients treated conservatively without hemodialysis. *Arch Intern Med* 1971;128:215–219.
20. Bailey D, Shaw R: Blood concentrations and clinical findings in nonfatal and fatal intoxications involving glutethimide and codeine. *Clin Toxicol* 1985;23:557–570.
21. Khajawall A, Sramek J: "Loads" alert. *West J Med* 1982; 137:166–168.
22. Preskorn S, Denner L: Benzodiazepines and withdrawal psychosis. *JAMA* 1977;237:36–38.
23. Parry H, Balter M, Mellnger G, et al: National patterns of psychotherapeutic drug use. *Arch Gen Psychiatry* 1973;28:769–783.
24. Rickels K, Case G, Downing R, et al: Long-term diazepam therapy and clinical outcome. *JAMA* 1983;250:767–771.
25. Brown S, Goenechea S: Methaqualone: metabolic, kinetic, and clinical pharmacologic observations. *Clin Pharmacol Ther* 1973; 14:314–321.
26. Mills D: Effects of methaqualone on blood platelet function. *Clin Pharmacol Ther* 1978;23:685–691.
27. Sanderson J, Corodele R, Higgins G: Fatal poisoning with methaqualone and diphenhydramine. *Lancet* 1966;2:803–804.
28. Inaba D, Gay G, Newmeyer J, et al: Methaqualone abuse. *JAMA* 1973;224:1505–1509.
29. Pascarelli E: Methaqualone abuse: the quiet epidemic. *JAMA* 1973; 224:1512–1514.
30. Wetli C: Changing patterns of methaqualone abuse. *JAMA* 1983;249:621–626,
31. Garnier R, Guerault E, Muzard D, et al: Acute zolpidem poisoning—analysis of 344 cases. *J Toxicol Clin Tox* 1994;32:391–404.

ADDITIONAL SELECTED REFERENCES

Costello J, Poklis A: Treatment of massive phenobarbital overdose with dopamine diuresis. *Arch Intern Med* 1981;141:938–940.

Faulkner T, Hayden J, Mehta C, et al: Dose-response studies on tolerance to multiple doses of secobarbital and methaqualone in a polydrug abuse population. *Clin Toxicol* 1979;15:23–37.

Hall S: Apnea after intravenous diazepam therapy. *JAMA* 1977;238:1052.

Hancock B: Acute barbiturate poisoning in young epileptics. *Postgrad Med J* 1974;50:242–244.

Kaplan S, Jack M, Alexander K, et al: Pharmacokinetic profile of diazepam in man following single intravenous and oral and chronic oral administrations. *J Pharmacol Sci* 1973;62:1789–1796.

Korttila K, Linnoila M: Absorption and sedative effects of diazepam after oral administration and intramuscular administration into the vastus lateralis muscle and the deltoid muscle. *Br J Anaesth* 1975;47:857–862.

Lightman S: Phenobarbital dyskinesia. *Postgrad Med J* 1978;54:114–115.

Maes V, Huyghens L, Dekeyser J, et al: Acute and chronic intoxication with carbromal preparations. *Clin Toxicol* 1985;23:341–346.

McGuigan M, Lovejoy F: Overdose of Lomotil, editorial. *Br Med J* 1978;1:990.

Murphy J, Sawasky F, Marquardt K, et al: Deaths in young children receiving nitrazepam. *J Pediatr* 1987;111:145–147.

Roytblat L, Bear R, Gesztes T: Seizures after pentazocine overdose. *Isr J Med Sci* 1986;22:385–386.

Sato S, Baud F, Bismuth C, et al: Arterial-venous plasma concentration differences of meprobamate in acute human poisonings. *Hum Toxicol* 1986;5:243–248.

CHAPTER 50

Central Nervous System Stimulants

Stimulants have been used for thousands of years and are still popular as a class for abuse. Users, many of whom do not realize that they are abusing drugs, tend to rely on stimulants to wake up in the morning, to be more alert and attentive, or to feel stronger, more decisive, and self-possessed. Although the problem of physical withdrawal from the drugs is minimal, the psychological dependence is strong.

The most prevalent and socially acceptable stimulants are nicotine in tobacco products and caffeine in coffee, tea, soft drinks, and combination medicines. The most toxic drugs in this group are the amphetamines, cocaine, and the "look-alike" drugs (Table 50–1).

All the stimulant drugs cause many similar effects, the most obvious of which affect the central and peripheral nervous systems and the cardiovascular system. Some of the other effects from the stimulants include a temporary sense of exhilaration and euphoria, increased feelings of sexuality, hyperactivity, irritability, decreased fatigue, and extended wakefulness. Anorexia is also an effect of the stimulants, and it is this property that may initially attract some people to these drugs. At typical therapeutic doses, however, dysphoric reactions such as anxiety and apprehension can also occur.

Physical signs of stimulant use may include tremors, dizziness, dilated and reactive pupils, dry mouth, hyperreflexia, mild hypertension, and tachycardia. Many abusers "shoot" the drugs because, with intravenous administration, the effects are greatly intensified. Shortly after injection, a sudden sensation known as a "flash" or "rush" is felt. This feeling is described by users as a "total body orgasm." The protracted use of stimulants is usually followed by a period of depression known as "crashing." This depression can be relieved by more stimulants, thereby setting up a cycle for the abuser.

TABLE 50–1. *Abused stimulant drugs*

Nicotine
Caffeine
Amphetamines
Cocaine
Methylphenidate
Anorectic drugs
"Look-alike" drugs

Large doses may result in behavioral abnormalities such as repetitive grinding of the teeth, touching and picking the face and extremities, performing the same act over and over, preoccupation with one's own thought processes, suspiciousness, a feeling of being watched, and auditory and visual hallucinations. Physiologic abnormalities may include tachydysrhythmias, hypertensive crisis, cardiovascular collapse, renal failure, and death (Table 50–2).

Amphetamines and cocaine are similar in the effects that they produce, and both have the same toxic manifestations. The main difference between the two stimulants is the duration of action and the degree of withdrawal. Whereas the effects of amphetamines may last for several hours, cocaine may be active in the body for only a few minutes because it is metabolized extremely rapidly by the liver. In addition, tolerance to cocaine does not appear to develop in the same manner as tolerance to amphetamines, and withdrawal symptoms (manifested by sleep disorders and profound depression on abrupt cessation of use) are usually less severe than with amphetamines.

TABLE 50–2. *Clinical effects of stimulants*

Neurologic
Hyperactivity
Tremors
Dizziness
Xerostomia
Hyperreflexia
Psychological
Temporary sense of exhilaration
Euphoria
Decreased fatigue
Superabundant energy
Decreased appetite
Anxiety
Paranoia
Hallucinations
Cardiovascular
Hypertension
Tachycardia
Dysrhythmias
Cardiovascular collapse

This chapter will discuss amphetamines and their derivatives, the so-called "designer drugs," including methcathinone; the "look-alikes"; propylhexedrine; methylphenidate; the appetite suppressants; caffeine; as well as other sympathomimetics. Chapter 51 will discuss cocaine.

AMPHETAMINES

Amphetamines became a drug of abuse about 50 years ago when they were available in nasal decongestant inhalers and other over-the-counter preparations. In addition, there were many other nonmedical uses of amphetamines. Subsequent recognition of the limited therapeutic value and high abuse potential of amphetamines led to a marked reduction in their medical use. Current applications include treatment for narcolepsy, for appetite control, and to control hyperkinetic behavior in children. Many authorities believe that less toxic alternatives exist and that, even for these indications, amphetamines should not be employed (1).

Mechanism of Action

The mechanism of action of amphetamines on peripheral structures is thought to be a combination of an indirect action by a release of norepinephrine from stores in adrenergic nerve terminals and a direct action on both α and β receptor sites (2). Amphetamines cause a release of catecholamines into the synaptic cleft and decrease the rate of catecholaminergic neuronal firing. The main site of the CNS action appears to be the cerebral cortex. The neurotransmitters in the CNS that are affected are norepinephrine, dopamine, and 5-hydroxytryptamine (3).

Pharmacokinetics

Amphetamine (phenylisopropylamine) is a noncatechol sympathomimetic adrenergic agent that is structurally related to norepinephrine but that has greater central stimulant activity than norepinephrine and other catecholamines (4).

The amphetamines (Table 50–3) (3) can be divided into the *d*-isomer and the *l*-isomer. The *d*-isomer has 2 to 4 times the potency of the *l*-isomer for CNS stimulation, and the *l*-isomer has greater cardiovascular effects. The racemic mixture is marketed as Benzedrine or "bennies" and the *d*-isomer as Dexedrine or "dexies" (5). For all practical purposes, however, the effects of all these products are similar, the differences being relative potency, half-life, CNS activity or peripheral activity, and onset of action. Methamphetamine may be favored by the drug abuser for parenteral use because it is water-soluble and can be injected more readily than the other agents. In addition, it is favored because it has more pronounced central effects and less pronounced peripheral effects.

TABLE 50–3. *Amphetamine preparations and their trade names*

Preparation	Trade name(s)
Benzphetamine	Didrex
Dextroamphetamine	Dexedrine
	Dexampex
	Ferndex
	Oxydess
Diethylpropion	Tenuate
	Tepanil
Fenfluramine	Pondimin
Methamphetamine	Desoxyn
Methylphenidate	Ritalin
Phendimetrazine	Adipost
	Bontril
	Dyrexan
	Melfiat
	Plegine
	Trimstat
	Wehless
Phenmetrazine	Preludin
Phentermine	Adipex
	Fastin
	Teramine

Adapted from *Top Emerg Med* 1985;7(3):21. Aspen Publishers Inc.

Amphetamines are absorbed rapidly from the gastrointestinal tract. At therapeutic doses, blood concentrations reach their peak 1 to 2 hours after ingestion. The plasma half-life of amphetamines depends on the pH of the urine. With an alkaline urine the plasma half-life is 15 to 30 hours, whereas with an acidic urine the half-life is 8 to 10 hours.

Toxicity

Amphetamines may be taken on a short- or long-term basis by oral, respiratory, intravenous, or vaginal routes (2). The amount of amphetamine required to produce serious features of overdose (Table 50–4) depends to a large extent on the frequency of previous usage and the size of the doses. There is a relatively large margin of safety between therapeutic and lethal doses. Tachyphylaxis occurs with amphetamines, and after repeatedly taking amphetamines most users develop a tolerance to the drug, and larger amounts can be taken with each dose (4).

The symptoms produced by cocaine and amphetamines are similar and may be difficult to differentiate clinically. The sole distinguishing clinical feature may be the longer half-life of amphetamines, which may be up to eight times longer than cocaine (1).

At average oral doses, amphetamines produce euphoria, a feeling of superabundant energy, extended wakefulness, and decreased appetite (2). An increase in blood

TABLE 50–4. *Clinical features of amphetamine intoxication*

Cardiovascular
Hypertension
Bradycardia
Tachycardia
Palpitations
Hypertensive crisis
Dysrhythmias
Central nervous system
Delirium
Euphoria
Mydriasis
Coma
Status epilepticus
Superabundant energy
Extended wakefulness
Hyperpyrexia
Anxiety
Seizures
Cerebrovascular accident
Psychosis
Hallucinations
Nonspecific
Anorexia
Myoglobulinemia
Rhabdomyolysis
Sweating

pressure with reflex bradycardia may also be noted, along with a relaxation of bronchial muscles and CNS stimulation. These are the desired effects of the amphetamines that are sought after by the user.

A patient who ingests amphetamine in moderate amounts may become symptomatic within 30 minutes. These symptoms may last for several hours and may include tachycardia, flushing, sweating, palpitations, and headache (6). A significant overdose of amphetamines may cause dilated, reactive pupils, hyperpyrexia, profound anxiety, and seizures. Severe overdosage may be followed by cardiac dysrhythmias, delirium, hypertensive crisis, cerebral vascular accidents (7), circulatory collapse, coma, and status epilepticus. Ischemic chest pain has occurred and may be secondary to vasospasm. Hyperthermia and disseminated intravascular coagulation have also been observed (3). In addition, acute renal failure associated with rhabdomyolysis is a well-recognized entity secondary to amphetamine overdose (8–10). Evidence of rhabdomyolysis and myoglobinuria usually consists of myalgia, muscle tenderness, myoedema, elevated creatinine phosphokinase concentrations, and myoglobinuria (3).

The intravenous injection of amphetamine produces a sudden "flash" or "rush" that is described as exhilarating; although transient, this experience is often the primary motive for parenteral abuse. The rush is followed by a persistent, invigorating sense of euphoria, clear thinking, gregariousness, self-confidence, excitement, and invulnerability (11).

Continued high-dose intravenous use induces mental disturbances such as confusion, delirium, and an acute psychosis that may be indistinguishable from schizophrenia. The individual may appear confused with disorganized behavior or may exhibit compulsive repetition of meaningless acts, such as picking at the bed sheets. The patient may become irritable, fearful, or suspicious of his or her surroundings and experience delusions and hallucinations. The hallucinations may be both visual and auditory. In addition to these findings, any of the complications of intravenous use discussed earlier may be noted (see Chapter 42).

"Ice"

Illicitly produced methamphetamine, the *N*-methyl homologue of amphetamine, is the newest "designer drug" on the street. Known as "ice," "zip," or "cristy" on the street, it appears to be methamphetamine freebase or methamphetamine hydrochloride upon analysis. Illegally, the drug resembles crystals or chunks (12). Smoking delivers a rapid bolus of drug to the brain, somewhat similar to intravenous administration. Because the duration of action of methamphetamine is much longer than that of cocaine, intoxication may last for several hours after a single smoke. It remains to be seen whether "ice" will replace "crack" or merely add another form of abusable drug.

Treatment

There is no specific antidote for amphetamine overdose, and most of the treatment is supportive (Table 50–5). Life-threatening overdoses are rare. If the drug has been ingested orally, then emesis or lavage and administration of activated charcoal and a cathartic should be performed. Alpha-adrenergic blocking agents can be lifesaving in patients with hypertensive crisis or for the hyperpyrexia associated with amphetamine toxicity (11).

TABLE 50–5. *Treatment of amphetamine overdose*

Indication	Treatment
Oral ingestion	Gastric lavage Activated charcoal and sorbitol
Hypertensive crisis, hyperpyrexia	Labetalol Nifedipine Nitroprusside Urine acidification (not recommended)
Acute psychosis, agitation	Haloperidol (2 to 5 mg IM)
Seizures	Diazepam (5 to 15 mg IV)

It has been suggested that, because the rate of renal excretion of amphetamines is dependent on the pH of the urine and is more than doubled in the presence of an acid urine, the patient should be given agents that will acidify the urine (13,14). This is discouraged, however, because if myoglobinuria is present acidifying the urine may favor the development of acute renal failure (10). Aggressive extracellular volume repletion and attempts to avert acute renal failure, as well as prophylaxis against or treatment of acute hyperkalemia, should be instituted (15). For treatment of acute psychotic manifestations, haloperidol or phenothiazines are commonly used. Chlorpromazine is believed by some investigators to prolong the half-life of amphetamines, and thus haloperidol (2 to 5 mg intramuscularly) is the preferred drug for treating the acute psychotic reactions. Diazepam can be administered for seizures (11).

Hyperthermia is a frequent complication, especially in fatal overdoses. Temperatures above 40°C are not uncommon, and require urgent therapy. The most effective way to lower temperature is by application of tepid water and fanning. If this procedure is not effective then muscle paralysis with pancuronium, with proper airway protection, is recommended. Dantrolene may be administered if the preceding measures are ineffective. Salicylates, acetaminophen, and cooling blankets are too slow to be effective, although they may be used as an adjunctive measure (16).

THE AMPHETAMINE-LIKE "DESIGNER DRUGS"

Mescaline–methamphetamine analogues were initially synthesized in the early 1900s. They recently have been rediscovered and produced as street drugs (17). These are considered "designer drugs" (Table 50–6).

The phenylethylamine molecule is the basic chemical structure for endogenous catecholamines and neurotransmitters as well as several therapeutic agents. It is also the structure from which are derived many substances of abuse, such as mescaline, MDA, and others (16). The prototype psychoactive phenylethylamine derivative is mescaline (3,4,5-trimethoxyphenylethylamine), an alkaloidal component of the peyote cactus. Structural modifications of the mescaline molecule have resulted in a plethora of psychoactive compounds.

TABLE 50–6. *Amphetamine-like designer drugs*

MDA (Methylenedioxyamphetamine)
MDMA (Methylenedioxymethamphetamine; Ecstasy, Adam)
MDEA (Methylenedioxyethamphetamine; Eve)
TMA (Trimethoxyamphetamine)
DOM (Dimethoxyamphetamine; STP)
PMA (*Para*-methoxyamphetamine)

Phenylethylamine derivatives exert a variety of direct and indirect effects upon the aminergic system of the brain. These properties include agonist effects at serotonin, noradrenaline, and dopamine receptors. The degree to which a given compound affects these various neurotransmitter systems varies such that each compound can have its own spectrum of activity.

The term *hallucinogenic amphetamine*, although commonly used, is in fact, a misnomer. At nominal psychoactive doses, these compounds exhibit neither true hallucinogenic activity (visualization of unreal objects) nor amphetamine-like stimulation. What are often referred to as "hallucinations" are actually alterations in color, color intensity, texture, or the elaboration of "fantasy" states. At larger doses, as in overdose, the hallucinogenic and/or sympathomimetic potential of these agents may be expressed, sometimes with serious consequences.

MDA (Methylenedioxyamphetamine)

MDA was initially synthesized in 1920. Proposed uses reflected the anorectic, antitussive, and tranquilizing activities of the drug (17).

MDA and its metabolites release norepinephrine and block norepinephrine reuptake (18). Its mild euphoric and intoxicating effects earned it the street name "love drug." Ingestion of MDA produces a heightened need for interpersonal relationships. Those under the influence of the drug have an increased desire to be with and talk to people. Effects occur within 30 to 60 minutes of ingestion and last 6 to 10 hours.

Signs and symptoms of MDA toxicity resemble those of amphetamine intoxication. The sympathomimetic effects of MDA derive from the phenylisopropylamine portion, and the psychoactive properties derive from the methyleneoxy group. Several deaths have been attributed to MDA overdose (17).

MDMA (Methylenedioxymethamphetamine)

MDMA was first synthesized in 1914 and was developed as an appetite suppressant, though it was never marketed as such. Even though it has had a long history, it is considered one of the new designer drugs (19,20). Some psychiatrists advocate the use of MDMA because they feel that communication is enhanced and anxiety and defenses are eliminated with patients in their clinical practice (20,21). Despite this claim, MDMA has no accepted medical use (22). Until 1985, MDMA was not a controlled substance and was legally available for use. Since that time, it has been placed on Schedule I (21,23).

MDMA synthesized clandestinely is sold as a beige powder, a clear unmarked gelatin capsule, or a beige or white unmarked tablet. A typical oral dose may be 75 to 150 mg. Best known as "Ecstasy" or "Adam" on the street, it is structurally similar to methamphetamine and mescaline. Consequently, it stimulates the CNS and produces hallucinogenic effects.

MDMA is popular because it produces positive changes in state of mind, which have been variously described as elevated mood, increased self-esteem, and increased sense of intimacy with others. However, because MDMA is closely related to the amphetamines, it may cause acute psychiatric disturbances, including panic, anxiety, and paranoid thinking. MDMA has recently been widely abused on college campuses for its alleged aphrodisiac effects.

The effects are primarily sympathomimetic in nature. The majority of acute or chronic users state that the effects, initially at least, are pleasurable. Users usually progress through three stages, beginning with disorientation, moving onto tingling and spasmodic jerking, and ending with "happy sociability."

Some of the less desirable effects are bruxism, jaw clenching, and myalgias. Confusion, depression, and anxiety have been reported by some users for several weeks after a single dose. High doses have contributed to dysphoria, paranoia, and rarely, hallucinations. There is also a "hangover" phenomenon. Acute intoxication with MDMA may also produce life-threatening dysrhythmias, hypertension, hyperthermia, and seizures (24).

A number of deaths have been linked to its abuse. The cause of these deaths is uncertain, but it has been postulated that MDMA induced fatal cardiac dysrhythmias, hyperthermia with seizures, or intracranial hemorrhage in its victims.

Chronic abuse may produce a paranoid psychosis clinically indistinguishable from schizophrenia.

MDEA (Methylenedioxyethamphetamine)

Following the designation of MDMA as a Schedule I controlled substance by the Drug Enforcement Administration, MDEA, which is known on the street as "Eve," appeared on the market as an analogue. The effects of MDEA are similar to those of MDMA. Deaths associated with MDEA have been reported, though cause could not definitely be attributed to the drug (17).

TMA

The chemical structure and pharmacology of TMA (2,4,5-trimethoxyamphetamine) resembles both mescaline, with respect to the ring substituents, and amphetamine, due to the methylation of the basic phenylethylamine structure. It was first synthesized in 1933 but its psychoactive potential was not recognized until 1962. A more potent psychoactive drug than mescaline, TMA shows qualitatively similar effects on mood alterations and sensory enhancement as mescaline. The difference in the amount of drug causing the desired psychoactive effects and that resulting in toxicity is small.

DOM/STP

DOM (4-methyl-2,5-dimethoxyamphetamine) has also been called STP on the street. This is due to "serenity, tranquillity, and peace." High initial doses with attendant untoward responses gave the drug an unfavorable reputation on the street and limited its acceptance.

The therapeutic index of DOM is narrow. Low doses of 2 to 3 mg produce mild sympathetic stimulation, euphoria, and perceptual distortions. Amounts greater than 5 mg consistently produce a hallucinatory reaction and more significant sympathetic stimulation.

DOB

Laboratory research found that replacing a methyl-ring substituent of DOM with a bromo group dramatically increased the psychoactive potency of the compound, termed bromo-DOM or simply, DOB. One of the most potent phenylethylamine compounds yet synthesized, DOB exhibits at least 100 times the potency of mescaline. It is one of the few drugs, like LSD, that are sold as drug-impregnated pieces of paper.

The course of intoxication is quite prolonged. Onset of effect following 2 to 3 mg is about an hour; full intoxication requires about 3 to 4 hours. A fantasy state and mood enhancement with minimal visual distortions persist for about 10 hours, followed by a gradual resolution of effects over 12 to 24 hours.

PMA

Para-methoxyamphetamine (PMA) appeared as a recreational drug in the early 1970s and was quickly associated with several fatalities. The drug exhibits potent hallucinatory and stimulatory properties. Overdoses with PMA have been characterized by marked adrenergic excess. It appears from the history of these exposures that PMA was a contaminant or substitute for what was often thought to be MDA. It is not generally a sought-after drug, but rather an example of a misrepresented street drug.

Methcathinone

Methcathinone is a relatively new designer drug developed in the Great Lakes area of the U.S. The drug, known as cat on the street, became popular in 1991. Methcathinone is a derivative of cathinone, which is the most potent amphetamine-like constituent occurring naturally in the evergreen tree khat, *Catha edulis*. Clandestine laboratories synthesize methcathinone from ephedrine. Because sodium dichromate, sulfuric acid, acetone, and toluene are used in the synthesis, toxicities could also be attributed to these compounds (25).

Shortly after intranasal use, the user experiences onset of euphoria, color enhancement, with occasional visual hallucinations. This period is followed by a 5- to 8-hour period of feeling invincible, with increased libido and desire to be physical. If a second or third dose is taken within several hours after the first, more visual effects and hallucinations are noted (25).

Acute Toxicity of Stimulant "Designer Drugs"

In overdose, phenylethylamine derivatives act as sympathomimetic agents, stimulating α- and β-adrenergic receptors to various degrees, depending on the specific compound (Table 50–7). The differences in their psychoactive effects are blurred by the predominance of the sympathetic nervous system effects. Clinically, one sees anxiety, agitation, anorexia, nausea, bruxism, tremors, muscle rigidity, hyperreflexia, mydriasis, diaphoresis, tachycardia, hypertension, and hyperthermia. In severe cases, a hyperdynamic cardiovascular collapse may occur.

Further complications of acute overdose include seizures, arrhythmias, intracerebral hemorrhage, secondary to a sudden increase in blood pressure, muscle rigidity with rhabdomyolysis, hyperthermia, adult respiratory distress syndrome, acute renal failure, hepatocellular necrosis, and coma (16).

TABLE 50–7. *Clinical effects of stimulant designer drugs*

Psychological
Aphrodisiac
Elevated mood
Increased self-esteem
Increased feeling of intimacy
Paranoia
Systemic—mild
Anxiety
Agitation
Tremors
Muscle rigidity
Hyperreflexia
Mydriasis
Diaphoresis
Tachycardia
Hypertension
Systemic—moderate–severe
Bruxism
Hyperthermia
Cardiovascular collapse
Seizures
Arrhythmias
Intracerebral hemorrhage
Rhabdomyolysis
Adult respiratory distress syndrome

NUTMEG

Nutmeg and mace are derived from the seeds of *Myristica fragrans*. Mace comes from the fleshy scarlet covering of the seed; nutmeg comes from the seed itself. Nutmeg is grown commercially in Granada and is imported to the U.S. Nutmeg does not have a psychological effect once the volatile oil has been removed, and the considerable variation seen in cases of nutmeg ingestion may be due to the variable loss of this volatile oil component during the storage.

The chemical agents which are thought to give nutmeg its psychoactive effects are myristicin and elemicin, which are amphetamine-like compounds similar to MDMA. Ingestion of several tablespoons of ground nutmeg, or two to five whole nutmegs (approximately 30 g of the ground powder) results in intense nausea and vomiting, followed by visual distortions. The ingestion of as little as 1 to 2 tablespoonsful, which may contain 5 to 10 g in each tablespoon, is capable of producing psychoactive effects described as hallucinations, euphoria, and other distortions of reality as well as many undesirable effects.

The symptoms begin 3 to 6 hours after ingestion and generally resolve in 24 hours. The first CNS effects are giddiness, tingling, dizziness, apprehension, anxiety, and a generalized feeling of excitement. Later, euphoria, visual hallucinations, distortions in time and space, reality detachment, sensations of limb loss, and fear of death may occur. This may progress to extreme drowsiness and lethargy that persist for a day or more.

The treatment is largely supportive in nature.

THE "LOOK-ALIKE" DRUGS

The "look-alike" drugs and "speed" are included in a recent but growing category of drugs of abuse (2,26,27). Because many over-the-counter stimulants are inexpensive and less risky to sell than controlled substances, they are often sold singly or more commonly in combinations as speed or cocaine. The most common over-the-counter stimulants sold as look-alikes are phenylpropanolamine, ephedrine, caffeine, and pseudoephedrine. Phenylpropanolamine is also called norephedrine, and pseudoephedrine is an optical isomer of ephedrine (28). These drugs may be in the form of tablets or capsules that resemble prescription drugs in shape, size, color, and markings, but they do not contain the same ingredients or have the same effectiveness. Phenylpropanolamine is found in more than 75 over-the-counter preparations for relief of colds, in anorectic preparations, in appetite control remedies, and in nasal decongestants (26). It is the

TABLE 50–8. *Selected products containing phenylpropanolamine*

Product name	Phenylpropanolamine (mg)	Caffeine (mg)
Anorexin	25–50	100
Codexin	75	100
Dex-a-diet	75	
Dexatrim	50	200
Dietac	25–50	
EZ Trim	75	
PVM Appetite Control	25–75	
Prolamine	37.5	140
Super Odrinex	25	100

Adapted with permission from *Ann Emerg Med* 1982;11: 483. © 1982 American College of Emergency Physicians.

active ingredient in the plant *Catha edulis*, whose leaves are chewed to achieve an amphetamine-like effect. Phenylpropanolamine is a derivative of ephedrine (42). Both these drugs are noncatecholamines, or indirectly-acting sympathomimetics structurally resembling the amphetamines (29). Phenylpropanolamine and ephedrine act both peripherally and centrally because, unlike catecholamines, they readily cross the blood–brain barrier. Of the two, ephedrine has a more potent effect on the CNS (2).

The most common look-alikes are copies of amphetamine compounds, but instead of containing amphetamine they contain 100 to 200 mg of caffeine, 25 to 30 mg of ephedrine, and 25 to 50 g of phenylpropanolamine (Table 50–8). Such preparations are currently considered legal and are available as diet aids or "pick-me-ups" in pharmacies, grocery stores, and drug paraphernalia shops and can even be obtained by mail order (2).

Uses

The look-alikes are capable of producing mood elevations and an altered state of consciousness, as is seen with amphetamines. Patients have a generalized feeling of well-being and experience anorexia (an effect that is much weaker than that induced by amphetamines and decreases with time), decreased fatigue, enhanced sensory perceptions, and improved motor skills (2).

One of the problems associated with the look-alike drugs is that the margin of safety between therapeutic and toxic doses of these agents is small. This property exposes patients to potentially toxic amounts at single doses barely exceeding those found in a combination pill. The toxicity of the triple combination of phenylpropanolamine, ephedrine, and caffeine in abuse quantities may even be greater than the toxicity of amphetamines. In addition, an inexperienced drug user may inadvertently overdose because of the mistaken idea that these drugs will not produce a "high" equivalent to that of amphetamines (5). Such a user may also wrongly assume that the look-alikes are safer, less potent substances and take several pills at a time, causing even greater toxicity (26).

Mechanism of Action

Phenylpropanolamine has two modes of action: a direct α-adrenergic action and an indirect action by virtue of its ability to release norepinephrine from storage sites at nerve terminals (29). There is also a weak β-adrenergic stimulatory component that may cause orthostatic hypotension (28).

Pharmacokinetics

Absorption of oral phenylpropanolamine is rapid, with the maximal clinical effect occurring in 1 to 3 hours (28). Phenylpropanolamine is a weak base and is eliminated most rapidly in an acid urine. Although the half-life is approximately 2 hours, clinical effects may last for a longer period (29).

Toxicity

Phenylpropanolamine has a low therapeutic index, which means that there is not a great deal of difference between a therapeutic and a toxic dose. Life-threatening complications may therefore occur at approximately 3 times the over-the-counter dose (28).

Central Nervous System Effects

Phenylpropanolamine is a less potent CNS stimulant than amphetamine. This can be dangerous if individuals attempt to simulate an amphetamine-like "high" and take more than a normal dose of phenylpropanolamine (29). Intoxication can occur from both central and peripheral adrenergic stimulation. A higher than recommended dose can cause agitation, restlessness, altered sleep patterns, headache, disorientation, and confusion (Table 50–9). Grand mal seizures have also been reported in patients taking phenylpropanolamine together with caffeine (28). Hemorrhagic and nonhemorrhagic stroke and transient ischemic neurologic deficit have been reported.

Cardiovascular Effects

Because phenylpropanolamine affects the adrenergic receptors and may produce cardiac dysrhythmias, premature ventricular contractions, premature atrial contractions, and atrial and ventricular tachycardia may be noted (30). Because of the greater peripheral effect, hyperten-

TABLE 50–9. *Clinical features of intoxication from look-alike drugs*

Central nervous system
Agitation
Restlessness
Headache
Disorientation
Confusion
Intracerebral hemorrhage
Seizures
Altered sleep patterns
Mania
Psychosis
Cardiovascular
Dysrhythmias
Premature ventricular contractions
Premature atrial contractions
Ventricular tachycardia
Paroxysmal atrial tachycardia
Hypertension
Postural hypotension
Bradycardia
Miscellaneous
Rhabdomyolysis
Myoglobulinemia
Myoglobinuria

sion (both systolic and diastolic) may be more pronounced than with amphetamines and may lead to hypertensive encephalopathy and intracerebral hemorrhage (2,28). Occasionally, postural hypotension may be observed (31). Reflex bradycardia has also occurred after phenylpropanolamine ingestion (28).

Hypertensive crisis can result from even a single therapeutic dose of phenylpropanolamine. Intracerebral hemorrhage has occurred secondary to the severe hypertension. The hypertensive effect may be potentiated by various other drugs, including monoamine oxidase inhibitors, ephedrine, caffeine, anticholinergic drugs, antihistamines, and antihypertensive agents.

Electrocardiographic abnormalities have been reported with phenylpropanolamine and include ventricular dysrhythmias and repolarization abnormalities. Direct myocardial injuries associated with symptoms of chest pain with elevation of the MB fraction of creatine phosphokinase have been described.

Miscellaneous Effects

Renal failure with (26,32) or without (33–34) rhabdomyolysis and hypertension may occur with phenylpropanolamine overdose.

Laboratory Analysis

Qualitative identification of phenylpropanolamine in urine can be accomplished by using thin-layer chromatography or enzyme-modified immunoassay. These techniques may not be readily available, however. Therapeutic doses typically produce serum concentrations between 60 and 200 ng/mL (28). Qualitative identification in the urine can also be performed.

Treatment

Treatment of patients with a suspected overdose of a look-alike drug (Table 50–10) should comprise immediate and frequent monitoring of the vital signs for possible life-threatening sequelae such as cardiac dysrhythmias and hypertensive crisis. Therapy with emesis or lavage, and activated charcoal and a cathartic should then be instituted (29). Most episodes of hypertension subside within 3 to 4 hours without treatment or with the addition of a mild sedative such as a benzodiazepine. Hypertension should be treated if accompanied by signs or symptoms of myocardial ischemia or hypertensive encephalopathy (28); sodium nitroprusside beginning at 3 μg/kg/minute and titrated according to effect is suggested (28). If serious cardiac dysrhythmias are present, lidocaine should be administered. Beta-adrenergic blocking drugs, although potentially useful for the tachydysrhythmias, may be harmful if the hypertension causes a vagal stimulation, which produces a reflex bradycardia that may be potentiated by the β-adrenergic blocking drug (29). The psychosis, if not responsive to supportive care, can be managed with the use of haloperidol or diazepam. Seizures should be treated with intravenous diazepam.

Acidification of the urine accelerates clearance but entails additional risks such as precipitation of myoglobin in the kidneys with minimal clinical benefit. For this reason, acid diuresis is not suggested (28). Dialysis and diuresis are not effective because of the large volume of distribution of these drugs.

PROPYLHEXEDRINE

This compound is the active ingredient in Benzedrex inhalers and is extracted from the wicks of the inhalers by

TABLE 50–10. *Treatment of overdose look-alike drugs*

Indication	Treatment
Oral ingestion	Gastric lavage Activated charcoal and cathartic
Seizures	Diazepam (5 to 15 mg IV)
Severe hypertension	Sodium nitroprusside (3 μg/kg/minute)
Ventricular dysrhythmias	Lidocaine (1 mg/k by 1 to 4 μg/kg/minute) β-Adrenergic blocking drugs (use with caution)
Psychosis	Haloperidol (2 to 5 mg IM)

drug abusers for intravenous injection (35). Compounds of this type are called "crank" or homemade speed.

The mechanism of action of propylhexedrine has not been conclusively determined but appears to be similar to that of amphetamine. Propylhexedrine indirectly stimulates α-adrenergic receptors of the sympathetic nervous system and exerts a minor stimulant effect on β-adrenergic receptors.

Following nasal inhalation of propylhexedrine, local vasoconstriction usually occurs within 30 seconds to 5 minutes and may persist for 30 minutes to 2 hours. Occasionally, enough propylhexedrine may be absorbed to produce systemic effects.

METHYLPHENIDATE

Methylphenidate (Ritalin) is an amphetamine-like stimulant indicated for the treatment of narcolepsy and the attention-deficit disorder. The pharmacologic actions of methylphenidate include CNS and respiratory stimulation and weak sympathomimetic activity. The mechanism of action involved in the central effect of methylphenidate has not been determined. The main sites of CNS action appear to be the cerebral cortex and subcortical structures including the thalamus; stimulation by methylphenidate causes an increase in motor activity, mental alertness, diminished sense of fatigue, brighter spirits, and mild euphoria. Methylphenidate apparently produces an anorexigenic effect. In usual therapeutic oral dosage, methylphenidate exhibits only moderate effects on the peripheral circulatory system (36).

In recent years, the prescribing of methylphenidate as an adjunct to the management of the attention-deficit disorder has increased significantly. As with any Schedule II-controlled drug, an increase in clinical prescribing is accompanied by an increase in drug-seeking scams and by abuse of the agent by chemical-dependent individuals.

Methylphenidate, cocaine, and amphetamine have identical dopaminergic effects, and these drugs produce a similar toxic picture of inanition, personality changes, rapid development of tolerance leading to compulsive use in susceptible individuals, and withdrawal depression.

Pharmacokinetics

Methylphenidate hydrochloride appears to be well absorbed from the gastrointestinal tract; effects persist for 3 to 6 hours after oral administration of conventional tablets and about 8 hours after oral administration of extended-release tablets. Extended-release methylphenidate tablets are absorbed more slowly but to the same extent as the conventional tablets.

Methylphenidate is water-soluble, lending itself to IV abuse, with the resulting morbidity and mortality of IV drug abuse in general. In addition, the Ritalin-SR preparation contains water-insoluble incipient constituents, which have been recognized to cause accelerated peripheral vascular sclerosis and pulmonary fibrosis. The water-insoluble incipient constituents appear to be responsible for the striking excess in pulmonary morbidity and mortality seen in methylphenidate abusers, as compared with that seen in IV cocaine or heroin addicts.

Acute Toxicity

Acute toxicity due to methylphenidate overdosage results in symptoms similar to those of acute amphetamine intoxication and may be manifested by cardiovascular symptoms including flushing, palpitation, hypertension, cardiac arrhythmias, and tachycardia (Table 50–11). Mental disturbances such as confusion, delirium, euphoria, hallucinations, and toxic psychosis may also occur. Other symptoms of overdosage include agitation, headache, vomiting, dryness of mucous membranes, mydriasis, hyperpyrexia, sweating, tremors, hyperreflexia, muscle twitching, and seizures which may be followed by coma.

APPETITE SUPPRESSANTS

Drugs used in obesity are commonly known as "anorectics." It has not been established, however, that the action of such drugs in treating obesity is exclusively one of appetite suppression. Other central nervous system actions, or metabolic effects may be involved as well. The anorexigenic effect of sympathomimetic compounds used in the treatment of obesity is temporary, seldom lasting more than a few weeks and tolerance may occur. The agents include fenfluramine, diethylpropion, mazindol, and phendimetrazine (Table 50–12). All of these agents may be abused as CNS stimulants.

Tolerance to the effect of many anorectic drugs may develop within a few weeks; if this occurs, the recommended dose should not be exceeded in an attempt to increase the effect; rather, the drug should be discontinued.

TABLE 50–11. *Signs and symptoms of methylphenidate overdose*

Central nervous system
Confusion
Delirium
Hallucinations
Psychosis
Headache
Cardiovascular
Arrhythmias
Hypertension
Tachycardia
Palpitations

TABLE 50–12. *Appetite suppressants*

Fenfluramine (Pondimin)
Mazindol (Sanorex)
Diethylpropion (Tenuate)
Phendimetrazine (Phenazine)

Fenfluramine (Pondimin)

Cardiovascular and autonomic effects produced by fenfluramine appear to be qualitatively similar to those of amphetamine but as a pressor agent it is 10–20 times less potent than dextroamphetamine. In obese hypertensive patients fenfluramine may have hypotensive effects. EEG studies show fenfluramine to be qualitatively different from amphetamine and other amphetamine congeners and suggest that fenfluramine may be more similar to sedative psychotherapeutic drugs rather than CNS or cerebral stimulants.

Mazindol (Sanorex)

Although chemically unrelated to amphetamines, mazindol has pharmacologic activity similar to the amphetamines and, like the amphetamines, may produce CNS and cardiac stimulation. The mechanism of action of mazindol also has not been clearly defined. Although mazindol is used in the treatment of obesity as an anorexigenic, it has not been firmly established that the pharmacologic action is primarily one of appetite suppression; other CNS actions and/or metabolic effects may be involved.

Diethylpropion (Tenuate)

Adverse nervous system effects of diethylpropion may include overstimulation, nervousness, restlessness, jitteriness, anxiety, insomnia, dizziness, euphoria, dysphoria, mental depression, headache, tremor, and blurred vision. Rarely, psychotic episodes may occur in patients receiving recommended dosages. An increase in seizures has occurred in some patients with epilepsy who received the drug.

Phendimetrazine (Phenazine, Wehless)

Phendimetrazine tartrate is an amphetamine congener which is used as an anorexigenic agent. As with other amphetamine derivatives, no primary effect on appetite has been demonstrated with phendimetrazine and it is probable that its anorexigenic effect is secondary to CNS stimulation. Although animal studies indicate that the cardiovascular and respiratory effects of phendimetrazine are not as pronounced as those of phenmetrazine, the clinical importance of these findings is questionable. Phendimetrazine is readily absorbed from the GI tract and effects persist for about 4 hours after oral administration.

Acute Toxicity of Anorexigenic Agents

Acute toxicity with other anorexigenic agents may produce restlessness, agitation, tremors, confusion, assaultiveness, hallucinations, hyperreflexia and muscle twitching, rapid respiration, and dizziness followed by fatigue and CNS depression. Cardiovascular effects may include arrhythmias, tachycardia, palpitation, hypertension or hypotension, and circulatory collapse. GI symptoms include nausea, vomiting, diarrhea, and abdominal cramps. In patients with severe overdosage, convulsions, coma, and death may occur.

BOTANICAL DIETARY SUPPLEMENTS

There have been an increasing number of reports of adverse events associated with use of certain products marketed as dietary supplements for weight loss, energy, and ergogenics (performance-enhancing) and body-building purposes. These apparently diverse categories of products often contain a number of similar ingredients, including Ma huang, which is *Ephedra sinica* or Chinese ephedra, a botanical source of ephedrine, pseudoephedrine, and norpseudoephedrine as well as guarana or Kola nut, which is a caffeine source. These may also contain various amino acids, glandular products, or other nutrients. They are touted for their reported stimulant effects and their ability to enhance metabolism with subsequent weight loss.

The adverse reactions reported vary from mild adverse effects known to be associated with sympathomimetic stimulants to chest pain, myocardial infarction, hepatitis, stroke, seizures, psychosis, and death. These adverse effects have been reported in both young, otherwise healthy individuals and persons with complicating conditions such as hypertension.

Because these products are commonly marketed as dietary supplements, there is little or no premarket review made of these products, with no good dosing or monitoring information.

CAFFEINE

Caffeine (1,3,7-trimethylxanthine) belongs to a group of methylated xanthines found in a variety of plants throughout the world. The closely related alkaloids theobromine and theophylline (1,3-dimethylxanthine) are other methylxanthines with similar properties (37). Although each differs in its potency on a particu-

TABLE 50–13. *Caffeine content of various beverages*

Product	Average caffeine content per dose (mg)
Coffee	100–150
Tea	40–60
Cocoa	10–40
Carbonated drinks	35–65
Chocolate	25
Headache remedies	50–75
Anorectic agents	100–200
Cold preparations	30–75
Stimulants	75–200

lar organ system, they share many pharmacologic effects. Aqueous extracts of these plants have for centuries formed the basis of a number of popular beverages, from the coffee bean in Arabia, the tea leaf in China, the kola nut in West Africa, to the cocoa bean in Mexico (38).

Caffeine is widely consumed today in beverages such as coffee, tea, and cocoa. Coffee and tea have been the most popular beverages in Western society for several hundred years. Although the major source of caffeine on a weight-for-weight basis is tea, the highest dose per serving is found in coffee, which has approximately twice the amount of caffeine that is obtained from an equal amount of tea (39). Caffeine is also an ingredient in chocolate as well as many over-the-counter analgesics, headache remedies, anorectic agents, and stimulants (Tables 50–13 and 50–14). Soft drinks represent a major source of dietary caffeine, particularly for children. Ingestion of caffeine, therefore, is common for therapeutic purposes or from consumption of various beverages. It is therefore important for the practitioner to know the various soft drinks that do not contain caffeine (Table 50–15). Naturopathic therapies such as caffeine enemas have been linked to deaths (38,40).

TABLE 50–14. *Concentrations of caffeine in beverages and pharmaceuticals*

Beverage	**Amount per 12-oz serving (mg)**
Jolt	70
Mountain Dew	55
Mello Yellow	53
Coca-Cola	47
Cherry Coke	46
TAB	45
Dr. Pepper	40
Mr. Pibb	40
Pepsi Cola	38
Diet Pepsi	36
Slice Red	34
Cherry spice slice	35
Dr. Slice	35
Over-the-counter medications	**Amount (mg) containing caffeine**
Anacin	33
Aspirin-Free Excedrin	65
Caferfot	100
Dexatrim	200
Dristan	15

TABLE 50–15. *Soft drinks not containing caffeine*

Caffeine-free colas
Carbonated water
Fresca
Fruit punch
Ginger ale
Grape
Mineral water
Orange (most)
Root beer (most)
Seven-up
Slice lemon-lime
Sprite
Squirt
Tonic water

Guarana extracts have been used for their effects secondary to the caffeine content. Guarana (*Paullinia cupana*) is a plant native to Brazil, and is sold in the U.S. in health food stores as an appetite suppressant, as an aid to restore mental alertness as well as for quick energy. The commercially available product contains 3% to 5% caffeine. A 1-g tablet of guarana would contain approximately 30 to 50 mg of caffeine.

Pharmacokinetics

Caffeine is absorbed rapidly after oral administration, and serum concentrations reach their peak in 30 to 60 minutes (28,38,39). The presence or absence of food in the stomach does not influence the absorption of caffeine. It is freely and equally distributed throughout the total body water and has a volume of distribution in adults of 0.5 L/kg (28). Caffeine has a plasma half-life of 3 to 4 hours in adults, although, the half-life of the drug is dependent on numerous factors, including age, prior medical conditions, and the concomitant ingestion of other drugs (29,38,40,41). It is metabolized in the liver to methyluric acid and methylxanthine, both of which are inactive and are excreted in the urine (38). Caffeine is also metabolized to theophylline (29).

Actions

Caffeine has many pharmacologic effects, including phosphodiesterase inhibition, sensitization of dopamine receptors, adenosine inhibition, modification of calcium metabolism, and increases in the release of epinephrine, norepinephrine, and plasma renin activity (42).

Caffeine causes a translocation of intracellular calcium by increasing the permeability of calcium in the sarcoplasmic reticulum, which accounts for its action of increasing the contractility of skeletal and cardiac muscle. It also causes an increased accumulation of cyclic nucleotides, particularly cyclic AMP, by inhibiting the enzyme phosphodiesterase (28,39,43). This enzyme is necessary for the degradation of cyclic AMP (29). By inhibiting phosphodiesterase, the metabolic action of endogenous sympathomimetics is enhanced. Additionally, caffeine blocks adenosine receptors (44,45). Adenosine acts as a neurotransmitter in purinergic neurons, which have diverse functions throughout the body (39). Some actions of adenosine include dilation of blood vessels, slowing of the rate of cardiac pacemaker cells, and inhibition of the release of norepinephrine from autonomic nerve endings. Because caffeine antagonizes this effect, sympathomimetic effects occur (39).

Caffeine is a potent releaser of epinephrine and to a lesser extent of norepinephrine from the adrenal medulla (28,29,39). The cardiac toxic effects as well as the metabolic effects (hyperglycemia, ketosis, and metabolic acidosis) of caffeine are probably due to increasing circulating concentrations of epinephrine and norepinephrine. It has been shown that caffeine can be an effective bronchodilator, although its use is not recommended.

Several of the biochemical effects, such as phosphodiesterase inhibition, calcium mobilization, and prostaglandin antagonism, occur only at relatively high doses. At the doses encountered in foods and beverages, the probable mechanism is that of adenosine receptor antagonism (28,39).

Acute Toxicity

Caffeine is a widely abused drug that is often overlooked as a cause of acute reactions. Caffeine has a wider therapeutic index than theophylline, resulting in a lower incidence of toxicity (38). The xanthine derivatives stimulate the CNS, produce a mild diuresis, stimulate cardiac muscle, and relax smooth muscle (notably bronchial muscle) (Table 50–16). Considering the widespread consumption of caffeine in drinks and over-the-counter medicines, relatively few cases of acute serious caffeine poisoning have been reported. Nevertheless, death has been reported from oral (46), rectal, and parenteral administration of caffeine (47).

Although serious methylxanthine poisoning is much more often the result of theophylline intoxication than caffeine intoxication, the clinical presentation is similar.

TABLE 50–16. *Clinical features of caffeine intoxication*

Central nervous system
Increased alertness
Decreased drowsiness
Increased psychomotor coordination
Headache
Tremors
Nervousness
Muscle twitching
Transient psychosis
Delirium
Cardiovascular
Palpitations
Extrasystoles
Supraventricular tachycardia
Premature ventricular contractions
Bigeminy
Pulmonary edema

Central Nervous System Effects

The primary effect of caffeine is CNS stimulation (39). The cerebral cortex is particularly sensitive to the effects of caffeine, and small doses result in increased alertness, a more rapid and clear thought flow, decreased drowsiness, and improvement of psychomotor coordination (48). These effects are milder and of shorter duration than those of amphetamines. Larger doses may produce headache, tremors (49), nervousness, muscle twitching, insomnia (50), tachypnea, and irritability, which may be indistinguishable from anxiety neurosis (42). Transient psychosis and delirium have also been reported (51).

Neurologic disturbances include clonus, opisthotonus, seizures, hallucinations, agitation, insomnia, tinnitus, fever, delirium, tremor, hyperreflexia, and CNS depression ranging from drowsiness to coma (41).

Cardiovascular Effects

The positive inotropic effect on the myocardium and the positive chronotropic effect at the sinoatrial node may produce palpitations, extrasystoles, sinus or supraventricular tachycardia, and other more major ventricular dysrhythmias such as premature ventricular contractions and bigeminy (52). Death, although very rare, results from respiratory failure or cardiac arrest (41). Hypotension and circulatory failure is a late and often terminal complication of massive caffeine overdose. Severe pulmonary edema also appears to be a consistent feature of acute caffeine poisoning (38).

Gastrointestinal Effects

Gastrointestinal irritation, including vomiting, abdominal pain, and hematemesis have been frequently reported (41). This may eliminate a substantial portion of the dose. It is possible to consume and retain lethal amounts of caffeine, and it is important that medical professionals not be lulled into a false sense of security regarding the potential seriousness of this frequently encountered drug. High doses of caffeine can produce vagal, vasomotor, and respiratory center stimulation causing bradycardia, vasoconstriction, tachypnea, and tonic-clonic seizures.

Laboratory Analysis

Because caffeine and theophylline are both methylxanthines and because caffeine decreases the hepatic clearance of theophylline, serum concentrations of theophylline should be measured when large changes in caffeine intake are to be expected. In addition, theophylline is a known metabolite of caffeine but in typical doses is present in extremely low concentrations (53,54). Caffeine can be confirmed by either thin-layer or gas chromatography (38).

Treatment

Treatment of an acute overdose of caffeine usually is limited to support and abstention from the caffeine-containing substance because there is no specific antidote for caffeine (48). Emesis or lavage, or administration of activated charcoal and a cathartic should be performed in the acute overdose of caffeine tablets (29). Seizures should be controlled with a benzodiazepine such as diazepam (38). Although it may seem to be logical to use a β-adrenergic blocking drug to reverse the manifestations of the hyperadrenergic syndrome, an unopposed α-adrenergic effect may result (29). For this reason, α-adrenergic blockers may be necessary in the presence of a β-adrenergic blocking drug. Administration of lidocaine or phenytoin is recommended for treatment of cardiac dysrhythmias (38). In addition, the administration of antacids to neutralize gastrointestinal irritation may be effective.

REFERENCES

1. Derlet R, Rice P, Horowitz Z, et al: Amphetamine toxicity: experience with 127 cases. *J Emerg Med* 1989;7:157–161.
2. King P, Coleman J Stimulants and narcotic drugs. *Pediatr Clin North Am* 1987;34:349–362.
3. Linden C, Kulig K, Rumack B: Amphetamines. *Top Emerg Med* 1985;7:18–32.
4. Derlet R, Albertson T, Rice P: Protection against *d*-amphetamine toxicity. *Am J Emerg Med* 1990;8:105–108.
5. King J: Hypertension and cerebral hemorrhage after Trimolets ingestion. *Med J Aust* 1979;2:258–259.
6. Van Dyke C, Byck R: Cocaine. *Sci Am* 1982;246:128–141.
7. Goodman S, Becker D: Intracranial hemorrhage associated with amphetamine abuse. *JAMA* 1970;212:480–482.
8. Citron B, Halpern M, McCarron M, et al: Necrotizing angiitis associated with drug abuse. *N Engl J Med* 1970;283:1003–1011.
9. Ginsberg M, Hartzman M, Schmidt-Nowara W: Amphetamine intoxication with coagulopathy, hyperthermia, and reversible renal failure. *Ann Intern Med* 1970;73:81–85.
10. Scanling J, Spital A: Amphetamine-associated myoglobinuric renal failure. *South Med J* 1982;75:237–240.
11. Chan P, Chen J, Lee M, et al: Fatal and nonfatal methamphetamine intoxication in the intensive care unit. *J Toxicol Clin Toxicol* 1994;32:147–156.
12. Taliaferro E, Rund D, Brown C, et al: Substance abuse education in residency training programs in emergency medicine. *Ann Emerg Med* 1989;18:1344–1347.
13. Fann W: Some clinically important interactions of psychotropic drugs. *South Med J* 1973;66:661–665.
14. Lockett S: Poisoning by salicylates. paracetamol, tricyclic antidepressants, and a miscellany of drugs. *Practitioner* 1973;211:105–112.
15. Rhee K, Albertson T, Douglas J: Choreoathetoid disorder associated with amphetamine-like drugs. *Am J Emerg Med* 1988;6:131–133.
16. Buchanan J, Brown C: "Designer drugs": a problem in clinical toxicology. *Med Toxicol* 1988;3:1–17.
17. Sternbach G, Varon J: "Designer drugs": recognizing and managing their toxic effects. *Postgrad Med* 1992;91:169–176.
18. Dargon D: Cocaine. *Top Emerg Med* 1985;7:1–8.
19. Resnick R, Resnick E: Cocaine abuse and its treatment. *Psychiatr Clin North Am* 1984;7:713–728.
20. Gay G: You've come a long way, baby! Coke time for the new American lady of the eighties. *J Psychoactive Drugs* 1981;13:297–318.
21. Gay G, Inaba D, Rappolt R, et al: "An' ho, ho, baby, take a whiff on me": la dama blanca cocaine in current perspective. *Anaesth Analg* 1976;55:582–587.
22. Jerrard D: "Designer drugs"—a current perspective. *J Emerg Med* 1990;8:733–741.
23. Cohen S: Cocaine. *JAMA* 1975:231:74–75.
24. Callaway C, Clark R: Hyperthermia in psychostimulant overdose. *Ann Emerg Med* 1994;24:68–76.
25. Emerson T, Cisek J: Methcathinone: a Russian designer amphetamine infiltrates the rural midwest. *Ann Emerg Med* 1993;22:1897–1903.
26. Bernstein E, Diskant B: Phenylpropanolamine: a potentially hazardous drug. *Ann Emerg Med* 1982;11:311–315.
27. Dietz A: Amphetamine-like reactions to phenylpropanolamine. *JAMA* 1981;245:601–602.
28. Pentel P: Toxicity of over-the-counter stimulants. *JAMA* 1984;252:1898–1903.
29. Bayer M, Maskell L: Abuse and toxicity of over-the-counter stimulants. *Emerg Med Rep* 1983;4:127–132.
30. Peterson R, Vasquez L: Phenylpropanolamine-induced ventricular arrhythmias. *JAMA* 1973;223:324–326.
31. Sawyer D, Conner C, Rumack B: Managing acute toxicity from nonprescription stimulants. *Drug Intell Clin Pharmacol* 1982;1:529–533.
32. Swenson R, Golper T, Bennett W: Acute renal failure and rhabdomyolysis after ingestion of phenylpropanolamine-containing diet pills. *JAMA* 1982;248:1216.
33. Horowitz J, Lang W, Howes L, et al: Hypertensive responses induced by phenylpropanolamine in anorectic and decongestant preparation. *Lancet* 1980;1:60–61.
34. Norvenius G, Widerlov E, Lonnerholm G: Phenylpropanolamine and mental disturbance. *Lancet* 1979;2:1367–1368.
35. Mancusi-Ungaro H, Decker W: Tissue injuries associated with parenteral propylhexedrine abuse. *Clin Toxicol* 1983;21:359–372.
36. Parran T, Jasinski D: Intravenous methylphenidate abuse: prototype for prescription drug abuse. *Arch Intern Med* 1991;151:781–783.
37. Zimmerman P. Pulliam J, Schwengels J, et al: Caffeine intoxication: a near fatality. *Ann Emerg Med* 1985;14:1227–1229.
38. Dalvi R: Acute and chronic toxicity of caffeine: a review. 1986;28:144–150.
39. Abbott P: Caffeine: a toxicological overview. *Med J Aust* 1986;145:518–521.
40. Jarboe C, Hurst H, Rodgers G, et al: Toxicokinetics of caffeine elimination in an infant. *Clin Toxicol* 1986;24:415–428.
41. Mrvos R, Dean B, Krenzelok E: Massive caffeine ingestion resulting in death. *Vet Hum Toxicol* 1989;31:571–572.
42. Wrenn K, Oschner I: Rhabdomyolysis induced by a caffeine overdose. *Ann Emerg Med* 1989;18:94–97.
43. Kramer G, Wells J: Effects of phosphodiesterase inhibitors on cyclic nucleotide levels and relaxation of pig coronary arteries. *Molec Pharmacol* 1979;16:813–822.
44. Daly J, Bruns R, Snyder S: Adenosine receptors in the central nervous system: relationship to the central actions of methylxanthines. *Life Sci* 1981;28:2083–2097.
45. Fredholm B: Are methylxanthine effects due to antagonism of endogenous adenosine? *Trends Pharmacol Sci* 1980;1:29–132.
46. McGee M: Caffeine poisoning in a 19-year-old female. *J Forensic Sci* 1980;25:29–32.
47. Jokela S, Vartianen A: Caffeine poisoning. *Acta Pharmacol Toxicol* 1959;15:331–334.

48. Derlet R, Tseng J, Albertson T: Potentiation of cocaine and *d*-amphetamine toxicity with caffeine. *Am J Emerg Med* 1992;10:211–216.
49. Reimann H: Caffeinism: a cause of long continued low-grade fever. *JAMA* 1967;202:1105–1106.
50. Silver W: Insomnia, tachycardia and cola drinks. *Pediatrics* 1971;47:635.
51. McManamy M, Purcell S: Caffeine intoxication: a report of a case the symptoms of which amounted to a psychosis. *N Engl J Med* 1966;215:616–620.
52. Myers M: Caffeine and cardiac arrhythmias. *Ann Intern Med* 1991;114:147–150.
53. Benowitz N, Osterloh J, Goldschlager N, et al: Massive catecholamine release from caffeine poisoning. *JAMA* 1982; 248:1097–1098.
54. Sved S, Hossie R, McGilveray I: The human metabolism of caffeine to theophylline. *Res Commun Chem Pathol Pharmacol* 1976; 13:185–192.

ADDITIONAL SELECTED REFERENCES

Alsott R, Miller A, Forney R: Report of a human fatality due to caffeine. *J Forensic Sci* 1973;18:135–137.

Anderson R, Reed W, Hillis L, et al: History, epidemiology, and medical complications of nasal inhaler abuse. *J Toxicol Clin Toxicol* 1982;19:95–107.

Baldessarini RI: Symposium on behavior modification by drugs: pharmacology of the amphetamines. *Pediatrics* 1972;49:694–701.

Becker A, Simons K, Gillespie C, et al: The bronchodilator effects and pharmacokinetics of caffeine in asthma. *N Engl J Med* 1984;310:743–746.

Benchimol A, Bartall H, Desser K: Accelerated ventricular rhythm and cocaine abuse. *Ann Intern Med* 1978;88:519–520.

Bennett W: Hazards of the appetite suppressant phenylpropanolamine. *Lancet* 1979;2:42–43.

Blum A: Phenylpropanolamine: an over-the-counter amphetamine?, editorial. *JAMA* 1981;245:1346–1347.

Caruana D, Weinbach B, Goerg D, et al: Cocaine-packet ingestion. *Ann Intern Med* 1984;100:73–74.

Chambers H, Morris L, Tauber M, et al: Cocaine use and the risk for endocarditis in intravenous drug users. *Ann Intern Med* 1987:106:833–836.

Curatolo P, Robertson D: The health consequences of caffeine. *Ann Intern Med* 1983;98:641–653.

Duffy W, Senekjian H, Knight T, et al: Acute renal failure due to phenylpropanolamine. *South Med J* 1981;74:1548.

Edison G: Amphetamines: a dangerous illusion. *Ann Intern Med* 1971;74:605–610.

Egan D, Robinson D: Cocaine: recreational drug of choice? *Rocky Mt Med J* 1978;75:34–36.

Eisele J, Reay D: Deaths related to coffee enemas. *JAMA* 1980;244:1608–1609.

Escobar J. Karno M: Chronic hallucinosis from nasal drops. *JAMA* 1982;247:1859–1862.

Fishbain D, Wetli C: Cocaine intoxication, delirium, and death in a body packer. *Ann Emerg Med* 1981;10:531–532.

Foley R, Kapatkin K. Verani R, et al: Amphetamine induced acute renal failure. *South Med J* 1984;77:258–259.

Gary N, Saidi P: Methamphetamine intoxication. *Am J Med* 1977;64:537–540.

Haddad L: 1978: Cocaine in perspective. *JACEP* 1979;8.374–376.

Harrington H, Heller A, Kawson D, et al: Intracerebral hemorrhage and oral amphetamine. *Arch Neurol* 1983;40:503–507.

Insley B, Grufferman S, Ayliffe E: Thallium poisoning in cocaine abusers. *Am J Emerg Med* 1986;4:545–548.

Jekel J, Podlewski H, Dean-Patterson S, et al: Epidemic free-base cocaine abuse. *Lancet* 1986;1:459–462.

Josephson G, Stine R: Caffeine intoxication: a case of paroxysmal atrial tachycardia. *JACEP* 1976;5:776–778.

Koff R, Widrich W, Robbins A: Necrotizing angiitis in a methamphetamine user with hepatitis B: angiographic diagnosis, five-month follow-up results and localization of bleeding site. *N Engl J Med* 1973; 288:946–947.

Leikin J, Zell M, Hyrhorczuk K: PCP or cocaine intoxication. *Ann Emerg Med* 1987;16:235–236.

Madden J, Payne T, Miller S: Maternal cocaine abuse and effect on the newborn. *Pediatrics* 1986;77:209–211.

May D, Long R, Madden R, et al: Caffeine toxicity secondary to street drug ingestion. *Ann Emerg Med* 1981;10:549.

Patel R, Dutta D, Schonfeld S: Free-base cocaine use associated with bronchiolitis obliterans organizing pneumonia. *Ann Intern Med* 1987;107:186–188.

Perry D: Heroin and cocaine adulteration, editorial. *Clin Toxicol* 1975;8:239–243.

Post R, Kopanda R: Cocaine, kindling, and psychosis. *Am J Psychiatry* 1976;133:627–640.

Rumack B: Phenylpropanolamine: a potentially hazardous drug, editorial. *Ann Emerg Med* 1982;11:332.

Schatzman M, Sabbadini A, Forti L: Coca and cocaine: a bibliography. *J Psychedelic Drugs* 1976;8:95–128.

Schenck N: The case for cocaine. *Res Staff Physician* 1975;21:67–69.

Scott M, Mullaly R: Lithium therapy for cocaine-induced psychosis: a clinical perspective. *South Med J* 1981;74:1475–1477.

Silverstein W, Lewin N, Goldfrank L: Management of the cocaine-intoxicated patient. *Ann Emerg Med* 1987;16:234–235.

Warner A, Pierozynski G: Pseudocatatonia associated with abuse of amphetamine and cannabis. *Postgrad Med* 1977;61:275–276.

Weiss S, Raskind K, Morganstein N, et al: Intracerebral and subarachnoid hemorrhage following use of methamphetamine ("speed"). *Int Surg* 1970;53:123–127.

Wetli C, Mettleman R: The body packer syndrome: toxicity following ingestion of illicit drugs packaged for transportation. *J Forensic Sci* 1981;26:492–500.

Winek C, Eastly T: Cocaine identification. *Clin Toxicol* 1979;8:205–210.

CHAPTER 51

Cocaine

The use of cocaine (benzoylmethylecgonine) began about 3,000 years ago, according to Inca documents found in the area of what is now known as Peru and Bolivia (1,2). Cocaine is a naturally occurring alkaloid extracted from the coca shrub *Erythroxylon coca*, which grows abundantly in the West Indies, Central and South America, and Mexico (3–5). The coca plant should not be confused with the cocoa plant, which contains another stimulant, caffeine. The coca plant grows to a maximum of 7 or 8 feet in height, and the cocaine extracted represents roughly 1% of the dry weight of the coca leaf (6,7). During the time of the Incas, coca leaves were considered precious and were usually reserved for use by the nobility and for religious ceremonies, although they were used by others as well because of their energizing properties.

At the beginning of the 20th century, many patent medicines and soft drinks in the United States contained small amounts of cocaine. At one time Coca-Cola contained cocaine; but shortly after the turn of the century, the cocaine was replaced with caffeine (4,8–10). Cocaine was indiscriminately included in over-the-counter medicines, tonics, and wines (4,11). It has subsequently been deleted from all these products. Estimates today are that more than 4 million Indians in Peru and Bolivia use coca leaves on a regular basis. Illegally imported cocaine is usually in the form of the hydrochloride salt, which is produced by a process of alkaloid extraction and crystallization (12).

RECENT HISTORY

In the past, cocaine was expensive and its price served as a barrier to widespread use. In recent years, cocaine has become less expensive and its availability and purity have increased (4). Although it was once a drug for the wealthy, cocaine now pervades all strata of society. Thus, during the last 10 years the growing epidemic of cocaine abuse in the United States has resulted in widespread physical, psychiatric, and social problems. At one time, cocaine was considered a safe, nonaddicting euphoriant. Historical descriptions of cocaine dependence were dismissed as exaggerations similar to marijuana reports from earlier eras. Systemic, objective, clinical research on cocaine abuse did not exist, which led to the misinterpretation that cocaine dependence did not exist (13). Although cocaine was once thought to be a relatively safe street drug, the incidence of cocaine-related deaths has been steadily rising (4,14). The illicit use of cocaine in this country has evolved from a relatively minor problem to a major public health threat with important economic and social consequences. Cocaine is probably one of the most dangerous illicit drugs in common use today. In recent years the cost of cocaine has decreased, in some places by as much as 50%, and its availability and purity have increased (15).

MEDICAL USES

Despite its legal classification as a narcotic, cocaine is actually a tropane related to the belladonna alkaloids and is the only naturally occurring local anesthetic. Cocaine acts as a local anesthetic by virtue of a blockade of nerve initiation and conduction after local application; this effect can last from 20 to 40 minutes.

Although cocaine has had many medical uses in the past, its use is now limited to that of a topical anesthetic for rhinoplasty and intranasal surgery. Cocaine is particularly useful for this type of surgery because of its ability to anesthetize as well as to cause local vasoconstriction and thus limit bleeding (8,12,16). Although cocaine had been used in ophthalmic surgery as both a local anesthetic and vasoconstrictor, this use has now been discontinued.

PHARMACOKINETICS

Cocaine is an ester of benzoic acid and the amino alcohol base ecgonine (3). The volume of distribution is 1.2 to 1.9 L/kg (15).

Absorption

Cocaine is absorbed from most routes. It may be injected intravenously, swallowed, smoked, nasally insufflated, applied to oral or genital mucous membranes, or mixed with liquor to make a "liquid lady" (5,17,18). Although it is widely assumed that the drug is inactive when given orally because of hydrolysis by gastrointestinal acids, overwhelming evidence to the contrary exists (5). The oral route results in far less toxicity than other routes of administration, but toxic effects are still detected with large ingestions. Generally cocaine is not taken orally for recreational purposes, but toxic reactions and death have been reported from "body packing" (ingestion of drug-filled balloons to avoid police detection).

The abuser of street cocaine usually obtains a 5% mixture that may range from 10 mg to 200 mg of cocaine per dose. The average "line" of cocaine is 25 mg, and 10 to 15 mg is usually administered by the intravenous route. The latter provides the equivalent of 10 mg of dextroamphetamine.

Absorption through mucous membranes results in a slow onset but prolonged duration of activity of 1 to 1.5 hours. In contrast, cocaine's effects appear in 15 to 60 seconds when the drug is administered intravenously or through the lungs, and lasts approximately 20 minutes (19).

Metabolism

Cocaine is rapidly and extensively metabolized. It is hydrolyzed by plasma and liver cholinesterases to ecgonine methyl ester, and it undergoes nonenzymatic hydrolysis to benzoylecgonine. In addition, a small amount of cocaine is *N*-demethylated to norcocaine (20). Plasma cholinesterase activity is much lower in fetuses, infants, elderly men, patients with liver disease, pregnant women, and individuals who are homozygous for atypical cholinesterase activity (Table 51–1) (4,11,17). These individuals may be unusually sensitive to cocaine and have an exaggerated response to otherwise low doses because of their decreased ability to hydrolyze the drug (4,20).

Mechanism of Action

Cocaine blocks the sodium channel and inhibits impulse propagation along axons in a manner similar to lidocaine, procaine, and related local anesthetic drugs. Unlike all other local anesthetic drugs, however, cocaine has potent sympathomimetic actions. In addition to blocking reuptake of norepinephrine, serotonin, and dopamine, cocaine also stimulates the release of these transmitters (21).

Cocaine has a major effect on the sympathetic division of the autonomic nervous system by preventing neuronal uptake of catecholamines as well as by increasing the release of these substances from adrenergic nerve terminals (4). Cocaine, therefore, blocks the reuptake of dopamine and norepinephrine in the central nervous system (CNS), which results in euphoria, garrulousness, restlessness, and increased motor activity (17). This mechanism appears to be involved in the physical and psychological dependence noted. Cocaine causes an increase in heat production by stimulating muscular activity and decreasing heat loss through vasoconstriction. This can lead to marked hyperpyrexia (17).

Several lines of evidence indicate that dopamine, but not norepinephrine, is critical in maintaining self-administration of cocaine. Dopamine receptor blockers, but not noradrenergic blockers, disrupt cocaine self-administration (15). Dopamine reuptake is decreased, and repeated use of cocaine leads to decreased concentrations of dopamine in the brain. Initially, this may produce such effects as decreased appetite, hyperactivity, and sexual excitement; with long-term use, impotence can occur. Cocaine also decreases the concentrations of serotonin and serotonin metabolites. The need for sleep may be reduced, since serotonin is thought to mediate the sleep–wake cycle.

FORMS OF ADMINISTRATION

Nasal Insufflation

Typically, cocaine is distributed as a white crystalline powder cut into grams or "spoons" (a spoon is considered approximately 0.5 g). One gram of cocaine may produce 30 to 40 lines (4). A common method of administration is intranasally (Table 51–2) (22). The cocaine is chopped with a razor blade into lines or columns on a

TABLE 51–1. *Populations in which plasma cholinesterase activity is decreased*

Acute infections
Chronically debilitated
Congenitally deficient individuals
Elderly individuals
Fetuses
Infants
Liver disease patients
Malnourished (any age)

TABLE 51–2. *Routes of administration of cocaine*

Nasal insufflation (snorting)
Smoking
Freebasing
Crack
Busuco
Oral
Body packing
Body stuffing
Intravenous

smooth surface such as a piece of glass, and a line is inhaled or snorted through a plastic straw or rolled up currency (4,11). This process is usually repeated with the other nostril. After insufflation approximately 60% of the drug is absorbed, and cocaine may be detected on the nasal mucosa for as long as 3 hours after application (17,23). Cocaine administered by insufflation limits its own absorption by causing vasoconstriction of the nasal mucosa, and the plasma drug concentration usually rises relatively slowly.

Free Basing

Cocaine hydrochloride is not suitable for smoking because heat causes it to decompose. Free base melts at 98°C and is heat stable, making it desirable for smoking. To be smoked, the cocaine hydrochloride must be made into a free base, which is then more heat stable (5). Free base, or cocaine alkaloid, is a colorless, odorless, transparent substance that is soluble in alcohol, acetone, ether, oils, and water (17). This free base is absorbed from all sites but primarily from the lungs (19).

Technique of free basing. Free basing, or "baseballing," is performed by one of two methods. The more dangerous method involves taking the hydrochloride salt of cocaine, mixing it with an alkaline solution such as ammonium chloride to convert it to a free base, and using ether as a solvent (17). Street cocaine is dissolved in water, and then a base with a pH higher than that of cocaine is added (24). Ether is then added to this mixture, and the cocaine alkaloid remains in the ether layer. After the ether evaporates, the substance remaining contains purified alkaloid crystals, which are more volatile than the cocaine salt (4,25). The less dangerous method does not involve ether and is used to manufacture "crack" (26).

Technically, free base differs from crack in the production process. Free base is prepared by using a potentially dangerous extraction process with a highly volatile vehicle, such as ether, which produces a relatively pure alkaloid. Crack is prepared in a safer manner with a water-extraction process, which results in a less pure alkaloid.

Properties of free base. The free base thus formed is more stable to heat and more pure because the process removes many of the cutting substances. This free base can then be smoked with a special pipe or sprinkled on a tobacco or marijuana cigarette (27). Compared with insufflation, free basing is extremely dangerous. When the hydrochloride salt is used intranasally, the local vasoconstrictor action on the nasal mucosa acts to limit absorption. Free base cocaine, when smoked, offers no such protection and actually simulates the immediate effect of intravenous administration, and the user may inadvertently overdose (4,22). In addition, the ether used as a solvent can be a fire hazard.

The highly vascularized lung surface facilitates immediate absorption of free base cocaine, and after smoking the onset and progression of effects occur almost immediately. The effect is an intense euphoric experience that is often followed within minutes by a dysphoric "crash," leading to frequently repeated doses and rapid addiction in the susceptible individual (22). Large doses of cocaine taken by this route have caused death within minutes.

"Crack"

Cocaine has glutted the street market over the last several years; and despite a government crusade against its use, it has never been more plentiful, cheaper, purer, or more widely used. Cocaine suppliers have had to resort to new marketing techniques and packaging to stay competitive in the industry. The use of free base has been linked to a shift in cocaine distribution patterns as dealers have switched from selling cocaine powder to free base cocaine in tiny chunks known as "rocks" or "crack" (1). Crack is designed for individuals who wish to try free base cocaine but are unwilling to free base it themselves because they either do not know how or are frightened to try (18).

Crack is extracted from cocaine powder in a procedure that uses sodium bicarbonate, heat, and water. This eliminates the need for chemicals and glassware. The process is simple and relatively safe compared with the more volatile method of processing cocaine powder into free base (26).

Free base cocaine is called "crack" because of the sound made by crystals popping when it is heated (1) and "rocks" because of its appearance. Dealers prefer to sell crack rather than cocaine powder because of crack's high addiction potential, low unit cost, and ease of handling (28). Crack is usually in the form of a light brown or beige pellet or a small chunk and is sold in clear plastic or amber vials. There are approximately 300 to 500 mg per vial. One vial usually provides two to three inhalations, and the effects may last approximately 20 minutes (17).

"Basuco"

Cocaine may also be smoked in the form of coca paste, which is also referred to as "pasta," "bazooka," or "basuco" (29,30). This is a crude extract of the coca leaf that is heated with sulfuric acid, precipitated with sodium carbonate, and then converted to cocaine sulfate.

Oral Administration

As mentioned above, there is a common misconception that cocaine is hydrolyzed in the gastrointestinal tract and rendered inactive. An oral dose of cocaine, however, is at least as effective as the same dose taken intranasally.

"Body Packing"

Because of increased surveillance by narcotics agents, individuals who smuggle drugs must devise schemes of surreptitiously bringing cocaine through customs. "Body packing" is one such scheme, in which extremely large amounts (3 to 6 g) of cocaine are ingested in condoms, toy balloons, or in the fingers of latex gloves with the expectation that these packets will be excreted 1 to 2 days after the smuggler's entry into the country (2,11,31,32). Some individuals take a substance such as diphenoxylate (Lomotil) before boarding the plane to slow gastrointestinal motility and prevent passage of the cocaine packets before landing. They then take a laxative once they reach their destination (28).

Many deaths are associated with body packing because leakage or rupture can occur in one or more of the packets (2,33). The rupture of even one packet can cause death because of the large dose of pure cocaine that is suddenly absorbed through the intestinal mucosa (11,31,34). Often, a roentgenogram will show evidence of these condoms, depending on the type of material used, as multiple oval soft tissue densities surrounding a gas halo (27). Enteric septicemia caused by fecal contamination of subsequently injected cocaine has been reported (35).

Intravenous Administration

The effects of intravenous administration are similar to those of smoking because both routes of administration demonstrate almost immediate effects (24). The intravenous injection sites of cocaine users are noted to have prominent ecchymoses, sometimes with a central area of pallor (36). Multiple ecchymotic areas are probably due to a direct cytotoxic reaction of cocaine coupled with the ischemic vascular injury secondary to vasoconstriction.

CUTTING SUBSTANCES AND CONTAMINANTS

Various cutting substances may be added to cocaine, some of which may greatly add to its toxicity (Table 51–3). Adulteration of cocaine makes it impossible for cocaine users to know how much cocaine they are taking (4). The user may only be getting 5% to 40% pure cocaine. Most of the active ingredients used as cutting substances for cocaine come from three major drug categories: xanthine alkaloids, local anesthetics, or decongestants. The use of cutting substances increases the dealer's profit; these particular substances are used because their stimulant effects mimic those of the pure drug to unsophisticated users.

TABLE 51–3. *Cocaine cutting substances*

Local anesthetics
Benzocaine
Lidocaine
Procaine
Stimulants
Caffeine
Amphetamines
Phencyclidine
Sugars
Inositol
Lactose
Sucrose
Miscellaneous
Benzene
Quinine

Local anesthetics may be added to simulate the expected anesthetic effect ("freeze") of the cocaine. Procaine is by far the most common local anesthetic cutting agent, followed by lidocaine, benzocaine, and tetracaine. Procaine is also the least toxic; lidocaine is about 2 to 3 times more toxic than procaine (4). Methidrine, an amphetamine, may be added because it is a cheap alternative to cocaine and has many of the same effects. Phencyclidine, caffeine, and quinine have also been used. The sugars lactose, sucrose, and inositol (an isomer of glucose) may be added as adulterants because they act as fillers and add weight to the cocaine (22). The disaccharide lactose, which is similar to sucrose, is most commonly used. Quinine is also used for cutting cocaine, just as it is for heroin.

In addition to these substances, the mixture may be contaminated with bacteria, fungi, or viruses.

TOXICITY

Clinical Features

The clinical picture of cocaine poisoning can easily be confused with that of amphetamine or phencyclidine poisoning. In most instances, the distinctive clinical feature of cocaine poisoning is the more rapid return of the patient to a normal physical state.

Cocaine overdose is more common than previously thought. Contrary to popular belief, users can overdose by any route of administration, including insufflation. Serious overdose may occur particularly in those with pseudocholinesterase deficiencies and in body packers, smokers, and intravenous users (37).

Onset and Duration of Symptoms

Cocaine reaction in the body is of a biphasic nature, with initial sympathetic stimulation followed by abrupt generalized CNS depression. In cases of acute toxicity, if death occurs it does so usually within 2 to 3 minutes, but sometimes there is a delay of up to 30 minutes. Deaths have been reported after smoking, insufflation, intravenous injection, and oral use (27,32,38). Nevertheless, cocaine use rarely leads to death.

The predominantly positive feelings that are experienced during the initial phase of cocaine intoxication are of short duration and are commonly followed by dysphoric feelings characterized by anxiety, depression, irritability, fatigue, and a craving for more cocaine.

Central Nervous System Effects

Systemically, cocaine stimulates the CNS from above downward. The first recognizable action is on the cortex, and is manifested by excitement, euphoria, garrulousness, and restlessness (Table 51–4) (4,12). These are some of the effects sought by the user. There may also be an increased capacity for muscular work. Nausea, vomiting, and abdominal pain often occur. Other signs and symptoms may include headache, chills, fever, mydriasis, and formication, which is the sensation of insects crawling under the skin (also called Magnan's sign) (12); these tactile hallucinations may lead to serious degrees of self-excoriation (11). Cocaine causes mydriasis indirectly by blocking the reuptake of norepinephrine. It usually does not cause cycloplegia.

Cocaine can produce a variety of neurologic problems, including seizures, stroke, headache, and transient symptoms such as visual impairment, tremor, dizziness, vertigo, tinnitus, blurred vision, and ataxia. The pathogenesis of most of the neurologic problems remains unknown. Possible etiologic mechanisms include cerebral vasospasm or thrombosis. There does not appear to be a clear correlation between the risk of these complications and the amount of drug used, how it was administered, or the prior use pattern of the patient.

TABLE 51–4. *Central nervous system symptoms of cocaine intoxication*

Ataxia
Excitement
Euphoria
Garrulousness
Headache
Tremors
Seizures
Fever
Hyperthermia
Mydriasis
Stroke
Subarachnoid hemorrhage
Intracerebral hemorrhage
Ischemic stroke
Brain abscess
Fungal cerebritis
Central retinal artery occlusion
Visual impairment
Blurred vision
Transient focal neurologic deficits
Toxic encephalopathy
Coma

Seizures

As the dose is increased, lower motor centers are stimulated, causing tremors and seizures. In general, seizures are generalized tonic-clonic in nature, although focal seizures have been reported (39). Although most seizures occur soon after taking cocaine, the interval between the last use of the drug and the onset of seizures can be several hours (40). Seizures and death have been associated with a wide range of plasma concentrations.

Seizures following cocaine use have long been associated with the drug and are most likely related to its local anesthetic effects (15). Lidocaine has effects on brain electrical activity similar to cocaine, anticonvulsant activity at low doses but potent convulsant effects at high doses (41). Seizures can be complicated by acidosis, which has been reported to potentiate the effects of catecholamines on the heart (42). This potentiation may lead to arrhythmias if the seizure is not properly controlled.

Headache

The pathophysiology of cocaine-induced headaches is probably multifactorial. Headache may be a manifestation of hypertension, in which case, the headache should resolve as blood pressure is lowered. Cocaine-induced migraine headache may result from inhibition of serotonin uptake.

Stroke

Stroke associated with cocaine use is a recently recognized phenomenon. Strokes of all types have been reported, including subarachnoid hemorrhage, intracerebral hemorrhage, and ischemic stroke located in all of the major vascular territories of the brain (39).

Cocaine-related stroke is a disease that occurs primarily in young individuals (19). It can occur in the first-time user as well as the chronic abuser and can follow any route of administration. The frequency of intracranial hemorrhage exceeds that of cerebral infarction and appears to often be associated with intracranial aneurysms and arteriovenous malformations.

So far, no evidence has emerged of a relationship between a route of administration of cocaine and the type of stroke (43). Stroke may follow cocaine use within seconds or as many as 12 hours later.

Although most of the patients have evidence of underlying cerebrovascular disease, such as rupture of preexisting unsuspected aneurysms or arteriovenous malformations under the influence of cocaine-induced hypertension, reports have failed to demonstrate underlying disease in some patients. Other mechanisms have been proposed for stroke associated with cocaine use including increased coagulability, impaired cerebrovascular autoregulation, vasospasm, embolism of particulate matter, and immunologically mediated arteritis or vasculitis.

Cerebral vasoconstriction or vasospasm, or both, may indirectly result from cocaine's stimulation of the sympathetic nervous system and resultant elevation of blood pressure. The activity of serotonin, a potent vasoconstrictor in the cerebral circulation, may be potentiated by cocaine, as cocaine centrally blocks the reuptake of this neurotransmitter (43).

Cardiovascular Effects

Abuse of the drug has been associated with numerous cardiovascular complications including aortic dissection, pulmonary edema, left ventricular dysfunction, dilated cardiomyopathy, myocarditis, pneumopericardium, endocarditis, sudden death, and myocardial infarction (Table 51–5).

Dysrhythmias associated with cocaine use include sinus tachycardia, ventricular premature contractions, ventricular tachycardia and fibrillation, and asystole.

Cocaine represents a potential hazard to individuals with underlying fixed coronary artery disease because it causes predictable increases in heart rate, systolic blood pressure, and myocardial oxygen demand. Angina pectoris and myocardial infarction apparently due to coronary artery constriction have also been reported in young, otherwise healthy individuals who used cocaine.

TABLE 51–5. *Cardiovascular symptoms of cocaine intoxication*

Endocarditis
Aortic dissection
Hypertension
Hypotension
Dysrhythmias
- Sinus tachycardia
- Atrial fibrillation
- Idioventricular rhythm
- Premature ventricular contractions
- Ventricular tachycardia
- Ventricular fibrillation

Chest pain
- Myocardial infarction
- Angina pectoris

Pulmonary edema
Cardiomyopathy
Myocarditis

One proposed mechanism for the cardiac effects of cocaine on these individuals is coronary vasospasm due to sympathetic potentiation or to a direct effect on the vascular smooth muscle. A term for the process, contraction band necrosis, is classically associated with an excessive amount of circulating catecholamines, which increases the local tissue concentration of norepinephrine. In addition, some of the contaminants of cocaine may have cardiovascular effects. The occurrence of an acute myocardial infarction in any young patient should raise the suspicion of coronary artery spasm related to cocaine use. A combination of factors may also lead to dysrhythmias, such as scarring in the conduction system and elevated catecholamine concentrations, both of which develop over the course of time.

In the past decade, many case reports have appeared linking cocaine use to various cardiovascular disorders. The association between cocaine use and cardiovascular disorders remains temporal in nature, as most of the information in the literature is in case-report form. The quantity of cocaine that must be taken and the length of time that it must be used before cardiovascular disorders appear have not been determined. In most cases, the patient is unable to give an accurate account of how much cocaine has been ingested or when symptoms began relative to the time of ingestion. In addition, cocaine sold on the street is alkalinized with a variety of excipients, making its purity highly variable.

Hypertension

The cardiovascular complications of cocaine use occur as a consequence of intense sympathetic neural stimulation and inhibition of sodium conductance in excitable neural and cardiovascular tissues (local anesthetic effect). Sympathetic neural stimulation results in hypertension and tachycardia. The hypertension appears to be a consequence of both increased cardiac output and increased vascular resistance. Hypertension may result in intracranial and subarachnoid hemorrhage, acute aortic dissection with or without rupture, and acute pulmonary edema. The latter is likely not only a consequence of increased afterload but may also be contributed to by an increase in pulmonary endothelial permeability.

Arrhythmias

Arrhythmias are common during cocaine intoxication and may be the consequence of sympathetic stimulation, myocardial ischemia, or myocarditis. Sympathetic stimulation as a cause of arrhythmias is to be expected in the early phase of intoxication when there is clinical evidence of other pharmacologic actions of cocaine. Myocardial ischemia and myocarditis tend to manifest later in the course of intoxication, after cocaine has already been eliminated from the body.

Low-dose cocaine may result in bradycardias either because of central vagal stimulation or as a reflex response to the hypertension, whereas higher doses have been associated with virtually all other arrhythmias. Sinus tachycardia, atrial fibrillation, ventricular extrasystoles, accelerated idioventricular rhythms, and ventricular tachycardia and fibrillation may follow exposure to cocaine and be related directly to increased catecholamine levels from effects on the central and peripheral sympathetic nervous systems.

The most common arrhythmia during cocaine intoxication is sinus tachycardia. Of note is that the electrocardiogram (EKG) during cocaine intoxication occasionally shows wide complex tachycardia, which may represent sinus tachycardia with impaired cardiac conduction due to the local anesthetic effects of cocaine. Ventricular fibrillation is presumably the cause of many of the sudden deaths in cocaine users (44).

Myocardial Infarction

The first report of myocardial infarction temporally related to the recreational use of cocaine appeared in 1982 (45). Since then, myocardial infarction has become recognized as the most common cardiovascular consequence of cocaine use. Although at present it has not been conclusively shown that the cocaine itself rather than any adulterant is the agent responsible for the induction of ischemia, both circumstantial and experimental evidence are mounting (46).

As the cocaine epidemic continues, many cocaine abusers are presenting to emergency departments (EDs) complaining of chest pain after cocaine use. Patients who complain of chest pain and have EKG evidence of myocardial injury or ischemia are easily identified (47). Of greater concern are patients who complain of chest pain after cocaine use and have a normal or nondiagnostic EKG. In these cases, the physician must decide whether to admit all patients with this complaint to determine whether myocardial infarction has occurred or to discharge patients with potential myocardial necrosis despite a normal or nondiagnostic EKG (48).

Demographics of Patient with Chest Pain

The typical patient is a young male smoker with a history of chronic cocaine abuse. Not infrequently, the patient has a history of prior episodes of chest pain, particularly following cocaine use. Myocardial infarction most commonly occurs soon after the use of cocaine, though it has also been reported during the period of withdrawal (47). The infarct is slightly more likely to occur in the anterior distribution and may be either Q wave or non-Q-wave in nature (46). Cocaine-induced myocardial infarctions have been documented in patients with normal, as well as abnormal, electrocardiograms (49).

There is no correlation between route of administration and incidence of myocardial infarction or ischemia; however, the majority of patients reported that they had used cocaine intranasally. In addition, there appears to be no correlation between habitual cocaine use and myocardial infarction or ischemia (50). The time of onset for infarction or ischemia has been variable, ranging from shortly after cocaine use to several hours later (48).

Proposed Mechanisms for Myocardial Infarction

Coronary artery spasm, in situ thrombus formation and platelet aggregation, direct myocardial toxicity, accelerated atherosclerosis, nonatherosclerotic intimal proliferation, and an increase in the myocardial oxygen demand have all been proposed as the mechanism of cocaine-induced myocardial infarction (Table 51–6) (51,52).

The analysis supports the view that a combination of these mechanisms may be active in any one patient and that the mechanism responsible for the development of ischemia in any individual patient may be somewhat dependent on whether the patient is a chronic abuser of cocaine, a smoker, or has underlying atherosclerotic heart disease (49).

A pathologic finding that has been cited to support the role of spasm in cocaine-related infarction is increased foci of contraction band necrosis in cases of cocaine-related deaths studied at necropsy (53). This finding is also consistent with the concept that myocardial damage resulting from cocaine abuse may be the result of cocaine-induced catecholamine excess, since contraction bands have been previously observed in association with pheochromocytoma and exogenous catecholamine administration. Contraction band necrosis is pathologically defined by the hypercontracted sarcomere and myofibrillar disruption (51). Myocyte necrosis occurs, and this tissue is ultimately replaced by fibrous tissue (54).

Another proposed mechanism is the following: Intranasal cocaine induces recurrent coronary vasoconstriction. The initial vasoconstriction, noted 30 minutes after drug administration, is temporally related to the peak blood concentration of cocaine (53). As the blood

TABLE 51–6. *Proposed mechanisms for myocardial infarction associated with cocaine use*

Coronary artery spasm
In situ thrombus formation
Direct myocardial toxicity
Accelerated atherosclerosis
Nonatherosclerotic intimal proliferation
Increased oxygen demand
Contraction band necrosis

concentration of cocaine declines, this vasoconstriction is alleviated. At 90 minutes after drug administration, however, coronary vasoconstriction recurs and is temporally related to increased blood concentration of cocaine's principal metabolites, benzoylecgonine and ethyl methyl ecgonine. It is thought by some that angina pectoris and myocardial infarction occurring hours after cocaine inhalation may be due to the coronary vasoconstrictive influence of cocaine's metabolites (54).

Regardless of the mechanism, there does not appear to be a relation between underlying heart disease and the risk of cocaine-related cardiac disorders. In addition, the cardiac events can occur regardless of the route of administration (15).

Organ Ischemia

Ischemic complications of cocaine, including myocardial infarction, renal infarction, intestinal infarction, and limb ischemia, a consequence of intense constriction of large arteries, have been well described in cocaine users (Table 51–7).

Renal and intestinal infarction may present with severe flank pain or diffuse abdominal pain. Intestinal infarction requires prompt diagnosis and surgical treatment, because without such treatment the mortality is likely to be substantial.

Pulmonary

The use of free base or crack cocaine has led to many reports of pulmonary complications. Pneumomediastinum and pneumothorax have been reported in patients who snort or smoke cocaine. These are probably caused by transiently increased airway pressure due to a forced Valsalva maneuver or coughing, which results in rupture of an alveolar bleb. Once the marginal alveolus ruptures, proximal dissection of air occurs along perivascular tissue planes. Once within the mediastinum, collections of air may outline mediastinal structures, including the aorta, trachea, vena cava, diaphragm, and occasionally the heart (Figure 51–1) (55).

A variety of symptoms have been reported by patients with pneumomediastinum after abusing cocaine. Patients with pneumomediastinum often experience the sudden onset of sharp, pleuritic chest pain; auscultation over the chest may reveal a crunching sound. Hamman's sign, or "crunch," is a crunching sound accentuated with systolic activity of the heart. Although this sign was considered pathognomonic of pneumomediastinum, an identical sound can be detected with patients with a pneumothorax (15). A pneumothorax can cause this crunching sound if air dissects centrally to a position adjacent to the heart (55).

Patients may smoke cocaine and note the immediate onset of chest pain, or pain may occur several hours later. The pain associated with pneumomediastinum is usually worse upon lying down and is somewhat alleviated by sitting forward. The chest roentgenogram is usually diagnostic, showing air surrounding the cardiac silhouette (19).

The possibility of a direct effect of cocaine on the pulmonary vasculature has not been evaluated thoroughly. This is extremely important in view of the highly concentrated heated cocaine alkaloid that is used frequently today and is delivered directly into the pulmonary circulation.

TABLE 51–7. *Miscellaneous effects of cocaine*

Organ infarction
Myocardial
Renal
Intestinal
Limb
Rhabdomyolysis
Myonecrosis
Acute tubular necrosis

Obstetric

Maternal cocaine use has recently been recognized as an increasing problem for the successful continuation of pregnancy as well as for subsequent fetal growth and development (56).

Infants born to cocaine-using mothers are at a higher risk for intrauterine growth retardation, lower birth weight, smaller head circumference, decreased length, lower Apgar scores, and neurobehavioral impairment than are infants of noncocaine–using mothers (Table 51–8) (57). Congenital malformations, including cardiac anomalies, skull defects, and genitourinary tract malformations have also been reported (58).

Women who use cocaine during pregnancy are at an increased risk for abruptio placentae, spontaneous abortion, and preterm labor and delivery (59). The increased incidence of spontaneous abortions and abruptio placentae with cocaine use appears to relate directly to placental vasoconstriction, which decreases placental vascular supply and increases uterine contractility. These factors, in addition to the marked hypertension associated with cocaine use, may precipitate abruptio placentae (57).

Cocaine exposure of the infant may continue after birth through breast milk.

Rhabdomyolysis

Numerous reports of cocaine-related rhabdomyolysis have demonstrated the association with massive creatine kinase levels, acute renal failure, profound hypotension,

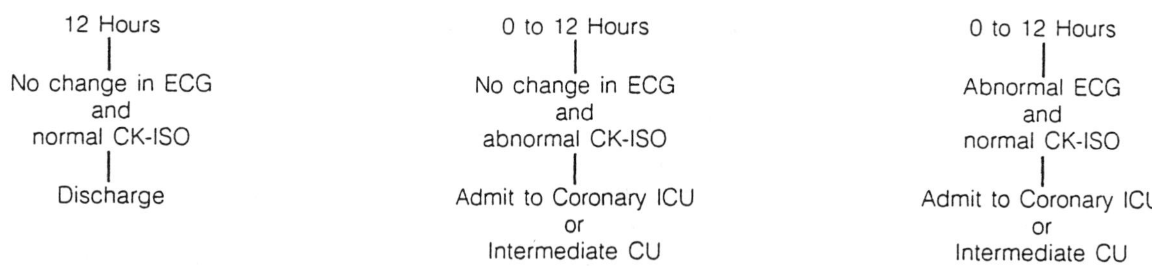

FIG. 51–1. Algorithm for disposition of patients based on ECG and creatine kinase (CK) and creatine kinase isoenzyme (CK-ISO) values. Reprinted with permission from *Ann Emerg Med* 1990;19:10.

and hyperthermia (60). A seizure, hypothermia, hypotension, or prolonged unconsciousness, however, was not necessary for the production of rhabdomyolysis, which suggests that cocaine may act as a direct muscle toxin (61,62). It has been postulated that rapid delivery of cocaine to the skeletal muscle vasculature leads to arterial vasoconstriction, tissue ischemia, and rhabdomyolysis (63).

Patients with rhabdomyolysis generally experience myalgias, including that of chest muscles, simulating acute myocardial infarction, and have elevated serum levels of creatine phosphokinase (CPK), creatinine, potassium, and uric acid (64). Myoglobinuria is detected by a positive reaction for heme on the urine dipstick in the absence of red cells microscopically (64).

COCAINE AND DEPENDENCE

Current data from animal studies suggest that cocaine may be more harmful than heroin because it is a powerful reinforcing drug (65). Self-administration leading to death has been noted in primates. In one study of laboratory animals, cocaine self-administration was accompanied by a substantially higher incidence of mortality than was heroin self-administration in a 30-day period (66,67). The number of fatalities occurring after unlimited access to cocaine was more than twice that after unlimited access to heroin. The mortality rate for 30 days of continuous testing was 36% for the heroin group and 90% for the cocaine group (66). The attempt to recapture the positive feelings and to relieve the abstinence syndrome appears to be an important factor underlying compulsive cocaine use (67).

TABLE 51–8. *Obstetrical problems associated with cocaine*

Congenital abnormalities
Skull defects
Cardiac abnormalities
Genitourinary tract malformations
Miscellaneous abnormalities
Intrauterine growth retardation
Lower birth weight
Small head circumference
Decreased Apgar score
Neurobehavioral impairment
Maternal problems
Abruptio placentae
Spontaneous abortion
Preterm labor

EFFECTS OF CHRONIC USE

In chronic users, septal atrophy, perforation, and ulcerations secondary to intense and repeated vasoconstriction may occur, although these are rare. In addition, reactive hyperemia leading to boggy nasal mucosa and a chronic stuffy nose or "cold" may develop. Atrophy of the nasal mucosa has been reported (12). These effects may lead individuals to abuse nasal sprays, which cause temporary vasoconstriction but have the same rebound phenomenon as cocaine.

DIFFERENTIAL DIAGNOSIS

Other drugs that may produce effects similar include amphetamines, phencyclidine, and anticholinergic agents.

Amphetamines produce identical physical and psychiatric effects but have no local anesthetic properties; because of their longer half-life, amphetamines may produce intoxicaton lasting several hours. Phencyclidine also produces sympathomimetic effects, but patients usually have normal or small pupil size, multidirectional nystagmus, and waxing and waning encephalopathy. Anticholinergic drugs and poisons often produce tachycardia, hyperpyrexia, agitated confusional state, and dilated pupils, but the skin is usually dry and flushed.

LABORATORY ANALYSIS

Patients suspected of cocaine use may undergo a toxicologic screen to confirm the presence of cocaine or its principal metabolite in the urine. Because of the usual acute nature of the overdose and the short half-life of the drug in the body, quantitative laboratory determinations of serum concentrations have no value in assessing the clinical state of the patient. Semiquantitative and qualitative immunoassays are available for detecting the inactive metabolite benzoylecgonine in the urine; such assays may be positive more than 24 hours after cocaine use (1,12,17). After a single nasal application of cocaine, metabolites may be detected in the urine within 4 hours and for as long as 27 hours.

None of the routine biochemical tests correlate with the clinical severity of cocaine intoxication. Electrocardiograms may be useful in assessing and monitoring cardiac abnormalities, and a chest roentgenogram may help rule out pulmonary edema.

Patients admitted with chest pain after using cocaine should be completely and expediently evaluated to exclude myocardial ischemia and infarction. All patients with serious intoxication should have frequent monitoring of the EKG, electrolytes, serum CPK, and urine myoglobin. A proposed algorithm for patients with chest pain is found in Figure 51–2 (48).

Radiographs of the abdomen may reveal swallowed radiopaque packets or drug-filled condoms in the gastrointestinal tract (GIT). These are not always radiopaque, so a negative roentgenogram does not guarantee their absence. Computed tomography (CT) scans of the head should be performed in any patient with severe headache, coma, or focal neurologic deficits.

All patients with abnormalities on neurologic examination require at a minimum consultation with a neurologist, and in any patient who presents with a stroke-like syndrome, complete evaluation with a cranial CT scan, lumbar puncture, cerebral angiography, and echocardiography should be considered.

TREATMENT

The treatment of acute reactions to cocaine is generally unnecessary because the reactions usually run their course before the patient arrives at the emergency department. For example, a patient undergoing a seizure due to cocaine will not usually have a second seizure or need seizure prophylaxis. Seizures caused by cocaine are usually brief and self-limited. Sustained or repeated seizures suggest hyperthermia, intracranial hemorrhage, metabolic abnormality, or massive intake as in the case of cocaine "body packers" (63). Generally, when treatment is necessary for cocaine overdose it consists of symptomatic and supportive care (Table 51–9). As usual, ingestion of an unknown substance requires the administration of glucose, thiamine, naloxone, and oxygen. If seizures occur, diazepam or a short-acting barbiturate can be administered (4). Paranoia can be treated with haloperidol. Lidocaine may be used for ventricular irritability unless the patient is having seizures (3,4). Gastrointestinal decontamination should be performed if the patient has ingested cocaine (68). Because of the potential for abrupt onset of seizures, ipecac-induced emesis is contraindicated.

TABLE 51–9. *Treatment of cocaine overdose*

Indication	Treatment
Agitation	Physical restraints Pharmacological Butyrophenones Benzodiazepines
Hypotension	Fluid therapy Vasoconstrictors
Seizures	Diazepam
Hypertension	Labetalol Nifedipine Nitroprusside
Hyperthermia	External cooling
Ventricular dysrhythmia	Lidocaine Sodium bicarbonate
Body packing	Surgical removal

Agitation

For agitated patients, physical restraints are necessary long enough to ensure that adequate pharmacologic sedation has taken effect. Either a benzodiazepine or haloperidol can be effective.

Ideally, if a restraining blanket is used, it should be constructed as a strong netting or mesh to avoid increasing the patient's temperature by preventing heat dissipation.

Hypotension

Hypotension from cocaine should be treated with fluid therapy and vasoconstrictors as necessary. The doses of pressor drugs should be low and titrated upward carefully, because the presence of cocaine may markedly enhance the potency of catecholamines.

Seizures

Agitation and seizures are managed in the standard manner with a focus on rapid control of motor activity while protecting the patient's airway and achieving adequate ventilation and oxygenation. Seizure management is vital, and intravenous diazepam remains the drug of choice of most clinicians. Seizures resistant to benzodiazepine therapy followed by loading doses of phenobarbital or phenytoin may require endotracheal intubation, neuromuscular blockade, and general anesthesia (15).

Hypertension

β-Adrenergic blocking drugs such as propranolol are rarely needed for hypertension, tachycardias, and dysrhythmias that are hemodynamically significant or for many of the minor symptoms associated with cocaine overdose. Propranolol may result in unopposed α-adrenergic-mediated vasoconstriction, possibly worsening hypertension. For this reason, labetalol, a combined α and β blocker, has been advocated for hypertension rather than the traditional blocker propranolol (69,70). Hypertensive crisis may also be treated with a short-acting antihypertensive preparation such as sublingual nifedipine or intravenous nitroprusside. Hypertension unresponsive to sedation should be managed with sodium nitroprusside (0.5 to 10 μg/kg/min) in a titrated fashion to achieve and maintain a normal blood pressure.

Phentolamine is also an effective vasodilator at doses of 5 to 10 mg IV and may improve perfusion. Phentolamine, however, has nonselective α-adrenergic properties that may intensify the reflex sympathetic stimulation of the heart; therefore, phentolamine should be used only in conjunction with a nonselective β blocker.

Calcium channel modulators may be an alternative to β blockers in treating hypertension cases of cocaine toxicity. Mechanistically, blocking the release of calcium in the smooth muscle of the vasculature counteracts the vasoconstrictive effects of norepinephrine.

Hyperthermia

Active external cooling maneuvers are suggested for hyperpyrexia, and core temperatures should be continuously monitored. Control of hyperthermia is best achieved by rapid cooling with an ice and water bath and a fan. Conduction and evaporation prove rapidly efficacious. For severe hyperthermia, it may be necessary to stop heat generation from muscles by neuromuscular paralysis as well as external cooling. This can be done with pancuronium (4).

Cardiac Arrhythmias

Tachyarrhythmias of atrial origin that have not responded to control of the central sympathetic agent should respond to labetalol, or verapamil. Use of these agents in a previously sedated individual limits both the risks of unmasking α-adrenergic effects and the theoretical concerns associated with the risks of seizures when calcium channel blockers are given.

Lidocaine may not be the agent of choice for the treatment of ventricular arrhythmias that develop immediately after cocaine use such as in an individual with a ruptured bag of cocaine in the GIT. These ventricular arrhythmias should be presumed to occur from catecholamine excess or from cocaine's direct effect on the myocardium. Because this latter effect may be due to cocaine's type I antiarrhythmic properties, the addition of a similar agent may exacerbate cardiac conduction abnormalities.

Recent evidence suggests that cocaine-induced, wide-complex arrhythmias may respond to administration of sodium bicarbonate, similar to arrhythmias produced during intoxication with type IA and type IC antiarrhythmics (45).

Myocardial Ischemia

Any patient, regardless of age, who is complaining of anginal-type symptoms temporally related to the use of cocaine should have an intravenous line in place, have continuous cardiac monitoring, and be admitted to a monitored area to rule out the possibility of an acute myocardial infarction. Once myocardial ischemia or infarction is suspected, these atypically young patients should be considered in the same manner as anyone else who is presumed to be at risk for coronary artery disease.

The use of thrombolytics in intravenous drug abusers is not well established, yet thrombolytic therapy probably has a role in the early management of cocaine-induced myocardial infarction (19). It should be noted though that the increased incidence of mycotic aneurysms and mass lesions may lead to a higher than normal incidence of hemorrhagic complications. At the present time, in the absence of a conventional contraindication to thrombolysis, it appears that patients with a cocaine-induced myocardial infarction should be considered as candidates for this therapy.

Body Packers

Body packing merits serious consideration of surgical removal of the cocaine packages (2). Some investigators have suggested a conservative approach of observation without surgery. If signs of toxicity are present, however, emergency surgery may be lifesaving after pharmacologic intervention. The longer these packages remain in the gastrointestinal tract, the greater the possibility of cocaine leakage. Endoscopic removal of the packages has caused their rupture (2), so surgery rather than endoscopy is recommended for removal of all intact packages (4). Syrup of ipecac-induced emesis has resulted in the successful removal of recently ingested drug packets. In patients who are not body packers but who have recently ingested drug packets to avoid police detection, emesis induced by syrup of ipecac has been successful in expelling the packets because they are still in the stomach.

For patients who have ingested cocaine-containing packets, balloons, or vials, cocaine release and toxicity may be delayed. Because these containers may carry huge doses of cocaine, careful observation is mandatory until the material has passed rectally. Repeated doses of activated charcoal and the use of whole bowel irrigation with an isosmotic bowel preparation solution such as

Golytely or Colyte, 1 to 2 L per hour orally or by nasogastric tube until the material has passed has been advocated. Radiographic contrast studies such as an upper GI series with small bowel follow-through may be required to outline suspected retained packets.

REFERENCES

1. Cregler L, Mark H: Medical complications of cocaine abuse. *N Engl J Med* 1986;315:1495–1500.
2. Suarez C, Arrango A, Lester L: Cocaine-condom ingestion: surgical treatment. *JAMA* 1977;238:1391–1392.
3. Dipalma J: Cocaine abuse and toxicity. *Am Fam Physician* 1981; 24:236–238.
4. Dargon D: Cocaine. *Top Emerg Med* 1985;7;1–8.
5. Resnick R, Resnick E: Cocaine abuse and its treatment. *Psychiatr Clin North Am* 1984;7:713–728.
6. Cohen S: Cocaine. *JAMA* 1975:231:74–75.
7. Cohen S: Amphetamine abuse. *JAMA* 1975; 231:414–415.
8. Gay G: You've come a long way, baby! Coke time for the new American lady of the eighties. *J Psychoactive Drugs* 1981;13:297–318.
9. Gay G, Inaba D, Rappolt R, et al: "An' ho, ho, baby, take a whiff on me": la dama blanca cocaine in current perspective. *Anaesth Analg* 1976;55:582–587.
10. Van Dyke C, Byck R: Cocaine. *Sci Am* 1982; 246:128–141.
11. Fairbanks D, Fairbanks G: *Ann Plast Surg* 1983;10:452–457.
12. Gay G: Clinical management of acute and chronic cocaine poisoning. Ann Emerg Med 1982;11:562–572.
13. Derlet R, Tseng J, Albertson T: Potention of cocaine and *d*-amphetamine toxicity with cocaine. *Am J Emerg Med* 1992;10:211–216.
14. Isenberg S, Spierer A, Inkelis S: Ocular signs of cocaine intoxication in neonates. *Am J Ophthalmol* 1987;103:211–214.
15. Mueller P, Benowitz N, Olson K: Cocaine. *Emerg Med Clin North Am* 1990;8:481–493.
16. Gay G, Inaba D, Sheppard C, et al: Cocaine: history, epidemiology, human pharmacology, and treatment: a perspective on a new debut for an old girl. *Clin Toxicol* 1975;8:149–178.
17. Cregler L, Mark H: Relation of acute myocardial infarction to cocaine abuse. *Am J Cardiol* 1985;56:794.
18. Merigan K, Roberts J: Cocaine intoxication: hyperpyrexia, rhabdomyolysis and acute renal failure. *Clin Toxicol* 1987;25:135–148.
19. VanDette J, Cornish L: Medical complications of illicit cocaine use. *Clin Pharm* 1989;8:410–411.
20. Hoffman R, Henry G, Howland M, et al: Association between life-threatening cocaine toxicity and plasma cholinesterase activity. *Ann Emerg Med* 1991;21:247–253.
21. Rich J, Singer D: Cocaine-related symptoms in patients presenting to an urban emergency department. *Ann Emerg Med* 1991;20:616–621.
22. Perez-Reyes M, DiGuiseppi S, Ondrusek G, et al: Free-base cocaine smoking. *Clin Pharmacol Ther* 1982;32:459–465.
23. Mathias D: Cocaine-associated myocardial ischemia. *Am J Med* 1986;81:67–78.
24. Derlet R, Albertson T: Emergency department presentation of cocaine intoxication. *Ann Emerg Med* 1989;18:182–186.
25. Shesser R, Davis C, Edelstein S: Pneumomediastinum and pneumothorax after inhaling alkaloidal cocaine. *Ann Emerg Med* 1981;10:213–315.
26. Snyderman C, Weissmann J, Tabor E, et al: Crack cocaine burns of the larynx. *Arch Otolaryngol Head Neck Surg* 1991;117:792–795.
27. Allred R, Ewer S: Fatal pulmonary edema after intravenous "freebase" cocaine use. *Ann Emerg Med* 1981;10:441–442.
28. Pollack C, Biggers D, Carlton F, et al: Two crack cocaine body stuffers. *Ann Emerg Med* 1992;21:1370–1380.
29. Siegel R: Cocaine hallucinations. *Am J Psychiatry* 1978; 135:309–314.
30. Siegel R: Treatment of cocaine abuse: historical and contemporary perspectives. *J Psychoactive Drugs* 1985;17:1–9.
31. McCarron M, Wood J: The cocaine "body packer" syndrome: diagnosis and treatment. *JAMA* 1983;250:1417–1420.
32. Wetli C, Wright R: Death caused by recreational cocaine use. *JAMA* 1979;241:2519–2522.
33. Bettinger J: Cocaine intoxication: massive oral overdose. *Ann Emerg Med* 1980;9:429–430.
34. Aks S, VanderHoek T, Hryhorczuk D, et al: Cocaine liberation from body packets in an in vitro model. *Ann Emerg Med* 1992; 21:1321–1325.
35. Marc B, Baud F, Maison-Blanche P, et al: Cardiac monitoring during medical management of cocaine body packers. *J Toxicol Clin Toxicol* 1992;30:387–397.
36. Mittleman R, Wetli C: Death caused by recreational cocaine use. *JAMA* 1984;252:1889–1893.
37. Drake T, Henry T, Marx J, et al: Severe acid-base abnormalities associated with cocaine abuse. *J Emerg Med* 1990;8:331–334.
38. Lundberg G, Garriott J, Reynolds P, et al: Cocaine related death. *J Forensic Sci* 1977;22:402–408.
39. Spivey W, Euele B: Neurologic complications of cocaine abuse. *Ann Emerg Med* 1990;19:1422–1428.
40. Tseng C, Derlet R, Albertson T: Cocaine-induced respiratory depression and seizures are synergistic mechanisms of cocaine-induced death in rats. *Ann Emerg Med* 1992;21:486–493.
41. Holland R, Marx J, Earnest M, et al: Grand mal seizures temporally related to cocaine use: clinical and diagnostic features. *Ann Emerg Med* 1992;21:772–776.
42. Ernst AA Sanders WM: Unexpected cocaine intoxication presenting as seizures in children. *Ann Emerg Med* 1989;18:774–777.
43. Rowbotham M, Lowenstein D: Neurologic consequences of cocaine use. *Ann Rev Med* 1990;41:417–422.
44. Nademanee K, Gorlick D, Josephson M, et al: Myocardial ischemia during cocaine withdrawal. *Ann Intern Med* 1989;111:876–880.
45. Goldfrank L, Hoffman R: The cardiovascular effects of cocaine. *Ann Emerg Med* 1991;20:165–175.
46. Lange R, Cigarroa R, Yancy C, et al: Cocaine-induced coronary-artery vasoconstriction. *N Engl J Med* 1989;321:1557–1562.
47. Brogan W, Lange R, Glamann B, et al: Recurrent coronary vasoconstriction caused by intranasal cocaine: possible role for metabolites. *Ann Intern Med* 1992;116:556–561.
48. Tokarski G, Paganussi P, Urbanski R, et al: An evaluation of cocaine-induced chest pain. *Ann Emerg Med* 1990:19:1088–1092.
49. Hollander J, Hoffman R: Cocaine-induced myocardial infarction: an analysis and review of the literature. *J Emerg Med* 1992;10:169–177.
50. Minor R, Scott B, Brown D, et al: Cocaine-induced myocardial infarction in patients with normal coronary arteries. *Ann Intern Med* 1991;115:797–806.
51. Smith H, Liberman H, Brody S, et al: Acute myocardial infarction temporally related to cocaine use. *Ann Intern Med* 1987;107:13–18.
52. Isner J, Chokshi S: Cocaine and vasospasm. *N Engl J Med* 1989; 321:1604–1606.
53. Zimmerman J, Dellinger R, Majid P: Cocaine-associated chest pain. *Ann Emerg Med* 1991;20:611–615.
54. Gitter M, Goldsmith S, Dunbar D, et al: Cocaine and chest pain: clinical features and outcome of patients hospitalized to rule out myocardial infarction. *Ann Intern Med* 1991;115:277–282.
55. Brody S, Anderson G, Gutman J: Pneumomediastinum as a complication of "crack" smoking. *Am J Emerg Med* 1988:241–243.
56. Ellis J, Byrd L, Sexson W, et al: In utero exposure to cocaine: a review. *South Med J* 1993;86:725–731.
57. Volpe J: Effect of cocaine use on the fetus. *N Engl J Med* 1992;327:399–407.
58. Kain Z, Kain T, Scarpelli E: Cocaine exposure in utero: perinatal development and neonatal manifestations—review. *J Toxicol Clin Toxicol* 1992;30:607–636.
59. Bates C: Medical risks of cocaine use. *West J Med* 1988; 148:440–444.
60. Lombard J, Wong B, Young J: Acute renal failure due to rhabdomyolysis associated with cocaine toxicity. *West J Med* 1988; 148:466–468.
61. Singhal P, Rubin R, Peters A, et al: Rhabdomyolysis and acute renal failure associated with cocaine abuse. *J Toxicol Clin Toxicol* 1990;28:321–330.
62. Roth D, Alarcon F, Fernandez J, et al: Acute rhabdomyolysis associated with cocaine intoxication. *N Engl J Med* 1988;319:673–677.
63. Fritsma G, Leikin J, Maturen A, et al: Detection of anticardiolipin antibody in patients with cocaine abuse. *J Emerg Med* 1991;9: 37–43.
64. Brody S, Wrenn K, Wilber M, et al: Predicting the severity of

cocaine-associated rhabdomyolysis. *Ann Emerg Med* 1990;19: 1137–1143.
65. Gawin F: Cocaine dependence. *Ann Rev Med* 1989;40:149–161.
66. Bozarth M, Wise R: Toxicity associated with longterm intravenous heroin and cocaine self-administration in the rat. *JAMA* 1985; 254:81–83.
67. Pollin W: The danger of cocaine. *JAMA* 1985;254:98.
68. Tomaszewski C, Voorhees S, Wathen J, et al: Cocaine adsorption to activated charcoal in vitro. *J Emerg Med* 1992;10:59–62.
69. Sand I, Brody S, Wrenn K, et al: Experience with esmolol for the treatment of cocaine-associated cardiovascular complications. *Am J Emerg Med* 1991;9:161–163.
70. Gay G, Loper K: The use of labetalol in the management of cocaine crisis. *Ann Emerg Med* 1988;17:282–283.

ADDITIONAL SELECTED REFERENCES

Alsott R, Miller A, Forney R: Report of a human fatality due to caffeine. *J Forensic Sci* 1973;18:135–137.

Anderson R, Reed W, Hillis L, et al: History, epidemiology, and medical complications of nasal inhaler abuse. *J Toxicol Clin Toxicol* 1982; 19:95–107.

Baldessarini R: Symposium on behavior modification by drugs: pharmacology of the amphetamines. *Pediatrics* 1972;49:694–701.

Becker A, Simons K, Gillespie C, et al: The bronchodilator effects and pharmacokinetics of caffeine in asthma. *N Engl J Med* 1984;310: 743–746.

Benchimol A, Bartall H, Desser K: Accelerated ventricular rhythm and cocaine abuse. *Ann Intern Med* 1978;88:519–520.

Bennett W: Hazards of the appetite suppressant phenylpropanolamine. *Lancet* 1979;2:42–43.

Blum A: Phenylpropanolamine: an over-the-counter amphetamine?, editorial. *JAMA* 1981;245:1346–1347.

Caruana D, Weinbach B, Goerg D, et al: Cocaine-packet ingestion. *Ann Intern Med* 1984;100:73–74.

Chambers H, Morris L, Tauber M, et al: Cocaine use and the risk for endocarditis in intravenous drug users. *Ann Intern Med* 1987:106:833–836.

Curatolo P, Robertson D: The health consequences of caffeine. *Ann Intern Med* 1983;98:641–653.

Duffy W, Senekjian H, Knight T, et al: Acute renal failure due to phenylpropanolamine. *South Med J* 1981;74:1548.

Edison G: Amphetamines: a dangerous illusion. *Ann Intern Med* 1971;74:605–610.

Egan D, Robinson D: Cocaine: recreational drug of choice? *Rocky Mt Med J* 1978;75:34–36.

Eisele J, Reay D: Deaths related to coffee enemas. *JAMA* 1980;244: 1608–1609.

Escobar J, Karno M: Chronic hallucinosis from nasal drops. *JAMA* 1982;247:1859–1862.

Fishbain D, Wetli C: Cocaine intoxication, delirium, and death in a body packer. *Ann Emerg Med* 1981;10:531–532.

Foley R, Kapatkin K. Verani R, et al: Amphetamine induced acute renal failure. *South Med J* 1984;77:258–259.

Gary N, Saidi P: Methamphetamine intoxication. *Am J Med* 1977; 64:537–540.

Haddad L: 1978: Cocaine in perspective. *JACEP* 1979;8.374–376.

Harrington H, Heller A, Kawson D, et al: Intracerebral hemorrhage and oral amphetamine. *Arch Neurol* 1983;40:503–507.

Insley B, Grufferman S, Ayliffe E: Thallium poisoning in cocaine abusers. *Am J Emerg Med* 1986;4:545–548.

Jekel J, Podlewski H, Dean-Patterson S, et al: Epidemic free-base cocaine abuse. *Lancet* 1986;1:459–462.

Josephson G, Stine R: Caffeine intoxication: a case of paroxysmal atrial tachycardia. *JACEP* 1976;5:776–778.

Koff R, Widrich W, Robbins A: Necrotizing angiitis in a methamphetamine user with hepatitis B: angiographic diagnosis, five-month follow-up results and localization of bleeding site. *N Engl J Med* 1973; 288:946–947.

Leikin J, Zell M, Hyrhorczuk K: PCP or cocaine intoxication. *Ann Emerg Med* 1987;16:235–236.

Madden J, Payne T, Miller S: Maternal cocaine abuse and effect on the newborn. *Pediatrics* 1986;77:209–211.

May D, Long R, Madden R, et al: Caffeine toxicity secondary to street drug ingestion. *Ann Emerg Med* 1981;10: 549.

Patel R, Dutta D, Schonfeld S: Free-base cocaine use associated with bronchiolitis obliterans organizing pneumonia. *Ann Intern Med* 1987;107:186–188.

Perry D: Heroin and cocaine adulteration, editorial. *Clin Toxicol* 1975;8:239–243.

Post R, Kopanda R: Cocaine, kindling, and psychosis. *Am J Psychiatry* 1976;133:627–640.

Rumack B: Phenylpropanolamine: a potentially hazardous drug, editorial. *Ann Emerg Med* 1982;11:332.

Schatzman M, Sabbadini A, Forti L: Coca and cocaine: a bibliography. *J Psychedelic Drugs* 1976;8:95–128.

Schenck N: The case for cocaine. *Res Staff Physician* 1975;21:67–69.

Scott M, Mullaly R: Lithium therapy for cocaine-induced psychosis: a clinical perspective. *South Med J* 1981;74:1475–1477.

Silverstein W, Lewin N, Goldfrank L: Management of the cocaine-intoxicated patient. *Ann Emerg Med* 1987;16:234–235.

Warner A, Pierozynski G: Pseudocatatonia associated with abuse of amphetamine and cannabis. *Postgrad Med* 1977;61:275–276.

Weiss S, Raskind K, Morganstein N, et al: Intracerebral and subarachnoid hemorrhage following use of methamphetamine ("speed"). *Int Surg* 1970;53:123–127.

Wetli C, Mettleman R: The body packer syndrome: toxicity following ingestion of illicit drugs packaged for transportation. *J Forensic Sci* 1981;26:492–500.

Winek C, Eastly T: Cocaine identification. *Clin Toxicol* 1979;8:205–210.

CHAPTER 52

Phencyclidine

Phencyclidine (phenylcyclohexylpiperidine, PCP) is chemically related to the phenothiazines, and consists of a benzene ring, a cyclohexyl ring, and a piperidine ring (1). Phencyclidine is a synthetic drug and one of a large family of arylcyclohexylamines developed more than 20 years ago as possible anesthetic agents with structures different from those of other psychomimetic drugs and neurotransmitters (2,3). More than 30 phencyclidine analogs have been developed through minor modifications of the manufacturing process. Many investigators have attempted to classify PCP, and although it is sometimes classified as an atypical hallucinogen it appears to fall into a class of its own. It produces both (central nervous system) (CNS) stimulation and depression, hallucinations, analgesia, and cholinergic-like symptoms along with many other effects.

Phencyclidine was developed for use in humans for general anesthesia and as a short-acting analgesic under the trade name Sernyl (4–7). Because of postoperative side effects, however, such as postanesthetic excitement, visual disturbances, and delirium, the drug was withdrawn for human use (2). Its use continued as a veterinary anesthetic under the trade name Sernylan, but this was also withdrawn from the market. Since 1978, all legal manufacture and sale has been stopped, and PCP is now classified as a Schedule II controlled substance. Federal reporting of the sale of piperidine, which is necessary for the synthesis of PCP, became mandatory in 1978 (8).

Phencyclidine is structurally similar to ketamine and was first seen as a street drug in San Francisco in 1967, as the Peace Pill. It is misrepresented as many other drugs of abuse, such as tetrahydrocannabinol (THC), cocaine, mescaline, psilocybin, peyote, and LSD. It has since replaced other drugs as the most readily available street drug and is difficult to control, probably because it is simple and inexpensive to make. Early in its history, PCP developed a negative reputation among the drug-using community, but it no longer carries such a stigma because it is more of an accepted drug of abuse. Today, there are a great many analogs of phencyclidine available on the street. At least 60 precursors, derivatives, and analogs of PCP have been prepared and nearly all cause pharmacologic effects similar to those of PCP (9).

TABLE 52–1. *Actions of phencyclidine*

Analgesic
Local anesthetic
Sympathomimetic
Anticholinergic
Cholinergic
Dopaminergic
Antidopaminergic

ACTIONS

Phencyclidine appears to alter the association pathways in the brain, thus interfering with the ability to process and react appropriately to sensory stimuli (3). PCP is believed to affect multiple neurotransmitter receptors in the brain. Evidence suggests involvement of the noradrenergic, dopaminergic, cholinergic, α-aminobutyric acid, and serotonergic systems as well as the opiate receptors and the endorphins (3,10). Because PCP affects so many neurotransmitters, the clinical picture of intoxication can vary greatly (11).

Phencyclidine is an analgesic with local anesthetic properties that are twice as effective as those of procaine and half as potent as those of cocaine (Table 52–1). In addition, PCP appears to have sympathomimetic activity, causing both CNS stimulation and depression (12). Although an anticholinergic action may explain many of the manifestations that appear to be adrenergic, there are, in addition, many cholinergic-like effects seen with the drug. PCP also appears to both stimulate and block the dopaminergic receptors in the brain to cause marked psychomimetic actions (12).

PCP-intoxicated patients may be brought to the emergency department (ED) because of alterations in mental status, bizarre or violent behavior, or injuries sustained while intoxicated. They are also at risk for significant medical complications such as rhabdomyolysis, seizures, and hyperthermia.

PHARMACOKINETICS

Absorption

Phencyclidine can be absorbed from most routes. Although it can be ingested orally in the form of tablets, this is rarely seen in the sophisticated drug user. Oral ingestion may be employed, however, in a suicide attempt. Smoking of a "joint" is the usual route. The user may sprinkle powdered PCP ("Angel Dust") on dried parsley, mint, or low-grade marijuana and smoke it, thus allowing maximum control over the dose ingested. Rarely has the intravenous administration of PCP been attempted. In addition, leaf mixtures, rock crystals, and capsules containing the crystalline or granular powder are used, or the user may insufflate the powder.

Phencyclidine enters the bloodstream rapidly by all routes and, because it is highly lipid-soluble, quickly distributes to tissues with a high lipid content such as adipose and brain tissues (13). Metabolism of adipose tissue may cause the release of PCP, contributing to the recurrence of symptoms and fluctuations in clinical status. The half-life varies widely, from 7 hours to more than 3 days. Also, because it is a basic compound, it achieves high concentrations in body compartments that have an acidic pH, such as the cerebrospinal fluid and gastric secretions (3). Phencyclidine's volume of distribution is 6.2 L/kg (8).

Onset of Action

The effects of PCP are noted immediately with parenteral administration. If smoked, effects may begin as early as 2 to 5 minutes. The onset of symptoms with oral administration occurs within 15 minutes. Although the "high" may last 4 to 6 hours, the user generally requires 24 to 48 hours to return to a normal state. This is thought to be attributable to some binding of the drug in the CNS as well as to enterohepatic circulation of the drug. In the stomach PCP is in a substantially ionized form because the pKa of the stomach is 8.5 (3). Because it is not very lipid-soluble in the stomach, there is little absorption from that area. Most of the drug is absorbed in the alkaline small intestine (14). The compound undergoes enterogastric reabsorption, whereby it is secreted back into the stomach from the systemic circulation and is then reabsorbed as it proceeds into the more alkaline portions of the intestinal tract. This recirculation may account for the drug's prolonged systemic course and the fact that it continues to be excreted in the urine for several days (13).

Metabolism

The primary site of PCP metabolism is the liver; hydroxylated metabolites are excreted by the kidneys. Approximately 10% of absorbed PCP is excreted unchanged in the urine. Because phencyclidine is a weak base, with a pKa of approximately 8.5, it is ionized and trapped in an acid environment. This is the basis for some of the strategies that have been proposed in attempts to enhance drug elimination (13).

TOXICITY

The signs and symptoms of PCP intoxication are related to the dose, the route of administration, and the individual's idiosyncratic response to the drug (12). Because the signs and symptoms of PCP intoxication vary greatly, classification according to dose is confusing and difficult to use. Indeed, dose can rarely be determined; in many cases, patients are not aware that they have taken PCP.

Effects of PCP can be divided into five areas: behavioral, neurologic, cardiovascular, renal, and gastrointestinal. PCP may act as a depressant, a stimulant, or a hallucinogen depending on such variables as route of administration and dosage. Because of this, it is difficult to predict the clinical effects of the drug. Patients may display rapid and unpredictable fluctuations in their clinical state of intoxication. Low-dose intoxications may become behavioral emergencies but rarely represent a true medical emergency.

Behavioral Effects

Phencyclidine can cause behavioral changes secondary to either CNS stimulation or depression and may vary markedly depending on individual factors as well as the dose. The risk of dysphoric reactions from PCP may be increased in the presence of previous underlying psychiatric illness (Table 52–2) (11,15).

The behavioral effects at low doses may include euphoria, a pleasurable "high," amnesia, anxiety, agitation, a disordered thought process, and hallucinations. Many times users experience a sense of strength (16).

TABLE 52–2. *Behavioral effects of phencyclidine*

Euphoria
Amnesia
Body image distortion
Feeling of dissociation
Anxiety
Agitation
Depersonalization
Disordered thought process
Hallucinations
Feeling of superhuman strength
Psychosis
Catatonia
Blank stare

Although frank hallucinations are not common, illusions or delusions are common. The dissociation of somatic perception, and therefore the lack of experienced pain, leads to illusions of superhuman strength, power, and invulnerability. Most deaths result from aberrant behavior rather than from the drug itself.

Phencyclidine is unique in that it may produce a psychosis indistinguishable from schizophrenia. Many similarities exist between the hyperdopaminergic state of schizophrenia and intoxication with PCP. Depersonalization and distortions of body image and perceptions of all sensory modes are the psychological effects most frequently reported. Users describe a sense of distance and estrangement from their surroundings. Time seems to expand, and body movements seem to be slowed. Users report that feelings of immobility, numbness, and detachment are among the desired effects of the drug. Individuals may have fluctuating levels of consciousness, in which at one moment they are mute and at the next propelled into action. This action can take the form of agitated pacing, unprovoked aggression, or loss of impulse control. Other individuals feel paralyzed, off-balance, or restrained. Still others may seem to be catatonic, and although they appear to be awake, with eyes open in a blank stare, they have no response to any external stimuli, and may be unable to speak. Catatonic patients characteristically display catalepsy, posturing, mutism, rigidity, staring, and negativism.

Because of PCP-induced behavioral abnormalities and analgesic effects, intoxicated patients are prone to sustaining significant injuries. Analgesia and alterations in mental status can mask these injuries, which may only be discovered on careful physical examination.

Most deaths in PCP-intoxicated patients occur not because of direct effects of the drug but because of its behavioral toxicity. The bizarre and violent behavior induced by PCP, along with analgesic effects and the lack of muscular coordination, may cause drowning or significant trauma.

Neurologic Effects

The neurologic manifestations of PCP intoxication result from cerebellar dysfunction and may include dizziness, ataxia, slurred speech, dysarthria, and nystagmus (Table 52–3). The nystagmus, which is commonly seen, is first horizontal and then vertical or rotatory and can occur at low or moderate doses (17). It is first noted only with appropriate stimuli but later may occur spontaneously. The nystagmus has irregular burst-like features and can be helpful in establishing a definitive diagnosis (18,19). Miotic pupils are typically seen, although the pupil size can be variable (12). In addition, blurred vision, decreased pain perception, decreased proprioception, and unusual temperature response are attributable to the anesthetic action of the drug. Tremors, muscle weakness, slurred speech, drowsiness, salivation, and drooling may also be noted. High-dose intoxication may cause coma or generalized intense muscle rigidity. Intracranial hemorrhage associated with PCP abuse has also been reported (20). Opisthotonic or decerebrate posturing may be present along with myoclonus and generalized tonic-clonic seizures, which can progress to status epilepticus (13).

TABLE 52–3. *Neurologic manifestations of phencyclidine intoxication*

Dizziness
Ataxia
Slurred speech
Dysarthria
Nystagmus
Miosis
Lack of experienced pain
Decreased proprioception
Tremors
Muscle weakness
Coma
Muscle rigidity
Seizures

Cardiovascular Effects

The cardiovascular manifestations of PCP intoxication (Table 52–4) may include tachycardia and hypertension. Although the blood pressure elevation can be significant, it usually is mild and transitory and does not lead to serious consequences (12). Ordinarily, hypertension occurs in the early phases of intoxication (especially when the patient is hypertonic) or as a dopaminergic crisis in the recovery phase. On occasion, accelerated hypertension may result in serious complications, including intracerebral hemorrhage and other cerebrovascular accidents; careful monitoring of the vital signs is therefore essential (13). Tachyphylaxis to the pressor effects of PCP develops rapidly, and hyper-

TABLE 52–4. *Cardiovascular, renal, and gastrointestinal manifestations of phencyclidine intoxication*

Cardiovascular
Tachycardia
Hypertension
Renal
Antidiuresis
Rhabdomyolysis
Gastrointestinal
Nausea
Vomiting
Salivation
Drooling
Abdominal pain
Hematemesis

tension is not of major consequence in the long-term PCP user (8).

Renal Effects

One of the major renal consequences of PCP intoxication is myoglobinuria leading to acute tubular necrosis (Table 52–4) (21). The mechanism for muscle injury is thought to be related to a number of factors, including increased and excessive isometric muscle activity and the generalized hypertonicity associated with the severe agitation or as a result of grand mal seizures. There is no evidence that PCP has a direct toxic effect on skeletal muscle (22). If significant rhabdomyolysis has occurred, myoglobinuria may be present and may lead to acute renal failure (13).

It is important to recognize that rhabdomyolysis is not a rare complication of PCP abuse and that it is often clinically inapparent. Most patients with rhabdomyolysis have had no history of exaggerated muscle activity and no physical evidence of muscle injury. The mechanism of acute renal failure in acute rhabdomyolysis is not clearly understood, and several mechanisms have been suggested (23,24). Tubular obstruction by myoglobin casts, passive back-diffusion of glomerular filtration through damaged tubular epithelial cells, myoglobin nephrotoxicity, renal ischemia, and a decreased glomerular permeability have all been implicated. Urinary acidification enhances myoglobin and uric acid precipitation in the renal tubules, which could increase the likelihood of acute renal failure (23). An elevation of the serum uric acid concentration above the normal range and a moderate increase in the serum creatine kinase concentration are indicative of rhabdomyolysis (24), although these changes may occur without an elevation in serum creatine concentration. A positive urine dipstick test for blood, with no red blood cells on the microscopic examination of the urine, may indicate myoglobinuria secondary to rhabdomyolysis.

The potential for rhabdomyolysis should be considered in all patients intoxicated with PCP. At a minimum, urine should be screened for myoglobin by dipstick testing for heme. Serum creatine phosphokinase (CPK) should be measured in patients with heme-positive urine. Because the presence of urinary myoglobin may be transient, serum CPK should be measured when rhabdomyolysis is strongly suspected on clinical grounds, even with heme-negative urine.

Gastrointestinal Effects

Gastrointestinal manifestations of PCP intoxication may include nausea, vomiting, salivation, and drooling (Table 52–4). Abdominal cramps and hematemesis, seen in users of illicit preparations of PCP, may be secondary to the by-products produced during the synthesis of the drug (25).

Major Complications

Major complications of PCP intoxication include respiratory depression and apnea (which can occur abruptly), seizures and status epilepticus (26), intracerebral hemorrhage (27), hypertensive encephalopathy (12), rhabdomyolysis and myoglobinuria with renal failure, hyperpyrexia, psychosis, adrenergic crisis, laryngospasm, and cardiac arrest (Table 52–5). Trauma injuries are a large part of the major problems associated with PCP abuse. Unrecognized and painless self-injury, automobile accidents, violent behavior, falls, and drowning, sometimes in very shallow water (11) are associated with PCP overdose. The injuries are due to the anesthetic action of the drug coupled with the user's overconfidence, disorientation, and ataxia and the muscle rigidity, prolonged reaction time, and sensory aberrations induced by the drug (16).

In the low-dose range, deaths are usually attributable to behavioral disturbances, and result from impaired perception or delusional beliefs in addition to the marked tendency that the user has toward violence. In the high-dose range, deaths may be secondary to the physiologic changes from sympathetic hyperstimulation (25).

Pediatric Intoxications

Children often become intoxicated by ingesting the butts of used PCP-impregnated cigarettes. Also, sidestream smoke may contain enough PCP to be responsible for the intoxication of pediatric patients by passive inhalation (8).

Children usually present with alterations in consciousness or abnormal neurologic signs; aggressive behavior and violence are unusual.

The most common clinical findings in PCP-intoxicated children are lethargy or more severe depression of consciousness, ataxia, nystagmus, and staring episodes (25). PCP-intoxicated children may present with apnea,

TABLE 52–5. *Major complications of phencyclidine intoxication*

Respiratory depression and apnea
Seizures and status epilepticus
Intracerebral hemorrhage
Hypertensive encephalopathy
Rhabdomyolysis and renal failure
Hyperpyrexia
Psychosis
Adrenergic crisis
Laryngospasm
Cardiac arrest
Trauma

seizures, opisthotonus, or choreoathetosis. Miosis is found more commonly in children than in adults.

Laboratory Analysis

Although a tentative diagnosis of PCP intoxication can be made on clinical grounds, confirmation requires a positive assay of urine, blood, or gastric contents. For the most part, quantitatively measured PCP concentrations do not provide clinically useful information beyond what could be obtained from a qualitative screen. PCP can be rapidly and inexpensively identified by thin-layer chromatography, but gas chromatography with mass spectroscopy and ultraviolet detection have also been used successfully. Gas chromatography with nitrogen detection is a sensitive but time-consuming technique. Gas chromatography with flame ionization is less sensitive and may yield a negative result even when PCP is identified by other means. The enzyme-multiplied immunoassay is a rapid and sensitive technique. Analysis of serum for PCP may be misleading, however, because blood concentrations may be unmeasurable several hours after exposure, whereas the urine may still be positive.

In the emergency department various functions should be monitored (Table 52–6), including the respiratory rate and depth (because of acute apnea), blood pressure (because of hypertension or hypotension), muscle tone (because of rhabdomyolysis), renal function (because of acute renal failure secondary to rhabdomyolysis), and temperature (because of hyperthermia) (8).

TREATMENT

There is no agent known that is specific in antagonizing the toxic effects of PCP, so that the treatment for intoxicated patients is primarily supportive medical and psychiatric care (Table 52–7) (28). Routine emesis and gastric lavage are not generally necessary because the drug is usually not ingested. Nevertheless, if there is any question about the amount taken or, more important, about the concomitant ingestion of other drugs, the stomach should be emptied and activated charcoal and a cathartic administered. Sensory isolation with frequent monitoring and avoidance of unnecessary instrumentation is best for the mildly intoxicated patient (29).

TABLE 52–6. *Physiologic functions to monitor in phencyclidine overdose*

Respiratory rate and depth
Blood pressure
Muscle tone
Renal function
Cardiac monitor
Psychiatric condition

TABLE 52–7. *Treatment of phencyclidine overdose*

Indication	Treatment
Agitation	Physical restraints
	Pharmacological
	Butyrophenones
	Benzodiazepines
Hypotension	Fluid therapy
	Vasoconstrictors
Seizures	Diazepam
Hypertension	Labetalol
	Nifedipine
	Nitroprusside
Hyperthermia	External cooling
Ventricular dysrhythmia	Lidocaine

Control of the Airway

Intubation with ventilatory assistance may be required, possibly for an extended period, because of the prolonged and delayed hypoventilation and apnea that may occur with PCP intoxication (29). These effects usually occur only at high doses. Intubation, if required, may be difficult because of the increased muscle rigidity. Because laryngeal reflexes are maintained, attempted endotracheal intubation may precipitate laryngospasm. In some cases, it has been necessary to use a neuromuscular blocking agent for successful endotracheal intubation.

Nasogastric Suction

Attempts to increase elimination may include intermittent nasogastric suction. As mentioned before, because PCP is a weak base, it is highly ionized in the acid medium of the stomach. Ionized drugs do not pass through biologic membranes, so that PCP is not well absorbed in the stomach. If nasogastric suction is used, drug that is secreted back into the stomach from the small intestine is removed before it returns to the small intestine (12,30). Multiple-dose activated charcoal has also been advocated because it can adsorb any compound secreted into the stomach and be removed by nasogastric suction. Although these methods may be effective, the potential benefit must be weighed against the risk of the procedure in an uncooperative patient predisposed to rhabdomyolysis. Many investigators hold that the risks of these procedures in this group of patients outweigh the potential benefit (31).

Control of Seizure Activity

Small doses of diazepam can be administered slowly to control muscle spasticity, opisthotonus, and seizures unless there is an associated closed head injury. Diazepam can be followed by intravenous phenytoin for seizure prophylaxis. The use of barbiturates is not recommended because a synergistic depressant effect may occur (16). If seizures are persistent, then consideration should be given to the use of a neuromuscular blocking agent and institution of mechanical respiratory support. Although seizures are rare, they should be treated immediately to decrease the risk of rhabdomyolysis (3).

Acidification of Urine

Urinary elimination of PCP is significantly dependent on urinary pH, and measures aimed at lowering the pH of the urine have been recommended to facilitate excretion of the drug. Although acidification of the urine has been shown to increase excretion (30), it is not recommended because of the possibility of decreased myoglobin excretion and the development of acute tubular necrosis (3). Moreover, by reducing uric acid solubility an acid urine may predispose the patient to the development of acute uric acid nephropathy.

Control of Hypertension

Often, hypertension is not severe enough to require treatment but blood pressure monitoring is vital. If treatment is required, nifedipine or nitroprusside is suggested for severe or malignant hypertension. A β blocker may be administered if the adrenergic crisis is severe.

Control of the Violent Patient

Violent and combative patients must be protected from injuring themselves and others. "Talk down" therapy, which may be effective for other drugs, not only is ineffective for PCP but may aggravate the patient's condition. Initially, these patients should be restrained. Physical restraints should be soft in order not to traumatize the patient further. Physical restraints should be used for the shortest possible period of time because they intensify isometric muscle tension, which directly correlates with muscle toxicity and the development of rhabdomyolysis. Pharmacologic therapy may be instituted after the patient has been physically restrained.

The most widely used tranquilizing agents are benzodiazepines and haloperidol. Haloperidol given intramuscularly is rapidly effective in most patients. Theoretically, it may lower the seizure threshold, cause dystonic reactions, and interfere with temperature-regulatory mechanisms. Nonetheless, clinical experience with haloperidol in PCP-intoxicated patients and in patients with psychosis, agitation, and violence resulting from various other etiologies has been quite favorable; adverse effects are uncommon (29).

Haloperidol, rather than chlorpromazine, should be used and is an excellent agent for sedation of the uncontrollable patient (15,19,32 34). The phenothiazines should be avoided because they may increase the likelihood of severe hypotension as well as decrease the seizure threshold and thus increase the likelihood of seizures. Neuromuscular blocking agents in a controlled setting may be useful if muscular rigidity remains a problem. Psychiatric intervention is begun only after the patient is clinically stable and no longer profoundly agitated.

Methods to Avoid

The use of sympathomimetics should be avoided because these drugs have the potential to exacerbate tachycardia and hypertension. Dialysis is ineffective in enhancing the removal of PCP.

Criteria for Hospitalization

The signs and symptoms of PCP intoxication may wax and wane; patients should be observed until their mental status has remained normal for several hours. Most patients with mild to moderate symptomatology will improve rapidly and can be discharged from the ED. Patients with severe poisoning often have a more prolonged course and require admission. Patients with complications such as seizures, rhabdomyolysis, hyperthermia, and significant injuries require hospitalization.

OTHER PHENCYCLIDINE-LIKE SUBSTANCES

Many other arylcyclohexylamines have appeared on the street (Table 52–8) and are similar structurally to PCP. Intoxication with these substances should be considered in a patient having a "bad trip" (9).

Piperidinocyclohexane carbonitrile (PCC) is an intermediary in the synthesis of PCP and is difficult to separate from the final product. PCC appears to be strongly psychoactive and causes unpleasant reactions, including severe psychological side effects, nausea, vomiting, hematemesis, and abdominal cramping. Other by-products of PCP synthesis are of concern in the PCP-intoxicated patient. PCP can be manufactured with piperidine, cyclohexane, and potassium cyanide. The cyano group in PCC is labile, especially with heating, and decomposes to release hydrogen cyanide. The amount of PCC contaminating PCP is probably not sufficient to cause serious complications in moderate to low doses but may worsen

TABLE 52–8. *Selected phencyclidine analogs*

PCC—Piperidinocyclohexane carbonitrile
PHP—Phenylcyclohexylpyrrolidine
TCP—Thienylcyclohexylpiperidine
PCE—Cyclohexamine ketamine

the effects of an overdose. On this basis it may be worthwhile to determine blood concentrations of cyanide in patients suspected of having used PCP chronically or in excessive doses (35).

Phenylcyclohexylpyrrolidine (PHP) is another analog of PCP. It is similar chemically and pharmacologically, has the same effects on ingestion or smoking, and is much easier to synthesize. The chemicals for its manufacture are easier to obtain than piperidine, which is now a controlled substance. PHP has also become popular because it has been difficult to detect its presence with the thin-layer chromatographic examination generally used by hospital and police toxicology laboratories. The patient may therefore show a negative PCP screen and still be intoxicated with a PCP-like substance (33,36).

Thienylcyclohexylpiperidine (TCP) is the thiophene analog of PCP and produces similar effects. It was first seen in San Francisco and is considered more potent than PCP but is sold on the same weight basis as PCP (37,38).

Cyclohexamine Ketamine (PCE) first appeared in Los Angeles in 1969. This analog is considered somewhat more potent than PCP but has similar effects (39).

Ketamine (Ketalar, Ketaject) is a dissociative anesthetic that has found use in medicine and abuse in the street (2). Ketamine is considered somewhat less potent than PCP in producing depersonalization and intoxication, and it is considered superior to PCP by some users. It may be administered intranasally, intramuscularly, and intravenously and by inhalation (2).

REFERENCES

1. Fauman B, Baker F, Coppleson L, et al: Psychosis induced by phencyclidine. *JACEP* 1975;4:223–225.
2. Felser J, Orban D: Dystonic reaction after ketamine abuse. *Ann Emerg Med* 1982;11:673–675.
3. Hartness C, Buchan J, Bayer M: Phencyclidine. *Top Emerg Med* 1985;7:33–38.
4. Owens S, Mayersohn M: Phencyclidine-specific Fab fragments alter phencyclidine disposition in dogs. *Drug Metab Disp* 1986;14:52–58.
5. Burns R, Lerner S: Phencyclidine: an emerging problem. *Clin Toxicol* 1976;9:473–475.
6. Bayer M, Norton R: Solving the clinical problems of phencyclidine intoxication. *ER Rep* 1983;4:7–12.
7. Done A, Aronow R, Miceli J: Pharmacokinetic bases for the diagnosis and treatment of acute PCP intoxication. *J Psychedelic Drugs* 1980;12:253–258.
8. Baldridge E, Bessen H: Phencyclidine. *Emerg Med Clin North Am* 1990;8:541–549.
9. Jerrard D: "Designer drugs"—a current perspective. *J Emerg Med* 1990;8:733–741.
10. Price W, Giannini A: Management of PCP intoxication. *Am Fam Physician* 1985;32:115–118.
11. Burns R, Lerner S: Perspectives: acute phencyclidine intoxication. *Clin Toxicol* 1976;9:477–501.
12. Krenzelok E: Phencyclidine: a contemporary drug of abuse. *Crit Care Q* 1982;4:55–63.
13. Jackson J: Phencyclidine pharmacokinetics after a massive overdose. *Ann Intern Med* 1989;111:613–615.
14. Rhee K, Albertson T, Douglas J: Choreoathetoid disorder associated with amphetamine-like drugs. *Am J Emerg Med* 1988;6:131–133.
15. Balster R, Chait L: The behavioral pharmacology of phencyclidine. *Clin Toxicol* 1976;9:513–528.
16. Johnson K, Jones S: Neuropharmacology of phencyclidine: basic mechanisms and therapeutic potential. *Annu Rev Pharmacol Toxicol* 1990;30:707–750.
17. McCarron M, Schulze B, Thompson G, et al: Acute phencyclidine intoxication: incidence of clinical findings in 1000 cases. *Ann Emerg Med* 1981;10:237–242.
18. Hershowitz J: More about poisoning by phencyclidine. *N Engl J Med* 1977;297:1405.
19. Showalter C, Thornton W: Clinical pharmacology of phencyclidine toxicity. *Am J Psychiatry* 1977;124:1234–1238.
20. Bessen H: Intracranial hemorrhage associated with phencyclidine abuse. *JAMA* 1982;248:585–586.
21. Hoogwerf B, Kern J, Bullock M, et al: Phencyclidine-induced rhabdomyolysis and acute renal failure. *Clin Toxicol* 1979;14:47–53.
22. Kunel R, Metzler H: Pathologic effect of phencyclidine and restraint on rat skeletal muscle: prevention by prior denervation. *Exp Neurol* 1974;45:387–402.
23. Patel R, Das M, Palazzolo M, et al: Myoglobinuric acute renal failure in phencyclidine overdose: report of observations in eight cases. *Ann Emerg Med* 1980;9:549–553.
24. Patel R, Connor G: A review of thirty cases of rhabdomyolysis-associated acute renal failure among phencyclidine users. *Clin Toxicol* 1986:23:547–556.
25. Young J, Crapo L: Protracted phencyclidine coma from an intestinal deposit. *Arch Intern Med* 1992;152:859–860.
26. Kessler G, Demus L, Berlin C, et al: Phencyclidine and fatal status epilepticus. *N Engl J Med* 1974;291:979–984.
27. Eastman J, Cohen S: Hypertensive crisis and death associated with phencyclidine poisoning. *JAMA* 1975;231:1270–1272.
28. Owens S, Hardwick W, Blackall D: Phencyclidine pharmacokinetic scaling among species. *J Pharmacol Exp Ther* 1987;242:96–101.
29. Milhorn H: Diagnosis and management of phencyclidine intoxication. *Am Fam Physician* 1991;43:1293–1302.
30. Aronow R, Miceli J, Done A: A therapeutic approach to the acutely overdosed PCP patient. *J Psychedelic Drugs* 1980;12:259–267.
31. Callaway C, Clark R: Hyperthermia in psychostimulant overdose. *Ann Emerg Med* 1994;24:68–76.
32. Fox S: Haloperidol in the treatment of phencyclidine intoxication. *Am J Hosp Pharmacol* 1979;36:448–451.
33. Giannini A, Castellani S: A case of phenylcyclohexylpyrrolidine (PHP) intoxication treated with physostigmine. *J Toxicol Clin Toxicol* 1982;19:505–508.
34. Castellani S, Giannini A, Boeringa J, et al: Phencyclidine intoxication: assessment of possible antidotes. *J Toxicol Clin Toxicol* 1982;19:313–319.
35. Skinner M, Thompson D: Pharmacologic considerations in the treatment of substance abuse. *South Med J* 1992;85:1207–1219.
36. Dulik D, Soine W: Color test for detection of 1-piperidinocyclohexane carbonitrile (PCC) in illicit phencyclidine. *Clin Toxicol* 1981;18:737–742.
37. Shulgin A, MacLean D: Illicit synthesis of phencyclidine (PCP) and several of its analogs. *Clin Toxicol* 1976;9:553–560.
38. Lundberg G, Gupta R, Montgomery H: Phencyclidine: patterns seen in street drug analysis. *Clin Toxicol* 1976;9:503–511.
39. Beebe D, Walley E: Substance abuse: the designer drugs. *Am Fam Physician* 1991;43:1689–1698.

ADDITIONAL SELECTED REFERENCES

Aronow R, Done A: Phencyclidine overdose: an emerging concept of management. *JACEP* 1978;7:56–59.

Barton C, Sterling M, Vaziri N: Phencyclidine intoxication: clinical experience in twenty-seven cases confirmed by urine assay. *Ann Emerg Med* 1981;10:243–246.

Brown J, Malone M: Status of drug quality in the street drug market: an update. *Clin Toxicol* 1976;9:145–168.

Budd R: PHP: a new drug of abuse. *N Engl J Med* 1981;303:588.

Burns R, Lerner S: Phencyclidine deaths. *JACEP* 1978;7:135–141.

Castellani S, Adams P: Effects of dopaminergic and cholinergic agents on phencyclidine-induced behaviors in rats. *Neurosci Abstr* 1980; 6:311–314.

Fallis R, Aniline O, Weiner L, et al: Massive phencyclidine intoxication. *Arch Neurol* 1982;89:316.

Fauman B, Aldinger G, Fauman M, et al: Psychiatric sequelae of phencyclidine abuse. *Clin Toxicol* 1976;9:513–528.

Garey R, McQuitty S, Tootle D, et al: The effects of apomorphine and Haldol on PCP-induced behavioral and motor abnormalities in the rat. *Life Sci* 1980;26:277–284.

Giannini A, Price W, Loiselle R, et al: Treatment of phenylcyclohexylpyrrolidine (PHP) psychosis with haloperidol. *Clin Toxicol* 1985;23:185–189.

Goldfrank L, Osborn H: Phencyclidine (angel dust). *Hosp Physician* 1978;14:18–21.

Gupta R, Lu I, Oei G, et al: Determination of phencyclidine (PCP) in urine and illicit street drug samples. *Clin Toxicol* 1975;8:611–621.

Karp H, Kaufman N, Anand S: Phencyclidine poisoning in young children. *J Pediatr* 1980;97:1006–1009.

Liden C, Lovejoy F, Costello C: Phencyclidine: nine cases of poisoning. *JAMA* 1975;234:513–516.

Luisada P, Brown B: Clinical management of phencyclidine psychosis. *Clin Toxicol* 1976;9:539–545.

McCann D, Smith C, Winter J: A caution against use of verapamil in phencyclidine intoxication. *Am J Psychiatry* 1986;143:679.

Munch J: Phencyclidine: pharmacology and toxicology. *Bull Narcotics* 1974;26:9–17.

Nicholas J, Lipshitz J, Schreiber B: Phencyclidine: its transfer across the placenta as well as into breast milk. *Am J Obstet Gynecol* 1982; 143:143–146.

Pearlson G: Psychiatric and medical syndromes associated with phencyclidine (PCP) abuse. *Johns Hopkins Med J* 1981;148:25–33.

Picchioni AL, Consroe P: Activated charcoal: a phencyclidine antidote, in hogs or dogs. *N Engl J Med* 1979;300:202.

Price W, Giannini A, Krishen A: Management of acute PCP intoxication with verapamil. *Clin Toxicol* 1986;24:85–87.

Rainey J, Criwder M: Prolonged psychosis attributed to phencyclidine: report of three cases. *Am J Psychiatry* 1975;132:1076–1078.

Rappolt R, Gay G, Farris R: Emergency management of acute phencyclidine intoxication. *JACEP* 1979;8:68–76.

Rappolt R: Phencyclidine (PCP) intoxication: diagnosis in stages and algorithms of treatment. *Clin Toxicol* 1980;16:509–529.

Reed A, Kane A: Phencyclidine (PCP): another illicit psychedelic drug. *J Psychedelic Drugs* 1972;5:8–12.

Reynolds R: Clinical and forensic experiences with phencyclidine. *Clin Toxicol* 1976;9:547–552.

Rumack B: Phencyclidine overdose: an overview, editorial. *Ann Emerg Med* 1980;9:595.

Russ C, Wong D: Diagnosis and treatment of phencyclidine psychosis: clinical considerations. *J Psychedelic Drugs* 1979;11:277–282.

Sidoff M: Phencyclidine: syndromes of abuse and modes of treatment. *Top Emerg Med* 1979;1:111–119.

Siegel R: PCP and violent crime: the people vs peace. *J Psychedelic Drugs* 1980;12:317–330.

Smith D, Wesson D: PCP abuse: diagnostic and psychopharmacological treatment approaches. *J Psychedelic Drugs* 1980;12:293–299.

Soine W, Vincek W, Agee D: Phencyclidine contaminant generates cyanide. *N Engl J Med* 1979;301:438.

Stillman R, Petersen R: The paradox of phencyclidine (PCP) abuse. *Ann Intern Med* 1979;90:428–430.

Thompson T: Malignant hyperthermia from PCP. *J Clin Psychiatry* 1979;40:327.

Tong T, Benowitz N, Becker C, et al: Phencyclidine poisoning. *JAMA* 1975;234:512–513.

Varipapa R: PCP treatment, editorial. *Clin Toxicol* 1977;10:353–355.

Walker S, Yesavage J, Tinklenberg J: Acute phencyclidine (PCP) intoxication: quantitative urine levels and clinical management. *Am J Psychiatry* 1981;138:674–675.

Welch M, Correa G: PCP intoxication in young children and infants. *Clin Pediatr* 1980;19:510–514.

CHAPTER 53

Volatile Inhalants

Abuse of volatile inhalants has been practiced since earliest recorded history (1). This is sometimes referred to as volatile substance abuse. The substances inhaled represent a group of diverse chemicals that produce psychoactive vapors and include a wide variety of gases, smokes, powders, and fluids. The abuse of these substances has been slowly but steadily increasing among adolescents. An extremely wide range of volatile fat-soluble compounds is used; in the vapor phase, these compounds pass easily through the lungs and into the blood (2). The efficient pulmonary absorption of the substance bypasses the detoxifying enzymes of the liver, thus avoiding the first-pass metabolism seen with oral administration of some of these compounds (3). Once within the brain, compounds with a wide variety of chemical structures can cause disturbances of consciousness ranging from mild intoxication through hallucinatory states to coma with cardiorespiratory depression (4).

Inhaling volatiles is called glue sniffing, solvent sniffing, solvent abuse, and inhalant abuse (2). Substances that are abused by inhalation can be categorized as aromatic and aliphatic hydrocarbons, alcohols, esters, ketones, aliphatic nitrites, anesthetic agents, halogenated solvents, and propellants (Table 53–1) (5). With aliphatic hydrocarbons, CNS depressant activity generally increases as the length of the chain increases. For the aromatics, however, CNS potency tends to decrease as the length of the side chain increases (6). Among the alkyl halides, CNS potency tends to increase as the number of halide substitutions increases. Any compound that is gaseous or that rapidly evaporates at room temperature and is psychoactive and not highly irritating is potentially subject to abuse by inhalation (7). All these substances are inhaled for the purpose of achieving a state of altered awareness (8), and most are easily available at home and in industry. Any volatile substance that has an intoxicating vapor has a potential for abuse, and often the clinical effects are due entirely to the solvent content and not to its other constituents (Tables 53–2 and 53–3) (9).

Solvents constitute a group of lipid-soluble substances widely used in industry. Although solvents make up a heterogeneous group, most are volatile, lipophilic, and have CNS depressant effects (a volatile substance is one that readily vaporizes at ambient temperatures). The selection of a particular intoxicant for abuse seems to follow well-defined trends, with one type of inhalant becoming popular and being widely abused for a time and then giving way to another substance (10).

There are more than 50 commonly abused solvents of widely different properties cited in the literature (11).

TABLE 53–1. *Substances with abuse potential by inhalation*

Classification	Examples
Aerosols	Fluorocarbons (see halogenated hydrocarbons, below)
	Isobutane
Aliphatic hydrocarbons	*n*-Hexane
	Ethane
	Acetylene
	Butane
	Isopentane
Anesthetic agents	Nitrous oxide
	Ether
	Chloroform
Aromatic hydrocarbons	Benzene
	Toluene
	Xylene
	Styrene
	Naphthalene
Esters	Ethyl acetate
	Isopropyl acetate
Fuels	Gasoline
	Naphtha
Halogenated hydrocarbons	Carbon tetrachloride
	Trichloroethylene
	Trichloroethane
	Perchloroethylene
	Methylene chloride
	Methylchloroform
	Fluorocarbons (dichlorodifluoromethane, trichlorofluoromethane)
Ketones	Acetone
	Methyl-*n*-butyl ketone
	Methylethyl ketone
Nitrites	Amyl nitrite
	Isobutyl nitrite
	Butyl nitrite

TABLE 53–2. *Solvents contained in commercial products commonly abused by inhalation*

Commercial product	Solvent
Acrylic paints	Toluene
Acrylic spray paints	Toluene
Adhesives	Acetone
	Toluene
	n-Hexane
	Trichloroethylene
Aerosol propellants	Freon
Anesthetic agents	Nitrous oxide
	Ether
Cleaning fluid	Carbon tetrachloride
	Benzene
	Trichloroethylene
	Trichloroethane
Coronary vasodilator	Amyl nitrite
Degreasers	Trichloroethylene
Dry cleaning fluid	Trichloroethane
	Trichloroethylene
Nail polish remover	Acetone
Gasoline	Hydrocarbons
	Tetraethyl lead
	Paraffins
	Olefins
Glues and adhesives	Benzene
	Xylene
	Acetone
	Naphtha
	n-Hexane
	Trichloroethylene
	Tetrachloroethylene
	Trichloroethane
	Carbon tetrachloride
Indelible ink	Methylethyl ketone
	Methyl-*n*-butyl ketone
	Acetone
Lacquer thinner	Toluene
	Aliphatic acetates
	Ethyl alcohol
	Propyl alcohol
Lighter fluid	Naphtha
	Perchloroethylene
	Carbon tetrachloride
	Trichloroethane
Liquid solder	Benzene
Model cement and glue	Acetone
	Toluene
	Naphtha
	Methylisobutyl ketone
Paint thinner	Trichloroethylene
Plastic cement	Acetone
	Toluene
	n-Hexane
	Ethylacetate
Refrigerants	Freon
Room deodorizers	Amyl nitrite
	Isobutyl nitrite
	Butyl nitrite
Rubber cement	Benzene
	n-Hexane
	Trichloroethylene
Shoe polish	Toluene
	Chlorinated hydrocarbons
Spot remover	Trichloroethane
	Trichloroethylene
	Carbon tetrachloride
Tube repair kits	Benzene
Typewriter correction fluid	Trichloroethane
	Trichloroethylene
	Perchloroethylene

Some of the more popular inhalants include or have included glue, coolants, paint thinner, nail polish remover, petroleum fuels such as gasoline, transmission fluid, and many aerosolized substances such as hair spray, room deodorizers, deodorants, insecticides, glass chillers, and vegetable oil frying–pan lubricants (12,13). Typewriter correction fluid now appears to be a popular item of abuse by inhalation. The volatile nitrites ("poppers") and nitrous oxide are also popular. The use of multiple agents is the rule rather than the exception (14).

OVERVIEW

Methods of Abuse

Inhaling of volatile substances of abuse is usually limited to a brief period of experimentation but may occasionally become regular or even chronic. Abusers are typically urban adolescent males who use volatile substance abuse as an inexpensive, legal, and readily available substitute for other intoxicants. The inhalation of volatile substances is generally a group activity (15).

Three of the most common methods for inhalation are called "huffing," "bagging," and "sniffing." In "huffing" a cloth sprayed or soaked with an inhalant is placed in front of the mouth and nose, and the vapors are inhaled (16). Breathing through a dust protection mask or gas mask with its filters replaced with volatile substance of abuse–soaked cotton balls is a variant of this method. "Bagging" is much more dangerous and involves pouring the material into a plastic bag, shaking the bag so that it is vaporized, inflating the bag by breathing into it, and then inhaling the vapors (17,18). Placing a volatile substance of abuse in a large can and breathing directly over its open end is another form of this technique. "Sniffing" describes the simple inhalation of the substance directly from the container. The preferred method is "bagging" because the direct inhalation of the vapor from the air or a bottle may not ensure a high concentration. Because the concentration of inspired volatile substances generally increase from sniffing to huffing to bagging, it is common for abusers to begin with sniffing and progress to bagging as the duration and intensity of abuse increases. Because of the potential for abuse of materials containing

TABLE 53–3. *Solvents and their commercial products*

Solvent	Commercial product
Acetone	Plastic cement
	Model cement
	Fingernail polish remover
Carbon tetrachloride	Degreasers
Benzene	Gasoline
Ether	Anesthetic
Freons	Aerosol propellant
	Refrigerant
Gasoline	Motor fuel
Hexane	Plastic cement
	Rubber cement
Hydrocarbons	Gasoline
Naphtha	Lighter fluid
	Model cements
Nitrites	Room deodorizers
	Coronary vasodilator
Nitrous oxide	Anesthetics
	Degreaser
Styrene	Adhesives
Tetraethyl lead	Gasoline
Toluene	Acrylic sprays and paints
	Plastic cement
	Indelible marking ink
	Lacquer thinner
Trichloroethane	Spot remover
	Dry cleaner
	Typewriter correction fluid
Trichloroethylene	Degreaser
	Dry cleaner
	Anesthetic agent
	Rubber cement
	Paint thinner
	Typewriter correction fluid
Xylene	Indelible inks

solvents, many manufacturers add oil of mustard (allyl isothiocyanate), a mucosal irritant, to products in an effort to deter abusers (19).

Toxicity

General Considerations

Because of the lipid solubility and high vapor pressure of solvents, these materials gain rapid access to the bloodstream across the alveolar–capillary membrane in the lungs when inhaled. Pulmonary absorption circumvents the first-pass hepatic extraction and metabolism that occurs following ingestion (14). Hence, the dose necessary to produce toxic effects by inhalation is typically quite small. Once absorbed, the compounds are distributed to tissues with high lipid content, particularly brain tissue (3). The onset of effects generally occurs within seconds to minutes. Peak blood levels are usually noted in 15 to 30 minutes but because of relatively slower diffusion into tissues, peak effects occur somewhat later. Excretion occurs primarily through exhalation, with a small fraction metabolized in the liver or excreted through the kidneys (6).

The early clinical effects of abuse of inhalants, regardless of the substance involved, are similar to those of alcohol consumption or anesthesia and may vary from mild alcohol-like inebriation to frank chemical psychosis and gross behavioral disturbances. With sufficient exposure, drunkenness, dizziness, perceptual changes, and euphoria are seen almost universally (20).

Users may present to the emergency department with paint around the face or white typewriter correction fluid around the mouth, have a solvent odor on their breath, or with glue on their hands or face. Erythematous spots around the nose and mouth, called "glue sniffer's rash," may be observed when a plastic bag is used for inhalation (5,18).

Although their potency is variable, all volatile substances of abuse have the ability to cause neurologic dysfunction, asphyxia, cardiovascular abnormalities, and tissue irritation. The alkyl halides, aromatic hydrocarbons, alkyl nitrites, and ketones have additional toxicity that is unique to their structural class. Although altered states of consciousness may be perceived as pleasurable and hence psychologically reinforcing, there is no evidence that volatile substances of abuse are physical addicting (21).

Acute Effects

Patients with acute volatile substance of abuse intoxication usually present with altered mental status, gastrointestinal complaints, cyanosis, respiratory symptoms, trauma, syncope, or cardiac arrest. Patients are usually brought in by friends, relatives, or the police. They may be mistakenly triaged for psychiatric evaluation.

Central Nervous System

The clinical effects of solvent inhalation develop rapidly and peak quickly. After several deep inhalations, a state of intoxication is produced that may last from 30 minutes to 3 hours (4,16,17). Volatile substances of abuse are CNS depressants. However, because the inhibition of cortical function generally precedes the inhibition of brain stem activity, initial or low-dose effects may include euphoria and hyperactivity. As stated above, clinical manifestations resemble those of ethanol intoxication except that the solvents often produce a greater degree of excitation with exhilaration, euphoria, restlessness, incoordination, and delirium (Table 53–4). Mild CNS depression may follow the stage of exhilaration with symptoms of confusion, disorientation, tinnitus, blurred vision,

TABLE 53–4. *Acute clinical effects of volatile inhalants*

Central nervous system
Confusion
Euphoria
Exhilaration
Hallucinations
Restlessness
Incoordination
Confusion
Disorientation
Ataxia
Nystagmus
Delirium
Coma
Death
Cardiovascular
Ventricular fibrillation

TABLE 53–5. *Long-term sequelae from inhalation abuse*

Aplastic anemia
Hepatic damage
Renal damage
Renal tubular acidosis
Neurologic sequelae
Optic atrophy
Cognitive impairment
Corticospinal tract dysfunction
Deafness
Dementia
Encephalopathy
Oculomotor abnormalities
Cerebellar degeneration
Disorders of equilibrium
Peripheral neuropathies
Tremor
Electrolyte disturbances
Lead poisoning
Weight loss

headache, and analgesia. Many patients develop ataxia and nystagmus. Other manifestations include diplopia, incoordination, lethargy, mydriasis, and slurred speech. Massive exposure can lead to greater degrees of CNS depression, coma, and death (22). Psychomimetic effects have been reported and include both visual and auditory hallucinations. These effects have been noted with gasoline, lighter fluid, and toluene inhalation.

Cardiovascular

The fluorinated hydrocarbons used as propellants in aerosol sprays and refrigerants have been implicated in sudden death. Typically, the individual looks startled, jumps up and runs for a few hundred feet, and then collapses (23). Although previous theories suggested suffocation as the cause of death, it is probably attributable to a cardiac dysrhythmia such as ventricular fibrillation, which occurs by sensitization of the patient's myocardium to endogenous circulating epinephrine (10,24 27) as well as by depression of myocardial contractility and consequent reduction in cardiac output. "Sudden sniffing death," as it has been termed in the literature, may occur from any of the volatile inhalants and does not appear to be related to one type of chemical such as the fluorinated hydrocarbons (28,29). The ability to sensitize myocardial tissue to epinephrine seems to be characteristic of many lipid-soluble chemicals. The most recent reports of sudden sniffing death have occurred after inhalation of trichloroethane, trichloroethene, and gasoline (26,30,31). Aliphatic hydrocarbons and alkyl halides are particularly notorious for this activity (6).

Long-Term Effects

The physical sequelae of prolonged solvent abuse have included aplastic anemia and acute hepatic and renal damage (Table 53–5) (5,32,33). Other long-term sequelae include cardiac dysrhythmias, peripheral neuropathies, electrolyte disturbances, and lead poisoning (16,34).

Neurologic

Neurologic abnormalities attributable to solvent inhalation vary from mild isolated cognitive impairment to severe dementia associated with elemental neurologic signs such as corticospinal tract dysfunction, oculomotor abnormalities, tremor, and deafness (35). Cognitive dysfunction, optic atrophy, encephalopathy, cerebellar degeneration, and equilibrium disorders have also been reported.

Renal

A characteristic renal lesion of renal tubular acidosis is associated with long-term inhalation of toluene (36,37). The non-anion gap metabolic acidosis is due to the loss of bicarbonate rather than the addition of any exogenous acid (38). Patients may exhibit diffuse weakness associated with hypokalemia and hypophosphatemia, often with accompanying rhabdomyolysis (39). There may also be markedly elevated serum creatine phosphokinase. Deaths from these electrolyte disturbances have been reported (24).

Lead Poisoning

Although lead poisoning is an extremely rare sequela of solvent abuse, repeated intoxication by prolonged, deliberate inhalation of leaded gas may lead to organic lead encephalitis (22,40–44). Tetraethyl lead is an entity separate and distinct from the inorganic leads that cause lead poisoning and is significantly more toxic than inorganic lead. This is because the molecular species as a whole is involved rather than the metallic constituent alone (39). Although tetraethyl lead is not by itself toxic, it is converted to the toxic derivative triethyl lead in the liver. Both tetraethyl and triethyl lead are more lipid-soluble than inorganic lead and can therefore rapidly accumulate in the CNS, causing early neurologic dysfunction (16). The most noticeable clinical sign of tetraethyl lead poisoning is encephalopathy.

Laboratory Analysis

In cases of suspected solvent abuse, arterial blood gases and electrolytes may demonstrate either a hyperchloremic metabolic acidosis or an anion gap metabolic acidosis. Tests for renal and liver function may document the status of these organ systems. In the case of a suspected volatile organonitrite, methemoglobin concentrations should be measured (45).

Laboratory testing for solvents is required in cases of glue sniffing only when medical complications occur or for medicolegal purposes. Volatile substances of abuse and their metabolites can be detected in biologic specimens using various types of gas chromatography. This technology is not widely available, however, and volatile substances are not detectable by routine screening methods; thus, special precautions should be used to improve the likelihood of recovery, such as the use of volatile analysis containers. Although solvents are relatively inert to biologic degradation, their volatile nature may lead to inaccurate or negative studies if they are not collected properly. Sensitive methods of analysis such as gas chromatography with mass spectrophotometry may be required for the accurate characterization of these compounds. Chromatographic methods are available for the detection of compounds such as acetone, trichloroethene, isopropanol, methylethyl ketone, benzene, trichloroethane, toluene, and many others (46). Blood concentrations of many of these volatiles may correlate with the depth of narcosis. The blood concentrations may be biphasic, with an initial peak followed by a trough; this reflects lipid binding by the CNS and a subsequent slow release into the blood.

Although blood is the specimen of choice for the detection of the agents abused, the analysis of urine may provide useful additional or corroboratory information in some instances. This applies particularly when abused substances may have cleared the circulation before a blood specimen can be obtained (33).

Methemoglobinemia should be considered in the cyanotic patient who is unrelieved with oxygen or whose blood appears brown. Methemoglobinemia may be secondary especially to the volatile nitrites (47,48).

Treatment

Symptomatic, conservative treatment is called for in cases of acute solvent intoxication. Generally, no further intervention is needed except psychiatric evaluation and follow-up. Fluid, electrolyte, and acid-base disturbances should be corrected. Hypotension should be treated with volume expansion rather than vasopressors because the latter may promote cardiac arrhythmias. Treatment of toluene inhalation includes fluid and electrolyte replacement. Patients presenting with distal renal tubular acidosis and marked metabolic acidosis should be admitted and treated with bicarbonate. Serum electrolyte abnormalities such as hypokalemia, hypophosphatemia, and hypochloremia are common and must be corrected. Seizures may be treated with usual doses of a benzodiazepine or phenytoin (6).

Patients with extreme agitation or hallucinations may require treatment with benzodiazepine or a neuroleptic agent. Treatment for methemoglobinemia secondary to the nitrites should follow the protocol outlined in Chapter 35. In cases of nitrous oxide abuse, vitamin B_{12} and thiamine supplements may correct the mixed neuropathic abnormalities (49).

The treatment of ventricular fibrillation secondary to inhalation of volatile drugs sometimes presents a dilemma. If an inhalation were known to have occurred, ventricular fibrillation should be treated with a β-blocking agent, since the dysrhythmia is secondary to myocardial sensitization to endogenous epinephrine. Most of the time, though, practitioners are not fortunate enough to know the full circumstances preceding the arrest. It is therefore of the utmost importance that a history of inhalant abuse prior to the arrest be acertained, so as to accurately treat the underlying cause of the dysrhythmia.

Patients with acute volatile substances of abuse intoxication whose symptoms do not resolve during a 4- to 6-hour period of observation or who require active interventions should be admitted. Those with signs and symptoms limited to behavioral or psychiatric disturbances can be admitted to a detoxification unit or psychiatric ward. Patients with physical, laboratory, EKG, or x-ray abnormalities should be admitted to a medical service.

AROMATIC HYDROCARBONS

Benzene

The aromatic hydrocarbons most frequently abused are benzene, toluene, and xylene. Benzene is lipophilic and may serve as a vehicle for penetration of other neurotoxic solvents into the nervous system. For example, benzene is a constituent of gasoline and may contribute to the cerebral toxicity noted after chronic inhalation of lead-based gasoline (4).

TABLE 53–6. *Compounds containing benzene*

Rubber cement, glues, and adhesives
Cleaning fluid
Tube repair kits
Liquid solder
Gasoline

Formerly, benzene was the major organic hydrocarbon in paints, lacquers, and thinners (Table 53–6). Because benzene is toxic to bone marrow and liver, however, it has been replaced by toluene (methylbenzene) and aliphatic hydrocarbons, which nevertheless have toxicities of their own (19).

Toluene

Toluene is probably the most popular of the solvents abused and is also the best described. It is a common constituent of paints, paint and spot removers, varnishes, lacquers, adhesives (glues and cements), and transmission fluid (Table 53–7) (50).

Toluene is a hydrocarbon that is insoluble in water. On inhalation it is absorbed by the lungs and bound to lipoproteins. Toluene is metabolized in hepatic microsomes by oxidation to benzoic acid, which is conjugated with glycine to form hippuric acid and is eliminated by the kidneys (36).

The effects of toluene on the CNS may be depression or excitation, with euphoria in the induction phase followed by disorientation, tremulousness, mood lability, tinnitus, dysarthria, diplopia, pleasant hallucinations, and ataxia that may last from 1 to 2 hours (37). Large doses may produce seizures and coma (25).

Blood concentrations of toluene may be biphasic. An initial peak is followed by a trough, reflecting lipid binding by the CNS, and by subsequent slow release into the blood (50).

Long-term toluene abuse may cause certain symptom complexes such as muscle weakness; gastrointestinal complaints, including abdominal pain and hematemesis; and neuropsychiatric disorders, including an altered mental status, cerebellar abnormalities, and peripheral neuropathy (Table 53–8). Renal tubular damage has been noted in many individuals, with potassium, phosphorus, and bicarbonate wasting (39). Pyuria, hematuria, proteinuria, and membranous glomerulonephritis have also been described (50). Both hyperchloremic metabolic acidosis and an elevated anion gap metabolic acidosis have been noted with toluene sniffing (37,51). The latter is possibly secondary to accumulation of metabolites of toluene (36). Long-term exposure may also lead to hepatomegaly with impaired liver function. Aplastic anemia and severe erythroid hypoplasia may occur.

TABLE 53–7. *Compounds containing toluene*

Plastic cement
Model glue
Lacquer thinner
Shoe polish
Model cement
Acrylic spray paints
Acrylic paints
Indelible ink
Cleaning fluid

TABLE 53–8. *Clinical effects of toluene intoxication*

Gastrointestinal
Abdominal pain
Hematemesis
Central nervous system
Altered mental status
Cerebellar abnormalities
Peripheral neuropathy
Muscle weakness
Renal
Renal tubular acidosis
Pyuria
Hematuria
Proteinuria
Membranous glomerulonephritis
Electrolyte abnormalities
Hypokalemia
Hypophosphatemia
Hyperchloremic metabolic acidosis
Anion gap metabolic acidosis
Miscellaneous
Hepatomegaly
Aplastic anemia

The dose-related neurotoxicity of hydrocarbons, especially toluene, is known (52). The legally allowed maximum concentration of pure toluene vapor to which an individual may be exposed is 200 parts per million (ppm); at higher concentrations, fatigue, headache, paresthesias, and slowed reflexes appear. Exposure to concentrations greater than 600 ppm causes confusion or delirium. Long-term abusers are exposed to concentrations well above 1,000 ppm for prolonged periods and often to other compounds as well.

HALOGENATED HYDROCARBONS

Chlorinated or fluorinated hydrocarbons have been used for years as active compounds or inert solvents (16). The fluorinated hydrocarbons, or freons, have been implicated in many deaths from inhalation, but chlorinated hydrocarbons such as methylene chloride, trichloroethylene, and methylchloroform are also considered dangerous. As mentioned above, the most recent substance of popular abuse appears to be typewriter correction fluid (9).

The aliphatic fluorinated hydrocarbons are no longer widely used as propellants and refrigerants in over-the-counter preparations; they have been replaced by propane, isobutane, and carbon dioxide.

The halogenated hydrocarbons are potentially toxic to the lungs, bone marrow, liver, kidney, and heart. Dysrhythmias may be a significant problem after exposure to these agents.

Typewriter Correction Fluid

Typewriter correction fluid (Liquid Paper, Wite-Out, Snopake) is a solvent-containing liquid used to eradicate typing errors. The inhalation of these products is known as getting "whited out" (9,52). Most of these substances contain trichloroethylene, trichloroethane, or perchloroethylene either singly or in combination. These compounds are also used industrially as degreasers and solvents. Typewriter correction fluid is found in offices, schools, and hospitals (52). It is easily available in many retail outlets and is inexpensive to purchase. All three of the active agents have been associated with seizures, CNS depression, confusion, loss of consciousness, euphoria, and incoordination. In addition, trichloroethylene has been associated with visual disturbances, multiple nerve palsies, and peripheral neuropathies (30). Trichloroethylene and perchloroethylene have been associated with massive hepatic necrosis (9). These agents have caused cardiac dysrhythmias as a result of sensitization of myocardial tissue to epinephrine with subsequent ventricular fibrillation (52).

Many of the new typewriter correction fluids have been reformulated with mustard oil to discourage intentional inhalation (19).

Other Aliphatic Hydrocarbons

n-Hexane is a principal component of gasoline and naphtha fractions as well as over-the-counter glues and cements. Individuals who inhale the vapors of these products may therefore be exposed to high concentrations of this aliphatic agent. Severe peripheral neuropathy has been attributed to *n*-hexane (8,19). Other aliphatic hydrocarbons such as ethane, acetylene, propane, propylene, isobutane, butane, and isopentane are toxic to the heart and may produce narcosis.

GASOLINE

Gasoline sniffing was first noted in the 1950s and was most popular among teenagers in remote rural areas, where access to alcohol and other more commonly used drugs was restricted (39). Gasoline sniffing is more commonly performed by males than females and often begins during childhood; it is done in groups as a social activity along with friends or siblings (53). Fifteen to twenty breaths of gasoline vapor are sufficient to produce an intoxication that can last for 5 to 6 hours (19,53).

The toxicity of inhaled gasoline is complex because gasoline is a mixture of alkanes, cycloalkanes, alkenes, and aromatic hydrocarbons. The toxicity of gasoline is related to the composition of the mixture (4).

Benzene, a known bone marrow depressant, constitutes a small percentage of gasoline. Gasoline may also have organic lead as an ingredient. The most common organolead compound in gasoline is tetraethyl lead. Chronic inhalation of these compounds may lead to organolead intoxication. The symptomatology of organolead poisoning differs from that of inorganic lead poisoning and is discussed in Chapter 62.

ALCOHOLS, KETONES, AND ESTERS

Ketones are largely produced industrially from petrochemicals by dehydrogenation of two alcohols. They are widely used in industrial operations and are components of various household products. They are used as solvents for inks, paints, and resins, as intermediates in organic synthesis, and in some perfumes. Acetone, methyl-*n*-butyl ketone, methylisobutyl ketone, and methylethyl ketone are among the ketones abused by inhalation.

Methylethyl ketone, a highly volatile solvent, is a component in aerosolized paints and coatings, adhesives and cements, sealers, liquid holders, primers, lacquers, varnishes, and brush cleaners. It is abused because of its hypnotic effects, which are considered greater than those of ethanol (19). The ketones produce sharp irritation that is usually sufficient to prevent acute overexposure. Because of the irritating effects on the nose and mouth, the abuse of these agents is reduced. Both methyl-*n*-butyl ketone and methylethyl ketone may cause peripheral neuropathies.

ANESTHETIC AGENTS

Anesthetics commonly abused by inhalation include ether, chloroform and related gases, and nitrous oxide. Nitrous oxide is the most widely abused member of this class.

Nitrous oxide is produced from ammonium nitrate; extensive commercial purification removes toxic byproducts such as ammonia and oxides of nitrogen, principally nitric oxide and nitrogen dioxide (54). Nitrous oxide is an analgesic-anesthetic gas popularly known as "laughing gas." It has marked analgesic properties in subanesthetic concentrations. Its onset of action is rapid, and its effects disappear in 2 to 3 minutes. The populations at greatest risk for nitrous oxide include health professionals, particularly dentists; medical and dental students; and susceptible members of the general population (55).

Abuse of nitrous oxide was widespread for many years (56). It is a commonly used industrial agent, particularly in the food industry, because it is nonflammable and bacteriostatic and has no flavor. For these reasons, it has been used as a propellant in whipped cream dispensers. Inhalation of some of these pressurized sources without the use of reducing valves has led to alveolar rupture with dissection of the gas, resulting in pneumomediastinum (57). Other gases have replaced nitrous oxide as an aerosol propellant in most products.

Inhalation of 50% to 75% nitrous oxide produces an exhilarating "rush" within 15 to 30 seconds that is followed by a sense of euphoria and detachment for 2 to 3 minutes. The most common early symptom reported after inhalation is numbness or tingling of the extremities (Table 53–9). Some long-term abusers present with loss of finger dexterity, ataxia, and leg weakness. Ataxia may also be secondary to sensory loss. Neuropsychiatric symptoms such as depression, impaired memory, or confusion have been noted; these symptoms improve after cessation of abuse.

Nitrous oxide inactivates vitamin B_{12} by oxidizing it. Because this vitamin is a cofactor for enzymes involved in DNA synthesis, repeated exposure can cause suppression of mitotic activity of frequently dividing cells (6).

Chronic abusers may present with manifestations of vitamin B_{12} deficiency such as pernicious anemia, leukopenia with impaired white cell chemotaxis and phagocytosis, decreased sperm counts, and a sensorimotor peripheral polyneuropathy combined with posterior and lateral column signs of spinal cord involvement (7).

Polyneuropathies from the inhalation of nitrous oxide have been reported, although some signs suggest a possible cerebellar disorder (58). The neuropathology has been linked to the inactivation of vitamin B_{12}, which is the coenzyme for methionine synthesis. This neurologic disorder, which may be similar to subacute combined degeneration, includes early sensory complaints, loss of balance, impaired gait, impotence, and sphincter sensorimotor polyneuropathy often combined with signs of involvement of the posterior and lateral columns of the spinal cord. Vitamin B_{12} deficiency may also lead to megaloblastic anemia. In cases of nitrous oxide abuse, vitamin B_{12} and thiamine supplements may correct the mixed neuropathic abnormalities.

TABLE 53–9. *Signs and symptoms of nitrous oxide abuse*

Neurologic
Ataxia
Numbness or tingling of extremities
Loss of finger dexterity
Leg weakness
Impotence
Neuropsychiatric
Depression
Impaired memory
Confusion
Miscellaneous
Megaloblastic anemia

VOLATILE ALKYL NITRITES

The volatile alkyl nitrites, predominantly amyl, butyl, and isobutyl nitrite, are formed by combining the corresponding alcohol with sodium nitrite and sulfuric acid. They are powerful oxidizing agents and are also flammable. In the body, the nitrites are hydrolyzed to nitrite ion and the corresponding alcohol.

History of Nitrite Abuse

Amyl Nitrite

Amyl nitrite was introduced into medical practice as a coronary vasodilator more than a century ago (59). It has been abused since at least the 1930s, but recently it has been displaced by the organic nitrites.

Amyl nitrite is a yellowish, volatile, flammable liquid with a fruity odor (60). It is unstable and decomposes in the presence of air and light. Amyl nitrite has been marketed in fragile glass "perles." The glass is covered with a woven absorbent material, so that the perles can be safely crushed in the hand and the vapors from the liquid inhaled. The terms "snappers" and "poppers" are used for these agents because of the sound made by the perles when they are broken. Although amyl nitrite is rapidly absorbed through the lungs, gastric secretions decompose it, and it is thus ineffective when swallowed (59).

Isobutyl Nitrite

Because amyl nitrite perles are prescription items and somewhat difficult to obtain, new products have appeared and are sold at adult bookshops. These include various isomers of the nitrites (61). Since the late 1960s, butyl and isobutyl nitrite have been commercially available as "liquid incense" and "room deodorizers." Isobutyl nitrite is marketed in drug paraphernalia stores under such trade names as Rush, Bolt, Hardware, Quick Silver, and Satan's Scent (61,62).

Volatile nitrites are increasingly abused as stimulants, aphrodisiacs, and psychedelic agents. Currently available products are more than 90% nitrites and contain small quantities of the corresponding alcohol and vegetable oil to render them less volatile (29).

Clinical Effects of Nitrites

Alkyl nitrites produce relaxation of smooth muscle in vessels, including the coronary arteries, thereby produc-

TABLE 53–10. *Clinical effects of the alkyl nitrites*

Hypotension
Tachycardia
Nausea
Dizziness
Weakness
Syncope
Slowed perception of time
Headache
Methemoglobinemia

ing tachycardia; the meningeal vessels, thereby producing throbbing headache; and the subcutaneous vasculature, thereby producing a cutaneous blush in the upper torso and head (11). Increased intraocular pressure has also been noted. Hemodynamic effects of the nitrites include a decrease in blood pressure and an increase in heart rate within 10 seconds of inhalation (Table 53–10) (63). Nausea, dizziness, and weakness may also be noted as a result of the hypotension. Syncope, especially if the patient is standing, can occur. Peak effects occur within 30 seconds, with a return to normal by 90 seconds.

The perceived slowing of time, which is one of the drug's experienced effects, is what gave rise to a modest amount of its nonmedical use. For example, if the vapors are inhaled just before sexual climax, the sensation of orgasm is prolonged and allegedly enhanced (63).

Methemoglobin concentrations from inhalation of the volatile nitrites average less than 5% in normal individuals and are higher in reductase-deficient individuals (13,48). Inhaling isobutyl nitrite theoretically can lead to significant methemoglobin accumulation even in normal subjects if the exposure is intense or if inadequate time is allowed between inhalations for methemoglobin reduction. When the alkyl nitrites are ingested, however, they carry the risk of profound and potentially lethal methemoglobinemia (12,13,63).

Burns can result from hydrolysis of the nitrite to nitrous acid on the skin. The use of the alkyl nitrites can be dangerous in individuals with cerebral hemorrhage, recent head injury, hypotension, or glaucoma (47).

REFERENCES

1. Novak A: The deliberate inhalation of volatile substances. *J Psychedelic Drugs* 1980;12:105–122.
2. Anderson H, Dick B, Macnair R, et al: An investigation of 140 deaths associated with volatile substance abuse in the United Kingdom (1971–1981). *Hum Toxicol* 1982;1:207–221.
3. Sourindrhin I: Solvent misuse. *Br Med J* 1985;290:94–95.
4. Polkis A, Burkett C: Gasoline sniffing: a review. *Clin Toxicol* 1977;11:35–41.
5. Davies B, Thorley A, O'Connor D: Progression of addiction careers in young adult solvent misusers. *Br Med J* 1985;290:109–110.
6. Linden C: Volatile substances of abuse. *Emerg Med Clin North Am* 1990;8:559–578.
7. Miller N, Gold M: Organic solvent and aerosol abuse. *Am Fam Physician* 1991;44:183–189.
8. Edwards I: Solvent abuse. *N Z Med J* 1982;95:880–883.
9. Akerman H: The constitution of adhesives, and its relationship to solvent abuse. *Hum Toxicol* 1982;1:223–230.
10. Greer J: Adolescent abuse of typewriter correction fluid. *South Med J* 1984;77:297–298.
11. Garriott J, Petty C: Death from inhalant abuse: toxicological and pathological evaluation of 34 cases. *Clin Toxicol* 1980;16:305–315.
12. Shesser R, Mitchell J, Edelstein S: Methemoglobinemia from isobutyl nitrite preparations. *Ann Emerg Med* 1981;10:262–264.
13. Shesser R, Dixon D, Allen Y, et al: Fatal methemoglobinemia from isobutyl nitrite ingestion. *Ann Intern Med* 1980;92:131–132.
14. Seaman M: Barotrauma related to inhalational drug abuse. *J Emerg Med* 1990;8:141–149.
15. Alldredge B, Lowenstein D, Simon R: Seizures associated with recreational drug abuse. *Neurology* 1989;39:1037–1039.
16. Barnes G: Solvent abuse: a review. *Int J Addict* 1979;14:1–26.
17. Goldfrank L, Kirstein R, Bresnitz E: Gasoline and other hydrocarbons. *Hosp Physician* 1979;15:32–38.
18. Saxena K: Glue sniffing and other deliriants. *Top Emerg Med* 1985;7:55–62.
19. Prockop L: Neurotoxic volatile substances. *Neurology* 1979; 29:862–865.
20. Beebe D, Walley E: Substance abuse: the designer drugs. *Am Fam Physician* 1991;43:1689–1698.
21. Jerrard D: "Designer drugs"—a current perspective. *J Emerg Med* 1990;8:733–741.
22. Coulehan J, Hirsch W, Brittman J, et al: Gasoline sniffing and lead toxicity in Navajo adolescents. *Pediatrics* 1983;71:113–117.
23. Francis J, Murray V, Ruprah M, et al: Suspected solvent abuse in cases referred to the poisons unit, Guy's hospital, July 1980–June 1981. *Hum Toxicol* 1982;1:271–280.
24. Kirk L, Anderson R, Martin K: Sudden death from toluene abuse. *Ann Emerg Med* 1984;13:68–69.
25. Taher S, Anderson R, McCartney R, et al: Renal tubular acidosis associated with toluene "sniffing." *N Engl J Med* 1974;290:765–768.
26. Boon N: Solvent abuse and the heart. *Br Med J* 1987;294:722.
27. Reinhardt C, Azor A, Maxfield M, et al: Cardiac arrhythmias and aerosol "sniffing." *Arch Environ Health* 1971;22:265–279.
28. Clark D, Tinston D: Acute inhalation toxicity of some halogenated and non-halogenated hydrocarbons. *Hum Toxicol* 1982;1:239–247.
29. Wason S, Setsky A, Platt O, et al: Isobutyl nitrite toxicity by ingestion. *Ann Intern Med* 1980;92:637–638.
30. King M, Day R, Oliver J, et al: Solvent encephalopathy. *Br Med J* 1981;283:663–665.
31. King M: Neurological sequelae of toluene abuse. *Hum Toxicol* 1982;1:281–287.
32. Cordes D, Brown W, Quinn K: Chemically induced hepatitis after inhaling organic solvents. *West J Med* 1988;148:458–460.
33. Mizutani T, Oohashi N, Naito H: Myoglobinemia and renal failure in toluene poisoning: a case report. *Vet Hum Toxicol* 1989;31:448–449.
34. Ron M: Volatile substance abuse: a review of possible long-term neurological, intellectual and psychiatric sequelae. *Br J Psychiatry* 1986;148:235–246.
35. Hormes J, Filley C, Rosenberg N: Neurologic sequelae of chronic solvent vapor abuse. *Neurology* 1986;36:698–702.
36. Streicher H, Gabow P, Moss A, et al: Syndromes of toluene sniffing in adults. *Ann Intern Med* 1981;94:758–762.
37. Patel R: Renal disease associated with toluene inhalation. *Clin Toxicol* 1486;24:213–223.
38. O'Brien E, Yeoman W, Hobby J: Hepatorenal damage from toluene in a "glue sniffer." *Br Med J* 1971;2:29–30.
39. Moss M. Cooper P: Gasoline sniffing and lead poisoning. *Acta Pharmacol Toxicol* 1986;59:48–51.
40. Boeckx R, Postl B, Coodin F: Gasoline sniffing tetraethyl lead poisoning in children. *Pediatrics* 1977;60:140–145.
41. Hanson K, Sharp F: Gasoline sniffing, lead poisoning, and myoclonus. *JAMA* 1978;240:1375–1376.
42. Law W, Nelson E: Gasoline sniffing by an adult: report of a case with the unusual complication of lead encephalopathy. *JAMA* 1968; 204:1002–1004.
43. Seshia S, Rajani K, Boeckx R, et al: The neurological manifestations of chronic inhalation of leaded gasoline. *Dev Med Child Neurol* 1978;2:323–324.

44. Valpey R, Sumi S, Corass M, et al: Acute and chronic progressive encephalopathy due to gasoline sniffing. *Neurology* 1978;28: 507–510.
45. Schwartz R: Urine testing in the detection of drugs of abuse. *Arch Intern Med* 1988;148:2407–2412.
46. Ramsay J, Flanagan R: The role of the laboratory in the investigation of solvent abuse. *Hum Toxicol* 1982;1:299–311.
47. Munjack D: Sex and drugs. *Clin Toxicol* 1979;15:75–89.
48. Horne M, Waterman M, Simon L, et al: Methemoglobinemia from sniffing butyl nitrite. *Ann Intern Med* 1979;91:417–418.
49. Skinner M, Thompson D: Pharmacologic considerations in the treatment of substance abuse. *South Med J* 1992;85:1207–1219.
50. Cohr K. Stokholm J: Toluene: a toxicologic review.*Scand J Work Environ Health* 1979;5:71–90.
51. Fischman C, Oster J: Toxic effects of toluene: a new cause of high anion gap metabolic acidosis. *JAMA* 1979;241:1713–1715.
52. King G, Smialek J, Troutman W: Sudden death in adolescents resulting from inhalation of typewriter correction fluid. *JAMA* 1985; 253:1604–1606.
53. Edminster S, Bayer M: Recreational gasoline sniffing: acute gasoline intoxication and latent organolead poisoning. *J Emerg Med* 1985; 3:365–370.
54. Sterman A, Coyle P: Subacute toxic delirium following nitrous oxide abuse. *Arch Neurol* 1983;40:446–447.
55. Rosenberg H, Orkin F, Springhead J: *Anesth Analg* 1979;58:104–106.
56. Layzer R: Myeloneuropathy after prolonged exposure to nitrous oxide. *Lancet* 1978;2:1227–1230.
57. LiPuma J, Wellman J, Stern H Nitrous oxide abuse: a new cause for pneumomediastinum. *Radiology* 1982;145:602.
58. Layzer R, Fishman R, Schafer J: Neuropathy following abuse of nitrous oxide. *Neurology* 1978;28:504–506.
59. Cohen S: The volatile nitrites. *JAMA* 1979;241:2077–2078.
60. Haley T: Review of the physiological effects of amyl, butyl, and isobutyl nitrites. *Clin Toxicol* 1980;16:317–329.
61. Fisher A, Brancaccio R, Jelinek J: Facial dermatitis in men due to inhalation of butyl nitrite. *Cutis* 1981;27:146–153.
62. Smith M, Stair T, Rolnick M: Butyl nitrite and a suicide attempt. *Ann Intern Med* 1980;92:719–720.
63. Dixon D, Reisch R, Santinga P: Fatal methemoglobinemia resulting from ingestion of isobutyl nitrite, a "room odorizer" widely used for recreational purposes. *J Forensic Sci* 1981;26:587–593.

ADDITIONAL SELECTED REFERENCES

Barnes G, Vulcano B: Bibliography of the solvent abuse literature. *Int J Addict* 1979;14:401–421.

Blyth A: Solvent abuse: summary of a paper presented on behalf of the DHSS. *Hum Toxicol* 1982;1:347–349.

Cherry N, McArthy T, Waldron H: Solvent sniffing in industry. *Hum Toxicol* 1982;1;289–292.

Dossing M, Aren-Soborg P, Petersen L, et al: Liver damage associated with occupational exposure to organic solvents in house painters. *Eur J Clin Invest* 1983;13:151–157.

Evans M: Solvent misuse; educational implications. *Hum Toxicol* 1982;1:337–343.

Gay M, Meller R, Stanley S: Drug abuse monitoring: a survey of solvent abuse in the county of Avon. *Hum Toxicol* 1982;1:257–263.

Hershey C, Miller S: Solvent abuse: a shift to adults. *Int J Addict* 1982;17:1085–1089.

Jones R, Winter D: Two case reports of deaths on industrial premises attributed to 1,1,1-trichloroethane. *Arch Environ Health* 1983;38:59–61.

Kalf G, Post G, Snyder R: Solvent toxicology: recent advances in the toxicology of benzene, the glycol ethers, and carbon tetrachloride. *Annu Rev Pharmacol Toxicol* 1987;27:299–327.

Klein B, Simon J: Hydrocarbon poisonings. *Pediatr Clin North Am* 1986;33:411–419.

Lewis J, Moritz D, Mellis L: Long-term toluene abuse. *Am J Psychiatry* 1981;138:368–370.

Lindstrom K: Behavioral effects of long-term exposure to organic solvents. *Acta Neurol Scand* 1982;66:131–141.

Lynn E, Walter R, Harris L, et al: Nitrous oxide: it's a gas. *J Psychedelic Drugs* 1972;5:1–7.

Massengale O, Glaser H, LeLievre R, et al: Physical and psychologic factors in glue sniffing. *N Engl J Med* 1963;269:1340–1344.

McLeod A, Marjot R, Monaghan M, et al: Chronic cardiac toxicity after inhalation of 1,1,1-trichloroethane. *Br Med J* 1987;294:727–729.

Messina F, Wynne J: Homemade nitrous oxide: no laughing matter. *Ann Intern Med* 1982;96:333–334.

O'Conner D: The use of suggestion techniques with adolescents in the treatment of glue sniffing and solvent abuse. *Hum Toxicol* 1982;1:313–320.

Oliver J, Watson J. Abuse of solvents "for kicks." *Lancet* 1977;1:84–86.

Panson R, Winek C: Aspiration toxicity of ketones. *Clin Toxicol* 1980;17:271–317.

Ramsay A: Solvent abuse: an educational perspective. *Hum Toxicol* 1982;1:265–270.

Riihimaki V, Pfaffli P: Percutaneous absorption of solvent vapors in man. *Scand J Work Environ Health* 1978;4:73–85.

Roberts D: Abuse of aerosol products by inhalation. *Hum Toxicol* 1982;1:231–238.

Skuse D, Burrell S: A review of solvent abusers and their management by a child psychiatric out-patient service. *Hum Toxicol* 1982;1:321–329.

Tarsh M: Schizophreniform psychosis caused by sniffing toluene. *J Soc Occup Med* 1979;29:131–133.

Watson J: Morbidity and mortality statistics on solvent abuse. *Med Sci Law* 1979;19:246–252.

Watson J: Solvent abuse: presentation and clinical diagnosis. *Hum Toxicol* 1982;1:249–256.

Woodcock J: Solvent abuse from a health education perspective. *Hum Toxicol* 1982;1:331–336.

CHAPTER 54

Hallucinogens

Hallucinogens, also known as psychedelic drugs, are chemicals that produce changes in perception, thought, and mood. These drugs are also referred to as psychomimetic agents, psycholytics, or psychotogens and include lysergic acid diethylamide (LSD), morning glory seeds, mescaline, psilocybin, and some of the "designer drugs" (1,2). Hallucinogens can be derived from natural products or produced synthetically. Although tetrahydrocannabinol, the psychoactive ingredient in marijuana, may cause hallucinations or illusions, these properties are not noted in the typical dosage that is smoked. Marijuana is discussed in Chapter 55.

HALLUCINOGENIC SUBSTANCES: GENERAL CONSIDERATIONS

Substances in this group are perhaps more properly called "illusionogenic" because they produce a distortion of an actual stimulus rather than create a new stimulus where none exists (1).

Mechanism of Action

All the hallucinogenic agents affect the pons, which is the bridge between the higher and lower cortical centers. The mechanism by which the hallucinogens produce psychedelic action is not known, although they appear to interact with serotonin synapses (1). The emotional response to a hallucinogen can vary from an ecstatic, blissful feeling to a miserable, hopeless dysphoria.

Actions

The hallucinogens produce a flooding of sensation by inhibiting the usual dampening of sensory input. There is a heightened awareness of colors, sounds, and textures, distortion of object contours, a diminished sense of reality, increased suggestibility, and occasionally a sense of anxiety or panic. Distortion of ego functions causes depersonalization. Subjective time appears to be slowed. Illusions are common, but true hallucinations are infrequent (3). Changes in self-image are substantial. Overflow from one sensory modality to another, or synesthesia, may occur, so that the user may "hear" colors or "feel" sounds. Hallucinations of this type are not typically encountered in any form of functional psychosis (4).

Toxicity

The uncomplicated hallucinogenic experience rarely comes to the attention of the physician (5). It is the untoward effects such as acute anxiety, panic, and psychotic episodes that bring the user to the emergency department. Death due directly to an unadulterated hallucinogen is infrequent. When it has occurred, it is usually accidental and a result of misinterpretation of the environment.

Diagnosis and Treatment

Diagnosis of hallucinogen intoxication is generally based on a history of recent ingestion along with appropriate symptomatology.

An individual under the influence of a hallucinogenic drug is in a state of extreme hypersensitivity, and a hostile environment is harmful. Most cases of hallucinogen intoxication resolve without incident (5). Panic, acute anxiety, and psychotic episodes may require some form of therapy. Psychological support and reassurance can be helpful for the individual experiencing a "bad trip." A quiet environment is usually sufficient to reduce the dysphoria. The patient should not be left alone but be accompanied by someone familiar or who can provide reassurance. Usually after a period of observation the patient improves (1). For severe agitation, minor tranquilizers such as diazepam may be used. Major tranquilizers such as haloperidol should be reserved for the most disturbed and agitated patients. Attempts at gastrointestinal decontamination will probably not be useful if the patient is already symptomatic (1). "Flashbacks" should be managed by support and reassurance (6).

Withdrawal

A withdrawal syndrome does not occur with hallucinogenic drugs, and physical dependence has not been reported.

TYPES OF HALLUCINOGENS

Indolalkylamines

The indolalkylamines comprise the prototypical drug LSD, psilocybin, and psilocin.

Lysergic Acid Diethylamide

LSD is the most commonly abused drug in the indolalkylamine class. It was first synthesized in the 1930s from the ergot fungus that grows in heads of rye and wheat and from morning glory seeds. This compound was discovered accidentally when a European chemist tasted a small amount of the fungus extract and experienced hallucinogenic effects. It is the most potent psychoactive drug known, producing effects at doses as low as 20 μg (7).

How Supplied

LSD is a colorless, tasteless substance usually sold in the form of capsules or pills, as a white powder, in thin squares or gelatin ("windowpane"), and in liquid form absorbed onto paper ("blotter acid"), or sugar cubes. The amount of the drug in each dose may vary greatly. Although LSD can be found in naturally occurring ergot, most of the drug that is currently used is synthetic and derived from ergonovine (8).

Pharmacokinetics

The dose of LSD that produces hallucinogenic effects is 100 to 250 μg (1 to 2 μg/kg), which usually produces an experience lasting 8 to 12 hours. Effects usually begin 20 minutes to 1 hour after ingestion and peak at 2 to 3 hours. LSD is 100 times more potent than psilocybin and 4,000 times more potent than mescaline in producing altered states of consciousness.

Clinical Effects

LSD affects both the sympathetic and parasympathetic nervous system, but sympathetic activities predominate. Initial physical symptoms are sympathomimetic in nature and include mydriasis, hypertension, hyperthermia, tachycardia, and piloerection. Psychological effects soon follow (9).

TABLE 54–1. *Signs and symptoms of LSD*

Sympathomimetic
Mydriasis
Hypertension
Hyperthermia
Tachycardia
Piloerection
Psychological
Synesthesia
Short attention span
Ego detachment
Flashbacks

Although LSD acts on the auditory, tactile, olfactory, and gustatory senses, the most marked effects are visual (Table 54–1). Colors of objects are perceived as more intense than usual, and fixed objects seem to undulate and flow. Because of the disruption of neuronal mechanisms that inhibit sensory input, the user is unable to experience stable, clear sensations. Synesthesia occurs, the attention span is short, and the user may experience poor judgment. Ego dissolution and detachment may occur, and experiences may seem to have increased meaningfulness (8).

Toxicity and Treatment

LSD has low toxicity, and deaths due directly to overdose have not been reported (1). Fatalities are usually secondary to trauma incurred when users attempt unreasonable feats. The greatest danger from the use of LSD and related drugs is to borderline psychotic and depressed patients because suicide and prolonged psychotic behavior have been precipitated in some groups.

Pharmacotherapy of the LSD-intoxicated individual is usually unnecessary. For severe agitation in which patients may be a danger to themselves, diazepam is recommended. Haloperidol may be used in cases of extreme agitation or hallucinosis. Phenothiazines have been advocated in the past for the treatment of LSD delirium, but because of reported adverse reactions they are no longer recommended.

Flashbacks

A "flashback," or the recurrence of some aspect of the hallucinogenic experience days to months after ingestion of the hallucinogen, is another characteristic of LSD. The phenomenon of flashbacks is not completely understood. Users describe flashbacks as transient, spontaneous recurrences of a previous hallucinogenic experience after a period of apparent normalcy. The effects are usually unpleasant and often involve visual distortions and altered self-perception (8). Flashbacks appear to occur more frequently in those who previously experienced a "bad trip." There is no set pattern of frequency or intensity of flashbacks. Ordinarily they tend to disappear with time and reassurance if the drug is not taken again (5).

Morning Glory Seeds

Morning glory seeds are from the *Ipomoea* species and have been abused for their hallucinogenic potential. The seeds contain lysergic acid–like compounds which are similar to LSD. Commercially purchased seeds for garden use are coated with a noxious fungicide, which allegedly dissuades prospective abusers from ingesting large quantities.

The number of seeds necessary to achieve the desired effects will vary, but in general, the greater the number of seeds, the greater the effect. Typically, a user may ingest 20 to 400 seeds, and the effects may take up to 3 hours to manifest.

Treatment should consist of supportive care and sedation, if necessary.

Psilocybin

Psilocybin and psilocin ("magic Mexican mushroom," "silly putty") are derived from several species of mushrooms, notably *Psilocybe mexicana*, which has been used for centuries in Native American ceremonies. Other mushrooms in the genera *Panaeolus* and *Conocybe* also contain these agents. Psilocin and psilocybin are chemically related to LSD.

Psilocybin is the phosphorylated ester of psilocin (4-hydroxydimethyltryptamine). After psilocybin is ingested the phosphoric acid is removed, producing psilocin. Psilocin and psilocybin are 100 to 200 times less potent than LSD. Both substances are found in various hallucinogenic substances (5).

The hallucinations and distortions of time and space produced by these two drugs are similar to those produced by LSD, but the duration of action is much shorter, between 2 and 4 hours. A dose of 20 to 60 mg produces effects similar to those of LSD. Usually one or two dried mushrooms are ingested to produce the psychedelic effects. CNS effects include an initial anxiety followed by a dreamy state, visual distortions, and feelings of depersonalization. Treatment is supportive (see Chapter 70).

Phenylisopropylamines

Compounds in this class are more numerous than the indolalkylamines and include hundreds of natural and synthetic compounds (5).

TABLE 54–2. *Signs and symptoms of mescaline*

Nausea
Vomiting
Ataxia
Nystagmus
Altered sensations
Sight
Smell
Touch
Hearing

Mescaline and Peyote

The main representatives of the phenylethylamine group are mescaline (3,4,5-trimethoxyphenylethylamine) and peyote, which are derived from the Mexican peyote cactus (*Lophophora williamsii*) once used in religious ceremonies by the Aztecs. The peyote cactus is common to the Southwestern United States and Mexico; it has a small crown, a long root, and small pink or red flowers. The crown is cut from the cactus and dried to form a hard brown disk; this is frequently referred to as a mescal "button," which is the street name for mescaline. Each button contains from 6 to 45 mg of mescaline.

Mescaline is the least active of the hallucinogens and a close chemical relative of epinephrine. It achieves its effects by stimulating adenylate cyclase activity at central dopaminergic receptors in anterior limbic structures. The effects of mescaline cannot be differentiated from those of LSD, but LSD is approximately 4,000 to 5,000 times more potent than mescaline.

Mescaline is usually ingested orally in doses of 300 to 500 mg. The drug is completely absorbed from the gastrointestinal tract, and effects appear 1 to 2 hours after ingestion, peak at 5 to 6 hours, and may last 8 to 12 hours. Besides the psychedelic effects, nausea and vomiting occur 30 to 60 minutes after ingestion with subsequent mydriasis, hyperreflexia, ataxia, nystagmus, and tremors. Psychological effects are essentially identical to those of LSD and may include altered sensations of sight, smell, touch, and hearing. (Table 54–2). There is less mental reorganization with mescaline than with LSD.

REFERENCES

1. Strassman R: Adverse reactions to psychedelic drugs. *J Nerv Ment Dis* 1984;172;577–595.
2. Sternbach G, Varon J: "Designer drugs": recognizing and managing their toxic effects. *Postgrad Med* 1992;91:169–176.
3. Harrison D, Walls R: "Cotton fever": a benign febrile syndrome in intravenous drug abusers. *J Emerg Med* 1990;8:135–139.
4. Sloan M, Kittner S, Rigamonti D, et al: Occurrence of stroke associated with use/abuse of drugs. *Neurology* 1991;41:1358–1364.
5. Cohen S: The hallucinogens and the inhalants. *Pediatr Clin North Am* 1984;7:681–688.
6. Beebe D, Walley E: Substance abuse: the designer drugs. *Am Fam Physician* 1991;43:1689–1698.
7. Kulig K: LSD. *Emerg Med Clin North Am* 1990;8:551–557

8. Behan W, Bakheit A, Behan P, et al: The muscle findings in the neuroleptic malignant syndrome associated with lysergic acid diethylamide. *J Neurol Neurosurg Psychiatry* 1991;54:741–743.
9. Maslanka A, Scott S: LSD overdose in an eight-month old boy. *J Emerg Med* 1992;10:481–483.

ADDITIONAL SELECTED REFERENCES

Genest K, Farmilo C: The identification and determination of lysergic acid diethylamide in narcotic seizures. *J Pharm Pharmacol* 1964; 16:250–257.

Greenland S, Staisch K, Brown N, et al: The effects of marijuana during pregnancy. *Am J Obstet Gynecol* 1982;143:408–413.

Satinder K, Black A: Cannabis use and sensation-seeking orientation. *J Psychol* 1984;116:105–105.

Schwartz R, Hawks R: Laboratory detection of marijuana use. *JAMA* 1985;254:788–792.

Wert R, Raulin M: The chronic cerebral effects of cannabis use: part I: methodological issues and neurological findings. *Int J Addict* 1986; 21:605–628.

Wert R, Raulin M: The chronic cerebral effects of cannabis use: part II: psychological findings and conclusion. *Int J Addict* 1986;21: 629–642.

CHAPTER 55

Marijuana

Marijuana is an ancient drug that was first described as early as 2700 BC (1,2). It is the most widely abused drug in American society after tobacco, alcohol, and caffeine (3,4); and it is the most commonly used illegal substance in the United States. Its use has increased dramatically in the United States during the last decade. Marijuana and related drugs are sedative-hypnotics, tranquilizers, hallucinogens, or narcotics. Although they have properties in common with all these classes of drugs, they are in a class by themselves.

The name marijuana is derived from the Mexican Spanish word *maraguana*, which is a general term indicating any substance that can cause intoxication, but refers specifically to a mixture of cut, dried, and ground flowers, leaves, and stems of the leafy green hemp plant *Cannabis sativa*. Marijuana is the principal drug produced from the hemp plant, although biochemists have identified approximately 400 drug constituents in the plant resin. Approximately 60 are known collectively as the cannabinoids. Of these, delta-9-tetrahydrocannabinol (THC) is by far the most active and is considered the main psychoactive agent in marijuana. Although the concentration of THC in a plant depends on genetic and environmental factors, selective breeding now yields marijuana with a much higher concentration than was previously available (5). THC is a lipid-soluble, water-insoluble compound. It has been synthesized, but because it is expensive to produce, material sold on the street as synthetic THC is likely to be phencyclidine, mescaline, LSD, or other drugs.

Marijuana is frequently classified as a hallucinogen, but these effects are not noted at the doses most commonly taken. The cannabinoids in marijuana have a multitude of effects, including psychotropic, hypnotic, tranquilizing, antiemetic, anticonvulsant, and analgesic effects. They also lower intraocular pressure, increase the appetite, and affect the cardiovascular, respiratory, reproductive, and immune systems.

Marijuana is prepared from all portions of the *Cannabis* plant that are capable of producing psychoactive effects (the stems and seeds are virtually inactive). The most potent type of marijuana is sinsemilla, which is prepared from unpollinated female hemp plants (5). In general, the concentration of THC in marijuana is 1% to 2%.

Hashish is a concentrated preparation of the resinous secretions collected from the flowering tops and leaves of high-quality hemp plants. The resin is dried and compressed into balls or cakes (2). The concentration of THC in hashish is 5% to 15%.

The potency of drug-quality marijuana has been steadily increasing, averaging 3.65% THC in 1987 versus 1.5% THC a decade ago. Sinsemilla, the highly potent seedless variety of marijuana preferred by many users, averages 7% THC; as such, it is approximately twice as potent as the hashish available in the U.S. (6).

METHODS OF ADMINISTRATION

Smoking

Marijuana is typically rolled into a cigarette (called a "joint") and smoked. The amount of THC per puff varies widely and increases toward the butt of the marijuana cigarette. The average marijuana cigarette weighs 0.5 to 1 g and may contain 20 to 35 mg of THC. Approximately 25% to 50% of the THC content is delivered to the lungs and brain, and approximately 25% collects in the butt of the cigarette (known as a "roach"). The remainder is destroyed by pyrolysis. Sidestream smoke losses of 40% to 50% and pyrolytic destruction of 23% to 30% of the active drug have been documented. Water pipes (bongs) or regular pipes may also be used (7).

Usual effects after inhalation are noted within 5 to 10 minutes of smoking, reach a peak within 20 minutes, and may last for 2 to 3 hours. Intrapatient variability in smoking dynamics contributes to the uncertainty in dose delivery. The number, duration, and spacing of puffs, hold time, and inhalation volume greatly influence the degree of drug exposure (Table 55–1) (8).

Ingestion

Marijuana and hashish may be ingested orally in brownies or other foods. With oral ingestion there is usually a delay in the onset of symptoms from 30 minutes to more than 2 hours. Effects from oral ingestion are more

Table 55–1. *Pharmacokinetics of marijuana*

Absorption	
Inhalation	10% to 50%
Oral	1% to 10%
Peak levels	
Inhalation	7 to 8 min
Oral	45 min
Peak effect	
Inhalation	20 to 30 min
Oral	2 to 3 hours
Vd	10 liters per kg
Protein binding	>99%
Metabolism	Hepatic microsomal enzymes hydroxylate delta-9-THC to various alcohols (some active), Which are then metabolized by dehydrogenase to inactive end products.
Elimination	
Urine	13% to 16% after 3 days
Feces	30% to 50% after 3 days
Plasma elimination half-life	
Non-user	25-57 hours
Chronic user	20-28 hours

prolonged than those from smoking but are usually not as intense. This is in part due to decreased bioavailability after oral ingestion.

METABOLISM

Because THC is lipid-soluble, once it enters the bloodstream it is distributed to organs and fatty tissue and readily enters the brain. Inhaled THC is not excreted by the lungs, in contrast to volatile inhalants.

THC undergoes a complex and extensive transformation in the body, and less than 0.2% of the dose is excreted unchanged. It is stored in body fat, where it has a half-life of 7 to 8 days (9). Approximately two thirds of the cannabinoid metabolites are excreted in the feces and the remainder in the urine. Urinary metabolites consist primarily of delta-9-carboxy-THC and 11-hydroxy-delta-9-THC, the latter of which is oxidized to 11-nor-delta-9-carboxylic acid. There are also some 20 other similar acid metabolites, whose concentrations may remain high enough to be detected in some individuals up to 30 days after the last use.

Because of the long half-life of THC and its metabolites, repeated use of marijuana or hashish at intervals shorter than the half-life (7 to 8 days) results in accumulation in the body tissues.

CLINICAL EFFECTS

General Considerations

The quality, intensity, and duration of effects from marijuana and related substances are influenced by many factors, including the route and speed of administration, the experience of the user, the social setting, and the potency of the preparation. Users report feelings of relaxation and well-being, mild euphoria, relief of anxiety, heightened sexual arousal, and a keen sense of hearing (Table 55–2). The senses of taste, touch, and smell may seem to be enhanced or altered. Ideas may appear to be disconnected, rapid flowing, and altered in emphasis and importance. Time seems to pass slowly, with little activity needed and no sense of boredom. Individuals often spend long periods listening to music or reading. Increased desire to eat, especially sweets, is characteristic of the individual under the influence of marijuana. Short-term memory, learning ability, and psychomotor performance may be impaired after long-term use (9).

Cardiovascular Effects

Marijuana exposure produces rapid changes in some physiologic effects. The most constant cardiovascular effect of marijuana is sinus tachycardia with increased peripheral blood flow probably mediated by β-adrenergic stimulation. Continuous EKG monitoring has demonstrated increased heart rate soon after smoking. Maximum heart rates have been noted within 4 minutes of the last inhalation. The sinus tachycardia is dose-dependent and may be blocked by propranolol, suggesting a sympathetic nervous system response. Blood pressure is not altered significantly. Premature atrial contractions, premature ventricular contractions, T wave and S-T segment changes, P wave and second-degree heart block may occur with acute and chronic marijuana use. The actual frequency of these EKG abnormalities is not known.

Ocular Effects

Conjunctivitis may be noted after the use of marijuana from engorgement of the blood vessels in the eye (5). This effect appears to be dose-related. Pupillary changes

TABLE 55–2. *Clinical effects of marijuana*

Psychological
Relaxation
Feeling of well-being
Heightened sexual arousal
Craving for sweets
Cardiovascular
Sinus tachycardia
Ocular
Conjunctivitis
Decreased intraocular pressure
Respiratory
Bronchodilation
Miscellaneous
Antiemetic

tend to be mild and inconsistent. THC has been noted to decrease intraocular pressure.

Respiratory Effects

Other physiologic effects of marijuana use include bronchodilation (10). Whereas the delta-9-THC in smoked marijuana initially relaxes airway smooth muscle in both healthy persons and stable asthmatic patients, causing bronchodilation, this bronchodilator effect is relatively short-lived and diminishes with the repeated use of marijuana. In contrast to its acute bronchodilator effect, regular marijuana smoking has been shown to cause abnormal decrements in lung function, most likely due to damaging effects on airways having long-term exposure to noxious components within the smoke (11).

Contamination of marijuana with *Aspergillus fumigatus* can cause lung disease and an allergic bronchopulmonary aspergillosis as well as an invasive *Aspergillus* pneumonitis in patients with impaired immunity (12).

Miscellaneous Effects

At the usual doses there are no constant effects on respiration or body temperature (13). THC has been shown to be an effective antiemetic in patients receiving cancer chemotherapy.

Pneumomediastinum has been reported to occur after marijuana smoking. This was most likely caused by increased intrathoracic pressure due to Valsalva maneuvers during the breath-holding after deep inhalation of the smoke, leading to alveolar rupture with dissection of air along the vessels and bronchi to the mediastinum.

Hydrocarbon components within the smoke of marijuana, like that of tobacco, can induce hepatic mixed oxidases to accelerate the metabolic clearance of theophylline. As a consequence, the serum theophylline half-life is shortened in habitual marijuana smokers receiving theophylline.

TOXICITY

A novice user may experience fearfulness, confusion, and panic attacks. This is especially true if the setting is unfamiliar. Psychologically predisposed individuals are more susceptible to these adverse reactions. High doses may produce such a state even in experienced users.

Although high doses can induce disorientation, delusion, feelings of paranoia, and frank hallucinations, these effects are rarely noted in the United States because the concentrations of THC necessary to induce them are not usually found in marijuana grown in or brought into this country (14). At the usual doses there is little cognitive or motor dysfunction, but the drug may affect the ability to drive or operate machinery safely.

EFFECTS OF LONG-TERM USE

Heavy smokers of marijuana may experience varying degrees of respiratory tract irritation leading to bronchitis, pharyngitis, sinusitis, and uvular edema (Table 55–3). In addition, there may be a reduction in testosterone levels and some degree of suppression of the immune system (15). Marijuana cigarettes do not contain filters and generate about twice as much tar as tobacco per unit of weight, assuming a similar smoking profile. Marijuana smoke contains larger amounts of carcinogenic hydrocarbons than tobacco smoke, and this may be a problem in long-term heavy users. The techniques for smoking marijuana and tobacco differ substantially: on the average, with marijuana the inhalation, or "puff" volume is about two thirds larger, the depth of smoke inhalation about 40% greater, and breath-holding about four times longer than those characteristic of tobacco smoking. These differences in filtration and smoking technique can result in about a fourfold greater amount of tar delivered to and retained in the lungs from the smoking of marijuana than from a comparable amount of tobacco, thus potentially amplifying the harmful effects of marijuana on the lungs. Although THC freely crosses the placental barrier and is distributed to the fetus, at present there is no sound evidence to indicate that THC causes genetic abnormalities in humans. Most individuals who use marijuana in moderation for a time are unlikely to suffer any lasting harmful effects (16). The available evidence suggests strongly that there are no gross structural or neurologic defects attributable to the use of marijuana, and current research does not support the contention that use results in permanent cerebral impairment.

Physical and psychological dependence on marijuana and related substances are suggested but not documented in numerous reports (17). Although there may not be a true withdrawal syndrome after cessation of smoking and although physical dependence has not been documented in long-term heavy users, irritability, restlessness, nervousness, and insomnia have been noted in individuals who abruptly discontinue use (4,18).

MARIJUANA AND PARAQUAT

A number of years ago there was some concern that the herbicide paraquat, which was sprayed on marijuana

TABLE 55–3. *Long-term effects of marijuana*

Bronchitis
Pharyngitis
Sinusitus
Uvular edema
Reduced testosterone levels

fields in Mexico, would lead to poisoning of marijuana users. Despite the fact that paraquat was detected on marijuana from sprayed fields, lung damage, the major manifestation of paraquat poisoning, has not been reported in human cases (19). This is probably because paraquat is changed by pyrolysis to bipyridine, a nontoxic by-product (19,20).

LABORATORY ANALYSIS

The most widely used techniques for measuring marijuana in samples include immunoassay, gas chromatography, gas chromatography with mass spectrometry, thin-layer chromatography, and high-performance liquid chromatography (21). The two most widely used screening procedures are enzyme immunoassay and radioimmunoassay. With few exceptions, the specimen used to test for marijuana is urine.

Plasma concentrations of THC reach a maximum within 1 hour after marijuana is smoked and fall rapidly to about one-tenth the peak plasma concentrations shortly thereafter (5). The metabolites of THC that account for a positive urine test may remain in the body for up to 21 to 30 days after the last dose in a long-term heavy user (5). This is because THC is stored in adipose tissues of long-term users and is released back into the circulation (22). In the occasional user, a urine test may be positive for several days up to 1 week after a single exposure, depending on the method of screening.

TREATMENT

Treatment of effects from the use of marijuana and related substances is usually limited to supportive care. Treatment of panic and paranoid episodes depends on the characteristics and severity of the episode. Reassurance is usually sufficient to calm a distressed patient. Medicating the patient is usually not necessary.

REFERENCES

1. Strassman R: Adverse reactions to psychedelic drugs. *J Nerv Ment Dis* 1984;172;577–595.
2. Tashkin D, Soares J, Hepler R, et al: Cannabis,1977. *Ann Intern Med* 1978;89:539–549.
3. Charles R, Holt S, Kirkham N: Myocardial infarction and marijuana. *Clin Toxicol* 1979;14:433–438.
4. Millman R, Shriglio R: Patterns of use and psychopathology in chronic marijuana users. *Psychiatr Clin North Am* 1986;9:533–545.
5. Schwartz R: Marijuana; a crude drug with a spectrum of underappreciated toxicity. *Pediatrics* 1984;73:455–458.
6. Schwartz R, Gruenewald P, Klitzner M, et al: Short-term memory impairment in cannabis-dependent adolescents. *Am J Dis Child* 1989;143:1214–1219.
7. Huestis M, Sampson A, Holicky B, et al: Characterization of the absorption phase of marijuana smoking. *Clin Pharmacol Ther* 1992;52:31–41.
8. Selden B, Clark R, Curry S: Marijuana. *Emerg Med Clin North Am* 1990;8:528.
9. Zachariah S: Stroke after heavy marijuana smoking. *Stroke* 1991;22:406–409.
10. Tashkin D: Pulmonary complications of smoked substance abuse. *West J Med* 1990;152:525–530.
11. Selden B, Clark R, Curry S: Marijuana. *Emerg Med Clin North Am* 1990;8:527–539.
12. Friedman G, Hartwick W, Ro J, et al: Allergic fungal sinusitis. Report of three cases associated with dematiaceous fungi. *Am J Clin Pathol* 1991;96:368–372.
13. Wu H, Wright R, Sassoon C, et al: Effects of smoked marijuana of varying potency on ventilatory drive and metabolic rate. *Am Rev Respir Dis* 1992;146:716–721.
14. Beaconsfield P. Ginsburg J, Rainsbury R: Marihuana smoking: cardiovascular effects in man and possible mechanisms. *N Engl J Med* 1972;287:209–212.
15. Hollister L: Marijuana and immunity. *J Psychoactive Drugs* 1992;24:159–164.
16. Azorlosa J, Heishman S, Stitzer M, et al: Marijuana smoking: effect of varying delta-9-tetrahydrocannabinol content and number of puffs. *J Pharmacol Exper Ther* 1992;261:114–122.
17. Zweben J, O'Connell K: Strategies for breaking marijuana dependence. *J Psychoactive Drugs* 1992;24:165–170.
18. Miller N, Gold M: The diagnosis of marijuana (cannabis) dependence. *J Subst Abuse Treat* 1989;6:183–192.
19. Landrigan P, Powell K, James L, et al: Paraquat and marijuana: epidemiologic risk assessment. *Am J Public Health* 1983;73:784–788.
20. Fairshter R, Wilson A: Paraquat and marihuana. *Chest* 1978;74:357.
21. Moyer T, Palmen M, Johnson P, et al: Marijuana testing—how good is it? *Mayo Clinic* 1987;62:413–417.
22. Silber T, Getson P, Ridley S, et al: Adolescent marijuana use: concordance between questionnaire and immunoassay for cannabinoid metabolites. *J Pediatr* 1987;111:299–302.

ADDITIONAL SELECTED REFERENCES

Genest K, Farmilo C: The identification and determination of lysergic acid diethylamide in narcotic seizures. *J Pharm Pharmacol* 1964;16: 250–257.

Greenland S, Staisch K, Brown N, et al: The effects of marijuana during pregnancy. *Am J Obstet Gynecol* 1982;143:408–413.

Satinder K, Black A: Cannabis use and sensation-seeking orientation. *J Psychol* 1984;116:105–105.

Schwartz R, Hawks R: Laboratory detection of marijuana use. *JAMA* 1985;254:788–792.

Wert R, Raulin M: The chronic cerebral effects of cannabis use: part I: methodological issues and neurological findings. *Int J Addict* 1986;21:605–628.

Wert R, Raulin M: The chronic cerebral effects of cannabis use: part II: psychological findings and conclusion. *Int J Addict* 1986;21:629–642.

PART IX

AGENTS FOR PAIN

CHAPTER 56

Acetaminophen

Acetaminophen (*N*-acetyl-*p*-aminophenol; APAP) was first synthesized in the United States in 1877 (1). Its use did not become extensive until 1949, when it was recognized as the principal active metabolite of phenacetin (2–4). Acetaminophen (paracetamol in the United Kingdom) is one of three *para*-amino compounds still in use (5). The other two, acetanalid and phenacetin, owe their analgesic and antipyretic properties to the metabolic generation of acetaminophen (6).

The status of acetaminophen as a prescription drug is similar to that of the nonsteroidal anti-inflammatory agent ibuprofen in that acetaminophen was a prescription drug for a short period but since 1960 has been marketed in the United States without a prescription (7,8). It is now sold under approximately 50 trade names and in 200 proprietary combinations with other drugs (Table 56–1) (5,9). Its use has dramatically increased over the past 20 years (10,11), and it is one of the most commonly used over-the-counter analgesic and antipyretic agents in the United States, primarily because it is generally considered safer than aspirin and has none of aspirin's undesirable side effects when taken in therapeutic doses (12–14). In addition to the regular-strength acetaminophen (325 mg) that is available, it is marketed in extra-strength (500-mg) tablets as well as a new, extended release preparation.

TABLE 56–1. *Selected preparations of acetaminophen by trade name*

Aceta	Halenol
Actamin	Liquiprin
Amphenol	Neopap
Anacin-3	Oraphen-PD
Anuphen	Panex
APAP	Pedric
Bayapap	Phenaphen
Bromo Seltzer	SK-APAP
Conacetol	Sudoprin
Dapa	Tapar
Datril	Tempra
Dolanex	Tenol
Febrigesic	Tylenol
Febrinol	Valadol

Toxic effects of acetaminophen overdose were first noted in 1966. At that time overdose with this substance was one of the most common causes of hepatic necrosis in the United Kingdom (1,7,15). Toxic effects of overdosage were not seen in the United States until 1971 (16–18). Because acetaminophen poisoning is a common toxicologic problem that clinicians can expect to encounter even more in the future, a thorough discussion of the pharmacology and toxicology of the compound is warranted

ACTIONS

Analgesia

Acetaminophen relieves mild to moderate pain. A number of studies comparing acetaminophen with salicylate have shown that both drugs have equal effects on pain when given in equivalent doses if the pain is noninflammatory in origin (19). For inflammatory pain, salicylates have been shown to be superior to acetaminophen.

The mechanism of action of acetaminophen appears to be related to the inhibition of brain cyclo-oxygenase (prostaglandin synthetase) (5), with much less of an effect on the peripheral enzyme. The peripheral action appears to be blockade of pain impulse generation. In addition to inhibiting cyclo-oxygenase centrally, salicylates also inhibit this enzyme peripherally, which appears to result in anti-inflammatory activity (20).

Antipyresis

Acetaminophen is also an antipyretic agent, altering the response of the heat-regulating center in the hypothalamus and leading to a lowering of the set point by vasodilation and sweating (21). This central antipyretic action probably involves inhibition of prostaglandin synthesis in the hypothalamus. Studies comparing acetaminophen and salicylates have shown no significant difference in temperature response, time of onset, time of peak action, or duration of antipyretic action (22).

TABLE 56–2. *Effects caused by other analgesics not seen with acetaminophen*

Gastric irritation
Gastric erosion
Platelet function interference
Oral anticoagulant potentiation
Methemoglobinemia
Hemolytic anemia
Mood and mentation changes
Renal damage

ADVANTAGES OF ACETAMINOPHEN

Acetaminophen has several advantages over many of the other analgesic agents. It has relatively few side effects and drug interactions when ingested in therapeutic amounts (Table 56–2). Unlike aspirin, acetaminophen is stable in solution, so that a liquid formulation is available. Hypersensitivity to acetaminophen rarely occurs but when present is manifested by erythema or urticaria. Because acetaminophen and aspirin have completely different chemical structures, there is no cross-sensitivity between the two drugs (23).

Acetaminophen also has advantages over other analgesics in that it does not share many of their adverse effects (24). Acetaminophen does not cause gastric irritation or erosion, as do the salicylates (25–27), nor does it interfere with platelet function or platelet aggregation or have any delayed effects on small vessel hemostasis as measured by bleeding time (5,28,29). Short-term therapy causes no interaction with oral anticoagulants (30), but there does appear to be some alteration in prothrombin time with doses of acetaminophen administered over a period of weeks (30). This has not been found to be clinically significant. Occasional or small doses of acetaminophen have little effect on coumarin action. Acetaminophen does not cause methemoglobinemia, hemolytic anemia, or changes in mood, energy, and mentation, as do phenacetin and acetanalid.

PHARMACOKINETICS

Acetaminophen is rapidly absorbed from the gastrointestinal tract, with peak concentrations noted between 60 and 120 minutes after oral administration of tablets and more quickly after ingestion of liquid preparations (31–33). Therapeutic concentrations occur much earlier; a therapeutic concentration is usually less than 9 μg/mL at 4 hours (34). The rate of absorption of acetaminophen is even more rapid from an alcoholic solution than from tablets or suspensions. Bezoar formation has not been reported with acetaminophen overdose, as it has with salicylate overdose (35). Approximately 10% of acetaminophen is bound to plasma proteins (36). The volume of distribution for both children and adults is approximately 1 to 1.2 L/kg (37).

The half-life of acetaminophen is 2 to 3 hours and appears to follow first-order, noncumulative, log-linear kinetics in therapeutic situations (38). Because its metabolism is largely enzymatic, toxic amounts of acetaminophen are eliminated by zero-order kinetics, and as the concentration increases the half-life also increases. Most investigators believe that the prolonged half-life seen in patients intoxicated with acetaminophen results from impaired metabolism due to ensuing liver damage (39). It may, however, also be a consequence of the limited capacity of the major biotransformation pathways, namely sulfate and glucuronic acid, because the metabolic conversion of large doses of acetaminophen eventually depletes the free sulfate needed to convert it to acetaminophen sulfate, a nontoxic by-product (32).

The extended release preparation is a bi-layered product that contains 650 mg of acetaminophen per caplet. One layer provides an immediate release while the second layer provides a slow and continuous release of acetaminophen from the surface of the layer. The time to peak blood levels following a 1,300-g dose is between 1–2 hours.

METABOLISM

Acetaminophen is a major metabolite of phenacetin, another derivative of *p*-aminophenol, but does not share some of its pharmacologic properties. Phenacetin can cause methemoglobinemia by forming an aniline derivative (*p*-phenitidin) (Fig. 56–1) (40), but acetaminophen lacks the ability to cause methemoglobinemia because of an alternate metabolic pathway in the liver. Phenacetin has also has been associated with analgesic nephropathy, including renal papillary necrosis with subsequent chronic interstitial nephritis, and no longer is commercially available in the U.S.

A small amount of acetaminophen is excreted unchanged in the urine. Most of a dose is conjugated with either glucuronic acid or sulfate and then excreted by the kidneys. This accounts for 80% to 90% of the metabolic by-product. The toxicity of acetaminophen is not due to either of these pathways (41,42). The cytochrome P-450 microsomal mixed-function oxidase system metabolizes a small (4%) but clinically significant portion of acetaminophen to an active intermediate apparently by first-order kinetics (Fig. 56–2) (39,43,44). Normally, this minor metabolite of hydroxylation, which is an iminodoquinone, *N*-acetyl-*p*-benzoquinonimine (NAPQI) (45–47), is detoxified by conjugation with hepatic glutathione when it is present; and the end products (mercapturic acid and cysteine) are then excreted (48–50). When acetaminophen is ingested in pharmacologic doses, 5% to 10% is excreted in the urine as mer-

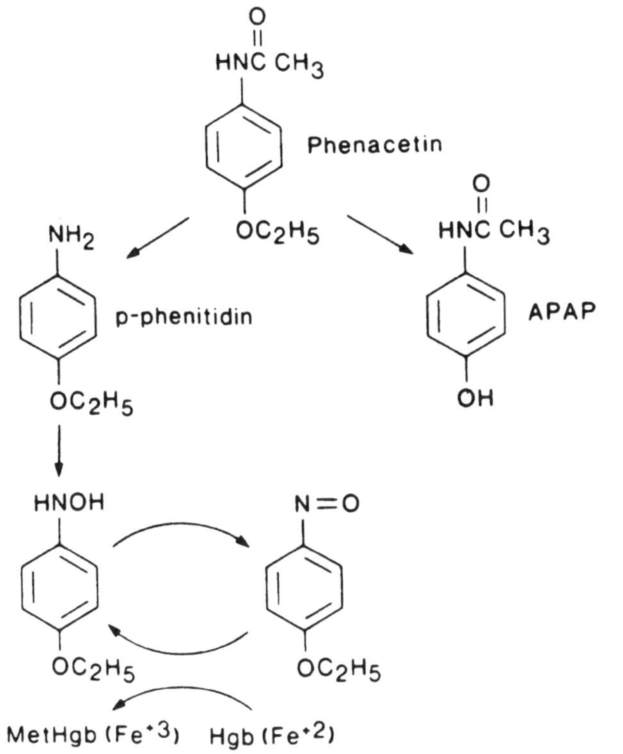

FIG. 56–1. Metabolic pathway of phenacetin. Reproduced from *Pediatrics* 1978;62:877 by permission of the American Academy of Pediatrics.

capturic acid (10,11). When large doses of acetaminophen are ingested, both the glucuronidation and the sulfation processes become saturated, shunting more acetaminophen toward the P-450 enzyme system and increasing NAPQI formation (46,51,52). Once glutathione is depleted to less than 30% of normal, NAPQI accumulates (36,49,53). When this occurs, NAPQI arylates to proteins of the cytosol and endoplasmic reticulum in the centrilobular zone of the liver and produces cell necrosis and death (Fig. 56–3) (14,34,54). In other words, NAPQI is neutralized by glutathione, which contains a sulfhydryl group. If all the glutathione is used up, other sulfhydryl groups in the liver are attacked, and the cells are damaged or destroyed (Fig. 56–3) (44,54,55).

TOXICITY

Acute

There are essentially four phases in an acute acetaminophen overdose (Table 56–3). There are no specific early signs or symptoms, and the true gravity of the situation is often not appreciated when the patient is first seen (34).

Phase 1 occurs within hours after an ingestion and may persist for 24 to 48 hours (12). Most patients are anorectic, nauseated, and vomiting. This is especially true with children. Diaphoresis may also be noted as a result of the effects of acetaminophen on the heat-regulating center in the hypothalamus (35). The early symptoms are due to the local action of acetaminophen; the more severe the overdose, the more likely these symptoms are to be present. An important feature of this phase is that there are no specific symptoms to indicate how serious the intoxication may eventually become. Some patients may be completely asymptomatic during the initial phase of intoxication, even after ingesting large doses. As a rule,

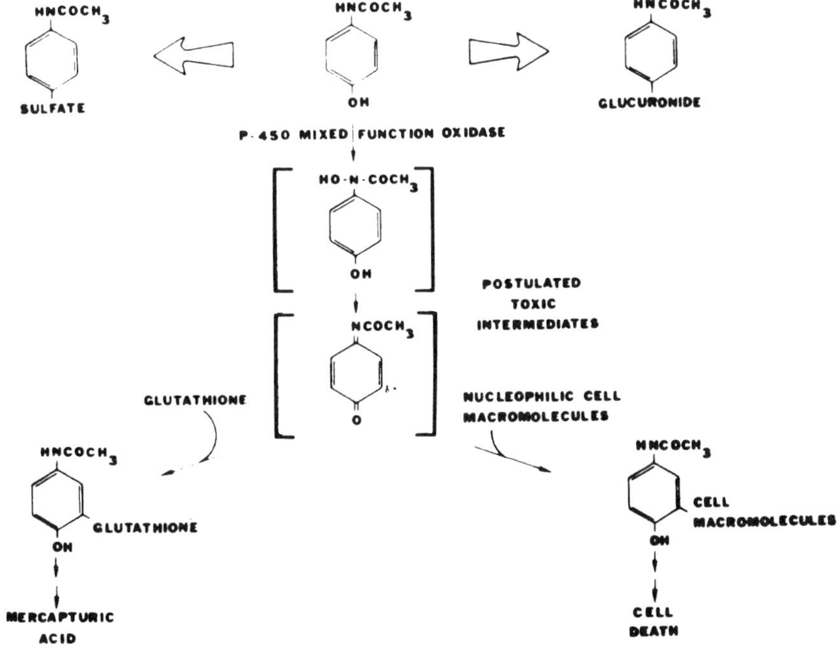

FIG. 56–2. Metabolic pathway of acetaminophen. Reprinted from *Clin Pharmacol Ther* 1974;16:677 with permission of CV Mosby Company.

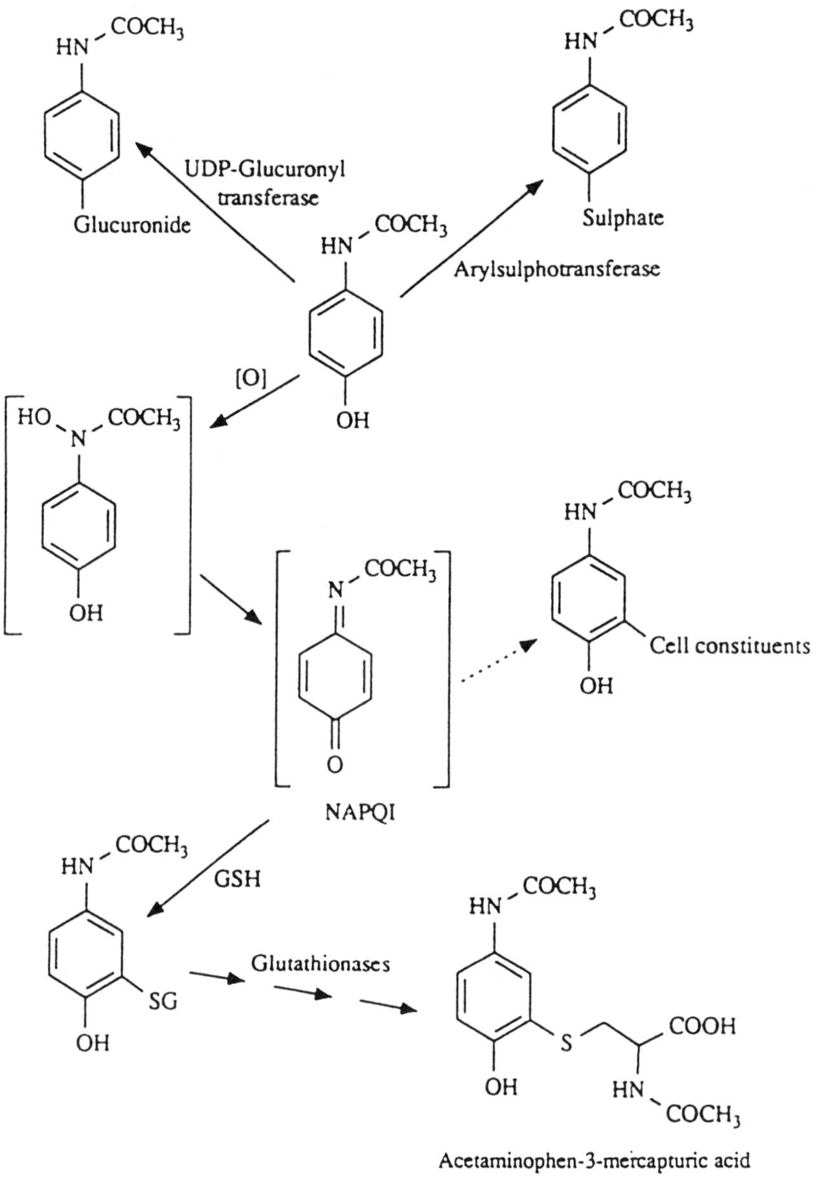

FIG. 56–3. Summary of acetaminophen (paracetamol) metabolism.

liver enzyme abnormalities do not occur during this period (10,11).

CNS depression is not usually a feature during this phase unless the patient has also ingested other depressant-type drugs, such as codeine, propoxyphene, alcohol, antihistamines, or decongestants (11). On rare occasions, lethargy, coma, and significant metabolic acidosis may occur with massive APAP ingestions. However, these symptoms are so uncommon during Phase 1, that they can be attributed to acetaminophen only when co-ingestion of depressant-type drugs and other etiologies for CNS depression have been excluded (16).

Phase 2 occurs between 24 and 72 hours after ingestion, and although the previously described symptoms may lessen in severity they may continue for up to 48 hours. Laboratory evidence of abnormal liver function (bilirubin, alkaline phosphatase, serum glutamic-oxaloacetic transaminase, serum glutamic-pyruvic transaminase, and lactic acid dehydrogenase) may now appear. In general, the elevations of serum transaminase concentrations do not correlate well with the clinical outcome. The patient may complain of right upper quadrant pain at this time.

Phase 3 occurs 3 to 5 days after an ingestion; there may be evidence of hepatic necrosis in patients who have ingested a significant overdose (56). Symptoms consist of jaundice, hypoglycemia, and encephalopathy. In acute hepatic necrosis, coagulation disorders may be severe and may include disseminated intravascular coagulation and bleeding diathesis (18,57). Liver enzyme abnormalities may peak during this phase; a concentration of aspartate aminotransferase (AST) (also known as serum glu-

TABLE 56–3. *Phases of acute acetaminophen intoxication*

Phase 1 (30 minutes to 4 hours)
Anorexia
Nausea
Vomiting
Diaphoresis
Phase 2 (24 to 72 hours)
Abatement but continuation of Phase 1 symptoms
Liver function abnormalities
Right upper quadrant pain
Phase 3 (3 to 5 days)
Jaundice
Coagulopathy
Hypoglycemia
Encephalopathy
Renal failure
Myocardiopathy
Phase 4 (7 to 8 days)
Abnormalities return to normal, or
Condition continues to deteriorate

tamic-oxaloacetic transaminase [SGOT, AST]) greater than 1,000 IU/L is taken to define hepatotoxicity (see Fig. 56–4) (10,11,41).

Phase 4 occurs 7 to 8 days after an ingestion. In most patients, this is usually the period in which the abnormal laboratory values return to normal. In a small number of patients, liver abnormalities continue, leading to liver failure and death.

Renal Toxicity

The kidneys are the second most common major organ involved in acute APAP toxicity. Although renal failure and myocardiopathy have been reported in association with liver disease, they appear to occur only as secondary events if the overdose results in severe hepatic failure (58); it has not been definitively determined whether they are primary events (59). Acetaminophen metabolites accumulate in the renal medulla, where reactive free radicals may cause direct nephrotoxicity. Acute renal failure secondary to severe hepatic failure manifests itself as the hepatorenal syndrome. The renal lesion is acute tubular necrosis and is usually associated with death (2,14,58).

Chronic

Case reports have previously described hepatic injury in patients taking APAP chronically in therapeutic and near-therapeutic dosages (60). The literature concerning this mode of toxicity is controversial and confusing. The majority of these reports involve alcoholics as subjects and allude to alcohol's ability in long-term abuse to potentiate APAP hepatotoxicity by induction of the cytochrome P-450-dependent enzyme pathway (61). Despite the large number of these reports, convincing metabolic evidence for this is lacking (62).

Nevertheless, persons with alcoholism are known to be at increased risk for APAP toxicity (62). The molecular basis for these persons' enhanced susceptibility to APAP toxicity is not known but two complementary theories have been proposed (63). The first is that the livers of persons with alcoholism are depleted in glutathione and are therefore incapable of detoxifying the electrophilic metabolites of APAP produced by the liver's mixed-function oxidase system that appears to generate the toxic metabolites (64). The second mechanism involves induction of liver cytochrome P-450-IIE1, which has recently been isolated in humans (62). This cytochrome P-450-IIE1 can catalyze the oxidation of a number of xenobiotics including ethanol, acetaminophen, isoniazid, ace-

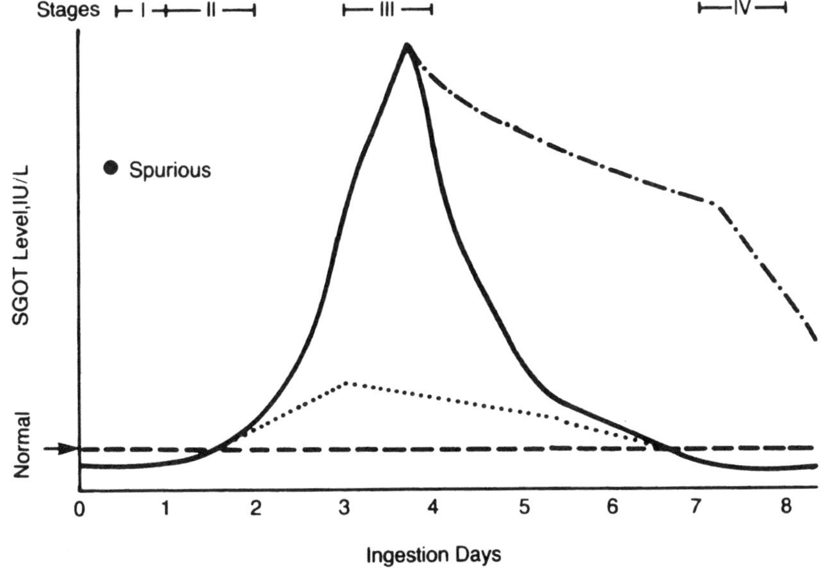

FIG. 56–4. Course of those who received acetylcysteine (*dotted line*); those with natural course (*solid line*); and those with severe course (*dotted-and-dashed line*). Reprinted from *Arch Intern Med* 1981;141:385 with permission of the American Medical Association.

tone, and others. Alcoholics metabolize APAP rapidly via cytochrome P-450-IIE1 where its oxidation produces an increased amount of NAPQI (60).

Clinical Presentation of Chronic Toxicity

Although APAP hepatotoxicity in chronic alcoholics involves the same metabolic pathways as APAP hepatotoxicity in suicide ingestions, the clinical presentation is distinct in several regards. First, the suicide ingestion patient arrives at the emergency department (ED) with normal liver tests. If hepatotoxicity develops, it appears 2 to 3 days after hospitalization. The chronic alcoholic arrives at the ED only after, and because, hepatotoxicity has fully developed. Second, the suicide ingestion patient has high blood APAP levels on presentation. The chronic alcoholic typically has discontinued APAP use several days before admission and has low or absent APAP levels on presentation (Table 56–4). Thus, the clinician can only make the diagnosis by recognizing the clinical picture and taking appropriate history, and should not be dissuaded by low or normal APAP levels. Third, the suicide ingestion patient who develops hepatotoxicity demonstrates high elevations of AST (SGOT) and ALT (SGPT), whereas the chronic alcoholic has a lower ALT and maintains the high AST/ALT ratio seen in alcoholic liver disease. The important features that allow early recognition of the clinical syndrome of APAP hepatotoxicity in chronic alcoholics are as follows: (a) There are very high elevations of hepatic aminotransferases with serum AST elevation typically greater than twice that of ALT; (b) the prothrombin time is sometimes remarkably elevated; and (c) the APAP level in the blood is typically low or normal at presentation (65).

Evaluation of Multiple-Dose Ingestions

Currently, there are no standard guidelines for the evaluation and treatment of multiple-dose APAP ingestions occurring over a period of time. The APAP nomogram is applicable for acute APAP ingestion and is not accurate for repeated or prolonged ingestion. However, because of the potentially beneficial action of *N*-acetylcysteine (NAC), therapy with this agent appears reasonable in this setting. NAC should be considered if the total dose of APAP ingested over a 24-hour period exceeds 50 mg/kg, if the APAP half-life is greater than 4 hours, or if liver enzymes are elevated (36).

TABLE 56–4. *Acute vs. chronic APAP ingestion*

Condition	Acute	Chronic
Liver function tests (LFTs)	Normal	Abnormal
Clinical hepatotoxicity	No	Yes
Serum level	High	Low

PREDICTING HEPATOTOXICITY

A number of factors should be taken into account in predicting whether liver disease may occur (Table 56–5). One factor is the total quantity of drug ingested. It has been shown in laboratory animals that liver necrosis occurs after an ingested dose of acetaminophen sufficient to deplete more than 70% of the glutathione in the liver (12,51). Because approximately 4% of the acetaminophen ingested is metabolized by this pathway, it has been estimated that approximately 15 g of acetaminophen is required to cause liver toxicity in a 70-kg person (5,66,67). Many clinicians accept 7.5 g as the toxic dose to take into account those individuals with liver disease from any cause or those individuals with decreased glutathione stores. The minimum toxic dose in children is considered 150 mg/kg. Since the widespread availability of rapid serum APAP analysis, the history of the amount ingested is less important in predicting toxicity.

Correlating the ingested dose with degree of liver damage is problematic because information obtained regarding the amount of drug ingested or eliminated by vomiting may be inexact, or there may be a lack of information regarding whether other drugs were taken that could affect the metabolic disposition of the acetaminophen. A history, then, should only be used as a rough guide. It has been suggested that the 4-hour plasma acetaminophen concentration (C_p) in a patient seen at any point between 2 to 16 hours after ingestion may be predicted from the following formula:

$$C_p = 0.59 \times \text{dose (in milligrams per kilogram)}$$

Although there are many factors that are not taken into account by this formula (such as degree of emesis), it may enable an early assessment to be made of the relative severity of the overdose until laboratory results are available. It should not be used as an indication for treatment.

Spontaneous Emesis

Whether the patient has undergone a spontaneous emesis before arriving in the emergency department influ-

TABLE 56–5. *Factors involved in predicting hepatotoxicity from acetaminophen*

Total quantity of ingested material
History of spontaneous emesis
Time from ingestion to medical attention
Activity of the cytochrome P-450 system
Age of the patient
Serum concentration in relation to nomogram (see Fig. 56–5)

ences the course of the intoxication. Vomiting is an early effect of acetaminophen, and its occurrence lessens the likelihood of a severe toxic reaction.

Metabolic Activity of Cytochrome System

The metabolic activity of the cytochrome P-450 pathway is a factor in the extent of toxicity of an overdose. Certain drugs, such as phenobarbital and ethyl alcohol, stimulate the cytochrome P-450 pathway when chronically administered (68). A patient taking such drugs on a long-term basis may have an increased likelihood of intoxication because that pathway is metabolizing a greater percentage of the acetaminophen to the potentially toxic intermediate (51).

On the other hand, use of cimetidine may afford protection against a toxic dose of acetaminophen (69,70). It has been shown that standard therapeutic doses of cimetidine can reduce cytochrome P-450 metabolism of some drugs, including acetaminophen, because they appear to have a lower affinity for cytochrome P-450 than cimetidine (71). Metabolism of these drugs through this pathway is therefore inhibited, and in the case of acetaminophen a smaller amount of the toxic intermediary is formed (69,72). The acute ingestion of ethyl alcohol appears to decrease the toxicity of acetaminophen in the same manner.

In animals, prior administration of high doses of inhibitors of oxidative metabolism, such as cimetidine, reduces NAPQI formation and thus the frequency and severity of hepatotoxicity. This approach is not appropriate for the treatment of poisoning in humans, for an inhibitor would have to be given before APAP overdose (71). Because cimetidine has not proved to affect the metabolism of APAP in humans, there is no established role for cimetidine in the treatment of APAP toxicity (36,73,74).

Other known inhibitors of the cytochrome P-450 system, such as piperonylbutoxide (51), cobaltous chloride, and metyrapone, either have not been clinically effective or have shown undesirable side effects. Although in animals prior administration of inhibitors of oxidative metabolism such as cimetidine can reduce the formation of NAPQI, research has concentrated on the use of other sulfur-containing compounds with the aim of detoxifying this metabolite.

Pediatric Ingestion

Children appear to be less vulnerable than adults to the toxic effects of acetaminophen. Although there are a few reports, it is extremely rare for clinical intoxication or death to occur in the pediatric age group even when toxic blood concentrations are found (12,75–77). The reasons for this phenomenon are still unclear. The plasma half-life of acetaminophen in adults and children is nearly identical, and the volume of distribution is similar (40,78,79). The only difference appears to be the major pathway for conjugation in adults and children (80). In adults, glucuronide conjugation is the major pathway, and in children between 3 and 9 years of age the sulfate conjugate is the major pathway (40). This factor should not, however, account for the difference in toxicity because the conjugated pathways do not have an effect on toxicity, the intermediary formed from the cytochrome P-450 pathway being the entity that leads to liver toxicity. Other proposed mechanisms suggest that decreased toxicity in young children may be due to smaller amounts of the drug being metabolized through the cytochrome P-450 system (76). Children older than 6 years of age can be considered similar to adults with regard to elimination of acetaminophen as well as the proportion of sulfate and glucuronide metabolites excreted (76).

Acetaminophen Nomogram

The single most important prognostic indicator of acetaminophen hepatotoxicity is obtained from a serum concentration, which is placed on the acetaminophen nomogram (Fig. 56–5) (81,82). Serum concentration has been shown to be a more accurate indicator of the possibility of liver toxicity than the amount of drug ingested. The nomogram that was first described in 1976 is based on the correlation between liver toxicity and plasma concentration of acetaminophen measured between 4 and 24 hours after ingestion (83). This nomogram is accurate to a high confidence level. The nomogram has been modified to include a second elimination curve 25% lower than the standard curve, which allows for errors in the history of the time of ingestion. Those patients whose plasma acetaminophen concentrations fall between 150 and 200 μg/mL at 4 hours after ingestion, or between the two lines at any later time, are considered at "possible" risk for toxicity. Concentrations higher than those indicated by the standard nomogram line are considered at "probable" risk (11,37,72). To avoid confusion, values should always be reported in micrograms per milliliter (or μmol/L). Serious illness and death have resulted from the withholding of treatment because of confusion as to the units used to report plasma concentrations.

To properly interpret the serum acetaminophen concentration, the time of ingestion must be established as accurately as possible. As an example, a concentration greater than 150 μg/mL at 4 hours is considered potentially toxic, and concentrations greater than this indicate antidotal therapy (40). The nomogram begins 4 hours after ingestion, which is considered the time when peak concentration is attained. Before 4 hours concentrations may be falsely low but can be used if they are high because they may indicate that a significant amount was

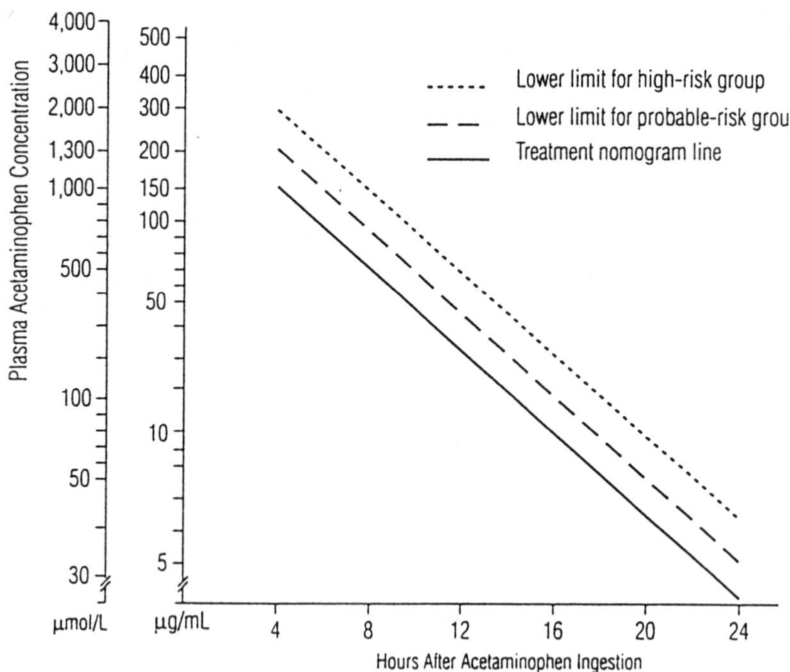

FIG. 56–5. Nomogram lines used to define risk groups, according to initial plasma acetaminophen concentration. Adapted from Smilkstein et al., *Ann Emerg Med* 1991;20:1058–1063.

ingested earlier than suspected. A single APAP level obtained at least 4 hours after ingestion is usually sufficient to determine toxicity (84). Repeated APAP levels are usually not helpful and are therefore unnecessary except in the rare instance when the result obtained is close to the toxic line on the nomogram. In that instance, it could be beneficial to obtain a second level after 2 to 4 hours (85).

There are two potential errors that should be noted in determining acute APAP toxicity. First, the units in which the APAP level is reported should be confirmed. Some laboratories may report the result in µg/dL instead of µg/mL, which may lead to a tenfold underestimation error. The second source of error involves the method of APAP assay. The most reliable methods for determining APAP levels are radioimmunoassays, high-pressure liquid chromatography, and gas chromatography. Assays using rapid colorimetric techniques may be unreliable in the presence of hyperbilirubinemia, salicylates, methyldopa, and renal failure (36).

Extended Release Caplets and the Nomogram

At present, there is insufficient clinical experience with the situation of overdose of the extended release preparation, but the manufacturer suggests that an initial plasma acetaminophen level be drawn at least 4 hours after ingestion and an additional level be drawn 4–6 hours following the initial level. These levels would be plotted on the nomogram. If either of the two levels is above the line of toxicity on the nomogram, the entire course of NAC should be administered, or if initiated, completed.

Serum Half-Life

Serum half-life, although used in the past, is not as reliable in predicting toxicity as a laboratory determination of serum concentration (14,72,83). If the estimated time of ingestion cannot be obtained, making prognosis from the nomogram impossible, then the half-life may be helpful (11). The half-life of acetaminophen at therapeutic plasma concentrations is 2 to 3 hours (83). Because its metabolism is largely enzymatic, elimination is according to zero-order kinetics as concentrations increase. It has been shown that, if the half-life is greater than 4 hours, liver damage is likely and appropriate treatment should be instituted (72). The half-life has been observed to increase to 8 hours in individuals who have ingested hepatotoxic quantities of acetaminophen (11).

Histologic Findings

The histologic abnormalities associated with acetaminophen overdose include centrilobular hemorrhagic hepatic necrosis. The sinusoids are often congested and dilated centrally. This location coincides with the centrilobular location of the enzymes responsible for the main metabolism of the drug. Tissue regeneration and repair are normally rapid and complete (45).

LABORATORY DETERMINATIONS

Venous blood samples should be drawn for a complete blood cell count and for evaluation of platelets, prothrombin time, electrolytes, blood urea nitrogen, glucose,

TABLE 56–6. *Laboratory determinations in acetaminophen overdose*

Toxicology screen with acetaminophen level
If toxic then serial
Complete blood count
Platelet count
Prothrombin time
Liver function tests
Serum glutamic-oxaloacetic transaminase
Serum glutamic-pyruvic transaminase
Alkaline phosphatase
Bilirubin

and liver function such as serum glutamic-oxaloacetic transaminase, serum glutamic-pyruvic transaminase, bilirubin, and alkaline phosphatase. A toxicology screen should also be performed. If the acetaminophen concentration is found to be within the toxic range, then evaluation of liver function should be performed at 24-hour intervals for at least 4 days (Table 56–6).

Prompt determination of serum acetaminophen concentrations can have a significant impact on the patient's treatment and prognosis (86). Therefore, rapid and reliable techniques for measuring the drug are required. Laboratory methods may include colorimetric techniques, radioimmunoassay, high-performance liquid chromatography, and gas chromatography (5,39,87). The preferred method of analysis for acetaminophen is high-performance liquid chromatography, but this has a high initial cost and requires a trained technician for operation (88). Another successful method is enzyme-modification immunoassay, but this may also be expensive and is not feasible for use by a small laboratory because of reagent instability (87). Spectrophotometric methods, such as those involving nitration and ferric reduction, may be unreliable because of the presence of interfering substances (88).

In a patient being treated with *N*-acetylcysteine, serial liver function tests should be performed. These should include the tests described in Table 56–6 as well as serum blood urea nitrogen and serum creatinine determinations (81).

TREATMENT

Effective Methods

Effective treatment and management of the acetaminophen-intoxicated patient consists of measures as in Table 56–7.

TABLE 56–7. *Treatment of acetaminophen overdose*

Gastric lavage
Activated charcoal and cathartic
N-Acetylcysteine
Supportive measures (after 24 hours)
Neomycin enema
Fresh frozen plasma
Glucose

Gastric lavage should be performed with the proper-sized tube and an adequate amount of lavage fluid (88). This method should be performed in a timely fashion. Activated charcoal is an effective adsorbent for acetaminophen (25), and its use is suggested to adsorb the remaining acetaminophen or to adsorb any other compound ingested in conjunction with the acetaminophen (89,90). There is controversy concerning its role, however, because an orally administered antidote may be also absorbed by the activated charcoal (25,91). If oral *N*-acetylcysteine as an antidote (see below) is deemed necessary, an attempt could be made to remove the charcoal by gastric lavage before its administration (91). Even so, co-administration of activated charcoal and oral *N*-acetylcysteine has not been shown to affect peak *N*-acetylcysteine concentrations, absorption rate, time to peak concentration, or half-life (92,93). A cathartic should be administered in conjunction with the activated charcoal to decrease the transit time in the gastrointestinal tract.

Specific Treatment

A protocol for treatment of acetaminophen intoxication based on the drug's metabolism was tested in 1973. It was demonstrated that hepatotoxicity could be decreased by the administration of cysteine, which is a sulfhydryl precursor of glutathione (6). The protocol was based on the observation that when glutathione is present in sufficient quantity there is no toxic effect of acetaminophen on the liver, but when glutathione is depleted because of an overwhelming amount of acetaminophen metabolized through the cytochrome P-450 pathway, liver toxicity may occur (19). Attempts have been made to find a glutathione substitute that offers protection to the liver by virtue of supplying sulfhydryl groups for use in the detoxification of acetaminophen's metabolic intermediary. Glutathione, the obvious choice, is synthesized intracellularly and is not readily taken into cells when administered orally; it is also expensive and so has not met with success. A number of smaller sulfhydryl substances, however, can be taken into hepatocytes and have been found to be effective. Methionine, a precursor of glutathione, had been tried in the past but was abandoned because of some of the adverse reactions associated with its use (59,72,89,94). For the same reason cysteamine, a glutathione substitute, was tried and abandoned (95,96).

N-Acetylcysteine

The antidote of choice for acetaminophen overdose in the last few years has been *N*-acetylcysteine (NAC;

Mucomyst, *N*-acetyl-3-mercaptoalanine), an *N*-acetyl derivative of the naturally occurring amino acid L-cysteine (11,34,97,98). *N*-Acetylcysteine has been in clinical use as a mucolytic agent since the mid-1950s. There is a relatively wide margin of safety between therapeutic and toxic doses (54). This compound has been shown to offer protection against liver toxicity when administered within the first 24 hours after an acute acetaminophen overdose (79,98). Statistically significant differences in severity of hepatotoxicity have been observed between patients treated within 16 hours after ingestion and those treated between 16 and 24 hours after ingestion (11). Because of this, it is suggested that treatment begin within the first 16 hours after an acute ingestion (41,76). Initiating therapy after 24 hours appears not to be effective (54).

Mechanism of Action

N-Acetylcysteine is metabolized to cysteine and is taken up by cells, where it acts as a glutathione substitute, combining directly with the hepatotoxic metabolite to detoxify it (99). There may be other mechanisms by which *N*-acetylcysteine is effective, as evidenced by studies showing an increase in the rate of elimination of acetaminophen after administration of *N*-acetylcysteine (100). This finding suggests that it may also serve as a biologic source of inorganic sulfate, enhancing the formation of acetaminophen sulfate and thereby allowing metabolism through nontoxic routes (43,83,98,101). Another proposed mechanism for this compound is that it may stabilize cellular constituents against the possible deleterious effects of the covalent binding of the reactive metabolite (45,102).

Route of Administration

N-Acetylcysteine may be administered orally or intravenously. It has been approved for intravenous use in Canada and Europe (76) and is the therapy of choice in the United Kingdom, where it has been shown to be well tolerated and effective (95,96). In the United States, a special pyrogen-free preparation is available for investigational use. In the U.S., only the oral form of NAC is approved by the FDA (103). Oral NAC is slightly different from the intravenous form used in Canada and great Britain in that it is sterile but not pyrogen-free.

Dosage

Oral Protocol

The current recommended dosage regimen for *N*-acetylcysteine is to administer a loading dose of 140 mg/kg and then a maintenance dose of 70 mg/kg every 4 hours for 17 additional doses or for a total of 72 hours (Table 56–8). This is given as a 10% or 20% solution diluted to 5% with a soft drink or juice to disguise the unpleasant taste (36). If the patient refuses to ingest the material, it can be administered down a nasogastric tube. If the drug is administered orally and the patient has an emesis within 1 hour, the dose should be repeated (11,76). If emesis persists, insertion of a weighted tube such as a Miller-Abbott or Cantor tube and administration directly into the duodenum are suggested. Occasionally, an antiemetic agent such as metoclopramide (0.1–1.0 mg/kg intravenously) may help relieve gastrointestinal side effects (104).

TABLE 56–8. *Oral NAC protocol for treatment of acetaminophen overdose*

Oral 72 Hour—Oral administration protocol
Loading dose: 140 mg/kg diluted one part Mucomyst with 4–5 parts diluent. Dilutions should be freshly prepared and used within 1 hour.
Maintenance doses: 70 mg/kg every 4 hours starting 4 hours after the loading dose. The same dilutions should be used.
Total dose of NAC is 1,330 mg/kg over 72 hours.

Although the efficacy of NAC in treating APAP intoxication is a function of the length of time between APAP ingestion and NAC administration; the sooner NAC therapy is initiated after a significant ingestion, the more effective it will be. There is no difference in efficacy whether NAC is started 0 to 4 hours or 4 to 8 hours after APAP ingestion (62). This finding suggests that delays due to gastric emptying, to the administration of activated charcoal, or to the return of laboratory results do not adversely affect the outcome if NAC is started within 8 hours of APAP ingestion (103). During this period and regardless of the amount ingested and the APAP level, NAC is uniformly effective. After the 8-hour postingestion period, the efficacy of NAC decreases progressively.

Intravenous Protocol

The intravenous protocol under investigation in the United States differs considerably from that used in Europe and Canada (Table 56–9). The rationale for intravenous administration is that, because vomiting is a frequent effect in most patients receiving oral *N*-acetylcysteine, administering it parenterally would ensure complete absorption (94,95). Some investigators believe that there are theoretical advantages to the oral administration of *N*-acetylcysteine because of a significant first-pass effect, which would cause a significant portion of the drug to be extracted by the liver (the organ requiring

TABLE 56–9. *Intravenous NAC protocol for treatment of acetaminophen overdose*

20 Hour—IV administration protocol	48 Hour—IV administration protocol
Loading dose: 150 mg/kg in 200 mL of 5% dextrose in water (D5W) over 15 min, immediately followed by 50 mg/kg in 500 mL. D5W over next 4 hours, immediately followed by 100 mg/kg in 1,000 mL of D5W over next 16 hours. *Total dose of NAC is 300 mg/kg over 20 hours.*	**Loading dose:** 140 mg/kg diluted one part Mucomyst with 4–5 parts D5W and infused over 1 hour. **Maintenance doses:** 70 mg/kg every 4 hours after the loading dose for an additional 12 doses. Each infusion is over a 1-hour period. *Total dose of NAC is 980 mg/kg over 48 hours.*

protection) because of direct entry through the portal vein (46,76,92).

The intravenous protocol used in the United States consists of the same loading and maintenance doses as are used in the oral route (105). The preparation for intravenous use is administered for only 2 days (76). Overall, when treatment is started 10 to 24 hours after overdose, this protocol appears as effective as the 72-hour oral NAC treatment used in the U.S. and more effective than the 20-hour IV NAC currently used in Europe and Canada (81).

Pediatric Overdoses

Even though children less than 6 years of age with confirmed toxic blood concentrations of acetaminophen are unlikely to develop significant toxic effects, the recommendation is that any child with a plasma acetaminophen concentration in the toxic range on the nomogram should be offered the same treatment as adults.

Acetaminophen and Pregnancy

APAP can cross the placenta and cause fetal liver toxicity and fetal demise. APAP overdose is the most common overdose in pregnancy and has been associated with fetal death. This is independent of maternal mortality and is thought to be due to a direct toxic effect of APAP on the fetal liver. Because NAC appears to be safe in pregnancy, and because delaying therapy can lead to dire consequences, NAC should be started early in the pregnant patient with APAP toxicity.

Special Considerations

N-Acetylcysteine is administered on the basis of a potentially toxic plasma concentration of acetaminophen obtained from the nomogram. Once treatment has begun, subsequent measurements of plasma concentration should be of interest only and should not be used to determine whether treatment should continue. Even if a second concentration shows a decrease below the nomogram line, treatment should continue for the entire course. If treatment is started before a measurement of plasma acetaminophen concentration is available, it should be terminated in patients subsequently found not to be at risk.

Side Effects

N-Acetylcysteine does not have some of the adverse effects seen with other antidotes, such as increasing the likelihood of liver failure if administered too late in the course of an ingestion. It is relatively free from major adverse reactions when administered orally. When given parenterally, allergy and anaphylaxis have been reported 15 to 60 minutes after the onset of infusion; symptoms include angioedema, bronchospasm, flushing, hypotension, nausea, vomiting, rash, pruritus, and tachycardia (106). These reactions are rare and are not associated with oral use (37).

In special circumstances when NAC is indicated and oral administration is not possible, NAC may be given intravenously using the same dosing regimen. The NAC preparation should be infused over 60 minutes using a micropore filter attachment to the intravenous tubing. It is advisable to obtain patient consent and to consult with the local poison center if this route is necessary (36).

Other Methods

In patients who are treated more than 24 hours after an overdose of acetaminophen, *N*-acetylcysteine appears to be less effective. Such patients may still be treated by with NAC as well as supportive measures such as reduction of protein intake and neomycin enemas to reduce the degree of liver toxicity (10,11). In addition, fresh frozen plasma, vitamin K, and glucose may be administered if the patient shows signs of hypoprothrombinemia or hypoglycemia. If the prothrombin time is greater than 1.5 times the control value, phytonadione should be administered; if the prothrombin time is greater than 3 times the control value, fresh frozen plasma should be given (65).

Role of Liver Transplantation

Liver transplantation may be the last viable option in patients with fulminant hepatic failure from APAP. However, the shortcomings of this practice include deciding the optimal timing for referral and the relatively limited experience with liver transplantations for APAP hepatic damage (36). A serum bilirubin concentration greater than 4 mg/dL and a prothrombin time greater than 2.2 times the control value may indicate impending hepatic encephalopathy.

Despite the known potential for toxicity in massive overdose of acetaminophen, the great majority of cases do not result in fatalities, serious liver toxicity, or long-term complications. Mortality rates in patients with toxic plasma concentrations who do not receive antidotal therapy have been in the range of 2% to 4%.

Ineffective Methods

Several studies seem to have demonstrated that hemoperfusion removes acetaminophen (57,107–109). Nevertheless, because the toxic metabolite is formed relatively rapidly, and because the drug has such a short half-life, there appears to be little point in trying to remove the drug by this method (107,110). Hemodialysis reduces the half-life of acetaminophen and readily removes it from circulation, but because hepatic injury is an early event there is no strong evidence that this procedure will alter the clinical course (111,112). Peritoneal dialysis is also ineffective because of the strong protein-binding properties of acetaminophen (113). Forced diuresis is not indicated because only 5% of the unaltered drug is excreted in the urine (45).

SUMMARY

In summary, an overdose of acetaminophen may overwhelm the liver stores of glutathione and cause a rise in liver enzymes, which reflects the hepatic toxicity that may ensue. The patient can be protected from this by the timely administration of *N*-acetylcysteine, which supplies sulfhydryl groups to the toxic intermediary. Therapy should ideally be instituted as soon as possible, but significant protection is achieved if the antidote is administered within the first 24 hours (11).

REFERENCES

1. Black M, Raucy J: Acetaminophen, alcohol, and cytochrome P-450. *Ann Intern Med* 1986;104:427–428.
2. Prescott L, Matthew J: Cysteamine for paracetamol overdosage. *Lancet* 1974;1:998.
3. Proudfoot A, Wright N: Acute paracetamol poisoning. *Br Med J* 1970;3:557–558.
4. Hinson J: Reactive metabolites of phenacetin and acetaminophen: a review. *Environ Health Perspect* 1983;49:71–79.
5. Ameer B, Greenblatt D: Acetaminophen. *Ann Intern Med* 1977;87: 202–209.
6. Mitchell J: Acetaminophen toxicity. *N Engl J Med* 1988;319: 1601–1602.
7. Spooner J, Harvey J: The history and usage of paracetamol. J *Int Med Res* 1976;4:1–6.
8. Levy G, Khanna N, Soda D, et al: Pharmacokinetics of acetaminophen in the human neonate. *Pediatrics* 1975;55:818–824.
9. Heaver W: Aspirin and acetaminophen as constituents of analgesic combinations. *Arch Intern Med* 1981;141:293–300.
10. Rumack B, Matthew H: Acetaminophen poisoning. *Pediatrics* 1975;55:871–876.
11. Rumack B, Meredith T, Peterson R, et al: Panel discussion: Management of acetaminophen overdose. *Arch Intern Med* 1981;141: 401–403.
12. Temple A: Emergency treatment of acetaminophen overdose. *Curr Top Emerg Med* 1981;3:1–5.
13. Gerber J, MacDonald J, Harbison R, et al: Effect of IV-acetylcysteine on hepatic covalent binding of paracetamol (acetaminophen). *Lancet* 1977;1:657–658.
14. Prescott L, Sutherland G, Park J, et al: Cysteamine, methionine, and penicillamine in the treatment of paracetamol poisoning. *Lancet* 1976;2:109–113.
15. Clark R, Thompson R, Borirakchanyavat V, et al: Hepatic damage and death from overdose of paracetamol. *Lancet* 1973;1:66–69.
16. Goldfrank L, Kerstein R, Weisman R: Acute acetaminophen overdose. *Hosp Physician* 1980:16;52–60.
17. McJunkin B, Barwick K, Little W, et al: Fatal massive hepatic necrosis from acetaminophen overdose. *JAMA* 1976;236:1874–1875.
18. Gazzard B, Davis M, Spooner J, et al: Why do people use paracetamol for suicide? *Br Med J* 1976;1:212–213.
19. Cooper S: Comparative analgesic efficacies of aspirin and acetaminophen. *Arch Intern Med* 1981;141:282–285.
20. Levy G: Comparative pharmacokinetics of aspirin and acetaminophen. *Arch Intern Med* 1981;141:279–281.
21. Manoguerra A: Acetaminophen intoxication. *Clin Toxicol* 1979;14: 151–155.
22. Yaffe S: Comparative efficacy of aspirin and acetaminophen in the reduction of fever in children. *Arch Intern Med* 1981;141:286–292.
23. Hansten P: Acetaminophen interactions. *Drug Interact Newslett* 1983;3:55–59.
24. Hayes A: Therapeutic implications of drug interactions with acetaminophen and aspirin. *Arch Intern Med* 1981;141:301–304.
25. Levy G, Houston B: Effect of activated charcoal on acetaminophen absorption. *Pediatrics* 1976;58:432–435.
26. Goulston K, Shyring A: Effect of paracetamol (*N*-acetyl-*p*-aminophenol) on gastrointestinal bleeding. *Gut* 1964;5:463–466.
27. Jick H: Effects of aspirin and acetaminophen on gastrointestinal hemorrhage. *Arch Intern Med* 1981;141:316–321.
28. Mielke C: Comparative effects of aspirin and acetaminophen on hemostasis. *Arch Intern Med* 1981;141:305–310.
29. Mielke C, Herden D, Britten A, et al: Hemostasis, antipyretics and mild analgesics. *JAMA* 1976;235:613–616.
30. Antlitz A, Awalt L: A double-blind study of acetaminophen used in conjunction with oral anticoagulant therapy. *Curr Ther Res* 1969;11: 360–361.
31. Clements J, Heading R, Nimmo W, et al: Kinetics of acetaminophen absorption and gastric emptying in man. *Clin Pharmacol Ther* 1978; 24:420–431.
32. Slattery J, Koup J, Levy G: Acetaminophen pharmacokinetics after overdose. *Clin Toxicol* 1981;18:111–117.
33. Slattery J, Levy G: Acetaminophen kinetics in acutely poisoned patients. *Clin Pharmacol Ther* 1979;25:184–185.
34. Prescott L, Roscoe P, Wright N, et al: Plasma paracetamol half-life with hepatic necrosis in patients with paracetamol overdosage. *Lancet* 1971;1:519–522.
35. Rose S, Gorman R, Oderda G, et al: Simulated acetaminophen overdose: pharmacokinetics and effectiveness of activated charcoal. *Ann Emerg Med* 1991;20:1064–1068.
36. Chiang W, Wang R, Hoffman R, et al: Evaluation and management of acute acetaminophen toxicity. *Emerg Med Rep* 1993;14:83–90.
37. Rumack B, Peterson R: Acetaminophen overdose: incidence, diagnosis and management in 416 patients. *Pediatrics* 1978;62(Suppl.):901.
38. Piletta P, Porchet H, Dayer P: Central analgesic effect of acetaminophen but not of aspirin. *Clin Pharmacol Ther* 1991;49:350–354.

39. Ferguson D, Snyder S, Cameron A: Hepatotoxicity in acetaminophen poisoning. *Mayo Clin Proc* 1977;52:246–248.
40. Peterson R, Rumack B: Pharmacokinetics of acetaminophen in children. *Pediatrics* 1978;62 (Suppl.):877–879.
41. Rumack B, Peterson R, Koch G, et al: Acetaminophen overdose: 662 cases with evaluation of oral acetylcysteine treatment. *Arch Intern Med* 1981;141:380–385.
42. Gillette J: An integrated approach to the study of chemically reactive metabolites of acetaminophen. *Arch Intern Med* 1981;141:375–379.
43. Mitchell J, Thorgeirsson S, Potter W, et al: Acetaminophen-induced hepatic injury: protective role of glutathione in man and rationale for therapy. *Clin Pharmacol Ther* 1974;16:676–684.
44. Mitchell J, Jollow D, Potter W, et al: Acetaminophen-induced hepatic necrosis—part 1: role of drug metabolism. *J Pharmacol Exp Ther* 1973;187:185–201.
45. Prescott L: Paracetamol overdose: pharmacological considerations and clinical management. *Drugs* 1983;25;290–314.
46. Flanagan R: The role of acetylcysteine in clinical toxicology. *Med Toxicol* 1987;2:93–104.
47. Flanagan R, Mant T: Coma and metabolic acidosis early in severe acute paracetamol poisoning. *Hum Toxicol* 1986;5:179–182.
48. Hinson J, Nelson S, Mitchell J: Studies on the microsomal formation of arylating metabolites of acetaminophen and phenacetin. *Mol Pharmacol* 1977;13:625–633.
49. Gemborys M, Gribble G, Mudge C: Synthesis of *N*-hydroxyacetaminophen, a postulated toxic metabolite of acetaminophen, and its phenolic sulfate conjugate. *J Med Chem* 1978;21:649–652.
50. Mitchell J, Jollow D: Metabolic activation of drugs to toxic substances. *Gastroenterology* 1975;68:392–410.
51. Mitchell J, Lauterburg B: Drug-induced liver injury. *Hosp Pract* 1978;13:95–106.
52. Potter W, Thorgeirsson S, Jollow D: Acetaminophen induced hepatic necrosis: part V: correlation of hepatic necrosis, covalent binding and glutathione depletion in hamsters. *Pharmacology* 1974;12:129–143.
53. Abramowicz M: Acetaminophen hepatotoxicity. *Med Lett Drug* Ther 1978;20:61–63.
54. Flanagan R, Meredith T: Use of *N*-acetylcysteine in clinical toxicology. *Am J Med* 1991;91:131S–139S.
55. Jollow D, Thorgeirsson S, Potter W, et al: Acetaminophen-induced hepatic necrosis: part VI: metabolic disposition of toxic and nontoxic doses of acetaminophen. *Pharmacology* 1974;12:251–271.
56. Black M: Acetaminophen hepatotoxicity. *Annu Rev Med* 1984; 35:577–593.
57. Gazzard B, Willson R, Weston M, et al: Charcoal hemoperfusion for paracetamol overdose. *Br J Clin Pharmacol* 1974;1:271–274.
58. Boyer T, Rouff S: Acetaminophen-induced hepatic necrosis and renal failure. *JAMA* 1971;218:440–441.
59. Maxwell L, Cotty V, Marcus A, et al: Prevention of acetaminophen poisoning. *Lancet* 1975;2:610–611.
60. Kumar S, Rex D: Failure of physicians to recognize acetaminophen hepatotoxicity in chronic alcoholics. *Arch Intern Med* 1991;151: 1189–1191.
61. Henretig F, Selbst S, Forrest C, et al: Repeated acetaminophen overdosing. *Clin Pediatr* 1989;28:525–528.
62. Mathis R, Walker J, Kuhns D: Subacute acetaminophen overdose after incremental dosing. *J Emerg Med* 1988;6:37–40.
63. Eriksson L, Broome U, Kalin M, et al: Hepatotoxicity due to repeated intake of low doses of paracetamol. *J Intern Med* 1992;231:567–570.
64. Murphy R, Swartz R, Watkins P: Severe acetaminophen toxicity in a patient receiving isoniazid. *Ann Intern Med* 1990;113:799–800.
65. Watson W: Identifying the acetaminophen overdose. *Ann Emerg Med* 1989;18:1126–1127.
66. Clark P, Clark J, Wheatley J: Urine discoloration after acetaminophen overdose. *Clin Chem* 1986;32:1777–1778.
67. Prescott L: Treatment of severe acetaminophen poisoning with intravenous acetylcysteine. *Arch Intern Med* 1981;141:386–389.
68. Wootton F, Lee W: Acetaminophen hepatotoxicity in the alcoholic. *South Med J* 1990;83:1047–1049.
69. Jackson J: Cimetidine protects against acetaminophen hepatotoxicity. *Vet Hum Toxicol* 1981;23:7–9.
70. Ruffalo R, Thompson J: Cimetidine and acetylcysteine as antidotes for acetaminophen overdose. *South Med J* 1982;75:954–958.
71. Slattery J, McRorie T, Reynolds R, et al: Lack of effect of cimetidine on acetaminophen disposition in humans. *Clin Pharmacol Ther* 1989;46:591–597.
72. Prescott L, Newton R, Swainson C, et al: Successful treatment of severe paracetamol overdosage with cysteamine. *Lancet* 1974;1: 588–592.
73. Critchley J, Scott A, Dyson E, et al: Is there a place for cimetidine or ethanol in the treatment of paracetamol poisoning? *Lancet* 1983;1: 1375–1376.
74. Rolband G, Marcuard S: Cimetidine in the treatment of acetaminophen overdose. *J Clin Gastroenterol* 1991;13:79–82.
75. Nogen A, Bremme J: Fatal acetaminophen overdosage in a young child. *J Pediatr* 1978;95:832–833.
76. Rumack B: Acetaminophen overdose in children and adolescents *Pediatr Clin North Am* 1986;33:691–701.
77. Miller R, Roberts R, Fisher L: Acetaminophen elimination kinetics in neonates, children and adults. *Clin Pharmacol Ther* 1976;19:284–294.
78. Peterson R, Rumack B: Toxicity of acetaminophen overdose. *JACEP* 1978;7:202–205.
79. Peterson R, Rumack B: Age as a variable in acetaminophen overdose. *Arch Intern Med* 1981;141:390–393.
80. Spyker D: Expediting accurate assessment and specific therapy in acetaminophen poisoning. *Emerg Med Rep* 1987;8:1–8.
81. Smilkstein M, Bronstein A, Linden C, et al: Acetaminophen overdose: a 48 hour intravenous *N*-acetylcysteine treatment protocol. *Ann Emerg Med* 1991;20:1058–1063.
82. Atwood S: The laboratory in the diagnosis and management of acetaminophen and salicylate intoxications. *Pediatr Clin North Am* 1980:27:871–879.
83. Prescott L. Park J, Proudfoot A: Cysteamine for paracetamol poisoning. *Lancet* 1976;1:357.
84. Chamberlain J, Gorman R, Oderda G, et al: Use of activated charcoal in a simulated poisoning with acetaminophen: a new loading dose for *N*-acetylcysteine? *Ann Emerg Med* 1993;22:1398–1402.
85. Tighe T, Walter F: Delayed toxic acetaminophen level after initial four hour nontoxic level. *J Toxicol Clin Toxicol* 1994;32:431–434.
86. Ashbourne J, Olson K, Khayam-Bashi H: Value of rapid screening for acetaminophen in all patients with intentional drug overdose. *Ann Emerg Med* 1989;18:1035–1038.
87. Bridges R, Kinneburgh D, Keehn B, et al: An evaluation of common methods for acetaminophen quantitation for small hospitals. *J Toxicol Clin Toxicol* 1983;20:1–17.
88. Osterloh J: Limitations of acetaminophen assays. *J Toxicol Clin Toxicol* 1983;20:19–22.
89. Klein-Schwartz W, Oderda G: Adsorption of oral antidotes for acetaminophen poisoning (methionine and *N*-acetlylcysteine) by activated charcoal. *Clin Toxicol* 1981;18:283–290.
90. Spiller H, Krenzelok E, Grande G, et al: A prospective evaluation of the effect of activated charcoal before oral *N*-acetylcysteine in acetaminophen overdose. *Ann Emerg Med* 1994;23:519–523.
91. Watson W, McKinney P: Activated charcoal and acetylcysteine absorption: issues in interpreting pharmacokinetic data. *DICP Ann Pharmacother* 1991;25:1081–1084.
92. Renzi F, Donovan J, Marten T, et al: Concomitant use of activated charcoal and *N*-acetylcysteine. *Ann Emerg Med* 1985;14:568–572.
93. Rose S, Gorman R, Oderda G, et al: Simulated acetaminophen overdose: pharmacokinetics and effectiveness of activated charcoal. *Ann Emerg Med* 1991;20:1064–1068.
94. Vale J, Meredith T, Crome P, et al: Intravenous *N*-acetylcysteine: the treatment of choice in paracetamol poisoning?, editorial. *Br Med J* 1979;2:1435–1436.
95. Prescott L, Illingworth R, Critchley J, et al: Intravenous *N*-acetylcysteine: still the treatment of choice for paracetamol poisoning, editorial. *Br Med J* 1980;1:46–47.
96. Prescott L, Illingworth R, Critchley J, et al: Intravenous *N*-acetylcysteine: the treatment of choice for paracetamol poisoning. *Br Med J* 1979;2:1097–1100.
97. Peterson R, Rumack B: Treating acute acetaminophen poisoning with acetylcysteine. *JAMA* 1977;237:2406–2407.
98. Galinsky R, Levy G: Effect of *N*-acetylcysteine on the pharmacokinetics of acetaminophen in rats. *Life Sci* 1979;5:693–700.
99. Selden B, Curry S, Clark R, et al: Transplacental transport of *N*-acetylcysteine in an ovine model. *Ann Emerg Med* 1992;20: 1069–1072.

100. Flanagan R, Meredith T: Use of *N*-acetylcysteine in clinical toxicology. *Am J Med* 1991;91:131S–139S.
101. Pond S, Tong T, Kaysen G, et al: Massive intoxication with acetaminophen and propoxyphene: unexpected survival and unusual pharmacokinetics of acetaminophen. *J Toxicol Clin Toxicol* 1982;19: 1–16.
102. Labadarios D, Davis M, Portmann B, et al: Paracetamol-induced hepatic necrosis in the mouse: relationship between covalent binding, hepatic glutathione depletion and the protective effect of α-mercaptopropionylglycine. *Biochem Pharmacol* 1977;26:31–35.
103. Smilkstein M, Knapp G, Kulig K, et al: Efficacy of oral *N*-acetylcysteine in the treatment of acetaminophen overdose. *N Engl J Med* 1988;319:1557–1562.
104. Tobias J, Gregory D, Deshpande J: Ondansetron to prevent emesis following *N*-acetylcysteine for acetaminophen intoxication. *Pediatr Emerg Care* 1992;8:345–346.
105. Keays R, Harrison P, Wendon J, et al: Intravenous acetylcysteine in paracetamol induced fulminant hepatic failure: a prospective controlled trial. *Br Med J* 1991;303:1026–1029.
106. Walton N, Mann T, Shaw K: Anaphylactoid reaction to *N*-acetylcysteine. *Lancet* 1979;2:1298.
107. Gazzard B, Clark R, Borirakchavyavat V, et al: A controlled trial of heparin therapy in the coagulation defect of paracetamol-induced hepatic necrosis. *Gut* 1974;15:89–93.
108. Widdop B, Medd R, Braithwaite R, et al: Experimental drug intoxication: treatment with charcoal hemoperfusion. *Arch Toxicol* 1915;34:27–32.
109. Willson R, Winch J, Thompson R, et al: Rapid removal of paracetamol by hemoperfusion through coaled charcoal. *Lancet* 1973;1: 77–82.
110. Helliwell M, Essex E: Hemoperfusion in "late" paracetamol poisoning. *Clin Toxicol* 1981;18:1225–1233.
111. Farid N, Glynn J, Kerr D: Hemodialysis in paracetamol self-poisoning. *Lancet* 1972;2:396–398.
112. Winchester J, Gelfand M, Helliwell M, et al: Extracorporeal treatment of salicylate or acetaminophen poisoning—is there a role? *Arch Intern Med* 1981;141:370–374.
113. Maclean D, Peters T, Brown P, et al: Treatment of acute paracetamol poisoning. *Lancet* 1968;2:849–852.

ADDITIONAL SELECTED REFERENCES

Gilligan J, Kemp R, Pain R, et al: Paracetamol concentrations, hepatotoxicity, and antidotes. *Br Med J* 1980;280:114.

Hamlyn A, James O, Douglas A: Treatment of paracetamol overdose. *Lancet* 1976;2:362.

Heading R, Nimmo J, Prescott L, et al: The dependence of paracetamol absorption on the rate of gastric emptying. *Br J Pharmacol* 1973;47: 415–421.

Hinson J, Pohl L, Monks T, et al: Acetaminophen-induced hepatotoxicity. *Life Sci* 1981;29:107–116.

James O, Lesna M, Roberts S: Liver damage after paracetamol overdosage. *Lancet* 1975;2:579–581.

Koch-Weser J: Acetaminophen. *N Engl J Med* 1976;295:1297–1300.

Manor E, Marmor A, Kaufman S, et al: Massive hemolysis caused by acetaminophen. *JAMA* 1976;236:2777–2778.

Meredith T, Vale J, Goulding R: The epidemiology of acute acetaminophen poisoning in England and Wales. *Arch Intern Med* 1981;141:397–400.

Mitchell M, Schenker S, Avant G, et al: Cimetidine protects against acetaminophen hepatotoxicity in rats. *Gastroenterology* 1981;81: 1052–1060.

Pearson H: Comparative effects of aspirin and acetaminophen on hemostasis. *Pediatrics* 1978;62(Suppl. 1):926–929.

Plotz P, Kimberly R: Acute effects of aspirin and acetaminophen on renal function. *Arch Intern Med* 1981;141:343–348.

Schreiner G, McAnally J, Winchester J: Clinical analgesic nephropathy. *Arch Intern Med* 1981;141:349–357.

Seeff L, Cuccherini B, Zimmerman H, et al: Acetaminophen hepatotoxicity in alcoholics. *Ann Intern Med* 1986;104:399–404.

Stewart M, Barclay J: Emergency estimation of plasma paracetamol. *Lancet* 1976;1:362–363.

Vale J, Meredith T, Goulding R, et al: Treatment of acetaminophen poisoning: the use of oral methionine. *Arch Intern Med* 1981;141: 394–396.

Wilson J, Kasantikul V, Harbison R, et al: Death in an adolescent following an overdose of acetaminophen and phenobarbital. *Am J Dis Child* 1978;132:466–473.

Zimmerman H: Effects of aspirin and acetaminophen on the liver. *Arch Intern Med* 1981;141:333–342.

CHAPTER 57

Salicylates

Salicylates in rudimentary form have been known since ancient times and were first described by Hippocrates (1). Toxicity was described much later, after aspirin (acetylsalicylic acid) was synthesized by the Bayer company in the 1850s. For many decades salicylate intoxication was the leading cause of accidental poisonings and deaths among children (2–4). Although recently there has been a substantial reduction in these accidental poisonings and deaths (5–7), salicylate poisoning continues to be relatively common because of accidental ingestion in children, intentional overdose in adults, and therapeutic intoxication in persons of all ages (8–10). The great decrease in the number of accidental pediatric salicylate ingestions and deaths over the last few years is due primarily to the introduction of safety lids on containers, the restriction on the number of flavored aspirin to 45 grains or 36 1.25-grain tablets per container, and the decreased use of salicylates in children (5–7,10). More than 20 billion tablets of salicylate are consumed per year, and more than 200 aspirin-containing products are available. Salicylates probably exist in more different formulations than any other drug (11).

Salicylates are nonsteroidal, anti-inflammatory, synthetic derivatives of salicylic acid (12). Salicylic acid is not used systemically because of its severe irritating effect on gastrointestinal mucosa and other tissues. Because of these side effects, better tolerated chemical derivatives have been prepared for systemic use (Table 57–1). Acetylsalicylic acid (ASA, aspirin) is the prototypical salicylate found in most compound analgesics. Aspirin is metabolized by hydrolysis into the active salicylate and acetate. Sodium, choline, and magnesium salts of salicylate are also used as antipyretics and are hydrolyzed into salicylic acid. Salsalate is the salicylate ester of salicylic acid and hydrolyzes to two molecules of salicylate. All these drugs distribute rapidly throughout all tissues and are bound to serum proteins, especially to albumin. Pepto-Bismol contains bismuth subsalicylate (13,14).

A topical preparation, methyl salicylate (also known as oil of wintergreen), is the most toxic salicylate compound because of the high content of salicylate (7 g per 5 mL). This is equivalent to 21 325-mg tablets of aspirin and can be rapidly lethal in young children (12). Its pleasant odor and its use as an agent to flavor candies often causes its potential as a poison to be underestimated. Many lay persons do not realize the potential harm from what often seems an innocent topical ointment or candy flavoring. Methyl salicylate is also an ingredient in Ben-Gay. Salicylic acid ointment, a topical preparation used for removing scales of psoriasis and corns, can also cause salicylate intoxication. Aspercreme and kerolytic agents (12) are examples of this salicylic compound.

TABLE 57–1. *Commonly used salicylates by trade name*

Type of salicylate	Trade name(s)
Aspirin	Anacin
	Alka-Seltzer
	ASA
	Ascriptin
	Bufferin
	Easprin
	Measurin
	Ecotrin
	Zorprin
Choline magnesium trisalicylate	Arthropan
	Trilisate
Magnesium salicylate	Durasal
	Magan
	Mobidin
	Trilisate
Methyl salicylate	Oil of wintergreen
Salsalate	Disalcid
	Arcylate
Salicylic acid	Calicylic
	Fomac
	Keralyt
	Mediplast
	Debucare

Although related to the salicylates structurally and pharmacologically, salicylamide and sodium thiosalicylate are not hydrolyzed to salicylate. Salicylamide is a weak analgesic and is a substance in some over-the-counter preparations. It was once commonly used for the pediatric population. Salicylamide has a different toxicity than aspirin and is relatively ineffective and unreliable as an antipyretic. Diflunisal is a salicylic acid derivative that is not metabolized to salicylic acid and has less of an effect than aspirin on platelet function (15). For this reason these compounds are not considered true salicylates.

ACTIONS

All the salicylates have analgesic, anti-inflammatory, and antipyretic actions. The salicylates act as antipyretics by altering the response of the hypothalamus to pyrogens, which then causes vasodilation and sweating (16).

These effects are due to the actions of both the acetyl and the salicylate portions of the molecule as well as the active salicylate metabolite.

The irreversible inhibition of platelet aggregation that is one of aspirin's effects specifically involves its ability to act as an acetyl donor to the platelet membrane; the nonacetylated salicylates have no clinically significant effect on platelet aggregation. Salicylates other than aspirin may therefore be particularly useful in patients with gastrointestinal intolerance to aspirin or in patients in whom interference of normal platelet function by aspirin or other nonsteroidal anti-inflammatory agents is undesirable. The anti-inflammatory and toxic effects of the drug are produced by the hydrolysis product, salicylic acid.

Peripherally, salicylates inhibit the synthesis of prostaglandins in inflamed tissues and thus prevent the sensitization of pain receptors to mechanical stimulation or to chemicals such as bradykinin that appear to mediate the pain response.

PHARMACOKINETICS

Salicylic acid is a weak acid with a pKa of 3 and thus tends to ionize to a greater degree at an alkaline pH and to a lesser degree at an acidic pH (17,18). Although the volume of distribution of salicylates increases with increasing plasma concentration, in the therapeutic range it is usually between 0.15 and 0.2 L/kg. In toxic states the volume of distribution can increase to more than 0.6 L/kg; this is due to decreased binding of salicylate to plasma proteins. The practical implication of this phenomenon is that high serum concentrations result in disproportionately high tissue concentrations.

It is this changing V_d that makes it difficult to interpret serum salicylate levels. Because patients can have different V_ds, patients can have tremendous differences in total body burdens and in tissue levels of salicylate while having the same serum salicylate concentrations. When elevated serum salicylate levels are decreasing in a patient, they can be decreasing not only from metabolism and renal excretion but also because salicylate is leaving blood, moving into tissues, and causing more toxicity as the V_d increases. At toxic levels, renal excretion becomes a major route of elimination. Un-ionized salicylate is reabsorbed by the renal tubules, prolonging elimination. Alkaline urine favors the formation of ionized salicylate, which cannot be reabsorbed and is excreted in the urine.

The biologic half-life of aspirin in the therapeutic situation is about 15 minutes, and the half-life of salicylic acid is 2 to 4 hours except in an overdose situation, when it can be more than 20 hours. In therapeutic situations, plasma concentrations of salicylate greater than 30 mg/dL are often associated with adverse systemic effects (18).

After absorption, salicylate distributes throughout body tissues. At higher salicylate concentrations, a lesser percentage of the drug is protein-bound. As a metabolic acidosis develops, a greater percentage of the free drug is un-ionized and is able to move into tissue. In fact, a drop in pH from 7.4 to 7.2 almost doubles the amount of un-ionized drug which is able to diffuse out of the plasma. The decreased protein binding and increased un-ionized fraction of the drug at lower pHs cause a change in the volume of distribution of salicylate. Depending on various factors, the V_d can vary over twofold. Those suffering from chronic salicylate toxicity have large volumes of distribution.

Absorption

The absorption of salicylate is quite rapid under normal circumstances, and serum concentrations are measurable in 15 to 30 minutes (2). The oral absorption of salicylate is limited by the rate of dissolution of the particular preparation. When antacid is added to the salicylate, absorption is increased (18).

Aspirin is not stable in solution and must be dissolved just before use. This usually requires the addition of a base, typically sodium bicarbonate, because the weakly acidic aspirin is not readily water-soluble.

The absorption of enteric-coated tablets is erratic, delayed, and sometimes incomplete; such tablets may be found many hours later still undissolved in the gastrointestinal tract (17,19). Clinical toxicity and peak plasma salicylate levels may not appear for as long as 12 hours or even longer (12). Patients who retain these enteric-coated preparations in the stomach are at risk for multiple gastric perforations and rapid death. Rectal suppositories are also absorbed very slowly and incompletely. The viscous preparation of methyl salicylate may take as long as 6 to 8 hours to be absorbed in significant amounts (12).

Even though therapeutic amounts of aspirin are absorbed rapidly, large doses of aspirin may be absorbed slowly partly because of the inhibitory effect of aspirin on gastric emptying and the impaired dispersion of the salicylate in gastrointestinal fluids. It has been shown that large doses of salicylates can result in delayed absorption from salicylate-induced pylorospasm. Because of these factors, in the acutely overdosed patient the plasma salicylate concentration may rise continually for as long as 24 hours after an ingestion. In addition, the formation of concretions (or bezoar) has been reported with aspirin overdose and may result in continued absorption for several days even after charcoal and cathartics have been administered.

Metabolism

Salicylate is metabolized principally in the liver by the microsomal enzyme system and is predominately conjugated with glycine to form salicyluric acid (7,20). Salicylate is also conjugated with glucuronic acid to form salicylphenolic glucuronide and salicylacyl glucuronide (21). In addition, small amounts of salicylate are hydrolyzed to form gentisic acid, which is an active metabolite and a potent inhibitor of prostaglandin synthesis. Renal excretion of the unmetabolized drug also occurs.

Two of these pathways, those involved in the formation of salicyluric acid and salicylphenolic glucuronide, are of limited capacity and are rapidly saturated even at therapeutic plasma salicylate concentrations (7,19). This is an example of Michaelis-Menten kinetics, which leads to possible accumulation and intoxication at therapeutic doses (10,21). Therefore, a 50% increase in the daily dose of aspirin may produce a 300% increase in the concentration of salicylate in the serum (18).

As a consequence of the saturation of the salicylurate and salicylphenolic glucuronide pathways, the renal excretory pathway contributes even more to the elimination of salicylate as the dose increases, giving urinary pH a much greater role in either enhancing or retarding excretion (18,21). For example, renal excretion of unmetabolized drug is usually less than 19% at low doses, but it could account for 50% or more at high doses or in an overdose if the pH of the urine is properly adjusted. Renal excretion of salicylate and formation of salicylic acid glucuronides become relatively more important elimination pathways for large single doses and for multiple doses that produce high plasma salicylate concentrations (Fig. 57–1) (19,22).

At some therapeutic plasma concentrations, salicylate follows first-order kinetics, so that as more is ingested more is excreted in a linear fashion. At high therapeutic doses and for toxic concentrations, excretion changes to zero-order kinetics, allowing only a certain quantity to be excreted hourly regardless of the amount present in the plasma (23). When a steady state from repeated doses occurs, as in the long-term administration of salicylates, then saturation kinetics may take effect, and relatively small increases in dose result in large increases in plasma concentration (17). Chronic salicylism, therefore, occurs

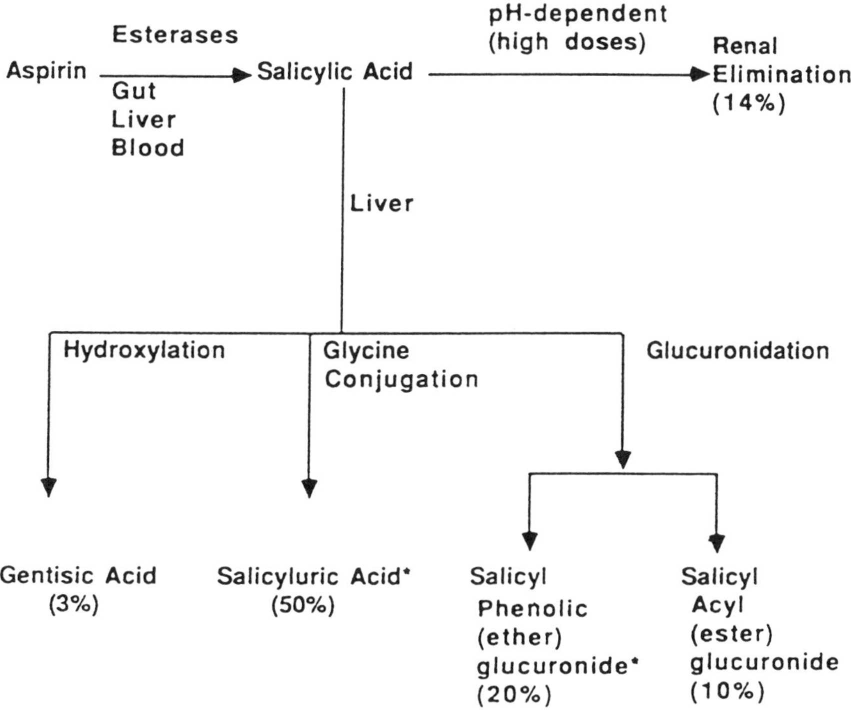

FIG. 57–1. Metabolism of aspirin and salicylates. The percentage of administered dose (3 g) metabolized to each metabolite appears in parenthesis. Asterisks indicate that formation of these metabolites is capacity-limited and thereby saturable. Compiled using data from Levy G, Tsuchiya T, Amsel LP: Limited capacity for salicyl phenolic glucuronide formation and its effect on the kinetics of salicylate elimination in man. *Clin Pharmacol Ther* 1972:13:258–268.

because of the early saturation of these enzymes and a switch in the kinetics from first-order to zero-order elimination (18).

In the situation of long-term maintenance aspirin therapy, the plateau level of salicylate may increase more than proportionately with increasing dosages. For these reasons, small upward changes in the maintenance dosage can have pronounced effects (24).

TABLE 57–2. *Disorders associated with salicylate overdose*

Acid-base disturbance
Hyperpyrexia
Electrolyte disorder
Dehydration
Clotting disorder
Gastrointestinal bleeding
Acute renal failure
CNS depression
Pulmonary edema

TOXICITY

There are many causes of intoxication by salicylates (salicylism), such as the administration of aspirin in too large a dose (10,25), the administration of adult aspirin or adult rectal suppositories to a child (9,10), and concomitant administration of salicylate with other salicylate-containing medicines (10,26). This last is common because many over-the-counter preparations contain aspirin and may be taken for various reasons. In addition to these causes of acute salicylism, chronic salicylate intoxication can occur after the prolonged routine administration of aspirin to a dehydrated patient or to one with other alterations in body homeostasis. Chronic salicylism may also occur in young children with an acute illness who are receiving salicylate too frequently or in elderly patients who, because of the chronicity of their problems, may be taking salicylate over a long period of time and become intoxicated in an insidious manner (26). Serious salicylate poisonings now seem to be most commonly associated with long-term or therapeutic administration of aspirin because of the peculiar metabolism of the salicylates, which change kinetics and begin to accumulate even with therapeutic doses (20,27).

Clinical Features

The pathophysiology of salicylate overdose is complex because of the range of toxic effects produced and their manifestations (Table 57–2). The principal toxic effects are extensions of the drug's pharmacologic actions and include direct CNS stimulation of respiration; uncoupling of oxidative phosphorylation leading to hyperpyrexia, electrolyte disturbances, and dehydration; altered glucose metabolism through inhibition of Krebs cycle enzymes; interference with hemostatic mechanisms leading to clotting disorders; and local gastrointestinal irritation leading to gastrointestinal bleeding (4,6,10). Acute renal failure, CNS dysfunction, and pulmonary edema are the more serious consequences of salicylism (7,28).

Respiratory Alkalosis

Early acid-base disturbances occur because aspirin increases medullary sensitivity to carbon dioxide, directly stimulating the CNS respiratory center in the medulla oblongata and resulting in hyperpnea and tachypnea (7). This leads to a decreased PCO_2, an increased pH, and respiratory alkalosis (Table 57–3) (10,29,30). Because of the excretion of the acidic carbon dioxide through the lungs, a compensatory increase in the renal excretion of bicarbonate occurs, which then causes loss of potassium and sodium in the urine (31). Many intoxicated adults and older children present with respiratory alkalosis with early bicarbonate excretion (19). This alkalosis fortuitously slows the entrance of salicylate into tissues and organs, including the brain (Fig. 57–2) (32).

It has been shown that the effects of CNS depressants may blunt the hypocapneic effect of salicylates, thereby reducing the incidence of respiratory alkalosis (31). Ingestion of CNS depressant drugs with aspirin, however, may not only diminish salicylate-induced hyperventilation in some patients but may also cause hypoventilation and respiratory acidosis, thus worsening the patient's condition (29).

Metabolic Acidosis

A metabolic acidosis (Table 57–4) may follow the physiologic compensation of respiratory alkalosis for a number of reasons. Acidosis develops principally from accumulation of organic acids. Salicylate and its metabolic by-products represent a large acid load but do not fully account for the metabolic acidosis (30). Pyruvic and lactic acids accumulate from the inhibition of α-ketoglutaric and succinic acid dehydrogenases of the Krebs cycle. In addition, inhibition of aminotransferases causes an increase in the amount of amino acids, and increased lipid metabolism leads to increased amounts of ketones such as acetoacetic acid, β-hydroxybutyric acid, and ace-

TABLE 57–3. *Pathophysiology of respiratory alkalosis*

Stimulation of respiratory center
Increased respirations
Increased carbon dioxide excretion
Decreased PCO_2
Increased plasma pH
Increased renal excretion of bicarbonate

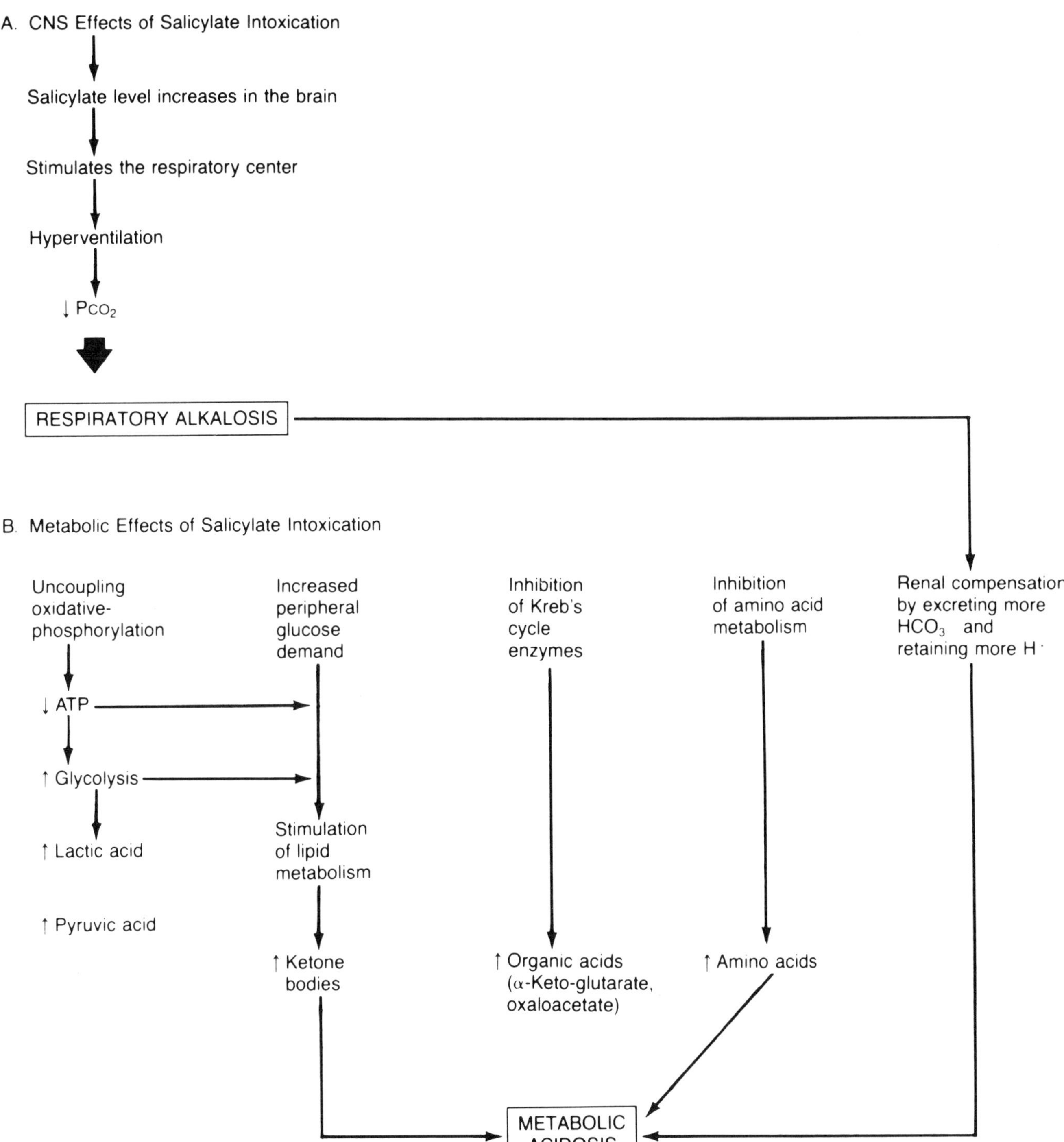

FIG. 57–2. Pathophysiologic consequences of salicylate intoxication.

TABLE 57–4. *Pathophysiology of metabolic acidosis*

Inhibition of Krebs cycle
Increased amounts of pyruvic and lactic acids
Increased peripheral demand for glucose
Stimulation of lipid metabolism
Increased formation of ketones

tone (10,31). Inorganic phosphoric and sulfuric acids accumulate secondary to salicylate-induced renal impairment (29). Depletion of buffer capacity as a result of the initial compensatory increase in renal excretion of bicarbonate also contributes to the development of metabolic acidosis. Together these changes produce a decrease in plasma pH and a metabolic acidosis (30,31).

Metabolic acidosis, however, may not occur until 12 to 24 hours after an acute ingestion of salicylate in an adult (33,34). The severity of the metabolic acidosis increases with decreasing age, and thus infants and children younger than 5 years of age are more susceptible to the development of ketosis with subsequent acidosis (12). A more rapid metabolic acidosis occurs in children because their ability to increase alveolar ventilation is quickly overcome by the accumulated acids (19). As a result, children quickly pass through the respiratory alkalosis stage to metabolic acidosis.

The likelihood of metabolic acidosis increases with the severity of salicylate intoxication (10). Chronic salicylism, too, may present with a compensated metabolic acidosis. The acutely salicylate-intoxicated adult usually exhibits a simple or compensated respiratory alkalosis and seldom proceeds to acidosis unless the poisoning is severe or salicylate was taken together with a respiratory depressant.

Uncoupling of Oxidative Phosphorylation

Salicylates have been shown to uncouple oxidative phosphorylation (4,35), resulting in failure to produce high-energy phosphates such as adenosine triphosphate while at the same time increasing oxygen utilization and carbon dioxide production, which increases heat production (12). In other words, because of the uncoupling energy normally conserved as a nucleotide, triphosphate (adenosine triphosphate) is dissipated as heat. In addition, salicylates in toxic doses decrease the efficiency of the normal cooling mechanisms. Hyperthermia may be striking, resulting in temperatures as high as 41°C to 42°C (105.8°F to 107.6°F) (35,36).

Hyperglycemia and Hypoglycemia

Salicylate causes mobilization of glycogen stores, resulting in hyperglycemia. However, salicylate is also a potent inhibitor of gluconeogenesis. Therefore, normoglycemia, hyperglycemia, or hypoglycemia may be noted in salicylate poisoning. Children are more likely than adults to develop hypoglycemia. Hypoglycemia, which can be severe, may occur late in the course of an acute intoxication after sufficient time has passed for glycogen stores to be depleted (8). Hyperglycemia can also occur early in the course of intoxication as a result of interference with tissue utilization of glucose (10). Hypoglycemia may be life-threatening and is most likely to occur in infants.

TABLE 57–5. *Pathophysiology of fluid and electrolyte disturbances*

Increased metabolism and heat production
Increased cutaneous insensible water loss through sweating
Organic aciduria and increased solute excretion
Increased renal output of water
Loss of gastric contents by emesis
Increased respiratory rate
Increased pulmonary insensible water loss
Increased renal excretion of bicarbonate
Increased excretion of sodium and potassium

Uncoupling of oxidative phosphorylation also leads to increased cerebral glycolysis (37). CNS glucose may be depleted even when the rest of the body is maintaining normal glucose concentrations (37) because the rate of glucose utilization from cerebrospinal fluid may exceed the rate of supply by the blood (10). Hypoglycemia should therefore be considered in a salicylate-intoxicated patient with seizures, coma, or altered mental status; and appropriate treatment should be initiated (37). Concurrent administration of glucose with salicylate overdose has been associated with striking improvement.

Fluid and Electrolyte Disorders

Dehydration and electrolyte loss occur early in salicylate intoxication as a result of a number of factors (Table 57–5). Because salicylates cause diaphoresis, water and sodium are lost. Further, because of the hyperventilation that occurs directly from salicylate ingestion, there is greater than normal insensible water loss from the lungs, which contributes to dehydration (8). Salicylates are an irritant to the gastrointestinal tract, causing vomiting and resultant fluid and electrolyte losses. Sodium and potassium are lost through the kidneys during respiratory alkalosis because the kidneys attempt to excrete bicarbonate and to conserve hydrogen ion (4). Dehydration may also be enhanced by decreased intake of fluids.

Hypokalemia is caused by both renal and extrarenal factors. The renal factor is excretion of bicarbonate, sodium, and potassium to compensate for the respiratory alkalosis. The extrarenal factors are loss of potassium from cells and an accumulation of sodium and water in cells due to the inhibition of the active cellular system for sodium–potassium transport caused by the uncoupling of oxidative phosphorylation. Hypokalemia may be a significant clinical finding, so that special attention may be required to normalize potassium during treatment.

Patients can be assumed to have total body potassium depletion even though normal serum potassium concentrations are present.

Clotting Disorders

Salicylates have important long-lasting effects on hemostasis. Clotting disorders occur because salicylates decrease the production of factor VIII, which results in a warfarin-like action of increasing prothrombin time. Clotting disorders can be treated by the administration of vitamin K (10). Other disorders include decreased prothrombin formation, decreased platelet adhesiveness, increased capillary fragility, and even decreased platelet amounts (29). The last effect is thought to be an autoimmune response. The effects of interference with platelet function remain for the life span of the platelets, which is 7 to 10 days. The result of this defect in platelet function is increased bleeding time and is due to irreversible acetylation of platelet prostaglandin cyclo-oxygenase. It has been shown that aspirin doses as low as 5 grains interfere with platelet aggregation (38). This effect is of possible therapeutic benefit in the prophylaxis of ischemic heart disease and cerebral transient ischemic attacks (39). Hypoprothrombinemia is considered secondary to inhibition of the vitamin K–dependent synthesis of factor VIII and, as stated above, can be reversed by administration of vitamin K (38).

Although bleeding can occur for many reasons, it is rarely secondary to the inhibition of clotting mechanisms in acute salicylate overdose. If bleeding does occur, it is usually from the gastrointestinal tract because salicylates exert a local effect on the mucosal lining: particulate aspirin in contact with the gastric mucosa dissolves the protective mucous lining, resulting in superficial erosions (40,41).

Central Nervous System Dysfunction

Patients who die from salicylate poisoning in spite of intensive supportive care frequently die a cerebral death (10,42). There appears to be a critical concentration of salicylate in brain tissue, at which death occurs, that is achieved over a wide range of serum salicylate concentrations. Confusion, lethargy, convulsions, respiratory arrest, and coma can all be seen in severe poisoning. Decreased adenosine-5'-triphosphate (ATP) production from uncoupling of oxidative phosphorylation results in acute brain failure and cerebral edema (43).

Except in severe cases, coma usually does not develop after acute ingestions. CNS depression is common in those with chronic toxicity. Symptoms of CNS dysfunction may include disorientation, hallucinations, and irritability or the more serious symptoms of coma, seizures, and cerebral edema. CSF glucose concentrations can be very low compared with serum glucose levels, and can mimic those of bacterial meningitis (Table 57–6) (44). The severity of CNS symptoms is directly related to the concentration of salicylate in the brain.

TABLE 57–6. *Central nervous system effects of salicylate overdose*

Cerebral edema
Coma
Confusion
Disorientation
Hallucinations
Irritability
Lethargy
Seizures

Acidosis increases the permeability of brain tissue to salicylate from the intravascular space because a low pH shifts the ratio of ionized to nonionized salicylate in favor of the nonionized form. Because the blood–brain barrier is more permeable to this nonionized salicylate, more of salicylate will enter the brain if the pH is lowered (43,45). As an example, a decrease in blood pH from 7.4 to 7.2 will double the amount of nonionized salicylate acid crossing the blood–brain barrier into the CNS (46). Therefore, one of the major therapeutic goals is to correct or avoid an acidosis.

Seizures may be a result of hypoglycemia or hypocalcemia, both of which can occur secondary to alkalosis or may be due to a direct effect of salicylate on the brain (43). Because seizures lead to a metabolic acidosis, their presence indicates a grave prognosis.

Another factor altering the distribution of salicylate is plasma protein binding. With high serum concentrations of salicylate, proportionately more is unbound and free to cross the blood–brain barrier.

Cardiac Dysfunction

Cardiac dysfunction may manifest as congestive heart failure, dysrhythmias, or sudden cardiac arrest. There are many factors contributing to cardiac abnormalities (47). The patient may be acidotic, hypokalemic, and hyperpyrexic, all of which may exacerbate any potential cardiac dysfunction and lead to decreased cardiac output and cardiac dysrhythmias.

Noncardiogenic Pulmonary Edema

Noncardiogenic pulmonary edema due to salicylate overdose is more common than has generally been realized (6,28,33,48–53). Pulmonary edema, although rare in children, appears to be a significant complication of salicylate intoxication in adults older than 30 years of age (54). Although pulmonary edema may occur from an acute overdose of salicylates, an increased risk for its development appears to be associated with chronic aspirin ingestion (55). In addition, pulmonary edema may be precipitated or aggravated by forced alkaline diuresis, but volume overload is not necessary for its occurrence (28,29).

The exact mechanism of salicylate-induced pulmonary edema remains unclear. Salicylates may cause pulmonary edema by increasing alveolar capillary membrane permeability (56). Most experimental evidence indicates that salicylates induce pulmonary edema by damaging the pulmonary vascular endothelium, thereby increasing permeability to fluid and protein in the pulmonary vascular bed (54,55), possibly mediated by inhibition of prostaglandin synthesis (10,57). Inappropriate secretion of antidiuretic hormone resulting in fluid retention has also been implicated as a possible mechanism triggering pulmonary edema (49). Some investigators have suggested that the edema may be centrally mediated and related to brain salicylate concentrations, secondary to hypoxia or myocardial failure, or due to a direct toxic effect of salicylate on the lungs or lung vasculature (10,52).

Salicylate-induced noncardiogenic pulmonary edema is usually manifested by tachypnea or dyspnea and hypoxemia (6). Physical examination usually reveals diffuse rales without signs of congestive heart failure such as gallop rhythm, cardiomegaly, peripheral edema, or jugular venous distension (49). Diffuse, bilateral alveolar infiltrates may be seen on the chest roentgenogram. Because the edema is noncardiogenic, the cardiac silhouette is not enlarged unless coincidental cardiac dysfunction is present (56). Proteinuria and adverse neurologic effects such as lethargy or confusion, profound respiratory failure, and the adult respiratory distress syndrome are often associated with pulmonary edema (58). Typically, patients with pulmonary edema may have a normal pulmonary capillary wedge pressure and are normotensive with normal cardiac output (6). Pulmonary edema appears to occur more frequently when the serum salicylate concentration exceeds 40 mg/dL; but in general, serum salicylate concentration correlates poorly with the subsequent development of pulmonary edema. With early diagnosis and prompt therapy, most patients survive and there is clearing of the chest roentgenogram in 1 to 7 days.

TABLE 57–7. *Signs and symptoms of chronic salicylism*

Gastrointestinal
Gastrointestinal hemorrhage
Gastric ulcer
Nausea
Vomiting
Neurologic
Tinnitus
Mental deterioration
Personality changes
Seizures
Coma
Hallucinations
Confusion
Disorientation
Slurred speech
Stupor
Hyperpyrexia
Miscellaneous
Pulmonary edema
Hypotension
Diaphoresis
Tachypnea
Abnormal bleeding diathesis

Chronic Salicylism

Although chronic salicylate poisoning frequently occurs, it may be occult and difficult to diagnose unless there is a high degree of suspicion (12,19). Chronic salicylism usually occurs accidentally and unknowingly from ingestion of moderate doses of aspirin prescribed for coexisting medical conditions (59). Chronic salicylism is usually associated with significant mortality (42). A 25% mortality has been reported in chronic salicylate intoxication when the diagnosis was delayed (46). Many times an elderly patient who is on various medications containing salicylates may present with atypical clinical features (24). Because of the cumulative kinetics of salicylate intoxication, these symptoms may include tinnitus, gastric ulcer with a gastrointestinal hemorrhage, abnormal bleeding parameters, weight loss, and mental deterioration or signs of "senility" (Table 57–7). The possibility of salicylate intoxication should always be kept in mind when attempting to diagnose the cause of these abnormalities (12).

Although serum salicylate concentrations are not reliable for an estimation of severity of intoxication or prognosis, they should be determined in all patients suspected of having chronic salicylism (60). A serum concentration in the therapeutic range does not rule out salicylate toxicity because the metabolic acidosis results in redistribution of salicylate from serum to tissue (42). The protean manifestations of chronic salicylate intoxication necessitate that medical practitioners maintain a high degree of clinical suspicion for this disorder in ill elderly patients (1).

ACUTE VERSUS CHRONIC POISONING

Acute and chronic poisoning have several distinct characteristics. The adult patient with acute salicylate toxicity usually presents with vomiting, abdominal pain, hyperventilation, diaphoresis, dehydration, ketonuria, and a respiratory alkalosis. As the poisoning progresses, acidemia, lethargy, cardiovascular abnormalities, coagulation disorders, hyperthermia, and serious neurotoxicity develop. Pulmonary edema can occur but is not common. Children frequently present with acidemia.

In contrast to acute poisoning, patients with chronic salicylate toxicity usually do not have significant gastroenteritis, although dehydration can be severe. They are usually brought in by family members because of changes in mentation, including lethargy, disorientation,

TABLE 57–8. *Features of acute salicylate intoxication*

Gastrointestinal
Nausea
Vomiting
Neurologic
Dizziness
Confusion
Vertigo
Tinnitus
Disorientation
Hallucinations
Coma
Seizures
Hearing loss
Miscellaneous
Acid-base disorder
Electrolyte disorder
Hyperpnea
Hyperpyrexia
Diaphoresis
Dehydration
Oliguria
Pulmonary edema

and hallucinations. Even adults are frequently but not always acidemic on presentation. Adult respiratory distress syndrome (ARDS) is common in chronic toxicity. Because patients with chronic toxicity have a large V_d, they present with more serious toxicity at a given serum salicylate concentration compared with an acutely poisoned patient.

Chronic salicylate toxicity must be considered in any patient with unexplained CNS dysfunction, especially in the presence of a mixed acid/base disturbance. Many patients with chronic salicylate toxicity are incorrectly diagnosed at the time of hospital admission (60).

SUMMARY OF SIGNS AND SYMPTOMS OF INTOXICATION

The possibility of salicylate poisoning should be considered in any patient who presents with unexplained hyperpnea in association with vomiting, confusion, lethargy, fever, coma, or convulsions (Table 57–8) (7,42). Nausea and vomiting commonly occur after salicylate overdose from the direct irritative effect on the gastric mucosa and the direct central effect, which is independent of the route of absorption. Tinnitus is also common in a significant overdose. As discussed, hyperpyrexia is a result of the uncoupling of oxidative phosphorylation. Hyperpnea is a reflection of the direct effect of salicylate on the respiratory center, causing a respiratory alkalosis (Table 57–9). Disorientation, coma, and seizures are ominous findings that suggest a serious overdose (6).

TABLE 57–9. *Metabolic abnormalities associated with salicylate overdose*

Hypoglycemia and hyperglycemia
Respiratory alkalosis
Metabolic acidosis
Hypokalemia
Hyponatremia and hypernatremia
Hypoprothrombinemia
Increased bleeding time
Ketosis
Altered renal function

Morbidity

The causes of morbidity from salicylate overdose are CNS dysfunction, cardiac dysfunction, and noncardiogenic pulmonary edema (36). It is clear that the plasma salicylate concentration is not the sole indicator of morbidity or a fatal outcome. Some patients with high levels are no more ill than others with concentrations only half as high. It is probable that the severity of salicylate intoxication depends more on the ratio of the plasma salicylate concentration to that in cerebrospinal fluid than to that in plasma alone, and, consequently, upon factors that increase penetration of the drug to the brain, foremost among which are acid-base abnormalities (61).

Assessment of Severity of Salicylate Overdose

History

In acute salicylate ingestions, the severity of intoxication can be roughly estimated by obtaining a history of the amount ingested (Table 57–10), evaluating the clinical condition of the patient, and measuring serum salicylate concentration in relation to the time since ingestion (20). As determined from the history, if the patient has ingested less than 150 mg/kg of salicylate, the likelihood of any serious symptoms developing is negligible. Patients who ingest 150 to 300 mg/kg may experience mild to moderate toxic reactions. At doses in excess of 300 mg/kg, patients may show prolonged and severe effects (Table 57–10) (62).

Salicylate Nomogram

Even though there may be an accurate history of the quantity ingested, laboratory evidence of the drug in the blood should be relied on to make a prognosis and therapeutic decision. In the past, laboratory determinations

TABLE 57–10. *Assessing severity of salicylate overdose by history*

Ingested dose (mg/kg)	Estimated severity
<150	Asymptomatic
150—300	Mild to moderate
300—500	Serious
>500	Potentially lethal

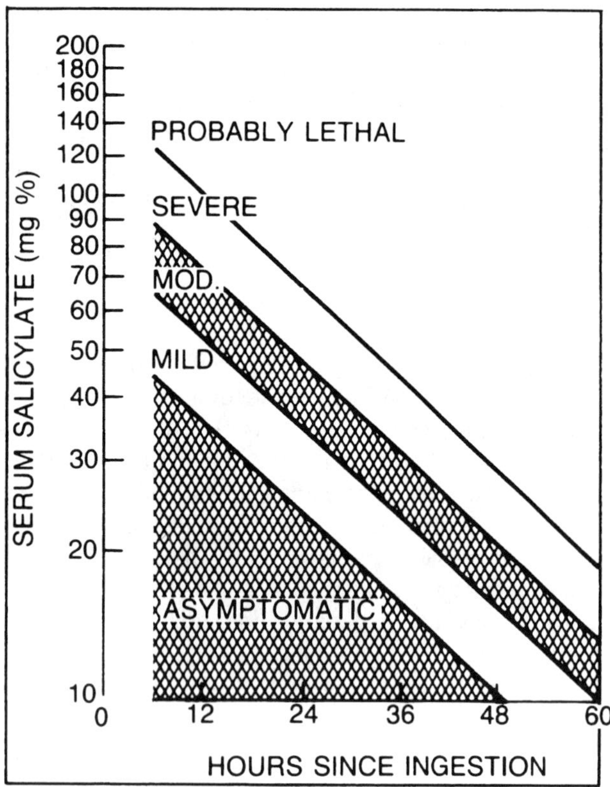

FIG. 57–3. Salicylate nomogram for acute salicylate toxicity. Reproduced from *Pediatrics* 1960;26:800 by permission of the American Academy of Pediatrics.

were problematic because of the poor correlation between serum salicylate concentration and clinical severity. Efforts to resolve this problem gave rise to the salicylate nomogram (Fig. 57–3), which is based on the stronger correlation between serum salicylate concentrations and the severity of symptoms when the time of ingestion is used as a point of reference (20,27). Severity is determined on the basis of the magnitude of the peak concentration, whenever it may have occurred (63).

The nomogram may be helpful in deciding the need for hospitalization and the type of therapy that may be required (62). Nevertheless, it can only be used with single, acute ingestions and has no relevance to chronic or multiple ingestions (44). It is also not applicable to overdoses with liquid salicylate preparations or enteric-coated tablets, for which peak concentrations may occur earlier (liquids) or later (enteric preparations) than for uncoated tablets (20). Other factors that may delay salicylate absorption must be considered when using the nomogram, including concomitant use of narcotics or anticholinergic agents or preexisting peptic ulcer disease.

The nomogram can be used for the acute ingestion of salicylates beginning at 6 hours after ingestion. Because absorption and distribution of salicylate may continue during the first 6 hours, blood concentrations measured before 6 hours should not be used to predict toxicity, although they may be useful in confirming an overdose (20). More than one measurement should always be made to ensure that a peak concentration is obtained (7), and a patient should never be released from the hospital on the basis of a single measurement. A concentration measured before 6 hours can be used if more than one measurement is made to establish that the concentration is declining.

For the patient who is within the asymptomatic range on the nomogram, there are usually no objective signs of salicylate poisoning. The patient who falls within the mild range may eventually experience some hyperpnea, lethargy, vomiting, and a small degree of hyperthermia. Acidosis is not usually noted. The patient in the moderate range has a greater degree of hyperpnea and may develop prominent neurologic disturbances, such as marked lethargy or perhaps excitability. More severe neurologic disturbances such as seizures or coma usually do not occur. Hypoglycemia may develop, and later in the course a compensated metabolic acidosis may ensue. The patient in the severe range may present in coma or become comatose, undergo seizures, and eventually develop a partially compensated metabolic acidosis. Usually, patients with readings of moderate or severe on the salicylate nomogram require hospitalization.

In massive overdoses, plasma salicylate concentrations may continue to increase up to 24 hours after ingestion. Bezoar formation should be considered in a patient who does not respond to therapy as predicted or in whom serum salicylate concentrations continue to increase after therapy has been instituted.

LABORATORY ANALYSIS

A number of laboratory tests are recommended for the patient intoxicated with salicylate (Table 57–11). As discussed above, the plasma salicylate concentration is the single most important prognostic indicator for the salicylate-intoxicated patient. Arterial blood gases should be measured to confirm the patient's acid-base status, especially if bicarbonate therapy is to be instituted. A urine specimen should be obtained for pH measurement, and a complete blood cell count and prothrombin time studies should be performed for baseline analysis. Electrolyte studies should be performed because of the potential for acid-base and fluid and electrolyte imbalances.

Bedside tests may aid in the detection of salicylism in a qualitative manner (19). The ferric chloride test can be performed on urine. This test is positive in the presence of any amount of salicylic acid, acetoacetic acid, or phenylpyruvic acid. Ferric chloride (10%) is added to a small amount of boiled urine, which removes any interfering substances such as ketones. A purple color indicates the presence of salicylates. A false-positive result may be produced by some phenothiazines (20,64).

Phenistix can be used in a semiquantitative manner (12); this test is used in the diagnosis of phenylketonuria. Development of a color when a stick is dipped into serum or urine indicates that salicylate or phenothiazines are present. The addition of one drop of sulfuric acid bleaches out the color from phenothiazines but not from salicylate. If a tan color develops, the salicylate concentration is considered less than 40 mg/dL. A deeper brown indicates a concentration in the range of 40 to 90 mg/dL, and a purple color indicates a concentration greater than 90 mg/dL. A gray-green to blue color develops if the test is positive for phenylketonuria (20,27).

TABLE 57–12. *Treatment of salicylate intoxication*

Indication	Treatment
Acute overdose	Lavage Activated charcoal and cathartic
Dehydration	Correction of fluid losses with normal saline and potassium chloride
Acidosis	Alkali therapy with sodium
Coagulopathies	Vitamin K
Hyperthermia	Sponge baths
Hypoglycemia	Glucose (25 g IV)
Seizures	Antiseizure medicines(diazepam or short-acting barbiturates)
Pulmonary edema	Oxygen or positive end-expiratory pressure

TREATMENT

A specific antidote for salicylate is not available; consequently, treatment of intoxication is limited to symptomatic, supportive care (Table 57–12), which is not always adequate (12). The emphasis should be on removing and adsorbing or decontaminating the remaining drug, controlling hyperthermia, correcting the metabolic disturbances and dehydration, and hastening excretion of the drug (10,12). Avoiding systemic acidosis is a primary therapeutic goal in salicylate intoxication because acidemia has been shown to be associated with increased neurologic abnormalities and a grave prognosis. Care must be taken that there is no interference with carbon dioxide excretion through the lungs, so that adequate ventilation must be maintained (65).

Decontamination should be attempted if the intoxicant is a topically absorbed preparation such as salicylic acid or oil of wintergreen. Lavage and administration of activated charcoal and a cathartic should be performed for orally ingested salicylate even late after ingestion because there may be decreased absorption of salicylate when it is taken in large amounts in addition to the concretions that sometimes form (66).

Multiple-Dose Activated Charcoal

Salicylates have a small volume of distribution and are dialyzable, so that multiple-dose activated charcoal (MDAC) has been suggested as a noninvasive approach to increasing clearance by an intestinal dialysis (67). The most favored hypothesis for the effectiveness of multiple-dose charcoal therapy is that it is a type of internal dialysis procedure (68). The repetitive charcoal administration lowers the concentration of free drug within the gastrointestinal tract, thus favoring back-diffusion from the bloodstream across the gastrointestinal epithelium, hence the term *gastrointestinal dialysis* (69,70). Some investigators have found no increase in the excretion of salicylate after MDAC (65).

TABLE 57–11. *Suggested laboratory tests for salicylate overdose*

Plasma salicylate concentration
Arterial blood gases
Complete blood cell count
Urinalysis
Electrolytes
Prothrombin time

Fluid Repletion

Almost all symptomatic patients with salicylate poisoning are dehydrated. Appropriate fluid challenges using saline or colloids should be given rapidly to replenish intravascular volume and produce adequate urine flow. Correction of fluid loss should be vigorous, with fluid administered in volume to compensate for the great amounts that may have been lost (71). Repletion may be performed at a rate of as much as 10 to 15 mL/kg/hour for the first 1 to 2 hours and then 4 to 8 mL/kg/hour. Potassium chloride (20 to 40 mEq/L) should be added.

Diuresis

There is controversy concerning the role of forced diuresis in the treatment of salicylate overdose. Proponents of forced diuresis have argued that it provides a safe and effective method of enhancing salicylate elimination, with clearance rates comparable to those achieved by hemodialysis (72–74). Opponents have questioned its efficacy and emphasized possible side effects, including hypernatremia and fluid overload (7). Large amounts of crystalloid solutions have the potential to increase lung microvasculature pressure and the transfer of fluid across the injured pulmonary vascular bed and to decrease colloid oncotic pressure, which is a factor that may be important in the pathogenesis of noncardiogenic pulmonary edema (6).

Urinary Alkalinization

Another concern is whether diuresis is effective in producing an alkaline urine in the severely intoxicated patient with electrolyte abnormalities (7). Recently, sodium bicarbonate without a diuresis was shown to be at least as effective as bicarbonate diuresis in enhancing elimination of salicylate but, unlike the diuresis regimens, did not cause fluid retention or any noticeable biochemical abnormalities (19,74). Until further work is done, a conservative approach, with the use of bicarbonate and administration of fluids for the massive fluid losses and without the use of diuresis, is recommended (6,74,75).

As a rule of thumb, a concentration of 30 mg/dL in adults indicates that renal excretion of salicylate should be enhanced by alkalinization (19). Because acidemia carries such an ominous prognosis, it should be corrected as rapidly as possible to minimize the entry of salicylate into CNS and other tissues (10,76). Furthermore, the acidotic state promotes retention of the drug because it reduces the effectiveness of the salicylate excretory mechanism of the kidney (65). Parenteral alkalinization with sodium bicarbonate, which is almost solely an extracellular alkalinizer, should be attempted for plasma ion trapping effects and to raise the pH of the urine for enhancement of excretion (70). The rate at which salicylate is removed from the body is augmented by making the urine alkaline, and a change in urine pH from 6.5 to 7.5 will enhance urinary excretion tenfold (72).

Oral alkalinization enhances gastrointestinal salicylate absorption and should not be used in therapy. Also, attempts to reduce hyperventilation through the use of CNS depressant drugs should never be made because they may depress the respiratory center and induce or exacerbate a potentially fatal metabolic acidosis (74).

The Role of Acetazolamide

Acetazolamide (Diamox), a carbonic anhydrase inhibitor, causes a loss of bicarbonate in the urine and so may be considered a logical choice for increasing salicylate excretion (77); it should not be used alone, however, because it also causes retention of hydrogen ions and thereby a metabolic acidosis and because salicylate becomes trapped in the brain and other tissues as a result of its use (78). There are reports of severe intoxication resulting from the combined therapeutic use of aspirin and a carbonic anhydrase inhibitor. This is probably due to the acidemia induced by the carbonic anhydrase inhibitor, which increases the concentration of freely diffusable nonionized salicylic acid and thereby enhances the ability of salicylate to penetrate into the CNS.

The frequent monitoring of arterial blood gases, serum electrolytes, and urine pH cannot be overemphasized. The acid/base and electrolyte status of the patient suffering from serious salicylate poisoning is constantly changing (68). Small changes in serum potassium levels or arterial pH can have dramatic effects on the degree of toxicity and on salicylate clearance.

Alkalinization should be attempted only in patients who require this therapy; and because salicylate can cause an alkalosis, care must be taken not to overalkalinize these patients, which may exacerbate hypokalemia or cause tetany or cardiac dysrhythmias (6). In severely intoxicated patients, however, it may be important to administer bicarbonate to replace that lost in the urine; loss of bicarbonate can lead to a metabolic acidosis and ultimately worsen the patient's condition (79). This is especially true for children who go through a transient stage of respiratory alkalosis. Vigorous potassium repletion may be required to ensure adequate alkalinization of the urine.

An alkaline urine may not be possible to achieve in the patient who needs it most (74). Such a situation is most probably due to marked metabolic acidosis, potassium depletion, and consequent aciduria. The potassium deficit may be severe because of the preexisting acidosis, which leads to intracellular penetration of hydrogen ion and displacement of potassium ion. Potassium is thereby lost in the urine. These underlying disorders may require correction before an alkaline urine can be obtained (12).

Both bicarbonate and potassium are needed to produce an alkaline urine and large doses of both may be required. Even if arterial pH is 7.5, if the serum potassium level is normal, and if the urine is acidic, more potassium is needed. Furthermore, an alkaline urine will not be produced if, when reabsorbing sodium, the kidney is preferentially secreting hydrogen ions into the tubular lumen rather than potassium ions.

Hyperthermia

Sponge baths and cooling blankets can be used for hyperthermia, and the use of salicylates should be avoided if the patient is hyperthermic for an unknown reason.

Pulmonary Edema

When measured, pulmonary capillary wedge pressure has been found to be normal during acute manifestations of salicylate-induced pulmonary edema (56). Treatment of pulmonary edema therefore is generally supportive and includes adequate oxygenation (28). Early hemodynamic monitoring, including arterial and pulmonary artery catheter placement, may be highly desirable (6,7). Ventilation management for these patients is similar to that recommended for patients with other forms of adult respiratory distress syndrome (28). Positive end-expiratory pressure may be necessary if oxygenation is not adequate, but diuretics have not been shown to be helpful. Resolution of roentgenographic abnormalities is frequent in 3 to 8 days, but fatal outcome has also been reported (56).

Hemorrhage

The intravenous administration of vitamin K (10 to 50 mg) is suggested only if hemorrhagic complications occur or if bleeding parameters are markedly abnormal.

Hypoglycemia

The possibility of hypoglycemia should be considered in any patient with salicylate poisoning who deteriorates unexpectedly. Therefore, glucose should be administered if coma, seizures, or an altered mental status occurs (8,10). If seizures continue, short-acting barbiturates or diazepam can be administered.

Role of Extracorporeal Removal

Although hemodialysis and hemoperfusion are effective in removing salicylate from the body, their role in the acute salicylate overdose is limited. Hemodialysis is preferred over hemoperfusion because acid-base and electrolyte disturbances are corrected more rapidly with the former (Table 57–13). For the most part, however, neither dialysis nor hemoperfusion is necessary in the care of the overdosed patient. Hemodialysis may be particularly useful in chronically intoxicated patients with high serum salicylate concentrations (19). Regardless of serum salicylate concentrations, hemodialysis may be especially useful for patients with an unresponsive acidosis, impaired renal function, pulmonary edema, persistent CNS manifestations, or progressive deterioration despite appropriate therapy, or for patients who have a preexisting disease that prohibits usual therapeutic measures (10,19). If the drug is present in a significant amount and if renal failure occurs, dialysis is necessary to remove the drug.

TABLE 57–13. *Indications for hemodialysis in salicylate overdose*

Renal failure
Clinical findings
Persistent CNS manifestations
Seizures
Coma
Pulmonary edema
Failure to respond to other therapy
Worsening acid-base disorder
Worsening electrolyte disorder

REFERENCES

1. Spitalnic S: Wang R: Updating salicylate toxicity. *Emerg Med Rep* 1993;14:174–180.
2. Andrews H: Salicylate poisoning. *Am Fam Physician* 1973;8: 102–106.
3. Temple A: Pathophysiology of aspirin overdosage toxicity, with implications for management. *Pediatrics* 1978;62(Suppl.):873–876.
4. Temple A: Acute and chronic effects of aspirin toxicity and their treatment. *Arch Intern Med* 1981;141:364–369.
5. Sherz R: Safely packaging impact on childhood poisoning in the United States. *Vet Hum Toxicol* 1979;21(Suppl.):127–129.
6. Fisher C, Albertson T, Foulke G: Salicylate-induced pulmonary edema. *Am J Emerg Med* 1985;3:33–37.
7. Henry J, Volans G: ABC of poisoning: analgesic poisoning. Part I: salicylates. *Br Med J* 1984;289:820–823.
8. Hill H: Current concepts: salicylate intoxication. *N Engl J Med* 1973; 288:1110–1112.
9. Griffith R, Decker W, Wright C: Iatrogenic salicylate poisoning of an infant by adult rectal aspirin suppositories. *J Fam Pract* 1981;12: 757–760.
10. Snodgrass W, Rumack B, Peterson R, et al: Salicylate toxicity following therapeutic doses in young children. *Clin Toxicol* 1981;18: 247–259.
11. Leist E, Banwell J: Products containing aspirin. *N Engl J Med* 1974;291:710–712.
12. Sullivan J, Lander D: Planning an effective therapeutic strategy in salicylate poisoning. *Emerg Med* 1986;7:89–96.
13. Mendelowitz P, Hoffman R, Weber S: Bismuth absorption and myoclonic encephalopathy during bismuth subsalicylate therapy. *Ann Intern Med* 1990;112:140–141.
14. Soriano-Brucher H, Avendano P, O'Ryan M, et al: Bismuth subsalicylate in the treatment of acute diarrhea in children: a clinical study. *Pediatrics* 1991;87:18–27.
15. Brogden R, Heel P, P Pakes G, et al: Diflunisal: a review of its pharmacological properties and therapeutic use in pain and musculoskeletal strains and sprains and pain in osteoarthritis. *Drugs* 1980;19: 81–106.
16. Lovejoy F: Aspirin and acetaminophen: a comparative view of their antipyretic and analgesic activity. *Pediatrics* 1978;62(Suppl.):904–909.
17. Levy G: Clinical pharmacokinetics of aspirin. *Pediatrics* 1978; 69(Suppl.):867–872.
18. Levy G, Tsuchiya T: Salicylate accumulation kinetics in man. *N Engl J Med* 1972;287:430–432.
19. Skiendzielewski J, Parrish G, Harrington T: Mental confusion in an elderly chronically ill patient. *Ann Emerg Med* 1986;15:571–575.
20. Done A, Temple A: Treatment of salicylate poisoning. *Mod Treat* 1971;8:528–551.
21. Netter P, Faure C, Regent M, et al: Salicylate kinetics in old age. *Clin Pharmacol Ther* 1985;38:6–11.
22. Murray M, Brater D: Nonsteroidal anti-inflammatory drugs. *Clin Geriatr Med* 1990;6:365–397.
23. Beveridge G, Forshall W, Munro J, et al: Acute salicylate poisoning in adults. *Lancet* 1964;1:1406–1412.
24. Shkrum M, Gay R, Hudson P: Fatal iatrogenic salicylate intoxication in a long-term user of enteric-coated aspirin. *Arch Pathol Lab Med* 1989;113:89–90.
25. Mitchell I: "Therapeutic" salicylate poisoning in children. *Br Med J* 1979;1:1081.
26. Cline M, Williams H: The clinical pharmacology of salicylates: medical staff conference. *Calif Med* 1969;110:410–422.
27. Done A: Aspirin overdosage: incidence, diagnosis, and management. *Pediatrics* 1978;62(Suppl.):890–897.

28. Davis P, Burch R: Pulmonary edema and salicylate intoxication. *Ann Intern Med* 1974;80:553–554.
29. Smith M: The metabolic basis of the major symptoms in acute salicylate intoxication. *Clin Toxicol* 1968;1:387–392.
30. Bartels P, Lund-Jacobsen H: Blood lactate and ketone body concentrations in salicylate intoxication. *Hum Toxicol* 1986;5:363–366.
31. Gabow P, Anderson R, Potts D, et al: Acid-base disturbances in the salicylate-intoxicated adult. *Arch Intern Med* 1978;138;1481–1484.
32. Gossel TA, Bricker JD. *Principles of clinical toxicology,* 3rd ed. New York: Raven Press; 1994.
33. Tashima C, Rose M: Pulmonary edema and salicylates. *Ann Intern Med* 1974;81:274–279.
34. Goldfrank L, Bresnitz X: Salicylism. *Hosp Physician* 1979;15(3): 50–60.
35. Miyahara J, Karlei R: Effect of salicylate on oxidative phosphorylation of mitochondrial fragments. *Biochem J* 1965;97:194–198.
36. Segar W, Holliday M: Physiologic abnormalities of salicylate intoxication. *N Engl J Med* 1958;259:1191–1194.
37. Thurston J. Pollack P, Warren S, et al: Reduced brain glucose with normal plasma glucose in salicylate poisoning. *J Clin Invest* 1970;49:2139–2142.
38. Pearson H: Comparative effects of aspirin and acetaminophen on hemostasis. *Pediatrics* 1978;62(Suppl):926–929.
39. Krasnoff S, Bernstein M: Acetylsalicylic acid poisoning. *JAMA* 1947;135:712–714.
40. Robins J, Turnbull J, Robertson C: Gastric perforation after acute aspirin overdose. *Hum Toxicol* 1985;4:527–528.
41. Ashworth C, McKemie J: Hemorrhagic complications, with death probably from salicylate therapy. *JAMA* 1944;126:806–810.
42. Anderson R, Potts D, Rumack R, et al: Unrecognized adult salicylate intoxication. *Ann Intern Med* 1976;85:745–748.
43. Fink M, Irwin P: Central nervous system effects of aspirin. *Clin Pharmacol Ther* 1982;32:362–365.
44. Wortzman D, Grunfeld A: Delayed absorption following enteric-coated aspirin overdose. *Ann Emerg Med* 1987;16:434–436.
45. Reed J, Palmisano P: Central nervous system salicylate. *Clin Toxicol* 1975;8:623–631.
46. Paul B: Salicylate poisoning in the elderly: diagnostic pitfalls. *J Am Geriatr Soc* 1972;20:387–390.
47. Berk W, Andersen J: Salicylate-associated asystole: report of two cases. *Am J Med* 1989;86:505–506.
48. Granville-Grossman K, Sergeant H: Pulmonary edema due to salicylate intoxication. *Lancet* 1960;1:575–577.
49. Greenstein S: Pulmonary edema due to salicylate intoxication: report of a case. *Dis Chest* 1963;44:552–553.
50. Hrnicek G, Skelton J, Miller W: Pulmonary edema and salicylate intoxication. *JAMA* 1974;230:866–867.
51. Hefner J: Noncardiogenic pulmonary edema: a complication of salicylate toxicity. *Respir Care* 1982;27:1215–1218.
52. Karliner J: Noncardiogenic forms of pulmonary edema. *Circulation* 1972;46:212–216.
53. Sorensen S: Adult respiratory-distress syndrome in salicylate intoxication. *Lancet* 1979;1:1025–1028.
54. Greenbaum D, Togba J, Blecker M, et al: Salicylate intoxication: an unusual presentation. *Chest* 1974;66:575–576.
55. Bowers R, Brigham K, Owen P: Salicylate pulmonary edema: the mechanism in sheep and review of the current literature. *Am Rev Respir Dis* 1977;115:261–268.
56. Shanies H: Noncardiac pulmonary edema. *Med Clin North Am* 1977; 61:1319–1337.
57. Hyman A, Spannhoke E, Kadowitz P: Prostaglandins and the lung. *Ann Rev Respir Dis* 1978;117:111–136.
58. Leventhal L, Kuritsky L, Ginsburg R, et al: Salicylate-induced rhabdomyolysis. *Am J Emerg Med* 1989;7:409–410.
59. Perrault J, Fleming R, Dozois R: Surreptitious use of salicylates: a cause of chronic recurrent gastroduodenal ulcers. *Mayo Clin Proc* 1988;63;337–342.
60. Bailey R, Jones S: Chronic salicylate intoxication: a common cause of morbidity in the elderly. *JAGS* 1989;37:556–561.
61. Chapman B, Proudfoot A: Adult salicylate poisoning: deaths and outcome in patients with high plasma salicylate concentration. *Quart J Med* 1989;72:699–707.
62. Dugandzic R, Tierney M, Dickinson G, et al: Evaluation of the validity of the Done nomogram in the management of acute salicylate intoxication. *Ann Emerg Med* 1989;18:1186–1190.
63. Brown S, Cameron J, Matthew H: Plasma salicylate levels in acute poisoning in adults. *Br Med J* 1967;2:738–739.
64. Trinder P: Rapid determination of salicylate in biological fluids. *Biochem J* 1954;57:301–303.
65. Mayer A, Sitar D, Tenenbein M: Multiple-dose charcoal and whole-bowel irrigation do not increase clearance of absorbed salicylate. *Arch Intern Med* 1992;152:393–396.
66. Boxer L, Anderson F, Rowe D: Comparison of ipecac-induced emesis with gastric lavage in the treatment of acute salicylate ingestion. *J Pediatr* 1970;74:800–803.
67. Hillman R, Prescott L: Treatment of salicylate poisoning with repeated oral charcoal. *Br Med J* 1985;291:1472.
68. Keller R, Schwab R, Krenzelok E: Contribution of sorbitol combined with activated charcoal in prevention of salicylate absorption. *Ann Emerg Med* 1990;19:654–656.
69. Kirshenbaum L, Mathews S, Sitar D, et al: Does multiple-dose charcoal therapy enhance salicylate excretion? *Arch Intern Med* 1990;150:1281–1283.
70. Vertrees J, McWilliams B, Kelly H: Repeated oral administration of activated charcoal for treating aspirin overdose in young children. *Pediatr* 1990;85:594–598.
71. Sallis R: Management of salicylate toxicity. *Am Fam Pract* 1989;39: 265–268.
72. Cumming G, Dukes D, Widdowson G: Alkaline diuresis in treatment of aspirin poisoning. *Br Med J* 1964;4:1033–1036.
73. Lawson A, Proudfoot A, Brown S, et al: Forced diuresis in the treatment of acute salicylate poisoning in adults. *Q J Med* 1969;38: 31–48.
74. Elenbaas R: Critical review of forced alkaline diuresis in acute salicylism. *Crit Care Q* 1982;4:89–95.
75. Prescott L, Balali-Mood M, Critchley J, et al: Diuresis or urinary alkalinization for salicylate poisoning? *Br Med J* 1982;285: 1383–1386.
76. Prowse K, Pain M, Matston A, et al: The treatment of salicylate poisoning using mannitol and forced alkaline diuresis. *Clin Sci* 1970; 38:327–337.
77. Morgan A, Polak A: Acetazolamide and sodium bicarbonate in treatment of salicylate poisoning in adults. *Br Med J* 1969;1:16–19.
78. Sweeney K, Chapron D, Brandt L, et al: Toxic interaction between acetazolamide and salicylate: case reports and a pharmacokinetic explanation. *Clin Pharmacol Ther* 1986;40:518–524.
79. McCain H, Teague R: Metabolic complications of salicylate overload. *Drug Ther* 1979;20:70–80.

ADDITIONAL SELECTED REFERENCES

Cabooter M, Elewaut A, Barbier F: Salicylate-induced pancreatitis. *Gastroenterology* 1981;80:214–215.

Cooper S. Needle S, Kruger G: Comparative analgesic potency of aspirin and ibuprofen. *J Oral Surg* 1977;35:898–903.

Hefner J, Sahn S: Salicylate-induced pulmonary edema: clinical features and prognosis. *Ann Intern Med* 1981;95:405–409.

Kahn A, Blum D: Fatal respiratory-distress syndrome and salicylate intoxication in a two-year-old. *Lancet* 1979;2:1131–1132.

McGuigan M: A two-year review of salicylate deaths in Ontario. *Arch Intern Med* 1987;147:510–512.

Miller R, Jick H: Acute toxicity of aspirin in hospitalized medical patients. *Am J Med Sci* 1977;274:271–279.

Paynter A, Alexander F: Salicylate intoxication caused by teething ointment. *Lancet* 1979;2:1132.

Proudfoot A, Brown S: Acidemia and salicylate poisoning in adults. *Br Med J* 1969;2:547–550.

Wallers J, Woodring J, Stelling C, et al: Salicylate-induced pulmonary edema. *Radiology* 1983;146:289–293.

Zimmerman G, Clemmer T: Acute respiratory failure during therapy for salicylate intoxication. *Ann Emerg Med* 1981;10:104–106.

CHAPTER 58

Nonsteroidal Anti-Inflammatory Agents

The adverse effects of aspirin, especially the gastric irritation that occurs when large doses are employed, have led to the search for alternative compounds. Starting with ibuprofen in 1974, several drugs with aspirin-like properties, designated nonsteroidal anti-inflammatory drugs (NSAIDs), have been approved for use in the U.S. for the treatment of rheumatoid arthritis or osteoarthritis. Nonsteroidal anti-inflammatory drugs have become the most frequently prescribed drugs, and within the last 10 years there has been a proliferation in the number of new NSAIDs (1,2). These drugs make up a heterogenous group of compounds that share certain therapeutic actions and side effects but that may be structurally dissimilar (Table 58–1) (3). Although aspirin is an NSAID, this term is usually used to designate the newer aspirin substitutes.

TABLE 58–1. *Nonsteroidal anti-inflammatory drugs (NSAIDs)*

Acetic acid derivatives
Etodolac (Lodine)
Indomethacin (Indocin)
Ketorolac (Toradol)
Sulindac (Clinoril)
Tolmetin (Tolectin)
Fenamate derivatives
Flufenamic acid
Meclofenamate (Meclomen)
Mefenamic acid (Ponstel)
Oxicam derivatives
Piroxicam (Feldene)
Propionic acid derivatives
Fenbufen
Fenoprofen (Nalfon)
Ibuprofen (Motrin, Rufen, Advil, Nuprin, Mediprin)
Indoprofen
Ketoproten (Orudis)
Naproxen (Naprosyn, Anaprox)
Nabumetone (Relafen)
Oxaprozin (Daypro)
Pyrazole derivatives
Oxyphenbutazone (Tandearil)
Phenylbutazone (Azolid, Butazolidin)

CLINICAL USES

The NSAIDs are used extensively as antiarthritics, analgesics, and antigout and pseudogout agents as well as for pain and inflammation associated with bursitis, tendonitis, costochondritis, pericarditis, and dysmenorrhea (Table 58–2) (3). NSAIDs have also been used to treat venous thrombosis, cerebrovascular disease, patent ductus arteriosus in premature infants, and hypercalcemia associated with certain malignancies (4). The NSAIDs produce their antipyretic effects by acting on the hypothalamus, with heat dissipation being increased as a result of vasodilation and increased peripheral blood flow.

PHARMACOKINETICS

Absorption

All the NSAIDs are absorbed rapidly and almost completely following oral administration. Absorption occurs by passive diffusion in the stomach and upper small intestine and is influenced by pH. Because NSAIDs are weak acids, they are un-ionized in the highly acid gastric environment. In this state, NSAIDs are lipid-soluble and easily diffuse into gastric cells, where the pH is higher and the drug dissociates. In this manner, NSAIDs become "ion-trapped" within the gastric cells. Such locally high concentrations contribute to the gastrointestinal side effects of NSAIDs (5).

Co-administration of aluminum or magnesium antacid may delay absorption of NSAIDs. Although prior antacid or food ingestion may delay NSAID absorption, the same amount of drug is absorbed. A larger fraction of the NSAID dose is absorbed in the small intestine under these circumstances. Rectal suppositories of NSAIDs do not confer any advantage because absorption is erratic and incomplete (4).

Protein Binding

All the NSAIDs are highly protein-bound, and only the unbound drug is biologically active. In general, less than 10% of a dose is excreted unchanged by the kidney; the

TABLE 58–2. *Indications for NSAIDs*

Analgesia and anti-inflammation
Arthritis
Gout
Pseudogout
Bursitis
Tendonitis
Costochondritis
Sprain or strain
Pericarditis
Dysmenorrhea
Antipyresis
Patent ductus arteriosus
Venous thrombosis
Hypercalcemia

drug is metabolized predominantly by the liver (2). This high degree of binding restricts these drugs to the plasma compartment, accounting for the small volumes of distribution. Most of the NSAIDs bind only to albumin. Once the albumin binding sites are saturated, the concentration of free drug rapidly increases (6). This accounts for the relatively speedy efficacy of most NSAIDs and for their self-prophylaxis: the free drug is rapidly excreted by the kidney, so that drug accumulation is prevented (5).

Because the NSAIDs are so strongly protein-bound, they can be displaced from binding sites or can displace other protein-bound drugs, including sulfonylurea agents, some β blockers, oral anticoagulants, hydantoins, salicylates, and sulfonamides (Table 58–3). This can potentiate the effects of the other agent (2).

Mechanism of Action

The generation of inflammatory reactions appears to require the action of a number of mediators, but the class of mediators most directly linked to the action of anti-inflammatory drugs is the prostaglandins (7). This group of biologically active molecules is now known to be a part of a broad class of lipids referred to as the eicosanoids (8).

The Prostaglandins (Table 58–4)

The prostaglandins are unsaturated fatty acid compounds derived from 20-carbon essential fatty acids (1).

TABLE 58–3. *Protein-bound drugs whose concentrations may increase with concomitant NSAID therapy*

β-Adrenergic blocking agents
Oral anticoagulants
Phenytoin
Salicylates
Sulfonamides
Sulfonylurea agents

They are found in tissue membranes, primarily phospholipids (2). These are synthesized from the dietary essential fatty acids linoleic acid and linolenic acid. The most important of the precursors to prostaglandin synthesis is arachidonic acid (8,9). Prostaglandins participate in a variety of activities, including mediation of inflammatory responses, protection of the gastrointestinal mucosa against injury, and regulation of renal blood flow.

Collectively, the prostaglandins, thromboxanes, and leukotrienes are called eicosanoids. Of the cyclo-oxygenase products, PGE_2 and prostacyclin play the most important roles in inflammation. Both are potent vasodilators and hyperalgesic agents and are presumed to contribute significantly to the erythema, swelling, and pain associated with inflammation (5).

Synthesis of Prostaglandins

Prostaglandin synthesis is initiated within the cell by cleavage of arachidonic acid from membrane phospholipids through the action of a phospholipase. Synthesis is initiated by a stimulus that damages or distorts the cell membrane, such as infection, trauma, fever, or platelet aggregation (11). Because the prostaglandins have an effect on target cells in the immediate vicinity of their site of biosynthesis, they are called “local hormones” (1). The prostaglandins appear in minute quantities, have a short half-life (seconds to minutes), are not stored in appreciable quantities in either cells or tissues, and are ubiquitous in their distribution throughout the body. In this respect the prostaglandins differ from circulating hormones (9).

NSAIDs and Prostaglandins

Prostaglandins not only have direct proinflammatory effects but also synergize with other inflammatory mediators such as bradykinin and histamine. NSAIDs block prostaglandin production, and hence their actions, by

TABLE 58–4. *Characteristics of the prostaglandins*

Composed of unsaturated fatty acids
Synthesized from linoleic, linolenic, and arachidonic acids
Physiologic stimulation of synthesis
Infection
Trauma
Fever
Platelet aggregation
Properties
Short half-life
Located in tissue membranes
Not stored in the body
“Local hormones”
Distributed throughout body

inhibition of the enzyme cyclo-oxygenase. Through the blockade of prostaglandin-derived mediators, NSAIDs reduce inflammation (11). Because NSAIDs bind reversibly to cyclo-oxygenase, both the beneficial and the toxic effects of the prostaglandins recede when the drug is stopped.

Corticosteroids, which are the most potent of the anti-inflammatory drugs, are also potent inhibitors of prostaglandin synthesis (9). The mechanisms of other anti-inflammatory drugs such as gold salts, penicillamine, and antimalarials are unknown at present, but they differ from NSAIDs and seem to have no important effects on prostaglandin synthesis.

The inhibition of prostaglandin biosynthesis may only partly explain the therapeutic effects of NSAIDs (11). Another postulated mechanism is interaction with the adenylate cyclase system. Some NSAIDs inhibit phosphodiesterase, thereby increasing the intracellular concentration of cyclic AMP. Cyclic AMP has been shown to stabilize membranes, including lysosomal membranes in polymorphonuclear leukocytes, thus preventing the release of enzymes that appear to play a major role in the inflammatory response (11).

Side Effects

Although the NSAIDs are among the most widely used drugs in medicine and are generally well tolerated, toxic effects have been noted, some of which may be quite severe (3). Side effects of NSAIDs are largely consequences of prostaglandin inhibition. Affected tissues are those in which NSAIDs tend to accumulate. In rare instances, these drugs can cause allergic reactions, peptic ulcer disease, elevation of liver enzymes, and kidney failure (Table 58–5). Problems with zomepiric (Zomax) and benoxaprofen (Oraflex) are extreme examples of known side effects (12,13); both compounds have been removed from the market. The voluntary withdrawal of these drugs by their manufacturers as well as recent reports of hepatic and renal toxicity have drawn attention to the potential toxicities of NSAIDs (14).

TABLE 58–5. *Side effects of NSAIDs*

Gastrointestinal
Dyspepsia
Epigastric pain
Gastritis
Peptic ulceration
Gastrointestinal bleeding
Hematologic
Impairment of platelet function
Mild bleeding diathesis
Renal
Acute renal failure
Chronic renal failure
Nephrotic syndrome
Interstitial nephritis
Hepatic
Hepatotoxicity (rare)

Unfortunately, all currently available NSAIDs appear to be nonselective inhibitors of cyclo-oxygenase, at least clinically. In addition to inhibiting unwanted prostaglandin synthesis, they also inhibit desirable prostaglandin synthesis as in gastric mucosa and the renal medulla (15).

Gastrointestinal

Gastrointestinal symptoms are the most common adverse effects reported. Most gastrointestinal side effects are mild, consisting of nausea, vomiting, abdominal pain, or upset (16). However, acute ulcer disease and massive life-threatening bleeding can occur, even without warning symptoms (17). NSAIDs can cause injury visible at endoscopy. These drugs produce three types of lesions in the stomach and duodenum: petechiae, erosions, and ulcers (18).

Mechanism of Action of Gastric Effects

Gastrointestinal damage associated with NSAIDs is thought to be a result of both the systemic and local effects of these drugs. Systemic effects are caused by NSAIDs' interference with the production of mucosal prostaglandins by inhibiting the activity of cyclo-oxygenase (19).

Several of the protective mechanisms thought to be important for normal health of the gastric and duodenal mucosa are regulated by the prostaglandins (20). Such mechanisms include mucus production, epithelial bicarbonate production, mucosal blood flow, and possibly cell restitution. Use of NSAIDs thus interferes with local protection of the mucosa and can result in an ulcer (18). There are thought to be other systemic mechanisms of injury, including generation of oxygen-free radicals and other products resulting from the lipoxygenase pathway (10). NSAIDs also directly affect the integrity of the gastric and duodenal mucosal barrier, permitting back-diffusion of hydrogen ions that may cause mucosal injury (18).

The prodrugs, such as fenbufen and sulindac, are not active until they are absorbed and metabolized by the liver and consequently are of low ulcerogenicity yet sulindac is still associated with gastrointestinal bleeding from solitary ulcers (16).

Drugs Used in Conjunction with NSAIDs

Misoprostol, a synthetic prostaglandin E_1 analog, decreases gastric acid secretion, stimulates the production and release of bicarbonate and mucus, and maintains mucosal blood flow. Misoprostol has been shown to be effective in the prevention of NSAID-induced gastric ulcers in patients with arthritis. This agent has also been shown to prevent the development of NSAID-induced duodenal lesions both in normal subjects and in arthritic patients (21).

Sucralfate is an effective anti-ulcer drug that has been shown to increase the release of endogenous prostaglandins from the gastric mucosa, suggesting that stimulation of prostaglandin synthesis may be a mechanism for its action (17). Despite the fact that sucralfate is widely used to prevent NSAID-induced gastrointestinal mucosal damage, no study has evaluated the efficacy of sucralfate in the prevention of NSAID-induced mucosal damage in chronic NSAID users.

Hematologic

NSAIDs impair platelet aggregation through inhibition of platelet cyclo-oxygenase–induced synthesis of thromboxane. Although this effect produces at most a mild bleeding diathesis in hematologically normal patients, bleeding may be severe in patients with coagulation defects caused by anticoagulants or hereditary clotting factor deficiencies.

Renal

The NSAIDs have been known to produce a wide array of untoward renal effects, including acute interstitial nephritis, acute papillary necrosis, nephrotic syndrome, and acute and chronic renal failure (1). This may develop insidiously and is neither dose-dependent nor related to duration of drug use (22). Patients rarely have symptoms suggestive of a hypersensitivity reaction, so the conditions may go undetected until advanced (23).

Prostaglandins are potent vasodilators in the kidney, and it appears that renal disease occurs by the inhibition of renal prostaglandin (24). Under basal conditions, inhibition of renal prostaglandin synthesis has little effect on renal function, but under conditions of ineffective circulatory volume, angiotensin II and catecholamine levels rise, stimulating prostaglandin production. The introduction of an NSAID in these circumstances may lead to unopposed vasoconstrictor activity by inhibiting prostaglandin production (25). The renal insufficiency that occurs under those conditions is generally reversible within 24–72 hours (23). This phenomenon occurs rarely with virtually all the NSAIDs that are primary prostaglandin inhibitors. The reaction is reversible if the drug is discontinued and appropriate supportive measures are taken. In addition, abnormalities of water metabolism and of sodium and potassium homeostasis have been noted (26).

Interstitial nephritis and nephrotic syndrome have been reported in patients on NSAID therapy (27). These patients do not necessarily have antecedent renal disease, and the duration of NSAID therapy may range from weeks to months. With discontinuation, clinical manifestations usually resolve.

Sodium retention represents a much more universal side effect of NSAID therapy and essentially all NSAIDs have been implicated. The etiology of the sodium retention is probably multifactorial, but the promotion of sodium uptake by the renal tubules as a result of prostaglandin synthesis inhibition is the major influence.

Severe hyperkalemia has been reported in patients who had mild renal insufficiency and who were given indomethacin for gout. Decreased renin activity has been demonstrated essentially with all NSAIDs, with the possible exception of sulindac.

Hepatic

Because the liver plays a central role in metabolism of NSAIDs, it is not surprising that there has been associated hepatotoxicity (2). Liver toxicity is rare with most NSAIDs but has been noted with phenylbutazone and oxyphenbutazone, which are the most hepatotoxic of the NSAIDs. To date, Reye's syndrome has not been associated with NSAID therapy (5).

CHARACTERISTICS OF THE NSAIDS

The NSAIDs can be divided into several chemical groups (see Table 58–1). Some of the NSAIDs are considered prodrugs, which are precursor drugs requiring metabolism to an active metabolite.

NSAIDs differ in a variety of ways: potency of cyclooxygenase inhibition, lipophilicity, pKa, absorption characteristics, half-life, and side effect profiles. Despite these differences, no one NSAID has been shown to be therapeutically superior.

Acetic Acid Derivatives

Etodolac (Lodine)

Etodolac is an indole acetic acid derivative used for anti-inflammatory and analgesic effects in the acute and chronic symptomatic treatment of osteoarthritis.

Etodolac is well absorbed from the gastrointestinal tract; serum concentrations of the drug reach a peak 1 to 2 hours after ingestion. Antacids and food decrease the peak concentration but do not affect the extent of absorption. As with other NSAIDs, more than 99% of the drug is bound to plasma proteins. Etodolac is metabolized in the liver to inactive metabolites, which are excreted in the urine, with an elimination half-life of 6 to 7 hours.

Abdominal pain, gastrointestinal ulceration, and dyspepsia have been the most frequent adverse effects of etodolac. Headache, dizziness, rash, and pruritus have also occurred in patients taking etodolac. Drug-associated hepatic and renal dysfunction and neutropenia have been reported.

Indomethacin

Indomethacin (Indocin) is rapidly absorbed from the upper gastrointestinal tract and may be absorbed even more quickly when given as a rectal suppository (11). Indomethacin is highly protein-bound, and its apparent volume of distribution ranges from 0.39 to 1.5 L/kg (7).

The elimination half-life of a therapeutic dose varies from 2.6 to 11.2 hours and is similar in duration to the half-life reported in the overdosed patient. Biotransformation is the major elimination pathway (3).

Acute intoxication with indomethacin may cause nausea, vomiting, anorexia, abdominal pain, headache, tinnitus, dizziness, lethargy, drowsiness, confusion, paresthesia, aggressive behavior, disorientation, restlessness, gastrointestinal bleeding, electrolyte imbalance, coma, and seizures (Table 58–6) (3). Although blood dyscrasias such as leukopenia, thrombocytopenia, and agranulocytosis have occurred, they are usually a consequence of chronic administration (11).

Sulindac

Sulindac (Clinoril) is a prodrug that is converted to active sulfide and sulfone metabolites by the cytochrome P-450 enzyme system (7). Sulindac and its metabolites undergo extensive enterohepatic circulation (3). The enterohepatic cycling prolongs the duration of action to about 16 hours. Sulindac bears a chemical resemblance to indomethacin but is a substituted indene rather than an indole. It was synthesized as the result of a search for a compound as effective as indomethacin but with less ulcerogenic potential (11).

The elimination half-lives of sulindac and its active metabolites are 7 and 16 hours, respectively. Because it is metabolized slowly, it can be given in twice-daily doses. The plasma protein binding of sulindac is approximately 95% (3).

The indications and adverse reactions are similar to those of other NSAIDs. Stevens-Johnson epidermal necrolysis syndrome, thrombocytopenia, agranulocytosis, and nephrotic syndrome have all been observed.

TABLE 58–6. *Clinical features of acute indomethacin overdose*

Gastrointestinal
Nausea
Vomiting
Anorexia
Abdominal pain
Hematemesis
Neurologic
Headache
Tinnitus
Dizziness
Lethargy
Drowsiness
Contusion
Paresthesia
Disorientation
Restlessness
Coma
Seizures

Tolmetin

Tolmetin (Tolectin) has a structural resemblance to indomethacin and sulindac but has an action and toxicity similar to those of the propionic acid derivatives (7). It is well absorbed from the gastrointestinal tract and is highly protein-bound (3). The plasma half-life of tolmetin is approximately 1 hour, and the drug has an apparent volume of distribution of 0.10 to 0.14 L/kg.

The side effects that may be seen after long-term administration of tolmetin may also be noted in the acute overdose and may consist of nausea, vomiting, epigastric pain, headache, dizziness, and tinnitus (Table 58–7). Central nervous system manifestations such as anxiety, nervousness, insomnia, drowsiness, and visual disturbances have also been reported (11).

Fenamate Derivatives

Meclofenamate

Meclofenamate (Meclomen) is highly protein-bound and undergoes significant enterohepatic circulation. The

TABLE 58–7. *Clinical features of acute tolmetin overdose*

Gastrointestinal
Nausea
Vomiting
Epigastric pain
Neurologic
Headache
Dizziness
Tinnitus
Anxiety
Nervousness
Insomnia
Drowsiness
Visual disturbances

half-life is approximately 3 hours (3,7). After acute massive overdose, CNS stimulation (manifested as irrational behavior, marked agitation, and generalized seizure) may occur. This initial phase may be followed by renal toxicity, including decreased urine output and increased serum creatinine concentration, and may be accompanied by oliguria or anuria and azotemia (3).

Mefenamic Acid

Mefenamic acid (Ponstel) is rapidly absorbed from the gastrointestinal tract. The plasma half-life of this highly protein-bound drug is 2 to 4 hours. Although it is eliminated by biotransformation, enterohepatic recirculation of metabolites also appears to occur (7).

The major side effect of mefenamic acid is diarrhea (3). This is a special problem in the elderly, and renal insufficiency has been reported in patients who became dehydrated as a result of the diarrhea (Table 58–8) (11). In addition, dyspepsia, upper gastrointestinal tract discomfort, and occasional ulceration with hemorrhage have been reported (28). Other findings in the acute overdose include coma, hypoprothrombinemia, and acute renal failure. Unlike overdosage with other NSAIDs, overdosage with mefenamic acid appears to be characterized by a relatively high incidence of seizures (3). Patients who have taken overdoses of mefenamic acid must be closely observed, particularly during the first few hours, when seizures are most likely to occur (28). The drug is usually eliminated very quickly, with rapid recovery noted (3).

Oxicam Derivatives

Piroxicam

Piroxicam (Feldene) is structurally distinct from other NSAIDs. It is a potent anti-inflammatory agent that is extensively bound to plasma protein. At therapeutic doses piroxicam has an elimination half-life of 45 hours (3). Piroxicam is one of the most widely used NSAIDs in the world because of its long half-life (29). Pharmacokinetic studies in the elderly and in patients with renal impairment show no evidence of drug accumulation.

TABLE 58–8. *Clinical features of acute mefenamic acid overdose*

Gastrointestinal
Diarrhea
Dyspepsia
Gastric ulceration
Miscellaneous
Renal insufficiency
Coma
Hypoprothrombinemia
Seizures

Acute overdose may cause nausea, vomiting, diarrhea, abdominal pain, gastrointestinal bleeding, dizziness, blurred vision, excitability, coma, seizures, hematuria, proteinuria, and acute renal failure.

Propionic Acid Derivatives

Fenbufen

Fenbufen is a prodrug with no anti-inflammatory activity of its own (3). Thus, there is a low incidence of gastrointestinal side effects associated with its use. After absorption, it is converted in the liver to its active metabolite (7). Fenbufen is highly protein-bound, and plasma concentrations reach their peak 1 to 2 hours after ingestion of therapeutic doses. The elimination half-life of the parent drug and that of its two principal metabolites after administration of therapeutic doses are approximately 10 hours.

Fenoprofen

Fenoprofen (Nalfon), as either the sodium or the calcium salt, is rapidly and completely absorbed from the gastrointestinal tract. Plasma concentrations reach a peak 2 hours after a single oral dose. Fenoprofen has a plasma half-life of 2 to 3 hours (11). It is bound extensively to human serum albumin and has a low apparent volume of distribution of 0.8 to 0.10 L/kg (3). It is metabolized extensively, and less than 5% of a dose is excreted unchanged in the urine. When substantial quantities of fenoprofen are ingested in acute overdose, hematuria and acute renal failure may occur.

Adverse effects and drug interactions of fenoprofen are similar to those of ibuprofen, i.e., nephrotoxicity, jaundice, nausea, dyspepsia, peripheral edema, rash, pruritus, central nervous system and cardiovascular effects, and tinnitus.

Ibuprofen

Ibuprofen (Motrin, Rufen, Advil, Nuprin, Mediprin) was the first phenylpropionate to be marketed in the United States. Although ibuprofen has shown anti-inflammatory, antipyretic, and analgesic activity, higher doses are required for anti-inflammatory effects than for analgesia. Ibuprofen is now available in several over-the-counter preparations (7,30).

Pharmacokinetics

The drug is well absorbed from the gastrointestinal tract, and plasma concentrations reach their peak about 1 to 2 hours after a single oral dose (31). Ibuprofen is highly bound to plasma proteins and is eliminated chiefly by biotransformation. The half-life is about 2 to 4 hours (11). There is no evidence of accumulation after multiple doses, and in the overdose setting the elimination half-life does not appear to be prolonged (32).

Adverse Effects

Since its introduction to the United States in 1974, ibuprofen has been shown to be relatively safe and effective for the treatment of inflammatory disorders. It is generally well tolerated, although mild and transient gastrointestinal discomfort may occasionally occur. Central nervous system complaints such as headache and giddiness may also occasionally occur. Diarrhea, vomiting, stomatitis, erythematous or urticarial skin rashes, constipation, deafness, and edema have been reported less frequently.

As with other propionic acid derivatives, acute overdose with ibuprofen causes nausea, vomiting, abdominal pain, drowsiness, nystagmus, diplopia, headache, tinnitus, impaired renal function, coma, and hypotension (Table 58–9). In addition, serious effects associated with a single large ingestion have included profound metabolic acidosis, hypotension, acute renal failure, acute liver cell injury, and acute cholestasis (30,32).

Ibuprofen is known to be extensively metabolized by oxidation of the isobutyl group and eliminated primarily by the kidney. Because ibuprofen and its metabolites are acidic compounds, their accumulation in the blood could be responsible for a metabolic acidosis (30). The ability of ibuprofen to inhibit renal prostaglandin synthesis may explain the renal toxic effects noted. In 1984, ibuprofen became available without a prescription in the U.S. (33). Greater availability and aggressive media marketing dramatically increased its use, with a corresponding increase in the number of reported cases of acute ibuprofen overdose (34).

TABLE 58–9. *Clinical features of acute ibuprofen overdose*

Gastrointestinal
Nausea
Vomiting
Abdominal pain
Neurologic
Tinnitus
Coma
Nystagmus
Diplopia
Headache
Miscellaneous
Metabolic acidosis
Hypotension
Acute renal failure
Acute liver cell injury
Acute cholestasis

Because there is no definitive treatment or antidote other than supportive care for patients with ibuprofen overdose, as there is for acetaminophen, there is no apparent need for routine use of ibuprofen serum concentrations as an adjunct in the management of ibuprofen overdose patients. The ibuprofen nomogram has not been noted to be useful in clinical overdoses due to the poor correlation between ibuprofen serum concentrations and toxicologic effect.

Ketoprofen (Orudis)

Ketoprofen, a propionic acid derivative, is a nonsteroidal anti-inflammatory agent. The drug is structurally related to fenoprofen, ibuprofen, and naproxen.

Ketoprofen is rapidly and almost completely absorbed from the gastrointestinal tract. The absolute bioavailability of commercially available ketoprofen capsules is approximately 90%. Food and milk decrease the rate of absorption of the drug, resulting in delayed and reduced peak plasma concentrations, but the extent of absorption is not affected. Following single 50-mg oral doses, average peak plasma ketoprofen concentrations of 4.1 μg/mL occur after about 1 hour in the fasted state compared with 2.4 μg/mL after 2 hours in the nonfasted state. Concomitant administration of an aluminum and magnesium hydroxides antacid or an aluminum phosphate antacid does not appear to affect absorption of the drug.

Although the relationship between plasma ketoprofen concentrations and therapeutic effect has not been precisely determined, a therapeutic range of 0.4–6 μg/mL has been suggested. Ketoprofen is approximately 99% bound to plasma proteins, mainly albumin. In geriatric patients and in patients with alcoholic cirrhosis, protein binding of the drug appears to be reduced.

Limited information is available on the acute toxicity of ketoprofen. Drowsiness, vomiting, and abdominal pain have been reported in a few individuals following acute overdosage of ketoprofen.

Ketorolac (Toradol)

Ketorolac is an intramuscular NSAID indicated for the treatment of acute pain. It is a compound chemically and structurally related to tolmetin, zomepirac, and indomethacin (35).

Ketorolac is a potent inhibitor of the cyclo-oxygenase pathway of arachidonic acid metabolism, resulting in a decrease in prostaglandin and thromboxane production (35). Ketorolac does not appear to have significant CNS effects or opioid-like effects nor does it enhance infection by inhibiting macrophage phagocytosis as do corticosteroids (36).

Pharmacokinetics

Ketorolac tromethamine is rapidly and completely or almost completely absorbed following intramuscular administration, with a maximum plasma concentration achieved in 45–50 minutes. Bioavailability has been reported to range from 80% to 100% following oral administration. The rate of absorption appears to be slower following intramuscular administration than following oral administration of the drug in fasting, healthy adults; however, the extent of absorption is similar following both routes of administration. Food decreases the rate, but not the extent, of absorption of orally administered ketorolac tromethamine. The rate of absorption from the gastrointestinal tract also may be decreased in patients with hepatic or renal impairment and in geriatric individuals (35).

The mean peak plasma concentration with a 30-mg dose is 2.24 μg/mL. It exhibits a high degree of protein binding with about 99% being protein-bound in plasma. Ketorolac has a volume of distribution of 0.11 L/kg. Ketorolac, like other NSAIDs, has the potential for causing gastric mucosal injury (35).

Toxicity

Tolerance, psychological dependence, or physical dependence do not appear to occur in patients receiving chronic oral ketorolac tromethamine (37). There also is no evidence of manifestations of withdrawal following abrupt discontinuance of intramuscular ketorolac tromethamine. The drug does not appear to affect opiate receptors and does not appear to exhibit opiate agonist or antagonist activity (38).

Acute and Chronic Toxicity

Limited information is available on the acute toxicity of ketorolac tromethamine. The acute lethal dose of ketorolac is not known. There have been no reports to date of overdosage with ketorolac tromethamine, and the potential efficacy of various management modalities has not been elucidated.

The most frequent adverse effects observed during chronic toxicity studies in animals were gastrointestinal irritation and/or ulceration, which at high dosages resulted occasionally in peritonitis, anemia, and death. Renal toxicity also was evident after prolonged therapy at relatively high dosages.

Naproxen

Naproxen (Naprosyn, Anaprox) is a propionic acid derivative with a long half-life (12 to 15 hours) (11). It is well absorbed from the upper gastrointestinal tract, and plasma concentrations reach a peak in 2 to 4 hours (39). Naproxen is highly bound to plasma albumin (3). Because of the long half-life, it is suitable for twice-daily administration; approximately 3 days are required to reach equilibrium. The apparent volume of distribution of naproxen is 0.1 L/kg. Large doses result in a disproportionate increase in renal excretion without evidence of saturation of the excretory mechanism. Therefore, it is a safer drug when taken in larger amounts than, for example, aspirin. Like ibuprofen, naproxen competes with aspirin for plasma protein binding sites. It also prolongs prothrombin time. Naproxen sodium is the salt of naproxen and has a faster rate of absorption than that of the parent acid (40).

Adverse effects and drug interactions of naproxen are similar to those of ibuprofen, i.e., nephrotoxicity, jaundice, nausea, dyspepsia, peripheral edema, rash, pruritus, central nervous system and cardiovascular effects, and tinnitus. Side effects after therapeutic dosing or overdosage may also include stomatitis, headache, vertigo, drowsiness, lightheadedness, dyspepsia, nausea, and vomiting. Severe effects are rare (3,11,41).

Long-term administration has been associated with pulmonary edema, congestive heart failure, pulmonary alveolitis, renal impairment, and cholestasis (40).

Nabumetone (Relafen)

Nabumetone, a naphthylalkanone derivative, is a nonsteroidal anti-inflammatory agent. Nabumetone is a prodrug and has little pharmacologic activity until it undergoes oxidation in the liver and forms 6-methoxy -2-naphthylacetic acid (6-MNA). This active metabolite is structurally similar to naproxen.

Pharmacokinetics

Nabumetone is absorbed mainly in the duodenum and converted in the liver to 6-MNA. Taking the drug with food increases the rate of absorption. Serum concentrations of the active metabolite reach a peak in 5 hours after a single dose or in 2.5 hours at steady state. 6-MNA has a terminal half-life of about 24 hours and undergoes little enterohepatic recirculation; it is degraded in the liver to inactive metabolites, which are excreted mainly in urine and bile. In the elderly and in patients with severe renal dysfunction, the half-life of 6-MNA may be prolonged and plasma concentrations may increase.

Toxicity

The most important adverse effects of NSAIDs are peptic ulceration and sometimes fatal gastrointestinal bleeding. As an inactive nonacidic prodrug, nabumetone theoretically should cause less locally mediated gastric irritation than other NSAIDs, but the relative contributions of local and systemic effects to NSAID-associated gastrointestinal bleeding are not clear.

The most common adverse effects reported with nabumetone have been abdominal pain, dyspepsia, nausea, and diarrhea. Photosensitivity reactions, headache, dizziness, rash, edema, tinnitus, and nightmares have also occurred. Pulmonary fibrosis has been reported in three patients taking the drug

Oxaprozin (Daypro)

Oxaprozin, a propionic acid derivative, is a nonsteroidal anti-inflammatory agent. Oxaprozin usually is administered once daily; however, administration of the drug in divided doses daily may improve tolerance in some patients.

Because pharmacokinetics of oxaprozin are altered in patients with renal impairment and in those undergoing hemodialysis, the manufacturer states that oxaprozin should be initiated at 600 mg daily in such patients. If an adequate response is not achieved, dosage may be increased with caution. Supplemental doses for patients undergoing hemodialysis are not necessary because the drug is highly protein-bound.

Pyrazalone Derivatives

Phenylbutazone and Oxyphenbutazone

Phenylbutazone (Butazolidin, Azolid) and oxyphenbutazone (Tandearil), which is a major metabolite of phenylbutazone, are two of the oldest and most potent NSAIDs but are also two of the most toxic (7). Phenylbutazone and oxyphenbutazone are both highly protein-bound. The apparent volume of distribution of phenylbutazone is 0.17 L/kg and that of oxyphenbutazone is 0.14 L/kg. Phenylbutazone is extensively metabolized; the major metabolites are formed by oxidation and conjugation with glucuronic acid. The elimination half-life of phenylbutazone is approximately 75 hours (3).

Both compounds have a high incidence of unpleasant side effects associated with long-term therapy (Table 58–10), which has limited their use in this setting. A serum-sickness reaction can be alarming but is usually self-limiting. Ulcerative stomatitis, hepatitis, and blood dyscrasias such as agranulocytosis and aplastic anemia occasionally occur during prolonged therapy. These hematologic effects are dose-related and are more likely to occur in the elderly. Although they are very uncommon, mortality due to aplastic anemia is significant.

Acute poisoning from phenylbutazone and oxyphenbutazone may produce myriad abnormalities (Table 58–11). Because the margin of safety between therapeutic and toxic doses is narrow, acute overdose is quite common, and the toxic effects may be severe. Toxicity is most frequently associated with serum phenylbutazone concentrations exceeding 100 μg/mL.

Gastrointestinal symptoms include nausea, vomiting, diarrhea, abdominal pain, peptic ulceration, and hematemesis. Neurologic findings may include euphoria, restlessness, psychosis, disorientation, nystagmus, tinnitus, trismus, hallucinations, ataxia, drowsiness, coma, and tonic–clonic seizures.

Metabolic disturbances reported with overdose of pyrazalone derivatives resemble those of salicylate overdose and may include a respiratory alkalosis due to hyperventilation and metabolic acidosis, which may occur either alone or after the respiratory alkalosis.

Hepatic dysfunction usually results in elevated liver enzymes and occasionally in jaundice and hepatomegaly. Acute renal failure together with sodium and water retention have also been described. This may be substantial and may lead to hypertension and peripheral edema. Hematuria has been noted as well as red discoloration of

TABLE 58–10. *Side effects of pyrazalone derivatives*

Serum-sickness reaction
Ulcerative stomatitis
Hepatitis
Blood dyscrasias
Agranulocytosis
Aplastic anemia

TABLE 58–11. *Clinical features of pyrazalone overdose*

Gastrointestinal
Nausea
Vomiting
Abdominal pain
Hematemesis
Peptic ulcer
Neurologic
Euphoria
Restlessness
Psychosis
Disorientation
Tinnitus
Trismus
Hallucinations
Ataxia
Drowsiness
Seizures
Coma
Miscellaneous
Respiratory alkalosis
Metabolic acidosis
Acute renal failure
Hepatotoxicity
Sodium retention
Peripheral edema
Cardiovascular collapse

the urine due to a phenylbutazone metabolite. In addition, proteinuria, oliguria, and, rarely, nephritis may be noted. Cardiovascular collapse with subsequent cardiac arrest has occurred (3).

TOXICITY OF NSAIDS

Despite the widespread availability of NSAIDs, relatively few cases of acute poisoning have been reported. Unless a substantial overdose is ingested, clinical features of acute NSAID poisoning are usually confined to the gastrointestinal tract and central nervous system and are mild (34). Symptoms following acute NSAID overdose are usually limited to lethargy, drowsiness, nausea, vomiting, and epigastric pain, which are generally reversible with supportive care (Table 58–12). Gastrointestinal bleeding can occur and coma has occurred following massive ibuprofen or mefenamic acid overdose. Hypertension, acute renal failure, and respiratory depression may occur, but are rare. Anaphylactoid reactions have been reported with therapeutic ingestion of NSAIDs and may occur following overdose. Serious complications such as seizures, cardiovascular collapse, acute renal failure, coma, and respiratory distress may complicate a major overdose. Acid-base disturbances have been described with ibuprofen and phenylbutazone (40).

Other than for confirming a diagnosis of acute NSAID overdose, the routine determination of plasma concentrations of these agents is neither clinically useful nor easily performed (3).

TREATMENT OF NSAID OVERDOSE

Supportive Care

Management of acute NSAID poisoning is essentially supportive and symptomatic. Gastric emptying procedures may be of benefit if instituted soon after the ingestion. Emptying should be followed by the administration of activated charcoal and a cathartic (32).

It is essential to maintain adequate respirations, so that an artificial airway may be required. Rarely, mechanical ventilation is necessary in severely poisoned patients who develop respiratory depression. If marked hypotension occurs, for example after phenylbutazone poisoning or after gastrointestinal bleeding, fluid therapy (including blood) may be necessary (3). Seizures induced by NSAIDs tend to occur only once and are short-lived. In adults, intravenous diazepam (5 to 10 mg or 0.1 to 0.3 mg/kg), if necessary, may be an effective treatment.

TABLE 58–12. *Clinical features of acute NSAID overdose*

Gastrointestinal
Nausea
Vomiting
Epigastric pain
Gastrointestinal bleeding
Central nervous system
Lethargy
Drowsiness
Coma
Miscellaneous
Hypertension
Acid-base disturbance
Severe
Acute renal failure
Respiratory distress
Seizures
Cardiovascular collapse

H_2 Receptor Antagonists

H_2-Receptor antagonists such as cimetidine and ranitidine have been used to minimize or prevent gastrointestinal irritation, ulceration, and hemorrhage. Although this treatment is expensive and its efficacy has not been shown, it is unlikely to be harmful.

The acid-base disturbances seen with phenylbutazone and ibuprofen overdose are rare and usually transient. They do not usually require active treatment except in the case of renal failure, but the patient should be closely monitored and appropriate treatment begun if deemed necessary (3).

Extracorporeal Removal

Most NSAIDs are highly protein-bound and extensively metabolized, so that it is both pharmacologically inappropriate and clinically unnecessary to undertake forced diuresis, dialysis, or hemoperfusion because such methods are unlikely to enhance elimination significantly.

Alkalinization of Urine

As in salicylate poisoning, the rate of excretion of some of the NSAIDs is increased if the urine is alkaline, but the difficulty of alkalinizing urine in a seriously poisoned patient may militate against the value of the procedure.

Multiple-Dose Activated Charcoal

Many of the NSAIDs undergo enterohepatic circulation, so that repeated doses of activated charcoal may be useful in reducing their elimination half-life. Although this remains to be shown, it is not a harmful procedure (32).

REFERENCES

1. Clive D, Stoff J: Renal syndromes associated with nonsteroidal anti-inflammatory drugs. *N Engl J Med* 1984;310;563–572.
2. Corre K: Nonsteroidal antiinflammatory drugs. *Top Emerg Med* 1986;8:12–25.
3. Vale J, Meredith T: Acute poisoning due to nonsteroidal anti-inflammatory drugs. *Med Toxicol* 1986;1:12–31.
4. Murray M, Brater D: Nonsteroidal anti-inflammatory drugs. *Clin Geriat Med* 1990;6:365–397.
5. Mortensen M, Rennebohm R: Clinical pharmacology and use of nonsteroidal anti-inflammatory drugs. *Pediatr Clin North Am* 1989;36: 1113–1139.
6. Fries J, Williams C, Bloch D: The relative toxicity of nonsteroidal antiinflammatory drugs. *Arthritis Rheum* 1991;34:1353–1360.
7. Kantor T: Control of pain by nonsteroidal anti-inflammatory drugs. *Med Clin North Am* 1982;66:1053–1059.
8. Metz S: Anti-inflammatory agents as inhibitors of prostaglandin synthesis in man. *Med Clin North Am* 1981;67:713–757.
9. Robinson D: Prostaglandins and the mechanism of action of anti-inflammatory drugs. *Am J Med* 1983;73:26–31.
10. Cryer B, Feldman M: Effects of nonsteroidal anti-inflammatory drugs on endogenous gastrointestinal prostaglandins and therapeutic strategies for prevention and treatment of nonsteroidal anti-inflammatory drug-induced damage. *Arch Intern Med* 1992;152:1145–1155.
11. Simon L, Mills J: Nonsteroidal antiinflammatory drugs. *N Engl J Med* 1980;302:1179–1243.
12. Panush R, Yonker P: Practical points on nonsteroidal antiinflammatory drugs. *Am Fam Physician* 1984;29:258–262.
13. Warren S, Mosley C: Renal failure and tubular dysfunction due to zomepirac therapy. *JAMA* 1983;249;396–397.
14. Patmas M, Wilborn S, Shankel S: Acute multisystem toxicity associated with the use of nonsteroidal anti-inflammatory drugs. *Arch Intern Med* 1984;144:519–521.
15. Allison M, Howatson A, Torrnae C, et al: Gastrointestinal damage associated with the use of nonsteroidal antiinflammatory drugs. *N Engl J Med* 1992;327:749–754.
16. Soll A, Weinstein W, Kurata J, et al: Nonsteroidal anti-inflammatory drugs and peptic ulcer disease. *Ann Intern Med* 1991;114:307–319.
17. Gabriel S, Jaakkimanien L, Bombardier C, et al: Risk for serious gastrointestinal complications related to use of nonsteroidal anti-inflammatory drugs. *Ann Intern Med* 1991;115:787–796.
18. Gibson G, Whitacre E, Ricotti C: Colitis induced by nonsteroidal anti-inflammatory drugs. Report of four cases and review of the literature. *Arch Intern Med* 1992;152:625–632.
19. Silverstein F: Nonsteroidal antiinflammatory drugs and peptic ulcer disease. *Postgrad Med* 1991;89:33–40.
20. Griffin M, Piper J, Daugherty J, et al: Nonsteroidal anti-inflammatory drug use and increased risk for peptic ulcer disease in elderly persons. *Ann Intern Med* 1991;114:257–263.
21. Agrawal N, Roth S, Graham D, et al: Misoprostol compared with sucralfate in the prevention of nonsteroidal anti-inflammatory drug-induced gastric ulcer. *Ann Intern Med* 1991;115:195–200.
22. Sandler D, Burr R, Weinberg C: Nonsteroidal anti-inflammatory drugs and the risk for chronic renal disease. *Ann Intern Med* 1991;115:165–172.
23. Lindsley C, Warady B: Nonsteroidal antiinflammatory drugs: renal toxicity. *Clin Pediatr* 1990;29:10–13.
24. Wagner E: Nonsteroidal anti-inflammatory drugs and renal disease—still unsolved. *Ann Intern Med* 1991;115:227–228.
25. Gurwitz J, Avorn J, Ross-Degnan D, et al: Nonsteroidal anti-inflammatory drug-associated azotemia in the very old. *JAMA* 1990;264:471–475.
26. Bakris G, Kern S: Renal dysfunction resulting from NSAIDs. *Am Fam Physician* 1989;40:199–204.
27. Perazella M, Buller G: Can ibuprofen cause acute renal failure in a normal individual? A case of acute overdose. *Am J Kidney Dis* 1991;18:600–602.
28. Balali-Mood M, Proudfoot A, Critchley J, et al: Mefenamic acid overdosage. *Lancet* 1981;1:1354–1356.
29. Nuki C: Non-steroidal analgesic and anti-inflammatory agents. *Br Med J* 1983;287:39–43.
30. Lee C, Finkler A: Acute intoxication due to ibuprofen overdose. *Arch Pathol Lab Med* 1986;220:747–749.
31. Steinmetz J, Lee C, Wu A, et al: Tissue levels of ibuprofen after fatal overdosage of ibuprofen and acetaminophen. *Vet Hum Toxicol* 1987;29:381–383.
32. Hall A, Smolinske S, Conrad F, et al: Ibuprofen overdose: 126 cases. *Ann Emerg Med* 1986 15:1308–1313.
33. Le H, Bosse G, Tsai Y: Ibuprofen overdose complicated by renal failure, adult respiratory distress syndrome, and metabolic acidosis. *J Toxicol Clin Toxicol* 1994;32:315–320.
34. McElwee N, Veltri J, Bradford D, et al: A prospective, population-based study of acute ibuprofen overdose: complications are rare and routine serum levels not warranted. *Ann Emerg Med* 1990;19: 657–662.
35. Resman-Targoff B: Ketorolac: a parenteral nonsteroidal antiinflammatory drug. *DICP Ann Pharmacother* 1990;24:1098–1104.
36. Quan D, Kayser S: Ketorolac induced acute renal failure following a single dose. *J Toxicol Clin Toxicol* 1994;32:305–310.
37. Lewis S: Ketorolac in Europe. *J Toxicol Clin Toxicol* 1994;32: 311–312.
38. Dube J: Ketorolac. *J Toxicol Clin Toxicol* 1994;32:313–314.
39. Alun-Jones E, Williams J, Clwyd G: Hyponatremia and fluid retention in a neonate associated with maternal naproxen overdose. *Clin Toxicol* 1986;24:257–260.
40. Martinez R, Smith D, Frankel L: Severe metabolic acidosis after acute naproxen sodium ingestion. *Ann Emerg Med* 1989;18: 1102–1104.
41. Fredell E, Strand L: Naproxen overdose. *JAMA* 1977:238:938.

ADDITIONAL SELECTED REFERENCES

Goodwin J: Toxicity of nonsteroidal anti-inflammatory drugs. *Arch Intern Med* 1987;147:34–35.

Roth S: Nonsteroidal anti-inflammatory drug gastropathy. *Arch Intern Med* 1986;146:1075–1076.

PART X

METALS AND ANTAGONISTS

CHAPTER 59

Metals

There are 72 elements in the periodic table that are classified as metals; of these, iron, mercury, lead, arsenic, barium, bismuth, and aluminum are of interest in toxicology and are discussed in this section. Metals may exist in the elemental, inorganic, and organic forms. Some are essential for life, being vital parts of life processes, and significant disease results when they are deficient from body systems; others have no known biologic function (1). Many are potent toxins. Metals that are essential nutrients can also exert toxic actions if the homeostatic mechanism maintaining them within physiologic limits is unbalanced (2).

Heavy metals in the environment pose a hazard to biologic organisms. Some of the oldest diseases of humans can be traced to heavy metal poisoning associated with the development of metal mining, refining, and use. Even with the present recognition of the hazards of heavy metals, the incidence of intoxication remains significant and the need for effective therapy remains high.

All organic poisons are eventually destroyed in the body through various metabolic processes, but no organism is capable of transforming toxic metals into harmless compounds. They therefore persist in the body and exert their toxic effects by combining with one or more reactive groups essential for normal physiologic function.

Although metals were once important therapeutic agents, their use in this area has declined. This is particularly true with the advent of more effective organic drugs in the treatment of infectious diseases (1). Present interest in the metals lies primarily in the toxic reactions they are capable of producing. The problems created by food contamination, water and air pollution from industrial and exhaust fumes, and the widespread use of agricultural chemicals are largely attributable to these toxins (3).

Most metals can be divided into two classes. Those in the first class bind preferentially to oxygen and nitrogen atoms; these include calcium, barium, and strontium (Table 59–1) (1). Those in the second class bind preferentially to sulfur and phosphorus atoms; these include mercury, arsenic, and gold. Most toxic metals fall into the second class. Lead is in a separate class because it binds to all four atoms (1).

TABLE 59–1. *Metals and elements to which they bind*

Elements	Oxygen/Nitrogen	Sulfur/Phosphorus
Metals	Calcium	Mercury
	Barium	Arsenic
	Strontium	Gold
	Lead	Lead

It is generally recognized that the absorption of inorganic compounds depends heavily on the compound's water solubility. Metals coming in contact with the body in elemental form are usually poorly absorbed. In compound form they vary considerably in the ease with which they cross biologic membranes. Soluble salts of metals dissociate readily in the aqueous environment of biologic membranes, which facilitates their transport as metal ions.

Some metals occur in the environment as alkyl (organometallic) compounds, in which the metal is firmly bonded to carbon. These alkyl compounds remain largely intact in the biologic environment. They are lipid-soluble and pass readily across biologic membranes unaltered by the surrounding medium. The most notable examples of organometallic compounds of interest in toxicology are methyl mercury and tetraethyl lead.

SOURCE OF HEAVY METAL EXPOSURE

Heavy metal poisonings can be grouped as occupational, community, and individual. Occupational heavy metal exposures are seen in a variety of industries, particularly mining, smelting, metal refining, and alloy production. Exposure often occurs from inhalation of metal dusts or vapors produced during the extraction or refining process. The smelting and refining process used in producing one metal may expose workers to a variety of other metals. For example, the smelting of copper can expose workers to toxic levels of arsenic and zinc.

Workers can also have contact with finished products containing high concentrations of heavy metals. For example, zinc and lead poisoning occurs in workers who produce, repair, or recycle automobile batteries; arsenic and zinc exposure may occur during the production of fertilizers and pesticides; and chromium poisoning may result from accidental ingestion of photographic solutions.

Community or societal exposures to heavy metals can be due to accidental ingestion of manufactured materials (Table 59–2). Acidic liquids, juice beverages placed in improperly glazed pottery, pewter plates and utensils, and inadequately galvanized iron cooking vessels can induce the release of trace amounts of copper, lead, and zinc. Fortunately, these exposures are uncommon and episodic (4).

Individuals may be exposed to toxic concentrations of heavy metals through malicious intent, accidental ingestion, or medicinal use. Many individual poisonings are the result of homicidal or suicidal ingestion. In an accidental poisoning, the cause may be difficult to find if the individual and his/her physician are not aware of the content of reportedly innocuous manufactured materials. For example, burning of batteries in a home stove or burning wood with fungicides can cause zinc or arsenic poisoning through inhalation of toxic fumes. Occasionally, exposure may result from medical therapy, for example, almost all cases of clinical gold toxicity are a consequence of therapy for rheumatoid arthritis. In this era of holistic medicine and megadose vitamin and mineral therapy, the physician will see increasing numbers of patients suffering from the toxic effects of heavy metal compounds about which little is known.

TABLE 59–2. *Metals and exposure*

Occupational
Mining
Smelting
Metal refining
Alloy production
Repair/recycling batteries
Fertilizer production
Photographic solutions
Community
Accidental ingestion
Inadequately galvanized cooking vessels
Improperly glazed pottery
Individual
Malicious intent
Homicidal
Suicidal
Accidental
Ingestion
Inhalation
Medicinal use
Gold therapy—rheumatoid arthritis
Natural or homeopathic remedies

MECHANISM OF ACTION

Once absorbed into the body, inorganic metals are capable of being taken up at various binding sites. Metals exert their toxic effects by combining with one or more reactive groups of enzymes that are essential for normal physiologic functions. An example of this is the binding of many metals to sulfhydryl groups, which are essential for the activity of certain enzymes. Other complexes are to amino, phosphate, carboxylate, imidazole, and hydroxyl radicals of enzymes and other essential biological proteins. The sensitivity of the particular system attacked by the metal and the degree of interference with cellular activity caused by the metal–protein complex determine the clinical effects and course of an intoxication.

ROUTES OF EXCRETION

The main routes by which the human body rids itself of small amounts of toxic metals are the excretory routes. The sloughing off of the skin, the growth of the hair, and, for volatile poisons, the breath can also be minor routes for elimination of toxic metals.

Gastrointestinal Toxicity

Any heavy metal poisoning can cause nausea, vomiting, diarrhea, and abdominal pain that may last for 24 hours after exposure (Table 59–3). Chronic exposure produces anorexia, weight loss, fatigue, and cachexia. Gastrointestinal (GI) side effects are common with all of the heavy metals, though the severity of clinical manifestations may vary. The gastrointestinal side effects of arsine inhalation may be sudden, whereas those of lead poisoning are usually chronic. Gold poisoning causes significant mucocutaneous toxicity with minimal gastrointestinal side effects.

The pathogenic effect of heavy metals on the GI system may be related to a direct toxic effect of ingested metal compounds on the intestinal mucosa. Heavy metals may cause bleeding through dilatation of small blood vessels, and ulceration and necrosis in the mucosa and submucosa of the stomach and small intestine.

Neurologic

Poisoning with lead, zinc, and arsenic produces peripheral nervous system manifestations, including paresthesia, loss of deep tendon reflexes, ataxia, and paralysis, which are the result of segmental demyelination of the nerve sheaths. Because this side effect may be particularly pronounced in the longest nerves, wrist drop or ankle drop may be observed.

TABLE 59–3. *General toxicity of heavy metals*

Gastrointestinal
Nausea
Vomiting
Diarrhea
Abdominal pain
Anorexia
Neurologic
Peripheral nervous system
Paresthesia
Loss of deep tendon reflexes (DTRs)
Ataxia
Paralysis
Central nervous system
Memory loss
Loss of consciousness
Tremors
Stupor
Coma
Renal
Oliguria
Uremia
Renal tubular acidosis
Renal tubular necrosis
Hematologic
Aplastic anemia
Hemolysis
Immunologic reactions

In other heavy metal poisonings, peripheral nervous system function is only moderately impaired, and neurologic side effects are manifested primarily as loss of memory, loss of consciousness, tremors, stupor, and coma. In milder, earlier cases, fatigue, lethargy, and somnolence are evident, with impaired cognitive capabilities. These effects have been attributed to interference with metabolism of neurotransmitters such as acetylcholine and catecholamine.

Renal

Heavy metals may be toxic to the proximal renal tubules, resulting in renal tubular acidosis and impairment of renal tubular absorption and secretion of organic compounds such as amino acids and uric acid. The early effects are impaired urine concentration, aminoaciduria, and hyperuricemia. Chronic or severe poisoning may lead to oliguria and uremia due to renal tubular necrosis. Heavy metals have been shown to damage renal tubular membrane transport mechanisms by interfering with disulfide bonds within the cellular membrane.

Hematologic

Heavy metals may induce hematologic effects by direct toxicity to marrow precursors, inhibition of enzymatic processes essential for cell division and maturation, impairment of red cell membrane transport, and immune-mediated cell destruction (5).

Heavy metals can be stored in bone marrow, where they may induce aplasia or an immunologic reaction. Many heavy metals impair normal metabolic pathways. Lead inhibits several enzymes essential to the synthesis and degradation of porphyrin by binding to thiol- and sulfhydryl-containing enzymes, causing disruption of disulfide bonds. Heavy metals, with the exception of lead, can inhibit glutathione synthetase and impair the ability of the cell to tolerate oxidant stresses, leading to hemolysis.

LABORATORY ANALYSIS

In suspected metal poisoning, both blood and urine should be obtained. Quantitative 24-hour urine collections are preferred because concentrations in random samples of urine may sometimes be misleading.

Differential Diagnosis

Whenever the clinical picture indicates involvement of several organ systems, metal poisoning should be considered in the differential diagnosis. The clinical picture can also vary depending on whether exposure is acute or chronic. The skin, gastrointestinal tract, liver, kidney, blood-forming organs, and peripheral and central nervous systems may be involved (Table 59–4). The digestive tract is involved because of its part in absorption; the liver is affected by virtue of its role as blood filter and detoxifier; and the kidney glomeruli and tubular cells are damaged through their function in excretion.

TREATMENT

The use of chelating agents in the treatment of heavy metal toxicity will be discussed in the following chapter. More specific treatment of heavy metal toxicity is discussed in the appropriate chapter.

TABLE 59–4. *Organs affected by metal intoxication*

Skin
Gastrointestinal tract
Liver
Kidney
Hematologic organs
Central and peripheral nervous systems

REFERENCES

1. Chisolm J: Poisoning due to heavy metals. *Pediatr Clin North Am* 1970;17:591–615.
2. Greenhouse A: Heavy metals and the nervous system. *Clin Neuropharmacol* 1982;5:45–92.
3. Oehme F: Mechanism of heavy metal toxicities. *Clin Toxicol* 1972;5:151–167.
4. Kosnett M: Unanswered questions in metal chelation. *J Toxicol Clin Toxicol* 1992;30:529–547.
5. Ringenberg Q, Doll D, Patterson W, et al: Hematologic effects of heavy metal poisoning. *South Med J* 1988;81;1132–1139.

ADDITIONAL SELECTED REFERENCES

Anseline P: Zinc-fume fever. *Med J Aust* 1972;2:316–318.

Day A, Golding J, Lee P, et al: Penicillamine in rheumatoid disease: a long-term study. *Br Med J* 1974;1:180–183.

Hughes R, Gazzard B, Murray-Lyon I, et al: The use of cysteamine and dimercaprol. *J Int Med Res* 1976; 4(Suppl.):123–129.

Oehme F: British anti-lewisite (BAL): the classic heavy metal antidote. *Clin Toxicol* 1972;5:215–222.

CHAPTER 60

Heavy Metal Antagonists

Because metals persist in the body, a major therapeutic objective in poisoning is the administration of drugs that enhance their excretion. This is done with the aid of chelating agents (1), which take up and firmly bind metallic ions (2,3). Chelation is a common chemical reaction that takes place in a large number of compounds. Among the familiar and important endogenous chelating agents are vitamin B_{12} (for cobalt), hemoglobin (for iron), chlorophyll (for magnesium), and cytochrome oxidase (for iron and copper).

Chelating agents are generally nonspecific with regard to their affinity for metals. To varying degrees they mobilize and enhance the excretion of a wide range of metals, including essential metals such as calcium and zinc. Some chelating agents may not be useful because they are rapidly metabolized to inactive forms in the body. Others bind tightly to a toxic metal but at the same time remain immobilized.

Because chelating agents have the common property of reacting with metals to form tightly bound complexes, they can prevent or reverse the binding of toxic metals in biologic substrates (2). This can only be achieved when the chemical affinity of the complexing agent for the metal ions is higher than the affinity of the metal for the sensitive biologic molecules (4). When two or more ligands (such as sulfhydryl groups) in a molecule simultaneously form bonds with a metal atom by giving up protons or electrons, the donor molecule is properly referred to as a chelating agent. The resultant compound is more stable than others with just one binding site. The product of such a reaction is a heterocyclic ring, which can be excreted in urine, feces, or both. Chelators are generally less stable at low pH, so that control of the pH of body fluids may be an important consideration during treatment (5).

Drugs that function as chelating agents include dimercaprol (British anti-lewisite; BAL), calcium ethylene diamine tetra-acetate (calcium EDTA), penicillamine (Cuprimine, Depen), 2,3-dimercaptosuccinic acid (DMSA, succimer), and deferoxamine (Desferal). Some of the newer agents not yet approved by the FDA are dimercaptopropanesulfonic acid (DMPS), and *N*-acetyl-D,L-penicillamine (1). Calcium EDTA is used in acute lead poisoning; dimercaprol is widely used in poisoning with mercuric, arsenic, and occasionally lead salts; penicillamine is used in copper, lead, and mercury poisoning; deferoxamine is used for acute iron poisoning; and succimer is used in lead poisoning (4).

DIMERCAPROL

Dimercaprol is a dithiol compound that was developed as an antidote for the organoarsenic war gas lewisite (2,4), which is a deadly gas that acts on the lungs and skin (6). Because arsenic is known to be poisonous by inhibiting sulfhydryl groups in essential enzymes, an effort was made to find sulfhydryl substances that had a stronger attraction for arsenic than endogenous body constituents (1,2).

Indications

Dimercaprol forms a poorly dissociable chelate with a number of metals and is effective for arsenicals, mercurials, and gold salts; it reduces the toxicity of chromium and nickel more than that of other metals (Table 60–1). It is of little value in alkyl lead and cadmium poisonings. In general, with the exception of copper, less depletion of trace metals is observed during therapy with dimercaprol than with calcium EDTA and penicillamine (6).

Dimercaprol is the antidote of choice in the treatment of acute mercury, arsenic (except arsine), and gold poisoning (2). When treating acute poisoning by mercury salts, dimercaprol is more effective if administered within 2 hours of ingestion because renal damage caused by mercury cannot be reversed. Dimercaprol is ineffective for alkyl mercury compounds, and the drug is only minimally effective in long-term mercury poisoning.

Even though dimercaprol chelates lead, other chelators such as calcium EDTA or penicillamine are preferred in treating lead poisoning. Dimercaprol, however, is useful as an adjunct to calcium EDTA in the treatment of acute lead encephalopathy or when blood lead concentration is greater than 70 μg per deciliter of whole blood. Dimercaprol is not useful in acute poisoning with alkyl lead compounds (tetraethyl lead), antimony, and bismuth. It should not be used in iron, cadmium, or selenium poi-

TABLE 60–1. *Characteristics and effects of dimercaprol*

Metals well chelated	
	Arsenic
	Mercury (except alkyl mercury)
	Gold
	Lead (encephalopathy, as adjunct to calcium EDTA)
	Chromium
	Nickel
Metals poorly chelated	
	Alkyl lead
	Alkyl mercury
	Antimony
	Iron
	Cadmium
	Selenium
Dosage	
	2.5 mg/kg IM every 4 hours for 2 days, then 2.5 mg/kg IM twice daily for 1 day, then 2.5 mg/kg IM once or twice daily for 5 to 10 days
Side effects	
	Vomiting
	Tremors
	Hypertension
	Tachycardia
	Local pain
	Sterile abscess
	Burning sensation (lips, mouth, throat, penis)
	Abdominal pain
	Seizures
	Rhinorrhea
	Coma
	Death

soning because the resulting dimercaprol–metal complexes are more toxic than the metal alone, especially to the kidneys (1).

Dimercaprol not only protects sulfhydryl enzymes from inactivation by metals but reactivates enzyme systems. The degree to which the enzyme can be reactivated is inversely proportional to the length of time it has been inactivated. Therefore, in the treatment of metal poisoning, especially of the acute type, therapy with dimercaprol is most effective if provided early in the course of poisoning (2).

If the affinity of the metal for dimercaprol is greater than that for enzymes, a mercaptide is formed and can be excreted from the body. The dimercaprol–metal complex can dissociate or be oxidized, however, thus releasing the metal to exert its toxic effects again.

Pharmacokinetics

Because of the instability of dimercaprol in aqueous solutions, peanut oil is the solvent employed in pharmaceutical preparations (2). Dimercaprol is administered by deep intramuscular injection. After injection of therapeutic doses, blood concentrations reach their peak in 30 to 60 minutes. On absorption, dimercaprol is distributed to all tissues including brain, with highest concentrations in liver and kidney. Elimination is complete within 4 hours. Dimercaprol can be administered in the presence of renal impairment because it is predominantly excreted in bile (6).

Dosage

Dimercaprol is available as a 10% preparation in peanut oil. The recommended dosage for mercury, arsenic, and gold poisoning is approximately 2.5 mg/kg administered at 4-hour intervals during the first 2 days, twice on the third day, and once or twice daily thereafter for 5 to 10 days or until the patient has recovered. In acute mercury poisoning, an initial dose of 5 mg/kg is given and then is followed by the above regimen. For acute lead encephalopathy, 4 to 5 mg/kg is given alone in the first dose and is followed by the same regimen in combination with calcium EDTA.

Adverse Effects

Reactions to dimercaprol are common but not cumulative and may occur in approximately 50% of patients (2). Dimercaprol has a strong mercaptan-like odor, which may be noted on the patient's breath. The outstanding side effects are on the central nervous and the cardiovascular systems. Toxic doses may cause vomiting, tremors, seizures, hypertension, and tachycardia beginning 15 to 30 minutes after injection (1). In addition, frequent pain and occasional sterile abscesses occur at the injection site, particularly if the drug is not administered deeply enough. A burning sensation around the lips, mouth, throat, and penis, tingling in the hands, abdominal pain, blepharal spasm, rhinorrhea, fever, transient elevation of hepatic transaminase, coma, and death may also occur. Most side effects are transient and rapidly subside as the drug is metabolized and excreted (2).

Dimercaprol should not be given concurrently with iron therapy because intensification of vomiting and reduction of lead excretion may occur. Renal damage is not a contraindication to its use. On the other hand, dimercaprol is potentially nephrotoxic. Because the chelate dissociates and breaks down in an acid medium, the urine should be kept alkaline during dimercaprol therapy to protect the kidneys. In patients with glucose-6-phosphate dehydrogenase (G-6-PD) deficiency, dimercaprol would be used only in life-threatening situations because it may induce hemolysis.

CALCIUM EDTA

Calcium EDTA (edathamil calcium disodium, calcium disodium versenate), a polyaminocarboxylic acid, can chelate any divalent or trivalent metal that has a higher binding affinity for it than calcium. It forms a stable soluble complex with the metal by displacement of the calcium on the molecule. This complex can then be excreted in the urine. In the past, the rapid intravenous administration of various sodium salts of EDTA produced precipitous decreases in the serum concentration of ionized calcium and symptoms of hypocalcemia. Unlike sodium EDTA, calcium EDTA is saturated with calcium and therefore can be administered intravenously in relatively large quantities without causing any substantial changes in serum or total body calcium. The drug is usually administered to adults by intravenous infusion, and intramuscular administration is also suggested for children and in patients with incipient or overt lead encephalopathy.

Indications

Calcium EDTA is the treatment of choice for lead poisoning (1) (Table 60–2). It may also be useful in acute cadmium poisoning. Calcium EDTA may also be beneficial in the treatment of poisoning from other metals such as chromium, manganese, nickel, zinc, and possibly vanadium (2). It may also be useful in the treatment of poisoning by radioactive and nuclear fission products such as plutonium, thorium, uranium, and yttrium (7). The drug is not effective in the treatment of mercury, gold, or arsenic poisoning (2). Although calcium EDTA was once administered orally to increase the excretion of lead, this route of administration is no longer recommended because the drug enhances absorption of lead in the gastrointestinal tract. In addition, orally administered calcium EDTA is poorly absorbed from the gastrointestinal tract and is therefore considered ineffective (1).

TABLE 60–2. *Characteristics and effects of calcium EDTA*

Metals well chelated
Lead
Cadmium
Metals somewhat chelated
Chromium
Manganese
Nickel
Zinc
Vanadium
Plutonium
Thorium
Uranium
Yttrium
Metals poorly chelated
Mercury
Gold
Arsenic
Dosage
50 mg/kg/day in 6 doses for 5 days
Side effects
Lacrimation
Nasal congestion
Sneezing
Muscular pain
Hypotension
Hypercalcemia
Renal tubular necrosis

Pharmacokinetics

Calcium EDTA has a plasma half-life of 20 to 60 minutes with intravenous administration and 1.5 hours with intramuscular administration (7). Fifty percent of a dose is excreted in the urine in 1 hour and 95% in 6 hours. When calcium EDTA is administered intravenously in the treatment of lead poisoning, urinary excretion of chelated lead begins within about 1 hour and peak excretion occurs within 24 to 48 hours.

Calcium EDTA is not metabolized. After parenteral administration it is rapidly excreted by glomerular filtration in urine either unchanged or as the metal chelate (1). Calcium EDTA does not enter the cells, and thus it removes metals such as lead from the extracellular compartment; indirectly, the remainder of the metal is reduced in soft tissues, CNS tissue, and red blood cells (7). When EDTA is used for lead poisoning, the amount of metal eliminated after an initial maximum in urine tends to decline and then again increases. This is because lead that is weakly bound to body constituents is eliminated initially and lead from intracellular locations is removed after a fairly long interval (2).

Dosage

Calcium EDTA is available commercially as a 20% solution that is diluted before injection. For intravenous use, calcium EDTA should be diluted with 5% dextrose or normal saline to a concentration of less than 0.5%. This solution should be infused over a matter of hours. In mildly and moderately ill patients, a dosage of 50 mg/kg per 24 hours should not be exceeded. Administration takes place over a 5-day period, after which treatment is stopped for 2 to 5 days before a second dose, if necessary, is administered. Adequate urine flow must be established before the drug is given, and renal failure is a contraindication to its use. For acute lead intoxication, calcium EDTA used alone without concomitant dimercaprol therapy may aggravate symptoms. Combined chelation therapy with dimercaprol is therefore warranted in patients with acute encephalopathy or high blood lead concentrations. After the course of therapy, penicillamine can be administered orally.

During chelation with EDTA, urinalysis, blood urea nitrogen, serum creatinine, and liver function tests should be carefully monitored.

Adverse Effects

In general, calcium EDTA is an agent of relatively low toxicity. Hypocalcemia has occurred with disodium EDTA injected in too rapid a fashion. Because calcium EDTA has produced electrocardiographic changes, such as inversion of the T wave, patients should be monitored for cardiac rhythm irregularities during parenteral therapy.

Mild side effects are common and include histamine-like reactions such as lacrimation, nasal congestion, and sneezing. Muscular pains, hypotension, and hypercalcemia may also occur. Calcium EDTA is potentially nephrotoxic, the principal lesion being renal tubular necrosis. Nephrotoxicity can usually be prevented by careful dosage regulation and use of intermittent therapy.

PENICILLAMINE

Penicillamine (Cuprimine, Depen, dimethylcysteine), a monothiol agent, is a hydrolysis product of penicillin (8). It has no antibacterial activity. It is an effective chelating agent for copper, mercury, iron, zinc, lead, and gold (Table 60–3) (9). The primary use of this drug as a chelating agent is to remove copper from individuals suffering from Wilson's hepatolenticular degeneration. Penicillamine is also effective in the treatment of rheumatoid arthritis and cystinuria (8).

Penicillamine is well absorbed from the gastrointestinal tract; therefore, one of its advantages is that it can be administered orally (1). Blood concentrations reach a peak approximately 1 hour after ingestion. Penicillamine is rapidly excreted in the urine. The drug is currently available in capsules of 125 and 250 mg. The usual dosage is 30 mg/kg/day or 250 mg 4 times a day in adults.

TABLE 60–3. *Characteristics and effects of penicillamine*

Metals well chelated	
	Copper
	Mercury
	Iron
	Zinc
	Lead
	Gold
Dosage	
	250 mg 4 times a day, or 30 mg/kg/day
Side effects	
	Hypersensitivity
	Nausea
	Vomiting
	Nephrotic syndrome
	Optic neuritis
	Systemic lupus erythematosus
	Leukopenia
	Neutropenia
	Pyridoxine deficiency
	Autoimmune hemolytic anemia
	Stevens-Johnson syndrome

Penicillamine is relatively nontoxic. Adverse effects include hypersensitivity reactions, rash, fever, nausea, vomiting, nephrotic syndrome, optic neuritis, drug-induced systemic lupus erythematosus, leukopenia, neutropenia, and coagulation deficits (9). Reactions are usually mild. Rarely, severe and even life-threatening reactions such as autoimmune hemolytic anemia and Stevens-Johnson syndrome have been observed. In addition, penicillamine is a pyridoxine antagonist because pyridoxal-dependent enzyme systems are inhibited. Dietary supplementation of pyridoxine is therefore recommended. Penicillin allergy is not usually a problem, but the possibility of an allergic reaction exists.

SUCCIMER

Succimer is a water-soluble chemical analog of dimercaprol but, in contrast to dimercaprol, has less toxicity, greater water solubility, and limited lipid solubility, and is effective when given orally (4). Succimer is the stable meso isomer of 2,3 dimercaptosuccinic acid; it also has been known as DMSA (10). Succimer forms stable complexes with lead and it also chelates other toxic heavy metals, such as arsenic and mercury (Table 60–4) (11). DMSA has no effect on the elimination of iron, calcium, or magnesium (12). When used in therapeutic doses, neither DMSA nor DMPS appears to have any marked effect on trace metals in the body except for a small increase in urinary excretion of zinc and copper. DMSA has recently been shown to be highly effective for the treatment of occupational plumbism as well as childhood lead intoxication, occupational mercurialism, and possibly methyl mercury poisoning (13–15).

Indications

Succimer was marketed in 1991 for the treatment of lead poisoning, specifically in children with blood lead

TABLE 60–4. *Characteristics and effects of DMSA*

Metals well chelated	
	Lead
	Mercury
	Lead
Metals poorly chelated	
	Iron
	Calcium
	Magnesium
Dosage	
	10 mg/kg orally every 8 hours for 5 days, then 10 mg/kg orally every 12 hours for 14 days.
Side effects	
	Nausea
	Vomiting
	Loose stools

concentrations higher than 45 μg/dL (11). Treatment with the drug should be accompanied by identification and removal of the source of lead exposure (4,12). Succimer should not be used prophylactically for the prevention of lead poisoning in a lead-containing environment. The decision to treat patients with blood lead concentrations of 70 μg/dL or higher using succimer rather than parenteral chelation therapy should be made with the understanding that experience with succimer in such patients is limited (16). Currently, there are no data on the efficacy of succimer for the treatment of lead encephalopathy in children, although several adults with this condition have been treated successfully with the drug (17). Pending further accumulation of data, the Centers for Disease Control currently considers oral succimer an alternative to generally preferred parenteral chelation therapy for patients with blood lead concentrations exceeding 45 μg/dL.

Clinical studies indicate that succimer is a relatively selective and a highly effective medication that lowers blood lead concentrations. Succimer reverses the adverse metabolic effects of lead on heme synthesis while increasing urinary lead output without adversely affecting essential mineral excretion at the recommended dosage regimen (18). The primary indicators of drug efficacy in the controlled trials of oral succimer were lowered blood lead concentrations and increased urinary lead excretion.

No controlled, randomized clinical studies of succimer have been conducted in cases of poisoning with other heavy metals. A limited number of patients have received succimer for mercury poisoning or arsenic poisoning through compassionate-use protocols (18).

Succimer is rapidly but variably absorbed and probably confined to the extracellular space. Most of the drug and the metals it binds are excreted in the urine; functioning kidneys are apparently required for the drug to be effective (12,16).

Adverse Reactions

Few adverse events have been observed in clinical trials and compassionate-use cases, and those that have been observed have generally been mild and transient. The most common adverse effects reported in clinical trials were primarily gastrointestinal and included nausea, vomiting, diarrhea, appetite loss, and loose stools. At times, these events have been believed to be related to the unpleasant mercaptan odor of succimer; administration in such a way as to minimize the odor may overcome some of these reactions (19). Rashes, some necessitating discontinuation of therapy, have been reported (20).

Because transient elevations of serum aminotransferase levels have been observed in some patients, primarily adults, during the course of succimer therapy, serum aminotransferases should be monitored before the initiation of therapy and at least weekly during therapy, particularly in patients with a history of liver disease.

The possibility of allergic or other mucocutaneous reactions to the drug should be considered when succimer is readministered. Patients requiring repeated courses of succimer should be monitored during each treatment course. As with any type of chelation therapy, succimer is not indicated for the prophylaxis of lead poisoning in a lead-containing environment.

Succimer-heavy metal chelates are excreted in the urine; therefore, all patients undergoing treatment should be adequately hydrated. Caution should be exercised when succimer therapy is considered in patients who have compromised renal function. Limited data suggest that succimer is dialyzable but that the lead chelates are not.

Dosage

The recommended initial dosage in children is 10 mg/kg or 350 mg/sq m every 8 hours for 5 days. After the initial 5 days of therapy, the dosage is reduced to 10 mg/kg or 350 mg/sq m every 12 hours for an additional 2 weeks of therapy. A course of treatment lasts 19 days. Repeated courses may be necessary when indicated by weekly monitoring of blood lead concentrations after each course. The manufacturer states that initiation of succimer therapy with higher dosages is not currently recommended. Depending on the blood lead concentration, additional courses of therapy with succimer may be necessary. Intervals of not less than 2 weeks are recommended between courses of succimer therapy unless blood lead concentrations require more prompt drug therapy. Patients who have received edetate calcium disodium (calcium EDTA) therapy, with or without dimercaprol, may receive succimer after an interval of 4 weeks; concomitant administration of succimer with calcium EDTA (with or without dimercaprol) currently is not recommended because the safety and efficacy of such combined therapy are not known.

Succimer should not be administered to women who are pregnant or who may become pregnant during therapy unless the potential benefit outweighs the potential risk to the fetus.

No cases of overdosage have been reported.

N-ACETYL-D,L-PENICILLAMINE

N-Acetyl-D,L-penicillamine is formed by the acetylation of the amine group of penicillamine. It is not active as a substrate for the amino acid oxidases and cysteine desulfhydrase, which allows for metal binding by its sulfhydryl groups (3).

Thus far, experience with *N*-acetyl-D,L-penicillamine has been encouraging. Toxicity is low and therapeutic effectiveness relatively high. Nevertheless, it is still classified as a "chemical" and not as an experimental drug; this classification impairs its use. Although a number of investigators have advocated the use of this agent, it is not currently available in North America.

Most patients treated with *N*-acetyl-D,L-penicillamine experienced urinary excretion of mercury, and those with neurologic impairment improved.

REFERENCES

1. Chenoweth M: Clinical uses of metal-binding drugs. *Clin Pharmacol Ther* 1968;9:365–387.
2. Greenhouse A: Heavy metals and the nervous system. *Clin Neuropharmacol* 1982;5:45–92.
3. Kostyniak P, Clarkson T: Role of chelating agents in metal toxicity. *Fundam Appl Toxicol* 1981;1:376–380.
4. Aaseth J: Recent advances in the therapy of metal poisoning with chelating agents. *Hum Toxicol* 1983;2:257–272.
5. Kosnett M: Unanswered questions in metal chelation. *J Toxicol Clin Toxicol* 1992;30:529–547.
6. Oehme F: Mechanism of heavy metal toxicities. *Clin Toxicol* 1972;5: 151–167.
7. Craven P, Morelli H: Chelation therapy. *West J Med* 1975;122: 277–278.
8. Silva A, Fleshman D, Shore B: The effects of penicillamine on the body burdens of several heavy metals. *Health Phys* 1973;24:535–539.
9. Halverson P, Kozin F, Bernhard C, et al: Toxicity of penicillamine. *JAMA* 1978;240:1870–1871.
10. Graziano J, Cuccia D, Friedheim E: The pharmacology of 2,3-dimercaptosuccinic acid and its potential use in arsenic poisoning. *J Pharmacol Exp Ther* 1978;20:1051–1055.
11. Mann K, Travers J: Succimer, an oral lead chelator. *Clin Pharm* 1991;10:914–922.
12. Lenz K, Hruby K, Druml W, et al: 2,3-Dimercaptosuccinic acid in human arsenic poisoning. *Arch Toxicol* 1981;47:241–243.
13. Graziano J, Leong J, Friedheim E: 2,3-Dimercaptosuccinic acid: a new agent for the treatment of lead poisoning. *J Pharmacol Exp Ther* 1978;206:696–700.
14. Friedheim E, Corvi C: Meso-dimercaptosuccinic acid: a chelating agent for the treatment of mercury poisoning. *J Pharm Pharmacol* 1975;27:624–626.
15. Bentur Y, Brook C: Meso-2,3-dimercaptosuccinic acid in the diagnosis and treatment of lead poisoning. *Clin Toxicol* 1987;25:39–51.
16. Aposhian H: DMSA and DMPS—Water-soluble antidotes for heavy metal poisoning. *Annu Rev Pharmacol Toxicol* 1983;23:193–215.
17. Aposhian H, Aposhian M: Meso-2,3-dimercaptosuccinic acid: chemical, pharmacological and toxicological properties of an orally effective metal chelating agent. *Annu Rev Pharmacol* 1990;30:279–306.
18. Graziano J: Role of 2,3-dimercaptosuccinic acid in the treatment of heavy metal poisoning. *Med Toxicol* 1986;1:155–162.
19. Gerr F, Frumkin H, Hodgins P: Hemolytic anemia following succimer administration in a glucose-6-phosphate dehydrogenase deficient patient. *J Toxicol Clin Toxicol* 1994;32:569–576.
20. Aposhian H, Maiorino R, Rivera M, et al: Human studies with the chelating agents, DMPS and DMSA. *J Toxicol Clin Toxicol* 1992;30: 505–528.

ADDITIONAL SELECTED REFERENCES

Anseline P: Zinc-fume fever. *Med J Aust* 1972;2:316–318.

Day A, Golding J, Lee P, et al: Penicillamine in rheumatoid disease: a long-term study. *Br Med J* 1974;1:180–183.

Hughes R, Gazzard B, Murray-Lyon I, et al: The use of cysteamine and dimercaprol. *J Int Med Res* 1976;4(Suppl.):123–129.

Oehme F: British anti-lewisite (BAL): the classic heavy metal antidote. *Clin Toxicol* 1972;5:215–222.

CHAPTER 61

Mercury

Mercury is a highly toxic metal that is slightly volatile at ordinary temperatures and has been used for 3,000 years. Because every known compound of mercury is potentially dangerous, the opportunity for accidental intoxication is widespread. Mercury is a relatively freely available toxin and poisoning has occurred by most routes, from oral to intra-arterial. Throughout the years mercury has been used in medicine, agriculture, and industry.

TABLE 61–1. *Sources of mercury exposure*

Industrial paper production
Chlorine manufacturing
Vinyl production
Folk remedies
Fungicides
Fingerprinting procedures
Medical laboratories
Dental laboratories
Mine ore reduction

SOURCES OF MERCURY EXPOSURE

The main industrial sources of inorganic mercury pollutants are the paint, chemical, and paper manufacturing industries (Table 61–1) (1,2). Mercury-containing paint can raise the total indoor air mercury concentration by 1,000 times the level before painting (3). Paint manufacturers agreed to stop using mercury in interior paint after 1990; however, sale of existing stocks of interior latex paints was allowed until 1991. Because many people keep partly used cans of paint, pre-1990 paint may continue to be a source of mercury exposure for years (4,5).

Mercury nitrate was used by the felt hat industry in France, and the resulting poisoning gave rise to the term "mad as a hatter" (6–8). The chemical industry requires organic mercury compounds for the production of vinyl chloride, which is important in the synthesis of many plastics. As with many other pollutants, mercury contamination of the environment has paralleled increasing industrial activity. The largest contribution to atmospheric mercury contamination is the burning of coal and other fossil fuels.

Mercury is used in dental laboratories in amalgam fillings, and the continual handling of amalgam by technicians may be a cause of chronic mercury poisoning (mercurialism) that may go unrecognized (9–12). Silver dental amalgams, which have been used for the past 150 years to fill cavities in teeth, can be 50% elemental mercury by weight. The mechanical action of chewing on a filling releases trace quantities of mercury vapor, which is partially absorbed. Typically, exposure to mercury from dental amalgams is less than exposure from foods such as tuna or swordfish that contain methyl mercury, a more toxic form of mercury. It is estimated that people with many amalgam fillings receive less than 1% of the daily mercury vapor dose that is considered occupationally safe. A National Institutes of Health expert panel recently concluded that amalgam fillings pose no significant risk of side effects.

Mercury is used in thermometers, barometers, mercury electrical switches, direct current meters, and in the vapor lamps that illuminate traffic arteries (Table 61–2) (13). Polyvinyl alcohol preservative used in hospitals as a mounting medium for ova and parasites contains mercuric chloride in various concentrations (14). Mercuric oxide is used for making dry batteries for hearing aids, small flashlights, and a number of electronic products (15,16). Mercury is also used in photoengraving. Contraceptives, bacteriostatic agents, and diuretics make use of both inorganic and organic mer-

TABLE 61–2. *Uses of mercury*

Thermometers
Barometers
Small batteries
Electrical switches
Vapor lamps
Photoengraving chemicals
Medicinals
Contraceptives
Bacteriostatic agents
Diuretics

cury salts (17,18). Mercury has been popular in agricultural use because of its ability to counteract fungi and mold, and therefore it has been widely used to prevent grain spoilage.

Metallic mercury has been used in folk remedies by Mexican-American and Asian populations for chronic stomach disorders and by Latin-American and Caribbean natives in occult practices (19).

TYPES OF MERCURY COMPOUNDS

Mercury compounds are divided into three chemical classes: elemental mercury, inorganic mercury compounds, and organic mercury compounds (Table 61–3). The inorganic mercury salts also exist either in the mercurous or mercuric state; mercuric salts are more toxic than mercurous salts. Within each class there are also subgroups with significantly different toxicologic properties (Table 61–4). The biologic half-life of inhaled elemental mercury is about 60 days and mercury salts have a shorter biologic half-life (about 40 days) than inhaled elemental mercury.

Elemental Mercury (Quicksilver)

Elemental mercury is a silver-gray liquid at room temperature that vaporizes readily when heated (20). Commonly referred to as quicksilver or metallic mercury, it is used in thermometers (21), thermostats, switches, barometers, batteries, and other products (22). Elemental mercury (free or metallic mercury) exists in the un-ionized form and is the most volatile of all forms of mercury (23). It is the only metal known that remains in liquid form at 0°C (24).

TABLE 61–3. *Types of mercury compounds*

Elemental mercury (metallic mercury)
Inorganic mercury compounds
Mercurous salts
Mercurous acetate
Mercurous chloride
Mercurous nitrate
Mercurous oxide
Mercuric salts
Mercuric chloride
Mercuric cyanide
Mercuric oxide
Mercuric nitrate
Organic mercury compounds
Alkoxyalkyl mercury compounds
Methoxyethylmercuric chloride
Aryl mercury compounds
Alkyl mercury compounds
Ethylmercury
Methylmercury

Effects of Ingestion

Typically, elemental mercury has no toxic effects when swallowed because it is poorly absorbed from the gastrointestinal tract (see Table 61–4). Patients who swallow mercury from a thermometer or from rupture of a Cantor or Miller–Abbott tube do not experience toxicity from absorption of mercury (10). The surface of the metal probably becomes coated rapidly with endogenous sulfur-laden compounds, and this coating impairs diffusion across the gastrointestinal mucosa. To effect systemic absorption of mercury requires the conversion of metallic mercury to the divalent form. If the integrity of the intestinal mucosa is preserved, metallic mercury normally passes through the gastrointestinal tract rapidly enough to preclude significant conversion to the divalent state. In some circumstances, increased or enhanced absorption after a relatively small dose may occur in patients with inflammatory bowel disease. Rarely, mercury becomes trapped in the appendix or intestine and requires surgical removal. If a site for mercury stasis exists, oxidation–reduction may occur slowly in the presence of water and chloride at body temperature, ultimately transforming metallic mercury into divalent mercuric compounds (25,26)

Effects of Inhalation

Elemental mercury has a high vapor pressure, and significant poisoning occurs when the substance is inhaled because it is almost completely absorbed through the alveolar membranes (17). As a result of its high lipid solubility and lack of charge, elemental mercury easily crosses the blood–brain barrier and accumulates in the cerebral and cerebellar cortex (10). As a result, central nervous system (CNS) changes are most prominent with intoxication. The term *erethism* (insomnia, loss of appetite, shyness, emotional lability, memory loss) is applied to the syndrome (Table 61–5). Severe intoxications can result in permanent CNS damage and death (23). There it is quickly oxidized to the divalent or mercuric ion, which forms a highly undissociated bond to sulfhydryl radicals on various protein molecules and leads to neurologic and behavioral abnormalities (27). Elemental mercury vapor accounts for most occupational exposures (28).

Inorganic Mercury Compounds

Inorganic mercury compounds contain mercury in the oxidized or ionized form and readily form salts and complexes with sulfhydryl groups (29). The monovalent (mercurous) form is highly insoluble, and the divalent (mercuric) form is highly soluble (30). Partly because of

TABLE 61–4. *Characteristics of mercury compounds*

Type	Absorption	Excretion	Systems affected
Elemental	Inhalation	Kidney	Pulmonary and central nervous systems
Inorganic	Gastrointestinal absorption	Kidney	Gastrointestinal and renal systems
Organic	Dermal and gastrointestinal absorption	Kidney	Gastrointestinal and renal systems
Alkyl	Inhalation, dermal and gastrointestinal absorption	Bile	Central nervous system

the divalent form's high degree of solubility, one of the most common and most toxic salts of mercury is mercuric chloride, which is also known as bichloride of mercury or corrosive sublimate (31).

Mercury salts are usually colorless or white crystals, or intensely colored yellow or red powders (32). They include mercuric chloride (antiseptic and disinfectant), mercuric cyanide and mercuric oxide (topical antiseptics), and mercuric nitrate (used in felt working).

Mercurous salts are typically colorless, white or yellow powders. They include mercurous acetate (antibacterial agent), mercurous chloride or calomel (cathartic, diuretic, antiseptic and antisyphilitic agent), mercurous nitrate (used to blacken brass), and mercurous oxide (used to make electrical batteries).

Inorganic mercury compounds are absorbed through the gastrointestinal tract or, if aerosolized, through inhalation. Little inorganic mercury is absorbed by skin contact (33). Oral ingestion of inorganic mercury can cause severe inflammation of the mouth, esophagus, stomach, and small intestine. Inorganic mercury is distributed preferentially to the kidney; secondarily, it accumulates in the liver. It is excreted mainly through the urine (10).

Although the mercuric salts can be extremely toxic, the mercurous salts, because of their low solubility, represent a minimal hazard (32). Nevertheless, children who ingested mercurous chloride (calomel) in teething powder developed a syndrome known as acrodynia (painful extremities) or pink disease (1,30).

TABLE 61–5. *Signs and symptoms of chronic mercury vapor inhalation*

Psychological disturbance—erethism
Anorexia
Anxiety
Depression
Emotional lability
Insomnia
Irritability
Memory loss
Nervousness
Regressive behavior
Shyness

Organic Mercury Compounds

Organic mercury compounds, in contrast to elemental and inorganic mercury, are environmental contaminants and pollutants (10). These compounds contain mercury bound covalently to at least one carbon atom; examples are dimethyl mercury and phenylmercuric acetate (24).

For toxicologic purposes, organic mercury compounds are divided into two classes on the basis of their toxic clinical effects (30). Differences in toxicity among the organic mercurials are due to the ease of dissociation of the organic moiety from the anion (27). Compounds in the first class break down readily in the body to yield inorganic mercury; these are primarily the alkoxyalkyl mercurials and the aryl compounds. Phenylmercuric salts such as methoxyethylmercuric chloride are examples of the alkoxyalkyl salts. In the aryl mercurials, mercury is bound to a carbon on an aromatic ring such as benzene, toluene, phenol, cresol, or nitrophenol (34). Compounds in the second class are short-chain alkyl mercury compounds in which the integrity of the carbon–mercury bond is maintained. These compounds demonstrate greater toxicity than those in the first class.

In view of these features, it is a mistake to differentiate inorganic from organic mercury, at least from a toxicologic point of view, because the mammalian body handles aromatic mercury compounds and some long-chain alkyl mercury compounds by breaking the mercury–carbon bond, thus rendering the mercury inorganic. In the methyl and ethyl forms of mercury, the mercury–carbon bonds are extremely stable; the attachment of the alkyl radical makes the compound more lipid-soluble, enabling it to cross the blood–brain barrier more easily.

Alkoxyalkyl Mercury Compounds

Alkoxyalkyl mercury compounds are salts of phenyl and methoxyethyl mercury. The physical properties of these compounds render them more easily absorbable than inorganic salts (27). Hence, their distribution throughout the body may be more widespread initially, but as they undergo biotransformation with splitting of the carbon–mercury bond and release of inorganic mercury, their distribution pattern becomes similar to that of the inorganic mercury compounds. These compounds therefore act as inorganic mercury in the body (35).

Aryl Mercury Compounds

The aryl compounds have distributional patterns different from those of the short-chain alkyl derivatives. The aryl compounds are not well absorbed, and being relatively unstable they are excreted mainly as mercuric ion through the kidneys (1). Phenylmercuric salts therefore are much safer than alkyl compounds because they are less volatile, much less able to enter the brain, much more readily metabolized, and more rapidly excreted (35).

Alkyl Mercury Compounds

The short-chain alkyl mercury compounds behave differently from the other organic mercurials. Chemically, these are organic compounds in which the mercury has at least one strong covalent bond with a carbon atom (36). This bond does not dissociate readily either within or outside the body, and toxic effects are attributed to the action of the intact molecule (27).

Under appropriate conditions, Hg^{+2} can covalently bind carbon to form organomercury compounds. The most important of these compounds in terms of human exposure is methyl mercury. Methyl mercury is the form most frequently involved in mercury food poisoning. Elemental mercury and methyl mercury compounds have a greater ability to cross cell membranes than do the mercurous or mercuric salts and, consequently, are more neurotoxic than mercury salts (37).

Methyl mercury compounds are biologically the most significant of the short-chain alkyl compounds because of their potential to enter the food chain. They become concentrated as they move up the phylogenetic chain and thus become considerably toxic pollutants. These compounds are soluble in organic solvents and lipids, pass readily through biologic membranes, and in the body bind to sulfhydryl groups of proteins. Methyl mercury poisoning is usually accidental and unrecognized until 4 to 6 weeks, after which time neurologic symptoms appear.

Alkyl mercury compounds are absorbed through the gastrointestinal tract, respiratory system, and skin (38). On ingestion, approximately 90% of a dose is absorbed directly from the intestine, in contrast to the considerably lower absorption shown by inorganic or phenyl mercury compounds. Alkyl mercury compounds distribute themselves more uniformly in the body than the inorganic compounds, concentrating in the liver, blood, brain, hair, and epidermis. The biologic half-life is 70 to 90 days, and the major clinical effects occur in the CNS (39).

The main excretion route of methyl mercury is through the bile to the intestine, where it is almost immediately reabsorbed into the blood; this internal recycling process partially accounts for the long half-life of methyl mercury in the body. Less than 10% is excreted in the urine (27).

MECHANISM OF ACTION

In general, mercury can be described as a potent, nonspecific enzyme poison. It produces its detrimental actions by releasing mercuric ions, which readily form covalent bonds with sulfhydryl groups (7,40). This results in the inactivation of metabolic enzymes, denaturation and precipitation of structural proteins, and disruption of cell membranes in the cells of the target organs (41). The inhibition of sulfhydryl enzymes is reversible after removal of mercury. Although this is a major mechanism of toxicity, it is probably not the only means by which mercury may interfere with metabolic processes (17). There are other ligands such as amine, phosphoryl, and carboxyl groups, also present in any living cell, with which mercury can form strong bonds. Mercury may also act by a local corrosive action on the gastrointestinal tract.

GENERAL EFFECTS OF MERCURY

Effects of mercury toxicity manifest primarily in the CNS and kidneys, where mercury accumulates after exposure. The duration, intensity, and route of exposure and the form of mercury influence the systems affected (34). The nervous system is primarily affected by chronic exposure to elemental mercury and organomercury compounds; the kidneys are primarily affected by chronic exposure to mercury salts. In acute poisoning, the respiratory system is affected by inhaled elemental mercury and the gastrointestinal, by ingested mercury salts. The cardiovascular system may be affected secondarily.

SYMPTOMS AND SIGNS OF INTOXICATION

Depending on the compound, mercury can be locally irritating or corrosive and damage the skin and mucous membranes, or it may cause systemic toxicity, or both. In addition, toxicity can result from acute or chronic exposure to agents that release the mercuric ion or to the alkyl mercuric compounds, which have different toxicities. The diagnosis is difficult during the earliest phases of mercury intoxication because the manifestations are nonspecific and could arise from causes other than mercury exposure.

Neurologic

CNS effects result primarily from exposure to elemental mercury vapor and to methyl mercury. These forms of mercury cross the blood–brain barrier readily and can produce irreversible brain damage. Methyl mercury ingestion leads to delayed CNS symptoms, which may not manifest until months after the initial exposure (24). Early symptoms are often nonspecific, such as malaise, blurred vision, or hearing loss. The peripheral nervous system also may be affected.

Renal

After inorganic salts or phenylmercury compounds are ingested, a large amount of mercury may accumulate in the kidneys, producing a generalized increase in the permeability of the tubular epithelium.

Exposure to mercury vapor or to mercury salts produces an apparently dose-dependent proteinuria or nephrotic syndrome. Acute tubular necrosis with resultant renal failure may occur.

Acute

Inhalation

Acute mercury inhalation exposure tends to occur in three settings: industrial accidents, accidents within the home, and in association with novice attempts to extract precious metals from mercury amalgam.

Respiratory absorption of mercury vapor is rapid because of the vapor's excellent diffusion through alveolar membranes (10). Whereas the CNS is the target organ after chronic exposure to mercury vapor, the lung is the critical organ in acute inhalational exposure (10,42). The mercury is oxidized in vivo to mercurous and mercuric ions, which are toxic. The kidney then becomes the elimination site, and buildup of mercury concentrations in this organ eventually causes renal damage (27).

Symptoms of acute mercury poisoning by inhalational exposure include an immediate salivation, a burning sensation in the mouth and throat, a paroxysmal dry cough, dysphagia, nausea, vomiting, substernal chest pain with subsequent shallow respiration, tachypnea, a necrotizing bronchiolitis, bronchitis, and interstitial pneumonitis (Table 61–6) (17). Chronic bronchiolitis may ensue and is suggested by the persistence of severe dyspnea despite negative radiographic findings and by the advent of airway obstruction in pulmonary function testing. Diffuse interstitial pulmonary fibrosis has also been reported in patients with acute mercury poisoning who survived for several weeks (43). Complications such as interstitial emphysema, pneumomediastinum, and pneumothorax can occur (17). In addition to the severe lung damage that may occur as a result of mercury vapor inhalation, the lung also serves as a site from which mercury is absorbed (22). It is widely distributed throughout the body and passes across the blood–brain barrier, with subsequent neurologic and behavioral abnormalities noted. Fine muscle tremors are among the early signs of mercurialism. Tremors usually begin in the fingers, eyes, or tongue. Mercury is largely ionized to mercuric ion in erythrocytes and other tissues (39).

TABLE 61–6. *Signs and symptoms of acute mercury vapor inhalation*

Gastrointestinal
Salivation
Burning
Mouth
Throat
Dysphagia
Nausea
Vomiting
Abdominal pain
Pulmonary
Dyspnea
Cough
Chest pain
Tachypnea
Bronchiolitis
Bronchitis
Pneumonitis
Interstitial fibrosis
Pneumomediastinum
Pneumothorax

Ingestion

When ingested, inorganic mercury is rapidly absorbed by the gastrointestinal tract; this should be considered an emergency of the highest priority. Ingestion is rarely encountered in industry but in other settings may be accidental or purposeful (7).

Ionizable mercuric salts are corrosive. Necrosis begins immediately in the mucosa of the mouth, throat, esophagus, and stomach. Gastrointestinal symptoms consist of local pain, nausea, profuse vomiting with hematemesis, violent abdominal pain, and hematochezia (Table 61–7). The patient may note a metallic taste in the mouth. Volume loss may lead to shock and vascular collapse, which can result in death within a few hours. The alimentary effects of many mercury compounds are so rapid that the course and prognosis are determined largely by events within the first 10 to 15 minutes, particularly by the intervention of vomiting or a therapeutic lavage. Albuminuria and skin lesions may also be noted, although these lesions are more commonly associated with organic than with inorganic mercury exposure. Renal tubular injury occurs with an initial diuresis and subsequent renal shutdown. CNS symptoms may also be noted.

TABLE 61–7. *Clinical features of acute ingestion of inorganic and aryl mercuric compounds*

Early
Necrosis of mucosa
Mouth
Throat
Esophagus
Gastrointestinal
Local pain
Nausea
Vomiting
Hematemesis
Abdominal pain
Hematochezia
Metallic taste in the mouth
Shock
Vascular collapse
Subsequent
Stomatitis
Salivation (ptyalism)
Membranous colitis
Renal abnormalities
Tubular necrosis
Albuminuria
Hematuria
Anuria

If death does not intervene, subsequent effects noted with both corrosive and noncorrosive mercurials develop within 1 to 3 days after the exposure and may include mercurial stomatitis, marked salivation (ptyalism), membranous colitis, and necrosis of the renal tubules with resultant polyuria, albuminuria, hematuria, and anuria. Death is usually the result of complete and irreversible renal failure. Psychological and CNS symptoms are uncommon in acute mercury poisoning, in contrast to chronic mercury poisoning (35).

Chronic

Inorganic, Elemental, and Aryl Compounds

Long-term, low-level exposure to mercury vapor is a common hazard in various industries. With the exception of alkyl mercury poisoning, the signs and symptoms of inorganic and aryl mercury poisonings are identical because of the rapid metabolic breakdown of these mercurials to mercuric ion (21). The CNS is affected more than any other system in chronic mercury poisoning, and the predominant manifestations are neurologic. The violent gastrointestinal reactions elicited in acute poisonings are absent, but excessive salivation, anorexia, digestive disturbances, vague abdominal distress, and mild diarrhea are common. At chronic low doses, the body oxidizes most of the elemental mercury to mercuric ions (Hg^{+2}), which do not readily cross the blood–brain barrier. At high doses, the body is not able to metabolize the mercury rapidly enough and more elemental mercury reaches the brain.

TABLE 61–8. *Signs and symptoms of chronic exposure to inorganic, elemental, and aryl mercury compounds*

Oral cavity disorders
Gingivitis
Stomatitis
Salivation
Tremor
Hands
Feet
Tongue
Psychological disturbances (erethism)
Anorexia
Anxiety
Depression
Emotional lability
Insomnia
Irritability
Memory loss
Nervousness
Regressive behavior
Timidity
Renal
Proteinuria
Edema
Miscellaneous
Weakness
Fatigue
Pallor
Anorexia
Weight loss
Gastrointestinal disturbances

Initial symptoms of inorganic, elemental, or aryl mercury poisoning may be insidious in onset and appear after only a few weeks, or they may not be evident for several years despite continuing exposure (Table 61–8). A triad of manifestations has become associated with the diagnosis of chronic mercurialism: (a) oral cavity disorders, such as gingivitis, stomatitis, or excessive salivation; (b) a fine involuntary tremor of the hands, feet, and tongue that is aggravated by voluntary movements (this "intention" or ataxic tremor occurs only when there is purposeful movement of a limb, especially when the limb approaches its intended object); and (c) psychological disturbances, called *erethism*, manifested as anxiety, irritability, depression, regressive behavior, timidity, or nervousness (the term *erethism* refers to the blushing and sweating that also occurs) (33). Renal involvement is well documented and may be evidenced by proteinuria and edema. Additionally, nonspecific symptoms such as weakness, fatigue, pallor, anorexia, weight loss, and gastrointestinal disturbances have also been reported (44).

Alkyl Compounds

Methyl, ethyl, propyl, and butyl mercury derivatives are potent neurotoxins on either acute or chronic exposure (36). They are especially hazardous because of their volatility, their ability to penetrate epithelial cells and the blood–brain barrier, and their persistence in the body (37).

Chronic exposure to organic mercurials primarily affects the CNS (Table 61–9). Whereas the effects of elemental mercury are neuropsychiatric, those of short-chain organic mercury compounds are sensorimotor (10,42). These compounds produce no biochemical or physiologic disturbances, such as proteinuria, that are clearly associated with exposure. At present, reliance on the neurologic examination or on subjective complaints by the patient is necessary.

The clinical picture may be gradual and delayed, with a latent period of as much as 2 months or more from exposure to the development of symptoms. Loss of sensation and paresthesias of the mouth, lips, tongue, hands, and feet may occur (38). Dysarthria, inability to concentrate, extreme fatigue, difficulty in swallowing, ataxia, and concentric constriction of the visual fields or "tunnel vision" may be noted (36). Tremors occur, but motor effects such as incoordination, paralysis, and abnormal reflexes are a result of defects in sensory input. Hearing impairment, coma, and death have also been noted in severe poisonings (38). Fetuses and neonates are most sensitive to methyl mercury, which can produce severe derangement of the developing CNS.

Epidemic methyl mercury poisoning has occurred among populations where fish or shellfish is the major dietary staple. This was described in the 1960s in Minamata Bay, Japan, and was due to contamination by nearby industrial wastes discharged into public waters (7,36). Although inorganic mercurials may have been discharged into the water, methylation of the mercury by microorganisms subsequently consumed by fish may have occurred. Other contaminations have been reported in Iraq, Pakistan, and Guatemala as a result of the ingestion of flour and wheat seed treated with methyl and ethyl mercury fungicide compounds (36,38,45).

TABLE 61–9. *Signs and symptoms of intoxication with alkyl mercury compounds*

Central nervous system
Neurasthenia
Headache
Paresthesia
Ataxia
Intention tremor
Hearing loss
Visual field loss
Paralysis
Coma
Nonspecific
Weakness
Fatigue
Apathy
Dysphagia

LABORATORY DETERMINATIONS

A complete history should be obtained in a patient with possible mercury toxicity. The nervous system and kidney should be carefully examined. Recent behavioral changes, such as increased irritability and shyness and changes in short-term memory should be documented. In children, developmental milestones should be evaluated.

Because of the often vague clinical picture, confirmatory laboratory tests are desirable (Table 61–10). Unlike the situation for lead poisoning, there are no specific biochemical tests that can be used to determine whether mercury exposure has occurred. The only indicator available is the concentration of mercury in the blood, urine, or hair. Determinations of mercury concentrations in blood or urine are most commonly used, although both are subject to wide variation. Urinary or blood concentrations may be nondiagnostic in many cases because they may vary among symptomatic patients and in individual patients on a daily basis. Findings of higher than normal concentrations of mercury in blood or urine may confirm exposure to mercury, but they correlate poorly with the appearance of clinical symptoms.

Because mercury has a short half-life in blood (3 days), blood analysis is typically performed shortly after an acute exposure. Urine is the best biologic specimen when chronic mercury exposure is suspected. Hair analysis can provide evidence of methyl mercury exposure.

For acute high-level mercury exposure, whole blood is a valid indicator of body burden; for low-level exposure, plasma should be analyzed separately. Blood samples should be collected in vacutainers containing heparin and refrigerated.

Because the mercuric ion is excreted by the kidney, poisoning from elemental, aryl, or long-chain organic mercury or mercuric salts can be best assessed by measuring the 24-hour urinary excretion of mercury. Although monitoring urinary concentration of mercury is the most common method for determining acute exposure and is helpful after chelation therapy (27), it is not useful after a chronic mercury exposure. A first-morning void can provide a close approximation of a 24-hour collection, particularly if it adjusted for the concentration of the urine.

TABLE 61–10. *Laboratory determinations in mercury exposure*

Inhalation
Chest roentgenogram
Arterial blood gas values
Blood mercury concentrations
24-Hour urinary sampling
Urinalysis
Ingestion
Serum electrolytes
Blood mercury concentrations
24-Hour urinary sampling
Urinalysis

Because organic mercury is usually excreted through the biliary system, urine levels are not useful in evaluating methyl mercury exposure. A urinary mercury concentration of less than 20 μg/L (100 nmol/L) in adults is considered background. Urine mercury concentrations from 20 to 100 μg/L (100 to 499 nmol/L) are associated with subtle changes on some tests, even before overt symptoms occur. If a 24-hour collection shows mercury in the range of 100 to 300 μg/L, either before or after therapy, then significant exposure has occurred. Symptoms may appear when the 24-hour collection contains more than 300 μg/L.

There is a considerably larger variability of the mercury concentrations in urine than in blood. Possible explanations may be difficulty in adequately controlling urine sampling, variations in renal mercury excretion during the day, and the influence of variations in kidney function on mercury excretion. Blood sampling is easier to control, and blood mercury concentrations are not affected in a misleading way by disturbed renal function.

In contrast to the other mercury compounds, the short-chain alkyl organic mercury compounds are mainly excreted in bile (28). Although they form a tight carbon bond, preferentially to red blood cells, they are uniformly distributed throughout the body. Because urinary excretion accounts for only 10% of total excretion, urinary measurements are not reliable in the assessment of poisoning by these compounds. In general, levels of mercury in hair are not useful in evaluating a patient clinically. A properly handled hair sample can provide evidence of methyl mercury exposure, however, because methyl mercury accumulates in hair, where its concentration remains constant. There is excellent correlation between the average mercury concentration in 1 cm of hair and the blood concentration at the time of formation of the hair sample. Measurement of concentrations in either red blood cells or hair correlates accurately with symptoms. In unexposed adults, the blood mercury level rarely exceeds 1.5 μg/dL (0.07 μmol per L); a blood concentration of 5 μg/dL (0.25 μmol per L) or greater is considered the threshold for symptoms of toxicity. Although whole blood mercury levels are considered the best measure of acute elemental mercury vapor absorption, the correlation with toxicity in chronically exposed individuals is variable.

As a rough guideline, a mercury concentration of 3.5 μg/dL in blood is approximately equivalent to 150 μg/L in a 24-hour urine collection. The concentration in hair is approximately 250 to 300 times the concentration in blood.

TREATMENT

Inorganic and Organic Compounds (Excluding Alkyl Compounds)

The treatment of acute mercury poisoning aims at removal of mercury from the gastrointestinal tract, the inactivation of absorbed mercuric ions, and general supportive measures to maintain electrolyte and fluid balance (Table 61–11). To be successful, treatment must be prompt and intensive. Gastric lavage should be performed, with subsequent administration of charcoal and a cathartic. Shock due to peripheral vascular collapse is treated with volume repletion.

Elemental

Patients who have experienced acute elemental mercury inhalation should receive supportive care. Patients exposed to high concentrations of mercury vapor should be removed from the contaminated environment. Supplemental oxygen should be given as needed, and patients should be monitored closely for the development of acute pneumonitis and pulmonary edema. If pulmonary toxicity is suspected, careful monitoring of chest roentgenograms and arterial blood gas values is indicated. Positive end-expiratory pressure may be required to assist ventilation (35). Chelation may be required.

Mercury Salts

Inorganic mercury can be removed from the gastrointestinal tract by lavage and catharsis. It is imperative that adequate intravenous fluids be administered to prevent dehydration and to reduce the concentration of mercury in the kidneys. Dimercaprol (British anti-lewisite, BAL) or another appropriate chelating agent should be administered immediately; usefulness depends on rapid administration.

Chelation Therapy

Elimination of the toxic mercuric ion is the specific objective in therapy for mercury poisoning. This is done with the use of chelating agents. A chelating agent is indicated in all mercury poisonings except those due to short-chain alkyl compounds. Treatment of mercury poisoning is limited to two commercially available agents, dimercaprol and penicillamine (30).

TABLE 61–11. *Treatment of mercury poisoning*

Lavage
Activated charcoal and cathartic
Volume repletion
Chelation therapy
Dimercaprol (acute inorganic mercury)
  3 to 5 mg/kg IM every 4 hours for 2 days, then
  3 to 5 mg/kg IM every 6 hours for 1 day, then
  3 to 5 mg/kg IM once or twice a day for 10 days
Penicillamine (chronic intoxication and mercury vapor)
  250 mg 4 times a day for 3 to 10 days, or 30 mg/kg per 24 hours not to exceed 1 g/day

Dimercaprol (BAL) was the first chelating agent used for mercury toxicity and is still widely used for inorganic mercury poisoning. BAL is contraindicated for methyl mercury poisoning, however, because it has been shown to increase the concentration of methyl mercury in the brain and therefore exacerbates symptoms. BAL is anticipated to be effective in treating phenylmercury poisoning, because phenylmercuric acetate is rapidly oxidized to Hg^{+2} in the body; hence, phenylmercury is similar to inorganic mercury.

Dimercaprol

Extensive clinical experience with dimercaprol has established it as the antidote of choice in acute poisonings due to inorganic mercuric salts, in which the critical target organ is usually the kidney. Dimercaprol is maximally effective when given early in the course of an acute episode and can often be lifesaving under those circumstances. If dimercaprol is given within 3 hours after ingestion, severe renal damage may be prevented. Dimercaprol enhances the renal excretion of mercury, so that caution is indicated in cases of acute renal insufficiency, in which the drug may aggravate the renal damage or manifest its own toxicity.

Dimercaprol is much less effective in chronic mercurialism, in which the brain is the critically diseased organ. Although it often provokes an increase in urinary mercury, the rise is usually small in terms of estimated body burden, and the clinical improvement is typically marginal.

The currently suggested treatment schedule for dimercaprol is intramuscular administration as a 10% solution in oil. Dosage is 3 to 5 mg/kg injected every 4 hours for 2 days, the same dose every 6 hours on the third day, and then daily or twice daily for 10 days. The dimercaprol–mercury complex is excreted in both the feces and urine (30).

Some hazard is attendant on the use of dimercaprol. The mobilization of large quantities of mercury from the body after its administration may impose an overwhelming mercury load on the kidneys with some risk of damage. Redistribution of body stores of mercury after injection of dimercaprol may also result in excessive deposition in the brain (27).

Penicillamine

Penicillamine appears to be preferable to dimercaprol in treating acute poisoning by mercury vapor and chronic mercurialism of almost any form (17). Penicillamine is preferable for mercury inhalation because of the tendency for absorbed mercury vapor to enter the brain and for dimercaprol therapy to increase mercury concentration in the brain.

Penicillamine is marketed as 125-mg and 250-mg capsules and is orally administered on an empty stomach in a dose of 250 mg 4 times a day for 3 to 10 days. A dosage of 30 mg/kg/day divided every 6 hours up to 1 g/day should be given for 5 to 10 days. A repeated 5-day course of treatment with a 2-day rest period between courses is indicated until the 24-hour urine mercury excretion is less than 50 μg/L. Although *N*-acetyl-D,L-penicillamine appears to be more effective and less toxic than penicillamine, it is not approved for use in the United States. Doses suggested have been equal to those of penicillamine.

Dimercaprol is preferable to oral penicillamine for acute mercury ingestion because vomiting may prevent retention of penicillamine and because penicillamine may enhance the gastrointestinal absorption of mercury.

Alkyl Compounds

Methyl and other alkyl derivatives of mercury pose more formidable problems in therapy than other mercurials because they are rapidly absorbed and penetrate quickly into the brain, where they are bound to plasma and cellular proteins. There is no specific therapy for alkyl mercury poisoning, and treatment is symptomatic (27). The use of chelating agents has been of limited value in aiding the elimination of short-chain organic mercury, probably because little of the organic mercury compounds dissociates to yield inorganic mercury ions. Dimercaprol is contraindicated for methyl mercury poisoning because it increases mercury accumulation in the brain. Several newer agents have been clinically evaluated, including *N*-acetylcysteine (46), *N*-acetyl-D,L-penicillamine (6), and dimercaptopropanesulfonic acid (DMPS) (47–49). Results have been promising with these water-soluble, orally active agents.

Succimer

Succimer is an orally active, heavy-metal chelating agent that forms stable, water-soluble complexes with lead and consequently increases the urinary excretion of lead (50). Succimer also has been found to chelate other toxic heavy metals, such as arsenic and mercury.

Succimer is rapidly but variably absorbed and probably confined to the extracellular space. It binds lead, mercury, or arsenic to a much greater extent than zinc or copper, and does not bind any significant amount of iron, calcium, or magnesium, avoiding depletion of essential minerals. Most of the drug and the metals it binds are excreted in the urine; functioning kidneys are apparently required for the drug to be effective. The efficacy of succimer in the treatment of other heavy metal poisonings has not been established by controlled studies, although the drug has increased urinary excretion of the metals and produced varying degrees of symptomatic improvement in a limited number of patients with mercury or arsenic poisoning.

The Role of Dialysis

Hemodialysis and peritoneal dialysis may be helpful in renal insufficiency, but they have little or no value for removing mercury because it is bound tightly to plasma and tissue proteins (51).

REFERENCES

1. Aronow R, Fleischmann L: Mercury poisoning in children. *Clin Pediatr* 1976;15:936–945
2. Duffield D, Paddle G, Woolhead G: Mortality study of non-malignant genitourinary tract disease in electrolyte mercury cell room employees. *J Soc Occup Med* 1983;33:137–140.
3. McLauchlan G: Acute mercury poisoning. *Anaesthesia* 1991;46: 110–112.
4. Janus C, Klein B: Aspiration of metallic mercury: clinical significance. *Br J Radiol* 1982;55:675–676.
5. Snodgrass W, Sullivan J, Rumack B, et al: Mercury poisoning from home gold ore processing. *JAMA* 1981;246:1929–1931.
6. Kark R, Poskanzer D, Bullock J, et al: Mercury poisoning and its treatment with *N*-acetyl-D,L-penicillamine. *N Engl J Med* 1971;285: 10–16.
7. Winek C, Fochtman F, Bricker J, et al: Fatal mercuric chloride ingestion. *Clin Toxicol* 1981;18:261–266.
8. Markowitz L, Schaumburg H: Successful treatment of inorganic mercury neurotoxicity with *N*-acetylpenicillamine despite an adverse reaction. *Neurology* 1980;30:1000–1001.
9. Brodsky JB, Cohen EN, Whitcher C, Brown BW Jr, Wu ML: Occupational exposure to mercury in dentistry and pregnancy outcome. *J Amer Dent Assoc*1985;111:779–780.
10. Bauer J: Action of mercury in dental exposures to mercury. *Oper Dent* 1985;10:104–113.
11. Mackert J: Hypersensitivity to mercury from dental amalgams. *J Am Acad Dermatol* 1985;12:877–879.
12. Abraham J, Svare C, Frank C: The effect of dental amalgam restorations on blood mercury levels. *J Dent Res* 1984;63:71–73.
13. Hudson P, Vogl R, Brondum J, et al: Elemental mercury exposure among children of thermometer plant workers. *Pediatrics* 1987; 79:935–938.
14. Siedel J: Acute mercury poisoning after polyvinyl alcohol preservative ingestion. *Pediatrics* 1980;66:132–134.
15. Mant T, Lewis J, Mattoo T, et al: Mercury poisoning after disc-battery ingestion. *Hum Toxicol* 1987;6:179–181.
16. Adams C, Ziegler D, Lin J: Mercury intoxication simulating amyotrophic lateral sclerosis. *JAMA* 1983;250:642–643.
17. Lien D, Todoruk D, Rajani H, et al: Accidental inhalation of mercury vapor: respiratory and toxicologic consequences. *Can Med Assoc J* 1983;129:591–595.
18. Giunta F, DiLandro D, Chiaranda M, et al: Severe acute poisoning from ingestion of a permanent wave solution of mercuric chloride. *Hum Toxicol* 1983;2:243–246.
19. Kew J, Morris C, Aihie A, et al: Arsenic and mercury intoxication due to Indian ethnic remedies. *Br Med J* 1993;306:506–507.
20. Lin J, Lim P: Massive oral ingestion of elemental mercury. *J Toxicol Clin Toxicol* 1993;31:487–492.
21. Sau P, Solivan G, Johnson F: Cutaneous reaction from a broken thermometer. *J Am Acad Dermatol* 1991;25:915–919.
22. Rowens B, Guerrero-Betancourt D, Gottlieb C, et al: Respiratory failure and death following acute inhalation of mercury vapor. *Chest* 1991;99:185–190.
23. Branches F, Erickson T, Aks S, et al: The price of gold: mercury exposure in the Amazonian rain forest. *J Toxicol Clin Toxicol* 1993;31:295–306.
24. Albers J, Kallenbach L, Fine L: Neurological abnormalities associated with remote occupational elemental mercury exposure. *Ann Neurol* 1988;24:651–659.
25. Bredfeldt J, Moeller D: Systemic mercury intoxication following rupture of a Miller-Abbott tube. *Am J Gastroenterol* 1978;69:478–480.
26. Geffner M, Sandler A: Oral metallic mercury. *Clin Pediatr* 1980;19: 435–437.
27. Joselow M, Louria D, Browder A: Mercurialism: environmental and occupational aspects. *Ann Intern Med* 1972;76:119–130.
28. Levin M, Jacobs J, Polos P: Acute mercury poisoning and mercurial pneumonitis from gold ore purification. *Chest* 1989;94:554–556.
29. Felton J, Kahn E, Salick B, et al: Heavy metal poisoning: mercury and lead. *Ann Intern Med* 1972;76:779–792.
30. Goldfrank L, Bresnitz E: Mercury poisoning. *Hosp Physician* 1980; 6:36–46.
31. Laundy T, Adam A, Kershaw J, et al: Deaths after peritoneal lavage with mercuric chloride solutions. *Br Med J* 1984;289:96–98.
32. Singer A, Mofenson H, Caraccio T, et al: Mercuric chloride poisoning due to ingestion of a stool fixative. *J Toxicol Clin Toxicol* 1994;32:577–582.
33. Rosenman K, Valciukas J, Meyers B, et al: Sensitive indicator of inorganic mercury toxicity. *Arch Environ Health* 1986;41:208–215.
34. Mant T, Lewis J, Mattoo T, et al: Mercury poisoning after disc-battery ingestion. *Hum Toxicol* 1987;6:179–181.
35. Greenhouse A: Heavy metals and the nervous system. *Clin Neuropharmacol* 1982;5:45–92.
36. Eyl T: Organic-mercury food poisoning. *N Engl J Med* 1971;284: 706–709.
37. Hamada R, Yoshida Y, Nomoto M, et al: Computed tomography in fetal methylmercury poisoning. *J Toxicol Clin Toxicol* 1993;31: 101–106.
38. Bakir F, Damluji S, Amin-Zaki L, et al: Methylmercury poisoning in Iraq. *Science* 1973;181:230–241.
39. Kanluen S, Gottlieb C: A clinical pathologic study of four adult cases of acute mercury inhalation toxicity. *Arch Pathol Lab Med* 1991;115: 56–60.
40. Oehme F: Mechanisms of heavy metal toxicities. *Clin Toxicol* 1972; 5:151–167.
41. Schwartz J, Snider T, Montiel M: Toxicity of a family from vacuumed mercury. *Am J Emerg Med* 1992;10:258–261.
42. Levine S, Cavender G, Langolf G, et al: Elemental mercury exposure: peripheral neurotoxicity. *Br J Ind Med* 1982;39:136–139.
43. Zelman M, Camfield P, Moss M, et al: Toxicity from vacuumed mercury: a household hazard. *Clin Pediatr* 1991;30:121–123.
44. Lilis R, Miller A, Lerman Y: Acute mercury poisoning with severe chronic pulmonary manifestations. *Chest* 1985;88:306–308.
45. Mattaffey K: Toxicity of lead, cadmium, and mercury: considerations for total parenteral nutritional support. *Bull N Y Acad Med* 1984;60: 196–209.
46. Lund M, Clarkson T, Berlin M: Treatment of acute methylmercury ingestion by hemodialysis with *N*-acetylcysteine (Mucomyst) infusion and 2,3-dimercaptopropane sulfonate. *Clin Toxicol* 1984;22: 31–49.
47. Graziano J: Role of 2,3-dimercaptosuccinic acid in the treatment of heavy metal poisoning. *Med Toxicol* 1986;1:155–162.
48. Aaseth I, Alexander J: Treatment of mercuric chloride poisoning with dimercaptosuccinic acid and diuretics: preliminary studies. *J Toxicol Clin Toxicol* 1982;19:173–186.
49. Aaseth J: Recent advances in the therapy of metal poisoning with chelating agents. *Hum Toxicol* 1983;2:257–272.
50. Mann K, Travers J: Succimer, an oral lead chelator. *Clin Pharm* 1991; 10:914–922.
51. Pellinen T, Karjalainen K, Haapanen E: Hemoperfusion in mercury poisoning. *J Toxicol Clin Toxicol* 1983;20;187–189.

ADDITIONAL SELECTED REFERENCES

Aposhian H: DMSA and DMPS—water soluble antidotes for heavy metal poisoning. *Annu Rev Pharmacol* 1983;23:193–215.

Cassar-Pullicino VN, Taylor DN, Fitz-Patrick JD: Multiple metallic mercury emboli. *Br J Radiol* 1985;58:470–474.

Chisolm J: Poisoning due to heavy metals. *Pediatr Clin North Am* 1970; 17:591–615.

Clarkson T, Cox L, Greenwood M, et al: Tests of efficacy of antidotes for removal of methylmercury in human poisoning during the Iraq outbreak. *J Pharmacol Exp Ther* 1981;218:74–83.

Dale I: An unusual case of mercury contamination. *J Soc Occup Med* 1985;35:95–97.

Gothe C, Langworth S, Carleson R, et al: Biological monitoring of exposure to metallic mercury. *Clin Toxicol* 1985;23:381–389.

Robillard J, Rames L, Jensen R, et al: Peritoneal dialysis in mercurial diuretic intoxication. *J Pediatr* 1976;88:79–81.

Smith P, Langold G, Goldberg J: Effects of occupational exposure to elemental mercury on short-term memory. *Br J Ind Med* 1983; 40:413–419.

Vermeiden I, Oranje A, Vuzevski V, et al: Mercury exanthem as occupational dermatitis. *Contact Dermatitis* 1980;6:88–90.

CHAPTER 62

Lead

Lead, one of the earliest metals used by humans, is poisonous in all forms. It is one of the most hazardous of the toxic metals because the poison is cumulative and because the toxic effects are many and severe (1). Lead is a naturally occurring bluish-gray metal found in small quantities in the earth's crust. The natural concentration of lead is less than 10 ppb in the earth's crust and less than 0.03 ppb in sea water. The inorganic form of lead is predominant in the environment.

In the body, lead is a trace element that has no known essential biological role (2). Because it is widespread in the environment, exposure to it is almost inevitable, even for fetuses, infants, and children (3). Lead poisoning (plumbism) usually results from cumulative absorption of small amounts of lead until toxic concentrations are reached in the body (4,5). Months or even years may pass before symptoms appear. Although there have been recent advances in the recognition and management of lead poisoning, it continues to be a significant problem (6,7).

TYPES OF COMPOUNDS

Metallic lead is stable in dry air. In moist air, it quickly forms lead monoxide, which in turn produces lead carbonate with carbon dioxide. The nitrate, chlorate, and acetate salts are water soluble; the chloride is slightly soluble. Sulfate, carbonate, chromate, phosphate, and sulfide salts are insoluble. The chromate, carbonate, nitrate, sulfide, and phosphate are soluble in acid, whereas the chloride is slightly soluble in acid. Lead forms stable tetralkyl compounds with the organic ligands—tetramethyl, tetraethyl, tetrapropyl, and tetrabutyl compounds. They are soluble in many organic solvents but are insoluble in water. The tetraorganolead compounds decompose to lead metal and free organic radicals at elevated temperatures or in the presence of light. In the presence of oxygen, the thermal decomposition of tetraethyl lead produces lead oxide rather than the free metal.

SOURCES OF LEAD POISONING

Usually, lead compounds are emitted into the atmosphere from three sources: gasoline-powered vehicles, industrial processes, and incineration (1,8,9). Exposure may occur from air, water, food, and dusts (Table 62–1). Besides the elemental form, lead may exist in both an inorganic and organic form. More than 95% of lead is inorganic and occurs as a lead salt; for practical purposes, all the inorganic forms of lead have the same action in the body (10). The carbonate and chromate salts and various oxides are found in paints and pottery glazes; the carbonate salt is known as *white lead*. Acidic foods have been found to leach lead from lead solder in cans and lead glazes used in making pottery and ceramic ware. Water from leaded pipes, soldered plumbing, or water coolers is another potential source of lead exposure. *Organic lead* (lead bound to carbon atoms in an organic molecule) is prevalent only in areas where leaded gasoline is combusted (11,12).

Today, the major environmental sources of metallic lead and its salts are paint, auto exhaust, food, and water. For children, the most important pathways are by ingestion of chips from lead-painted surfaces, inhalation of lead from automobile emissions, food from lead-soldered cans, drinking water from lead-soldered plumbing, and medications in the form of folk remedies. The major

TABLE 62–1. *Sources of lead poisoning*

Industrial
Ammunition manufacture
Battery manufacture
Lead refineries
Pigment manufacture
Printing
Shipbuilding
Smelting plants
Welding
Miscellaneous
Automobile exhaust
Contaminated alcohol
Firing ranges
Health foods
Intravenous drugs of abuse
Lead bullets
Lead-based paints
Leaded gasoline
Oriental herbal medicines
Pica
Pottery glaze

route of exposure to lead for the general population is food and beverage and, secondarily, through the air and breathing dust.

Lead paint also continues to be used on the exterior of painted steel structures, such as bridges and expressways (13). In addition to the obvious risk to workers, increased lead absorption has been reported in children exposed to chips or dust during the de-leading or maintenance of such structures (14).

Rather than occurring as trace ingredients or trace contaminants, various lead compounds are used as major ingredients of traditional medicines in numerous parts of the world. "Traditional healers," using non-Western pharmacopoeias, manufacture these products, which are often introduced to recent immigrant groups by friends and relatives. Examples of such exposures have been reported from Arab cultures, the Indo-Pakistan subcontinent, China, and Latin America.

Occupational Exposure

Lead toxicity continues to be a major health problem in many occupations because lead and its salts are used in a wide variety of processes. Most occupational exposures occur in the manufacturing or use of ammunition, brass, bronze pipes, storage batteries, lead shielding, pigments, chemicals, or processed metals (1,7). Most current exposures occur primarily through inhalation of lead dust during sanding, grinding, scraping, or powder mixing, or of lead fumes from burning, refining, pouring, or smelting (15,16). Studies have shown workers to be at risk in lead refineries, smelting plants, battery manufacturing plants, pigment manufacturing plants, shipyards, and other industries (8). These workers also risk transmitting the dust into their homes as a result of exposure to work clothes resulting in exposing their families to high ambient concentrations of lead. In addition, lead is used in printer's type, in welding or soldering of lead-coated steel, electric cable covering, and bearing alloys (7,17,18).

Household Exposure

Consumption of contaminated drinking water from lead-containing pipes, ingestion of lead-containing health foods, and Chinese herbal medicines are domestic sources of lead poisoning (8,17). In addition, cases of lead poisoning have been traced to illicit alcoholic beverages such as "moonshine," from burning color magazines containing leaded ink, and from paints and pottery glaze (1,19,20).

Several folk remedies used in this country have been shown to contain large amounts of lead. Two Mexican folk remedies are *azarcon* and *greta*, which are used to treat "empacho", a colic-like illness. Azarcon and greta are also known as liga, Maria Luisa, alarcon, coral, and rueda (21). These and other lead-containing remedies and cosmetics used by some Asian and Middle Eastern communities are listed in Table 62–2.

TABLE 62–2. *Folk remedies containing lead*

Hispanic
Azarcon
Greta
Liga
Maria Luisa
Alarcon
Coral
Rueda
Asian
Chuifong tokuwan
Pay-looah
Ghasard
Bali goli
Kandu
Middle Eastern
Alkohl
Kohl
Surma
Saoot
Cebagin

Environmental Exposure

The alkyl lead compounds (Table 62–3) are used primarily in gasoline; combustion of leaded gasoline accounts for most of the ambient air lead (9). organolead compounds are added to motor fuel to eliminate the "knock" or detonation in the internal combustion engine (8,17). After combustion, these compounds are oxidized and emitted in exhaust as a mixture of lead salts (7). Although local "fallout" from industrial plants processing lead can be severe, this is a minor contribution to regional pollution compared to automobile exhausts. Dust and soil may be contaminated principally by automobile exhaust and by the weathering and deterioration of old lead paint (15,22). Agricultural vehicles are not required to use unleaded gasoline; consequently, lead can be deposited on and retained by crops, particularly leafy vegetables.

Sniffing gasoline, both leaded and unleaded, is a problem of some magnitude within young age groups and in areas where there is local legal prohibition against alcohol because of the pleasurable effects of

TABLE 62–3. *Alkyl lead compounds*

Tetraethyl lead
Tetramethyl lead
Tetraethylmethyl lead
Diethyldimethyl lead
Ethyltrimethyl lead

acute inhalation and the availability and low cost of gasoline (see Chapter 72) (12).

Miscellaneous Exposures

Although cases of lead poisoning due to retained bullets are reported only rarely, they may represent potentially life-threatening reactions (13,23). Certain ammunition such as lead shot and .22-caliber bullets may provide a large surface area of lead dissolution and absorption (8,19,24,25). Inadequately ventilated firing ranges may also result in lead toxicity.

Illicit methamphetamine has been reported to contain substantial amounts of lead and acute lead toxicity has been reported in intravenous amphetamine users (26).

Many hobbies can result in substantial exposures to lead. For example, molten lead can be used in casting ammunition and making fishing weights or toy soldiers; leaded solder is used in making stained glass; leaded glazes and frits are used in making pottery; and artists' paints may contain lead. Furniture refinishing may also result in lead exposure (27).

Age-Related Exposure

In general, lead poisoning in children is a different health problem from that in adults (7,28). In children, it occurs as accidental poisoning whereas in adults it is usually a result of occupational exposure (29,30). Young children are exposed to lead in soil, air, house dust, food, and water. Childhood lead poisoning is one of the most common pediatric health problems in the United States today and it is entirely preventable (31).

In general, the main routes of lead exposure in children are inhalation and ingestion (18). Lead-based paint found on both interior and exterior housing surfaces remains the most common high-dose source of lead for preschool-aged children (4,17,32). A lead chip weighing only 2 g and containing 10% lead can deliver a potential dose of 100 mg; for comparison, the safe upper limit for daily intake of lead by children is 5 μg/kg (3,33). *Pica*, or the abnormal craving for and indiscriminate eating of non-food substances, is a frequent exposure factor in children in the development of chronic plumbism (15,28); however, a child does not have to eat paint chips to become poisoned. More commonly, children ingest dust and soil contaminated with lead from paint that flaked or chalked as it aged or that has been disturbed during home maintenance or renovation (34). This lead-contaminated house dust, ingested through normal repetitive hand-to-mouth activity, is now recognized as a major contributor to the total body burden of lead in children. This occurs most often in preschool children and is most prevalent among those 18 to 24 months old (8). Developing fetuses are also at risk from the exposure of the mother (10).

ABSORPTION

Lead enters the bloodstream through the gastrointestinal tract, respiratory tract, and to a lesser extent, mucous membranes (7,17). Absorption from the respiratory tract is rapid because of prompt phagocytosis and because lead enters directly into the general circulation instead of passing through the liver, as in gastrointestinal absorption (35).

Adults consume approximately 300 μg of lead per day, of which only 10% is absorbed (1,35). A larger percentage of ingested lead is absorbed by children (7). Deficiencies of other metals, such as iron, calcium, and zinc, all result in increased gastrointestinal absorption of lead. In the fetus, absorption of transplacental lead increases during the 12th week to 40th week of gestation.

In contrast to inorganic lead salts, which do not penetrate the skin, alkyl derivatives are capable of rapidly penetrating the intact skin.

DISTRIBUTION

Once in the blood, lead is distributed primarily among three compartments—blood, soft tissue (kidney, bone marrow, liver, and brain), and mineralizing tissue (bones and teeth) (7). Mineralizing tissue contains about 95% of the total body burden of lead in adults. Each compartment also has subcompartments. Once absorbed, about 99% of the lead circulating in blood is contained in the red blood cells of which about 50% is bound to hemoglobin A and the remaining 50% is bound to three compartments of red cell proteins (36).

The mean residence time of lead in blood is approximately 25 days. Most of the lead leaving the blood is excreted in urine, but about one fourth of the lead leaving blood goes to soft tissue, and a smaller fraction is deposited in bone. In soft tissue, such as the liver and kidney, lead has a mean residence time of about 40 days; it is then excreted in bile, hair, sweat, and nails, with a small portion returned to the blood. Bone is the largest compartment of body lead, comprising about 95% of the body burden of the metal and acting as a reservoir for endogenous intoxication; lead stored in bone is available for diagnosis by EDTA mobilization (17). The mean residence time of lead in bone varies from 3 years in trabecular bone to 30 years in cortical bone. Only a small quantity of inorganic lead accumulates in the brain, with most found in the gray matter and the basal ganglia (11).

TOXICITY OF ELEMENTAL AND INORGANIC LEADS

Lead has diverse biologic effects manifested at the subcellular level, none of which are beneficial (18). The basis of lead's toxicity is its ability as a metallic cation to bind with specific ligands such as sulfhydryl, amino, and carboxyl groups present in biomolecular substances that are crucial to various physiologic functions. These lead-containing complexes then interfere with normal function by competing with essential metals for binding sites, inhibiting enzyme activity, and inhibiting or altering energy metabolism and essential ion transport (16).

The critical target organelle for lead toxicity is the mitochondrion, with resultant structural changes and marked functional disturbance noted (35). Uptake of lead by mitochondria causes swelling, loss of cristae, and interference with oxidative phosphorylation and ion transport (7). Inhibition of mitochondrial respiration exerts obvious deleterious effects on cell function in various systems (4). In addition, intracellular lead metabolism overlaps considerably with that of calcium, which gives rise to a potential site of interaction between the elements and a plausible means by which lead impairs intracellular ion transport (17).

Lead may cause multisystem dysfunction in the gastrointestinal system (lead colic), the hematopoietic system (anemia), the CNS (lead encephalopathy), joints and ligaments (arthralgia and lead gout), the endocrine system (thyroid, adrenocortical, and testicular dysfunctions), and the kidneys (17).

Two clinically discrete syndromes of lead intoxication have been identified. In relatively acute intoxication, caused by brief exposure to high lead concentrations, the classic symptoms of colic, anemia, and encephalopathy are often seen (11). Chronic forms of intoxication, which occur after long-term exposure, may have few of the findings typical of classic lead intoxication. Both acute and chronic intoxications may be associated with organic brain disturbances and depression (4,17).

PEDIATRIC LEAD POISONING

Children show a greater sensitivity to lead's effects than do adults. The incomplete development of the blood–brain barrier in very young children up to 36 months of age, increases the risk of lead's entry into the developing nervous system, which can result in prolonged neurobehavioral disorders. Children absorb and retain more lead in proportion to their weight than do adults. Young children also show a greater prevalence of iron deficiency, a condition that can increase gastrointestinal absorption of lead (37).

Acute Intoxication

Intoxication from a single exposure is unusual but has resulted from both accidental and intentional ingestion of solutions of soluble lead salts (Table 62–4) (1). Initial clinical features of acute ingestion of large amounts of any soluble lead salt, especially acetate, carbonate, or chromate, are largely due to local irritation of the alimentary tract. The stool may be black if lead sulfide is ingested. Radiopaque flakes may be seen in the gastrointestinal tract after recent ingestion of lead-containing compounds (1,18). If sufficient lead is retained after a single exposure, a syndrome identical to that of chronic intoxication may develop with symptoms including leg cramps, muscle weakness, paresthesias, CNS depression, coma, and death within 1 or 2 days (2).

TABLE 62–4. *Signs and symptoms of acute lead intoxication*

Gastrointestinal toxicity
Leg cramps
Muscle weakness
Paresthesia
CNS depression
Coma
Death

Chronic Intoxication

For chronic lead poisoning to develop, major acute exposures to lead need not occur. The body accumulates this metal over a lifetime and releases it slowly, so even small doses over time, can cause lead poisoning. Long-term exposure to lead causes a wide range of systemic disorders (Table 62–5). The major systems affected are the gastrointestinal tract, hematopoietic, central nervous system, renal, oral cavity, and reproductive; each of which will be discussed.

Gastrointestinal Tract

The most common form of plumbism is gastrointestinal. After a prodromal stage of variable duration and associated with vague symptoms of anorexia, dyspepsia, constipation, and a metallic taste in the mouth, severe abdominal cramps or colic may occur (38). This is due to the intense spasm sometimes associated with rigidity of the abdominal wall. This colic is characteristically severe and paroxysmal (4).

Hematopoietic System

The lead in blood is mostly bound to the erythrocytes and the earliest demonstrated effect of lead poisoning is inhibition of heme formation. Lead at low blood concentrations can inhibit at least three enzymes that are important for heme synthesis (Fig. 62–1) (1,18). These enzymes are δ-aminolevulinic acid dehydratase (ALAD), coproporphyrinogen oxidase, and ferrochelatase (1,39). The erythrocyte ALAD activity is inhibited at blood lead concentrations of no more than 10 μg/dL in adults and, there-

TABLE 62–5. *Signs and symptoms of chronic inorganic lead intoxication*

Gastrointestinal		
	Anorexia	
	Dyspepsia	
	Constipation	
	Metallic taste in the mouth	
	Abdominal pain	
Hematopoietic		
	Anemia (hypochromic, normocytic)	
	Basophilic stippling	
Neurologic		
	Peripheral neuropathy	
	"Wrist drop" or "foot drop"	
	Lead encephalopathy	
		Vomiting
		Apathy
		Drowsiness
		Stupor
		Seizures
		Death
Renal		
	Albuminuria	
	Hematuria	
	Pyuria	
Oral cavity		
	Ulcerative stomatitis	
	"Lead line"	
Reproductive		
	Female	
		Abnormal ovarian cycle
		Infertility
Spontaneous abortion		
		Stillbirth
	Male	
		Chromosomal alterations
		Decreased sperm count
		Altered sperm morphology
		Decreased sexual drive
		Impotence
		Sterility
	Fetal	
		Macrocephaly
		Low birth weight
		Nervous system disorders
		Increased death rate during first year

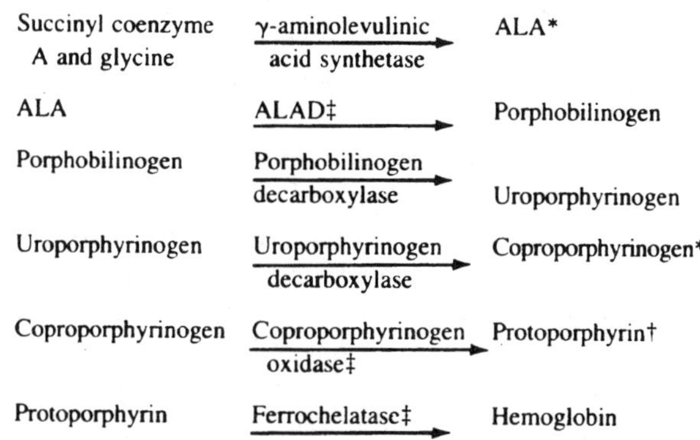

FIG. 62–1. Synthesis of hemoglobin and the effect of lead. *Increased concentration in urine; †Increased concentration in blood; ‡blocked by lead. Adapted with permission from *Medical Toxicology* (1986;1:387–410). © 1986 Adis Press International Inc.

fore, can act as a sensitive marker of lead intoxication. Lead prevents the conversion of δ-aminolevulinic acid (ALA) to porphobilinogen and the conversion of coproporphyrinogen to protoporphyrin by blocking the action of ALAD and coproporphyrinogen oxidase, respectively. This, in turn, causes ALA and corproporphyrin to accumulate in the urine, where they can be used as markers for lead poisoning (17).

Two effects are often seen in the human body when an enzyme is inhibited: first, the molecule on which the enzyme acts accumulates because it cannot undergo chemical reaction to produce the desired product; second, the amount of desired product decreases (11). With interference with heme synthesis, there is an increase in concentration of free erythrocyte protoporphyrin, erythrocyte zinc protoporphyrin, urinary ALA, and urinary coproporphyrin while erythrocyte ALAD activity and hemoglobin values are decreased (see Table 62–8) (39). Urinary ALA concentration may be elevated by other means so that it is not specific for lead exposure.

The hematologic effects are seen more commonly in children than in adults and may be helpful in arousing suspicion of lead poisoning (28).

Anemia. Lead can induce two types of anemia. Acute high-level lead poisoning has been associated with hemolytic anemia. In chronic lead poisoning, lead induces anemia by both interfering with erythropoiesis and by diminishing red blood cell survival.

Clinical anemia is an important finding in inorganic lead poisoning but not in organic lead poisoning (1,17). This is the most clear-cut functional defect caused by lead. The anemia is usually hypochromic and normocytic (7) because of a combination of decreased hemoglobin production and increased red blood cell destruction (17,40). To compensate, the marrow increases red blood cell production, releasing immature red blood cells. Reticulocytes and basophilic stippled cells also may appear in the blood (20,41). Macrocytosis may develop if anemia persists for any length of time. These symptoms of anemia may be nonspecific but are characteristic of the increased load on the cardiac system (17,42). They may include weakness, fatigue, pallor, waxy sallow complexion, headache, irritability, and others. It should be emphasized, however, that anemia is not an early manifestation of lead poisoning and is evident only when the blood lead level is significantly elevated for prolonged periods.

TABLE 62–6. *Conditions demonstrating basophilic hemolytic anemia*

Malaria
Thalassemia
Leukemia
Exposure to toxins
Lead
Aniline dyes
Benzene
Carbon monoxide
Copper

Basophilic Stippling. Because of the retardation of ribonuclease catabolism in maturing cells from lead poisoning, an accumulation of aggregates of incompletely degraded ribosomal fragments results in the phenomenon known as *basophilic stippling* (7,36,40). This is a nonspecific finding in many other conditions as well, such as hemolytic anemia, malaria, thalassemia, leukemia, and exposure to other toxins (1) and should be regarded as an unreliable index of lead intoxication (Table 62–6).

Central Nervous System

The most sensitive target of lead poisoning is the nervous system. In children, neurologic deficits have been documented at exposure levels once thought to cause no harmful effects. Adults also experience CNS effects at relatively low blood lead levels, manifested by subtle behavioral changes, fatigue, and impaired concentration. Peripheral nervous system damage, primarily motor, is seen mainly in adults.

The neurologic manifestations of acute or chronic lead intoxication are quite variable. Peripheral neuropathy is usually painless and limited to the extensor muscle groups. This may result in the classic picture of “wrist drop” or “foot drop” (7,17).

Lead Encephalopathy. The cerebral manifestations of lead poisoning have been called *lead encephalopathy*; this condition is less common in adults than in children (9). Lead encephalopathy constitutes the most severe consequence of lead intoxication (3). The most severe, often fatal form of encephalopathy may be preceded by lethargy, intermittent vomiting, apathy, drowsiness, irritability, stupor, poor memory, muscle tremors progressing to seizures, coma, and eventually death. Lead encephalopathy is almost always associated with a blood lead level exceeding 100 μg/dL, although occasionally, it has been reported at blood lead levels as low as 70 μg/L (7).

Renal System

Kidney disease due to lead exposure is far more prevalent than was previously believed (43). The hazard is compounded by the fact that, unlike the situation for the hematopoietic system, routine screening is ineffective in early diagnosis (7,44,45). In the adult, lead nephropathy is an insidious and progressive disease characterized by albuminuria, hematuria, pyuria, or a concentrating defect (in the early phases) (44,46). When less than two-thirds of kidney function is lost, blood urea nitrogen and serum creatinine may still be normal (47).

Impairment of proximal tubular function manifests in aminoaciduria, glycosuria, and hyperphosphaturia (a Fanconi-like syndrome). There is also evidence of an association between lead exposure and hypertension, an effect that may be mediated through renal mechanisms. Gout may develop as a result of lead-induced hyperuricemia, with selective decreases in the fractional excretion of uric acid before a decline in creatinine clearance.

Oral Cavity

Oral manifestations include ulcerative stomatitis, a blue gingival “lead line,” gray spots on the buccal mucosa, and a heavy coating on the tongue (1). A lead line is a great help in establishing exposure, but its presence does not mean that lead is being absorbed at that time. This blue line along the margin of the gums is caused by the action of hydrogen sulfide on the lead compound; hydrogen sulfide is a product of bacterial degradation in the gingival sulcus. This line is usually absent in edentulous patients or in patients who take care of their teeth.

Reproductive System

Exposure to lead has profoundly adverse effects on reproduction functions in both men and women, and lead is considered a potential human teratogen (48).

Exposure of women to lead is associated with abnormal ovarian cycles and menstrual disorders. An increased incidence of infertility, spontaneous abortion, stillbirth, and fetal macrocephaly has been associated with industrial lead exposure (49). Lead crosses the placenta and appears to be mobilized from maternal stores during pregnancy. Infants of mothers with lead poisoning have lower birth weights, slow growth, and nervous system disorders, and death is more likely in the first year of life.

Because lead readily crosses the placenta, the fetus is at greatest risk. Fetal exposure can cause potentially adverse neurologic effects in utero and during postnatal development.

Lead also affects the male gamete, and increased numbers of chromosomal alterations as well as abnormalities in sperm number, vigor, and morphologic features have been reported in lead workers. There may also be decreased sexual drive, impotence, and sterility. (50)

TOXICITY OF ORGANOLEAD COMPOUNDS

The signs and symptoms of organolead poisoning differ significantly from those of inorganic and elemental lead poisoning (Table 62–7). Like the organomercurials, tetraethyl and tetramethyl lead are lipid-soluble, highly volatile liquids that are absorbed quickly. The major effects of intoxication occur in the CNS.

The symptomatology of organic lead encephalopathy may be early in onset and correlate poorly with blood lead concentrations. Massive doses have caused death from cerebral and pulmonary edema (8). Small amounts of alkyl lead may cause sleep disturbances, including insomnia and nightmares, fatigue, headache, tinnitus, restlessness, irritability, weakness, ataxia, tremors, psychosis, delusions, suicidal tendencies, mania, and seizures (9). The most consistently observed neurologic manifestations are an abnormal jaw jerk, hyperactive deep tendon reflexes, stance and gait abnormalities, and an intention tremor (12). There may be a latent period which is variable in duration but usually ranges from 5 to 7 days; the more severe the exposure, the shorter the latent period.

Organolead poisoning is not associated with metaphyseal lead lines in the long bones, gingival lead lines, or nailbed changes. Hemoglobin synthesis does not appear to be greatly inhibited by organoleads and anemia and basophilic stippling generally do not occur (8).

TABLE 62–7. *Signs and symptoms of organolead intoxication*

Neurologic
Tinnitus
Headache
Weakness
Ataxia
Gait abnormalities
Tremors
Seizures
Coma
Cerebral edema
Psychiatric
Insomnia
Fatigue
Nightmares
Restlessness
Irritability
Psychosis
Delusions
Depression
Mania

DIAGNOSIS

Lead poisoning should be suspected in patients with nonspecific aches, pains, gastrointestinal symptoms, and subtle personality or CNS complaints, who are employed in an occupation susceptible to lead hazards. Lead encephalopathy should be suspected in patients with unexplained seizures that do not respond to conventional therapy and in patients with evidence of diffuse encephalopathy with or without focal signs in whom more common causes of encephalopathy have been excluded (51).

Childhood lead poisoning is an important differential diagnosis to keep in mind when a child presents with vomiting, abdominal pain, history of irritability, mood changes, or seizures.

The examination of a patient with a potential exposure to lead should include a work and medical history, a thorough physical examination, and appropriate laboratory studies. Once a diagnosis of increased lead absorption has been confirmed, the most important act of intervention is the prompt and complete termination of any further exposure to lead.

LABORATORY DETERMINATIONS

Laboratory determinations in suspected lead intoxication should include measurement of blood lead concentration, complete blood cell count with peripheral smear morphology and red cell indexes, a reticulocyte count, and if indicated and available, assays for serum iron and total iron-binding capacity and serum ferritin (Tables 62–8 and 62–9) (39). Because chelating agents that may be used in treatment are potentially nephrotoxic, a routine urinalysis for specific gravity and glucose and protein content should be performed first, together with microscopic examination and measurements of blood urea nitrogen and serum creatinine, to rule out occult renal disease (4). Long bone roentgenograms may be helpful in assessing chronic lead toxicity, and the diag-

TABLE 62–8. *Laboratory tests in elemental and inorganic lead poisoning*

Test	Finding
ALAD	Decreased
Urinary ALA	Increased
Blood ALA	Increased
Free erythrocyte protoporphyrin	Elevated
Zinc protoporphyrin	Elevated
Whole blood lead concentration	Elevated
Complete blood cell count	Anemia
Urinalysis	Abnormal
Blood urea nitrogen	Elevated
Serum creatinine	Elevated
Long-bone roentgenograms	Lead line

TABLE 62–9. *Laboratory tests in organolead poisoning*

Test	Finding
ALAD	Decreased
Urinary ALA	Increased or decreased
Blood AU	Decreased
Free erythrocyte	Increased or decreased protoporphyrin
Whole blood lead	Elevated concentration
Urine lead concentration	Elevated

nosis of acute lead intoxication may be aided by an abdominal roentgenogram (17).

Many screening tests for lead poisoning are based on the inhibition of heme synthesis, which, as just discussed, results in the buildup of heme precursors (11). A lead mobilization test may also be helpful in making the diagnosis in some patients (39).

In the early stages of lead intoxication, heme synthesis derangements may not be evident; the only abnormality may be an elevated blood lead concentration (52). Conversely, in chronic lead poisoning the various biochemical abnormalities may be noted but the circulating lead concentrations may often appear to be normal.

Blood Lead Concentrations

Blood lead concentration index is the most popular measure of recent exposure to lead because of its convenience and its accurate reflection of circulating lead concentration (Table 62–10) (52). In general, blood lead determination, even with its limitations, is accepted as the most valid and reliable indicator of recent excessive lead absorption (39). Because the half-life of circulating lead in blood is short, however, this measurement does not provide a realistic estimate of body burden (26). Unless exposure is constant and continuous, blood lead concentrations may not reflect previous uptake, absorption, or extent of biochemical injury (1). In other words, blood lead concentrations have no value in predicting excessive body stores of lead. In addition, the relationship between blood concentration and clinical effects varies. In general, adults tolerate high concentrations better than children (1).

TABLE 62–10. *Correlation between blood lead Concentration and symptoms of intoxication*

Lead concentration (mg per dL)	Symptoms
25–30	Subclinical (greater risk if pregnant)
40–50	Mild behavioral changes
50–70	Mild to moderate clinical symptoms
70–80	Severe symptoms
>80	Encephalopathy

Because 90% of the lead in circulating blood is fixed to red blood cell surfaces, it is critical that the assay for lead be done on whole blood (18). The value may fluctuate depending on current ingestion and metabolic shifts (5). A blood lead concentration greater than 25 μg/dL of whole blood and an erythrocyte protoporphyrin concentration greater than 35 μg/dL indicate undue absorption of lead (3). Blood lead should be well below this concentration especially in pregnant patients. These clinical standards have been lowered over the last 20 years with the growing awareness of the health risks associated with prolonged blood lead concentrations equal to or greater than 25 μg/dL; these include impaired heme synthesis, red blood cell nucleotide metabolism, and vitamin D and cortisol metabolism, decreased intelligence, and signs of subclinical alterations. The increased knowledge of the effects of low-level lead exposure has been reflected in changing definitions of toxic blood levels. Only 20 years ago the accepted threshold of undue lead absorption was a blood lead level of ≥60 μg/dL. Within 5 years, that threshold had been lowered twice by the Public Health Service and by 1975, stood at ≥30 μg/dL. In 1985, the CDC-defined lead toxicity as a blood level of ≥25 μg/dL. It is expected that these threshold levels will again be revised downward. New data indicate significant adverse effects of lead exposure in children at blood lead levels previously believed to be safe. Some adverse health effects have been documented at blood lead levels at least as low as 10 μg/dL of whole blood.

A lead concentration of 40 μg/dL of whole blood is considered the threshold for behavioral changes and mild CNS symptoms in adults (1). Patients whose blood lead concentrations are 50 to 70 μg/dL may have mild to moderate clinical symptoms. Concentrations of 70 to 80 μg/dL may indicate severe lead intoxication, and those in excess of 80 μg/dL are often associated with encephalopathy (see Table 62–8) (3).

Symptomatic plumbism (colic, seizures, acute encephalopathy) is usually associated with lead greater than 70 μg/dL, and chelation therapy should be administered promptly when presumptive laboratory tests are positive. In such cases, because the onset and course of encephalopathy are not predictable, the risk of delay outweighs the risks of a course of chelation.

Blood lead concentration should be interpreted with caution (41). A single elevated value may not indicate current excessive absorption, and a low value does not necessarily exclude a high bone burden of lead (39). A false impression of severity may be created by reliance on blood lead concentrations for the diagnosis of lead poisoning in adults. Serial determinations are needed to determine trends. Samples should be drawn by venipuncture rather than by fingerstick because of the possibility of skin contamination (53).

Normal Urinary Lead Excretion

Measurement of urinary lead excretion without chelation is unreliable in assessing lead stores because the lead concentration in urine depends on diuresis and specific gravity (1). Lead may also be in the soft tissues and not available for excretion until mobilized by a chelating agent.

Calcium EDTA Mobilization Test

The mobilization test is used to determine whether a child with an initial confirmatory blood lead level of 25 to 44 μg/dL will respond to chelation therapy with a brisk lead diuresis. Because of the cost and staff time needed for quantitative urine collection, this test is used only in selected medical centers where large numbers of lead-poisoned children are treated (54). Children whose blood lead levels are ≥45 μg/dL should not receive a provocative chelation test; they should be referred for appropriate chelation therapy immediately.

The outcome of the provocative chelation test is determined not by a decrease in the blood lead level but by the amount of lead excreted per dose of EDTA given. This test should not be done until the child is iron replete, since iron status may affect the outcome of the test (54).

An 8-hour mobilization test has been shown to be as reliable as a 24-hour mobilization test. An 8-hour test can be accomplished on an out-patient basis, but the patient should not leave the clinic during this test. To perform the test, a baseline blood lead level should be obtained. A dose of EDTA equal to 500 mg/m^2 in 5% dextrose is infused over 1 hour. All urine is then collected over the next 8 hours.

To obtain the total lead excretion in milligrams, the concentration of lead in the urine (μg/mL) is multiplied by the total urinary volume (mL). The total urinary excretion of lead (micrograms) is divided by the amount of EDTA given (mg) to obtain the lead excretion ratio (38).

An 8-hour EDTA chelation provocative test is considered positive if the lead excretion ration is >0.6. Children with blood lead levels 25 to 44 μg/dL and positive chelation test results should undergo a 5-day course of chelation (3). Because iron deficiency can enhance lead absorption and toxicity and often coexists with it, all children with blood lead levels ≥20 μg/dL should be tested for iron deficiency. Serum iron and iron binding capacity (transferrin saturation) and ferritin are the most sensitive indicators of iron status.

The utility and safety of the calcium EDTA diagnostic mobilization test to assess the body burden of lead have recently been questioned. (55)

Complete Blood Count

In a lead-poisoned patient, the hematocrit and hemoglobin values may be slightly to moderately low. The differential and total white count may appear normal. The peripheral smear may be either normochromic and normocytic or hypochromic and microcytic. Basophilic stippling is usually seen only in patients who have been significantly poisoned for a prolonged period. Eosinophilia may appear in lead-intoxicated patients but does not show a clear dose-response effects.

Tests for Biochemical Abnormalities

Most objective tests available for evaluating the adverse consequences of inorganic lead exposure depend on the disruption of the pathways of heme synthesis. As discussed, increased amounts of ALA in urine, decreased ALAD activity in red blood cells, and increased amounts of free erythrocyte protoporphyrin or zinc protoporphyrin are used as early warning signs of biochemical derangement produced by lead.

Concentrations of ALAD are consistently low in organolead poisoning, providing the most sensitive screening test; other markers of hemoglobin synthesis are not consistently altered. Because the amount of ALAD remaining is sufficient to synthesize hemoglobin, hemoglobin synthesis is not significantly inhibited by organolead compounds. There may, however, be a measurable increase in concentrations of ALA, and to a lesser extent, free erythrocyte protoporphyrin because of reduced activity of both ALAD and hemoglobin synthetase enzymes. Blood and urine concentrations of lead may also be moderately elevated (12).

Free Erythrocyte Protoporphyrin and Zinc Protoporphyrin

Historically, the terms *free erythrocyte protoporphyrin* (FEP) and *zinc protoporphyrin* (ZP) have been used interchangeably. This has since proven incorrect. Older, limited technology created the reasons for this unfortunate confusion owing to an inability to differentiate FEP from ZP (38). Although the chemical forms measured by the two methods differ slightly, on a weight basis they are roughly equivalent, so results reported as EP, ZPP, or FEP all reflect essentially the same analyte.

Until recently, the test of choice for screening asymptomatic children and other populations at risk was EP, commonly assayed as ZP. An elevated level of protoporphyrin in the blood is a result of accumulation secondary to enzyme dysfunction in the erythrocytes and reaches a steady state in the blood only after the entire population of circulating erythrocytes has turned over, about 120 days (56). Consequently, it lags behind blood lead levels and is an indirect measure of long-term lead exposure.

Lead inhibits ferrochelatase, the enzyme that catalyzes incorporation of iron into the porphyrin ring. There is an accumulation of protoporphyrin IX in the erythrocyte. If the pathway is interrupted as a result of lead poisoning or if adequate iron is not available, zinc is substituted for iron, resulting in an increase of ZP concentration. Monitoring of ZP is part of the proper screening for lead poisoning and is used in conjunction with blood lead levels to classify children as to risk category. Accumulation of EP (or ZP) occurs at thresholds of 25 to 30 μg/dL of lead in men and 15 to 20 μg/dL in women. For children, the threshold is approximately 15 μg/dL or even lower if there is iron deficiency (38).

Depending on the version of the test that is used, the EP test measures erythrocyte protoporphyrin either by (a) direct fluorescence of zinc protoporphyrin in intact red blood cells, or (b) by free erythrocyte protoporphyrin after it has been extracted from red blood cells that detect zinc protoporphyrin. They are commonly employed in field screening of large numbers of subjects. The instruments report ZPP values in EP equivalents.

Disadvantages

The major disadvantage of using EP and ZPP testing as a method for lead screening is that it is not sensitive at the lower levels of lead poisoning (15). Children can have lead levels above 30 μg/dL and EP levels within normal limits. An EP is still useful, however, in better identifying those patients whose blood lead levels are on the rise and in screening patients for iron-deficiency anemia.

Because the EP is not sensitive enough to identify more than a small percentage of children with blood lead levels between 10 and 25 μg/dL and misses many children with blood lead levels ≥25 μg/dL, measurement of blood lead levels has replaced the EP test as the primary screening method.

In current pediatric practice, if the EP or ZP is elevated, a blood lead quantification is carried out. Based on the result of that test, an appropriate medical intervention is pursued. Because EP levels take about 2 weeks to increase, EP levels may provide an indication of the duration of lead exposure.

The production of free erythrocyte protoporphyrin is not altered by environmental lead and is stable from day to day but its concentration is nonspecific, being elevated in iron deficiency, sickle cell anemia, and chronic infection (Table 62–11) (57).

TABLE 62–11. *Conditions that elevate blood concetrations of free erythrocyte protoporphyrin*

Chronic infection
Iron deficiency
Lead poisoning
Sickle cell anemia

Roentgenograms

Roentgenograms of the abdomen may reveal radiopaque material in the bowel if lead has been ingested during the preceding 72 hours (1). Neither negative nor positive x-ray results are diagnostic or definitive. A flat plate of the abdomen may, however, provide information about the source of lead if paint chips or other lead objects are found (34). Lines of increased density in the metaphyseal plate of the distal femur, proximal tibia, and fibula may be caused by lead which has disrupted the metabolism of bone matrix. Although these lines are sometimes called lead lines, they are areas of increased mineralization or calcification and not x-ray shadows of deposited lead (6). Lead lines may also be found at the ends of the metacarpals, ribs, tips of the scapulae, or over the iliac crests (34).

Hair Analysis

Hair analysis is not usually an appropriate assay for lead toxicity because no correlation has been found between the amount of lead in the hair and the exposure level (15). The probability of environmental lead contamination of a laboratory specimen and inconsistent sample preparation make the results of hair analysis difficult to interpret.

CDC CLASSIFICATION

As the concern for and knowledge about lead toxicity has increased, the amount of lead in the blood of children considered to warrant medical attention has progressively decreased.

The Centers for Disease Control (CDC) has recommended that annual screening for lead poisoning should be incorporated into general pediatric health care programs, especially for children from 6 months to 9 years of age. The latest CDC statement on the subject of lead toxicity is as follows: (a) A lead level of 25 μg/dL or greater defines an elevated blood lead; (b) A level of 35 μg/dL of blood EP plus an elevated blood lead concentration defines lead toxicity (Table 62–12) (38).

TREATMENT

Treatment of lead intoxication is aimed primarily at alleviating the acute symptoms and then at reducing the body lead stores (Table 62–13) (1). In the acute ingestion of lead, attempts at decreasing absorption should include gastric lavage and subsequent administration of activated charcoal and a cathartic.

In acute lead encephalopathy the management of intracranial hypertension is essential and may prove lifesaving if carried out rapidly and effectively (58). Reducing cerebral edema must be considered an urgent first step, especially because chelators do not work immedi-

TABLE 62–12. *CDC recommendations for lead toxicity*

Class	Blood Pb	Comment
I		A child in Class I is not considered to be lead-poisoned.
IIA	10–14	Many children (or a large proportion of children) with blood lead levels in this range should trigger community wide childhood lead poisoning prevention activities. Children in this range may need to be rescreened more frequently.
IIB	15–19	A child in Class IIB should receive nutritional and educational intervention and more frequent screening. If the blood lead level persists in this range, environmental investigation and intervention should be done.
III	20–44	A child in Class III should receive environmental evaluation an remediation and a medical evaluation. Such a child may need pharmacologic treatment of lead poisoning.
IV	45–69	A child in Class IV will need both medical and environmental interventions, including chelation therapy.
V	>70	A child with Class V lead poisoning is a medical emergency. Medical and environmental management must begin immediately.

ately. Volume replacement is restricted to basal requirements, and continuing losses must be carefully monitored. An adequate flow of urine must be established before intravenous chelation therapy is begun (53).

For initial control of seizures, diazepam is the preferred drug. Barbiturates and phenytoin are reserved for the long-term management of recurring seizures after the acute episode is managed and consciousness has been fully recovered (3).

There is no specific therapy for organolead poisoning. The efficacy of the therapeutic regimen for lead encephalopathy has not been adequately established for this type of intoxication (8). Although the therapeutic use of chelating agents in organolead poisoning has been somewhat disappointing compared with their effects on elemental and inorganic lead poisoning, these agents are not entirely without value (12).

Chelation Therapy

Chelating agents are the main modality of therapy in chronic inorganic lead poisoning (Table 62–14). Lead binds to all four sites on the chelator (oxygen, nitrogen, sulfur, and phosphorus) (17). The drugs approved for use as chelating agents are dimercaprol (BAL, British antilewisite), calcium EDTA, penicillamine, and succimer (8). Lead forms a complex with each of the chelating agents, and except for penicillamine, all are excreted in the urine. Penicillamine–lead complex is excreted in both urine and feces.

TABLE 62–13. *Treatment of lead intoxication*

Acute
Lavage
Charcoal and cathartic
Supportive care
Chelation therapy (see Table 61–12)
Chronic
Calcium EDTA mobilization test
Chelation therapy (see Table 61–12)

Calcium EDTA is the drug of choice for acute and chronic lead poisoning and lead encephalopathy. This compound forms a stable, soluble, nontoxic, nonionic complex with lead ions. Dimercaprol also forms a complex with lead, but for reasons that are not fully understood, dimercaprol by itself has seldom been useful in the treatment of clinical lead poisoning (17).

The lead-mobilizing patterns of dimercaprol and calcium EDTA differ and complement each other (8). Dimercaprol acts to chelate lead both intracellularly and extracellularly. Two molecules of dimercaprol combine with one atom of lead to form a complex that is excreted in the urine. Calcium EDTA removes lead from the extracellular compartment in soft tissues, CNS tissue, and red blood cells and increases its urinary excretion.

Calcium EDTA should be diluted to a concentration of less than 0.5% in dextrose and water or in a 0.9% saline solution. When administered intravenously as a single dose, it should be diluted similarly and administered by slow infusion over 15 to 20 minutes (3). Treatment with calcium EDTA should continue for no more than 5 days and should be followed by a rest period, usually of 5 to 7 days depending on patient response, to allow recovery from zinc depletion.

In the management of acute lead encephalopathy or when blood lead concentration is greater than 70 μg/dL, co-administration of dimercaprol and calcium EDTA is preferred (58). This therapy increases the rate of excretion of lead, lowers mortality, and may lower the incidence of brain damage compared with the use of calcium EDTA alone. The clinical deterioration seen with the use of calcium EDTA as the sole agent is thought to be due to partial dissociation of lead from the chelate, with release of lead into the brain. Dimercaprol, which penetrates the CNS, seems to protect against this effect. Treatment is, therefore, begun with a priming dose of dimercaprol only. Once urine flow is established, administration of calcium EDTA may begin. A second course of chelation therapy with EDTA alone may be

TABLE 62–14. *Indications for chelation therapy*

Clinically asymptomatic patients	
Blood lead, 40–70 μg/dL Negative calcium EDTA mobilization No encephalopathy Normal free erythrocyte protoporphyrin	No chelation
Blood lead, 40–70 μg/dL Positive calcium EDTA mobilization No encephalopathy	Calcium EDTA, 3–5 days Succimer
Blood lead, 25–50 μg/dL Metabolic evidence of poisoning Positive calcium EDTA mobilization	Calcium EDTA, 3–5 days or pennicillamine Succimer
Clinically symptomatic patients	
Blood lead, >70 μg/dL No encephalopathy Clinical evidence of poisoning	Calcium EDTA (50 mg/kg/day in six divided doses) and dimercaprol (4 mg/kg, then (16 mg/kg/day in six divided doses) Succimer
Blood lead, 56 to 69 μg/dL No encephalopathy Clinical evidence of poisoning	Calcium EDTA and penicillamine Succimer
Lead encephalopathy	Dimercaprol (24 mg/kg/day in six divided doses) and calcium EDTA (75 mg/kg/day in six divided doses)
Long-term therapy	Penicillamine (250 mg orally 4 times daily)

required if the blood lead concentration rebounds to a value ≥45 μg/dL within 5 to 7 days after treatment.

High-dosage therapy for lead encephalopathy consists of dimercaprol administered intramuscularly at 24 mg/kg/day in six divided doses and calcium EDTA administered intravenously at 75 mg/kg/day in six divided doses not to exceed 1.5 g/day (12). After the initial 5-day course of combined parenteral therapy, oral treatment should commence with 40 mg/kg/day of penicillamine 2 to 4 times per day until two consecutive measurements of blood lead concentration are less than 40 μg/dL and the 24-hour urine lead concentration is less than 100 μg per 24 hours (7,12).

Asymptomatic patients without encephalopathy and with blood lead concentrations greater than 70 μg/dL may receive low-dose therapy with calcium EDTA and dimercaprol or with calcium EDTA alone. Calcium EDTA is administered intravenously at 50 mg/kg/day in six divided doses, and dimercaprol is administered intramuscularly at an initial dose of 4 mg/kg and then 16 mg/kg/day in six divided doses. Symptomatic patients without encephalopathy and with blood lead concentrations between 56 and 69 μg/dL can be treated with low-dose calcium EDTA. Penicillamine may be used after completion of parenteral chelation therapy (7,12).

Only very minimal data exists about chelating children with blood lead levels below 25 μg/dL, and such children should not be chelated except in the context of approved clinical trials.

For blood lead levels from 25 to 44 μg/dL, the effectiveness of chelation therapy in decreasing the adverse effects of lead on children's intelligence has not been shown. Many experienced practitioners decide whether to use chelation therapy on the basis of the results of carefully performed EDTA mobilization tests.

Chelation therapy is advised for patients in groups III and IV of the CDC classification, including asymptomatic children. Such therapy before the onset of symptoms may lessen the risk and severity of injury to the brain. The standard course, for children in group III with venous blood lead of 50 to 69 μg/dl whole blood, has been calcium EDTA for 5 days at a dose of 1000 mg/m^2/day in two portions administered intramuscularly.

Use of the Calcium EDTA Mobilization Test

As discussed earlier, the calcium EDTA mobilization test is useful when blood lead concentration is elevated but there is uncertainty about the need for chelation, as in patients with blood lead concentrations of 25 to 50 μg/dL accompanied by erythrocyte protoporphyrin concentrations persistently greater than 35 μg/dL or in patients with free erythrocyte protoporphyrin concentration out of proportion to blood lead concentrations (38). This test provides an index of the mobile fraction of body lead and directly demonstrates whether a significant diuresis of lead will result from chelation (26). Patients with moderately elevated blood lead concentrations (25 to 50 μg/dL), no encephalopathy, and a positive mobilization test may be treated with penicillamine alone. Patients with blood lead concentrations less than 40 μg/dL, and those with moderately elevated blood concentrations (40 to 59 μg/dL) but negative mobilization tests and no encephalopathy require no chelation therapy.

Chelation Therapy in Renal Disease

Adults with lead nephropathy who have serum creatinine concentrations of 2 mg/dL or less may receive 1 g of calcium EDTA daily for 5 days (46). In patients with serum creatinine concentrations of 2 to 3 mg/dL, 500 mg every 24 hours for 5 days should be administered. In children, the dosage is 50 to 75 mg/kg daily with the total amount divided into two daily doses and each part dissolved in 500 mL of normal saline or 5% dextrose and water.

Role of Penicillamine

Penicillamine chelates lead but not to the same degree as dimercaprol or calcium EDTA (17). For this reason, it is not recommended for acute therapy but may be employed for long-term therapy (7). Because it can be given by mouth, penicillamine has found particular utility in mild and uncomplicated plumbism and for supplemental therapy (17).

Role of Succimer

For several decades, pharmacologic intervention for lead poisoning has relied on the parenteral administration of BAL plus CaNaEDTA. Both BAL and CaNaEDTA are unpleasant to use in the treatment of small children and both can evoke adverse effects (59). Succimer (Chemet) is an orally active, heavy metal chelating agent that is indicated for treatment of lead toxicity in children with blood lead levels ≥45 μg/dL. 2,3-Dimercaptosuccinic acid (Succimer) was first synthesized in 1954 and incorporated the molecule into the structure of an arsenical drug for the treatment of schistosomiasis (60–63). It was first proposed as an antidote for heavy metal poisoning by the Chinese and has been used fairly widely in China, the Soviet Union, and Japan. The drug is also potentially useful for the treatment of poisoning with arsenic and mercury.

Succimer is chemically similar to BAL but is more water soluble, has a high therapeutic index, and is absorbed from the gastrointestinal tract. It is effective when given orally and produces a lead diuresis comparable to that produced by EDTA. This diuresis lowers blood lead levels and reverses the biochemical toxicity of lead as indicated by normalization of circulating aminolevulinic acid dehydrase levels (64). Succimer appears to be more specific for lead than the most commonly used chelating agent, EDTA (65). Succimer is not indicated for prophylaxis of lead poisoning in a lead-containing environment.

The recommended initial dose is 350 mg/m^2 (10 mg/kg) every 8 hours for 5 days, followed by 350 mg/m^2 every 12 hours for 14 days (14). A course of treatment, therefore, lasts 19 days. If more courses are needed, a minimum of 2 weeks between courses is preferred unless blood lead levels indicate the need for immediate retreatment (66). In young children who cannot swallow capsules, succimer can be administered by separating the capsule and sprinkling the powder on soft food or by serving the drug in a spoon along with a fruit drink. Succimer is available in 100 mg capsules.

The most common adverse effects reported in clinical trials in children and adults were primarily gastrointestinal and include nausea, vomiting, diarrhea, and appetite loss. Rashes, some necessitating discontinuation of therapy, have been reported for about 4% of patients. Elevations in serum aminotransferase and alkaline phosphatase activities have also occurred (67).

Children with blood lead levels >45 μg/dL who are being treated with succimer, should, if possible, be hospitalized until their blood lead levels fall below 45 μg/dL and the lead hazards in their home are abated or alternative lead hazard-free housing has been identified.

REFERENCES

1. Ibels L, Pollock C: Lead intoxication.*Med Toxicol* 1986;1:387–410.
2. Lin-Fu J: Undue absorption of lead among children—a new look at an old problem. *N Engl J Med* 1972;286:702–710.
3. Piomelli S, Rosen J, Chisolm J, et al: Management of childhood lead poisoning. *J Pediatr* 1984;105:523–532.
4. Chisolm J: Treatment of acute lead intoxication—choice of chelating agents and supportive therapeutic measures. *Clin Toxicol* 1970;3: 527–540.
5. Sachs H, Blanksma L, Murray E, et al: Ambulatory treatment of lead poisoning: Report of 1155 cases. *Pediatrics* 1970;46:389–396.
6. Nelson M, Chisolm J: Lead toxicity masquerading as sickle cell crisis. *Ann Emerg Med* 1986;15:748–750.
7. Pincus D, Saccar C: Lead poisoning. *Clin Pharmacol* 1979;19: 120–124.
8. Greenhouse A: Heavy metals and the nervous system. *Clin Neuropharmacol* 1982;5:45–92.
9. Schottenfeld R, Cullen M: Organic affective illness associated with lead intoxication. *Am J Psychiatry* 1984;141:1423–1426.
10. Lin-Fu J: Vulnerability of children to lead exposure and toxicity. *N Engl J Med* 1973;289:1229–1233.
11. Chisolm J: Management of increased lead absorption and lead poisoning in children. *N Engl J Med* 1973;289:1016–1017.
12. Edminster S, Bayer M: Recreational gasoline sniffing: acute gasoline intoxication and latent organolead poisoning. *J Emerg Med* 1985;3: 365–370.
13. Tripathi R, Sherertz P, Llewellyn G, et al: Lead exposure in outdoor firearm instructors. *Am J Pub Health* 1991;81:753–755.
14. Meggs W, Gerr F, Aly M, et al: The treatment of lead poisoning from gunshot wounds with succimer (DMSA). *J Toxicol Clin Toxicol* 1994;32:377–386.
15. Bushnell P, Jaeger R: Hazards to health from environmental lead exposure: a review of recent literature. *Vet Hum Toxicol* 1986; 28:255–261.
16. Chisolm J: The use of chelating agents in the treatment of acute and chronic lead intoxication in childhood. *J Pediatr* 1968;73:1–38.
17. Gordon N, Brown S, Khosla V, et al: Lead poisoning. *Oral Surg* 1979;47:500–512.
18. Chisolm J, Mellits E, Keil J: A simple protoporphyrin assay microhematocrit procedure as a screening technique for increased lead absorption in young children. *J Pediatr* 1974;84:490–495.
19. Selbst S, Henretig F, Fee M, et al: Lead poisoning in a child with a gunshot wound. *Pediatrics* 1986;77:413–416.
20. Cohen G, Ahrens W: Chronic lead poisoning. *J Pediatr* 1959;54: 271–284.
21. Galazka S: Lead poisoning in a family. *J Fam Pract* 1990; 31:317–318.
22. Rose D, Cummings C, Molinaro J, et al: Screening for lead toxicity among autobody repair workers. *Am J Ind Med* 1982;3:405–412.
23. Manton W: Editorial comment: lead poisoning from gunshots—a five century heritage. *J Toxicol Clin Toxicol* 1994;32:387–390.
24. Dillman R, Crumb C, Lidsky M: Lead poisoning from a gunshot wound. *Am J Med* 1979;66:509–514.
25. Machle W: Lead absorption from bullets lodged in tissues. *JAMA* 1940;115:1536–1541.
26. Allcott J, Barnhart R, Mooney L: Acute lead poisoning in two users of illicit methamphetamine. *JAMA* 1987;258;510–511.
27. Hugelmeyer C, Moorhead J, Horenblas L, et al: Fatal lead encephalopathy following foreign body ingestion: case report. *J Emerg Med* 1989;6:397–400.

28. Cohen N, Modai D, Golik A, et al: An esoteric occupational hazard for lead poisoning. *Clin Toxicol* 1986;24:59–67.
29. Lin-Fu J: Vulnerability of children to lead exposure and toxicity. *N Engl J Med* 1973;289:1289–1293.
30. Hammer L, Ludwig S, Henretig F: Increased lead absorption in children with accidental ingestions. *Am J Emerg Med* 1985;3:301–304.
31. FriedmanJ, Weinberger H: Six children with lead poisoning. *Am J Dis Child* 1990;144:1039–1044.
32. Wiley J, Henretig F, Selbt S: Blood lead levels in children with foreign bodies. *Pediatrics* 1992;89:593–596.
33. Charney E, Kessler B, Farfel M, et al: Childhood lead poisoning. *N Engl J Med* 1933;309:1089–1093.
34. McElvaine M, DeUngria E, Matte T, et al: Prevalence of radiographic evidence of paint chip ingestion among children with moderate to severe lead poisoning, St. Louis, Missouri, 1989 through 1990. *Pediatrics* 1992;89:740–742.
35. Oehme F: Mechanisms of heavy metal toxicities. *Clin Toxicol* 1972; 5:151–162.
36. Pagliuca A, Mufti G, Baldwin D, et al: Lead poisoning: clinical, biochemical, and haematological aspects of a recent outbreak. *J Clin Pathol* 1990;43:277–281.
37. Kew J, Morris C, Aihie A, et al: Arsenic and mercury intoxication due to Indian ethnic remedies. *Brit Med J* 1993;306:506–507.
38. Gerson B: Lead. *Clin Lab Med* 1990;10:441–457.
39. Keate R, DiPietrantonio P, Randleman M: Occupational lead exposure. *Ann Emerg Med* 1983;12:786–788.
40. Cohen G: Lead poisoning. *Clin Pediatr* 1980;19: 245–250.
41. Alessio L, Castoldi M, Odone P, et al: Behavior of indicators of exposure and effect after cessation of occupational exposure to lead. *Br J Ind Med* 1981;38:262–267.
42. Green V, Wise C, Callenbach J: Lead poisoning. *Clin Toxicol* 1976; 9:33–51.
43. Wedeen R, Mallik D, Batuman V: Detection and treatment of occupational lead nephropathy. *Arch Intern Med* 1979;139:53–57.
44. Batuman V, Landy E, Maesaka J, et al: Contribution of lead to hypertension with renal impairment. *N Engl J Med* 1983;309:17–21.
45. Campbell B, Beattie A, Elliott H, et al: Occupational lead exposure and renin release. *Arch Environ Health* 1979;34:439–443.
46. Khan A, Patel U, Rafeeq M, et al: Reversible acute renal failure in lead poisoning. *J Pediatr* 1983;102:147–149.
47. Wedeen R: Lead and the gouty kidney. *Am J Kid Dis* 1983;2: 559–563.
48. Needleman H, Gunnoe C, Leviton A, et al: Deficits in psychologic and classroom performance of children with elevated dentine lead levels. *N Engl J Med* 1979;300:689–695.
49. Needleman H, Rabinowitz M, Leviton A, et al: The relationship between prenatal exposure to lead and congenital anomalies. *JAMA* 1984;251:2956–2959.
50. Needleman H, Landrigan P: The health effects of low-level exposure to lead. *Annu Rev Public Health* 1981;2:277–298.
51. Smith M: Recent work on low-level lead exposure and its impact on behavior, intelligence, and learning: A review. *J Am Acad Child Psychiatry* 1985;24:24–32.
52. Carton J, Maradona J, Arribas J: Acute-subacute lead poisoning: Clinical findings and comparative study of diagnostic tests. *Arch Intern Med* 1987;147:697–703.
53. Piomelli S, Davidow B, Guinee V, et al: The FEP test: a screening micromethod for lead poisoning. *Pediatrics* 1973;51:254–259.
54. Markowitz M, Rosen J: Need for the lead mobilization test in children with lead poisoning. *J Pediatr* 1991;119:305–310.
55. Markowitz M, Weinberger H: Immobilization-related lead toxicity in previously lead-poisoned children. *Pediatrics* 1990;86:455–457.
56. Berwick D, Komaroff A: Cost effectiveness of lead screening. *N Engl J Med* 1982;306:1392–1398.
57. Rosen I, Wildt K, Gullberg B, et al: Neurophysiological effects of lead exposure. *Scand J Work Environ Health* 1983;9:431–441.
58. Coffin R, Phillips J, Staples W, et al: Treatment of lead encephalopathy in children. *J Pediatr* 1966;69:198–206.
59. Graziano J, Lolacono N, Moulton T, et al: Controlled study of meso-2,3-dimercaptosuccinnic acid for the management of childhood lead intoxication. *J Pediatr* 1992;120:133–139.
60. Aposhian H: DMSA and DMPS-Water-soluble antidotes for heavy metal poisoning. *Annu Rev Pharmacol Toxicol* 1983;23:193–215.
61. Aaseth J: Recent advances in the therapy of metal poisonings with chelating agents. *Hum Toxicol* 1983:2:257–272.
62. Friedheim E, Graziano J, Kaul B: Treatment of lead poisoning by 2,3-dimercaptosuccinic acid. *Lancet* 1978;2:1234–1236.
63. Graziano J: Role of 2,3-dimercaptosuccinic acid in the treatment of heavy metal poisoning. *Med Toxicol* 1986;1:155–162.
64. Graziano J, Leong J, Friedheim E: 2,3-Dimercaptosuccinic acid: A new agent for the treatment of lead poisoning. *J Pharmacol Exp Ther* 1978;206:696–700.
65. Graziano J, Lolocono N, Meyer P: Dose-response study of oral 2.3-dimercaptosuccinic acid in children with elevated blood lead concentrations. *J Pediatr* 1988;113:751–757.
66. Graziano J, Siris E, Lolacono N, et al: 2,3-Dimercaptosuccinic acid as an antidote for lead intoxication. *Clin Pharmacol Ther* 1985;37: 431–438.
67. Cory-Slechta D: Mobilization of lead over the course of DMSA chelation therapy and long-term efficacy. *J Pharmacol Exp Ther* 1988;246:84–91.

ADDITIONAL SELECTED REFERENCES

Cohen A, Trotzky M, Pincus D: Reassessment of the microcytic anemia of lead poisoning. *Pediatrics* 1981;67:904–906.

Edwards E, Edwards E: Allergic contact dermatitis to lead acetate in a hair dye. *Cutis* 1982;30:629–630.

Ernhart C, Landa B, Schell N: Lead levels and intelligence. *Pediatrics* 1981;68:903–905.

Fischbein A, Cohn J, Ackerman G: Asbestos, lead, and the family: household risks. *J Fam Pract* 1980;10:989–992.

Glickman L, Valciukas J, Lilis R, et al: Occupational lead exposure. *Int Arch Occup Environ Health* 1984;54:115–125.

Gloag D: Sources of lead pollution. *Br Med J* 1981;282:41–44.

Mahaffey K, Annest J, Roberts J, et al: National estimates of blood lead levels: United States, 1976–1980. *N Engl J Med* 1982;307:573–579.

Miwa S, Ishida Y, Takegawa S, et al: A case of lead intoxication. *Am J Hematol* 1981;11:99–105.

Nathanson B, Nudelman H: Ambient lead concentrations in New York City and their health implications. *Bull NY Acad Med* 1980; 56:866–875.

Sixel-Dietrich F, Doss M, Pfeil C, et al: Acute lead intoxication due to intravenous injection. *Hum Toxicol* 1985;4:301–309.

Triebig G, Weltle D, Valentin H: Investigations on neurotoxicity of chemical substances at the workplace. *Int Arch Occup Environ Health* 1984;53:189–204.

Valciukas J, Lilis R: A composite index of lead effects. *Int Arch Occup Environ Health* 1982;51:1–14.

CHAPTER 63

Arsenic

GENERAL INFORMATION

Arsenic was first recorded as a medicinal agent in ancient Greece by Hippocrates. Although it is rarely part of the modern pharmacopeia, it is widely used in other applications.

Because arsenic is nearly tasteless and odorless, it was used extensively as a means of criminal poisoning, and although not as common, homicidal, suicidal, and accidental arsenic poisoning occur even today (1). Self-administration of arsenic by accident in children and as a suicide attempt in adults represent the most common types of ingestion. Purposeful self-administration of arsenic for the purpose of creating and maintaining a state of chronic invalidism has also been reported (2). Arsenic is second only to lead as a cause of chronic heavy metal poisoning.

TABLE 63–1. *Sources and uses of arsenic*

Fossil fuels
Pesticides
Insecticides
Rodenticides
Weed killers
Industry
Wallpaper
Paint
Ceramic
Glass
Wood preservation
Medicinal
Antiprotozoan
Homeopathic medicines
Veterinary Use

USES

In general, exposure to arsenic may come from environmental or industrial sources. As one of the elements making up the earth's crust, arsenic is ubiquitously distributed in nature. Rarely is it found occurring naturally in its elemental state. Arsenic is more widely distributed in a combined form with a variety of ores and minerals. Some of the more common arsenic compounds found in nature are the sulfide complexes, realgar (As_2S_2) and orpiment (As_2S_3), and arsenical pyrites (FeSAs).

For centuries, arsenic has played a role in medicine, industry, and criminal activities. Since ancient times, many physicians have believed in the medicinal value of arsenic and its effectiveness in a wide variety of disorders (3). Arsenic is present in fossil fuels, in air and water as an industrial byproduct, in food products (primarily seafood), in cosmetics, and in copper-smelting factories. Arsenic is a common ingredient in insecticides, rodenticides, weed killers, wallpaper, paint, ceramics, and glass (Table 63–1) (3). It is also used in wood preservation and as an additive to metal alloys to increase hardening and heat resistance (4). Organic arsenicals such as dimethylarsenic acid and monosodium methylarsenate are used in forestry as herbicides (5). Lead, calcium, and magnesium arsenate are the most common arsenicals; these are used primarily as pesticides in sprays of various kinds (6). Inorganic arsenic poisoning was fairly common in the United States before the Second World War (7) mainly because of the widespread use of medicinal arsenic and contamination of fruits and vegetables by arsenical sprays (8).

In some areas, organic arsenicals are still used in the treatment of certain protozoan diseases. Arsenic is also an ingredient in numerous homeopathic medicines (9). The use of penicillin for the treatment of syphilis drastically curtailed the medicinal importance of arsenicals, but they continue to have major agricultural and industrial importance, thereby affording innumerable opportunities for exposure (10). Arsenic-containing compounds are widely used in feed for poultry, cattle, and swine, purportedly to improve the nutritional status of the animals (Table 63–2) (3). Contamination of well water and of illicitly manufactured alcohol have been causes of arsenic poisoning.

Although the lethal adult dose ranges from 120 to 200 mg, acute ingestion of 9 to 14 mg of arsenic by a young child can produce classic gastrointestinal signs and symptoms of arsenic poisoning (10).

TABLE 63–2. *Common arsenic compounds*

Name		Chemica formula	Comments
Inorganic	+3 oxidation state		
Arsenic trioxide		As_2O_3	"White arsenic," most commercially important arsenic compound; used in the manufacture of most other arsenic compounds
Sodium arsenite		$NaAsO_2$	Pesticide
Potassium arsenite		$KAsO_2$	Constituent of Fowler's solution
Arsenic trichloride		$AsCl_3$	"Butter of arsenic," used in industry
Inorganic	+5 oxidation state		
Arsenic pentoxide		As_2O_5	Insecticide
Arsenic acid		H_3AsO_4	Leaf desiccant used in cotton production
Lead arsenate		$PbHAsO_4$	Insecticide
Calcium arsenate		$Ca_3(AsO_4)_2$	Insecticide
Organic	+3 oxidation state		
Arsphenamine (Salvarsan)		HO–C₆H₃(H₂N)–As=As–C₆H₃(NH₂)–OH	Anti-syphilitic drug
Melarsoprol (Mel B)		(H₂N)₂-triazinyl–NH–C₆H₄–As(S–CH₂)(S–CH–CH₂OH)	Still used in the treatment of African trypanosomiasis
Organic	+5 oxidation state		
Sodium arsanilate (Atoyxl)		H₂N–C₆H₄–As(OH)(=O)–O⁻Na⁺	Once used to treat African trypanosomiasis
Tryparsamide		NH₂COCH₂NH–C₆H₄–As(OH)(=O)–O⁻Na⁺	Less toxic than Atoyxl, also was used to treat African trypanosomiasis
Arsanillic acid		H₂N–C₆H₄–As(=O)(OH)₂	Livestock feed additive

From Malachowski M. *Clin Lab Med*, 1990;10:459–472, with permission from WB Saunders Company.

TYPES OF ARSENIC COMPOUNDS

Arsenic occupies the position between phosphorus and antimony, and many of its physiochemical properties closely resemble those of phosphorus. Arsenic is classified as a metalloid, having chemical properties intermediate between typical metals and nonmetals. Thus, arsenic is capable of forming alloys with metals but also readily forms covalent bonds with carbon, hydrogen, and oxygen.

The chemistry of arsenic is complex and the compounds it forms are numerous. This is because arsenic possesses several different valences or oxidation states, which result in the markedly different biologic behavior of its compounds.

From the toxicologic standpoint, the important compounds of arsenic fall into three major groups: (a) inorganic arsenicals, such as white arsenic, and the arsenate and arsenite salts; (b) organic arsenicals, which differ in the valence state of the arsenic atom (trivalent and pentavalent); (c) arsine gas.

In general, inorganic arsenic compounds are more toxic than organic arsenic compounds of similar valency. Arsine gas is the most toxic form of arsenic (Table 63–3) Next, are the commercially important trivalent arsenic compounds or arsenites in which arsenic is in its +3 oxi-

TABLE 63–3. *Toxicity of arsenic compounds (in decreasing order of toxicity)*

Arsine gas
Arsinites (As +3)
Arsenates (As +5)
Elemental arsenic (As°)

TABLE 63–4. *Biochemical effects of arsenicals*

Blockade of oxidative phosphorylation
Inhibition of acetyl and succinyl coenzyme A transformation
Inhibition of other enzymes
Monoamine oxidase
Lipase
Acid phosphatase
Liver arginase
Cholinesterase
Adenylcyclase

dation state. Least toxic are the pentavalent or arsenate compounds, which contain arsenic in its +5 oxidation state. Elemental arsenic (0 oxidation state) is considered to be nontoxic because it is insoluble.

Pentavalent arsenate, which is the naturally occurring environmental form of arsenic, is less toxic than trivalent arsenite because pentavalent compounds are relatively physiologically inactive; they are water soluble and are rapidly absorbed through mucous membranes. This leads to rapid penetration into all body tissues, most of which are capable of reducing arsenate to toxic arsenite. This mechanism has not been completely determined, however (8).

Although arsenic trioxide is less toxic than some of the more soluble herbicidal arsenicals, the dust can cause poisoning through ingestion, inhalation, or skin contact. Trivalent arsenic compounds are less readily absorbed through mucous membranes because of their lipid solubility but are better absorbed through the skin (8). Trivalent arsenicals such as phenylarsenoxide are more potent inhibitors of certain sulfhydryl enzymes than inorganic arsenites.

PHARMACOKINETICS

Absorption

Arsenic may enter the body through the gastrointestinal tract (GIT), lungs, or skin surface. Under normal circumstances, approximately 1 mg of arsenic is ingested daily (11). The extent of absorption depends on both the chemical form of the arsenic and its physical state. Thus, less water-soluble compounds, such as AsO_3, are poorly absorbed through mucous membranes compared to more water-soluble species, such as the arsenite salts. In addition, compounds in the form of fine powders are more readily absorbed than coarse substances, which may be eliminated in the feces before dissolving. In general, both the trivalent and pentavalent inorganic arsenic compounds are well absorbed from the gastrointestinal tract. Organic arsenicals, on the other hand, are more variably absorbed.

Distribution

Once in the bloodstream, arsenic initially becomes associated with the red blood cells, binding to the globin portion of hemoglobin. It does not readily penetrate the blood–brain barrier. Redistribution is said to occur within 24 hours, primarily to the liver, kidneys, spleen, lungs, and GIT. Any arsenic remaining intravascularly becomes bound to plasma proteins. A biologic half-life of only about 10 hours is commonly cited for arsenic (12).

Characteristically, within 2 to 4 weeks of absorption, arsenic begins to be incorporated into hair, nails, and skin owing to its predilection for sulfhydryl groups which are common in keratin (8). Within 4 weeks, arsenic can be detected in bone, in which it substitutes for phosphate. It has also been found that arsenic can readily cross the placenta and, thus, be transferred from the mother to the fetus.

Elimination

The biotransformation of arsenic in humans is not completely understood. It is generally believed that some trivalent inorganic arsenic compounds are oxidized to the less toxic pentavalent state. In addition, some reduction of pentavalent inorganic arsenic compounds to the trivalent state is also thought to occur. However, both the trivalent and pentavalent forms are transformed primarily into methylated compounds before excretion. Thus, the major metabolites of inorganic arsenic are methylarsinic acid, dimethylarsinic acid, and trimethylarsenic compounds.

The major route of arsenic elimination is through the kidney. Small amounts may also be excreted in feces, bile, sweat, and breast milk.

MECHANISM OF TOXICITY OF ARSENICALS

There are several mechanisms by which arsenic exerts its toxic effects (Table 63–4) . One mechanism by which arsenic exerts its toxic effects is through impairment of cellular respiration by the reversible inhibition of dehydrolipoate, a necessary cofactor of pyruvate dehydrogenase and the uncoupling of oxidative phosphorylation. This inhibition of the oxidation of dehydrolipoate to lipoate blocks the Krebs cycle, thus, interrupting oxidative phosphorylation, resulting in depletion of cellular energy stores, particularly adenosine triphosphate, disruption of multiple metabolic systems, and eventually cell death. Much of the toxicity of arsenic results from its ability to interact with sulfhydryl groups of proteins and enzymes and to substitute for phosphorus in a variety of biochemical reactions. Because sulfhydryl groups are present in many enzyme systems, it is not surprising that many enzyme systems are vulnerable; the pyruvate and succinate oxidation pathways are especially sensitive to disruption by arsenic.

In another major form of toxicity from arsenic, termed *arsenolysis*, arsenic acts as an anion and can substitute for phosphate in many reactions. This also disrupts oxidative phosphorylation by replacing the stable phosphoryl group with the less stable arsenyl group (11). The arsenyl decomposes, resulting in a loss of high-energy phosphate bonds and eventual stimulation of cellular respiration to restore lost energy.

Arsenic poisoning results in a clinical picture similar to that of thiamine deficiency because of prevention of the transformation of acetyl and succinyl coenzyme A (8). This blockade of thiamine-related metabolism accounts for the similarities in arsenic encephalopathy and Wernicke–Korsakoff's syndrome. Many other enzymes are susceptible to deactivation by arsenic, including monoamine oxidase, lipase, acid phosphatase, liver arginase, cholinesterase, and adenylcyclase, but these are less important clinically (6).

Systemic poisoning is the principal concern with all arsenic compounds, but arsenic trichloride and some organic derivatives such as lewisite are also strong local irritants that may penetrate the skin and act as vesicants (12).

TABLE 63–5. *Clinical features of acute arsenic intoxication*

Gastrointestinal
Metallic taste in the mouth
Garlic odor on the breath
Dysphagia
Abdominal pain
Vomiting
Diarrhea
Shock
Cardiac
Decreased force of contraction
Sinus tachycardia
Ventricular dysrhythmia
Nonspecific electrocardiographic changes
Neurologic
Headache
Muscle weakness
Muscle cramps
Peripheral neuropathy
Paresthesia
CNS depression
Coma
Cutaneous
Skin pigmentation changes
Aidrich-Mees lines
Exfoliative dermatitis
Dermatitis/keratosis
Facial edema

TOXICITY OF ARSENICALS

Acute

Acute arsenic poisoning is usually the result of suicidal or accidental ingestion, with occasional cases seen from industrial or environmental exposures (13). Clinical manifestations of acute arsenic poisoning usually occur within the first few hours after ingestion or exposure; symptoms may occur as soon as 30 minutes after exposure (14). The earliest clinical features reflect multi-organ involvement, which is manifested often as acute gastroenteritis and is variably associated with encephalopathy, pancytopenia, hepatitis, cardiomyopathy, and dermatitis (Table 63–5) (15). Death from acute arsenic poisoning is usually caused by irreversible circulatory insufficiency. If the patient survives the initial illness, recovery may be complicated by the development of nephritis, including hematuria, albuminuria, and glycosuria.

Acute massive intoxication, also referred to as *acute paralytic form*, occurs following the ingestion of large doses of soluble arsenic, usually on an empty stomach. In such instances, absorption of arsenic is rapid, causing an almost immediate onset of cardiopulmonary symptoms similar to shock. Gastrointestinal symptoms are usually not present, although, in some cases, the ingestion of huge doses of arsenic may produce immediate vomiting. The clinical presentation includes profound circulatory collapse with low blood pressure, weak pulse, shallow breathing, stupor, and occasionally, convulsions. Death from circulatory collapse or central nervous system depression typically occurs within a few hours of ingestion.

Gastrointestinal

Whatever the route of exposure, the presenting symptoms in most cases of acute arsenic poisoning are those of severe gastritis or gastroenteritis. Initially, the patient experiences a metallic taste in the mouth and a garlicky odor on the breath (6). Burning and dryness of the mouth and throat, dysphagia, colicky abdominal pain, projectile vomiting, and profuse watery diarrhea or "rice-water stools" are also early manifestations and occur within hours of exposure (16). Shock develops rapidly as a consequence of dehydration and generalized vasodilation. Because the lesions are usually due, not to local corrosion, but to vascular damage from absorbed arsenic, the first symptoms may be delayed for several hours. These complaints are invariably followed by a constellation of features reflecting multiple organ involvement.

Cardiac

Arsenic is a myocardial toxin that produces decreased contractile force of myocardial fibers secondary to inhibition of oxidative phosphorylation (17). Cardiac toxicity includes sinus tachycardia and ventricular dysrhythmias (11). Electrocardiographic changes include nonspecific ST segment changes, prolonged QT interval, and T–wave inversion (5).

Neurologic

Neurologic manifestations include pain in the extremities, headache, muscle weakness, CNS depression with coma, and polyneuropathies (13). The neuropathy is a late occurrence in the course of acute arsenic intoxication (18). It usually appears between 1 and 2 weeks after a single ingestion and involves both sensory and motor nerve fibers (19). Sensory changes are usually the initial manifestation (20). Paresthesias, aches, cramps, and tender muscles are common, and burning pain in the soles of the feet is a frequent complaint (21). The abnormal sensations increase in severity, and the areas of numbness extend rapidly and symmetrically through the limbs distally to proximally. Symptoms of severe neuropathy become more intense over the course of 1 to 2 weeks, reach a maximum, and then take weeks and sometimes months to abate. The degree of recovery depends on the severity of the neuropathy. Complete recovery occurs in purely sensory and in the mildest sensorimotor cases. Patients with severe degrees of motor disability take longer to recover, and permanent disability occurs in the most severe cases (20).

A great decline in mortality has resulted in a relative increase in the incidence of arsenical neuropathy. This is because patients who previously would have died from the effects of fluid loss during initial acute gastrointestinal illness now survive to develop neuropathies and other disorders formerly seen only in those with chronic exposure (21).

Cutaneous

Cutaneous involvement, including increased skin pigmentation, is considered a common characteristic of acute arsenic poisoning and may occur weeks after an acute ingestion. A variety of skin and nail changes occur with chronic arsenic poisoning. Initially, erythema develops due to dilatation of cutaneous capillary beds. This is followed by hyperpigmentation, hyperkeratosis, and desquamation of the skin. The changes in pigmentation characteristically are pronounced around the eyelids, temples, and neck, as well as the axillae, nipples, and groin. Dermatitis and keratosis of the palms and soles, in particular, commonly occur. In some instances, exfoliative dermatitis may be present. Varying degrees of alopecia also are seen frequently. Facial edema, particularly in the periorbital area, also may occur due to localized transudation of fluid.

TABLE 63–6. *Conditions associated with white nail striae*

Arsenic intoxication
Thallium intoxication
Trichinosis
Psoriasis
Leprosy
Malaria

Transverse white striae in the nails (Aldrich–Mees lines) are often seen. These lines are considered an actual deposit of arsenic and usually take 5 to 6 weeks to appear over the lunulae, so that a gross estimation of the time of exposure can be made by the distance of the line from the base of the nail. Aldrich–Mees lines are nonspecific for arsenic poisoning; they have also been noted in association with thallium intoxication and various nontoxic clinical conditions (Table 63–6).

Chronic Arsenic Poisoning

Chronic arsenic poisoning (Table 63–7) is insidious and often requires multiple hospitalizations before the correct diagnosis is discerned. In such instances, gastrointestinal disturbances may be slight or nonexistent. Nonspecific complaints of anorexia, weight loss, weakness, and general malaise predominate; however, dermatitis, stomatitis, peripheral neuropathy, and hematologic disorders may indicate arsenic poisoning (3).

Cutaneous

The cutaneous manifestations of chronic arsenic ingestion are characteristic but, for the most part, nonspecific. The earliest manifestation is persistent erythematous flushing caused by cutaneous capillary dilation (Table 63–7). Shortly thereafter, melanosis of nonexposed areas and hyperkeratosis occur. Desquamation of the skin and brittle nails with classic Aldrich–Mees lines may occur. In addition, there may be patchy or diffuse alopecia and edema of the face, periorbital region, or ankles from localized transudation of intravascular fluid. Aldrich–Mees lines may not be seen in chronic arsenic poisoning unless acute episodes have been superimposed.

Neurologic

In advanced arsenic poisoning, neurologic symptoms are prominent. Although encephalopathies have been described, peripheral neuritis is more common. Prolonged poisoning eventually leads to muscular atrophy, paralysis,

TABLE 63–7. *Clinical features of chronic arsenic intoxication*

Cutaneous
Acrocyanosis
Aldrich–Mees lines
Alopecia
Brittle nails
Desquamation of skin
Facial edema
Flushing
Hyperkeratosis
Melanosis of nonexposed areas
Pruritus
Raynaud's phenomenon
Gastrointestinal
Anorexia
Cirrhosis of liver
Diarrhea
Jaundice
Nausea
Vomiting
Neurologic
Ataxia
Diplopia
Muscular atrophy
Muscular paralysis
Optic neuritis
Hematologic
Anemia
Leukopenia
Thrombocytopenia
Miscellaneous
Cough
Conjunctivitis
Hoarseness
Salivation
EKG abnormalities
Renal tubular necrosis

and ataxia. Although cranial nerves are usually spared in chronic arsenic intoxication, diplopia and optic neuritis with dimming or concentric loss of vision are occasionally encountered. The manifestations of arsenical encephalitis may be similar to those of Wernicke's syndrome and Korsakoff's psychosis because of blockade of thiamine-associated metabolic reactions. Peripheral neuropathies may present with a "glove-and-stocking" distribution of sensory loss (18). Histologically, the nerves display a pattern consistent with axonal degeneration.

Hematologic

Chronic arsenic intoxication is also associated with severe hematopoietic disturbances (6). Anemia and leukopenia are almost universal and are frequently accompanied by thrombocytopenia. The anemia is usually normochromic and normocytic. Interference with folate metabolism may result in mild megaloblastic changes. Karyorrhexis, or fragmentation of the red blood cell nucleus, is characteristic of arsenic poisoning, and typical "cloverleaf" nuclei may be seen.

Gastrointestinal Tract

The gastrointestinal tract is more prominently involved in cases of acute arsenic intoxication; however, diarrhea may also be seen with chronic poisoning. In addition, loss of mucosal villi over time may result in the development of chronic malabsorption (8,22). Hepatic damage also may occur and is manifested by fatty infiltration, central necrosis, and, eventually, cirrhosis. In addition, liver enlargement may cause obstruction of bile ducts and results in clinical jaundice.

Cardiorespiratory

Myocardiotoxicity may be demonstrated by nonspecific electrocardiographic abnormalities, including prolongation of the QT interval, flat ST segment, and T-wave inversion. They usually subside in 6 to 8 weeks (10). Cardiac arrhythmias occur and may result in death.

Acute respiratory failure occurs because of severe weakness of the respiratory muscles. Bronchial pneumonia and upper respiratory tract inflammation commonly develop (10).

Miscellaneous

Among late symptoms and signs of chronic arsenical poisoning are anemia, cirrhosis of the liver, and jaundice (which may also be noted after an acute ingestion). Chronic arsenic poisoning may also be characterized by pruritis, soreness of the mouth, inflammation of the conjunctiva and nasal mucosa, salivation, loss of appetite, nausea, vomiting, and diarrhea (8,22). Renal tubular necrosis with resultant proteinuria, hematuria, and oliguria may occur (16). Acrocyanosis and Raynaud's phenomenon are common findings and may progress to enarteritis obliterans and frank gangrene of the extremities.

DIAGNOSIS

Acute Arsenical Intoxication

The diagnosis of acute arsenic intoxication should be considered in any patient presenting with gastrointestinal complaints as the hallmark, including epigastric burning, esophageal pain, colicky abdominal pain, and persistent vomiting and diarrhea, which may be bloody. The vomiting and diarrhea frequently manifest as profound dehydration, leading to cardiovascular collapse and possible seizures.

Arsenous oxide is as radiopaque as barium, and an alert clinician sometimes can make the diagnosis of arsenic ingestion from the plain film of the abdomen obtained during the work-up of a gastroenteritis.

In acute arsenic poisoning, a history of arsenic ingestion can occasionally be elicited. Particular difficulty may be encountered with pediatric patients or unsuspecting victims of homicide attempts (8).

Chronic Arsenical Intoxication

Chronic arsenic intoxication is more difficult to diagnose than acute intoxication. It should be considered in any patient who presents with combinations of neuropathy, skin rash, hematologic disturbances, and gastrointestinal complaints (8).

LABORATORY ANALYSIS

Blood or urine concentrations are valuable indicators of arsenic poisoning in instances of acute intoxication (23). However, urine concentrations decline rapidly after exposure has stopped; therefore, nails and particularly hair are the preferred specimens for the diagnosis of chronic exposure (16). Spot urine tests, though poorly sensitive and significant only if positive, are useful in identifying the causative agent in an acute poisoning. Because arsenic is rapidly cleared from the bloodstream, the preferred specimen for analysis is urine, ideally a sample from a 24-hour collection (3).

Hair Analysis

The analysis of sequential sections of hair provides reliable correlation to the pattern of arsenic exposure. In the hair follicle, arsenic circulating in the blood is deposited in the germinal cell matrix from blood vessels of the papilla. As the germinal matrix differentiates into keratin, the arsenic is trapped and carried up the follicle in the growing hair. The germinal cells are in relatively close equilibrium with the circulating arsenic, and as arsenic concentrations in blood increase or decrease, so does the amount of arsenic deposited in the growing hair vary. Hair analysis by neutron activation not only provides precise quantitation of arsenic concentration but also allows segmental analysis to determine when arsenic was ingested and the number of episodes. The analysis requires only a few hairs, and pubic hair is preferable because arsenic adsorption to exposed hairs may occur in an environment with elevated concentrations of atmospheric arsenic. In addition, arsenic persists longer in pubic hair because of its slower growth. Hair and nail samples containing more than 3 ppm of arsenic or 100 mg of arsenic per 100 g of specimen are diagnostic of arsenic intoxication (7). Hair grows at a rate of approximately 0.4 to 0.5 mm/day. Therefore, analysis of 1.0-cm segments provides a monthly pattern of exposure.

Normal arsenic concentration of hair varies with nutritional, environmental, and physiological factors; however, the maximum upper limit of normal arsenic concentration of hair, with 99% confidence limit in persons not exposed to arsenic, is approximately 5 mg/kg (16).

In some instances, the arsenic content may be falsely elevated due to external contamination. Arsenic in the environment also adheres firmly to these exposed tissues and is to easily removed by washing techniques. In some cases, the concentration of arsenic along the length of the hair is measured to obtain information about exposure over a extended period of time.

TABLE 63–8. *Treatment of arsenic poisoning*

Acute poisoning
Lavage
Charcoal and cathartic
Adequate intravenous volume replacement
Dimercaprol
2.5 to 3.0 mg/kg IM every 4 hours for 2 days then
2.5 to 3.0 mg/kg IM every 6 hours for 1 day then
2.5 to 3.0 mg/kg IM every 12 hours for 10 days
Chronic poisoning
Dimercaprol
Penicillamine (250 mg orally 4 times a day)

TREATMENT

After acute arsenic ingestion, residual arsenic should be removed from the stomach by gastric lavage and subsequent administration of activated charcoal and a cathartic (Table 63–8). Intravenous fluids must be provided because of the severe fluid and electrolyte losses that occur from profound emesis and diarrhea, as well as the extravascular fluid loss. Profound hypotension can initially be treated with fluids and by placing the patient in the Trendelenburg position. If the patient's condition does not respond to these measures, a dopamine or norepinephrine drip should be administered.

Urinary alkalinization is recommended to prevent deposition of red blood cell breakdown products in renal tubular cells. Enough sodium bicarbonate is used to maintain a urinary pH of at least 7.5. Adequate hydration, ensuring a urinary output of 1 to 2 mL per kg per hour, and administration of potassium supplements are necessary to adequately alkalinize the urine.

Chelation Therapy for Arsenic Intoxication

Measurement of the urinary excretion of arsenic during chelation therapy is important. When the 24-hour urinary arsenic excretion rate decreases to less than 50 μg per 24 hours, further chelation therapy is not necessary.

Acute Arsenical Intoxication

Dimercaprol is specific for arsenic and treatment should begin as soon as possible after diagnosis has been established; the earlier the dimercaprol is administered, the greater the possibility of avoiding serious intoxication. The use of dimercaprol to treat acute arsenic poisoning has been shown to be effective in preventing the occurrence of peripheral neuropathy if administered within 18 hours of ingestion.

Dimercaprol markedly enhances the urinary excretion of arsenic without damage to the excretory organs. The recommended dosage is 2.5 to 3.0 mg/kg intramuscularly every 4 hours for the first 2 days, every 6 hours during the third day, and every 12 hours for the next 10 days or until recovery is complete (7).

Chronic Arsenical Intoxication

The benefit of using dimercaprol to treat chronic arsenic poisoning is less certain than for acute poisoning, but a trial may be warranted because, once arsenic is bound to tissues, it is tightly held and cannot be displaced easily by chelators. Although dimercaprol may dramatically reverse the hematologic disturbance, it may have no effect on the neurologic lesions caused by arsenic poisoning.

ARSINE GAS

Arsine is the most dangerous form of arsenic and the most serious in terms of industrial hazard. Arsine is a colorless, nonirritating gas that can produce poisoning at less than 30 parts per million (ppm), a concentration that is far less than that at which its faint smell of garlic is detectable. Lewisite, a war gas, is an arsine derivative.

Arsine is liberated whenever hydrogen is generated in the presence of arsenic (24). Any ore contaminated with arsenic will also liberate arsine when treated with acid (25). Most industrial instances of arsine poisoning have occurred among metallurgical workers from the action of water or acid on arsenic-bearing metals. In addition, arsine gas may be encountered during electrolyte processes, the manufacture of zinc chloride and sulfate, and the smelting of metallic arsenical ore and in any setting where impure acids or metals are used.

TABLE 63–9. *Clinical features of arsine intoxication*

Gastrointestinal
Abdominal pain
Anorexia
Hematemesis
Jaundice
Nausea
Vomiting
Neurologic
Headache
Paresthesia
Miscellaneous
Anuria
Hemolysis
Myocardial damage
Nephrosis
Pulmonary edema

Mechanism of Toxicity of Arsine

A different mechanism of action is proposed to explain the pathogenesis of the toxic effects resulting from inhalation of arsine gas. A rapid and often severe intravascular hemolysis is characteristic of arsine poisoning. Like other arsenic compounds, which initially become bound to hemoglobin following their absorption, arsine also becomes localized in the erythrocytes. In the case of gaseous arsine, however, the association with hemoglobin results in its being fixed in a nonvolatile state, and lysis of the erythrocyte subsequently occurs. The mechanism of toxicity may relate to the inhibition of glutathione, which is necessary for red blood cell integrity (26). Glutathione is a peptide composed of glutamic acid, cysteine, and glycine and contains sulfhydryl or thiol groups, and it is thought that an irreversible complex with the arsenic atom is formed, causing hemolysis of the mature red blood cell (27).

Signs and Symptoms of Arsine Poisoning

The interval between exposure to arsine and the onset of symptoms is variable. There is usually a delay of 2 to 24 hours before manifestations of poisoning arise (Table 63–9).

Early symptoms of acute exposure may include headache, anorexia, nausea, vomiting, and paresthesia. Abdominal pain, chills, and hematemesis are common, and hemoglobinemia may appear as early as 4 hours after acute exposure. Frank jaundice and tenderness of the liver and spleen appear after 24 hours in acute cases. As with other conditions exhibiting acute massive hemolysis, anuria or hemoglobinuric nephrosis may result. Pulmonary edema and myocardial damage may also ensue.

Survivors of acute poisoning usually regain a normal state after about 2 weeks. If death occurs, it usually results from sudden myocardial failure or pulmonary edema.

Diagnosis of Arsine Gas Exposure

Arsine gas exposure produces a striking anemia of the hemolytic type (28). Arsine poisoning should be considered in the setting of an unknown gas causing a systemic reaction that includes anemia and hemolysis. Typical findings of arsenic poisoning may not be noted (29).

Treatment of Intoxication with Arsine Gas

Chelation therapy affords no protection against arsine intoxication. Because of the marked binding of the arsenic atom with hemoglobin arsine is poorly dialysable, and dialysis is primarily directed toward management of the associated renal failure (27). Survival of arsine poisoning depends on the degree of hemolysis and the course of the renal failure (29).

Role of Other Antidotes

Penicillamine also appears to promote the urinary excretion of arsenic in both acute and chronic poisonings, but it is not approved for this purpose by the FDA (5,30). The chelating agent penicillamine has fewer side effects and is considered as effective as dimercaprol but must be given orally. The dose is 25 mg per kg, given four times daily, up to 1 g per day. The daily dosage may be increased to 2 g if symptoms recur. Patients who are allergic to penicillin should be treated with dimercaprol for 5 to 10 days, with tapering of the dose after the first 5 days of treatment (10).

In a search for an effective antidote with fewer side effects than dimercaprol, a series of mercaptoalkanesulfonates was synthesized (31). Dimercaptopropanesulfonic acid (DMPS) and dimercaptosuccinic acid (DMSA) were two of these compounds. DMSA is now available as Succimer. It has been FDA-approved for use with lead poisoning and also should be of benefit for arsenic, although not yet approved for use. Succimer would not be of benefit for arsine poisoning.

REFERENCES

1. Arnando P: Attempted homicide with arsenic. *Clin Toxicol* 1979;14:575–577.
2. Petery J, Gross C, Victorica B: Ventricular fibrillation caused by arsenic poisoning. *Am J Dis Child* 1970;120:367–371
3. Malachowski M: An update on arsenic. *Clin Lab Med* 1990;10:459–472.
4. Beckett W, Moore J, Keogh J, et al: Acute encephalopathy due to occupational exposure to arsenic. *Br J Ind Med* 1986;43:66–67.
5. Peterson R, Rumack B: D-Penicillamine therapy of acute arsenic poisoning. *J Pediatr* 1977;91:661–666.
6. Vaziri N, Uphan T, Barton C: Hemodialysis clearance of arsenic. *Clin Toxicol* 1980;17:451–456.
7. Done A, Peart A: Acute toxicities of arsenical herbicides. *Clin Toxicol* 1971;4:343–355.
8. Schoolmeester W, White D: Arsenic poisoning. *South Med J* 1980;73:198–208.
9. Kersjes M, Maurer J, Trestrail J: An analysis of arsenic exposures referred to the Blodgett regional poison center. *Vet Hum Toxicol* 1987;29:75–78.
10. Campbell J, Alvarez J: Acute arsenic intoxication. *Am Fam Physic* 1989;40:93–97.
11. Petery J, Rennert O, Choi H, et al: Arsenic poisoning in childhood. *Clin Toxicol* 1970;3:519–526.
12. Tadlock C, Aposhian H: Protection of mice against the lethal effects of sodium arsenite by 2,3-dimercapto-1propane-sulfonic acid and dimercaptosuccinic acid. *Biochem Biophys Res Commun* 1980;94:501–507.
13. Fernandez-Sola J, Nogue S, Grau J, et al: Acute arsenical myopathy: morphological description. *J Toxicol Clin Toxicol* 1991;29:131–136.
14. Park M, Currier M: Arsenic exposures in Mississippi: a review of cases. *South Med J* 1991;84:461–464.
15. Kjeldsberg C, Ward H: Leukemia in arsenic poisoning. *Ann Intern Med* 1972;77:935–937.
16. Poklis A, Saady J: Arsenic poisoning: Acute or chronic? Suicide or murder? *Am J Foren Med Path* 1990;11:226–232.
17. Beckman K, Bauman J, Pimental P, et al: Arsenic-induced torsade de pointes. *Crit Care Med* 1991;19:290–293.
18. Hessl S, Berman E: Severe peripheral neuropathy after exposure to monosodium methyl arsonate. *J Toxicol Clin Toxicol* 1982;19:281–287.
19. Bansal D, Haldar N, Dhand U, et al: Phrenic neuropathy in arsenic poisoning. *Chest* 1991;100:878–880.
20. Lequensne P, McLeod J: Peripheral neuropathy following a single exposure to arsenic. *J Neurol Sci* 1977;32:437–451.
21. Freeman J, Couch J: Prolonged encephalopathy with arsenic poisoning. *Neurology* 1978;28:853–855
22. Greenberg C, Davies S, McGowan T, et al: Acute respiratory failure following severe arsenic poisoning. *Chest* 1979;76:596–598.
23. Grande G, Rogers A, Ling L, et al: Urine spot test as guide to treatment in acute pentavalent arsenic ingestion. *Vet Hum Toxicol* 1987;29:73–74.
24. Risk M, Fuortes L: Chronic arsenicalism suspected from arsine exposure: A case report and literature review. *Vet Hum Toxicol* 1991;33:590–594.
25. Fowler B, Weissberg J: Arsine poisoning. *N Engl J Med* 1974;291:1171–1174.
26. Leikin J, Goldman-Leikin R, Evans M, et al: Immunotherapy in acute arsenic poisoning. *J Toxicol Clin Toxicol* 1991;29:59–70.
27. Coles G, Davies H, Daley D, et al: Acute intravascular hemolysis and renal failure due to arsine poisoning. *Postgrad Med J* 1969;45:170–172.
28. Levinsky W, Smalley R, Hillyer P, et al: Arsine hemolysis. *Arch Environ Health* 1970;20:436–440.
29. Hocken A, Bradshaw G: Arsine poisoning. *Br J Ind Med* 1970;27:56–60.
30. Kuruvilla A, Bergeson P, Done A: Arsenic poisoning in childhood: An unusual case report with special notes on therapy with penicillamine. *Clin Toxicol* 1975;8:535–540.
31. Lenz K, Hruby K, Druml W, et al: 2,3-Dimercaptosuccinic acid in human poisoning. *Arch Toxicol* 1981;47;241–243.

ADDITIONAL SELECTED REFERENCES

Aposhian H, Hsu C, Hoover T: D,L- and meso-Dimercaptosuccinic acid: In vitro and in vivo studies with sodium arsenite. *Toxicol Appl Pharmacol* 1983;69:206–213.

Donofrio P, Wilbourn A, Alberg J, et al: Acute arsenic intoxication presenting as Guillain-Barre-like syndrome. *Muscle Nerve* 1987;10:114–120.

Kerr H, Saryan L: Arsenic content of homeopathic medicines. *Clin Toxicol* 1986;24:451–459.

Levin-Scherz J, Patrick J, Weber F, et al: Acute arsenic ingestion. *Ann Emerg Med* 1987;16:702–704.

CHAPTER 64

Iron

Iron is distributed throughout all life forms and is one of the most abundant and important of the biological trace metals. Although written reports of the toxic effects of iron have been known for more than 100 years, (1) iron has been used medicinally for several centuries (2,3). Iron and its compounds were once widely regarded as relatively harmless, and most adults and some medical personnel still may not be fully aware of iron's serious potential as a poison (3). Iron poisonings still occur each year in the United States. Although the mortality rate today is less than 5% (4,5), at one time, it was as high as 50% in serious poisonings (3,6–8). The decline in mortality rate is due, in part, to the use of the chelating agent deferoxamine (Desferal) but, in addition, better supportive medical care has become available (8).

Ferrous sulfate and ferrous gluconate are two of the most common preparations of iron. The accidental ingestion of preparations containing iron is still relatively common in children because of the multitude of such preparations (Table 64–1) (9); intentional overdose from iron is occasionally seen in adults (6,10). In addition, in homes with young children containers may be kept on the dining room table or the kitchen counter rather than in the medicine cabinet (11–13). The failure to dispense iron in child-resistant containers also may contribute to the problem (14). Factors contributing to the relatively high incidence of iron poisoning include widespread availability of iron-containing products, attractive packaging, and a benign reputation among the lay public. Iron is available without a prescription as brightly colored ferrous sulfate or ferrous gluconate salts, in children's pleasant-tasting chewable vitamins with iron, and within prescription prenatal vitamins. Most cases of serious toxicity occur with iron-only tablets or with the prenatal vitamins, both of which have large quantities of elemental iron per tablet. Because of such factors, the incidence of iron poisonings in children younger than 5 years of age appears to be greater than in adults.

Iron is capable of producing chronic poisoning as a result of dietary or medicinal overload, from various types of iron storage diseases, or secondary to occupational exposure. The emergency department physician, however, is most commonly confronted with the acute ingestion of iron.

TABLE 64–1. *Selected iron preparations by trade name*

Ferrous sulfate	Ferrous gluconate	Ferrous fumarate
Feosol	Fergon	Feco-T
Fer-In-Sol	Ferralet	Femiron
Fero-Gradumet	Ferrous-G	Feostat
Ferralyn		Fumasorb
Mol-Iron		Fumerin
		Ircon
		Laud-Iron
		Maniron
		Toleron

ABSORPTION

Iron crosses cell membranes only in the ferrous state; ferric ions in food are liberated in the stomach by acid digestion, reduced to the ferrous state, and absorbed. Typical daily intake of iron is approximately 15 to 40 mg (15), but because of an intestinal mucosal block, only 10% of ingested iron is absorbed (11,16). Even after massive iron ingestions, iron is absorbed by a first-order process, with the intestine regulating the amount of iron that is absorbed. In the routine daily absorption of dietary iron, the transport of ferrous compounds is energy-dependent. This saturable, carrier-mediated uptake process is dependent on the binding of iron in the lumen of the gastrointestinal tract and is the rate-limiting step for iron absorption. Absorption occurs mostly in the duodenum and upper jejunum, although the entire intestinal tract, including the colon, is able to absorb iron (17,18). The divalent (ferrous) iron is absorbed into the gastrointestinal mucosa and converted to the trivalent (ferric) form, which attaches to ferritin in the intestinal mucosal cell wall (2). The ferritin-ferric complex then passes into the bloodstream and is attached to transferrin (11). Iron is then carried to the reticuloendothelial cells of the bone marrow for hemoglobin synthesis or to the liver or spleen for storage as ferritin or hemosiderin (Fig. 64–1) (16).

Toxic amounts of iron in solution are rapidly absorbed in the large and small bowel in a concentration-dependent fashion. With toxic amounts the capacity of the normal

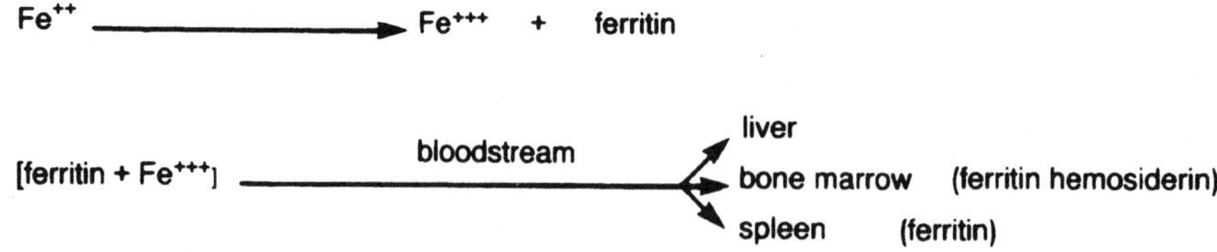

FIG. 64–1. Absorption of iron.

mechanisms of absorption is exceeded, and absorption becomes a passive, first-order process (11).

DISTRIBUTION

The body contains approximately 4 to 5 g of iron, of which approximately 60% is contained in hemoglobin, 25% is stored as ferritin and hemosiderin (mainly in the liver), 3% is in myoglobin, and 1% is distributed among various heme-containing enzymes such as cytochrome oxidase, xanthine oxidase, and catalase (15,18).

EXCRETION

Once iron is absorbed, its removal from the body is difficult. Although iron is lost through sweat, bile, and the desquamation of skin and mucosal surfaces, this loss only totals roughly 1.5 mg/day. In women, an additional 0.5 mg/day may be lost in the menses (11). There is no effective physiologic mechanism for iron excretion, which is a fact of great importance in iron intoxication (15,18). When iron accumulation occurs, iron excretion may double through the aforementioned pathways but cannot exceed a total of about 2 mg/day (19).

TOXICITY

When estimating toxicity of an acute ingestion of iron, the amount of elemental iron should be used in the calculation rather than the milligrams of a particular iron preparation (2). Ferrous sulfate contains approximately 20% elemental iron, ferrous gluconate 12%, ferrous fumarate 33%, and ferrocholinate 13% (2,20). Conversion factors for calculating the amount of elemental iron in an iron preparation are given in Table 64–2. For example, there is 60 mg of elemental iron in 300 mg of ferrous sulfate [the total mgs of prepared iron (300) divided by 5].

TABLE 64–2. *Amounts of elemental iron in various iron preparations*

Preparation	Percentage of iron	Conversion factor*
Ferrous sulfate	20	5
Ferrous gluconate	12	8.7
Ferrous fumarate	33	3
Ferrocholinate	13	7.7

*Conversion factor to calculate amount of elemental iron from milligrams of prepared iron.

Reduced or metallic iron in powder form is nontoxic unless it is oxidized and enters the metabolic cycles (21). A dose of 20 to 60 mg/kg of elemental iron is considered toxic and a lethal dose is within the range of 60 to 180 mg/kg (5,18,22).

The basic pathophysiologic effects of iron in toxic doses are of five types: (a) metabolic disorders, (b) hepatic dysfunction, (c) CNS dysfunction, (d) cardiovascular system dysfunction, and (e) gastrointestinal tract disturbances (11).

The symptoms of iron poisoning are due to both local and systemic effects and may be influenced by factors such as the chemical and physical forms of the iron, dose, route of administration, and duration of exposure (23). In general, the ferrous salts are more toxic than the ferric salts. Although a mucosal block or barrier to the absorption of iron exists with the normal intake of iron, in overdose situations, the mucosal barrier is less efficient and great amounts of iron may be absorbed (13). In this event, absorbed iron exceeds the binding capacity of transferrin and passes into various tissues, causing toxicity.

There are five phases of intoxication associated with the acute significant ingestion of iron (Table 64–3).

TABLE 64–3. *Phases of iron intoxication*

Phase
Phase 1: Gastrointestinal (30 minutes to 2 hours)
Vomiting
Hematemesis
Abdominal pain
Diarrhea
Lethargy
Shock
Hypotension
Metabolic acidosis
Phase 2: Recovery (2 to 24 hours)
Apparent response to therapy
Phase 3: Metabolic acidosis (12 to 48 hours)
Shock
Coma
Phase 4: Hepatic (2 to 4 days)
Hepatic necrosis
Bleeding diathesis
Phase 5: Gastrointestinal (2 to 4 weeks)
Gastric scarring
Pyloric stenosis
Achlorhydria
Hepatic cirrhosis
CNS abnormalities

These phases represent a rough guideline for the evolution of various toxic effects (24).

Phase 1

Phase 1 may begin 30 minutes to 2 hours after an acute ingestion. The first obvious signs of toxicity are gastrointestinal; this symptomatology not only is predominant but is considered the sine qua non of iron poisoning (24). Vomiting is invariably the first manifestation of toxicity and usually occurs within the first hour after ingestion. This may possibly proceed to hematemesis as a result of acute hemorrhagic gastritis, which may occasionally be life threatening (17). Other symptoms include colicky abdominal pain and diarrhea (which sometimes may be bloody and explosive). Lethargy (a common early symptom), coma, hypotension, and metabolic acidosis may ensue during this early phase (25).

Iron is a corrosive agent and, on direct contact, may produce lesions similar to those caused by acids, although generally they are more superficial in nature (26). Because iron is a solid, it spares the mouth, pharynx, and upper esophagus. Liquid preparations and tablets primarily affect the pyloric region of the stomach and the duodenum. Enteric-coated tablets may also involve the lower small intestine. Chewable tablets are associated with more proximal lesions (27).

The damage caused by the corrosive action of iron in the small intestine is variable and tends to decrease distally, with segmental infarction of the small bowel rarely occurring. The terminal ileum is rarely affected and the large intestine is usually unaffected. Some patients may also develop intestinal necrosis, perforation, and peritonitis (28).

Phase 2

Phase 2 may occur 2 to 24 hours after an ingestion; at this time, the patient appears to recover. This phase may be quite deceptive because the patient may seem to have responded to therapy or the condition may continue to go undiagnosed (26). An explanation for the disappearance of symptoms during phase 2 is that circulating free iron is being taken up by the reticuloendothelial system and, thus, is not yet available to cause cellular damage. The course of the intoxication proceeds directly to the next phase, however.

Phase 3

Phase 3 usually begins 12 to 48 hours after ingestion. A metabolic acidosis that may be particularly resistant to bicarbonate therapy, as well as shock and coma, may ensue. Metabolic acidosis from iron may be due to the hydrogen ion produced during conversion of ferrous to ferric iron in the blood, with the formation of ferric hydroxide complexes in the circulatory system (6,15,29). In addition, however, there is an interference with the Krebs cycle enzymes in the liver and other tissues, which causes a block in organic acid metabolism and a buildup of lactic and citric acids.

Shock is a cardinal feature of fatal acute iron poisoning in children. It may be diphasic, occurring within the first 6 to 8 hours and again approximately 36 hours after ingestion (20). The shock is thought to be due to peripheral circulatory failure induced by absorbed iron as well as to other factors such as ferritin, which may be acting as a vasodepressant. In addition, serotonin or histamine release may act to cause hypotension. The most likely explanation for shock is a combination of these factors in addition to the direct vasodilation effect of iron on blood vessels, which leads to shock. After acute ingestion of a large dose of iron, there is a dramatic decrease in circulating plasma volume, as reflected in increases in the hematocrit. Cardiac output is lowered on the basis of a decreased filling pressure.

Phase 4

Phase 4 may begin 2 to 4 days after an ingestion. The liver may rarely be a target organ for damage by direct uptake of iron, leading to hepatic necrosis. This may be evidenced by elevation of bilirubin, serum glutamic-oxaloacetic transaminase, and alkaline phosphatase concentrations and possibly manifested clinically by jaundice (31). In severe cases, hepatic coma with behavioral changes and elevated blood ammonia values have been reported. Damage is thought to be due to cellular injury from the direct action of iron on the mitochondrial cells of the liver. Another theory suggests that hepatic necrosis may be caused by depletion of sulfhydryl enzymes secondary to iron, which then allows another unknown toxin to produce necrotic changes (31,32).

A bleeding diathesis may also be noted during this phase. These changes, if present, are due to a direct effect of iron on the various proteins involved in blood coagulation and are not a consequence of acidosis, shock, or liver damage (21). Interference with these clotting mechanisms may contribute to severe hemorrhagic manifestations, which may include prolongation of the prothrombin time, reduction in thromboplastin generation, poor to absent clot retraction, and thrombocytopenia (5). All three stages of clotting may be involved: the generation of thromboplastin becomes impaired (first stage), the prothrombin time is prolonged (second stage), and the conversion of fibrinogen to fibrin becomes defective (third stage).

Phase 5

Phase 5 may occur 2 to 4 weeks after ingestion as a result of the early corrosive effect of iron on the gastrointestinal tract. It may be manifested by intractable nausea and vomiting secondary to gastric scarring as well as fibrosis leading to pyloric obstruction or stenosis (26). One report described a severe corrosive gastroduodenitis with subsequent fibrosis and scarring of the stomach and duodenum, necessitating abdominal surgery (33). Also, perforation and stricture formation are not uncommon. These lesions can be demonstrated by barium contrast studies. Because of this destruction, achlorhydria may supervene together with other nutritional problems caused by the destruction of the mucosa (18).

Hemodynamic Effects

Hemodynamic alterations, particularly the postarteriolar dilation and venous pooling, is postulated to be due to both a direct effect of the absorbed iron, as well as an increase in circulating ferritin. As a result, there is a compensatory increase in total peripheral resistance to maintain a normotensive state. Consequently, capillary leakage and plasma loss is encountered. This decreases venous return, cardiac output, and tissue perfusion, resulting in lactic acidosis, shock, and cardiac failure.

Metabolic Effects

Unbound iron distributes into cells, primarily in the liver. Iron is initially taken up by the Kupffer cells of the reticuloendothelial system and then moves rapidly to hepatic parenchymal cells, where it becomes localized in the area of the mitochondrial cristae.

Iron-induced mitochondrial dysfunction may be due to the potent catalytic effects of ferrous ions on the mitochondrial membrane composition and subsequent lipid peroxidation. Lipid peroxidation catalyzed by ferrous ions alters the membrane permeability of the mitochondria, allowing intramitochondrial accumulation of additional iron. Because an intact mitochondrial membrane is essential for the proper functioning of the electron transport system and for aerobic respiration, metabolic acidosis may occur as a result of anaerobic metabolism. In addition, iron may act as an electron sink, resulting in the shunting of electrons away from the electron transport system, thereby reducing adenosine triphosphate generation, leading to cellular dysfunction, metabolic acidosis, and ultimately, cell death.

The development of metabolic acidosis may also result from the release of hydrogen ions as iron is converted from the ferrous to the ferric state or from inhibition of enzymatic processes of the Krebs cycle and the resultant accumulation of organic acids.

Hepatic Effects

The hepatotoxic effects of iron are often realized in the unchecked or severe exposures, as this metal is known to be a potent catalyst of lipid peroxidation. Mitochondrial injury, swelling of hepatocytes, cirrhosis, and complete necrosis of the liver have all been reported (34).

Elevations in the prothrombin time, in combination with a direct effect on the coagulation factors, may result in clotting abnormalities and frank bleeding episodes.

Acute hepatic failure is a rare complication occurring after massive iron ingestion. Acute hepatic failure generally occurs in only those patients with severe iron poisoning and may be evidenced by jaundice and elevated bilirubin concentrations 3 to 4 days after acute iron ingestion.

Pathologically, hepatic injury may range from cloudy swelling of hepatocytes to complete necrosis. Whereas some areas of the liver may show no damage, others, most commonly the periportal parenchymal cells, show extensive necrosis, which is usually hemorrhagic in nature. This may progress to acute hepatic failure characterized by jaundice, hyperammonemia, hypoglycemia, coagulation defects, and encephalopathy.

Coagulopathy may aggravate early gastrointestinal blood loss associated with the corrosive effects of iron. Coagulation defects appear to be due to depression of vitamin K-dependent clotting factors.

Pregnancy

Normal fetal serum iron concentrations are higher than those of the mother. Serum iron levels in the newborn are higher than maternal values, and iron-binding capacities are about one half those of the mother. Iron normally does not diffuse through the placenta but is actively transported against a concentration gradient into the fetal circulation (35). It is not known whether toxic fetal serum iron levels are reached when maternal serum iron concentrations rise above maternal total iron-binding capacity and exceed fetal serum iron concentrations (36).

The human fetus must acquire about 500 mg iron during gestation. Iron transport across the placenta increases throughout pregnancy and the bulk of fetal iron acquisition occurs during the third trimester.

DIAGNOSIS AND LABORATORY ANALYSIS

History and Physical Examination

The diagnosis of acute iron poisoning in a young child is frequently complicated by an unreliable history and by the diphasic nature of the symptoms. Patients may present without a definite history of iron ingestion, but it should be suspected in any patient who is vomiting, has bloody diarrhea, or is lethargic, comatose, or in shock. If

TABLE 64–4. *Diagnostic work-up of iron poisoning*

Unknown poisoning
- Historical clues
- Lethargy
- Vomiting
- Hematemesis
- Shock
- Bloody diarrhea
- (If positive, proceed to suspected or confirmed poisoning)

Suspected poisoning
- Plain roentgenogram of abdomen
- Examination of emesis for iron
- Examination of stool for black color
- Provocative deferoxamine test of gastric aspirate
- (If positive, proceed to confirmed poisoning)

Confirmed poisoning
- Plain roentgenogram of abdomen
- Iron and total iron-binding capacity
- Fischer test (unreliable)
- Clotting studies
- Complete blood cell count
- Blood type and crossmatch
- Electrolyte studies
- Arterial blood gas analysis

iron poisoning is suspected, an examination of the patient's emesis may reveal iron tablets, and the stool should then be examined for a black color secondary to iron ingestion (Table 64–4) (37).

Plain Roentgenography

Plain roentgenography of the abdomen can be a useful diagnostic procedure in the management of iron overdose (38,39). Depending on the time after ingestion of iron-containing tablets, the preparation's solubility, and the degree of prior emesis or gastric lavage, the film can be a guide to the number of tablets taken and can indicate whether removal is necessary (40). A normal roentgenogram, however, does not rule out an ingestion because iron in solution is no longer radiopaque (33) and because iron-containing vitamins can be imaged for only a brief period and appear with low density. Ferrous sulfate, gluconate, and fumarate all have a high content of elemental iron, which results in a slower dissolution of the tablets and thereby renders the preparations radiopaque for a longer period of time.

Because of their higher content of elemental iron, ferrous sulfate tablets dissolve more slowly and remain radiopaque longer than a similar number of ferrous gluconate tablets, whereas chewable multivitamins with iron may not appear radiopaque. Chewed tablets would be expected to dissolve much more quickly than nonchewable iron supplements and thus should be absorbed faster (41).

Abdominal roentgenograms obtained more than 2 hours after ingestion or after ingestion of multivitamins should be interpreted with caution, as preparations with a greater solubility and lower iron content may have dissolved and may not appear as radiopaque densities on plain film, even though they remain in the gastrointestinal tract, available for absorption.

Colorimetric Tests

Colorimetric testing has serious limitations, and the results should not be relied on to make a diagnosis or to determine extent of injury (39). Two tests that have been employed in a suspected iron overdose involve the chelating agent deferoxamine. One test involves the oral administration of deferoxamine and is an attempt at diagnosis. The other involves intravenous administration of deferoxamine and is an attempt at determining whether free iron is in the blood, which is an indication for chelation therapy (42).

In the first test, a small amount of deferoxamine is mixed with gastric aspirate. If a red color is produced, the presence of iron in the gastrointestinal tract is confirmed (39). The major limitation of this test is that gastrointestinal bleeding is usually associated with a moderate to severe iron intoxication (38).

The second test is provocative and is not suggested for routine use; however, it may be helpful in the occasional situation where no laboratory analysis is available. This test involves the administration of deferoxamine intravenously (10 to 15 mg/kg). Production of a reddish-brown urine indicates that there is free iron circulating in the body that has been chelated with the deferoxamine (43). The value of this test may be limited because the characteristic color may not always develop despite the presence of chelated iron in the urine (38).

Serum Iron and Total Iron-Binding Capacity

Further work-up for suspected iron overdose should include a definitive test of the serum iron and iron-binding capacity, the results of which are crucial when deciding whether chelation treatment is to be instituted. As mentioned earlier, iron is considered toxic when the plasma concentration exceeds the total iron-binding capacity of transferrin because, once plasma transferrin has been saturated, the iron is distributed into cells and causes damage (44). Many hospitals do not perform serum iron and total iron-binding capacity tests as a "stat" procedure, but the importance of this test requires that there be some backup facility that can do so. Emergency serum iron measurements should be available around the clock to obviate the use of indirect methods (38).

The serum iron concentration must be measured after absorption is complete and before distribution and protein binding in the tissues have contributed to a significant decrease in the initial peak concentration (13). Although the kinetics of iron after overdose have not

TABLE 64–5. *Serum iron concentrations and toxicity*

Iron concentration (micrograms per deciliter)	Degree of toxicity
100	Nontoxic (normal value)
100–300	Minimal
350–500	Moderate
500–1000	Serious
1000	Potentially lethal

been thoroughly investigated, the limited evidence available indicates that serum iron concentration usually peaks 3 to 5 hours after ingestion and decreases rapidly thereafter (24,45,46); it is therefore advisable to obtain measurements during that time (38). Because of the rapid clearance of free iron, severely toxic conditions may be associated with only minimally elevated plasma iron concentrations if values are obtained after the peak period (46). Once the initial serum iron concentration has been determined to be in the toxic range, there is little value to continued measurements of the serum iron or total iron-binding capacity (44).

The normal serum iron concentration is 50 to 150 μg/dL in adults and children older than 5 years of age and 40 to 100 μg/dL for children younger than 5 years of age (Table 64–5). Total iron-binding capacity or plasma transferrin is roughly one-third saturated under normal conditions, with the total iron-binding capacity ranging from 300 to 450 μg/dL (18). Serum iron concentrations less than 350 μg/dL have rarely been associated with significant illness.

Most commonly used methods for the measurement of serum iron concentrations involve the liberation of ferric iron bound to transferrin by weak reducing agents followed by the formation of a colored complex with ferrous iron and a chromogenic agent such as ferrozine. If chelation therapy is instituted, these methods may reveal spuriously low serum iron concentrations because of the chelation of some of the iron liberated from transferrin (38).

Total Iron-Binding Capacity

Historically, the total iron-binding capacity (TIBC) was developed and used as an indirect measure of transferrin. Formulas have been derived to estimate the transferrin level from a colorimetric TIBC.

Traditionally, assessment of the severity of iron poisoning has been based on measurement of the total iron-binding capacity in addition to the serum iron concentration (47). A serum level greater than the TIBC was considered to reflect the presence of free iron in the serum and formed the basis for chelation treatment with deferoxamine, yet the TIBC may be falsely elevated in patients with high iron levels or in those given deferoxamine (44). Much of the rise in TIBC may be an aberration of the laboratory technique itself and not a physiological phenomenon (47,48).

Miscellaneous Laboratory Procedures

The Fischer test (49) or variations of the colorimetric test (22) that attempt to determine free iron are unreliable, and their results should not be substituted for serum iron and total iron-binding capacity (38,39). Clotting studies as well as a complete blood cell count, electrolyte studies, arterial blood gas analysis, and liver function tests should be obtained for baseline values (50). A blood type and hold should be performed because patients sometimes need blood transfusions. There is little value in obtaining indicators of hepatic function early in the course of iron intoxication other than for baseline values. It is reasonable to obtain transaminase values after the first 24 hours to assess baseline hepatic function. Prognosis is correlated with the presence of severe symptoms (shock, coma, or vasomotor instability) as well as the serum iron concentration in relation to the total iron-binding capacity within the first 3 to 5 hours after ingestion (38,51).

TREATMENT

Treatment must be vigorous and prompt and must consist of supportive measures, prevention of absorption of iron in the gastrointestinal tract, and chelation therapy (Table 64–6). Diuresis and dialysis have been shown to be ineffective. Although phlebotomy has been tried, the use of chelating agents is the preferred method of increasing excretion of iron.

Prevention of Absorption

Iron is notorious for its resistance to traditional stomach-emptying procedures probably because of its ability

TABLE 64–6. *Treatment of iron poisoning*

Indication	Treatment
Acute ingestion	Lavage
Fluid loss	Normal saline
Metabolic acidosis	Bicarbonate instillation
Shock	Sodium bicarbonate
	Military antishock trousers
	Parenteral fluids
	Vasopressors
Severe overdose	Deferoxamine
	IV: 1 g not to exceed 10 to 15 mg/kg/hour (or 6 g per 24 hours or 80 mg/kg per 24 hours) IM: 40 to 90 mg/kg every 8 hours

to clump together and form large aggregates. Initial treatment, however, should still consist of gastric lavage. Although the traditional methods of bowel decontamination are still considered the standard treatment for iron ingestions, whole-bowel irrigation with a polyethylene glycol-electrolyte lavage solution is being investigated as a possible safe and effective means of preventing absorption of iron from the gastrointestinal tract (52,53).

Intragastric Complexation

The use of intragastric complexation in iron intoxication is controversial (51); but, phosphates, deferoxamine, bicarbonate, and magnesium hydroxide have been suggested as complexing agents to decrease absorption of iron remaining in the gastrointestinal tract.

Phosphates

Sodium biphosphate (Fleet enema) solution combines with the ingested iron to form ferrous phosphate and ferric phosphate. Because maximum phosphate absorption occurs in the midgut, even if a small amount of the lavage solution is not retrieved it could present a significant phosphate load for absorption (13,38). In addition, the absorption of phosphate may be enhanced across an intestinal mucosal barrier that is disrupted by the direct irritant action of ingested iron. Because of reports of toxicity after the administration of phosphate in children, with ensuing hyperphosphatemia, hypocalcemia, and other disturbances (including dysrhythmias), this therapy is not recommended (54,55).

Deferoxamine

The oral administration of deferoxamine has been suggested to reduce the absorption of iron, but there is evidence that this complex is absorbed and may lead to further iron toxicity. Because deferoxamine is only effective in chelating ferric iron and all medicinal preparations contain ferrous salts, intragastric deferoxamine would seem to be of little value (38). In addition, deferoxamine is poorly absorbed from the gut when the mucosa is intact. Thus, its use is not recommended.

Bicarbonate

An alternative lavage solution is sodium bicarbonate, which when administered down the lavage tube, forms an insoluble complex of ferrous and ferric carbonate that is not absorbed from the gastrointestinal tract. Because sodium bicarbonate appears to be less dangerous than other intragastric complexing agents, its use is recommended. In addition, absorption of sodium bicarbonate could reduce the metabolic acidosis that occurs in iron intoxication (54). After gastric emptying, 100 mL of a 5% solution of sodium bicarbonate or sodium bicarbonate ampules can be instilled through the gastric lavage tube and then retrieved. Although the efficacy of this treatment has recently been questioned (51), there does not appear to be great potential for toxicity from this regimen.

Whole Gut Lavage

Whole gut emptying has been suggested if a slow-release iron formulation was ingested (53) or if an abdominal radiograph after gastric lavage shows persistence of tablets in the stomach or small intestine (38,56). When a large number of opacities are identified in a single location, it may be reasonable to consider surgical intervention (27). The clinician must consider the stability of the patient, the number of tablets seen on the radiograph, and the potential for other procedures such as lavage and emesis successfully to remove these tablets (52).

The suggested flow rate of the solution, administered at room temperature, is 0.5 L/hour for children up to 5 years of age and 2.0 L/hour for adolescents and adults (52).

Other Therapeutic Measures

An important part of therapy consists of adequately correcting any third-space fluid losses with appropriate crystalloid. Military antishock trousers may also be applied in an effort to increase venous return. An indwelling urinary catheter should be placed to measure the urine output and to observe the color of the urine for determining whether the chelating agent should be continued. Sodium bicarbonate should be administered for metabolic acidosis, and vasopressors may be necessary for shock if fluid administration and military antishock trousers are ineffective.

Chelation Therapy with Deferoxamine

Deferoxamine mesylate is a chelating agent that was originally obtained from a species of Streptomyces, one of the organisms that produce low-molecular weight chelators as part of their iron-transport systems. It was discovered as a result of the investigation of the antibiotic properties of the siderochromes, a class of naturally occurring compounds (29). Clinical use of deferoxamine mesylate for cases of acute iron poisoning was first reported in the early 1960s.

When deferoxamine chelates with iron, it forms a brownish-red complex with iron bound in the center (57). This stable ring, unlike free iron, is soluble in water and readily excreted by the kidneys. Theoretically, 100 mg of deferoxamine can bind 8 to 9 mg of elemental iron (21,46). Deferoxamine has an affinity for iron that is 10 times greater than that of any other known chelator and thus combines more firmly than other chelators, with resultant greater urinary excretion of iron (25). Deferoxamine also has the advantage of being specific for iron, with virtually no attraction to other metals. It, therefore, does not cause excretion of calcium, copper, magnesium, or zinc (13,21,46). Deferoxamine has a volume of distribution of about 60% body weight and a plasma half-life of 10 to 30 minutes. It is metabolized to inactive products by plasma and other tissues.

Indication for Chelation Therapy

Chelation therapy is indicated when iron concentrations exceed the total iron-binding capacity or if the serum iron concentration is greater than 350 μg/dL, (1,45) or in any patient who exhibits serious systemic toxicity when no measurements can be obtained (38). Chelation is not indicated if the patient is asymptomatic or has minor symptoms with no evidence of gastrointestinal bleeding or if the total iron-binding capacity is greater than the serum iron concentration and the patient has ingested approximately 150 to 300 mg/kg of elemental iron (48).

Method of Action

It is believed that the efficacy of deferoxamine involves the enhancement of iron elimination through the formation of water-soluble, renally excreted ferrioxamine (58). Several reports suggest that deferoxamine also exerts a protective effect at the cellular level by chelation of iron in the extracellular space (25). Another possibility is that deferoxamine enters cells and chelates extramitochondrial iron (38).

By chelating iron, deferoxamine also acts as an inhibitor of iron-dependent lipid peroxidation and iron-dependent hydroxy radical generation systems containing oxygen radicals or ascorbate. Deferoxamine is also a powerful scavenger of hydroxy radicals and a weak scavenger of oxygen radicals. Finally, deferoxamine prevents lipid peroxidation and reverses the functional impairment associated with iron toxicity in iron-loaded cells (35).

Route of Administration and Dosage

Various regimens and routes of administration of deferoxamine have been recommended. Deferoxamine is poorly absorbed from the gut if the mucosa is intact and, therefore, should be administered parenterally. Intravenous administration is preferred (1,46), but intramuscular administration was at one time suggested because of reports of hypotension from intravenous administration. It has been shown, however, that hypotension is a consequence of too rapid an intravenous administration. As long as deferoxamine is administered properly, there should be no significant side effects noted.

It has been shown that a dose of deferoxamine given by slow infusion results in more effective chelation and iron excretion than when the same dose is given as a single injection (29,59). In addition, maximal iron mobilization may require constant exposure of labile iron pools to deferoxamine (46). The pharmacodynamics of deferoxamine appear to support its use as a continuous infusion in acute iron overdosage to maximize net iron excretion. One gram should be administered in normal saline, with infusion rates not to exceed 10 to 15 mg/kg/hr (38). This rate can then be reduced to 5 mg/kg/hr after 4 to 6 hours. In severe cases, this therapy may be required for 48 to 72 hours (60). In view of the possible intracellular action of deferoxamine, it appears reasonable to continue treatment until after the pink color of the urine has disappeared and the patient is without signs and symptoms of iron poisoning for at least 24 hours (4). The total amount of deferoxamine should not exceed 6 g in any 24-hour period in an adult or 80 mg/kg in a child, whichever is lower (46). In the absence of toxicity, larger doses may be administered (38,58).

Although deferoxamine may be administered intramuscularly, the quantities required may cause pain at the site of injection, sterile necrosis, and local discoloration (57). The dose for intramuscular administration in a child ranges from 40 to 90 mg/kg, not to exceed 1 g every 8 hours (13,18,60). In an adult, 1 g is administered initially and is followed by 500 mg every 4 hours (45).

The endpoint of chelation therapy is not well defined (61). Some clinicians recommend continuing deferoxamine for 24 hours after the disappearance of the vin rose color from the urine, whereas others recommend continuation of therapy until the serum iron concentration is less than 100 μg/dL (62). Justification for longer therapy may be based on the lack of knowledge about iron toxicity at the mitochondrial level (42). The ability of clinicians to visually detect the vin rose color of the urine is questionable; the determination of a positive result depends on the concentration of iron as the iron-deferoxamine complex (63). Investigations indicate that physicians may not always be able to reliably detect this color change that indicates the amount of iron excreted in the urine and that this method should not be the sole indicator for therapy (61,62).

Toxicity

The toxicity of deferoxamine is minimal, but symptoms may include gastrointestinal discomfort after oral administration and hypotension after excessively rapid intravenous administration of a large dose, which is probably a result of venous dilation (26,46). If hypotension develops, the infusion should be temporarily stopped and begun again at a lower infusion rate (38). In addition, tachycardia as a result of the hypotension and urticaria as an allergic response may occur (64). Lens opacification has been reported in animals after long-term administration of deferoxamine, but this is not a problem in the acute overdose situation (29). Pregnancy is not considered a contraindication to the use of this antidote.

Dialysis

Although dialysis can be effective in removing the ferrioxamine complex or chelated iron, it is not as effective as renal excretion in iron removal. Dialysis is indicated only if renal shutdown occurs after chelation therapy has been instituted (38).

Miscellaneous Methods

Exchange transfusion has been used, but in view of the rapid intracellular movement of iron it is not an efficient therapeutic modality (65). Surgical intervention may be necessary for the patient who develops signs of perforation and peritonitis in the early stages of intoxication or subsequent stricture formation (26,66), and some investigators have recommended early laparotomy in patients with massive iron ingestion to resect potentially gangrenous bowel (33). Surgical intervention has been used occasionally in acute iron toxicity when gastric lavage has failed to remove iron concretions from the stomach. Operative findings suggest potential causes for the failure of emesis or lavage to empty the stomach. Iron has been found adhering to or embedded in the mucosa of the stomach, and in some cases, it has completely eroded through the stomach. Additionally, the sugar coating of iron tablets may partially dissolve and form a gelatinous mass in the stomach, thus, promoting the formation of large iron concretions. Individuals who recover from a significant iron overdose should have adequate follow-up for potential long-term complications (42).

REFERENCES

1. Greengard J: Iron poisoning in children. *Clin Toxicol* 1975;8: 575–597.
2. Crotty J: Acute iron poisoning in children. *Clin Toxicol* 1971;4: 615–619.
3. Aldrich R: *Iron in Clinical Medicine.* Berkeley, CA: University of California Press, 1958;58–65.
4. Leiken S, Vassough P, Mocher-Faterni F: Chelation therapy in acute iron poisoning. *J Pediatr* 1967;71:425–428.
5. Wasserman G, Martens V: Early aggressive treatment of iron poisoning. *Am Fam Physician* 1977;15:125–127.
6. Eriksson F, Johansson S, Mellstedt H, et al: Iron intoxication in two adult patients. *Acta Med Scand* 1974;196:231–236.
7. Ross F: Pyloric stenosis and fibrosis stricture of the stomach due to ferrous sulfate poisoning. *Br Med J* 1953;2:1200–1202.
8. Greenblatt D, Allen M, Koch-Weser J: Accidental iron poisoning in childhood: six cases including one fatality. *Clin Pediatr* 1976;15: 835–838.
9. Angle C: Symposium on iron poisoning. *Clin Toxicol* 1971;4: 525–527.
10. Wallack M, Winkelstein A: Acute iron intoxication in an adult. *JAMA* 1974;229:1333–1335.
11. Oderda G: Iron and vitamin toxicities. *Ear Nose Throat* 1983;62: 40–44.
12. Ng R, Perry K, Martin D: Iron poisoning: assessment or radiography in diagnosis and management. *Clin Pediatr* 1979;18(10):614–616.
13. Robertson W: Treatment of acute iron poisoning. *Med Treat* 1970;8:552–560.
14. Krenzelok F, Hoff J; Accidental childhood iron poisoning: a problem of marketing and labeling. *Pediatrics* 1979;63:591–596.
15. Harrison P: Biochemistry of iron. *Clin Toxicol* 1971;4:529–544.
16. Murray M: Iron absorption. *Clin Toxicol* 1971;4:545–558.
17. Murphy B: Hazards of children's vitamin preparations containing iron. *JAMA* 1974;229:324.
18. Haddad L: Iron poisoning. *JACEP* 1976;5:691–694.
19. Tenenbein M, Littman C, Stimpson R: Gastrointestinal pathology in adult iron overdose. *J Toxicol Clin Toxicol* 1990;28:311–320.
20. Erler M: Iron poisoning. *JEN* 1980;6:40–42.
21. Robertson W: Iron poisoning: a problem of childhood. *Top Emerg Med* 1979;1:57–63.
22. Cheng C, Sullivan T, Li P, et al: Iron toxicity screening. *JACEP* 1979;8:238–240.
23. Whitten C, Chen Y, Gibson G: Studies in acute iron poisoning: Part II: further observations on desferrioxamine in the treatment of acute experimental iron poisoning. *Pediatr Res* 1978;2:479–485.
24. Mann K, Picciotti M, Spevack T, et al: Management of acute iron overdose. *Clin Pharm* 1989;8:428–440.
25. Whitten C, Brough A: The pathophysiology of acute iron poisoning. *Clin Toxicol* 1971;4:585–595.
26. Whitten C, Chen Y, Gibson G: Studies in acute iron poisoning: further observations on desferrioxamine in the treatment of acute experimental iron poisoning. *Pediatrics* 1966;38:102–110.
27. Klein-Schwartz W, Oderda G, Gorman R, et al: Assessment of management guidelines: acute iron ingestion. *Clin Pediatr* 1990;29: 316–321.
28. Knasel A, Collins-Barrow M: Applicability of early indicators of iron toxicity. *J Nat Med Assoc* 1986;78:1037–1040.
29. Jacobs A: Iron chelation therapy for iron loaded patients. *Br J Haematol* 1979;43:1–5.
30. Jacobs J, Greene H, Gendel B: Acute iron intoxication. *N Engl J Med* 1965;273:1124–1127.
31. Gleason W, Demello D, Decastor F, et al: Acute hepatic failure in severe iron poisoning. *J Pediatr* 1979;95:138–140.
32. Witzleben C, Buck B: Iron overload hepatotoxicity: a postulated pathogenesis. *Clin Toxicol* 1971;4:579–583
33. Knoll L, Miller R: Acute iron intoxication with intestinal infarction. *J Pediatr Surg* 1978;13:720–721.
34. Vernon D, Banner W, Dean J: Hemodynamic effects of experimental iron poisoning. *Ann Emerg Med* 1989;18:863–866.
35. Lacoste H, Goyert G, Goldman L, et al: Acute iron intoxication in pregnancy: case report and review of the literature. *Obstet Gynecol* 1992;80:500–501.
36. Curry S, Bond G, Raschke R, et al: An ovine model of maternal iron poisoning in pregnancy.*Ann Emerg Med* 1990;19:632–638.
37. Lacouture P, Wason S, Temple A, et al: Emergency assessment of severity in iron overdose by clinical and laboratory methods. *J Pediatr 1981*;99:89–91.
38. Proudfoot A, Simpson D, Dyson E: Management of acute iron poisoning. *Med Toxicol* 1986;1:83–100.
39. McGuigan M, Lovejoy F, Marino S, et al: Qualitative deferoxamine color test for iron ingestion. *J Pediatr* 1979;94:940–942.
40. Everson G, Oudjhane K, Young L, et al: Effectiveness of abdominal radiographs in visualizing chewable iron supplements following overdose. *Am J Emerg Med* 1989;459–463.
41. Ling L, Hornfeldt C, Winter J: Absorption of iron after experimental overdose of chewable vitamins. *Am J Emerg Med* 1991;9:24–26.
42. Schauben J, Augenstein L, Cox J, et al: Iron poisoning: report of three

cases and a review of therapeutic intervention. *J Emerg Med* 1990;8:309–319.
43. Chyka P, Butler A: Assessment of acute iron poisoning by laboratory and clinical observations. *Am J Emerg Med* 1993;11:99–103.
44. Burkhart K, Kulig K, Hammond K, et al: The rise in the total iron-binding capacity after iron overdose. *Ann Emerg Med* 1991;20: 532–535.
45. James J: Acute iron poisoning: assessment of severity and prognosis. *J Pediatr* 1970;77:117–119.
46. Robotham J, Lietman P: Acute iron poisoning—A review. *Am J Dis Child* 1980;134:875–879.
47. Tenenbein M, Yatscoff R: The total iron-binding capacity in iron poisoning. Is it useful? *Am J Dis Child* 1991;145:437–439.
48. Dean B, Oehme F, Krenzelok, et al: A study of iron complexation in a swine model. *Vet Hum Toxicol* 1988;30:313–315.
49. Fischer DS: A method for the rapid detection of acute iron toxicity. *Clin Chem* 1967;13:6–11.
50. McEnery J: Hospital management of acute iron ingestion. *Clin Toxicol* 1971;4:603-613.
51. Dean B, Krenzelok E: In vivo effectiveness of oral complexation agents in the management of iron poisoning. *Clin Toxicol* 1987;25: 221–230.
52. Everson G, Bertaccini E, O'Leary J: Use of whole bowel irrigation in an infant following iron overdose. *Am J Emerg Med* 1991;9:366–369.
53. Tenenbein M, Wiseman N, Yatscoff R: Gastrotomy and whole bowel irrigation in iron poisoning.*Pediatr Emerg Care* 1991;7:286–288.
54. Bachrach L, Correa A, Levin R, et al: Iron poisoning: complications of hypertonic phosphate lavage therapy. *J Pediatr* 1979;94:147–149.
55. Geffner M, Opas L: Phosphate poisoning complicating treatment for iron ingestion. *Am J Dis Child* 1980; 134:509–510.
56. Fischer DS, Parkman R, Finch S: Acute iron poisoning in children: the problem of appropriate therapy. *JAMA* 1971;218:1179–1184.
57. Westlin W: Deferoxamine as a chelating agent. *Clin Toxicol* 1971;4: 597–602.
58. Peck M, Rogers J, Rivenbark J: Use of high doses of deferoxamine (Desferal) in an adult patient with acute iron overdosage. *J Toxicol Clin Toxicol* 1982;19:865–869.
59. Hussain M, Flynn D, Green N, et al: Effect of dose, time and ascorbate on iron excretion after subcutaneous desferrioxamine. *Lancet* 1977;1:977–979.
60. Chisholm J: Poisoning due lo heavy metals. *Pediatr Clin North Am* 1970;17:591–615.
61. Tenenbein M, Lowalski S, Sienko A, et al: Pulmonary toxic effects of continuous desferrioxamine administraton in acute iron poisoning. *Lancet* 1992;339:699–701.
62. Yatscoff R, Wayne E, Tenenbein M: An objective criterion for the cessation of deferoxamine therapy in the acutely iron poisoned patient. *J Toxicol Clin Toxicol* 1991;29:1–10.
63. Bentur Y, Louis P, Klein J, et al: Misinterpretation of iron-binding capacity in the presence of deferoxamine. *J Pediatr* 1991;118: 139–142.
64. Cohen A, Mizanin J, Schwartz E: Rapid removal of excessive iron with daily, high-dose intravenous chelation therapy. *J Pediatr* 1989; 115:151–155.
65. Movassaghi N, Purugganan G, Leikin S: Comparison of exchange transfusion and deferoxamine in the treatment of acute iron poisoning. *J Pediatr* 1969;75:604–608.
66. Peterson C, Fifield G: Emergency gastrotomy for acute iron poisoning. *Ann Emerg Med* 1980;9:262–264.

ADDITIONAL SELECTED REFERENCES

Gezernik W, Schmaman A, Chappell J: Corrosive gastritis as a result of ferrous sulphate ingestion. *S Afr Med J* 1980;57:151–153.

Henretig F, Karl S, Weintraub W: Severe iron poisoning treated with enteral and intravenous deferoxamine. *Ann Emerg Med* 1983;12: 306–309

Kleinman M, Linn W, Bailey R, et al: Human exposure to ferric sulfate aerosol: effects on pulmonary function and respiratory symptoms. *Am Ind Hyg Assoc J* 1981;42:298–304

Snyder R, Mofenson H, Greensher J: Acute iron poisoning in infancy: guide to treatment. *NY State J Med* 1974;74:2215–2217.

Tenenbein M: Whole bowel irrigation in iron poisoning. *J Pediatr* 1987;111:142–145.

CHAPTER 65

Miscellaneous Metals

Aluminum is the most abundant metal in the earth's crust. It is most commonly found in minerals as aluminum silicates and as aluminum oxides. Because of the widespread occurrence of aluminum in the environment and foodstuffs, it is virtually impossible for humans to avoid exposure to this metal ion (1).

There is no evidence that aluminum is an essential ion in any biochemical process or pathway. The metal is not a serious hazard for healthy individuals with average intake. Recent studies, however, suggest that aluminum toxicity may be linked to the pathogenesis of a number of clinical disorders associated with renal insufficiency. The toxic phenomena seen in chronic renal failure include a specific form of encephalopathy; dialysis encephalopathy, a metabolic bone disease; osteomalacia osteodystrophy, and anemia (2).

SOURCES

Aluminum has, until recently, been considered a benign metal. It has been, and in some parts of the world, continues to be used in water clarification. Some coffee pots and rice cookers are made of aluminum. Aluminum is sometimes used as an antacid preparation (3).

Aluminum is widely used as a building material and for other uses where light weight and corrosion resistance are important. Medically, various soluble salts of aluminum have been used as astringents, styptics, and antiseptics. The insoluble salts are used as antacids and as antidiarrheal agents. Inhalation of aluminum hydroxide has been used as a preventive and curative agent for silicosis.

Aluminum is naturally present in raw water, vegetation, and animal tissue (Table 65–1). Aluminum may be present in high concentrations in domestic tap water either naturally or, more commonly, because it has been added as a flocculating agent during the water purification process. Aluminum salts are widely used in foods and are also present in fluids and medications that are available either by prescription or as over-the-counter nonprescription items. The natural aluminum content of foods varies and appears to be dependent on the soil on which the food has been cultivated. Foods with naturally high aluminum content may have acquired aluminum during preparation, particularly if they are acidic, as a result of leaching from the cooking vessel. Aluminum salts, particularly aluminum hydroxide, are commonly used as antacid drugs. Aluminum hydroxide is also used as a buffer with aspirin to reduce the gastric irritation caused by this analgesic compound.

TABLE 65–1. *Sources of aluminum*

Foods
Food additives
Tap water
Antacids
Buffering agents

Aluminum salts are widely used as food additives. Sodium aluminum phosphates are added to commercial cake mixes and self-rising flour, where they act as leavening agents, and are added to processed cheeses, as emulsifying agents and to improve the texture, storage capability, and easy melting characteristics.

ABSORPTION

Aluminum is absorbed from the gastrointestinal tract in normal individuals and is excreted by the kidneys in the urine. The site of aluminum absorption in the gastrointestinal tract is not well defined although it is probably located in either the duodenum or proximal jejunum. In healthy individuals, absorption of aluminum following oral doses of aluminum-containing salts is associated with an increase in serum concentration followed by a rapid increase in urine excretion. A failure in the normal renal excretory mechanism accounts for the accumulation of aluminum in the tissues. Aluminum accumulation may also occur in nondialyzed patients, primarily infants and children with immature or impaired renal function, who have been on treatment with oral aluminum-containing phosphate-binding agents. Many aluminum salts are converted to the phosphate salt in the gastrointestinal tract and excreted in the feces as such. The simultaneous administration of aluminum salts with citrate enhances the intestinal absorption of aluminum and its subsequent tissue deposition.

LABORATORY

Aluminum, like many trace elements, is present in minute quantities in biologic fluids. The serum level for normal people, is in the range of 0 to 40 μg/L (0 to 1.5 μmol/L). Serum aluminum concentrations should never exceed 200 μg/L (7.4 μmol/L), and patients with values in excess of 100 μg/L (3.7 μmol/L) should be monitored frequently and subjected to close clinical surveillance for evidence of toxic phenomena (4).

The most reliable test for the diagnosis of aluminum related osteomalacia is histologic examination of a bone biopsy specimen.

ACUTE TOXICITY

Massive oral doses of aluminum are reported to be toxic and gastrointestinal irritation may occur following these large doses. The use of aluminum cooking utensils and cans is not enough to contribute significantly to either total body burden or toxic effects.

DIALYSIS ENCEPHALOPATHY

In the 1970s, the occurrence of a progressive fatal neurologic syndrome was reported in some patients with chronic renal failure on long-term treatment with intermittent hemodialysis (Table 65–2). It is now generally accepted that aluminum is the etiologic neurotoxic factor in the dialysis encephalopathy syndrome.

In the pathogenesis of dialysis encephalopathy, the patients develop evidence of progressive neurologic deterioration between 7 months and 6 years after beginning maintenance hemodialysis. The onset of the syndrome is manifested by a speech disturbance characterized by hesitancy and stuttering, followed by dysarthria, dyspraxia, and dysphasia. Later, patients develop myoclonic movements, seizure activity, and a progressive global dementia. Monitoring and maintaining the serum aluminum levels are essential for the well-being of these patients (2).

TABLE 65–2. *Signs and symptoms of dialysis encephalopathy*

Neurologic
Speech disturbance
Hesitancy
Stuttering
Dysarthria
Dyspraxia
Dysphasia
Myoclonus
Seizure
Global dementia

DIALYSIS OSTEODYSTROPHY

One of the characteristics of dialysis osteodystrophy is the development and progression despite the maintenance of plasma calcium and magnesium at concentrations that, in healthy persons, would not interfere with bone mineralization or be associated with the development of metabolic bone disease.

ANEMIA

Aluminum-related anemia is of the noniron-deficient, microcytic, hypochromic type and responds to the use of a low aluminum dialysate. Aluminum may cause a microcytic anemia by a direct effect on hemoglobin synthesis. Aluminum has been reported to inhibit ferrochelatase, the mitochondrial enzyme involved in the final step in the heme-biosynthetic pathway (5).

TREATMENT

The use of deferoxamine for the treatment of aluminum accumulation is well established. Deferoxamine provides symptomatic relief from dialysis encephalopathy and aluminum-related osteomalacia (6).

Deferoxamine acts by mobilizing aluminum from tissues by chelation, causing a significant increase in serum concentration with a decrease in the protein-bound fraction and renders the metal ion available for elimination from the body.

BARIUM

Barium is a heavy divalent alkaline earth metal that occurs in its natural form as barite ($BaSO_4$) and witherite ($BaCO_3$). These are the more common mineral forms of barium. Historically, barium was used between 1600 C.E. and 1900 C.E. as an emetic, diuretic, and depilatory in addition for its phosphorescent properties.

Sources and Uses

Barium salts are contained in some rodenticides, depilatories, and fireworks (Table 65–3). Oil and gas drillers are the principle industrial users of barium. Other activities with considerable use of barium include the manufacture of glass, paint, rubber, rat poison, fireworks, flares, and automotive lubricants. All water or acid-soluble barium salts are poisonous; currently, approximately 40 of these salts are used in industry. Medical contrast

TABLE 65–3. *Sources of barium*

Rodenticides
Depilatory agents
Fireworks
Industry
Oil and gas drilling
Glass manufacturing
Paint
Rubber
Automotive lubricants
Medical contrast media

media contain insoluble barium compounds and absorption normally is negligible.

Whereas human poisonings by soluble barium salts are uncommon, isolated accidental and suicidal ingestions are reported with surprising frequency. Epidemics provide most of the poisoning cases. Intoxication occurs most often when barium carbonate contaminates or is mistaken for flour or salt (7).

Pharmacokinetics

Intestinal absorption of barium is similar to calcium and excretion is mainly fecal. Stomach acid converts barium carbonate to its absorbable form, barium chloride; peak serum levels occur 2 hours after ingestion with an elimination half-life of 3.6 days. Over two thirds of absorbed barium is sequestered in bone. The toxic oral dose of barium in humans is approximately 200 mg, and the lethal dose reported in the adult falls between 11 and 15 g (7).

Clinical Manifestations

The insoluble forms of barium, particularly barium sulfate, are not toxic by the oral route because of minimal absorption. Accidental poisoning from the ingestion of soluble barium salts, however, has resulted in a myriad of clinical manifestations. The varied manifestations of barium poisoning are summarized by organ system (Table 65–4). Barium directly stimulates skeletal smooth and cardiac muscle resulting in myoclonus and cramping, hypertension, gastrointestinal hypermotility, and ventricular tachyarrhythmias. This has resulted in gastroenteritis, muscular paralysis, bradycardia, and ventricular fibrillation and extrasystoles (3).

Nervous system effects are diverse with paresthesias and progressive muscular paralysis occurring often. Motor disorders include stiffness and immobility of the limbs and sometimes of the trunk, leg cramps, twitching of facial muscles, and paralysis of the tongue and pharynx with attendant loss or impairment of speech and deglutition. Muscle paralysis follows initial muscular stimulation and is secondary to hypokalemia. There are no known long-term sequelae of acute barium poisoning (8).

TABLE 65–4. *Signs and symptoms of barium poisoning*

Gastrointestinal
Nausea
Vomiting
Abdominal pain
Increased peristalsis
Diarrhea
Musculoskelatal
Myoclonus
Cramping
Myalgia
Flaccid paralysis
Central nervous system
Paresthesia
Progressive muscle paralysis
Limb stiffness
Paralysis of tongue and pharynx
Cardiac
Hypertension
Premature ventricular contractions
QT prolongation
Ventricular tachycardia
Ventricular fibrillation
Asystole

Baritosis

Baritosis, a benign pneumoconiosis, is an occupational disease arising from the inhalation of barium sulfate dust and barium carbonate. It is not incapacitating but does produce radiologic changes in the lungs. The radiologic changes are reversible with cessation of exposure.

Barium and Hypokalemia

The hypokalemia of barium poisoning results from an intracellular potassium shift. Barium has no proven activity on the sodium-potassium pump; therefore, it is thought that the continued activity of this ion pump combined with blocked cellular potassium efflux produces intracellular potassium accumulation and a resultant extracellular hypokalemia (7).

Treatment

Most authorities recommend gastric lavage with magnesium or sodium sulfate to convert barium to the nontoxic sulfate when acute barium ingestion is recognized. Similarly, oral sulfates can be given without subsequent lavage to precipitate barium sulfate in the intestines. No adverse sequelae have been reported from this treatment. The mainstay of treatment for barium poisoning is aggressive administration of potassium. Potassium reverses the paralysis, diarrhea, and cardiac dysrhythmias in barium poisoning. When vomiting and hypokalemia are present, potassium replacement should be initiated intravenously, continued orally if possible, and followed with frequent serum levels.

Cardiac monitoring is suggested for patients with hypertension, paralysis, QT prolongation, and premature ventricular beats. Although lidocaine and procainamide have been reported to be useful in the treatment of ventricular arrhythmias, potassium replacement remains the therapy of choice for this complication.

COPPER

Copper is an essential trace metal that is widely distributed in nature and is an essential element. Copper is a constituent of many oxidative enzymes, including cytochrome oxidase, catalase, peroxidase, ascorbic acid oxidase, tyrosinase, and monoamine oxidase. Soluble and insoluble copper salts are used widely in fungicides and insecticides. In general, the soluble ionized salts of copper are much more toxic than the insoluble or slightly dissociated compounds. In the past, copper sulfate had been used as an emetic. Water purification processing has included the use of copper to remove algae. Many cases of copper poisoning result from the use of copper containers for food and drink (2).

Copper resembles many other heavy metals in its systemic toxic effects: widespread capillary damage, kidney and liver injury, and central nervous system excitement followed by depression.

Pharmacokinetics

The intestinal mucosa acts to some extent as a barrier to the absorption of ingested copper. The normal serum copper level is 120 to 145 μg/L. The bile is the normal excretory pathway and plays a primary role in copper homeostasis. The liver and bone marrow are the storage organs for excess copper.

Acute Poisoning

Acute poisoning from the ingestion of copper salts is rarely severe if the metal is removed promptly from the gastrointestinal tract, yet the acute poisoning from excessive amounts of copper sulfate has produced death. Emesis usually begins promptly after ingestion of the copper but would be delayed if food were in the stomach. The emesis sometimes has a blue-green color. Other symptoms may include hematemesis, hypotension, melena, coma, and jaundice (8).

Chronic Poisoning

Chronic copper poisoning due to excessive intake is rarely recognized. The characteristic clinical features of occult copper poisoning are hemolytic anemia with Heinz bodies, hemoglobinemia, and hemoglobinuria. Abdominal symptoms include pain, nausea, vomiting, and diarrhea.

TABLE 65–5. *Signs and symptoms of acquired copper poisoning*

Acute
Coma
Emesis
Hematemesis
Hypotension
Jaundice
Melena
Chronic
Abdominal pain
Diarrhea
Heinz body hemolytic anemia
Hemoglobinemia
Hemoglobinuria
Nausea
Vomiting

A type of chronic copper poisoning is recognized in the form of a metabolic disease called hereditary hepatolenticular degeneration or Wilson s disease. If dietary copper intake is reduced and urinary excretion promoted, the neurological signs and symptoms associated with Wilson s disease are alleviated.

Treatment is largely symptomatic. Further clinical trials are required to evaluate dimercaprol (British antilewisite) and penicillamine in both acute and chronic copper poisoning.

GOLD

Gold is rather widely distributed in small quantities, but the major economically usable deposits occur as the free metal in quartz veins. Gold is used for jewelry, for other ornamental uses, and for the special industrial purposes where its properties of electrical and heat conductivity and malleability outweigh its expense.

Although gold and its salts have been used for a wide variety of medicinal purposes, their present uses are limited to the treatment of rheumatoid arthritis and rare skin diseases. The toxicity of gold and its salts are largely associated with its therapeutic use rather than its industrial use. Gold salts are poorly absorbed from the gastrointestinal tract (2).

Toxicity

Dermatitis is the most frequently reported toxic reaction and stomatitis may accompany this reaction. Gold is the only heavy metal that commonly induces an immune-mediated hematologic effect. The clinical features most commonly observed are immune-mediated thrombocytopenia, occasionally with eosinophilia in the absence of other hematologic abnormalities. This thrombocytopenia may be caused by a platelet-associated IgG immunoglobulin, believed to be responsible for platelet destruction through phagocytosis of IgG-coated platelets by splenic macrophages (2).

Aplastic anemia is a rare though life-threatening complication of gold therapy. Generally, reversible hypoplasia occurs, starting with cumulative doses of 280 mg, irreversible marrow aplasia is more likely when the dose exceeds 400 mg. The etiology of gold-induced aplastic anemia is unknown. Gold accumulates in reticuloendothelial cells; accumulation in the marrow has a direct myelotoxic effect.

Nephritis with albuminuria, encephalitis, gastrointestinal damage, and hepatitis have also been reported but with less frequency.

ZINC

Zinc is ubiquitous and is considered an essential trace element. Zinc is omnipresent in the environment and is found in water, air, and all living organisms. It is necesary for normal growth and development and is present in a number of metalloenzymes including carbonic anhydrase, carboxypeptidase, alcohol dehydrogenase, and others. Therapeutically, zinc compounds are used as topical astringents, dermal products, antiseptics, and emetics (9).

Zinc chloride and zinc phosphide are highly corrosive salts and may produce severe hemorrhagic gastroenteritis. Although much less corrosive, zinc sulfate may also produce hemorrhagic gastroenteritis. The chloride salt of zinc is the most toxic of commonly occurring zinc compounds. Serious zinc ingestions have occasionally been reported in the toxicologic literature (10).

Zinc salts such as zinc chloride or zinc phosphide are acidic, and symptoms secondary to their corrosive effects on the gastrointestinal tract are seen within 30 minutes to 1 hour after ingestion (6). These compounds may produce gastroenteritis, gastric or substernal pain, vomiting, and diarrhea. These symptoms may result in sloughing of mucous membranes, ulcer formation, and later strictures. Symptoms may rapidly progress and the patient may suffer from gastrointestinal hemorrhage, shock, and cardiovascular collapse (1).

Zinc Phosphide

Zinc phosphide is a potent rodenticide rarely found in the household setting where its use is discouraged due to its high degree of toxicity and disagreeable odor.

The most common route of zinc phosphide intoxication is by oral ingestion. Zinc phosphide can also be inhaled as a dust or absorbed through broken skin. The substance is not known to penetrate the intact skin.

Mechanism of Toxicity

Zinc phosphide toxicity is mediated through the generation of phosphine gas. Phosphine is a colorless gas used as a fumigant in grain elevators and cargo ships, and in the manufacture of silicon chips for the computer industry. The gas smells of decaying fish and can be detected by humans at a concentration of 2 ppm (11).

Zinc phosphide has been noted to liberate phosphine gas rapidly when exposed to dilute acid and slowly when exposed to water. In patients who have ingested zinc phosphide, it is hypothesized that phosphine gas is released from the reaction of gastric acid with the zinc phosphide molecule (10). The reaction is catalyzed by the presence of elemental phosphorus, often found as a contaminant in these products. Both the immediate and delayed toxicities of zinc phosphide may be a direct result of the actions of phosphine gas on the body (9).

Signs and Symptoms

Early symptoms of toxicity from zinc phosphide poisoning include fatigue, nausea, cough, dizziness, and headache. Dyspnea or thirst suggests a more serious intoxication. Physical signs of toxicity include pulmonary edema, hypotension, putrid breath, black vomitus or stools, jaundice, ataxia, diplopia, and intention tremors (10).

Serious toxicity includes shock, oliguria, metabolic acidosis, hypocalcemic tetany, seizures, and coma. Hypertension, cardiac arrhythmias, purpura, and a thrombocytopenia have also been described (11).

A small number of patients who succumb to zinc phosphide toxicity die within the first few hours after ingestion from pulmonary edema, a direct result of the action of phosphine. The majority of deaths occur within 30 hours of ingestion from peripheral vascular collapse secondary to a direct toxic effect of phosphine on the myocardium. Fulminant pulmonary edema also plays a significant role in the demise of these patients (9).

Treatment

Treatment of zinc phosphide poisoning is primarily symptomatic and supportive. Gastric emptying techniques should be avoided due to the corrosive nature of the compound. Special attention should be paid to the patient's cardiopulmonary status and maintenance of adequate oxygenation and tissue perfusion is a paramount importance. Aggressive airway control, including intubation with mechanical ventilation, should be pursued if signs of pulmonary edema develop, and hypotension should be managed with volume replacement and vasopressor therapy as guided by the patient's central venous pressure (11).

Chelating Agents

Ca EDTA and BAL have been suggested for use as chelating agents in patients with significant zinc toxicity. EDTA is the preferred agent in zinc poisoning and can markedly increase urinary excretion of zinc. It should be administered as the calcium salt to avoid the complication of hypocalcemia, as EDTA reacts with calcium in the same way as with other metals.

The use of penicillamine is theoretically unwise in that the complex of zinc-penicillamine has been found to be lethal to laboratory animals. The postulated mechanism is said to be due to overproduction of prostaglandin.

METAL FUME FEVER

Metal fume fever is an industrial disease as old as the metallurgy of brass. The constellation of symptoms presently known as metal fume fever has been previously described as brass founder's ague, zinc chills, smelter shakes, and copper fever. Metal fume fever is an occupational syndrome that develops on exposure to fresh metal oxide fumes (12,13). This occurs when fumes from metals heated above their melting point are inhaled (14). Whereas zinc oxide fumes are the most common cause of metal fume fever, inhalation of other metal oxides may induce this reaction (15). Other metal oxides that can cause metal fume fever include copper, manganese, silver, tin, aluminum, magnesium, iron, selenium, cadmium, antimony, and nickel (Table 65–6) (12,13). Exposure is most common in the metal (steel and iron) industry, metal grinding and welding, zinc foundries, galvanizing, and chrome plating. Other activities that may emit potentially toxic fumes include soldering, brazing, cutting, metallizing, forging, melting, and casting. Zinc, copper, and iron remain the primary offending metals (16).

Although the symptoms of metal fume fever are recognized by welders and metal workers and are well known to physicians in occupational medicine, most primary care physicians are unaware of this disorder (17).

Originally, it was speculated that only freshly formed metal oxide fumes could induce metal fume fever. It is now generally accepted that particle size is the precipitating factor. The syndrome occurs mainly in nonatopic individuals who inhale an organometallic dust of particle size less than 1.5 g, which can penetrate the alveoli of the lungs (17). The pulmonary and subsequent systemic reactions occur when this material is retained and absorbed after exposure (13).

Clinical Features

The initial symptoms of metal fume fever are of sudden onset (usually within 4 to 8 hours of exposure) and begin with mild upper airway irritation that later resembles the onset of a viral or bacterial infection (Table 65–7). Workers present most often in the late afternoon or early evening with a variety of nonspecific complaints. The syndrome is heralded by a metallic or sweet taste and dry throat. Cough and dyspnea may follow, accompanied by malaise, myalgias, arthralgias, and nausea. A fever of 38°C to 39°C develops and peaks 10 to 12 hours after inhalation. Chills and sweats, myalgia and thirst are frequently reported (16).

Physical findings noted may be moist rales at the base of the lungs with or without wheezing. The chest film is usually normal. In addition, the precipitating antibodies and pulmonary infiltrates present in the occupational and vocational hypersensitivity pneumonitides are absent in metal fume fever (14).

The signs and symptoms of metal fume fever (Table 65–8) are self-limited and usually resolve within 24 to

TABLE 65–6. *Signs and symptoms of zinc poisoning*

Pulmonary
Dyspnea
Pulmonary edema
Neurologic
Ataxia
Diplopia
Intention tremors
Severe
Shock
Oliguria
Metabolic acidosis
Hypocalcemic tetany
Seizures
Coma
Hypertension
Cardiac dysrhythmias

TABLE 65–7. *Incriminators of metal fume fever*

Aluminum
Antimony
Cadmium
Copper
Iron
Magnesium
Manganese
Nickel
Selenium
Silver
Tin
Zinc

TABLE 65–8. *Signs and symptons of metal fume fever*

Arthralgia
Chills/sweats
Cough
Dry throat
Dyspnea
Fever
Malaise
Nausea
Sweet taste

48 hours after termination of exposure. No long-term sequelae or complications are known to exist.

Mechanism of Intoxication

The pathogenesis of metal fume fever remains controversial. The most commonly accepted theory involves a delayed hypersensitivity mechanism. The inhaled metal oxide particles cause inflammation of the respiratory tract and release of a histamine-like substance. Antigen-antibody complex formation then generates an allergic reaction producing metal fume fever.

Diagnosis

The diagnosis may be easily overlooked because of the mild, influenza-like symptoms. Historical data and clinical findings provide the only leads, because there are no specific tests for this syndrome. Diagnosis of metal fume fever is usually based on an occupational history of exposure to metal fumes. There is no specific test for metal fume fever. One must rely on the clinical picture when formulating a diagnosis. A moderate leukocytosis with a left shift may develop along with an elevated erythrocyte sedimentation rate. This will usually persist until approximately 12 hours after the patient becomes afebrile. Lactate dehydrogenase may be increased in the setting of a normal aspartate aminotransferase and alanine aminotransferase. Isoenzyme determination will often reveal an elevated lactate dehydrogenase, indicating damage to the pulmonary tissue. Arterial blood gases may show hypoxemia if pulmonary involvement is extensive. In addition, the complete resolution of symptoms and functional abnormalities by 24 to 48 hours favors the diagnosis of metal fume fever (16).

Treatment

The treatment of metal fume fever is supportive and includes bedrest, analgesics, and antipyretics. Metal fume fever usually resolves completely in 24 to 48 hours without the need for treatment and without causing permanent lung damage. Patients who present in a toxic state require immediate care in the emergency department. Oxygen should be administered to correct hypoxemia and bronchospasm can be treated with xanthine bronchodilators. A history of exposure to cadmium or zinc chloride fumes requires hospitalization for observation and supportive care (167).

REFERENCES

1. Kosnett M: Unanswered questions in metal chelation. *J Toxicol Clin Toxicol* 1992;30:529–547.
2. Chisolm J: Poisoning due to heavy metals. *Pediatr Clin North Am* 1970;17:591–615.
3. Greenhouse A: Heavy metals and the nervous system. *Clin Neuropharmacol* 1982;5:45–92.
4. Chan S, Gerson B: Technical aspects of quantification of aluminum. *Clin Lab Med* 1990;10:423–433.
5. Hewitt C, Savory J, Wills M: Aspects of aluminum toxicity. *Clin Lab Med* 1990;10:403–422.
6. Ringenberg Q, Doll D, Patterson W, et al: Hematologic effects of heavy metal poisoning. *South Med J* 1988;81;1132–1139.
7. Johnson C, Van Tassell V: Acute barium poisoning with respiratory failure and rhabdomyolysis. *Ann Emerg Med* 1991;220:1138–1142.
8. Oehme F: Mechanism of heavy metal toxicities. *Clin Toxicol* 1972;5:151–167.
9. Burkhart K, Kulig K, Rumack B: Whole-bowel irrigation treatment for zinc sulfate overdose. *Ann Emerg Med* 1990;19:1164–1170.
10. Chobanian S: Accidental ingestion of liquid zinc chloride: local and systemic effects. *Ann Emerg Med* 1981;10:91–93.
11. Zinc phosphide ingestion: a case report and review. *Vet Hum Toxicol* 1989;31:559–562.
12. Mueller E, Seger D: Metal fume fever—a review. *J Emerg Med* 1985;2:271–274.
13. Johnson J, Kilburn K: Cadmium-induced metal fume fever: results of inhalation challenge. *Am J Industr Med* 1983;4:533–540.
14. Dula D: Metal fume fever. *MCEP* 1978;7:448–450.
15. Anseline P: Zinc-fume fever. *Med J Aust* 1972;2:316–318.
16. Offermann P, Finley C: Metal fume fever. *Ann Emerg Med* 1992;21: 872–875.
17. Hopper W: Metal fume fever. *Postgrad Med* 1978;63:123–127.

ADDITIONAL SELECTED REFERENCES

Anseline P: Zinc-fume fever. *Med J Aust* 1972;2:316–318.

Day A, Golding J, Lee P, et al: Penicillamine in rheumatoid disease: a long-term study. *Br Med J* 1974;1:180–183.

Hughes R, Gazzard B, Murray-Lyon I, et al: The use of cysteamine and dimercaprol. *J Int Med Res* 1976;4(suppl):123–129.

Oehme F; British anti-lewisite (BAL): the classic heavy metal antidote. *Clin Toxicol* 1972;5:215–222.

PART XI

MISCELLANEOUS AGENTS

CHAPTER 66

Theophylline

Theophylline (1,3-dimethylxanthine) is a naturally occurring alkaloid closely related to caffeine. Like caffeine and theobromine, theophylline is structurally classified as a xanthine derivative (1–4). Xanthine is an intermediate in the normal catabolism of purines in humans and has no known pharmacologic activity. The most popular nonalcoholic stimulant beverages of the world are prepared from plants containing derivatives of xanthine. For example, tea contains theophylline and coffee contains caffeine (5).

Theophylline has been used for more than 40 years as a mainstay in the treatment of bronchoconstriction secondary to bronchial asthma and reversible bronchospasm that may occur in association with chronic bronchitis or emphysema (6,7). It has also been used to relieve periodic apnea in the newborn and in augmenting diaphragmatic contractility in respiratory failure. Adverse effects and nonpurposeful overdose from theophylline occur relatively often because this drug has a narrow therapeutic index (8,9). There is also a wide variability among individuals in the clearance of theophylline (8). Cases of deliberate overdose and accidental accumulation of theophylline have been increasing in recent years (10–12).

THEOPHYLLINE DERIVATIVES

Although theophylline is the reference compound, structural modifications of the theophylline molecule by chemical synthesis generally result in derivatives that are less potent than theophylline, that have pharmacologic and toxic activities similar to theophylline, and that have altered pharmacokinetic parameters. Notable among these are aminophylline (theophylline ethylenediamine) and theophylline sodium acetate or glycinate. Oxtriphylline is the choline salt of theophylline (Table 66–1) (1–3).

TABLE 66–1. *Selected theophylline xanthine compounds by trade name*

Compound	Trade name
Theophylline	Accurbron Aquaphyllin Asmalix Elixicon Lanophyllin Liquophylline Physpan Theolixir Theon Theostat
Theophylline, sustained release formulations	Aerolate Aminodur Dura-tab Bronkodyl Constant-T Elixophyllin Quibron-T Respbid Slo-Phyllin Sustaire Theobid Theo-Dur Theolair Theospan Theovent Uniphyl
Oxtriphylline	Choledyl*
Aminophylline	Lixaminol Phyllocontin* Somophyllin*

Note: (*)Sustained release preparation available

Aminophylline

Aminophylline is the ethylenediamine salt of theophylline. On exposure to air, aminophylline solutions gradually liberate free theophylline (13,14). The ethylenediamine increases the solubility of theophylline in water approximately fivefold, which decreases the likelihood of volume overload (15). In the past, aminophylline was the only parenteral theophylline preparation available but there is an IV theophylline preparation now available that is not aminophylline. In this product, the theophylline is dissolved in dextrose thus allowing parenteral administration of theophylline itself without the potential adverse effects of ethylenediamine (16).

Diphylline

Dyphylline (dihydroxypropyltheophylline) is a distinct chemical entity that is pharmacologically similar to theophylline. It is a nontheophylline xanthine bronchodilator that is marketed in the United States under various trade names and is sometimes advertised as a theophylline derivative. Diphylline is not metabolized to theophylline and is similar to theophylline with respect to bronchodilator activity but at a dose approximately twice that of theophylline. In contrast to theophylline, dyphylline has little effect in preventing exercise-induced bronchospasm.

Sustained Release Formulations

In addition to plain tablets and capsules, there are at least 30 sustained release formulations of theophylline whose pharmacokinetic properties are prolonged (17,18). These preparations offer the potential advantages of longer dosing intervals and less fluctuation of serum concentration during long-term therapy (6). Many clinicians prefer the sustained release formulations over the regular formulations for these reasons (19).

CLINICAL USE

Four major clinical uses of theophylline are (a) bronchodilatation in patients with acute symptoms of asthma with or without an inhaled or ingested β2-adrenergic agonist, (b) maintenance therapy for prevention of symptoms and signs of chronic asthma (3,20), (c) treatment of recurrent apnea of prematurity (21) (not FDA-approved for this use), and (d) augmenting diaphragmatic contractility in respiratory failure (not FDA-approved for this use).

PHARMACOKINETICS

Bioavailability

There are major differences in the bioavailability of various theophylline preparations. Theophylline is not very water soluble and preparations have been manufactured in an attempt to increase its solubility (22). Theophylline does not form stable compounds with the various strong bases such as ethylenediamine, choline, or calcium salicylate that are used to produce the so-called salts. For all practical purposes, these substances are simply mixtures of theophylline and an excipient. For example, ethylenediamine (aminophylline) serves the purpose of increasing the pH sufficiently to allow theophylline to dissolve at a convenient concentration. Aminophylline is 85% theophylline and oxtriphylline, the choline salt of theophylline and the ingredient in many theophylline preparations such as Choledyl contains 64% theophylline (10). The calcium salt is approximately 50% theophylline. In recent years, there has been a trend back toward the use of anhydrous theophylline in the treatment of chronic asthma (Table 66–2).

TABLE 66–2. *Theophylline preparations and anhydrous theophylline content*

Drug	Anhydrous theophylline (%)
Aminophylline (anhydrous)	85
Aminophylline (hydrous)	79
Diphylline	0
Oxtriphylline	64
Theophylline calcium salicylate	50
Theophylline monohydrate	90
Theophylline sodium glycinate	46

Route of Administration

Theophylline concentrations in the blood reach their peak almost immediately after intravenous and intramuscular administration of the drug and approximately 2 to 3 hours after oral administration of tablets (23). Administration of theophylline in the form of an oral elixir usually produces a peak serum concentration of theophylline within 45 minutes. Enteric-coated theophylline tablets produce variable serum concentrations that usually peak at about 5 hours (24). The absorption from these slow-release preparations can continue for up to 12 hours after a therapeutic dose and overdose, producing peak concentrations up to or later than 12 to 24 hours (5,25). Rectal theophylline suppositories require 3 to 5 hours to produce serum concentrations (11,24). Because rectal suppositories result in erratic absorption, the drug must be in solution if this route is to be used. This is due to an increased absorption lag time or a prolonged absorption half-life.

Theophylline and Age

The pharmacokinetics of theophylline changes with age. Maximal clearance is thought to be achieved in patients 1 to 9 years of age. Clearance decreases in adolescence and tends to stabilize in the mid-teen years (26). The average half-life for theophylline is approximately 5 hours in adults but this varies widely. In young children, the half-life is slightly shorter (3.5 hrs), and in the newborn it is approximately 30 hours (27,28). Prolonged half-life in neonates and premature infants may be due to incomplete neonatal development of the cytochrome P-450 monoxygenase system, which is responsible for the

N-demethylation of this compound (29). In addition, the neonate metabolizes 20–30% of theophylline to caffeine, which does not occur in adults. There is also reduced protein binding of theophylline in full-term infants, which may result in increased free or pharmacologically active drug in any given serum concentration (30). This increased free drug-to-serum concentration ratio may produce toxic manifestations at serum concentrations generally considered nontoxic.

Metabolism

Most of an administered dose of theophylline is biotransformed by the hepatic cytochrome P-450 microsomal mixed-function oxygenase system, with less than 10% being eliminated unchanged in the urine (31,32). In the liver, theophylline is demethylated and oxidized to methylxanthine, dimethyluric acid, and methyl uric acid (10,11,13,14). These metabolites are inactive and are excreted in the urine. Hepatic cellular dysfunction is the most important cause of delayed theophylline elimination (33).

Theophylline and Michaelis-Menten Elimination

The metabolic pathways of degradation, especially the N-demethylation processes, are capacity limited; that is, the rate of elimination cannot increase proportionately to increases in drug concentration (2,3,34–36). As a result, the biologic half-life increases with increasing dose or plasma concentration (28,31). Theophylline follows Michaelis-Menten kinetics where at low serum levels, theophylline exhibits first-order kinetics, and at high serum levels, theophylline switches to zero-order kinetics (37). Therefore, in the therapeutic range, a small increase in the amount of drug administered may result in a disproportionately large increase in the serum level (38). This is an important aspect of pharmacological dosing because the elimination pattern changes in the therapeutic range that can lead to inadvertent toxicity with long-term administration.

Theophylline Clearance

Factors Increasing Serum Theophylline Concentration

Factors increasing the plasma half-life of theophylline and, therefore, the serum theophylline concentration include upper respiratory infections (39), sustained high fever, obesity, and administration of cimetidine (Table 66–3) (17,40). Other drugs that increase the half-life include the macrolide antibiotics erythromycin and troleandomycin (40,41). Troleandomycin has been shown to slow elimination of theophylline sufficiently to double its serum concentration. Elderly patients and those with congestive heart failure or severe liver disease (13,14) have a markedly reduced capacity to eliminate or metabolize theophylline. This may, therefore, result in chronic accumulation of the drug (42). Elderly patients and neonates may also have reduced theophylline clearance as a result of decreased protein binding (7).

TABLE 66–3. *Factors affecting theophylline half-life*

Effect on Factor	Half-life
Smoking	Decrease
Upper respiratory infection	Increase
Sustained high fever	Increase
Old age	Increase
Liver disease	Increase
Congestive heart failure	Increase
Corpulmonale	Increase
Use of oral contraceptive	Increase
Obesity	Increase
Infections	Increase
Drug interactions	
Allopurinol	Increase
Caffeine	Increase
Cimetidine	Increase
Erythromycin	Increase
Propranolol	Increase
Troleandomycin	Increase
Isoproterenol	Decrease
Phenobarbital	Decrease
Phenytoin	Decrease

Factors Decreasing Serum Theophylline Concentration

Habitual smoking can double the elimination of theophylline so that the half-life of theophylline in smokers (1 to 2 packs a day) is 4 to 5 hours, whereas that in nonsmokers averages 7 to 9 hours (43). Smoking results in the induction of drug-metabolizing enzymes in the liver microsomes, which are responsible for the increased rate of theophylline metabolism (5). In addition, simultaneous administration of phenytoin, phenobarbital, and intravenous isoproterenol decreases the half-life of theophylline (Table 66–3) (7).

Volume of Distribution and Protein Binding

The apparent volume of distribution of theophylline in adults and children is relatively constant averaging 0.5 L/kg (10,11). It is elevated in premature neonates to 0.69 L/kg and decreased in obese patients, but otherwise it is not significantly affected by age, sex, smoking, heart failure, or airway obstruction (44).

Approximately 60% of theophylline is bound to plasma proteins. Because serum theophylline reflects both the bound and unbound drug, a patient with hypoalbuminemia may have toxic symptoms at normal serum levels (45).

Actions

Theophylline has actions resembling those of the other xanthine derivatives such as caffeine and theobromine (Table 66–4). These actions are central nervous system stimulation, cardiac muscle stimulation, relaxation of smooth muscle, and diuresis (2,34,46). Theophylline has greater potency as a dilator of bronchial smooth muscle and as a relaxant of involuntary muscle than the other two derivatives. Its diuretic action, although stronger than that of caffeine, is of shorter duration. The pharmacologic actions of theophylline also include stimulation of respiration, cerebral vascular constriction, and gastric acid secretion; augmentation of cardiac inotropy and chronotropy; relaxation of uterine smooth muscle which inhibit uterine contractions (11).

Because it is a methylxanthine, theophylline increases plasma and urinary catecholamine concentrations (46,47). Theophylline also increases the release of catecholamines from the sympathoadrenal medullary system, increases cyclic adenosine monophosphate concentration, and inhibits nonneuronal uptake and metabolism of catecholamines (48). In addition, theophylline is a potent glycogenolytic, gluconeogenic, and lipolytic agent and is synergistic in these respects with the catecholamines (47,49).

Mechanism of Action

The methylxanthines inhibit the enzyme phosphodiesterase, which is responsible for the degradation of cyclic AMP. Thus, the actions of theophylline are due to an inhibition of an enzyme that normally breaks down the mediator of adrenergic activity (28,50). This results in bronchial smooth muscle relaxation and in the inhibition of the release of histamine by mast cells.

Although the elevated concentration of cyclic AMP has been cited to explain how theophylline produces bronchodilation, the concentrations obtained do not appear to be sufficient to produce this effect, nor does this theory explain why other phosphodiesterase inhibitors do not result in bronchodilation (2,3,6,50,51). Many believe that at therapeutic concentrations, theophylline binds to adenosine receptors and functions pharmacologically either as an adenosine agonist or antagonist, depending on the tissue exposed to theophylline. It is the adenosine receptor that directly influences the activity of adenyl cyclase. Other proposed mechanisms of action of theophylline include inhibition of prostaglandin activity with consequent decreased contraction of bronchial smooth muscle, stimulation of catecholamine release, beta-adrenergic receptor agonism (2,6,51).

TABLE 66–4. *Actions of theophylline*

Diuresis
Relaxes involuntary smooth muscle bronchi (blood vessels, uterus)
Increases plasma catecholamines
Increases cyclic AMP
Stimulates respiration
Stimulates cerebrovascular constriction
Stimulates gastric acid secretion
Increases glycogenolysis
Increases lipolysis
Increases cardiac inotropy and chronotropy

Serum Theophylline Concentration

Serum theophylline concentrations are among the most clinically useful of all the serum drug concentrations that can be measured (38). Assays to measure the serum concentration of theophylline have improved the ability to diagnose theophylline intoxication and assess its prognosis (52). The immunoassay and HPLC techniques are specific and reliable for measuring serum theophylline levels. In the older spectrophotometirc methods, other methylxanthines contributed to a false positive.

It has been shown that theophylline concentrations of 10 μg/mL to 20 μg/mL (55 to 110 μmol/L) are needed to produce maximal bronchodilation; some patients with mild pulmonary disease experience relief of bronchospasm with serum theophylline concentrations of 5 μg/mL (7). Because of the low therapeutic index for theophylline, serum concentrations only slightly higher than the therapeutic range may be toxic. There is a wide variability among patients in the overlapping of the therapeutic and toxic serum ranges for theophylline. This overlapping can occur even in the conventional range of 10 to 20 μg/mL (18,31,53).

Each increase of 1 μg/mL in serum concentration requires a loading dose of approximately 0.5 mg/kg; in other words, each mg per kg of theophylline administered will result in an average increase of 2 μg/mL in serum theophylline concentration. As an example, if the patient has a known subtherapeutic serum level of theophylline, the loading dose of theophylline to produce a higher serum concentration can be calculated as follows:

Loading Dose = Desired level - Existing level × 0.5 L/kg

Plasma concentrations of theophylline may change as a result of a change in dosage interval of the drug, the rate of biotransformation, the rate of clearance from the body, or the volume of distribution (54,55). Because of the many factors that may account for different clearance rates of theophylline (see Table 66–3), it is difficult to design a safe and effective dosage regimen without monitoring plasma concentrations (8).

There is an important difference between chronic and acute theophylline intoxication because of the lag between the serum concentration and toxic effect (19).

Therefore, at a given serum concentration, patients with chronic theophylline intoxication may experience more severe symptoms than patients with acute theophylline intoxication.

TOXICITY

As with all drugs having a narrow therapeutic index, the potential for accidental poisoning with theophylline is, therefore, significant. Theophylline intoxication is a common problem that occurs in two distinct settings: chronic and acute intoxication (46,48,56). Patients who have been repeatedly administered standard doses of the drug may develop subacute or chronic intoxication that is often attributable to excessive dosage or decreased clearance due to heart failure, liver disease, or drug interactions. Such patients may have serious complications at blood concentrations that are just above the therapeutic range. Chronic theophylline intoxication may occur when the dose of theophylline administered on a repeated basis is excessive compared with the patients' capacity to metabolize and excrete it (24). Acute accidental or suicidal overdoses of theophylline may result in high blood concentrations that may be somewhat better tolerated initially than in the chronically intoxicated patient.

Sustained Release Preparations

Ingestion of an overdose of a sustained release theophylline preparation may cause dramatic late increases in serum theophylline concentration. The delay before the onset of symptoms may be as many as 10 hours and there may be a prolonging of toxic manifestations as well (17,18).

Clinical Manifestations of Toxicity

The clinical manifestations of theophylline intoxication (Table 66–5) result from an accentuation of the drug's pharmacologic effects. The systems mainly affected are the gastrointestinal system, the cardiovascular system, and the central nervous system (10,46,56). Because theophylline has been shown to stimulate catecholamine release, acute theophylline poisoning may produce a state of increased beta-adrenergic stimulation that accounts for many of the toxic effects, including cardiac dysrhythmias, hypotension, tremor, agitation, and metabolic disturbances (46).

The most frequently reported gastrointestinal symptoms are nausea, vomiting, dyspepsia, abdominal pain, and generalized gastrointestinal symptoms (10). Neurologic symptoms most frequently reported are anxiety, irritability, restlessness, seizures, and headache. Cardiovascular manifestations affect both the heart and the vasculature. In the heart, theophylline toxicity can produce both supraventricular and ventricular dysrhythmias (22). Among supra-ventricular dysrhythmias encountered are sinus tachycardia, multifocal atrial tachycardia, and atrial flutter and fibrillation. The most frequently reported metabolic disorders seen are dehydration, hypokalemia, and hyperglycemia (57).

TABLE 66–5. *Clinical manifestations of theophylline intoxication*

Mild
Anorexia
Abdominal pain
Vomiting
Moderate
Cardiac
Sinus tachycardia
Hypertension
Hypotension
Neurologic
Increased wakefulness
Restlessness
Irritability
Tremor
Hallucinations
Severe
Cardiac dysrhythmia
Neurologic
Seizures
Coma
Metabolic
Hyperthermia
Hypokalemia
Hyperkalemia
Hyperglycemia
Hypophosphatemia
Metabolic acidosis

Hemodynamic changes are dose dependent. At low doses, theophylline induces a transitory hypertension secondary to an increase in cardiac output and total peripheral resistance. At high doses, the direct effect of theophylline on the blood vessels predominates (58). This β_2-adrenergic effect reduces the total peripheral resistance, resulting in decreased blood pressure. Elderly patients have an inordinately greater risk of a life-threatening event than younger patients.

Mild Intoxication

Theophylline toxicity increases in parallel with serum theophylline concentration and increases notably at serum concentrations exceeding 20 μg/mL (18,31). Adverse effects observed with serum theophylline concentrations greater than 20 μg/mL include gastrointestinal reactions, an early sign of toxicity that may be misdiagnosed as evidence of a gastrointestinal abnormality not attributable to drug toxicity (59). Vomiting is a common early sign of toxicity from all routes of administration and reflects stimulation of the medulla oblongata (10,11). Vomiting may also be partly due to an irritation of the gastric mucosa and an increase in the volume of gastric secretions. Diarrhea may also be noted as a result of increased secretion of fluid by the intestinal mucosa (10,11). Vomiting is generally violent and persistent but may be slight or absent in poisonings from sustained-release preparations.

Other early signs of toxicity are restlessness and irritability, which are attributable to the stimulatory actions of theophylline on all parts of the central nervous system. These actions may progress to extreme agitation, tremors, delirium, seizures, and coma.

Moderate Intoxication

A moderate overdose of theophylline may produce symptoms of increased wakefulness, mild sinus tachycardia, tachydysrhythmias, and hypertension or hypotension (11). Hypotension is a common but poorly understood complication of massive theophylline ingestion. It is frequently refractory to conventional vasopressors and contributes significantly to mortality. Hyperthermia, albuminuria, and dehydration may also be noted. As toxicity increases, vomiting becomes more frequent and hematemesis may ensue. Manic behavior as well as hallucinations may be noted.

Severe Intoxication

Life-threatening theophylline toxicity includes cardiac dysrhythmias, seizures, dehydration, severe metabolic abnormalities, extreme hyperthermia, coma, and death. Although seizures have been associated with theophylline concentrations as low as 25 μg/mL, they are usually associated with concentrations of 40 to 50 μg/mL (46). Seizures are usually preceded by other signs of drug toxicity, although they have occurred without any prodromal signs (60). When seizures do occur in the low toxic range in chronically intoxicated patients, these patients often have cirrhosis, cor pulmonale, viral illnesses, prior history of seizures, congestive heart failure, or focal central nervous system lesions as well (41). Acutely intoxicated patients may not have seizures until a serum concentration of approximately 90 μg/mL is attained (47). The actual mechanism of action by which theophylline causes seizures is unknown. Once seizures have occurred, the outcome in cases of both acute and chronic theophylline poisoning is often poor regardless of the therapy used (21,48,61). For this reason, there has been considerable interest in using hemodialysis or hemoperfusion to remove the drug before seizures occur (62).

Metabolic Abnormalities

Metabolic abnormalities are an aspect of theophylline toxicity that has not been previously well recognized (63). Metabolic abnormalities include hyperglycemia, hypophosphatemia, leukocytosis, and, less commonly, hyperkalemia (10,11,48,63,64). Metabolic acidosis has also been reported and is probably due to accumulation of lactic acid secondary to increased glycolysis in muscles (48). These abnormalities are characteristic features of acute but not of chronic theophylline overdose and may be related to the adrenergic overdrive (65). Hypokalemia and hyperglycemia appear to result from hyperinsulinemia and glycogenolysis (11).

Hypokalemia

Hypokalemia is common after theophylline intoxication and distinct metabolic profiles appear depending on the method of intoxication (65). Hypokalemia is most severe in those with acute theophylline intoxication and can be correlated with serum theophylline concentrations. In chronic intoxication, hypokalemia is less common and does not correlate with the serum theophylline concentration. Elevated serum concentration of insulin and glucose promotes an intracellular shift of glucose and potassium that results in relative hypokalemia (47). This does not represent a total body depletion of potassium but results from various cellular shifts of fluid and electrolyte (10). Hypokalemia may also be a result of vomiting and diarrhea. These abnormalities are not usually associated with clinical or electrocardiographic changes (62).

ACUTE VERSUS CHRONIC RISK FACTORS

When compared with acute theophylline intoxication, chronic toxicity causes a lower frequency of vomiting, lower rate of hypokalemia, a greater frequency of seizures and cardiac arrhythmias, and a lack of correlation between peak serum theophylline concentrations and clinical course.

Seizures occur both in acute and chronic intoxications. Although unlikely at concentrations of less than 100 μg/mL after acute ingestion in adults, seizures are seen at much lower concentrations after chronic overmedication.

The risk of life-threatening theophylline toxicity depends on the chronicity of the overdose. Patients with acute single theophylline ingestion typically tolerate levels of up to 80 to 100 μg/mL without seizures or other serious complications. Older patients with a higher prevalence of underlying cardiopulmonary disease are also more susceptible to life-threatening complications. Acute overdose is, therefore, suggested by a history of suicidal or accidental single ingestion and the presence of hypotension, hypokalemia, and metabolic acidosis. With acute overdose, seizures and severe cardiovascular manifestations are unlikely to occur unless peak serum concentrations are high (greater than 80 μg/mL).

TABLE 66–6. *Laboratory determinations in theophylline overdose*

Toxicologic screen
Serum theophylline concentration
Serum electrolytes
Arterial blood gas
Electrocardiogram

LABORATORY DETERMINATIONS

The concentration of theophylline is important to measure, and a toxicologic screen may be necessary to rule out co-ingestants (Table 66–6). In the severely intoxicated patient, theophylline concentration should be measured at frequent intervals to ensure that clearance is not prolonged. In cases of a potentially toxic overdose with a sustained release formulation, early plasma theophylline concentrations will not reflect accurately the degree of intoxication; concentrations should be measured every 2 hours until a peak is reached, and then every 4 hours when the concentration is declining, until a therapeutic level is attained (19).

Because of the various electrolyte abnormalities that may ensue, serum electrolytes are also important to monitor (46). A determination of arterial blood gas may also be necessary. In addition to continuous cardiac monitoring, an electrocardiogram should also be obtained. Examination of the gastric contents and stool for blood may be necessary as well (46).

After an acute intoxication, serum theophylline concentrations correlate with the development of toxic manifestations. When patients are chronically intoxicated, the correlation between theophylline serum concentrations and the appearance of serious toxic manifestations is less obvious. Relatively low concentrations over a long period may result in more neurotoxicity and poorer outcome than high concentrations in acute intoxication. Peak serum theophylline concentration cannot predict which patients with chronic theophylline intoxication will have a life-threatening event.

Age is also an important factor to consider when interpreting theophylline serum concentrations. Older patients seem to experience serious toxic manifestations such as seizures and dysrhythmias at lower concentrations than those that induce such symptoms in children.

TREATMENT

Every theophylline overdose should be regarded as potentially fatal and all patients should be closely observed (Table 66–7). (12,47). Most patients with acute theophylline intoxication can be managed in a traditional manner that includes careful attention to serum electrolytes, acid-base balance, glucose, and neurologic complications. Cardiovascular monitoring should also be performed until theophylline concentration and the patient's clinical course have excluded the possibility of toxicity.

TABLE 66–7. *Treatment of theophylline overdose*

Indication	Treatment
Acute overdose	Gastric lavage Charcoal, and cathartic Pulse charcoal
Hypotension	Fluids
Hypotension	Pressor agents
Supraventricular tachycardia	Verapamil
Ventricular ectopy	Lidocaine
Ventricular ectopy	B_1 blocking agent
Seizures	Diazepam
Refractory seizures, refractory dysrhythmias, deterioration	Hemoperfusion or dialysis

Because of the differences in pharmacokinetic characteristics of sustained formulations, the approach to a patient who had an overdose with these preparations must be modified. In the absence of toxicity, observation on the basis of history alone may be necessary for a much longer period than for conventional formulations (18). It should be remembered that theophylline may still be in the stomach hours after ingestion because of a sustained-release preparation ingested or due to the formation of concretions (66). Pharmacobezoars have also been reported with sustained release theophylline preparations (57).

Standard techniques to reduce drug absorption such as emptying the stomach via gastric lavage should be performed in the acute overdose (11) followed by the administration of activated charcoal and a cathartic (66–70). This may be useful even late after an acute overdose, especially if a sustained release preparation has been ingested. Most theophylline overdoses respond to supportive measures (12). Whole-bowel irritation has also been suggested (57,71,72).

Treatment of Metabolic Abnormalities

Biochemical abnormalities respond to conservative management and resolve rapidly with fluid replacement and modest potassium supplementation (22). Administration of phenothiazines for intractable hyperthermia may be warranted in life-threatening situations (58). Conventional antiemetics do not appear to relieve vomiting (47), but the administration of H_2 antagonists such as ranitidine (50 mg every 6 hours) or droperidol (5 mg intravenously) has been successful in controlling vomiting (34). Ranitidine is a good choice because, unlike cimetidine, it does not interfere with the clearance of theophylline.

Supplementation of potassium is necessary in most cases; and in adults, up to 40 to 60 mmol/hr may be necessary in the first few hours, yet moderate supplements of potassium may suffice. Monitoring of serum potassium concentrations should be performed because as theophylline concentrations decrease, the initial intracellular shift of potassium may revert with spontaneous resolution of hypokalemia.

Treatment of Cardiac Abnormalities

Sinus tachycardia should be intensively observed rather than treated, unless there are significant adverse effects on the circulation. Although verapamil has been used effectively for the supraventricular tachycardia associated with theophylline overdose, there are reports of increased mortality with the use of this drug. Therefore, verapamil should not be used until further studies are performed (10,11). Lidocaine may be of benefit for ventricular ectopy. A cardiospecific β-adrenergic blocking agent may be useful in the treatment of serious tachydysrhythmias because catecholamine release has been implicated in their genesis.

Propranolol may prevent or reverse the metabolic and cardiovascular consequences of theophylline toxicity. The risk of precipitating bronchospasm with its administration to patients with asthma is uncertain, however, and caution should be exercised in this patient population. An ultra-short-acting parenteral β-blocking agent such as esmolol may be useful because it is easily titratable and disappears rapidly from the circulation. Hypotension should be initially treated with intravenous crystalloid. Hypotension that does not respond to intravenous fluids can be treated with the cautious administration of pressor agents (66–68).

Treatment of Seizures

Seizures may be treated with diazepam. As an alternative, the prophylactic administration of phenobarbital to prevent seizures and associated complications should be considered for patients with severe theophylline intoxication (10,11,66–68). Seizures secondary to theophylline toxicity are frequently refractory to diazepam, phenobarbital, and phenytoin; nevertheless, these agents should be tried (25,66–68). Status seizures that are unresponsive to those drugs may merit treatment with paralyzing drugs and general anesthesia.

Attempts To Enhance Elimination

Diuresis

Although theophylline is a weak base, there is probably little to be gained by acidification of the urine to enhance excretion. In addition, because theophylline is mainly metabolized by the liver with only a fraction excreted unchanged in the urine, it is unlikely that forced diuresis would significantly increase elimination.

Multiple-Dose Activated Charcoal

Multiple-dose activated charcoal can be administered in an attempt to increase elimination of theophylline by the gastrointestinal tract (34,72). This has been successful in the removal of other drugs, such as phenobarbital, carbamazepine, and phenylbutazone (52,61,74). Some studies have shown a twofold increase in the systemic elimination of theophylline when multiple-dose activated charcoal is administered.

Oral activated charcoal is, therefore, useful in the acute overdose because it adsorbs the drug and also because it may promote drug elimination, thereby shortening the duration of toxic symptoms (48,75). This latter action is due to gastrointestinal dialysis, whereby the charcoal absorbs the drug entering the intestine, which acts as a dialysis membrane (19,52,76,77) (see Chapter 3). Although biliary excretion of theophylline has not been demonstrated (72), activated charcoal appears to enhance the rate of diffusion into the intestines by absorbing theophylline in gastrointestinal fluids, thereby maintaining a constant diffusion gradient into the intestine (78). This method has been shown to reduce the serum half-life of theophylline that is administered both intravenously and orally (76).

Activated charcoal should be administered in dosages of 0.5 to 1 g/kg every 2 to 4 hours until serum theophylline concentrations are within normal limits (77). Unless there are specific indications, a cathartic should be administered only once.

Early treatment with orally administered activated charcoal, although it may enhance theophylline elimination, may not avert a large delayed elevation in serum theophylline concentrations in patients who have ingested sustained release preparations (18).

The efficacy of MDAC is comparable with that of hemodialysis, increasing theophylline clearance by approximately 50 ml/min (66).

Extracorporeal Removal

Because of the relatively low protein binding (about 40%) and small volume of distribution, theophylline is one of the few drugs commonly taken in overdose in which an extracorporeal technique can remove a large proportion of the total body burden of the drug (25). Yet, the role of extracorporeal means of removal of theophylline is controversial. Hemodialysis (79) and hemoperfusion (80,82) have been shown to increase plasma clearance of theophylline, yet no controlled studies of the use of these methods have been performed (17,47). Although there seems to be the potential for theophylline-intoxicated patients to benefit significantly from hemodialysis or hemoperfusion, these procedures are expensive and not without risks, including hypotension, bleeding, hemolysis (66), hypocalcemia, thrombocytopenia, and sepsis (10,11,48). In addition, both hemodialysis and hemoperfusion are invasive and require time and specialized facilities before they can be instituted. Peritoneal dialysis in the clinical situation does not produce a significant increase in total body clearance compared with endogenous removal of theophylline (83). Peritoneal dialysis or exchange transfusion cannot significantly increase theophylline clearance and thus have no place in therapy. Hemoperfusion is considered the definitive therapy for theophylline intoxication and is capable of increasing theophylline clearance by 150 to 200 ml/min (84).

Hemodialysis

Hemodialysis can be expected to double the rate of drug elimination, although it is far less effective than hemoperfusion, which increases clearance four- to sixfold. Hemodialysis may rarely be an alternative if hemoperfusion is not available or in series with hemoperfusion if significant rhabdomyolysis is present.

Hemoperfusion

Hemoperfusion has been recommended for serum theophylline levels of greater than 60 μg/ml for chronic overdose, and over 100 μg/mL for an acute overdose. However, all patients with intractable seizures or arrhythmias or clinical deterioration should be hemoperfused if their level is ≥20 mg/L (25,83). Hemoperfusion with a resin column or an activated charcoal column appears to be more effective than hemodialysis in removing theophylline (10,11,17,81,85,86). In most patients, a 4-hour hemoperfusion is long enough to allow significant clinical improvement (25). Also, a rebound effect is possible when hemoperfusion is completed (6,80,87) and, therefore, after hemoperfusion, drug concentrations should be further monitored for at least 12 hours (25).

Although hemoperfusion is the most efficient method for removing theophylline, multiple-dose activated charcoal is less expensive, more widely accessible, and probably safer (72,74). Because hemoperfusion is an extracorporeal system of removal, it should only be performed in a hemodialysis area or an intensive care unit by a physician and technical team familiar with the procedure. If hemoperfusion is performed because of signs of neurotoxicity such as seizures, it should be done as early as possible (88).

In the acute overdose with serum concentrations less than 80 μg/mL, patients have been managed with supportive care alone. In the chronic overdose, in patients with underlying cardiovascular disease, in clinically unstable patients, or in patients with a high serum concentration that is still increasing, extracorporeal means may be attempted early in the course.

Recommended levels should, however, remain as guidelines, and plasma concentrations alone should not determine whether or not hemoperfusion should be performed.

Conservative Management

The vast majority of theophylline overdoses can be managed in a traditional manner with careful monitoring, intensive supportive measures, and thorough evacuation of the remaining drug from the gastrointestinal tract (5). Repeated doses of activated charcoal should be administered at least until charcoal is visible in the stool. Patients may recover completely from a substantial overdose with conservative management (89–92).

REFERENCES

1. Weinberger M, Riegelman S: Rational use of theophylline for bronchodilatation. *N Engl J Med* 1974;291:151–153.
2. Weinberger M: Theophylline for treatment of asthma. *J Pediatr* 1978; 92:1–7.
3. Weinberger M: The pharmacology and therapeutic use of theophylline. *J Allergy Clin Immunol* 1984;73:525–541.
4. Labovita E, Spector S: Placental theophylline transfer in pregnant asthmatics. *JAMA* 1982;247:786–788.
5. Miech R, Stein M: Methylxanthines. *Clin Chest Med* 1986;7: 331–340.
6. Heath A, Knudsen K: Role of extracorporeal drug removal in acute theophylline poisoning: a review. *Med Toxicol* 1987;2:294–308.
7. Mountain R, Neff T: Oral theophylline intoxication. *Arch Intern Med* 1984;144:724–727.
8. Elenbaas R, Payne V: Prediction of serum theophylline levels. *Ann Intern Med* 1984;13:92–96.
9. Greenberg A, Piraino B, Kroboth P, et al: Severe theophylline toxicity. *Am J Med* 1984;76:854–860.
10. Gaudreault P, Guay J: Theophylline poisoning. *Med Toxicol* 1986;1: 169–191.
11. Gaudreault P, Wason S, Lovejoy F: Acute pediatric theophylline overdose: a summary of 28 cases. *J Pediatr* 1983;102:474–476.
12. Mant T, Cochrane M, Henry J: ABCs of poisoning: respiratory drugs. *Br Med J* 1984;289:1133–1135.
13. Piafsky K, Sitar D, Rangno R, et al: Theophylline disposition in patients with hepatic cirrhosis. *N Engl J Med* 1976;296:1495–1497.
14. Piafsky K, Ogilvie R: Dosage of theophylline in bronchial asthma. *N Engl J Med* 1973;292:1218–1222.
15. Terzian C: Aminophylline hypersensitivity apparently due to ethylenediamine. *Ann Emerg Med* 1992;21:312–317.
16. Wrenn K, Slovis C, Murphy F, et al: Aminophylline therapy for acute bronchospastic disease in the emergency room. *Ann Intern Med* 1991; 115:241–247.
17. Ahlemen C, Heath A, Herlitz H, et al: Treatment of oral theophylline poisoning. *Acta Med Scand* 1984;216:423–426.
18. Corser B, Youngs C, Baughman R: Prolonged toxicity following massive ingestion of sustained release theophylline preparation. *Chest* 1985;88:749–750.
19. Minocha A, Spyker D: Acute overdose with sustained release drug formulations. *Med Toxicol* 1986;1:300–307.
20. McFadden E: Methylxanthines in the treatment of asthma: the rise, the fall, and the possible rise again. *Ann Intern Med* 1991;115: 323–324.
21. Gal P, Roop C, Robinson H, et al: Theophylline induced seizures in accidentally overdosed neonates. *Pediatrics* 1980;65:547–549.

22. Sessler C: Theophylline toxicity: clinical features of 116 consecutive cases. *Am J Med* 1990;88:566–576.
23. Carrier J, Shaw R, Porter R, et al: Comparison of intravenous and oral routes of theophylline loading in acute asthma. *Ann Emerg Med* 1985;14:1145–1151.
24. Powell E, Reynolds S, Rubenstein J: Theophylline toxicity in children: a retrospective review. *Pediatr Emerg Care* 1993;9:129–133.
25. Heath A, Knudsen K: Role of extracorporeal drug removal in acute theophylline poisoning. *Med Toxicol* 1987;2:294–308.
26. Rangsithienchai R, Newcomb R: Aminophylline therapy in children: guidelines for dosage. *J Pediatr* 1977;91:325–330.
27. Rosen J, Danish M, Ragni M, et al: Theophylline pharmacokinetics in the young infant. *Pediatrics* 1979;64:248–251.
28. Rothstein R: Intravenous theophylline therapy in asthma: a clinical update. *Ann Emerg Med* 1980;9:327–330.
29. Simons F, Friesen F, Simons K: Theophylline toxicity in term infants. *Am J Dis Child* 1980;134:39–41.
30. Arwood L, Dasta J, Friedman C: Placental transfer of theophylline: two case reports. *Pediatrics* 1979;63:844–846.
31. Davis R, Ellsworth A, Justus R, et al: Reversal of theophylline toxicity using oral activated charcoal. *J Fam Prac* 1985;20:73–75.
32. Mangione A, Imhoff T. Lee R, et al: Pharmacokinetics of theophylline in hepatic disease. *Chest* 1978;73:616–622.
33. Spivey J, Laughlin P, Goss T, et al: Theophylline toxicity secondary to ciprofloxacin administration. *Ann Emerg Med* 1991;20: 1131–1134.
34. Amitai Y, Yeung A, Moye J, et al: Repetitive oral activated charcoal and control of emesis in severe theophylline toxicity. *Ann Intern Med* 1986;105:386–387.
35. Weinberger M, Matthay R, Ginchansky E, et al: Intravenous aminophylline dosage. *JAMA* 1976;235:2110–2113.
36. Weinberger M, Bronsky E, Bensch G, et al: Interaction of ephedrine and theophylline. *Clin Pharmacol Ther* 1975;17:585–592.
37. Kadlec G, Jarboe C, Pollard S, et al: Acute theophylline intoxication: biphasic first-order elimination kinetics in a child. *Ann Allergy* 1978;41:337–339.
38. Butts J, Secrest B, Berger R: Nonlinear thoephylline pharmacokinetics. A preventable cause of iatrogenic theophyllione toxic reactions. *Arch Intern Med* 1991;151:2073–2077.
39. Vozeh S, Powell R, Riegelman S, et al: Changes in theophylline clearance during acute illness. *JAMA* 1978;240:1882–1884.
40. Jackson J, Powell J, Wandell M, et al: Cimetidine decreases theophylline clearance. *Am Rev Respir Dis* 1981;123:615–617.
41. Bahls F, Ma K, Bird T: Theophylline-associated seizures with "therapeutic" or low toxic serum concentrations: risk factors for serious outcome in adults. *Neurol* 1991;41:1309–1312.
42. Tenenbein M: Theophylline toxicity due to drug interaction. *J Emerg Med* 1989;7:249–251.
43. Brown J, Hoffman R, Aaron C, et al: Theophylline therapy. *Ann Emerg Med* 1989;18:425–427.
44. Stine R, Marcus R, Parvin C: Aminophylline loading in asthmatic patients: a protocol trial. *Ann Emerg Med* 1989;18:640–646.
45. McGuigan M, Tenenbein M: Planning an effective strategy for theophylline poisoning in adults. *Emerg Med Rep* 1987;8:41–48.
46. Albert S: Aminophylline toxicity. *Pediatr Clin North Am* 1987;34:61–73.
47. Kearney T, Manoguerra A, Curtis G, et al: Theophylline toxicity and the β-adrenergic system. *Ann Intern Med* 1985;102:766–769.
48. Biberstein M, Ziegler M, Ward D: Use of beta-blockade and hemoperfusion for acute theophylline poisoning. *West J Med* 1984;141: 485–490.
49. Vaucher Y, Lightner E, Watxon P: Theophylline poisoning. *J Pediatr* 1977;90:827–83.
50. Marney S: Asthma: Recent developments in treatment. *South Med J* 1985;78:1084–1096.
51. Weinberger M, Hendeles L, Wong L, et al: Relationship of formulation and dosing interval to fluctuation of serum theophylline concentration in children with chronic asthma. *J Pediatr* 1981;99: 145–152.
52. Brashear R, Aronoff G, Brier R: Activated charcoal in theophylline intoxication. *J Lab Clin Med* 1985;106:242–245.
53. Olson K, Benowitz N, Woo O, et al: Theophylline overdose: acute single ingestion versus chronic repeated overmedication. *J Emerg Med* 1985;3:386–394.
54. Jacobs M, Senior R, Kessler G: Clinical experience with theophylline. *JAMA* 1976;235:1983–1986.
55. Jenne J, Wyze E, Rood F, et al: Pharmacokinetics of theophylline. *Clin Pharmacol Ther* 1972;13:349–360.
56. Bertino J, Walker J: Reassessment of theophylline toxicity. *Arch Intern Med* 1987;147:757–760.
57. Bernstein G, Jehle D, Bermaslo E. et al: Failure of gastric emptying and charcoal administration in fatal sustained-release theophylline overdose: pharmacobezoar formation.*Ann Emerg Med* 1992;21: 1388–1390.
58. Bernard S: Severe lactic acidosis following theophylline overdose. *Ann Emerg Med* 1991:20:1135–1137.
59. Anderson J, Poklis A, Slavin R: A fatal case of theophylline intoxication. *Arch Intern Med* 1983;143:559–560.
60. Zwillich C, Sutton R, Neff T, et al: Theophylline induced seizures in adults. *Ann Intern Med* 1975;82:784–787.
61. Gal P, Miller A, McCue J: Oral activated charcoal to enhance theophylline elimination in an acute overdose. *JAMA* 1984;251: 3130–3131.
62. Anderson W, Youl, B, Mackay I: Acute theophylline toxicity. *Ann Emerg Med* 1991;20:1143–1145.
63. Hall K, Dobson K, Dalton J, et al: Metabolic abnormalities associated with intentional theophylline overdose. *Ann Intern Med* 1984;101: 457–462.
64. Sawyer W, Caravati M, Ellison M, et al: Hypokalemia, hyperglycemia, and acidosis after intentional theophylline overdose. *J Emerg Med* 1985;3:408–410.
65. Amitai Y, Lovejoy F: Hypokalemia in acute theophylline poisoning. *Am J Emerg Med* 1988;6:214–218.
66. Goldberg M, Park G. Berlinger W: Treatment of theophylline intoxication.*J Allergy Clin Immunol* 1986;78:811–817.
67. Goldberg M, Spector R, Miller G: Phenobarbital improves survival in theophylline-intoxicated rabbits. *Clin Toxicol* 1986;24:203–211.
68. Goldberg M, Spector R, Park G, et al: The effect of sorbitol and activated charcoal on serum theophylline concentrations after slow-release theophylline. *Clin Pharmacol Ther* 1987;41:108–111.
69. Lim D, Sing P, Nourtsis S, et al: Absorption inhibition and enhancement of elimination of sustained-release theophylline tablets by oral activated charcoal. *Ann Emerg Med* 1986;15:1303–1307.
70. True R, Berman J. Mahutte K: Treatment of theophylline toxicity with oral activated charcoal. *Crit Care Med* 1984;12:113–114.
71. Buckley N, Dawson A: Whole-bowel irrigatio for theophylline overdose.*Ann Emerg Med* 1993;22:1774–1775.
72. Burkhart K, Wuerz R, Donovan J: Whole-bowel irrigation as adjunctive treatment for sustained-release theophylline overdose. *Ann Emerg Med* 1992;21:1316–1320.
73. Kulig K, Bar-Or D, Rumack B: Intravenous theophylline poisoning and multiple dose charcoal in an animal model. *Ann Emerg Med* 1987;16:842–846.
74. Berlinger W, Spector R, Goldberg M, et al: Enhancement of theophylline clearance by oral activated charcoal. *Clin Pharmacol Ther* 1982;33:351–354.
75. Park G, Spector R, Roberts R, et al: Use of hemoperfusion for treatment of theophylline intoxication. *Am J Med* 1983;74:961–966.
76. Ginoza G, Strauss A, Iskra M, et al: Potential treatment of theophylline toxicity by high surface area activated charcoal. *J Pediatr* 1987;1:140–143.
77. Shannon M, Amitai Y, Lovejoy F: Multiple-dose activated charcoal for theophylline poisoning in young infants. *Pediatrics* 1987;8: 368–370.
78. Levy G: Gastrointestinal clearance of drugs with activated charcoal. *N Engl J Med* 1982;307:676–678.
79. Levy C, Gibson T, Whitman W, et al: Hemodialysis clearance of theophylline. *JAMA* 1977;237:1466–1467.
80. Lawyer C, Aitchison J, Sutton J, et al: Treatment of theophylline neurotoxicity with resin hemoperfusion. *Ann Intern Med* 1978;88: 516–517.
81. Laggner A, Kaik G, Lenz K, et al: Treatment of severe poisoning with slow release theophylline. *Br Med J* 1984;288:1497.
82. Gallagher E, Howland M, Greenblatt H: Hemolysis following treatment of theophylline overdose with coated charcoal hemoperfusion. *J Emerg Med* 1987;5:19–22.
83. Russo M: Management of theophylline intoxication with charcoal-column hemoperfusion. *N Engl J Med* 1979;30:24–26.

84. Ohning B, Reed M, Blumer J: Continuous nasogastric administration of activated charcoal for the treatment of theophylline intoxication. *Pediatr Pharmacol* 1986;5:241–245.
85. Chang T, Espinosa-Melendez E, Francoeur T, et al: Albumin-Collodion activated charcoal hemoperfusion in the treatment of severe theophylline intoxication in a 3-year-old patient. *Pediatrics* 1980;65: 811–814.
86. Woo O, Pond S, Benowitz N, et al: Benefit of hemoperfusion in acute theophylline intoxication. *Clin Toxicol* 1984;22:411–424.
87. Connell J, McGeachie J, Knepil J, et al: Self-poisoning with sustained-release aminophylline: secondary rise in serum theophylline concentration after charcoal hemoperfusion. *Br Med J* 1982;284:943.
88. Kelly W, Parkin W: Charcoal hemoperfusion treatment of severe theophylline toxicity. *Aust N Z J Med* 1985;15:75–77.
89. Kossoy A, Weir M: Potentially toxic theophylline ingestions: are heroic measures indicated? *South Med J* 1985;78:1000–1002.
90. Hendeles L, Bighley L, Richardson R: Frequent toxicity from IV aminophylline infusions in critically ill patients. *Drug Intell Clin Pharmacol* 1977;11:12–18.
91. Weibert R: Theophylline. *Clin Toxicol* 1979;14:157–160.
92. Whyte K, Addis G: Treatment of theophylline poisoning. *Br Med J* 1984;288:1835–1838.

ADDITIONAL SELECTED REFERENCES

Baker M: Theophylline toxicity in children. *J Pediatr* 1986;109:538.

Cereda J, Scott J, Quigley E: Endoscopic removal of pharmacobezoar of slow release theophylline. *Br Med J* 1986;293:1143.

Jusko W, Koup J, Vance J, et al: Intravenous theophylline therapy: nomogram guidelines. *Ann Intern Med* 1977;86:400–404.

Kordash T, Van dellen R, McCall J: Theophylline concentrations in asthmatic patients. *JAMA* 1977;238:139–141.

Miceli J, Bidani A, Aronow R, et al: Peritoneal dialysis of theophylline. *Clin Toxicol* 1979;14:539–544

Mitenko P, Ogilvie R: Bioavailability and efficacy of a sustained-release theophylline tablet. *Clin Pharmacol Ther* 1974;16:720–726.

Mitenko P, Ogilvie R: Rational intravenous doses of theophylline. *N Engl J Med* 1973;289:600–603.

Scott P, Tabachnik E, MacLeod S, et al: Sustained-release theophylline for childhood asthma: evidence for circadian variation of theophylline pharmacokinetics. *J Pediatr* 1981;99:476–479.

Stine R, Marcus R, Parvin C: Clinical predictors of theophylline blood levels in asthmatic patients. *Ann Emerg Med* 1987;16:18–24.

Tattersfield A: Bronchodilator drugs. *Pharmacol Ther* 1982;17: 299–313.

Wyatt R, Weinberger M, Hendeles L: Oral theophylline dosage for the management of chronic asthma. *J Pediatr* 1977;92:125–130.

Yarnell P, Chu N: Focal seizures and aminophylline. *Neurology* 1975;25:819–822.

CHAPTER 67

Anticonvulsants

Although the administration of antiseizure medications remains the cornerstone of treatment of seizure disorders, it is recognized that the danger of toxicity is inherent in all pharmacologic agents, particularly those that require long-term administration (1).

Although many drugs such as barbiturates and benzodiazepines can be used for seizure disorders, they are discussed elsewhere in this text. This chapter includes a discussion of phenytoin, carbamazepine, valproic acid, and felbamate.

TABLE 67–1. *Classification of seizure disorders*

Partial seizures
Elementary symptomatology
Jacksonian
Complex symptomatology
Temporal lobe or psychomotor seizures
Secondarily generalized symptoms
Generalized seizures
Tonic-clonic seizures
Absence seizures (petit mal)
Myoclonic seizures
Akinetic seizures
Status epilepticus

CLASSIFICATION OF SEIZURE DISORDERS

The *International Classification of Epileptic Seizures* currently classifies seizure disorders into 4 major categories: partial seizures, generalized seizures, unilateral seizures, and unclassified epileptic seizures (Table 67–1) (2).

Partial seizures are subdivided into those with elementary symptomatology, those with complex symptomatology, and those that are secondarily generalized. Partial seizures with elementary symptomatology include those with motor symptoms (e.g., Jacksonian seizures) or with autonomic symptoms. Partial seizures with complex symptomatology are also known as temporal lobe or psychomotor seizures.

Generalized seizures include tonic–clonic (grand mal) seizures, absence (petit mal) seizures, myoclonic seizures, and akinetic seizures. Seizures that recur at a frequency which does not allow consciousness to be regained in the interval between seizures are known as *status epilepticus* (2).

MECHANISM OF ACTION OF ANTISEIZURE MEDICATIONS

The principal pharmacologic actions of the anticonvulsants are elevation of the seizure threshold of the motor cortex to electrical or chemical stimuli and/or limitation of propagation of the seizure discharge from its origin (focus) to the effector organ(s). Limitation of spread of the seizure discharge from its focus may be accomplished by depression of synaptic transmission, limiting posttetanic potentiation of synaptic transmission, or reducing nerve conductance.

The precise mechanism(s) of action of anticonvulsants has not been confirmed at the molecular level. The basic mechanism is probably stabilization of the cell membrane secondary to modification of cation (sodium, potassium, calcium) transport either by increasing sodium efflux or inhibiting sodium influx.

BARBITURATES

Barbiturate-derivative anticonvulsants, particularly phenobarbital, are used in the prophylactic management of various types of seizures. Phenobarbital is used principally in the management of tonic-clonic seizures and partial seizures. Phenobarbital is also used in the prophylaxis of febrile seizures. Although the therapeutic uses of primidone are similar to those of phenobarbital and include management of tonic–clonic seizures and various partial seizures, the drug is used mainly in the prophylactic management of partial seizures with complex symptomatology. Primidone may also be useful in the management of partial seizures with autonomic symptoms and akinetic seizures.

Barbiturates are discussed in Chapter 47.

BENZODIAZEPINES

Benzodiazepine anticonvulsants are used mainly in the management of absence seizures, akinetic seizures, and myoclonic seizures. Clonazepam is the most widely used benzodiazepine anticonvulsant. Clonazepam is used alone or with other anticonvulsants for the management of absence seizures, especially Lennox–Gastaut syndrome (petit mal variant epilepsy), and of akinetic or myoclonic seizures. Oral benzodiazepines have generally been used as adjuncts to other anticonvulsants in the management of seizures refractory to other drugs.

Benzodiazepines are discussed in Chapter 48.

PHENYTOIN

Phenytoin is the most common anticonvulsant in use today. Although it is not a barbiturate, it is related to the barbiturates in chemical structure. Phenytoin is useful in the treatment of generalized tonic–clonic and partial-complex seizures. The primary site of action appears to be the motor cortex, where it inhibits the spread of seizure activity (3). Phenytoin limits the development of maximal seizure activity from an active focus by stabilization of the excitable neuronal membrane (4). It does this by interfering with the movement of ions across the cell membrane. Specifically, phenytoin decreases resting fluxes of sodium ions as well as sodium currents that exist during action potentials in chemically induced depolarization (5). Although phenytoin is commonly advocated and used as an antidysrhythmic agent, it is not approved by the FDA for such use.

Phenytoin as Antiarrhythmic Agent

Phenytoin as an antiarrhythmic agent is thought to restore normal membrane responsiveness, conduction velocity, and automaticity. Thus, it acts to depress the action potential of ischemic cells while facilitating the activities of normal cells (6). This antiarrhythmic action is similar to that of quinidine, with major effects on partially depolarized fibers and reversal of the inactive state of the sodium fast channel. However, phenytoin has an opposite effect than that of quinidine, which decreases depolarization of Purkinje fibers and increases the stimulation threshold. Phenytoin has properties similar to those of lidocaine in that it enhances conduction at the Purkinje myocardial junctions and shortens the duration of the action potential in injured tissue, raising the threshold for ventricular fibrillation.

Pharmacokinetics

The pharmacokinetics of phenytoin are complicated and present a number of problems when dealing with toxicity. They are based on its limited aqueous solubility, dose-dependent elimination, and hepatic inactivation, all of which may be influenced by other drugs (7).

TABLE 67–2. *Side effects of intravenous phenytoin*

Neurologic
Nystagmus
Ataxia
Dizziness
Dermatologic
Local burning
Phlebitis
Cardiac
Hypotension
Bradycardia
Cardiac dysrhythmias
Increased PR interval
Increased QRS complex duration
Abnormalities of ST segment and T wave

Phenytoin may be administered orally or intravenously. Oral absorption is slow and sometimes variable or incomplete. Oral phenytoin is absorbed more slowly from the stomach and more rapidly from the small bowel. Peak concentrations after a single oral dose may occur approximately 6 hours after administration (8).

Although the drug has not been recommended for use in intravenous infusion because of the possibility that microcrystallization of phenytoin may occur, many clinicians suggest that intravenous infusions are feasible, provided that appropriate precautions are taken (9,10). The drug may be administered intravenously in normal saline no faster than 25 to 50 mg/minute to avoid undesirable side effects such as hypotension and cardiac dysrhythmias (Table 67–2). In neonates, the drug should be administered at a rate not exceeding 1 to 3 mg/kg/minute (5). The intravenous preparation of phenytoin is solubilized with 40% propylene glycol and 10% ethyl alcohol in addition to being adjusted to pH 12 with sodium hydroxide (11–13).

Intramuscular administration is not suggested because absorption by this route is erratic and plasma drug concentrations are unpredictable (14). In addition, intramuscular phenytoin can cause tissue necrosis and sterile abscesses due to the high alkalinity of the solution (10).

Some of the side effects that were previously recorded with intravenous phenytoin have been shown to be related to the solvent propylene glycol (13). These effects are hypotension, disturbances of cardiac rhythm, prolongation of PR intervals and QRS complexes, and alterations of ST segments and T waves in the electrocardiogram (12).

Elimination

Phenytoin is 90% protein bound, mainly to albumin. It has a volume of distribution of 0.6 to 0.7 L/kg (15). Phenytoin is eliminated largely by parahydroxylation of one of the phenol rings to 5-hydroxyphenyl-5-phenylhydantoin, which is an inactive metabolite (16). Within the therapeutic range of 10 to 20 μg/mL, phenytoin metabolism becomes capacity-limited and demonstrates Michaelis–Menten pharmacokinetics. Under these condition, the half-life of phenytoin increases as the serum concentration increases. This phenomenon creates a difficult situation in the patient with acute toxicity with a substantial prolongation of half-life (17). Phenytoin, therefore, exhibits nonlinear pharmacokinetics. In low doses, elimination appears to occur by a first-order process; with an increase in dose, the plasma concentration increases disproportionately. This change in kinetics from first-order to zero-order fits the Michaelis–Menten model of enzyme saturation (18). Consequently, a small change in dose may cause a great change in the observed plasma concentration (16). As an example, the steady-state plasma concentration may double or triple from a 10% increase in dose (19).

At therapeutic concentrations, phenytoin has a half-life of 7 to 24 hours; in healthy adults, it averages 22 hours. As concentrations increase and the enzymes become saturated, the half-life also increases (4). At concentrations greater than 30 μg/mL, the half-life ranges from 72 to 120 hours (15). Variations in half-life may be due to variations in hepatic function, enzyme self-induction, genetic factors affecting individual differences in substrate saturation of the rate-limiting enzyme, and variations in dose dependency.

This unique aspect of phenytoin among the antiepileptic drugs is often not appreciated by physicians and results in toxicity. Dosage is usually increased in increments of 100 mg, the size of the most commonly used capsule. Instead, once a plasma phenytoin level of 10 μg/mL is reached, the dose should be increased by 30 to 50 mg and a new steady-state should be attained before any additional increase in dose.

Drug Interactions

Various drugs may affect the serum concentration of phenytoin (Table 67–3) (20). Drugs that may decrease concentrations include chronically ingested alcohol, carbamazepine, and reserpine. Drugs that may increase concentrations include phenothiazines, diazepam, disulfiram, acutely ingested alcohol, salicylates, dicumerol, isoniazid, chlordiazepoxide, cimetidine, trazodone, and others. This may be due to the high protein binding by these drugs which compete for binding sites on albumin and displace phenytoin levels or inhibit its metabolism by the liver (16). Folic acid deficiency may result in an elevation of phenytoin levels in plasma because this cofactor is utilized in the metabolism of phenytoin (8).

There is a complicated interaction between phenytoin and sodium valproate. Valproate displaces phenytoin from protein-binding sites and, thus, changes the therapeutic range; it also inhibits phenytoin metabolism which makes it difficult to interpret plasma phenytoin concentrations in patients taking valproate.

TABLE 67–3. *Drugs that alter phenytoin serum concentration*

Increased phenytoin concentration
Chlordiazepoxide
Cimetidine
Diazepam
Dicumarol
Dimercaprol
Disulfiram
Ethyl alcohol (acute)
Isoniazid
Phenothiazines
Salicylates
Trazodone
Decreased phenytoin concentration
Carbamazepine
Ethyl alcohol (chronic)
Reserpine

Adverse Reactions

Since its introduction more than 50 years ago, phenytoin has been a remarkable safe anticonvulsant. Oral phenytoin can cause many uncommon adverse reactions (Table 67–4), including hematologic, reticuloendothelial, metabolic, gastrointestinal, neurologic, genitourinary, and cutaneous disorders (when chronically administered). Gingival hyperplasia is more common in young patients than in adults but has no predilection for either sex (21); it never occurs in edentulous patients (13). A period of 4 to 6 months is required for the changes to develop; if they are allowed to continue, they reach a maximum in 9 to 12 months. This phenomenon disappears spontaneously after withdrawal of phenytoin. Significant drug-induced side effects, although rare, do occur. These include Steven–Johnson syndrome, hepatic necrosis, polyarteritis nodosa, and serum sickness.

TABLE 67–4. *Adverse reactions to oral phenytoin*

Hematologic
Thrombocytopenia
Leukopenia
Agranulocytosis
Megaloblastic anemia
Cutaneous
Morbilliform rash
Stevens–Johnson syndrome
Gingival hyperplasia
Gastrointestinal
Nausea
Vomiting
Constipation

Plasma Concentrations

Therapeutic drug monitoring is routinely performed in patients who are receiving phenytoin because of its narrow therapeutic range, saturation pharmacokinetics, and the large interpatient variability in its maximum rate of metabolism. Blood concentrations of phenytoin are usually measured as the total (bound and unbound) drug; therefore, medical disorders or drugs that displace or prevent phenytoin from binding with albumin may cause an increase in the free phenytoin fraction and may lead to intoxication even if the total amount of drug is within the therapeutic range (4,22). In addition, phenytoin protein binding can be altered in patients with severe conditions, including hypoalbuminemia, hyperbilirubinemia, and uremia. These alterations in protein binding may have significant clinical consequences, because the unbound phenytoin concentration is a more useful indicator of the pharmacologic and toxic phenytoin effects than is the total drug concentration. Monitoring total phenytoin concentrations in such patients may provide a misleading estimate of the pharmacologically active drug concentration.

Therapeutic plasma concentrations usually are in the range of 10 to 20 μg/mL (23). Because the volume of distribution is relatively constant within the therapeutic range, it can be used to calculate appropriate doses for the attainment of desired serum concentrations (24). In general, steady-state therapeutic plasma concentrations are achieved about 7 to 10 days after initiation of therapy with a daily oral dose of 300 mg in adults. After intravenous administration, therapeutic plasma concentrations are attained within 1 to 2 hours (16). Because of the great variation in plasma concentrations that may occur, measurements should be performed when initiating therapy, changing the dose, or adding or deleting other drugs from the regimen (25).

Most laboratories use an enzyme-linked or fluorescent immunoassay. These methods measure the total (protein bound and unbound) plasma phenytoin concentration. In certain patients (neonates, those with chronic hepatic or renal disease, those in the third trimester of pregnancy, and those taking drugs such as sodium valproate), plasma protein binding may be reduced; and the total phenytoin concentration may greatly underestimate the concentration of unbound, pharmacologically active drug.

Toxicity

Following massive ingestion, serum levels of phenytoin are affected by altered pharmacokinetics. In acute intoxication the phenytoin metabolizing enzymes are saturated. With saturation, drug metabolism switches from first-order to zero-order pharmacokinetics and the drug is metabolized at a fixed rate (17).

TABLE 67–5. *Contributing factors in chronic phenytoin intoxication*

Change in kinetics
Hypoalbuminemia
Chronic renal failure
Hepatic dysfunction
Genetic defect in phenytoin metabolism
Concomitant administration of other drugs

Chronic phenytoin intoxication with typical therapeutic doses may result from several mechanisms (Table 67–5) (26,27). In patients with hypoalbuminemia, a large proportion of phenytoin remains unbound and, therefore, in active form (28). In patients with chronic renal failure, there is also a decreased ability to bind phenytoin (29).

The mixed-function oxidases responsible for phenytoin metabolism are located in the central area of the liver lobules and any damage to these areas can slow the rate of metabolism. Phenytoin intoxication may, therefore, result from hepatic dysfunction secondary to cirrhosis or hepatitis (16). In addition, it may result from a genetic defect in phenytoin metabolism, or as just mentioned, from the inhibition of its metabolism by other drugs (30,31). Intoxication may result from accumulation of the drug, which saturates the enzyme system and switches kinetics from first-order to zero-order (23).

In therapeutic doses, phenytoin does not exhibit sedative properties. Overdose by the oral route gives rise to symptoms referable primarily to the cerebellum and vestibular systems; these are usually dose-related. Because of the drug's long half-life, the major manifestations of intoxication may persist for 4 to 5 days after diagnosis (17).

Correlation Between Serum Concentration and Toxic Effects

Most patients tolerate phenytoin blood concentrations less than 25 μg/mL (Table 67–6). Nystagmus on lateral gaze usually appears at 20 to 25 μg/mL. Ataxia and diplopia may occur at 30 μg/mL (32). Although nystagmus and ataxia usually precede more severe symptoms, toxicity may remain unrecognized by the patient (4).

TABLE 67–6. *Phenytoin serum concentrations and corresponding toxic effects*

Concentration (μg/mL)	Symptoms
10 to 20	Therapeutic
20 to 30	Nystagmus, ataxia, diplopia
30 to 40	Dysarthria
40 to 50	Lethargy, drowsiness, asterixis
50 to 60	Stupor
60	Coma

When the blood concentration exceeds 30 μg/mL dysarthria may be noted (33). Concentrations greater than 40 μg/mL may cause lethargy, drowsiness, and rarely, asterixis. Extreme lethargy and occasionally coma may occur with concentrations greater than 50 μ/mL.

Clinical Features

Oral phenytoin overdose in adults is a serious, although rarely life-threatening, condition. The potential for morbidity is related principally to falls occurring as a result of ataxia and poor judgment stemming from phenytoin-induced obtundation. Appropriate precautions should, therefore, be taken to ensure that patients with severe ataxia and mental status changes remain at supervised rest until signs and symptoms resolve.

The common neurologic manifestations of phenytoin intoxication are nystagmus, ataxia, and dysarthria (Table 67–7). Nondose-related toxic effects appear in the gastrointestinal tract as nausea, vomiting, and constipation (11). Blurred vision and a skin rash have also been noted (13). Rarely, phenytoin may cause mental changes such as confusion and focal neurologic signs such as hemihyperesthesia and progressive hemiparesis (34–37).

Movement disorders or choreoathetosis have also been described with phenytoin intoxication and are characterized by hyperkinesis, limb chorea, ballismus, and dystonias (38,39). Most cases of phenytoin-induced chorea have been associated with either markedly elevated phenytoin concentrations or pre-existing brain damage or both (40,41). This type of movement disorder has also been reported in the acute administration of phenytoin at nontoxic doses (42). Orofacial dyskinesias similar to those caused by neuroleptic drugs have been reported with phenytoin toxicity. The exact mechanism by which phenytoin does this is unclear, but it may be related to its dopamine antagonistic properties (3,42).

A rare manifestation of phenytoin intoxication is generalized seizure activity, particularly when concentrations are high. Although seizures have occurred in this group of patients, a causal relationship has never been demonstrated (43).

TABLE 67–7. *Nondose-related toxic effects of phenytoin*

Gastrointestinal
Nausea
Vomiting
Constipation
Neurologic
Confusion
Hemihyperesthesia
Hemiparesis
Choreoathetosis
Dystonia
Dysarthria
Generalized seizures

Deaths from oral ingestion of an overdose of phenytoin are extremely rare; if death were to occur from oral administration, it would be from progressive neurologic depression and coma, not from cardiac toxicity (44). Most fatalities have been associated with intravenous preparations for the treatment of cardiac dysrhythmias (45,46).

The long duration of CNS effects and the potential for persistent neurologic sequelae exist (47). Peripheral neuropathies have been described in patients receiving long-term phenytoin therapy, primarily in those with histories of phenytoin intoxication (48). Degeneration of cerebellar Purkinje's cells in chronic phenytoin intoxication has also been documented (4).

Phenytoin is clearly identified as causing specific detrimental cardiac effects as a function of its membrane stabilizing properties. This feature necessitates intravenous administration with simultaneous EKG monitoring. This factor has led to the widespread use of cardiac monitoring for oral phenytoin overdose, yet data do not support the routine EKG monitoring in patients with an uncomplicated overdose (49). Concern about cardiovascular complications has prompted clinicians to manage patients with oral phenytoin overdose and high blood levels in monitored settings at considerable cost (50). This strategy reflects physician awareness of phenytoin's documented effects on cardiac conduction and contractility as well as incidents of cardiovascular collapse associated with IV administration of phenytoin (51). In case reports of fatalities caused by oral phenytoin overdose, however, neurologic complications have predominated and circulatory complications have been rare (52).

Propylene Glycol and Phenytoin Toxicity

Propylene glycol is the solvent used in the commercial preparation of phenytoin. Introduced in the 1930s, propylene glycol is now in widespread use as a solvent for food flavorings; preservative for syrups, and packaged foods, and vitamins; and emollient in cosmetics. Propylene glycol is an ingredient in at least 28 parenteral drug preparations with concentrations ranging from 0.45 to 0.725 g/mL. The commercially available parenteral preparation of phenytoin contains 400 mg propylene glycol and 50 mg phenytoin/mL.

It has been found that cardiodepression and hemodynamic collapse are characteristic of rapid injection of propylene glycol and that the detrimental cardiac effects of intravenous phenytoin administration, is actually due to the rapid administration of propylene glycol (53,54).

Treatment of Intoxication

Treatment of phenytoin intoxication is nonspecific because there is no antidote. In the acutely overdosed patient, treatment consists of gastrointestinal emptying and subsequent administration of activated charcoal and a cathartic (55). Repeated oral doses of activated charcoal may be given, even though the efficacy of this regimen has not been established (56,57,58). Generalized supportive care is usually all that is necessary. Ingestions of up to 300 mg/kg have been survived with conservative therapy. Management with continuous EKG monitoring is not mandatory in stable adult cases of severe oral phenytoin overdose (49).

Various adjunctive methods have been attempted to increase the clearance of phenytoin (59). Hemodialysis, peritoneal dialysis, and forced diuresis have been shown to be of no value in the treatment of phenytoin intoxication (60). Although the molecular size of phenytoin enables the drug to diffuse across a dialysis membrane, the protein binding appears to be a limiting factor. Charcoal hemoperfusion also does not result in significantly better clearance. In addition, exchange transfusion has been of little value in treatment (61).

The decision regarding when to recommence phenytoin therapy after an episode of acute intoxication depends on the availability of laboratory services for monitoring serum phenytoin concentrations (16,62). If these services are available, therapy can begin again when serum concentrations are in the therapeutic range (63).

CARBAMAZEPINE

Carbamazepine is a synthetic iminostilbene derivative that is chemically and structurally related to tricyclic antidepressants and spatially related to phenytoin. In overdose, carbamazepine often exhibits toxicities shared by these compounds. Carbamazepine is the drug of choice for the treatment of complex partial seizures and is one of the major drugs of choice for simple partial and secondarily generalized seizures. It is also the drug of choice for the treatment of trigeminal neuralgia. As a result of the increasing and widespread use of carbamazepine, intentional and accidental overdoses with carbamazepine have become much more common (64).

Actions

The pharmacologic actions of carbamazepine appear to be qualitatively similar to those of the hydantoin-derivative anticonvulsants. The anticonvulsant activity of carbamazepine, like phenytoin, principally involves limitation of seizure propagation by reduction of post-tetanic potentiation of synaptic transmission. Carbamazepine appears to provide relief of pain in trigeminal neuralgia by reducing synaptic transmission within the trigeminal nucleus. The drug has also demonstrated sedative, anticholinergic, antidepressant, muscle relaxant, antiarrhythmic, antidiuretic, and neuromuscular transmission-inhibitory actions. Carbamazepine has only slight analgesic properties (64).

Pharmacokinetics

Carbamazepine is slowly absorbed from the gastrointestinal tract. Following oral administration of carbamazepine tablets, peak plasma concentrations are reached in 2–8 hours. Two to 4 days of therapy may be required to achieve steady-state plasma concentrations. Although optimal therapeutic plasma concentrations suitable for all patients have not yet been determined, therapeutic plasma concentrations of carbamazepine are usually 3–14 μg/mL. Nystagmus may occur when plasma concentrations are greater than 4 μg/mL and ataxia, dizziness, and anorexia often occur when plasma concentrations are 10 μg/mL or greater. There appears to be a wide variation in steady-state plasma concentrations produced by specific daily dosages of carbamazepine (65).

The half-life of carbamazepine varies from about 36 hours in nonusers to 10 to 20 hours after enzyme induction, which occurs after about 3 to 6 weeks of therapy. The variability results, in part, because carbamazepine can induce its own metabolism (64). The plasma half-life generally ranges from 25–65 hours initially and from 12–17 hours with multiple dosing. Ingested carbamazepine can form a bolus in the gut, which in combination with reduced bowel motility, may result in delayed absorption for several days. Concomitant treatment with phenobarbital, phenytoin, or felbamate may further reduce the half-life of carbamazepine by heteroinduction (65).

Carbamazepine induces liver microsomal enzymes and, thus, may accelerate its own metabolism and that of other concomitantly administered drugs that are metabolized by these enzymes. Carbamazepine is a lipophilic substance that is metabolized via a number of routes in liver mitochondria. The major pathway is from carbamazepine to carbamazepine epoxide, which is the rate-limiting step, and then to carbamazepine transdiol. Carbamazepine-10,11-epoxide, the active metabolite of carbamazepine, has anticonvulsant activity and, in overdose, must be considered to possibly have toxic properties as well (66).

Mechanism of Action

The anticonvulsant properties of carbamazepine have, in part, been attributed to inhibition of sodium channels and interference with norepinephrine and glutamate metabolism (66).

Overdose

Signs and symptoms of overdose have included nausea, vomiting, dizziness, ataxia, drowsiness, respiratory depression, hypotension, hypersensitivity skin reactions, hypothermia, and cyanosis (Table 67–8).

Antimuscarinic symptoms may include decreased bowel sounds, tachycardia, hypertension, mydriasis, flushing, and urinary retention. The antimuscarinic effect of carbamazepine overdose decreases stomach motility, thus, prolonging absorption and half-life. A similar effect may result from a drug mass forming in the stomach.

Carbamazepine poisoning also causes CNS depression, with coma and respiratory compromise as the major sequelae. Other CNS effects have included stupor, opisthotonos, restlessness, agitation, disorientation, tremor, involuntary movements, adiadochokinesis, abnormal reflexes (hypoactive or hyperactive), and nystagmus. Several deaths associated with toxic carbamazepine ingestions have been reported (67). An antidiuretic effect can induce hyponatremia and complicate fluid resuscitation with crystalloid (68).

The constellation of antimuscarinic signs and stupor or coma with adventitious movements in a patient with a seizure disorder should alert the clinician to the possibility of serious carbamazepine overdose (67).

Laboratory

Concentrations are commonly assessed by fluorescence polarization immunoassay, liquid chromatography, or enzyme-multiplied immunoassay. Laboratory findings in some cases of overdosage have included leukocytosis, reduced leukocyte count, glycosuria, and acetonuria. EEG may show dysrhythmias (67).

Treatment

The general management principles for carbamazepine overdose are the same as for any case of toxic ingestion. This would include assisting ventilation, if necessary, emptying of stomach contents with lavage if appropriate, and treating toxic symptoms symptomatically. Treatment for carbamazepine overdose is largely supportive. Hypotension and respiratory failure are treated with pressors and ventilatory assistance. Because of the relationship of carbamazepine to the tricyclic antidepressants, the ECG should be monitored to detect cardiac dysfunction (65).

TABLE 67–8. *Signs and symptoms of carbamazepine overdose*

Antimuscarinic
Mydriasis
Flushing
Hypertension
Tachycardia
Absent bowel sounds
Urinary retention
Neurologic
Stupor
Opisthotonos
Restlessness
Agitation
Disorientation
Tremor
Adiadochokinesis
Abnormal reflexes

VALPROIC ACID

Valproic acid, valproate sodium, and divalproex sodium are carboxylic acid-derivative anticonvulsants. Valproic acid is primarily used to treat absence seizures. The anticonvulsant activity of valproic acid is believed to be related to its ability to increase the concentration of GABA in the brain, although the exact mechanism of antiseizure activity is unknown (69).

In addition to its anticonvulsant properties, valproic acid has been shown to have morphine-like analgesic properties, which are believed to be related to increased GABA concentrations and/or to its stimulation of the enkephalin system.

Pharmacokinetics

Following oral administration, valproate sodium is rapidly converted to valproic acid in the stomach. Valproic acid is rapidly and almost completely absorbed from the gastrointestinal tract. The bioavailability of valproate from divalproex sodium delayed-release tablets has been shown to be equivalent to that of valproic acid capsules. Administration of divalproex sodium with food would be expected to slow absorption but not affect the extent of absorption.

The peak level of valproic acid is achieved in 1–4 hours after single-dose ingestion of the acid or the sodium salt and 3–5 hours following a single oral dose of divalproex sodium (69). The half-life is approximately 7 to 8 hours. After a large overdose, the half-life may be prolonged to 20 hours. Some reports indicate that therapeutic plasma concentrations may be 50–100 μg/mL and that concentrations in this range are maintained in most adults receiving 1.2–1.5 g of valproic acid daily (70).

Valproic acid is eliminated by first-order kinetics and reportedly has an elimination half-life of 5–20 hours. Elimination half-lives in the lower portion of the range are usually observed in patients receiving other anticonvulsants concomitantly. Half-lives of up to 30 hours have been reported following overdosage of valproate sodium (70).

Toxicity

The most common manifestation of acute valproic acid overdose is central nervous system depression ranging

TABLE 67–9. *Signs and symptoms of valproic acid overdose*

Central nervous system
Drowsiness
Altered mental behavior
Confusion
Cerebral edema
Coma
Miscellaneous
Fever
Muscle spasms
Hypocalcemia
Liver damage
Thrombocytopenia
Pancreatitis
Metabolic acidosis
Hyperthermia

from altered behavior, confusion, and poor seizure control to cerebral edema (Table 67–9). Other recognized features of acute valproate poisoning include fever, coma, muscle spasms, hypocalcemia, liver damage, and thrombocytopenia. Drowsiness is common and toxic encephalopathy and optic atrophy have been described. Cerebral edema is uncommon but has been observed in postmortem examination following fatal acute and chronic overdose. Pancreatitis has been reported in both long-term and massive overdose of valproate (70). Other effects of acute toxicity include hypernatremia, hypocalcemia, metabolic acidosis, leukopenia, and hyperthermia. Acute toxicity seems less severe in patients who are chronically receiving valproate (69).

Long-term effects of valproic acid use include abdominal cramping, diarrhea, anorexia, drowsiness, hair loss, thrombocytopenia, and abnormal liver function tests. It is speculated that the long-term sedative effects of valproic acid may be attributed to elevated levels of ammonia.

Treatment

Treatment of valproic acid intoxication consists of general supportive therapy, particularly maintenance of adequate urinary output. Because the drug is rapidly absorbed, gastric lavage may be of limited value; because absorption of divalproex sodium delayed-release tablets is delayed, the value of gastric lavage or emesis will vary with time since ingestion if this form of the drug has been ingested. Naloxone has been reported to reverse the CNS depressant effects of valproic acid overdosage; however, naloxone should be used with caution because it could also theoretically reverse the anticonvulsant effects of valproic acid.

FELBAMATE (FELBATOL)

Felbamate, a dicarbamate, is an anticonvulsant agent. Felbamate is structurally related to, but pharmacologically distinct from, meprobamate. Felbamate is used as monotherapy or in combination with other anticonvulsant agents in the management of partial seizures.

Pharmacokinetics

Felbamate is available for oral use only. More than 90% is absorbed, even in the presence of food or antacids. Serum concentrations reach a peak in 1–3 hours. Felbamate circulates primarily as free drug; only 20–25% is bound to plasma proteins. It is partly metabolized in the liver and excreted in the urine. The half-life of the drug is about 20–23 hours.

Adverse Effects

Early on, felbamate was generally thought to be well tolerated. Most adverse effects of the drug usually are mild to moderate in severity and self-limiting, infrequently requiring dosage adjustment. Gastrointestinal tract and nervous system effects are the most frequent adverse effects of felbamate and the adverse effects most frequently requiring discontinuance of the drug.

In adults, the most frequent adverse effects of felbamate during monotherapy or adjunctive therapy are anorexia, nausea, vomiting, insomnia, and headache; dizziness and somnolence also are frequent during adjunctive therapy. In children, the most frequent adverse effects of the drug during adjunctive therapy are anorexia, vomiting, insomnia, headache, and somnolence. The frequency of most adverse effects associated with felbamate appears to be lower during monotherapy than adjunctive therapy.

There have been reports of a serious side effect from felbamate. Aplastic anemia discovered after 5–30 weeks of felbamate therapy has been reported during felbamate's use. This has lead to a suspension of the drug unless in the physician's judgment the patient's well-being is so dependent on continued treatment with felbamate that abrupt withdrawal is deemed to pose an even greater risk.

There are no clinical reports as of yet concerning an overdose of felbamate.

GABAPENTIN (NEUROTIN)

Gabapentin is a new antiepileptic drug indicated as an adjunct to current antiepileptic therapy in adults for the treatment of partial seizures with or without secondary generalization.

The mechanism of action of gabapentin remains unknown. Despite structural similarities to GABA, gabapentin does not appear to have significant interactions with GABA-A or GABA-B receptors, or affect GABA turnover.

The pharmacokinetic properties of gabapentin are significantly different from those of other antiepileptic agents. Peak plasma concentrations occur 2–4 hours after ingestion. Unlike most other antiepileptic agents, gabapentin does not bind to human plasma proteins and is not metabolized by the liver. Instead, gabapentin is primarily excreted by the kidneys entirely as unchanged drug.

Gabapentin is a well-tolerated antiepileptic agent that has some mild CNS effects when used as an adjunct with other antiepileptic agents. Significant side effects include drowsiness, nonspecific dizziness, ataxia, and fatigue. However, the incidence of these adverse effects are considered low in patients already treated with one of two standard antiepileptic drugs. It does not appear to interact with other antiepileptic drugs, is not bound to plasma proteins, is not metabolized, and does not induce liver enzymes.

No clinical experience with overdose has been described.

REFERENCES

1. Aronson J, Hardman M, Reynolds D: Phenytoin. *Br Med J* 1992;305: 1215–1218.
2. Dreifuss F: Anticonvulsant agents. *Crit Care Clin* 1991;7:521–531.
3. Murphy J, Motiwala R, Devinsky O: Phenytoin intoxication. *South Med J* 1991;84:1199–1204.
4. Cranford R, Leppik I, Patrick B, et al: Intravenous phenytoin: clinical and pharmacokinetic aspects. *Neurology* 1978;28:874–881.
5. Rivey M, Schottelium D, Berg M: Phenytoin-folic acid: a review. *Drug Intell Clin Pharmacol* 1984;18:292–301.
6. D'Souza S, Robertson I, Donnai D, et al: Fetal phenytoin exposure, hypoplastic nails, and jitteriness. *Arch Dis Child* 1990;65:320–324.
7. Katz A, Hoffman R, Silverman R: Phenytoin toxicity from smoking crack cocaine adulterated with phenytoin. *Ann Emerg Med* 1993; 22:1485–1487.
8. Campbell W: Periodic alternating nystagmus in phenytoin intoxication. *Arch Neurol* 1990;37:178–180.
9. Bauman J, Siepler J, Fitzloff, J: Phenytoin crystallization in intravenous fluids. *Drug Intell Clin Pharmacol* 1977;11:646–649.
10. Earnest M, Marx J, Drury L: Complications of intravenous phenytoin for acute treatment of seizures. *JAMA* 1983;249:762–765.
11. Atkinson A, Shaw J: Pharmacokinetic study of a patient with diphenylhydantoin toxicity. *Clin Pharmacol Ther* 1973;14:521–528.
12. Louis S, Kutt H: The cardiocirculatory changes caused by intravenous Dilantin and its solvent. *Am Heart J* 1967;74:523–528.
13. Olanow C, Finn A: Phenytoin: pharmacokinetics and clinical therapeutics. *Neurosurgery* 1981;8:112–117.
14. Rosen M, Lisak R, Rubin I, et al: Diphenylhydantoin in cardiac arrhythmias. *Am J Cardiol* 1967;20:674–678.
15. Dodson W: Phenytoin elimination in childhood: effect of concentration-dependent kinetics. *Neurology* 1980;30:196–199.
16. Adler D: Phenytoin. *Clin Toxicol* 1979;14:147–150.
17. Mellick L, Morgan A, Mellick G: Presentations of acute phenytoin overdose. *Am J Emerg Med* 1989;7:61–67.
18. Gugler R, Manion C, Azarnoff D: Phenytoin: pharmacokinetics and bioavailability. *Clin Pharmacol Ther* 1975;19:135–142.
19. Albani M: An unusual case of phenytoin intoxication. *Neuropadiatrie* 1978;9:185–188.
20. Moling J, Posch J: Acute diphenylhydantoin intoxication. Pediatrics 1957;20:877–880.
21. Brown C, Kaminsky M, Feroli E, et al: Delirium with phenytoin and disulfiram administration. *Ann Emerg Med* 1983;12:310–313.
22. Theodore W, Yu L, Price B, et al: The clinical value of free phenytoin levels. *Ann Neurol* 1985;18:90–93.
23. Leal K, Troupin A: Clinical pharmacology of antiepileptic drugs: a summary of current information. *Clin Chem* 1977;23:1964–1968.
24. Gill M, Kern J, Kaneko J, et al: Phenytoin overdose kinetics. *West J Med* 1978;128:246–248.
25. Matthews C, Harley J: Cognitive and motor-sensory performances in toxic and nontoxic epileptic subjects. *Neurology* 1975;25:184–188.
26. Pruitt A, Zwiren G, Patterson J, et al: *Clin Pharmacol Ther* 1975;18: 112–120.
27. Herberg K: Delayed and insidious onset of diphenylhydantoin toxicity. *South Med J* 1975;68:70–74.
28. Tibbs P, Bivins B, Rapp R, et al: Phenytoin-induced hypotension in animals receiving sympathomimetic pressor support. *J Surg Res* 1980;29:338–347.
29. Holcomb R, Lynn R, Harvey B, et al: Intoxication with 5,5-diphenylhydantoin (Dilantin). J Pediatr 1972;80:627–632.
30. Blum R, Wilton J, Hilligoss D, et al: Effect of fluconazole on the disposition of phenytoin. *Clin Pharmacol Ther* 1991;49:420–425.
31. Selhorst J, Kaufman B, Horowitz S: Diphenylhydantoin-induced cerebellar degeneration. *Arch Neurol* 1972;27:453–456.
32. Kuhn G: Serum theophylline and phenytoin levels: can we afford to do them? Can we afford not to? *Ann Emerg Med* 1986;15:344–348.
33. Osborn H, Zisfein J, Sparano R: Single-dose oral phenytoin loading. *Ann Emerg Med* 1987;16:407–412.
34. Findler G, Lavy S: Transient hemiparesis: a rare manifestation of diphenylhydantoin toxicity. *J Neurosurg* 1979;50:685–687.
35. Parker W, Shearer C: Phenytoin hepatotoxicity: a case report and review. *Neurology* 1979;29:175–178.
36. Parker W, Gumnit R: Diphenylhydantoin toxicity: dose-dependent blood dyscrasia. *Neurology* 1974;24:1178–1180.
37. Sandyk R: Transient hemiparesis–a rare complication of phenytoin toxicity. *Postgrad Med J* 1983;59:601–602.
38. Filloux F, Thompson J: Transient chorea induced by phenytoin. *J Pediatr* 1987;110:639–641.
39. Shuttleworth E, Wise C, Paulson C: Choreoathetosis and diphenylhydantoin intoxication. *JAMA* 1974;230:1170–1171.
40. Wilder B, Buchanan R, Serrano E: Correlation of acute diphenylhydantoin intoxication with plasma levels and metabolite excretion. *Neurology* 1973;23:1329–1332.
41. Wilder B, Ramsay E, Willmore L, et al: Efficacy of intravenous phenytoin in the treatment of status epilepticus: kinetics of central nervous system penetration. *Ann Neurol* 1977;1:511–518.
42. Wilson J, Huff J, Kilroy A: Prolonged toxicity following acute phenytoin overdose in a child. *J Pediatr* 1979;95:135–138.
43. Bazemore R, Zuckerman E: On the problem of diphenylhydantoin-induced seizures. *Arch Neurol* 1974;31:243–249.
44. Laubscher F: Fatal diphenylhydantoin poisoning. *JAMA* 1966;198: 194–195.
45. Gellerman G, Martinez C: Fatal ventricular fibrillation following intravenous sodium diphenylhydantoin therapy. *JAMA* 1967;2: 161–162.
46. Fulop M, Widrow D, Colmers R, et al: Possible diphenylhydantoin-induced arrhythmia in hypothyroidism. *JAMA* 1966;196:168–170.
47. Dobkin B: Reversible subacute peripheral neuropathy induced by phenytoin. *Arch Neurol* 1977;34:189–190.
48. Damato A: Diphenylhydantoin: Pharmacological and clinical use. *Prog Cardiovasc Dis* 1969;12:1–15.
49. Wyte C, Berk W: Severe oral phenytoin overdose does not cause cardiovascular morbidity. *Ann Emerg Med* 1991;20:508–512.
50. Osborn H, Zisfein J: Advocating single-dose phenytoin loading. *Ann Emerg Med* 1988;17:295–296.
51. Barclay L, McLean M, Hagen N, et al: Severe phenytoin hypersensitivity with myopathy: a case report. *Neurology* 1992;42:2303.
52. Mellick L, Morgan A, Mellick G: Presentations of acute phenytoin overdose. *Am J Emerg Med* 1989;7:61–67.
53. York R, Coleridge S: Cardiopulmonary arrest following intravenous phenytoin loading. *Am J Emerg Med* 1988;6:255–259.
54. Vukmir R, Stein K: Torsades de pointes therapy with phenytoin. *Ann Emerg Med* 1991;20:198–200.
55. Rowden A, Spoor J, Bertino J: The effect of activated charcoal on phenytoin pharmacokinetics. *Ann Emerg Med* 1990;19:1144–1147.
56. Dolgin J, Nix D, Sanchez J, et al: Pharmacokinetic simulation of the effect of multiple-dose activated charcoal in phenytoin poisoning—report of two pediatric cases. *DICP Ann Pharmacother* 1991;25: 646–649.

57. Ros S, Black L: Multiple-dose activated charcoal in management of phenytoin overdose. *Pediatr Emerg Care* 1989;5:169–170.
58. Mauro L, Mauro V, Brown D, et al: Enhancement of phenytoin elimination by multiple-dose activated charcoal. *Ann Emerg Med* 1987;16:1132–1135.
59. Spector R, Davidoff R, Schwartzman R: Phenytoin-induced ophthalmoplegia. *Neurology* 1976;26:1031–1034.
60. Curtis D, Piibe R, Ellenhorn M, et al: Phenytoin toxicity: predictors of clinical course. *Vet Hum Toxicol* 1989;31:162–163.
61. Larsen L, Sterrett J, Whitehead B, et al: Adjunctive therapy of phenytoin overdose–a case report using plasmapheresis. *Clin Toxicol* 1986; 24:37–49.
62. Jacobsen D, Alvik A, Bredesen J, et al: Pharmacokinetics of phenytoin in acute adult and child intoxication. *J Toxicol Clin Toxicol* 1987;24:519–531.
63. Curtis D, Piibe R, Ellenhorn M, et al: Phenytoin toxicity: a review of 94 cases. *Vet Hum Toxicol* 1989;31:164–165.
64. Macnab A, Birch P, Macready J: Carbamazepine poisoning in children. *Pediatr Emerg Care* 1993;9:195–198.
65. Hojer J, Malmlund H, Berg A: Clinical features in 28 consecutive cases of laboratory confirmed massive poisoning with carbamazepine alone. *J Toxicol Clin Toxicol* 1993;31:449–458.
66. Benassi E, Bo G, Cocito L, et al: Carbamazepine and cardiac conduction disturbances. *Ann Neurol* 1987;22:280–281.
67. Spiller H, Krenzelok E, Cookson E: Carbamazepine overdose: a prospective study of serum levels and toxicity. *J Toxicol Clin Toxicol* 1990;28:445–458.
68. Spiller H, Krenzelok E: Carbamazepine overdose: serum concentration less predictive in children. *J Toxicol Clin Toxicol* 1993;31:459–460.
69. Khoo S, Leyland M: Cerebral edema following acute sodium valproate overdose. *J Toxicol Clin Toxicol* 1992;30:209–214.
70. Alberto G, Erickson T, Pipiel R, et al: Central nervous system manifestations of a valproic acid overdose responsive to naloxone. *Ann Emerg Med* 1989;18:889–891.

ADDITIONAL SELECTED REFERENCES

Bridgers S, Ebersole J: Incidence of seizures with phenytoin toxicity. *Neurology* 1985;35:1767–1768.

Caracta A, Damato A, Josephson M, et al: Electrophysiologic properties of diphenylhydantoin. *Circulation* 1973;47:1234–1241.

Christiansen C, Kristensen M, Rodbro P: Latent osteomalacia in epileptic patients on anticonvulsants. *Br Med J* 1972;3:738–739.

Derby B, Ward J: The myth of red urine due to phenytoin. *JAMA* 1983;249:1723–1724

Durelli L, Mutani R, Sechi G, et al: Cardiac side effects of phenytoin and carbamazepine: a dose-related phenomenon? *Arch Neurol* 1985;42:1067–1068.

Flowers F, Araujo O, Hamm K: Phenytoin hypersensitivity syndrome. *J Emerg Med* 1987;5:103–108.

Gallagher B, Baumel I, Mattson R, et al: Primidone, diphenylhydantoin and phenobarbital *Neurology* 1973;23:145–149.

Gerber N, Lynn R, Oates J: Acute intoxication with 5,5-diphenylhydantoin (Dilantin) associated with impairment of biotransformation. *Ann Intern Med* 1972;77:765–771.

Gharib H, Munoz J: Endocrine manifestations of diphenylhydantoin therapy. *Metabolism* 1974;23:515–524.

Jones D, Helfer R: A teething lotion resulting in the misdiagnosis of diphenylhydantoin administration. *Am J Dis Child* 1971;122:259–260.

Kapur R, Girgis S, Little T, et al: Piphenylhydantoin induced gingival hyperplasia: its relationship to dose and serum level. *Dev Med Child Neurol* 1973;15:483–487.

Lindahl S, Westerling D: Detoxification with peritoneal dialysis and blood exchange after diphenylhydantoin intoxication. *Acta Paediatr Scand* 1982;71:665–666.

Marquis J, Carruthers S, Spence J, et al: Phenytoin-theophylline interaction. *N Engl J Med* 1982;307:1189–1190.

Matzke G, Cloyd J, Sawchuk G: Acute phenytoin and primidone intoxication: a pharmacokinetic analysis. *J Clin Pharmacol* 1981;21:92–99.

Rodbro P, Christiansen C, Lund M: Development of anticonvulsant osteomalacia in epileptic patients on phenytoin treatment. *Acta Neurol Scand* 1974;50:527–532.

Rosenblum E, Rodichok L, Hanson P: Movement disorder as a manifestation of diphenylhydantoin toxicity. *Pediatrics* 1974;54:364–366.

Stilman N, Masdeu J: Incidence of seizures with phenytoin toxicity. *Neurology* 1985;35:1769–1772.

Tichner J, Enselverg C: Suicidal Dilantin poisoning. *N Engl J Med* 1951; 245:723–725.

Vincent F: Phenothiazine-induced phenytoin intoxication. *Ann Intern Med* 1980;93:56–57.

Wallis W, Kutt H, McDowell F: Intravenous diphenylhydantoin in treatment of acute repetitive seizures. *Neurology* 1968;18:513–523.

Wit A, Rosen M, Hoffman B: Electrophysiology and pharmacology of cardiac arrhythmias: Part VIII: cardiac effects of diphenylhydantoin: Part A. *Am Heart J* 1975;90:265–272.

Wit A, Rosen M, Hoffman B: Electrophysiology and pharmacology of cardiac arrhythmias: Part VIII: cardiac effects of diphenylhydantoin: Part B. *Am Heart J* 1975;90:397–404.

Woodbury D: Phenytoin: introduction and history. *Adv Neurol* 1980;27:305–313.

Zoneraich S, Zoneraich O, Siegel J: Sudden death following intravenous sodium diphenylhydantoin. *Am Heart J* March 1976;91:375–377.

CHAPTER 68

Isoniazid

Since its introduction more than 35 years ago, isoniazid has been used worldwide as a synthetic antibiotic for the treatment of active pulmonary tuberculosis as well as prophylactically in patients with a positive tuberculin skin test (1). Isoniazid intoxication is most commonly encountered in groups where tuberculosis is prevalent. The wide availability of the drug has led to a number of reports regarding accidental or intentional acute poisonings after excessive ingestion (2).

PHARMACOKINETICS

Isoniazid (INH, Niconyl, Nydrazid) is a hydrazide of isonicotinic acid (3). It is absorbed rapidly from the gastrointestinal tract and from intramuscular administration. Plasma concentrations reach their peak 1 to 2 hours after oral administration and fall to 50% within 6 hours (4). It is not substantially protein-bound and diffuses into all body fluids. It is excreted mainly in the urine, partly unchanged and partly acetylated, and small amounts are excreted in the bile (5). The primary route of isoniazid inactivation is by acetylation and dehydrazination (6). In the presence of normal renal function, 75–95% of isoniazid is excreted within 24 hours mostly as metabolites (7).

The plasma half-life of isoniazid in patients with normal renal and hepatic function ranges from 1 to 4 hours depending on the rate of metabolism. The rate of disappearance of isoniazid from serum is the determining factor in the manifestation of toxicity and varies greatly among individuals; this variability is genetically determined, resulting from a relative deficiency of the hepatic enzyme N-acetyltransferase. Individuals may be identified as having slow, intermediate, or rapid rates of acetylation (2); the rate of acetylation is usually constant for each individual. In the former group, the plasma half-life of isoniazid is 2.5 to 3 times that in fast acetylators (140 to 200 minutes as opposed to 45 to 80 minutes). Approximately 50–60% of Caucasians and Blacks have slow rates of acetylation (8). Most Orientals and Eskimos have rapid rates of acetylation. Consequently, both a higher incidence and a more severe form of toxicity from isoniazid may be expected in Caucasians and Blacks (1).

TABLE 68–1. *Side effects of isoniazid*

Side effects
Peripheral neuropathy
Paresthesia
Psychosis
Depression
Hepatitis

Isoniazid has a comparatively wide margin of safety between therapeutic and toxic doses (9). Side effects are not uncommon but at small doses they are, for the most part, not severe (Table 68–1) (10). Peripheral neuropathy is the most common neurologic manifestation and is usually preceded by paresthesia of the feet and hands (11). Neurotoxic effects may be prevented or relieved with low doses of pyridoxine (vitamin B6) during therapy. Psychotic and depressive reactions associated with suicidal manifestations have also been reported (3). Severe and sometimes fatal hepatitis associated with isoniazid therapy has been reported and may develop even after many months of treatment (12). This risk appears to be age related, with older patients being at greatest risk (5).

MECHANISM OF ACTION

The metabolic abnormalities and CNS alterations caused by isoniazid overdose are thought to be a result of alterations in the metabolism of pyridoxine, which consequently affects the production of γ aminobutyric acid (GABA), an inhibitory synaptic neurotransmitter in the brain (Figure 68–1) (13). Glutamic acid decarboxylase (GAD) is the enzyme that converts glutamic acid to GABA; this enzyme requires pyridoxal-5'-phosphate, which is the active form of pyridoxine as a coenzyme (14). Isoniazid directly combines with pyridoxine and forms an isonicotinoylhydrazide complex that is excreted in the urine. It also is an inhibitor of pyridoxine kinase, the enzyme responsible for producing pyridoxal phosphate, the biologically active form of pyridoxine (15). Thus, isoniazid creates an absolute

Glutamic acid Glutamic acid
decarboxylase γ-Aminobutyric acid
(requires vitamin B_6)

Isoniazid + Vitamin B_6 ⟶ Isoniazid–pyridoxine hydrazone

FIG. 68–1. Mechanism of interference of isoniazid in metabolism of gamma-aminobutyric acid.

pyridoxine deficiency exacerbated by an interference with the ability to use any remaining stores of this vitamin.

Of particular significance is pyridoxal phosphate's coenzyme role in the synthesis of GABA by L-glutamic acid decarboxylase. GABA is the major inhibitory neurotransmitter of the CNS, and the blockage of its production secondary to a state of pyridoxine deficiency, which results in unopposed excitation, is a major factor in the pathogenesis of isoniazid-induced seizures.

At the molecular level, isoniazid interferes with nicotinamide adenine dinucleotide (NAD)-catalyzed reactions (8). NAD is recognized as an essential component of the energy-producing reactions of glycolysis and the tricarboxylic acid cycle (2). The introduction of isoniazid into the NAD molecule forms an inactive analog of NAD that seriously disrupts intermediary metabolism and inhibits the conversion of lactate to pyruvate (16).

TOXICITY

Typically, after ingestion of large amounts of isoniazid, the patient experiences a latent period of 30 minutes to 2 hours (Table 68–2) (9). Subsequently, there is the gradual development of nausea, vomiting, blurred vision, visual hallucinations (which may include colored lights, spots, or strange designs), dizziness, slurred speech, dilated pupils, ataxia, tachycardia, and hyperthermia (8). Within 90 minutes to 3 hours after ingestion, which corresponds roughly to the time at which peak isoniazid serum concentrations are attained, the patient may suddenly lapse into stupor and may also develop sudden tonic–clonic generalized or localized seizures (17,18). There may then be rapid progression to intractable coma, marked hyperreflexia or complete areflexia, severe hypotension, cyanosis, and death.

Metabolic alterations associated with isoniazid intoxication include severe metabolic acidosis, hyperglycemia, and glycosuria. In severe cases, pneumonitis and cardiorespiratory arrest may occur (16).

The underlying cause of the metabolic acidosis in isoniazid intoxication is not entirely understood. It has been suggested that the acidosis is related to the inhibition of the NAD, which consequently causes a buildup of lactic acid (8). Another proposed mechanism is that the metabolic acidosis is due to the lactic acidosis secondary to the prolonged seizure activity (16).

TABLE 68–2. *Signs and symptoms of isoniazid intoxication*

Gastrointestinal
Nausea
Vomiting
Neurologic
Blurred vision
Dizziness
Slurred speech
Mydriasis
Ataxia
Hallucinations
Hyperreflexia or areflexia
Stupor
Seizures
Coma
Metabolic
Metabolic acidosis
Hyperglycemia
Glycosuria
Hyperthermia
Miscellaneous
Hypotension
Cyanosis
Tachycardia
Pneumonitis
Death

INH has been associated with multiple neurologic toxicities, of which peripheral neuropathy secondary to distal axonopathy is most common. Sensory complaints are the most frequently described, however, muscle weakness, atrophy, and fasciculations, alterations in reflexes, autonomic dysfunction, mental status changes, and headache have also been described (19).

DIAGNOSIS

The diagnosis of isoniazid intoxication should be considered in patients presenting with unexplained seizures and metabolic acidosis (20). Often, these seizures are unresponsive and refractory to conventional antileptic therapy (2). Isoniazid as a cause of seizures should be considered in patients who have access to the drug and in anyone whose seizures are poorly controlled with the usual anticonvulsants and in whom isoniazid overdose could be suspected (13).

LABORATORY ANALYSIS

Although there are numerous methods for determining isoniazid concentrations in blood or urine, there are few laboratories that are able to make such measurements except in experimental situations (21,22). In a therapeutic situation, serum concentrations are usually between 1 and 7 μg/mL (4). Blood concentrations of isoniazid are usually

TABLE 68–3. *Laboratory abnormalities in isoniazid intoxication*

Hyperglycemia
Glucosuria
Ketonuria
Hyperkalemia (mild)
Elevated serum isoniazid concentration
Anion gap metabolic acidosis
Increased excretion of pyridoxine

TABLE 68–5. *Treatment for isoniazid overdose*

Medical observation (6 hours if asymptomatic)
Lavage
Charcoal and cathartic
Intravenous fluid therapy
Hypotension diuresis
Sodium bicarbonate (as necessary)
Pyridoxine (2 to 5 9 IV)
Forced (alkaline) diuresis
Dialysis (if renal failure present)

significantly higher in acute intoxications than those from therapeutic doses (6); toxic blood concentrations are considered greater than 20 μg/mL (23).

Laboratory tests usually reveal a severe metabolic acidosis (24), hyperglycemia, glycosuria, ketonuria, mild hyperkalemia, and increased urinary excretion of pyridoxine (Table 68–3) (22). Blood should, therefore, be drawn for arterial blood gases, serum electrolytes, blood urea nitrogen, and glucose concentration. Blood should also be typed and cross-matched in the event that hemodialysis is required (Table 68–4) (14).

TREATMENT

Because of severe morbidity and high mortality rates, patients who are asymptomatic after isoniazid overdose should be observed medically for at least 4 to 6 hours (Table 68–5) (21). It may also be safer to assume that absence of symptomatology reflects a latent period rather than lack of a toxic response to isoniazid (13).

Emergency treatment consists of attention to the airway, cardiorespiratory support, treatment of seizures, correction of the metabolic acidosis, enhancing excretion of the drug, and administration of pyridoxine (18).

Supportive care includes gastric lavage with subsequent administration of activated charcoal and a cathartic. Intravenous fluids should be given both to control hypotension and to induce a diuresis. Sodium bicarbonate is usually not needed for the metabolic acidosis if seizure activity is stopped with adequate doses of pyridoxine (23).

Pyridoxine

Therapeutic trials have shown the effectiveness of parenteral doses of pyridoxine to treat isoniazid intoxication, especially the associated seizure activity (4). Pyridoxine is thought to prevent the effects of isoniazid on GAD activity and thereby to prevent a decrease in brain GABA. Large doses of pyridoxine are given intravenously on the basis of a suspected milligram-per-milligram equivalency of ingested isoniazid (20). If the amount of isoniazid ingested is unknown, 5 g of pyridoxine (50 ml of a 10% solution) is given over a period of 3 to 5 minutes and may be followed in 30 minutes by an additional 5 g (18). Preferably, pyridoxine therapy should begin during the latent interval between ingestion and seizure activity (15).

Pyridoxine is commercially available in 10-mL vials containing 1 g of pyridoxine each. The danger of pyridoxine overdosage is slight, and although chronic intoxication can occur (25), acute intoxication occurs only if massive amounts are administered (18). Toxic effects of pyridoxine include tachypnea, postural reflex abnormalities, paralysis, and convulsions; these usually arise after more than 5 to 6 g/kg has been administered (Table 68–6). In INH, overdose up to 52 g of intravenous pyridoxine has been tolerated without adverse effect (15).

Animal studies suggest a synergistic effect of pyridoxine and diazepam in the suppression of isoniazid-induced seizures (18). Phenytoin and barbiturates do not appear to be effective for these seizures. Phenytoin may even be toxic to patients with a high serum isoniazid concentration because isoniazid is a potent inhibitor of phenytoin metabolism by inhibition of the parahydroxylation of phenytoin. This may lead to excessive concentrations of phenytoin and associated toxic symptoms (23).

TABLE 68–4. *Laboratory determinations in isoniazid intoxication*

Arterial blood gas
Serum electrolytes
Blood urea nitrogen
Serum glucose concentration
Blood type and cross-match
Serum isoniazid concentration (if available)

Bicarbonate

If seizure activity is allowed to continue before pyridoxine is given, a severe lactic acidosis can result (4). This reverses when seizures abate (24). Also, because the lactic acidosis seen after seizures resolves spontaneously

TABLE 68–6. *Side effects of pyridoxine (5 to 6 g/kg)*

Tachypnea
Postural hypotension
Paralysis
Seizures

and because metabolic alkalosis may result from metabolism of excess lactate, the administration of large amounts of bicarbonate may be potentially harmful (20).

Methods to Enhance Excretion

Forced diuresis has been shown to increase clearance of isoniazid (4). In addition, the physical properties of isoniazid, a small, water-soluble molecule that is poorly protein-bound and that has a small volume of distribution, suggest that it would be efficiently removed from the circulation by dialysis. Hemoperfusion or hemodialysis may be helpful to remove the systemic isoniazid and improve acid-base status if forced diuresis proves inadequate. If adequate doses of pyridoxine are given, dialysis does not seem to be required except in those patients who develop acute renal failure (16,20).

Renal excretion accounts for between 50–80% of INH elimination. However, most of the drug is excreted in an inactive form having first undergone acetylation in the liver. Slow acetylators will excrete more active drug. Consequently, uremic patients will not necessarily demonstrate a prolonged INH half-life or elevated serum concentrations unless they are also slow acetylators. Patients who have both renal failure and slow acetylation status will be at the greatest risk for the development of toxicity (24).

REFERENCES

1. Byrd R, Nelson R, Elliott R: Isoniazid toxicity. *JAMA* 1972;220: 1471–1473.
2. Cameron W: Isoniazid overdose. *Can Med Assoc J* 1978;118: 1413–1414.
3. Terman D, Teitelbaum D: Isoniazid self-poisoning. *Neurology* 1970;20:299–304.
4. Coyer J, Nicholson D: Isoniazid-induced convulsions. *South Med J* 1976;69:294–297.
5. Bahri A, Chiang C, Timbrell J: Acetylhydrazine hepatotoxicity. *Toxicol Appl Pharmacol* 1981;60:561–569.
6. Holdiness M: Neurological manifestations and toxicities of the antituberculosis drugs. *Med Toxicol* 1987;2:33–51.
7. Lewin P, McGreal D: Isoniazid toxicity with cerebellar ataxia in a child. *Can Med Assoc J* 1993;148:49–50.
8. Chin L, Sievers M, Herrier R, et al: Convulsions as the etiology of lactic acidosis in acute isoniazid toxicity in dogs. *Toxicol Appl Pharmacol* 1979;49:377–384.
9. Sievers M, Herrier R, Chin L, et al: Treatment of acute isoniazid toxicity. *Am J Hosp Pharmacol* 1975;32:202–206.
10. Blumberg E, Gil R: Cerebellar syndrome caused by isoniazid. *DICP Ann Pharmacother* 1990;24:829–831.
11. Miller J, Robinson A, Percy A: Acute isoniazid poisoning in childhood. *Am J Dis Child* 1980;134:290–292.
12. Bailey W, Weill H, DeRouen T, et al: The effect of isoniazid on transaminase levels. *Ann Intern Med* 1974;81:200–202.
13. Wason S, Lacouture P, Lovejoy F: Single high-dose pyridoxine treatment for isoniazid overdose. *JAMA* 1981;246:1102–1104.
14. Sievers M, Chin L: Treatment of isoniazid overdose. *JAMA* 1982;247:583–584.
15. Brent J, Vo N, Rumack B: Reversal of prolonged isoniazid-induced coma by pyridoxine. *Arch Intern Med* 1990;150:1751–1753.
16. Bear E, Hoffman P, Siegel S, et al: Suicidal ingestion of isoniazid: an uncommon cause of metabolic acidosis and seizures. *South Med J* 1976;69:31–32.
17. Bredemann J, Krechel S, Eggers G: Treatment of refractory seizures in massive isoniazid overdose. *Anesth Analg* 1990;71:554–557.
18. Yarbrough B, Wood J: Isoniazid overdose treated with high-dose pyridoxine. *Ann Emerg Med* 1983;12:303–305.
19. Torrent J, Izquierdo I, Cabezas R, et al: Theophylline–isoniazid interaction. *DICP Ann Pharmacother* 1989;23:143–145.
20. Cocco A, Pazourek L: Acute isoniazid intoxication—management by peritoneal dialysis. *N Engl J Med* 1963;269:852–853.
21. Brown A, Mallett M, Fiser D, et al: Acute isoniazid intoxication: reversal of CNS symptoms with large doses of pyridoxine. *Pediatr Pharmacol* 1984;4:199–202.
22. Scott E, Wright R: Fluorometric determination of isonicotinic acid hydrazide in serum. *J Lab Clin Med* 1967;70:355–360.
23. Brown C: Acute isoniazid poisoning. *Am Rev Respir Dis* 1972;105: 206–216.
24. Black L, Ros S: Complete recovery from severe metabolic acidosis associated with isoniazid poisoning in a young boy. *Pediatr Emerg Care* 1989;65:257–258.
25. Schaumburg H, Kaplan J, Windebank A, et al: Sensory neuropathy from pyridoxine abuse. *N Engl J Med* 1983;309:445–448.

PART XII

BOTANICAL AGENTS

CHAPTER 69

Plants

The ubiquity of plants in homes, fields, and gardens makes plant poisoning an ever-present potential health hazard. *Phytotoxicology* is the study of poisonings of humans and animals by plants (1). As both medicinal agents and poisons, plants have been prominent in history, in the healing arts, in religious rituals, and as homicidal and suicidal agents (2). The attractive appearance of many plants or plant parts often entices children and adults to sample them (3). With the increasing popular interest in horticulture and health foods and the recent surge in outdoor camping activity, the number of cases of plant intoxication is increasing and is likely to continue to rise (4).

Plant ingestion may extend the treating physician beyond the limits of existing sources of medical knowledge, but emergency department staff should be able to recognize toxic house plants and should to some extent know the symptoms produced by their ingestion as well as appropriate treatment (5). Although there are thousands of species of plants capable of producing moderate to severe and possibly fatal poisoning, relatively few cases of serious intoxication occur in the United States, and these are associated with a limited number of plants (6).

PLANT IDENTIFICATION

Common or vernacular names are an entirely inadequate means of specifying plants, and without reliable determination of the botanical name the existing toxicologic information concerning a given plant is unavailable for review. Definitive identification should be left to a professionally trained botanist. As an example, the common name *hemlock* may mean many different things. *Water hemlock* may cause seizures and is different from *poison hemlock*, which causes muscular paralysis (1,3). *Ground hemlock* is another name for the native American yew and causes completely different symptoms. The *hemlock tree*, a conifer, is not considered poisonous.

Making a clinical diagnosis of plant poisoning is often difficult. Characteristic structures and features of ingested plants are often distorted or lost while passing through the gastrointestinal tract. Ingested plants may be affected by physical factors such as mastication, muscular contractions, gastric acid, other ingestants, water and gases, and microbial agents.

This chapter identifies various classes of symptoms and signs caused by the various groups of plants and is not intended to provide detailed botanical classifications.

CLINICAL EFFECTS

Poisonous plants may produce a wide range of clinical effects, some relatively minor and others severe enough to be fatal (Table 69–1). The exact amounts required to produce toxic effects vary, depending on the type and part of the plant ingested, the age of the patient, and the season of the year. No botanical relationship exists to help localize toxicity in the plant kingdom (3). Nearly all major groups of plants from algae and fungi through gymnosperms and angiosperms have ample toxic representatives scattered among them. Some plants poison if they are chewed or swallowed. Others poison by causing allergies, dermatitis, or mechanical injury (5). Some plants are harmful if eaten or chewed at certain stages of their growth, and others are toxic at all stages. Parts of a plant can differ greatly in toxicity. A good example is rhubarb, which has a stalk that is commonly eaten but a leaf blade that is very toxic (2).

Patients poisoned by plant ingestion are asymptomatic in most cases. Rarely will a patient become mildly symptomatic (7). Most patients are admitted to the emergency

TABLE 69–1. *Plants and their clinical effects*

Alkaloids
Antimuscarinic alkaloids
Nicotine-like
Purine
Glycosides
Cardiac
Cyanogenic
Oxalate-containing
Seizure-producing
Phytotoxins
Skin-sensitizing
Gastroenteritis-producing

department shortly after their symptoms begin; and in plant poisoning, the symptoms at patient's admission usually dictate the appropriate therapy because in most instances there is neither a specific treatment nor an antidote. The initial approach to management of any plant ingestion should be the same as that for any toxic ingestion (8).

HISTORY

A detailed history may be critical for distinguishing a potentially lethal ingestion from a mildly noxious exposure. Elements important in the history include onset of symptoms from time of ingestion, parts and amount of the plant consumed, initial symptoms, and method of preparation of the plant. The type and onset of symptoms are the most important information and are more reliable than the presumed identification of the plant in gauging toxicity. Most symptoms will be apparent within 1 to 2 hours of ingestion; only rarely will evidence of significant toxicity begin more than 4 hours after ingestion.

PHYSICAL EXAMINATION

Physical examination is an important supplement to the patient's symptoms. Most symptomatic patients who have ingested toxic plants present with nausea, vomiting, and diarrhea. Skin flushing and pupil dilation can be important clues to toxicity. Cardiovascular abnormalities including dysrhythmias and bradycardia may be present and indicate the need for monitoring. Central nervous system depression or excitement and seizures can occur as a result of nicotinic and antimuscarinic poisonings.

LABORATORY

In symptomatic patients, the important baseline laboratory tests are dictated on the basis of the type of plant ingested. Laboratory tests may include complete blood cell count; measurements of serum electrolytes, blood urea nitrogen, and serum creatinine; and urinalysis. If oxalate has been ingested, serum calcium and phosphorus measurements may be necessary. If a hepatotoxin is suspected, liver function and coagulation studies are recommended. For suspected cardiac glycosides, an electrocardiogram is necessary (2).

The noxious chemicals in plants may be classified as alkaloids, glycosides, resins, phenols, alcohols, oxalates, and phytotoxins. Plants can also be grouped according to the symptoms produced on ingestion, which are based on the type of active compound in the plant or plant part. In this chapter, plants are divided into the alkaloids, which include the belladonna group as well as the group associated with nicotine; the glycosides, which include the cardiac glycosides and cyanogenic glycosides; plants that cause direct skin injury on contact, such as those that contain oxalate; the gastrointestinal irritants; the hallucinogens; plants that cause seizures; plants that contain pressor amines; and plants that contain miscellaneous compounds (3,5).

PLANTS THAT CONTAIN ALKALOIDS

Antimuscarinic Alkaloids

The tropane alkaloids are often called belladonna alkaloids (9). Plants that contain belladonna alkaloids produce their clinical effects by competitive inhibition of acetylcholine, whereby a dose-related blockade of the cholinergic nervous system develops (10). These plants may contain active ingredients such as atropine (hyoscyamine), scopolamine (hyoscine), stramonium alkaloids, and ecgonine compounds (Table 69–2).

The tropane alkaloids are rapidly absorbed from the gastrointestinal tract, mucosal surfaces, and respiratory tree (11). The drugs are hydrolyzed in the liver and excreted in the urine. Young children are more sensitive to atropine poisoning than adults because of their lower tolerance to elevated body temperature, which may be caused by these agents (12).

Jimson Weed

Datura species are the most commonly ingested antimuscarinic plants. Common names include Jamestown weed, jimson weed, loco weed, devil's weed, and thornapple (Fig. 69–1) (1). Jimson weed (*Datura stramonium*) is an abused substance with potentially serious clinical effects that is popular with adolescents and young adults, who ingest or smoke it to produce hallucinations. There are no legal controls or regulations on this plant.

Jimson weed is widely distributed in fields and waste areas throughout the United States, especially in the South but can also be grown as a garden ornamental. The plant has white to purplish flowers and prickly seed pods. Adult poisonings are usually the result of ingesting tea made from the flowers, seeds, or leaves of jimson weed (3). Some patients may ingest seeds intentionally for the CNS effects. Ingestion of the flowers, drinking teas from

TABLE 69–2. *Plants that cause antimuscarinic syndrome*

Datura species (jimson weed)
Atropa belladonna (deadly nightshade)
Cestrum sp (jasmine)
Hyoscyamus niger (henbane)
Lycium haliamifolium (matrimony vine)

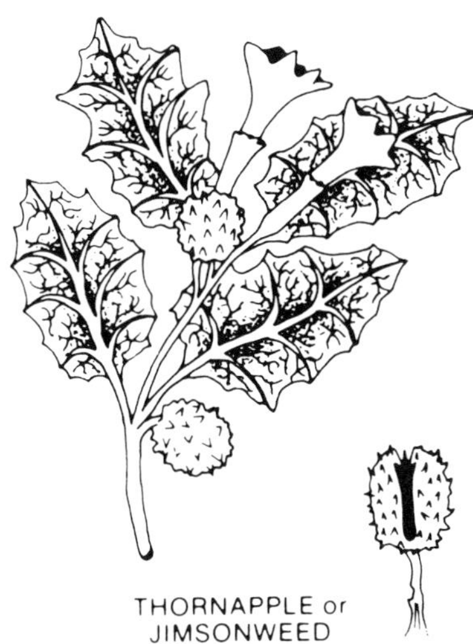

FIG. 69–1. Jimson weed. From Gossel TA and Bricker JD. *Principles of Clinical Toxicology, Third Edition,* New York: Raven Press, 1994, p. 251, with permission.

the plant parts, or smoking *stramonium* cigarettes also can induce CNS toxicity (10).

The flowers of *Datura stramonium* are generally light purple, but other members of the *Datura* family may have white, yellowish, or pink flowers all with the distinctive funnel shape. Although the entire plant is toxic, the seeds are most often used in abuse. The tan to black, kidney-shaped, 2- to 3-mm-long seeds are found inside a spiked ball-like capsule about the size of a golf or tennis ball, which may contain between 50 and 100 seeds. The seeds contain the highest concentration of alkaloids (0.40%); the leaves and flowers contain about 0.25%.

The active ingredients are solanaceous alkaloids; the primary alkaloid being hyoscyamine, with lesser amounts of atropine and scopolamine. The antimuscarinic effects are, therefore, similar to that seen with atropine ingestion.

Symptoms begin 2 to 6 hours after ingestion and resolve in 24 to 48 hours (Table 69–3). Patients typically present with tachycardia, dilated pupils, blurred vision, and hypertension. Delirium, hallucinations involving natural colors, and alterations of perception occur in almost all individuals. Hallucinations may be both auditory and visual (10). Patients communicate with invisible friends and pick things off walls or clothing. Seizures and tactile hallucinations may occur, but are uncommon. Traumatic death may occur, often as a result of errors in judgment while under influence of the plant. Similar effects are seen with ingestions of henbane (*Hyoscyamus niger)*, deadly nightshade (*Atropa belladonna*), and other plants containing antimuscarinic-like compounds.

Treatment of antimuscarinic poisoning is discussed in Chapter 10.

TABLE 69–3. *Signs and symptoms of solanaceous alkaloid toxicity*

Peripheral
Tachycardia
Pupillary dilatation
Blurred vision
Hypertension
Absent bowel sounds
Urinary retention
Central nervous system
Delirium
Hallucinations (visual, auditory, tactile)
Seizures

Solanine Alkaloids

The plant genus *Solanum* includes some 1,500 species, and most contain the alkaloid solanine (Table 69–4). Some common plants that contain solanine include the potato (*Solanum tuberosum*) and the Jerusalem cherry (*Solanum pseudo-capsicum*) (13). The common potato can cause intoxication from ingestion of leaves, all green parts of the plant, and the roots, which contain high concentrations of solanine. The Jerusalem cherry is a potted plant with attractive red berries that often appears in households during the Christmas season.

Solanine is a glycoalkaloid that, when hydrolyzed by gastric acid, yields a sugar and an alkamine (7). The intact glycoalkaloid is an irritant to the mucous membranes and the gastrointestinal tract. The alkamine primarily affects the CNS, and the cardiovascular system (1). Initial symptoms are burning of the mouth and oropharynx; gastrointestinal symptoms including nausea, vomiting, and diarrhea then develop. Neurologic symptoms include apathy, hallucinations, tremor, paralysis, and mydriasis (6). Patients with solanine poisoning may also develop concomitant signs of anticholinergic poisoning. Most symptoms resolve within 24 hours, and deaths are rare (2).

Nicotine-like Alkaloids

Plants containing nicotine, cytisine, and coniine all exert similar toxic actions. These are all pyridine or piperidine alkaloids; other substances of this type include lobeline, arecoline, and piperine (Table 69–5). The toxic effects of nicotine and treatment of intoxication are discussed fully in Chapter 83.

TABLE 69–4. *Plants containing solanine*

Solanum dulcamara (woody nightshade, European bittersweet)
Solanum nigrum (black nightshade, common nightshade)
Solanum pseudo-capsicum (Jerusalem cherry)
Solanum tuberosum (potato)

TABLE 69–5. *Nicotine-like alkaloids*

Common name	Botanical name	Alkaloid
Tobacco	*Nicotiana* sp	Nicotine
Golden chain	*Laburnum anagyroides*	Cytisine tree
Poison hemlock	*Conium maculatum*	Coniine

Fatalities from nicotine-containing plants have occurred with the ingestion of "salads" prepared from wild tobacco leaves (*Nicotiana* sp). Symptoms can also occur from the ingestion of cigarettes, cigars, cigarette butts, snuff, and Nicorette gum. The action of nicotine and its congeners on neuroeffector junctions is rapid and variable. There is an initial stimulation of autonomic ganglia with a subsequent depression of transmission. Nicotine similarly affects the neuromuscular junction, with a stimulatory phase that is followed rapidly by paralysis (3).

Cytisine poisoning is most commonly encountered in children who shell and eat the seeds from the pea-like pods of the golden chain tree (*Laburnum anagyroides).*

Coniine, which is the principal alkaloid in poison hemlock, is a pyridine derivative similar to nicotine. Coniine poisoning usually results from eating of the parsley-like leaves or seeds of poison hemlock (*Conium maculatum*) (1). Poison hemlock is a European plant that was introduced into North America and grows in marshy areas; it should not be confused with water hemlock (1). Poison hemlock and wild carrot both have a long, white, unbranched, turnip-like taproot. The white flowers bloom in flat clusters and emit a strong odor of urine when crushed. The entire plant contains coniine, especially the seeds and roots. Poison hemlock eventually acts by depressing the CNS and bringing on paralysis. Death ensues when the muscles of respiration become paralyzed (2).

Clinical Effects of Intoxication

Initial symptoms result from stimulation of autonomic ganglia. Clinical symptoms, however, are mixed because of the variability of the clinical response. Usually, there is a spontaneous emesis within 15 to 30 minutes after ingestion. Initial parasympathomimetic signs change to sympathomimetic signs, and bradycardia, miosis, and hyperventilation may change to tachycardia and mydriasis. Seizures and hypotension may ultimately occur, along with respiratory failure.

Treatment

Treatment consists of supportive measures. It may be a mistake to treat the initial bradycardia with atropine because this naturally progresses to a tachycardia. If treatment of the bradycardia is necessary, temporary cardiac pacing may be indicated.

Purine Alkaloids

The purine alkaloids caffeine and theobromine are found in various plants. The derivative beverages may represent a toxic risk.

Chapter 50 includes a discussion of caffeine toxicity.

PLANTS THAT CONTAIN GLYCOSIDES

Cardiac Glycosides (Fig. 69–2)

Plants that contain cardiac glycosides are the most widely used in standard medicine (Table 69–6). There are a number of varieties of these plants, including foxglove (*Digitalis purpurea*), oleander (*Nerium oleander*), and lily of the valley (*Convallaria majalis*) (14). Neither boiling nor drying affects the toxicity of these plants.

Glycosides in *Nerium oleander* include oleandrin, oleandroside, nerioside, and digitoxigenin. Yellow oleander contains thevetin and thevetoxin (1). Oleander is a shrub that grows up to 20 feet in height. It is an extremely hardy plant and is popular because of the ease with which it is grown and its attractive red, pink, or white clusters of

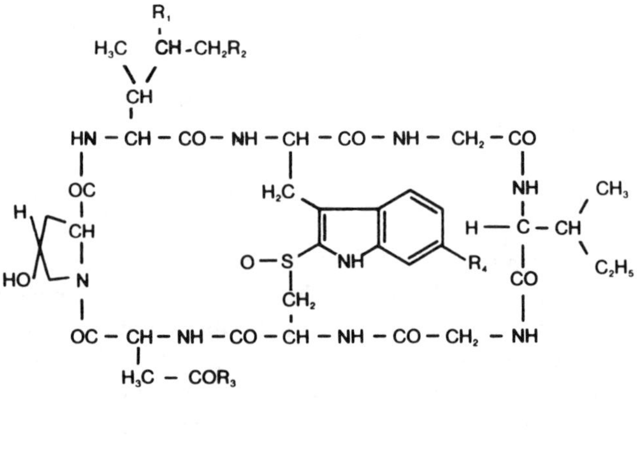

	R_1	R_2	R_3	R_4
α-Amanitin	OH	OH	NH_2	OH
β-Amanitin	OH	OH	OH	OH
γ-Amanitin	H	OH	NH_2	OH
ε-Amanitin	H	OH	OH	OH
Amanin	OH	OH	OH	H

FIG. 69–2. Plants containing cardiac glycosides. From Gossel TA and Bricker JD. *Principles of Clinical Toxicology, Third Edition,* New York: Raven Press, 1994, p. 251, with permission.

TABLE 69–6. *Cardiac glycoside–containing plants*

***Digitalis purpurea* (foxglove)**
Digoxin
Digitoxin
Gitoxin
Others
***Nerium oleander* (oleander)**
Oleandroside
Oleandrin
Nerioside
***Urginea maritima* (squill)**
***Convallaria majalis* (lily of the valley)**
Convallatoxins
***Thevetia peruviana* (yellow oleander)**
Thevetin A and B
Thevetoxin
Peruvoside
Fluvoside
Nerilifolin
***Rhododendron* sp (azalea)**
Andromedotoxins (grayanotoxins)
***Taxus* sp (yew)**

flowers. The entire plant is toxic; toxicity is also associated with smoke from burning cuttings and water in which the flowers are placed (2). In addition to causing cardiac toxicity, oleander also irritates mucous membranes, causing buccal erythema and burning of the mouth. Gastrointestinal effects include nausea, vomiting, increased salivation, abdominal pain, and diarrhea (14).

Several reports note a cross-reactivity between digitalis and oleander glycoside in radioimmunoassays, causing elevation of the reported digoxin concentration after ingestion of oleander. Because the amount of cross-reactivity is unknown, digitalis radioimmunoassay predicts only the presence of the glycoside, not the degree of toxicity.

A detailed discussion of signs, symptoms, workup, and treatment of the patient with cardiac glycoside intoxication is given in Chapter 21.

Andromedotoxin

Azaleas, rhododendrons, and laurels contain andromedotoxin, which has properties similar to those of the cardiac glycosides or *Veratrum* alkaloids. All 250 species of azalea (*Rhododendron occidental*) are poisonous, although this is an area of controversy (15). Andromedotoxin may cause hypotension and bradycardia. Other effects include salivation, nasal discharge, anorexia, vomiting, and diarrhea. These may progress to drowsiness, headache, seizures, paralysis, and coma (7).

Symptoms of poisoning usually begin within 1 to 2 hours of ingestion. Initially there is local irritation of the mouth and emesis (16). In contrast to poisonings with the pure cardiac glycosides, poisoning with these plants is associated with gastrointestinal manifestations and abdominal pain due to the presence of saponins and other irritants. Visual disturbances may also be noted. In a patient with a normal heart, toxicity is generally manifested by conduction defects rather than by increased automaticity, and an electrocardiogram may show atrioventricular conduction defects and sinus bradycardia. Hyperkalemia may occur in severe ingestions because of interference with the normal cellular sodium–potassium transport mechanism (14).

Yew

The yew (*Taxus* sp) is a popular ornamental evergreen shrub-like tree. It is the darkest green of all evergreen shrubs, and they flourish in different soil types. Their popularity has resulted in widespread cultivation along fences, borders, buildings, and yards for shade and screen (17). All *Taxus* species and all parts of the plant except the fleshy fruit are poisonous and can be lethal to human beings when ingested, yet the bitter taste of the leaves and berries probably prevents accidental ingestion of significant amounts. The seeds are not toxic if swallowed whole because the seed coat resists digestive enzymes (18).

Mechanism of Toxicity

The yew plant contains an alkaloid with powerful arrhythmogenic capabilities similar to the cardiac glycosides in foxglove and oleander. Intoxications are usually attributed to a group of 10 alkaloids, of which the cardiotoxic taxine A and taxine B are considered the primary toxicants. Once ingested, the alkaloids are rapidly absorbed and metabolized. The primary toxicity appears to be at the level of the myocardial cell (17). The specific mechanism is unknown; however, it is believed that the taxines produce a decrease in cardiac conduction, causing the heart to stop in diastole, followed by asphyxiation (18). The mechanism is thought to be by interference with the cardiac conduction system through effects on the sodium–potassium transport mechanism. Negative inotropic effects produce hypotension and cardiac unresponsiveness (17).

Clinical Effects

The clinical effects of yew toxicity resemble both digitalis and oleander toxicity and also produce lethargy, vomiting, confusion, and a variety of arrhythmias, including a broad complex, idioventricular rhythm. Acute poisoning is more common and is characterized by sudden death within a few hours of ingestion with no significant postmortem lesion. Most cases are fatal, but a few victims have spontaneously recovered (18).

Diagnosis

Diagnosis is based on identification of the plant in the gastrointestinal tract, clinical presentation, history of exposure, and absence of other diseases and toxicants.

Treatment

There is no specific treatment for taxine poisoning. Treatment is supportive and may include cardiovascular support in the form of intravenous fluids and antidysrhythmic agents. Poor outcomes have been reported with external transcutaneous pacing for patents with asystole, electromechanical dissociation, and pulseless idioventricular rhythms. External cardiac pacing for patients with bradyarrhythmias, however, has been more encouraging (17). Clinical experience suggests that digoxin-specific antibody fragments may be useful in patients who suffer cardiotoxic effects from naturally occurring plant toxins.

False Hellebore

Veratrum viride or false hellebore is a tall perennial herb that grows widely in low-lying areas of Canada and the eastern U.S. from New England to Georgia. All parts of *Veratrum* plants contain poisonous *Veratrum* alkaloids, which can produce vomiting, bradycardia, and hypotension (19). *Veratrum* species contain toxic alkaloids that are chemically similar to steroids.

Mechanism of Toxicity

The primary site of action of *Veratrum* alkaloids is on afferent receptors in the posterior wall of the left ventricle and coronary sinus baroreceptor area. The resulting activity of these afferents causes a reflex lowering of blood pressure by a decrease in peripheral α-adrenergic tone. This reflex lowering of blood pressure and associated bradycardia produced by *Veratrum* alkaloids is termed the Bezold-Jarisch reflex. The afferent information is transmitted by the vagus nerve and the reflex is abolished by vagotomy and reversed by atropine (19).

Treatment

Treatment of patients with *Veratrum* intoxication is supportive. The patient must be watched closely for changes in airway status if severe hypotension ensues. It is reasonable to administer charcoal and a cathartic after nausea subsides, but clinical data illustrating their efficacy are unavailable. Seizures are rare and may be treated with the usual anticonvulsant drugs. The bradycardia produced by *Veratrum* alkaloids responds to atropine, but the blood pressure response after atropine varies. A patient may remain hypotensive, achieve normal blood pressure, or become hypertensive. Rarely and perhaps only in the setting of preexisting cardiac disease or medication would β agonists or pacing be required.

TABLE 69–7. *Plants containing cyanogenic glycosides*

Pyrus sylvestris (apple)
Prunus armeniaca (apricot)
Prunus cerasus (cherry)
Prunus persica (peach)
Prunus virginiana (choke cherry)

Prognosis

The majority of patients can be expected to recover in 24 to 48 hours unless delay in treatment, preexisting cardiovascular illness, or metabolic derangement compromise the patient's ability to tolerate the intoxication (19).

Cyanogenic Glycosides

Glycosides that yield hydrocyanic acid on hydrolysis are known as cyanogenic glycosides. The most important glycoside in this group is amygdalin, which is abundant in plants of the Rosaceae family (Table 69–7). A full discussion of these glycosides is given in Chapter 21.

PLANTS THAT CONTAIN OXALATE

Many species of *Arum* contain calcium oxalate as a toxic ingredient (Fig. 69–3). Other genera of plants that contain oxalates include *Monstera* (Swiss cheese plant), *Colocasia* (elephant's-ear), *Caladium*, and *Xanthosoma* (Table 69–8) (20). Oxalates can be in the form of insoluble calcium oxalate crystals, called raphides, or soluble sodium and potassium oxalate. The raphides are located in ampule-shaped raphide ejector cells. Irritation or slight pressure on the cap causes swelling of the ejector cell contents, resulting in sudden expulsion of the raphides as well as free oxalic acid. The prototype of this species is the dieffenbachia (8).

The dieffenbachia are both indoor and outdoor plants and resemble sugar cane or the banana plant. The dieffenbachia have a thick green stem with oval leaves up to 15 inches long (20). Plants may grow 3 to 6 feet in height or more (21). All parts of the dieffenbachia are toxic, including the leaves, stem, and roots. The sap can produce corneal opacification if it comes in contact with the eye (2,21).

Plants of the genus *Philodendron* are extremely popular houseplants because they require little light and attention. Whereas the philodendron is a vine, the dieffenbachia usually grows vertically on a large cane-like stalk which often necessitates that it is placed on the floor in areas that are accessible to children. Like the philodendron, the dieffenbachia is a member of the

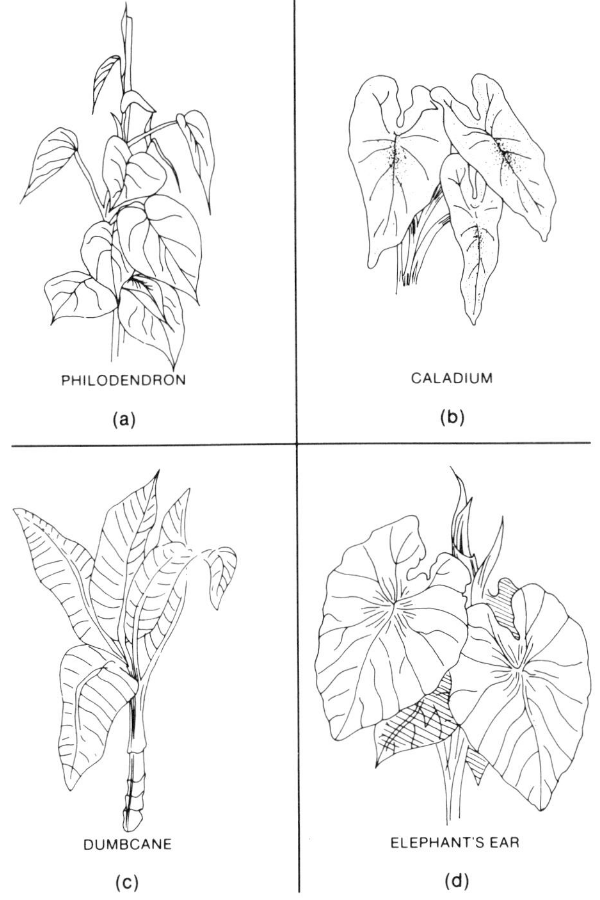

FIG. 69–3. Common household plants of the Arum family that cause poisoning. (From Gossel TA and Bricker JD. *Principles of Clinical Toxicology, Third Edition,* New York: Raven Press, 1994, p. 247, with permission.)

Araceae family and shares the same toxic principles. It is often referred to as "dumb" cane because individuals who have chewed on the stalk or cane have been unable to speak due to intense irritation and swelling in the oral cavity. The clinical symptoms are similar to those of oxalic poisoning (8).

The tuber of *Colocasia antiquorum* (elephant's-ear) is processed into a starchy food called poi, but the green parts contain oxalates and cause significant irritation when ingested. Rhubarb is a coarse perennial plant the leaf blade of which contains soluble oxalate (3).

Clinical Effects of Intoxication

Ingestion of calcium oxalate causes extreme irritation of the mucous membranes. Biting or chewing plants containing these chemicals rapidly produces severe pain, salivation, swelling of the oropharynx, and speech difficulties and inflammation (16). Increased salivation, difficulty in swallowing, and laryngeal irritation can also occur. Corrosive burns of the mouth, oropharynx, esophagus, and stomach may ensue. The airway may become obstructed as the tongue enlarges (8). On occasion, systemic toxicity may occur (14). This is especially true for the soluble oxalates as a result of their rapid absorption from the gastrointestinal tract.

TABLE 69–8. *Oxalate-containing plants*

Arum sp
Philodendron sp (philodendron)
Dieffenbachia (dumbcane)
Caladium sp (caladium)
Colocasia sp (elephant's-ear)
Rheum rhaponticum (rhubarb)
Arisaema triphyllum (jack-in-the-pulpit)
Symplocarpus foetidus (skunk cabbage)
Monstera sp (Swiss cheese plant)

Laboratory Analysis and Treatment

A measurement of serum calcium concentrations is indicated in all ingestions, although it is rare for the hypocalcemia to be a symptomatic problem. Symptomatic and supportive care is usually the extent of necessary treatment. A patent airway is the first concern, and patients should be observed for airway obstruction. Ice may be used to reduce swelling. A mixture of 2% viscous lidocaine with diphenhydramine elixir may be applied to the affected areas for local pain relief (22). Hypocalcemia should be treated by the parenteral administration of calcium gluconate or some other calcium salt. Neither antihistamines nor corticosteroids have been shown to be effective. If calcium oxalate crystals are present in the urine, maintenance of an adequate urine flow is mandatory (2).

Soluble Oxalates

Soluble oxalates are found in the leaves of rhubarb (*Rheum rhaponticum*) and other plants and may be rapidly absorbed through the gastrointestinal tract, causing systemic effects secondary to hypocalcemia. Unlike the raphides or crystal oxalates, this form of oxalate combines with calcium to form calcium oxalate and can lead to severe hypocalcemia with accompanying muscle fasciculations or generalized seizures. Acute renal failure may ensue as a result of obstruction of the renal tubules by the calcium oxalate crystals as well as by the chemical action of the oxalate ion. Oxalate crystals in the ureter, kidney, and bladder may also cause pain, oxaluria, oliguria, and hematuria (4).

Patients who ingest rhubarb leaves generally become symptomatic within 6 to 12 hours, although delays of up to 24 hours have been reported. Patients with gastrointestinal symptoms should have serum calcium measurements monitored for 24 hours.

Treatment and Disposition

Most ingestions cause only mild symptoms, with rapid onset and rapid resolution. Patients with significant oxalate exposure may develop oral ulcerations. If significant hypocalcemia occurs, calcium replacement with calcium gluconate or chloride may be necessary. Patients with severe oral burns or significant oral swelling should be admitted and observed for airway obstruction (4).

PLANTS CAUSING SEIZURES

The principal plants responsible for producing seizures as their primary toxic manifestation are water hemlock (*Cicuta* sp: beaver poison, wild carrot, wild parsnip, and cowbane) and chinaberry (*Melia azederach*); both are members of the carrot family (23). Water hemlock is possibly the most toxic plant that grows in the United States (1). It is found only in wet, swampy areas and is most often ingested by individuals who mistake it for wild parsnips because of the yellow oil that is produced when the plant is injured (23). All parts of the plant are toxic, including the roots, leaves, and stems. The toxin has been called cicutoxin and is a highly unsaturated alcohol. Although most cases of toxicity occur through ingestion, the toxin also can be absorbed through the skin.

Symptoms begin within 15 to 60 minutes of ingestion and initially consist of muscarinic effects such as salivation, abdominal pain, diarrhea, and vomiting. This prodrome may be followed quickly by multiple grand mal seizures. Other CNS effects such as obtundation and respiratory distress may occur. Death may be secondary to the prolonged anoxia encountered with the tonic contractions (23). Long-term sequelae, including impaired intellectual function, may result from ingesting water hemlock.

Treatment is symptomatic and supportive. Maintenance of a patent airway and seizure precautions should be the first priorities. Seizures may be controlled with diazepam. Vigorous fluid replacement with isotonic saline may be required (1).

PLANTS THAT CONTAIN PHYTOTOXINS

Toxalbumins are phytotoxins, which are the most potent toxins in existence. The two most lethal plants containing toxalbumins are the castor bean and the jequirity bean (Table 69–9). The castor bean contains the toxalbumin ricin, and the jequirity bean contains abrin (24).

TABLE 69–9. *Plants containing toxalbumins*

Ricinus communis (castor bean)
Abrus precatorius (jequirity bean, rosary pea. precatory bean)
Hura crepitans (sandbox tree)
Jatropha sp (bellyache bush, Barbados nut)
Robinia pseudoacacia (black locust)

Castor Bean

The castor bean, which is obtained from a woody shrub that grows up to 15 feet in height, is white, black, and brown in a variegated pattern somewhat resembling a tick (1). This bean is native to Asia and Africa but now grows in many uncultivated areas in the United States (20). Ricin is composed of large protein molecules and resembles bacterial toxins in its structure and antigenic ability. Ricin has both hemagglutinin and toxic hemolytic components (20). Ricin is found in greatest quantities in the seed and is released if the hard-shelled beans are chewed or chopped (25).

Toxicity

The beans should be identified, and it should be determined whether they were raw and chewed or otherwise unhusked. The clinical severity of the intoxication cannot be predicted on the basis of the number of beans ingested.

The dust of the castor bean plant and crushed castor beans contain glucoproteins that are extremely allergenic; numerous allergic reaction ranging from contact dermatitis to anaphylaxis have been reported (25). Gloves should be worn when handling raw castor beans.

Most commonly, castor bean toxicity causes nausea, vomiting, and colicky abdominal pain which begins 2 to 10 hours after ingestion and often progresses to hemorrhagic gastritis. The initial gastrointestinal symptoms may be followed by systemic toxicity, including hemolysis and multi-organ failure involving the kidney, liver, and pancreas. Hemolysis has been documented up to 12 days after ingestion (4).

Disposition

Asymptomatic

The lag time from ingestion of the beans to onset of symptoms ranges from 15 minutes to 10 hours, although most symptoms occur in less than 6 hours. Therefore, asymptomatic patients who have chewed raw beans should probably be observed for at least 4 to 6 hours before being discharged home with appropriate warnings to return immediately if symptoms develop. Patients who have not chewed the beans or sucked beans with disrupted husks may be discharged after gastric decontamination (25).

Symptomatic

All symptomatic patients should be hospitalized until they are asymptomatic and laboratory values are within or approaching normal limits. Serum glucose concentrations should be monitored to detect hypoglycemia, which may reflect depletion of liver stores or glucose or inadequate nutrition during severe vomiting (25). A second hematocrit reading or hemoglobin determination should be performed to rule out hemolysis. In cases with significant fluid and electrolyte disturbances, liver dysfunction, rhabdomyolysis, and renal insufficiency secondary to prolonged hypovolemia should be anticipated.

Although the ingestion of castor beans may result in serious clinical intoxication, most patients respond well to intravenous fluid and electrolyte replacement and recover without permanent sequelae (25). Because ricin is not dialyzable and very little ricin is excreted in the urine, hemodialysis or forced diuresis is not indicated.

Jequirity Beans

Jequirity beans are brought into the United States from Central and South America. The bean is small and red in color with a black "eye" at the hilus (13). Because of its intense colors, it has been used extensively in beadwork and jewelry in the West Indies. Recently jequirity beans have been used in necklaces, belts, moccasins and slippers, bead bags, and rosaries and for eyes in dolls (14). In addition to abrin, the jequirity bean contains an amino acid, abric acid, and glycyrrhiza (13). The mature bean, if ingested whole, is innocuous because the hard outer shell is unaffected by digestive secretions (16). Chewing destroys the shell and allows absorption of the toxin. The immature bean, whose shell is soft and easily broken, is equally poisonous (2).

Clinical Effects of Intoxication

The toxic effects of abrin are considered due to both the red cell agglutination and a direct toxic action on parenchymal cells. Ricin causes the same symptoms as abrin but does not cause local toxicity (1). Recently, there has been some question as to the actual toxicity of ricin.

Toxicity may be noted in two phases (Table 69–10). During the acute phase, which may last 2 to 24 hours, there is burning in the mouth and throat with subsequent gastroenteritis. Nausea, vomiting, and abdominal pain may also occur, and severe hemorrhagic gastroenteritis may ensue. Because of the fluid loss, severe dehydration may result in oliguria and cardiovascular collapse. During the second phase, stupor, seizures, and death have been reported. Systemic symptoms involving the CNS and the cardiovascular system may begin after a delay of up to several days and may persist for as long as 10 days.

TABLE 69–10. *Signs and symptoms of phytotoxin poisoning*

Acute phase
Burning in the mouth
Burning in the throat
Nausea
Vomiting
Abdominal pain
Hemorrhagic gastroenteritis
Delayed symptoms
Central nervous system
Stupor
Seizures
Coma
Cardiovascular
Hypotension
Retinal hemorrhage
Scleral hemorrhage
Hepatic necrosis
Renal failure

Patients may develop hypotension, CNS hemorrhage, and retinal and scleral hemorrhages. Hepatic necrosis and renal failure have also been described. Because these beans are highly allergenic, they may cause dermatitis, urticaria, or anaphylaxis after skin contact.

Treatment

Treatment is supportive (3). The patient who is symptomatic and appears to have local burns should be treated as for any caustic burn. Close monitoring of the electrocardiogram and fluid and electrolyte status is the mainstay of supportive care. Vigorous fluid replacement in severe cases may be required to keep up with fluid losses (26).

PLANTS AFFECTING THE SKIN

There is a long list of plants that are capable of causing dermatitis in sensitized individuals, but the most frequent offenders are plants of the family *Anacardiaceae*, which contains species of *Toxicodendron* (Table 69–11) (27). These include plants with the common names of poison ivy, poison oak, and poison sumac. At one time these plants were mistakenly classed in the genus *Rhus* (26).

The *Toxicodendron* species are vigorous woody vines or shrubs that have a characteristic trifolate pattern. All these plants contain urushiol, an oil that acts as a hapten and elicits a type IV cell-mediated delayed hypersensitivity (26).

TABLE 69–11. Toxicodendron *species causing dermatitis*

T. radicans (poison ivy)
T. quercifolium, T. diversiloba (poison oak)
T. vernix (poison sumac)

Poison ivy is found throughout the United States and appears as a short rope-like vine or small shrub. In the western United States poison oak is an upright spreading shrub with oak-like leaves that are hairy on both sides; it grows as a low shrub in the eastern United States. Poison sumac is predominantly found east of the Mississippi River and grows as a tall shrub or tree up to 15 feet in height.

Mechanism of Toxicity

About 50% of the adult population is sensitized to poison ivy, although the dose and time of exposure required to produce symptoms may vary. When sensitized individuals contact poison ivy or its relatives, a pruritic, erythematous, and often vesicular rash develops within hours to days and may persist up to 10 days.

The sensitizer, urushiol, is found in all parts of the poison ivy plant, including the remaining twigs found in the winter. In addition to handling the plant, dermal exposure also can occur from contaminated animal fur or camping gear. Urushiols are catechols with long carbon side chains; the differences among the urushiols in the various *Toxicodendron* species depend essentially on the length of the side chain. Catechol molecules from the urushiol enter the skin and bind to surface proteins in the epidermis and dermis to form complete antigens. These "presenter" cells (catechol molecules that enter skin) transfer the antigen to T4-inducer lymphocytes. After a second urushiol challenge, the lymphocytes elicit a cell-mediated cytotoxic immune response characterized by erythema, edema, and vesiculation.

The dermatitis associated with these plants results from a delayed hypersensitivity reaction; there is no reaction from the first exposure. Subsequent exposures may result in a reaction within 24 to 48 hours of contact, depending on the sensitivity of the individual. Some individuals never develop dermatitis despite frequent contact (5).

Contrary to popular belief, poison ivy cannot be spread from the fluid contained within the skin vesicles, but urushiol may be retained under nails and spread by scratching.

Treatment

Treatment consists of immediately washing the exposed areas with soap and water. Although this does not prevent the dermatitis, it does prevent spread of the toxic chemical to other parts of the body. Drug therapy may involve the use of topical or systemic steroids (3). The use of a potent topical steroid cream with an oral antipruritic agent may be all that is necessary in some individuals with minor, localized reactions. Topical application of freshly-made Dakin's solution (sodium hypochlorite 0.5%) may provide symptomatic relief and improve rash healing (4).

Role of Systemic Steroids

For severely affected patients, a course of high-dose oral steroids in addition to an antipruritic is necessary. Typically, a 10-day regimen of steroids is begun, with the dose being decreased every other day (26). Systemic steroids are indicated if the disease is of rapid onset, if the face or genitals are involved, or when large body surfaces are affected. Intramuscular steroids (methylprednisolone 40 mg IM) or tapering doses of oral steroids are often helpful. Rashes present for more than 24 hours generally are less responsive to steroids. Attempts at oral desensitization with extracts from these plants have not been shown to be effective (27).

Capsicum

Local oral irritation also may result from exposure to members of the hot pepper family, *Capsicum*, which includes the chili pepper, hot pepper, jalapeno, Christmas pepper, and cayenne. Children who chew these plants or handle hot peppers and then touch their mouth may develop severe, burning oral pain. Ocular irritation may occur from eye inoculation.

PLANTS CAUSING GASTROENTERITIS

Most plant intoxications in the United States occur from the ingestion of plants containing gastrointestinal irritants. The onset of the irritant response is variable and depends on the chemical nature of the toxin (16). Although almost all plants may cause some degree of gastroenteritis, two groups of toxic chemicals are more specific for causing gastrointestinal irritation. These are (a) ilicin and (b) phytolaccine, phytolaccotoxin, and saponins (3).

Pokeweed

Phytolaccine and phytolaccotoxin are two of the active compounds in pokeweed (*Phytolacca americana*) (28); saponins and glycoproteins are also concentrated in the root. This shrub-like plant is indigenous to the United States. Other names for pokeweed include pokeberry, Virginia poke, garget, and inkberry (Fig. 69–4). The plant measures from 3 to 10 feet in height and has stout, reddish-purple branched stems. In the fall, the plant dies down to the ground, and in late summer and early fall it produces white to purplish flowers and round clusters of dark purple berries with red juice; these may be attractive to young children. Stains from these berries may be on the hands of an intoxicated individual. Pokeweed root is often

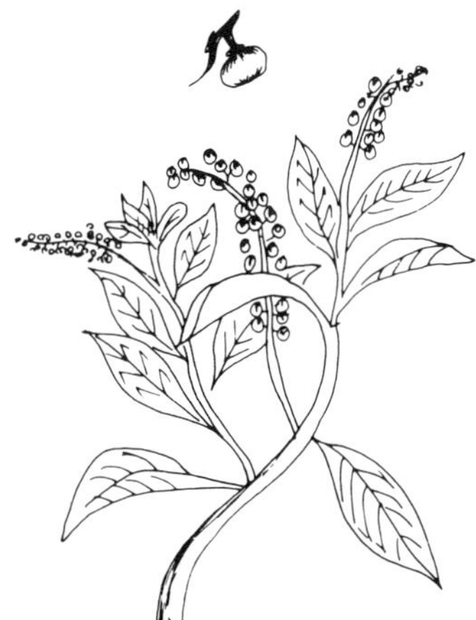

FIG. 69–4. Pokeweed. (From Gossel TA and Bricker JD. *Principles of Clinical Toxicology, Third Edition,* New York: Raven Press, 1994, p. 253, with permission.)

mistaken for horseradish, parsnips, or Jerusalem artichoke, and the shoots are sometimes substituted for asparagus. Native Americans have used the plant as an emetic and purgative, and the plant is still used today as a folk remedy for pruritus. Powdered pokeweed root is sold in health food stores as an herbal tea preparation (28).

The effects of pokeweed intoxication may arise from ingestion of any or all plant parts, with the root having the largest amount of toxin. Intoxications have also been reported from liquid preparations of plant extracts and through skin contact with the plant itself. This plant is a popular ingredient as a tea, or at times, is eaten like turnip greens. Correct preparation of pokeweed involves boiling it at least twice and discarding the water each time. Occasionally, gastrointestinal symptoms can occur when the preparation is not meticulous, or when the plant contains large quantities of the toxin despite "correct" preparation.

The main toxic agents of pokeweed are the glycoside saponins and a glycoprotein mitogen known as pokeweed mitogen (3); saponins are irritants when applied to the skin or mucous membranes (16). The saponin glycosides are found throughout the plant kingdom, for example in English Ivy (*Hedera helix*), ginseng (*Panax ginseng*), and licorice (*Glycyrrhiza glabra*). After hydrolysis, saponin glycosides yield an aglycone, sapogenin (which is responsible for the toxicity), and a sugar that may enhance solubility and absorption.

Saponins may induce lysis of erythrocytes, causing hemolytic anemia. Most saponins are found in combination with other toxins, including gastrointestinal irritants and phytotoxins, which contributes to the widely varying clinical picture (28).

As with many plant species, gastrointestinal symptoms predominate early after ingestion of pokeweed if it was not processed properly. Typically, the patient complains of an initial burning sensation in the mouth and throat

TABLE 69–12. *Clinical effects of pokeweed intoxication*

Gastrointestinal
Burning in the mouth
Burning in the throat
Nausea
Vomiting
Hematemesis
Abdominal pain
Diarrhea
Melena
Miscellaneous
Weakness
Decreased vision
Respiratory depression
Seizures
Cardiac dysrhythmias
Hypotension
Diaphoresis

(Table 69–12). A severe hemorrhagic gastroenteritis associated with nausea, vomiting, hematemesis, abdominal cramps, diarrhea, melena, weakness, diaphoresis, and hypotension may ensue. In severe cases, there may also be neurologic symptoms such as decreased vision, respiratory depression, seizures, and cardiac dysrhythmias. Nonfatal cases usually resolve in 24 to 48 hours. Deaths have been reported (28).

MISCELLANEOUS PLANT TOXINS

Christmas Tree Plants (Table 69–13)

Poinsettia (Fig. 69–5)

The poinsettia (*Euphorbia pulcherrima*) is a member of a family that comprises more than 7,000 herbs, shrubs, and trees. Although the family is morphologically diverse, the presence of latex or milky juice in these plants is common to all species. This latex is economically important as a natural rubber source (29).

The poinsettia plant is an ornamental plant that is popular during the Christmas season. Its flowers are small

TABLE 69–13. *Common ornamental Christmas plants*

Common name	Botanical name	Toxic substance
Holly	*Ilex* sp	Ilicin Saponins
Jerusalem cherry	*Solanum pseudo-capisicum*	Solanine Solanidine Solanocapsine
Mistletoe	*Phoradendron flavescens*	Viscotoxin Phoratoxin Viscumin
Poinsettia	*Euphorbia pulcherrima*	Latex soap

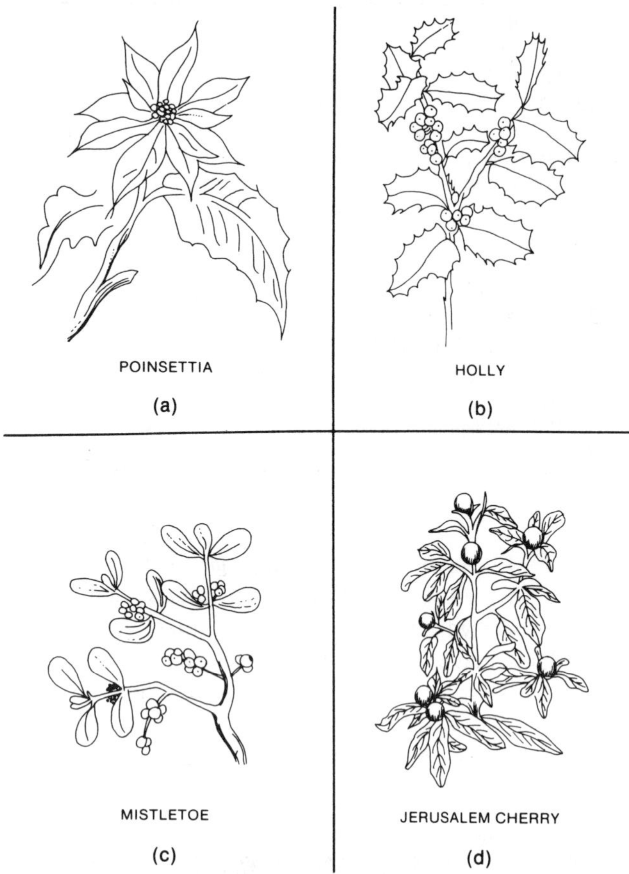

FIG. 69–5. Common Christmas tree plants. **B—D** cause poisoning. (From Gossel TA and Bricker JD. *Principles of Clinical Toxicology, Third Edition,* New York: Raven Press, 1994, p. 248, with permission.)

and yellow (29); it is the large colorful leaf that is responsible for the plant's popularity (16). For many years the poinsettia was considered a poisonous plant that could be fatal if ingested, but it probably is not as toxic as some reports have indicated because little documentation of these serious effects can be found. The plant is capable of causing varying degrees of irritation of the local mucosa as well as gastrointestinal distress. The ingestion of small amounts is not expected to produce any symptoms. Although uncommon, the latex-like sap which exudes from the damaged leaves may produce dermal irritation. Treatment, if necessary at all, is symptomatic (14).

Mistletoe

Mistletoe (*Phoradendron villasum, P. flavescens*) is a woody perennial that usually grows on oak trees; it is also widely available during the Christmas season as an ornament. Its small white berries contain β-phenylethylamine and tyramine, which can act as pressor amines. Mistletoe extracts have been used in teas sold in health food stores and have also been used as illegal abortifacients. The teas are particularly toxic and have been associated with fatalities.

TABLE 69–14. *Clinical effects of mistletoe poisoning*

Gastrointestinal
Gastritis
Nausea
Vomiting
Diarrhea
Neurologic
Hallucinations
Delirium
Coma
Seizures
Cardiovascular
Bradycardia
Heart blocks

Gastrointestinal, neurologic, and cardiovascular effects may be noted from ingestion of mistletoe berries (Table 69–14). Gastrointestinal effects include gastritis and gastroenteritis. Neurologic effects have included hallucinations, delirium, coma, and seizures. Cardiovascular depression presents much like that associated with cardiac glycoside toxicity, with bradycardia and heart block noted.

Treatment is supportive and symptomatic. Intravenous fluids may be necessary for gastroenteritis, and diazepam may be required for seizures (14).

Ilicin

Ilicin is contained in holly berries (*Ilex* sp) and causes severe gastroirritation including nausea, vomiting, and diarrhea. Rarely, it may also result in stupor, narcosis, and CNS depression.

Herbal Intoxication

An herb is a plant that has a fleshy stem as distinguished from the woody tissue of shrubs and trees. Many of these are aromatic plants used in medicine or seasoning of food. While the use of herbal medicines dates back to ancient Chinese and early Greek practices, recently, there has been a substantial increase in both the medical and nonmedical use of herbal products, including cigarettes, smoking mixtures, tea, and capsules. Although many herbal remedies are safe and may even be pharmacologically worthwhile, many others can be lethal if misused. Some of these products are often advertised as natural and legal drugs or herbal highs, and are readily available in health food stores and

Table 69-15. *Psychoactive substances used in herbal preparations*

Labeled ingredient	Botanical source	Pharmacologic principle	Suggested use	Reported effects
African yohimbe bark;	*Corynanthe yohimbe*	Yohimbe	Smoke or tea as stimulant	Mild hallucinogen
Broom; Scotch broom	*Cystisus* sp	Cytisine	Smoke for relaxation	Strong sedative–hypnotic
California poppy	*Eschscholtzia californica*	Alkaloids and glucosides	Smoke as marijuana substitute	Mild euphoriant
Catnip	*Nepeta cataria*	Nepetalactone	Smoke or tea as marijuana substitute	Mild hallucinogen
Cinnamon	*Cinnamomum camphora*	?	Smoke with marijuana	Mild stimulant
Damiana	*Turnera diffusa*	?	Smoke as marijuana substitute	Mild stimulant
Hops	*Humulus lupulus*	Lupuline	Smoke or tea as sedative and marijuana substitute	None
Hydrangea	*Hydrangea paniculata*	Hydrangin, saponin, cyanogenes	Smoke as marijuana substitute	Stimulant
Juniper	*Juniper macropoda*	?	Smoke as hallucinogen	Strong hallucinogen
Kavakava	*Piper methysticum*	Yangonin, pyrones	Smoke or tea as marijuana substitute	Mild hallucinogen
Kola nut; gotu kola	*Cola* sp	Caffeine, theobromine, kolanin	Smoke, tea, or capsules as stimulant	Stimulant
Lobelia	*Lobelia inflata*	Lobeline	Smoke or tea as marijuana substitute	Mild euphoriant
Mandrake	*Mandragora officinarum*	Scopolamine, hyoscyamine	Tea as hallucinogen	Hallucinogen
Mate	*Ilex paraguayensis*	Caffeine	Tea as stimulant	Stimulant
Mormon tea	*Ephedra nevadensis*	Ephedrine	Tea as stimulant	Stimulant
Nutmeg	*Myristica fragrans*	Myristicin	Tea as hallucinogen	Hallucinogen
Passion flower	*Passiflora incarnata*	Harmine alkaloids	Smoke, tea, or capsules as marijuana substitute	Mild stimulant
Periwinkle	*Catharanthus roseus*	Indole alkaloids	Smoke or tea as euphoriant	Hallucinogen
Prickly poppy	*Argemone mexicana*	Protopine, bergerine, isoquinillnes	Smoke as euphoriant	Narcotic–analgesic
Snakeroot	*Rauwolfia serpentina*	Reserpine	Smoke or tea as tobacco substitute	Tranquilizer
Thorn apple	*Datura stramonium*	Atropine, scopolamine	Smoke or tea as tobacco substitute or hallucinogen	Strong hallucinogen
Tobacco	*Nicotiana spp*	Nicotine	Smoke as tobacco	Strong stimulant
Valerian	*Valeriana officinalis*	Chatinine, velerine alkaloids	Tea or capsules as tranquilizer	Tranquilizer
Wild lettuce	*Lactuca sativa*	Lactucarine	Smoke as opium substitute	Mild narcotic–analgesic
Wormwood	*Artemisia absinthium*	Absinthine	Smoke or tea as relaxant	Narcotic–analgesic

From Siegel, *JAMA* 1976;236:474, with permission.

markets, as well as by direct mail order from suppliers and importers. Many preparations contain substantial amounts of psychoactive substances, and their use has resulted in a number of intoxications requiring clinical attention (Table 69–15). Physicians should be aware of the psychoactive effects of these compounds, particularly those effects resulting from long-term use, even when acute effects are minimal. Unfortunately, many of the users may be unprepared for these effects. They may not even suspect that these effects can occur, because herbs are often viewed as food rather than as drugs (30). Drug histories should therefore include information on the use of herbal preparations, and their possible role in the etiology of medical complaints should be consid-

Table 68–16 *Miscellaneous plants of abuse*

Plant	Part used	Toxic agent
Argyreia nervosa	Seed	Ergoline hallucinogens
Atropa belladonna	Seed	Tropane alkaloids
Banistereopsis species	Various	Harmaline (hallucinogen)
Cola nitida	Seed	Caffeine
Datura species	Seed	Tropane alkaloids
Hyoscysmus niger	Whole plant	Tropane alkaloids
Ilex paraguarensis	Leaf	Caffeine
Mandragora officinarum	Whole plant	Tropane alkaloids
Methysticodendron amesianum	Stems/leaf	Tropane alkaloids
Mimosa hostilis	Root	Phenylamine hallucinogens
Olmedioperebea sclerophylla	Fruit	Unknown hallucinogen
Passiflora incarnata	Stem/leaf	Harmaline (hallucinogens)
Pelganum harmala	Seed	Harmaline (hallucinogens)
Piper methysticum	Root	Methysticin/kawain
Piptadenia colubrina	Seed	Phenylamine hallucinogens
Piptadenia cexcelsa	Seed	Phenylamine hallucinogens
Piptadenia macrocarpa	Seed	Phenylamine hallucinogens
Piptadenia peregrina	Seed/bark	Phenylamine hallucinogens
Salva divinorum	Leaf	Unknown hallucinogen
Sophora secundiflora	Seed	Cytisine (stimulant)
Tabernanthe iboga	Root	Ibogaine (hallucinogen)
Trichocereus pachanoi	Cactus	Mescaline
Virola calophylla	Bark	Phenylamine hallucinogens

TABLE 69–17. *"Nontoxic" plants*

African violet (*Saintpaulia*)
Aluminum plant (*Pilea*)
Aphelandia
Baby's tears (*Helxine*)
Begonia (*Begonia*)
Bloodleaf (*Iresine*)
Boston fern (*Nephrolepis exaltata bostoniensis*)
Ceropegia
Christmas cactus (*Zygocactus*)
Coleus (*Coleus*)
Copperleaf (*Abutilon*)
Corn plant (*Dracaena*)
Dandelion
Dracaena (*Dracaena*)
Dusty miller (*Cineraria*)
False aralia (*Dizgotheca*)
Gardenia
Gynura
Hawaiian ti (*Cordyline*)
Hibiscus
Jade plant (*Crassula arborescens*)
Lipstick plant (*Aeschynanthus*)
Marigold (*Tagetes*)
Mother-in-law tongue (*Sansevieria*)
Palm
Peperomia (*Peperomia*)
Prayer plant (*Maranta*)
Rosary vine (*Ceropegia*)
Rose
Rubber plant (*Ficus elastica*)
Schefflera (*Brassaia*)
Sensitive plant (*Mimosa pudica*)
Snake plant (*Sansevieria*)
Spider plant (*Anthericum*)
Swedish ivy (*Plecthranthus*)
Umbrella plant (*Cyperus alternifolius*)
Velvet plant (*Hoya*)
Wax plant (*Hoya*)
Weeping fig (*Ficus*)
Zebra plant (*Aphelandia*)

(Scientific names).

ered. In addition, a search for plants with abuse potential should also be undertaken (Table 69–16).

"NONTOXIC" PLANTS

Although almost any substance taken in a large enough quantity may be toxic, there are a number of plants that when ingested mistakenly will result in little toxicity. Table 69–17 lists those plants that are associated with very little toxicity or are essentially nontoxic.

REFERENCES

1. Geehr L: Common toxic plant ingestions. *Emerg Med Clin North Am* 1984;2:553–562.
2. DiPalma J: Poisonous plants. *Am Fam Physician* 1994;29:252–254.
3. Spoerke D, Hall A, Dodson C, et al: Mystery root ingestion. *J Emerg Med* 1987;5:385–388.
4. Krenzelok E, Schneider S, Ellis M: Toxic plant ingestions: optimizing the course of treatment. *Emerg Med Rep* 1992:13:141–150.
5. Epstein W: The poison ivy picker of Pennypack Park: the continuing saga of poison ivy. *J Invest Dermatol* 1987;88:7s–11s.
6. Kingsbury J: Phytotoxicology: part I: major problems associated with poisonous plants. *Clin Pharmacol Ther* 1969;10:163–169.
7. Kingsbury J: Phytotoxicology: part II: poisonous plants and plant-caused emergencies. *Clin Toxicol* 1969;2:14:143–148.
8. Mrvos R, Dean B, Krenzelok E: Philodendron/dieffenbachia ingestions: are they a problem? *J Toxicol Clin Toxicol* 1991;29:485–491.
9. Bryson P, Watanabe A, Rumack B, et al: Burdock root tea poisoning. *JAMA* 1978;239:2157–2158.
10. Spoerke D, Hall A: Plants and mushrooms of abuse. *Emerg Med Clin North Am* 1990;8:579–593.
11. Rhoads P, Tong T, Banner W, et al: Anticholinergic poisonings associated with commercial burdock root tea. *Clin Toxicol* 1985;22: 581–584.
12. Bryson P: Burdock root tea poisoning. *JAMA* 1978;240:1586.
13. Hart M: Jequirity-bean poisoning. *N Engl J Med* 1963;268:885–886.
14. Yarbrough B: Plant poisoning: a comprehensive management guide. *ER Rep* 1983;4:19–24.
15. Klein-Schwanz W, Litovitz T: Azalea toxicity: an overrated problem? *Clin Toxicol* 1985;23:91–101.
16. Kunkel D, Spoerke D: Evaluating exposures to plants. *Emerg Med Clin North Am* 1984;2:133–144.
17. Cummins R, Haulman J, Guan L, et al: Near-fatal yew berry intoxication treated with external cardiac pacing and digoxin-specific FAB antibody fragments. *Ann Emerg Med* 1990;19:38–43.
18. Ogden L: *Taxus* (yews)—a highly toxic plant. *Vet Hum Toxicol* 1988; 30:563–564.
19. Jaffe A, Gephardt D, Courtemance L: Poisoning due to ingestion of *Veratrum viride* (false hellebore). *J Emerg Med* 1990;8:161–167.
20. Rauber A, Heard J: Castor bean toxicity re-examined: a new perspective. *Vet Hum Toxicol* 1985;27:498–502.
21. Drach G, Maloney W: Toxicity of the common houseplant dieffenbachia. *JAMA* 1963;184:113–114.
22. McIntire M, Guest J, Porterfield J: Philodendron—an infant death. *J Toxicol Clin Toxicol* 1990;28:177–183.
23. Landers D, Seppi K, Blauer W: Seizures and death on a White River float trip—report of water hemlock poisoning. *West J Med* 1985; 142:637–640.
24. Rauber A: Observations on the idioblasts of dieffenbachia. *Clin Toxicol* 1985;23:79–90.
25. Challoner K, McCarron M: Castor bean intoxication. *Ann Emerg Med* 1990;19:1177–1183.
26. Epstein W: Plant-induced dermatitis. *Ann Emerg Med* 1987; 16:950–955.
27. Marks J, Trautlein J, Epstein W, et al: Oral hyposensitization to poison ivy and poison oak. *Arch Dermatol* 1987;123:476–478.
28. Roberge R, Brader E, Martin M, et al: The root of evil—pokeweed intoxication. *Ann Emerg Med* 1986;15:470–473.
29. Edwards N: Local toxicity from a poinsettia plant: a case report. *J Pediatr* 1983;102:404–405.
30. Siegel R: Herbal intoxication: psychoactive effects from herbal cigarettes, tea, and capsules. *JAMA* 1976;236:473–476.

ADDITIONAL SELECTED REFERENCES

Giannini J, Castellani S: A manic-like psychosis due to khat (Catha edulis Forsk.). *J Toxicol Clin Toxicol* 1982;19:455–459.

Harrison T: Ergotaminism. *JACEP* 1978;7:162–169.

Haynes B, Bessen H, Wightman W: Oleander tea: herbal draught of death. *Ann Emerg Med* 1985;14:350–353.

Millet Y, Jouglard J, Steinmetz M, et al: Toxicity of some essential plant oils: clinical and experimental study. *Clin Toxicol* 1981;18:1485–1498.

Segelman A, Segelman F, Karliner J, et al: Sassafras and herb tea: potential health hazards. *JAMA* 1976;236:477.

Siegel R: Ginseng abuse syndrome: problems with the panacea. *JAMA* 1979;241:1614–1615.

Siegel R: Herbal intoxication: psychoactive effects from herbal cigarettes, tea, and capsules. *JAMA* 1976;236:473–476.

CHAPTER 70

Mushrooms

Mycology, or the study of mushroom fungi, was originated by the ancient Greeks who sought to distinguish poisonous mushrooms from the edible varieties (1). Today, the gathering and eating of mushrooms remain a popular pastime in Europe and has recently become popular in the United States, partly because of increased interest in "organic" foods (2). In the last decade, increased interest in the collection and consumption of uncultivated mushrooms has resulted in more frequent episodes of serious poisonings in the U.S. Increased mushroom foraging among organic food enthusiasts and various ethnic groups, as well as articles in the lay press describing these delicacies, has contributed to the increased incidence of mushroom poisoning (3,4).

Of the 5,000 known species of mushrooms, fewer than 100 are poisonous to humans (5–7) and only about 10 mushroom species have been associated with fatalities (2). Toxic and nontoxic species often grow in the same places and may resemble each other (8). Mushroom species for the most part are not unique in appearance, and most of the popular edible varieties have one or more poisonous look-alikes. Even a trained mycologist may not be able to distinguish edible from poisonous mushrooms without a microscopic examination (9).

Mushrooms are plant fungi; because they do not contain chlorophyll they must rely on dead organic material to survive (10,11). The mushroom is the reproductive fruit of the mycelium; its relation to the mycelium is analogous to the relation of any fruit to the tree. Mature mushrooms eject spores that are dispersed by wind to establish new mycelia.

MUSHROOM IDENTIFICATION

In a suspected case of mushroom poisoning, identification of species by morphologic characteristics is a formidable task because the appearance of the mushroom may be distorted, especially when parts are brought to the physician or after the mushroom has been ingested (4,9). Attempts to identify the mushroom by collecting specimens from the same area are of little value because poisonous species frequently grow in immediate proximity to nontoxic ones (12). Examination of fungus spores in the gastric contents may also be inconclusive (9). Only 800 of the 3,000 species found in Central Europe can be identified accurately without the aid of a microscope.

Mushroom Anatomy

The mushroom is comprised of the stipe or stalk; the pileus or cap; and the gills, the vertical plates that radiate from the stalk on the underside of the cap (Fig. 70–1) (7). Although these names are the important parts of the mushrooms, in actuality it is not necessary for either the patient or the physician to know this. The physician will make the diagnosis and treatment decision on other criteria.

Examination of Spores

Examination of mushroom spores is also a task that will not yield practical information a physician might uti-

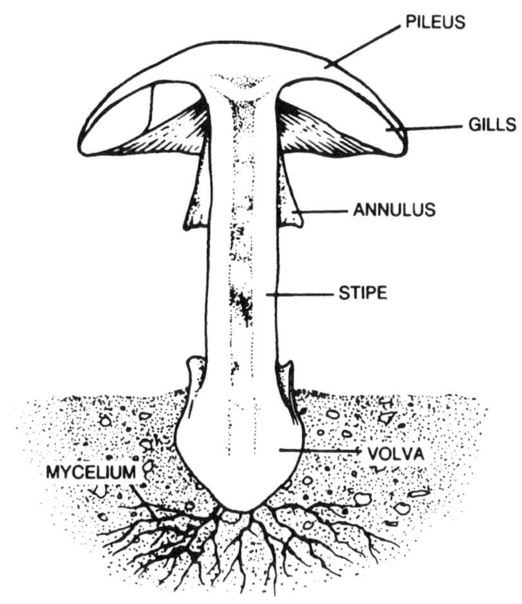

FIG. 70–1. Parts of a mushroom. Copyright © 1975 by Scientific American Inc.

lize. Nevertheless, a procedure is outlined for those interested in spore identification. To prepare spores, the gastric juice is filtered through cheesecloth and then centrifuged. The heavier layer contains the spores and can be placed under a microscope with an oil-immersion lens (3). Spores are generally the same size as a red blood cell (7). The physician should then use a textbook or handbook of mycology for identification of spores, as that discussion is beyond the scope of this text.

Mushroom Identification and the Emergency Department Physician

The emergency department physician must therefore have access to a simpler approach than species identification to the patient who has ingested a potentially toxic mushroom (6). This approach divides the toxic mushrooms into two major groups: those that cause symptoms immediately after ingestion and those that cause delayed symptoms (Table 70–1) (9,13). Under these major groups, mushrooms are divided into at least seven groups on the basis of the type of toxin and the symptoms elicited (8). Each group has a predictable target organ, incubation period, and clinical presentation (5). A diagnosis and treatment regimen based on these criteria will be accurate more than 90% of the time (3,13).

In general, the time of onset of symptoms from ingestion is inversely proportional to the overall severity of the mushroom ingested (14). An immediate response is one in which symptoms appear from a few minutes to 6 hours after ingestion; a delayed response shows symptoms arising beyond this time limit (8). The important considerations for mushrooms causing an immediate response are that poisoning is rarely serious and that treatment is conservative and symptomatic (6). A fatal outcome from poisoning by these mushrooms is extremely rare and may be attributed to inadequate fluid and electrolyte management in young children (13). Delayed symptoms from mushroom ingestion, appearing more than 6 hours after ingestion and generally after approximately 12 hours, are indicative of a serious poisoning with a potentially grave prognosis (14).

Toxins may be identified by radioimmunoassay from a sample of the mushrooms or in gastric juice, stool, urine, or blood. Laboratory tests are rarely needed for institution of appropriate patient management, however (5).

TABLE 70–1. *Toxicologic classification of mushrooms*

Delayed symptoms (more than 6 hours after ingestion)
Group I—Cyclopeptide-containing species
Group II—Monomethylhydrazine producers
Immediate symptoms (less than 6 hours after ingestion)
Group III—*Coprinus* sp
Group IV—Muscarine-containing species
Group V—Ibotenic acid–containing species
Group VI—Indole-containing species
Group VII—Gastrointestinal irritants

TABLE 70–2. *Factors influencing severity of symptoms of mushroom poisoning*

Season of the year
Maturity of mushroom
Location of mushroom
Amount of mushroom ingested
Method of preparation
Age of patient

Severity of symptoms depends on the season, the maturity of the mushroom when picked and eaten, the location of the mushroom, the amount ingested, the method of preparation of the mushroom, and the age of the patient (Table 70–2) (4). There is no simple test for distinguishing the edible species from the poisonous ones (6).

Mushrooms considered lethal belong for the most part to the cyclopeptide-containing species. In fact, almost all deadly mushrooms are members of a single genus: *Amanita*. The distinguishing feature between the cyclopeptide mushrooms and all of the other groups that may produce symptoms but rarely produce death is that, with the cyclopeptides, the symptoms commence after 6 hours after ingestion (15). All other poisonous but not deadly mushrooms will have symptoms that commence before 6 hours after ingestion. Although this generalization is not absolute, it is a worthwhile guide to the consideration of mushroom toxicity.

MUSHROOMS WITH DELAYED ONSET OF SYMPTOMS

The mushrooms in groups I and II account for more than the 95% of deaths associated with mushrooms (9,13,14).

Group I—Cyclopeptide-Containing Mushrooms

Almost all of fatal mushrooms are species in the genus *Amanita*; these include *A. phalloides* (destroying angel), *A. virosa*, *A. bisporigera*, and others (Table 70–3) (10,16). *Amanita phalloides* generally appears in late summer or fall and grows to a height of 3 to 8 inches (17). The cap varies in color from light yellow to greenish-brown, and the stalk is usually lighter, from a light greenish-yellow to pure white. *Amanita virosa* is pure white throughout.

Members of the genus *Galerina* also cause severe toxicity, but these mushrooms are not as likely to be chosen for ingestion (18).

Amanita phalloides was once thought to be strictly a European mushroom (9); it was first positively identified growing wild in the United States in 1970 (4). It is now

TABLE 70–3. *Cyclopeptide-containing mushrooms*

Amanita bisporigera
Amanita hydroscopica
Amanita ocreata
Amanita phalloides
Amanita suballiacea
Amanita tenuifolia
Amanita verna
Amanita virosa
Galerina autumnalis
Galerina marginata
Galerina venenata
Lepiota sp

found in all areas of the United States but to a greater degree in the Western coastal states (19). This mushroom may have been introduced into the United States by inadvertent transportation on the roots of imported ornamental trees (3).

The principal toxins of this group are complex proteins containing cyclic heptapeptides, called phallotoxins, and cyclic octapeptides, called amatoxins (20). These cyclopeptides consist of amino acids linked together by peptide bonds to form a continuous ring (16). *Amanita* species contain both these toxins, whereas *Galerina* species contain only amatoxins. Amatoxins are believed to be the major toxins responsible for the symptoms and pathology due to ingestion of *Amanita phalloides* and related mushrooms (19). Cooking, steaming, or drying do not materially affect the toxins in these species (9).

Phallotoxins include phalloidin, phalloin, phallisin, phallacidin, phalacin, and phallisacin (18). In vitro, the phallotoxins appear to disrupt hepatic cell membranes and to change the structure of the hepatic endoplasmic reticulum. The phallotoxins are not well absorbed from the gastrointestinal tract and therefore contribute little to toxicity. The major contributing toxins are the amatoxins (9).

Amatoxin is a collective term for a number of orally toxic cyclic octapeptides, of which five have been characterized. They have been designated as α, β-, γ-, and ε-amanitin and amanin. The amanitins have a delayed toxicity that commences about 16 to 24 hours after mushroom ingestion (16).

Amatoxins are taken up by hepatocytes, in which their primary action is to inhibit nucleoplasmic RNA polymerase II, which in turn interferes with the synthesis of messenger RNA (20). This effectively halts protein synthesis and causes cellular necrosis, which ultimately results in a severe acute hepatitis indistinguishable from acute viral hepatitis. Amanitin is also a direct-acting nephrotoxin that produces necrosis of the distal and proximal convoluted tubules (7,13). It appears that the effects of amatoxin are dose-dependent, with low doses producing solely renal involvement and high doses producing hepatic damage. In other words, the target organ appears to be dependent on the quantity of mushroom toxins ingested (3).

Clinical Effects

Because of the delayed onset of symptoms in poisonings with phallotoxic *Amanita* species, patients frequently may not associate their symptoms with the ingestion of the wild mushroom (6). Therefore, a careful history of the patient's activities before the onset of symptoms is imperative (8).

Symptoms of poisoning characteristically occur in three stages (Table 70–4). Although any type of eukaryotic cell can be damaged by amatoxin, the initial stage of the clinical picture is dominated by lesions of intestinal mucosal cells and the final stage by deterioration of liver cell function. The hepatic destruction noted is similar to that seen in poisonings with substances such as acetaminophen and carbon tetrachloride, which are converted in the liver into toxic metabolites (20).

Stage I. The first stage occurs abruptly 6 to 24 hours after ingestion. The patient may complain of abdominal pain and subsequent nausea, violent emesis, and diarrhea; occasionally, hematochezia and hematuria are noted (16). These symptoms are frequently accompanied by fever, tachycardia, hyperglycemia, hypotension, dehydration, and electrolyte imbalance (10). If a large amount was eaten or if medical care is not provided, death may occur from fluid and electrolyte loss (4). This can usually be avoided with vigorous intravenous therapy and other supportive measures (9).

Stage II. During the next 24 to 48 hours there appears to be remission of symptoms in the face of progressive deterioration of hepatic and renal function (6).

Stage III. The third stage occurs 3 to 5 days after ingestion of the mushroom and consists of increasing hepatocellular damage and renal impairment. This is noted by

TABLE 70–4. *Signs and symptoms of poisoning with* Amanita phylloides species

Stage I (6 to 24 hours)
Abdominal pain
Nausea
Emesis
Diarrhea
Hematochezia
Hematuria
Fever
Hyperglycemia
Tachycardia
Electrolyte imbalance
Stage II (24 to 48 hours)
Period of recovery
Stage III (3 to 5 days)
Hepatic dysfunction
Renal dysfunction
Myocardial dysfunction

massive elevations in the liver function tests and the development of jaundice and hepatic coma. Because amatoxins enter liver cells more rapidly than other organ cell types and because protein synthesis is active in liver cells, the hepatocyte is rendered vulnerable to the inhibitors of the transcription processes. In addition, myocardiopathy and coagulopathy may be present, and seizures, coma, and death may occur (21). Endocrine abnormalities, including hypocalcemia, decreased thyroid function studies, and elevated insulin levels despite hypoglycemia, may be noted but are rarely of clinical importance. Death from *Amanita phalloides* species is usually the result of hepatic or renal failure or both and may occur 4 to 7 days after ingestion (20).

Fatal outcomes have been correlated with age less than 10 years, a short latency between ingestion and onset of symptoms, and severity of coagulopathy. Although mortality from *Amanita* poisoning has decreased in recent decades with improved supportive care, fatalities are still reported in 20% to 30% of cases (22).

Laboratory Analysis

Baseline laboratory data should be obtained. Depending on the certainty of the diagnosis, laboratory studies may include a complete blood cell count, serum electrolytes, blood urea nitrogen, glucose concentration, creatinine concentration, urinalysis, liver function tests, prothrombin time, partial thromboplastin time, platelet count, and fibrinogen concentration (Table 70–5) (9,13). Serum or urine should be saved and sent for radioimmunoassay of amatoxins to an appropriate referral center (19); these tests are usually beyond the capabilities of most hospital laboratories (20). A urine sample may show identifiable quantities of amatoxins within 90 to 120 minutes of ingestion.

Treatment

Treatment consists of supportive care and vigorous intravenous fluid replacement to correct fluid loss.

TABLE 70–5. *Laboratory studies in poisoning with* Amanita phylloides *species*

Complete blood cell count
Serum electrolytes
Blood urea nitrogen
Blood glucose concentration
Serum creatinine concentration
Urinalysis
Liver function tests
Prothrombin time
Partial thromboplastin time
Platelet count
Fibrinogen concentration
Amatoxin radioimmunoassay

Attention must also be directed toward correcting any metabolic and coagulation disturbances (4). Although the cyclopeptide-containing mushrooms cause more than 95% of the deaths from mushroom poisoning, the overall survival rate is 75% to 80% with supportive therapy (13,16).

There is no satisfactory treatment for the hepatorenal phase of amatoxin poisoning (22). Neomycin is not recommended because of the associated renal damage from amatoxin. Dietary protein should be restricted and parenteral vitamin K and fresh frozen plasma provided as necessary (20).

Many treatment regimens have been advocated for poisonings with *Amanita phalloides* species, including thioctic acid, penicillin, cimetidine, silibinin, and extracorporeal methods. None of these has been shown to be of benefit, however (13,16).

Thioctic Acid. Thioctic acid (α-lipoic acid) is a component of coenzymes in the Krebs cycle that is necessary for oxidation of ketoacids such as pyruvate (23). This agent has been advocated for mushroom poisonings since the 1960s, but there has been no well-designed clinical trial to document its efficacy (3,16).

Penicillin. The proposed mechanism of action of intravenous penicillin is competition with amanitin for binding sites on serum proteins. This leaves more toxin free for renal excretion and less to be taken up into liver cells. This treatment has not been shown to be clinically effective, however (6).

Cimetidine. Cimetidine produces a competitive inhibition of the cytochrome P-450 system by binding of its imidazole ring to the heme moiety on the cytochrome (24). Although theoretically this compound may be protective or antidotal in poisonings with *Amanita phalloides* species, no clinical trials have shown this to be the case (24).

Silibinin. Silibinin is a water-soluble preparation of silymarin and has been advocated in Europe as an antidote in poisonings with *Amanita phalloides* species. Silymarin is the active ingredient of the milk thistle; it is thought to inhibit the penetration of the amatoxins into liver cells (16). There are not enough data to verify the benefit of silibinin, and it is not available in the United States.

Extracorporeal Methods. Both dialysis and hemoperfusion have been advocated in the past for poisonings with *Amanita phalloides* species, but there is no evidence that either procedure is protective. These procedures may actually worsen the patient's prospect of recovery, perhaps by unfavorably influencing the already compromised coagulation pattern. Hemodialysis has been used successfully to treat renal failure but not to remove amanitin, which is poorly dialyzable.

Liver Transplantation. The only effective definitive therapy may be orthotropic liver transplantation once fulminant hepatic failure occurs. Unfortunately, patient selection criteria and timing for transplantation in this setting are not clearly defined (9). There are no clear guidelines for transplantation, and there is no laboratory test or even combination of factors to predict which patients will recover and which will die. Early identification of potential candidates is important because hepatic failure can progress rapidly, and organ procurement may require several days (25).

The best studies suggest that most patients with SGOT levels ≥ 2,000, grade 2 hepatic encephalopathy, or a PT > 50 may die. In addition, a decrease in the thromboplastin time (Quick's test) to below 10% of normal after 48 hours has been strongly associated with mortality (22). These patients should be considered for hepatic transplantation (25). Because hepatic failure develops rapidly, it is imperative that these patients be considered for hepatic transplant prior to reaching these extreme stages (26).

Group II—Monomethylhydrazine Producers

The morels are one of the most highly prized of all edible mushrooms. Toxic *Gyromitra* species resemble this type of mushroom and are called "false morels." The false morel *Gyromitra esculenta* contains gyromitrin (also known as helvella), a protoplasmic toxin less dangerous than the amatoxins. The morels have a cap resembling a pine cone that is textured with ridges and pits and is attached at the base of the mushroom (27). *Gyromitra* species are called false morels because they have a wrinkled or saddle-shaped cap unattached at the base. Distinguishing between these two types of mushrooms is difficult. Most poisonings have occurred in Europe, although there have been occasional poisonings reported in North America (Table 70–6) (3). The toxin is somewhat heat-labile; therefore, cooking may decrease or eliminate it.

Mechanism of Toxicity

Mushrooms of the genus *Gyromitra* contain gryomitrin, which in most individuals is hydrolyzed to monomethylhydrazine after ingestion. Monomethylhydrazine acts as a competitive inhibitor of the coenzyme pyridoxal phosphate (vitamin B_6) (27), which serves as a coenzyme for many enzyme systems, including γ-aminobutyric acid, decarboxylases, deaminases, and transaminases. Inhibition of pyridoxal phosphate results in multiorgan dysfunction. Damage may extend to the liver, kidneys, CNS, and hematopoietic system (8).

TABLE 70–6. *Monomethylhydrazine producers*

Gyromitra ambigua
Gyromitra brunnea
Gyromitra caroliniana
Gyromitra esculenta
Gyromitra fastigiata

Clinical Effects of Intoxication

Because the toxic component of this group of mushrooms is highly volatile, it is inactivated by cooking. If the mushroom is not cooked, then symptoms are typically delayed for 6 to 12 hours after ingestion. Whether or not the mushroom was cooked is an important part of the history (2).

Initially, gastrointestinal symptoms predominate, with complaints of bloating, nausea, vomiting, diarrhea, cramping, and abdominal pain (Table 70–7). These symptoms are usually self-limited and resolve in 1 to 3 days (27). Other symptoms may be noted subsequently; these consist of hemolysis (which may also occur early), hemoglobinemia, clinical anemia, jaundice, and hemoglobinuria. The mechanism of the hemolysis is unknown. There appears to be a direct effect on the mixed-function oxidase systems in the liver with subsequent hepatotoxicity (18). Methemoglobinemia may also be noted. Because vitamin B_6 antagonists cause inhibition of the inhibitory neurotransmitter γ-aminobutyric acid, seizures are often noted in the symptomatic individual (3).

Laboratory Analysis

Baseline laboratory studies should include a complete blood cell count, urinalysis, serum free hemoglobin concentrations, blood urea nitrogen, creatinine and glucose concentrations, liver function tests, serum electrolytes, arterial blood gas values, and a methemoglobin concentration (if necessary) (8).

Treatment

Although *Gyromitra* species have the potential to cause death, ingestion of these mushrooms is rarely fatal. None of the toxins in these species is related chemically to those of *Amanita phalloides* species. In addition, the

TABLE 70–7. *Signs and symptoms of* Gyromitra *species poisoning*

Gastrointestinal
Bloating
Nausea
Vomiting
Diarrhea
Abdominal pain
Hematologic
Hemolysis
Hemoglobinemia
Anemia
Jaundice
Methemoglobinemia
Hepatotoxicity
Neurologic
Seizures

symptoms of poisoning by these mushrooms are not the same as those of *Amanita* species (14).

Treatment consists of supportive care with replacement of any fluid and electrolyte losses. Large parenteral doses of pyridoxine may be necessary to counteract the antagonistic effects of the monomethylhydrazine. Pyridoxine hydrochloride at a dose of 2 to 5 g in an adult or 25 mg/kg in a child should be administered intravenously. The urine should be alkalinized to prevent hemoglobin deposition. Dialysis is not recommended except for frank renal failure (27).

MUSHROOMS WITH IMMEDIATE ONSET OF SYMPTOMS

Mushrooms in groups III to VII (see Table 70–1) are rarely involved in major medical problems except for fluid and electrolyte changes, which may be severe.

Group III—*Coprinus Species*

Ingestion of mushrooms in the genus *Coprinus*, specifically *C. atramentarius*, and of *Clitocybe clavipes* produces no symptoms unless alcohol is ingested while the toxic components of the mushroom are still in the body. These mushrooms are considered both common and palatable; a characteristic is that at maturity the gills dissolve into an inky black fluid (8).

Mechanism of Toxicity

Many *Coprinus* species contain coprine, which is metabolized after ingestion to an acetaldehyde dehydrogenase inhibitor. Coprine is broken down to another active derivative, aminocyclopropanol, which acts like disulfiram (1). This reaction prevents the metabolism of acetaldehyde to acetate, thus allowing accumulation of acetaldehyde. There is some evidence that this reaction is due to β-receptor stimulation.

Clinical Effects

When a patient ingests certain mushrooms from the *Coprinus* family and subsequently drinks alcohol, symptoms nearly identical to the alcohol–disulfiram reaction may occur. The sensitivity to alcohol may begin 2 to 6 hours after the mushroom is ingested but may last up to 72 hours. Frequently, the patient will not correlate the mushroom ingestion with alcohol and the resulting reaction (28). The mushroom and alcohol need not be ingested at the same time, and because the toxin is not cleared from the body for several days an alcoholic drink during that period may precipitate the reaction. If no alcohol is ingested during that time, no toxic symptoms occur (18).

TABLE 70–8. *Signs and symptoms of* Coprinus–alcohol interaction

Gastrointestinal
Nausea
Vomiting
Skin
Diaphoresis
Flushing
Throbbing in neck veins
Cardiovascular
Chest pain
Palpitations
Supraventricular dysrhythmia
Hypotension
Neurologic
Paresthesia
Headache

Symptoms may commence 20 minutes to 2 hours after consuming alcohol. The patient may experience an increase in body temperature with flushing, nausea, vomiting, a feeling of fullness and throbbing in the neck veins, chest pain, palpitations, paresthesia in the hands and feet, diaphoresis, and headache (Table 70–8). Supraventricular dysrhythmias and hypotension have been reported in severe cases. No deaths have been reported (8).

Treatment

Most symptoms of poisoning resolve spontaneously within 3 to 6 hours, and treatment is symptomatic and supportive. There are anecdotal reports of success with parenteral antihistamines and ascorbic acid (14).

Group IV—Muscarine-Containing Species

Muscarine is a natural parasympathomimetic alkaloid first isolated from *Amanita muscaria*; this species contains clinically insignificant amounts of muscarine, however (8). It was subsequently found that mushrooms of the genera *Inocybe* and *Clitocybe* (Table 70–9) can cause muscarine poisoning, with cholinergic effects that can be blocked by atropine.

In the symptomatic individual, signs of cholinergic activity may be noted 15 minutes to 2 hours after ingestion and may last for 6 to 24 hours. The most common

TABLE 70–9. *Muscarine-containing mushrooms*

Clitocybe cerrusata
Clitocybe dealbata
Clitocybe nuulosa
Inocybe fastigiata
Inocybe geophylla
Inocybe rimosus

TABLE 70–10. *Signs and symptoms of muscarinic mushroom poisoning*

Diaphoresis
Abdominal pain
Nausea
Vomiting
Salivation
Miosis
Blurred vision
Bronchoconstriction
Bradycardia
Hypotension

feature is diaphoresis, which may be accompanied by abdominal pain, nausea, vomiting, salivation, miosis, blurred vision, bronchoconstriction, bradycardia, and hypotension (Table 70–10). Although atropine provides prompt and specific treatment for symptoms of muscarinic mushroom poisoning, it is only necessary in the substantially symptomatic individual. The dosage of atropine is related to the severity of symptoms and should be titrated to clinical effect.

Group V—Ibotenic Acid-Containing Species

The toxic ingredients in *Amanita muscaria* are ibotenic acid and muscimol (Table 70–11). Ibotenic acid is a derivative of glutamic acid, and muscimol is a derivative of γ-aminobutyric acid. Ibotenic acid is an unstable compound, especially in the presence of an acid (29). It acts as an insecticide; flies die on contact with *A. muscaria*, hence the name fly agaric. Muscimol is several times more active than ibotenic acid and is formed by decarboxylation of ibotenic acid. Muscimol and related compounds have been characterized as an anticholinergic by some authorities and as a γ-aminobutyric acid antagonist by others.

Clinical Effects

Amanita muscaria and *A. pantheria* ("the panther") are common mushroom species intentionally ingested for their psychoactive properties. *Amanita muscaria* is probably the most common poisonous mushroom ingested in the United States (29). Although the mushroom is called *Amanita muscaria*, there are actually insignificant amounts of muscarine in this mushroom.

TABLE 70–11. *Ibotenic acid–containing mushrooms*

Amanita cothurnata
Amanita gemmata
Amanita muscaria
Amanita pantherina

TABLE 70–12. *Signs and symptoms of poisoning by ibotenic acid–containing mushrooms*

Euphoria
Dizziness
Ataxia
Visual disturbances
Mydriasis
Agitation
Myoclonus
Seizures
Coma

Symptoms may occur 30 minutes to 2 hours after ingestion and include euphoria, dizziness, ataxia, and drunken behavior (Table 70–12). With severe intoxication, visual disturbances, mydriasis, agitation, myoclonus, seizures, and coma may occur. Contrary to some reports, no clear pattern of cholinergic or anticholinergic effects is observed (28). The ibotenic acid is similar to and mimics many of the effects of glutamic acid. It is metabolized to muscimol, which resembles γ-aminobutyric acid (GABA) and has a high affinity for GABA receptor sites.

Treatment

Treatment is supportive. Because vomiting is not a clinical feature, attempts should be made to empty the stomach. Unless severe anticholinergic symptoms and signs are present, physostigmine should not be administered. Barbiturates, atropine, and benzodiazepines should also not be administered because they may exacerbate toxicity (29).

Group VI—The Indole-Containing Mushrooms

The principal hallucinogenic mushrooms come from three genera found largely in the Pacific Northwest, Florida, and Hawaii. These are *Psilocybe*, *Paneolus*, and *Gymnophilus* (30).

Many species are found, usually within 24 hours of a spring or fall rain. They are found on cattle manure in pasture land. More commonly used terms may be "magic mushroom", "blue legs", or "liberty cap". These mushrooms are frozen or dried to preserve them for later use. Neither procedure affects their potency (28).

"Magic" mushrooms containing hallucinogens have been used for religious ceremonies for centuries and currently are popular with the drug-seeking population. These mushrooms contain the psilocybin toxin and similar hallucinogens. The ingestion of several mushrooms is often required to produce CNS excitation and hallucinations. The effects may vary among individuals but usually are more severe in children (28).

Signs and Symptoms of Psilocybin

The chemical nature of psilocybin, which is the toxic ingredient in these mushrooms, resembles that of 5-hydroxytryptamine and lysergic acid diethylamide (1,31). Onset of symptoms may begin 30 minutes after ingestion of the mushroom with a duration of usually less than 4 hours. Although early after ingestion there are symptoms of weakness and dizziness, this usually passes on to a euphoria and dreamlike state with visual perceptual distortions. Symptoms seen following ingestion may include facial flushing, mild tachycardia, mild hypertension, mydriasis, compulsive muscular movements, dizziness, paresthesia, ataxia, and vomiting. Seizures, tonic–clonic and intermittent in nature, have been reported, more commonly in children than in adults. Intoxications generally terminate with drowsiness, which progresses to sleep. Fatalities are unusual but have been reported in children who develop hyperpyrexia and status epilepticus (28).

Symptoms generally resolve spontaneously in 5 to 10 hours, but clinicians have documented flashbacks that have occurred in patients up to 4 months after ingestion (2).

Treatment

Treatment is supportive (30,32). As patients abusing these mushrooms generally do not reach medical attention until absorption of the active principle has occurred, it may be too late for gastric lavage to be of much value. The potential effectiveness of late administration of activated charcoal has not been evaluated (see Chapter 54).

Group VII—Gastrointestinal Irritants

The most common adverse reaction to eating mushrooms is gastrointestinal irritation. Little is known about the chemistry and pharmacologic activity of the mushrooms in this group (11). It appears that the toxin produced may be somewhat destroyed by heat, although cooking the mushrooms does not ensure safety (5).

Although the species encountered most frequently in this group is *Chlorophyllum molybdites*, many of the common "little brown mushrooms" found in the backyard are found in this group (Table 70–13) (11).

TABLE 70–13. *Genera of mushrooms that are gastrointestinal irritants*

Agaricus
Boletus
Chlorophyllum
Entoloma
Gomphus
Hebeloma
Lactarius
Lycoperdon
Morchella
Naematoloma
Paxillus
Pholiota
Polyphorus
Ramaria
Russula
Scleroderma
Tricholoma
Verpa

Clinical Effects

The onset of signs and symptoms generally begin within 2 hours of ingestion and consists of gastrointestinal irritation in the form of nausea, vomiting, diarrhea, and abdominal pain (Table 70–14). The diarrhea is often bloody. The profuse, watery diarrhea may lead to significant volume and electrolyte loss. The illness is self-limited, and most symptoms resolve in 3 to 4 hours (5). A characteristic of mushrooms in this group is the absence of intense diaphoresis, delirium, hallucinations, and hepatorenal damage.

One common mushroom family causing gastrointestinal upset is the *Boletus* family, which has characteristic minute pores on the undersurface of the cap surrounding the gills. As with other mushrooms, this family contains both edible and gastrointestinal irritating mushrooms, thereby complicating identification.

Treatment

Because symptoms are self-limiting, no specific treatment other than fluid and electrolyte replacement is necessary. The very young and the debilitated are most vulnerable to the fluid and electrolyte shifts and should be monitored closely. In some cases, fluid loss has been of sufficient magnitude to induce hypovolemic shock (5).

TABLE 70–14. *Signs and symptoms of ingestion of gastrointestinal irritant mushrooms*

Present
Nausea
Vomiting
Diarrhea
Abdominal pain
Absent
Diaphoresis
Delirium
Hallucinations
Hepatorenal damage

TABLE 70–15. *Summary of the features of various types of mushroom poisoning*

Toxin	Genus	Organ systems affected	Symptoms	Time of onset after ingestion	Possible antidote
Amanitin, phalloidin (cyclopeptides)	*Amanita* *Galerina*	Blood, liver, kidney, gastrointestinal tract	Hematuria proteinuria, gastroenteritis, jaundice	6–24 hours	Supportive care
Monomethylhydrazine (gyromitrin)	*Gyromitra*	Blood, liver, kidney, gastrointestinal tract	Hemolysis, abdominal pain, liver and kidney failure, weakness	6–24 hours	Pyridoxine, 25 mg/kg IV
Coprine	*Coprinus*	Autonomic nervous system	With alcohol ingestion, disulfiram-like reaction	20 minutes–5 days	Supportive care
Muscarine	*Clitocybe* (*Omphalotus*) *Inocybe*	Autonomic nervous system	Salivation, lacrimation, excessive urination, diarrhea	20 minutes–2 hours	Atropine 2 mg IV (as indicated)
Ibotenic acid, muscimol	*Amanita*	Central nervous system	Dry mouth, cycloplegia (anticholinergic effects), delirium, ataxia	20 minutes–2 hours	Physostigmine 2 mg IV (only when indicated)
Psilocybin, psilocin	*Psilocybe* *Panaeolus*	Central nervous system	Hallucinations, hyperkinetic state (anticholinergic effects)	15–30 minutes	Supportive care

From Lincoff G, Mitchell DH: *Toxic and hallucinogenic mushroom poisoning.* Litton Educational Publishing; 1977.

SUMMARY

Although mushroom identification is a formidable task, even for the professional mycologist, it is not necessary for the emergency department physician to identify the exact mushroom that is causing toxic symptoms to diagnose the patient's condition and to plan a treatment regimen that will be successful most of the time. This regimen consists of knowing when symptoms began after ingestion of the mushroom as well as characterizing the symptoms present (Table 70–15). If symptoms began within 6 hours of ingestion, it is unlikely that they will progress to serious toxicity, and the signs and symptoms present dictate treatment necessary (14). For the most part, treatment consists of fluid and electrolyte replacement. For those mushrooms that present with symptoms 6 hours after ingestion and generally after 12 hours, there is a good possibility of a serious poisoning with a potentially grave prognosis. Because there are no effective antidotes available for poisonings with *Amanita phalloides* and related species, the management consists of the same fluid and electrolyte support as well as monitoring for signs of hepatic and renal involvement. When mixed ingestions are suspected, early symptoms should be treated, and when the patient is asymptomatic he or she may be discharged with instructions to return if gastrointestinal symptoms arise again. Alternatively, the patient may be instructed to return for daily liver function tests (14).

REFERENCES

1. Hanrahan J, Gordon M: Mushroom poisoning. *JAMA* 1984;251:1057–1061.
2. Schneider S, Cochran K, Krenzelok E: Mushroom poisoning: recognition and emergency management. *Emerg Med Rep* 1991;12:81–87.
3. Becker C, Tong T, Boerner U, et al: Diagnosis and treatment of *Amanita phalloides*-type mushroom poisoning. *West J Med* 1976;125:1–109.
4. Parish R, Doering P: Treatment of *Amanita* mushroom poisoning: a review. *Vet Hum Toxicol* 1986;28:318–322.
5. Blayney D, Rosenkranz E, Zettner A: Mushroom poisoning from *Chlorophyllum molybdites*. *West J Med* 1980;132:74–77.
6. Page L: Mushroom poisoning. *West J Med* 1980;132:66–68.
7. Litten W: The most poisonous mushrooms. *Sci Am* 1975;232:90–101.
8. DiPalma J: Mushroom poisoning. *Am Fam Physician* 1981;23:170–172.
9. Bivins H, Knopp R, Lammers R, et al: Mushroom ingestion. *Ann Emerg Med* 1985;14:1099–1104.
10. Mitchel D: *Amanita* mushroom poisoning. *Ann Rev Med* 1980;31:51–57.
11. Levitan D, Macy J, Weissman J: Mechanism of gastrointestinal hemorrhage in a case of mushroom poisoning by *Chlorophyllum molybdites*. *Toxicol* 1981;19:179–180.
12. Trestrail J: Mushroom poisoning in the United States—an analysis of 1989 United States Poison Center data. *J Toxicol Clin Toxicol* 1991;29:459–465.

13. Lampe K: Current concepts of therapy in mushroom intoxication. *Clin Toxicol* 1974;7:115–121.
14. Hanrahan J, Gordon M: Treatment of mushroom poisoning. *JAMA* 1984;252:3130–3133.
15. Jaeger A, Jehl F, Flesch F, et al: Kinetics of amatoxins in human poisoning: therapeutic implications. *J Toxicol Clin Toxicol* 1993;31: 63–80.
16. Floersheim G: Treatment of human amatoxin mushroom poisoning: myths and advances in therapy. *Med Toxicol* 1987;2:1–9.
17. Kelner M, Alexander N: Endocrine hormone abnormalities in *Amanita* poisoning. *Clin Toxicol* 1987;25:21–37.
18. Lampe K, McCann M: Differential diagnosis of poisoning by North American mushrooms, with particular emphasis on *Amanita phalloides*-type intoxication. *Ann Emerg Med* 1987;16:956–962.
19. Pond S, Olson K, Woo O, et al: Amatoxin poisoning in Northern California, 1982–1983. *West J Med* 1986;145:204–209.
20. Bartoloni F, Omer S, Giannini A, et al: *Amanita* poisoning: a clinical-histiopathological study of 64 cases of intoxication. *Hepato-Gastroenterol* 1985;32:229–231.
21. Cappell M, Hassan T: Gastrointestinal and hepatic effects of *Amanita phalloides* ingestion. *J Clin Gastroenterol* 1992:15:225–226.
22. McClain J, Hause D, Clark M: *Amanita phalloides* mushroom poisoning: a cluster of four fatalities. *J Forens Sci* 1989;34:83–87.
23. Plotzker R, Jensen D, Payne J: *Amanita virosa* acute hepatic necrosis: treatment with thioctic acid. *Am J Med Sci* 1982;283:79–82.
24. Schneider S, Borochovitz D, Krenzelok E: Cimetidine protection against α-amanitin hepatotoxicity in mice: a potential model for the treatment of *Amanita phalloides* poisoning. *Ann Emerg Med* 1987; 16:1136–1140.
25. Pinson C, Daya M, Benner K, et al: Liver transplantation for severe *Amanita phalloides* mushroom poisoning. *Am J Surg* 1990;159: 493–499.
26. Galler G, Weisenberg E, Brasitus T: Mushroom poisoning: the role of orthotopic liver transplantation. *J Clin Gastroenterol* 1992;15: 229–232.
27. Coulet M, Guillot J: Poisoning by *Gyromitra*: a possible mechanism. *Med Hypotheses* 1982;8:325–334.
28. Spoerke D, Hall A: Plants and mushrooms of abuse. *Emerg Med Clin North Am* 1990;8:579–593.
29. Gilad E, Biger Y: Paralysis of convergence caused by mushroom poisoning. *Am J Ophthalmol* 1986;102:124–125.
30. Curry S, Rose M: Intravenous mushroom poisoning. *Ann Emerg Med* 1985;14:900–902.
31. Peden N, Pringle S, Crooks J: *Hum Toxicol* 1982;1:417–424.
32. Peden N, Bissett A, Macaulay K, et al: Clinical toxicology of magic mushroom ingestion.*Postgrad Med J* 1981;57:543–545.

ADDITIONAL SELECTED REFERENCES

Homann J, Rawer P, Bleyl H, et al: Early detection of amatoxins in human mushroom poisoning. *Arch Toxicol* 1986;59:190–191.

Schumacher T, Hoiland K: Mushroom poisoning caused by species of the genus *Cortinarium fries*. *Arch Toxicol* 1983;53:87–106.

Vesconi S, Langer M, Iapichino G, et al: Therapy of cytotoxic mushroom intoxication. *Crit Care Q* 1985;13:402–406.

PART XIII

TOXINS IN FOOD

CHAPTER 71

Sulfites and Monosodium Glutamate

Thousands of chemicals are used to preserve, color, and flavor foods and drugs. Reactions to foods or substances in foods may occur with disturbing frequency (1). Many times, the reactions may go undiagnosed. Adverse reactions to foods whose pathogenesis involves an immunologic response to the food components, primarily glycoproteins, are appropriately called *food-hypersensitivity reactions*, a term generally considered to be synonymous with *food allergy*, although the latter term is often used to denote any unusual response to food (2).

Food *intolerance* is an abnormal, nonimmunologic response to an ingested food that may be pharmacologic, toxic, or metabolic. Pharmacologic reactions to foods are the result of natural or added chemicals that produce an effect like that of a drug. Metabolic reactions result from the effect of the food on the metabolism of the recipient, and food toxicity is caused by toxins contained in the food or released by microorganisms contaminating the food product (3).

Food *hypersensitivity* encompasses a number of distinct clinicopathologic entities. These include anaphylaxis and other immediate reactions, eosinophilic gastroenteritis, eczema, and food protein–induced gastroenteropathy in infants and children. Gluten-sensitive enteropathy, attributed to immunologic responses to gluten, is technically a food allergy, although it is usually considered in a separate category because of its unique features (4).

There have been numerous reports of allergic reactions after the ingestion of food additives such as yellow dye and tartrazine, food preservatives and antioxidants such as sulfites, and flavor enhancers such as monosodium L-glutamate (MSG) (5). This chapter discusses the toxicity associated with the sulfites and MSG.

SULFITES

Sulfur dioxide and various sulfites have been used for centuries as preservatives, sanitizing agents, and selective inhibitors of growth of microorganisms in the food industry (6,7). During Roman times, sulfur wicks were burned to prevent further fermentation of wines and to inhibit the growth of yeast and mold (6,8). Because ingestion of sulfites, even in large amounts, does not have apparent ill effects in normal individuals, they are listed on the FDA's schedule of substances generally recognized as safe (9,10). Nevertheless, asthmatic patients are highly susceptible to bronchospasm following sulfite ingestion (6). Recently, the FDA has banned use of sulfites as preservatives in raw fruits and most vegetables (8).

Uses

Sulfites prevent microbial spoilage and browning of foods and are also used as preservatives and antioxidants in a number of medications. Sulfites include potassium and sodium metabisulfite, potassium and sodium bisulfite, sodium sulfite, and sulfur dioxide (Table 71–1). All the sulfites contain sulfur in the 4^+ oxidation state and function as strong reducing agents (11). The choice of a particular sulfite is made primarily on the basis of convenience because all are chemically equivalent, and a reaction reportedly provoked by a specific sulfite can generally be attributed to any of these closely related compounds (6). The solid form, metabisulfite, is readily converted on hydration to the active component bisulfite, which under appropriate conditions can form sulfite or sulfuric acid (11).

Sulfites in Foods

Sulfites can react with foods by reducing sugars, proteins, lipids, and their components to form combined sulfites. The antioxidant properties of sulfites keep fruits

TABLE 71–1. *Sulfites*

Potassium metabisulfite
Potassium bisulfite
Sodium metabisulfite
Sodium bisulfite
Sodium sulfite
Sulfur dioxide

TABLE 71–2. *Partial list of foods that may contain sulfites*

Alcoholic beverages (beer, cocktail mix, red wine, white wine)
Nonalcoholic beverages (colas, fruit drinks)
Baked goods (baking mixes, cookies, crackers, crepes, pie crust, pizza crust, soft pretzels, quiche crust, tortillas, waffles)
Coffee and tea, including instant tea
Condiments (olives, relishes, pickles, salad dressing mixes, wine vinegar)
Confections (brown sugar, raw sugar, powdered sugar)
Dairy analogs (filled milk)
Seafoods (clams, crab, dried cod, lobster, scallops, shrimp)
Fresh seafoods (clams. crab, lobster, scallops, shrimp)
Fresh fruits (fruit salads, grapes, other)
Fresh vegetables (avocado salad, guacamole, cabbage, mushrooms, salad bars, tomatoes)
Gelatins/puddings/fillings (fruit filling, gelatin, pectin jelling agents)
Grain products (batters, breadings, corn starch, food starches, noodle/rice mixes)
Gravies/sauces (milk-based gravy, others)
Hard candies
Commercial jams and jellies
Nuts
Protein isolates
Processed fruits (dietetic fruit or juice, dried fruit, fruit juice, glaced fruit, juice)
Processed vegetables (avocado mix, canned vegetables, dried vegetables, green vegetables, hominy, pickled vegetables, potatoes, spinach, vegetable juice)
Snack foods (apple bits, dried fruit, filled crackers, tortilla chips, trail mix, potato chips)
Soft candies (caramel, others)
Soups (canned soups, dry soup mix)
Sugar (white granulated)
Sweet sauces (corn syrup, dextrose monohydrate, fruit topping, glucose syrup, maple syrup, molasses, pancake syrup)

Reprinted, with permission, from *Ann Allergy* 1985;54:421. American College of Allergists.

and vegetables looking fresh; oxygen is unavailable to promote bacterial growth, so that there is inhibition of enzyme-catalyzed oxidative discoloration and browning of these foods (11). Because of this, their use in restaurant salad bars has increased in the last few years (12).

Sulfites are also used in many processed foods, including beer and wine, fruit drinks, baked goods, and dried fruits and vegetables (Table 71–2) (6). They are used in the processing of food ingredients such as gelatin, beet sugar, corn sweeteners, and food starches (1). Sulfites are also used in industry as sanitizing agents for food containers and fermentation equipment (9).

Sulfites in Medicine

Exposure to sulfites may also occur through many medications; thus, sulfites may inadvertently be administered to sulfite-sensitive individuals (10,11). Medications containing sulfites include adrenergic bronchodilator solutions, steroids (14), antiemetics, cardiovascular preparations, antibiotics, analgesics, local anesthetics, psychotropic drugs, and intravenous solutions (Table 71–3). Because sulfites destroy thiamine, they are no longer used in thiamine-containing foods (7,11,15). Sulfites are commonly used in parenteral emergency drugs, including dopamine, dobutamine, epinephrine, dexamethasone, phenylephrine, physostigmine, and procainamide (16).

Life-threatening adverse reactions to sulfite preservatives in parenteral medications are infrequent and are not easily predicted by patient history. Many sulfite-sensitive individuals may be able to tolerate the low doses of sulfites contained in local anesthetics for dental use. A subpopulation of exquisitely sulfite-sensitive patients who react to oral challenges of 5–10 mg or less may be at increased risk for parenteral reactions.

Daily Intake of Sulfites

The average daily diet is estimated to contain from 2 to 15 mg of naturally occurring sulfites (15). Dehydrated fruits and vegetables may contain up to 75 to 80 mg per serving, fruit drinks up to 30 mg per serving, and sausages up to 60 mg (6,10,15). Alcoholic beverages such as wine and beer may contain 5 to 10 mg per ounce. A single restaurant meal may contain more than 150 to 200 mg of sulfite (9,11).

Metabolism

Sodium and potassium sulfites are stable salts. When added to water, they hydrolyze to sodium and potassium cations and bisulfite radicals. Acid pH, as in gastric contents, and increased temperature enhance these events (1). The free bisulfite is then oxidized to sulfate by the enzyme sulfite oxidase and is excreted in the urine (Fig. 71–1). Sulfite oxidase is widely distributed in the body, with the highest activity found in the liver and kidney. Defects in sulfite oxidase activity may potentially be of importance in the pathogenesis of adverse reactions to sulfites (6).

Sulfites are also formed during normal metabolism, particularly of cysteine (17). Sulfite radicals are present in cells and plasma but are quickly converted by sulfite oxidase (9).

Toxicity

The prevalence of sensitivity to sulfiting agents in the general population is unknown. Only a relatively small number of vulnerable individuals appear to develop sys-

TABLE 71–3. *Partial list of medications that may contain sulfites*

Nebulized bronchodilators	**Antiemetics (parenteral)**
Isoetharine (Bronkosol)	Metoclopramide (Reglan)
Isoproterenol (Isuprel)	Promethazine (Phenergan)
Metaproterenol (Alupent, Metaprel)	Prochlorperazine (Compazine)
Cardiovascular drugs (parenteral)	**Antibiotics (aerosolized, parenteral)**
Dopamine	Sulfonamides (Gantrisin, Bactrim, sulfadiazine, Septra, sulfacetamide)
Epinephrine (EpiPen Auto Injector, Anakit, etc.)	Tetracyclines
Procainamide	Aminoglycosides (tobramycin, kanamycin, gentamicin, streptomycin)
Norepinephrine (Levophed)	**IV Solutions**
Metaraminol (Aramine)	ISolyte, Aminosyn, Travamin, Amigen, Inpersol, Ionosol, Alba-Dex, Intropin, ascorbic acid, Travert, FreAmine HBC, HepatAmine, parenteral nutrition, Travasol, etc
Isoproterenol	**IV Contrast solutions**
Methoxamine (Vasoxyl)	**Local anesthetics**
Psychiatric drugs (parenteral)	Mepivacaine (Carbocaine)
Chlorpromazine	Chloroprocaine (Nesacaine)
Prochlorperazine	Procaine (Novocain)
Imipramine (Tofranil)	Bupivacaine (Marcaine)
Perphenazine (Trilafon)	Tetracaine (Pontocaine)
Phenothiazines (e.g., Torecan)	Lidocaine
Analgesics	Mericaine
Codeine	**Muscle relaxants (parenteral)**
Morphine	Orphenadrine (Norflex)
Acetaminophen (Tylenol, etc.)	Methocarbamol (Robaxin)
Pentazocine (Talwin)	Tubocurarine
Nalbuphine (Nubain)	
Meperidine	
Oxymorphone (Numorphan)	
Peritoneal dialysis solutions	
Dialyte, Inpersol, etc	
Steroids, parenteral	
Betamethasone	
Dexamethasone	
Prednisolone	
Hydrocortisone	
Miscellaneous	
Otic preparations	
Ophthalmic preparations	
Liver injections	
Ergoloid mesylates	
B complex	
Edrophonium (Tensilon)	
Sodium thiosulfate	

Reprinted, with permission, from *Ann Allergy* 1985;54:422. American College of Allergists.

temic reactions to sulfites. The first documented report of a reaction to sulfites was in 1976. Since that time, sulfites have been reported to produce a wide spectrum of severe adverse reactions, including urticaria, angioedema, asthma, abdominal pain, and diarrhea. Few reactions have been directly attributed to sulfites in drugs, which contain much smaller amounts of sulfites than foods (11).

After exposure through inhalation, intravenous injection, or ingestion of sulfites, the onset of symptoms is rapid, usually occurring within 2 to 15 minutes; onset tends to be more rapid when the sulfiting agents are ingested in solution. When sulfites are ingested in solid food, the onset of symptoms is generally within 15 to 30 minutes, although some reactions to solid foods have occurred immediately.

A number of signs and symptoms have been ascribed to sulfite sensitivity (Table 71–4); besides those mentioned above, symptoms may include flushing, tingling, pruritus, tachypnea, wheezing, tachycardia, dizziness, and weakness. Rhinitis, conjunctivitis, and nausea (9) and dysphagia (15) have also been reported (9). Swelling of the tongue may also occur in sulfite-sensitive individuals (15). The most commonly reported reaction to sulfites is bronchospasm; this occurs most frequently in asthmatics. Bronchoconstriction has also occurred in asthmatics after inhalation of sulfite-preserved bronchodilator solutions. The most serious reactions from large amounts of sulfites are loss of consciousness, anaphylactic shock, central nervous system stimulation, seizures, and death (11).

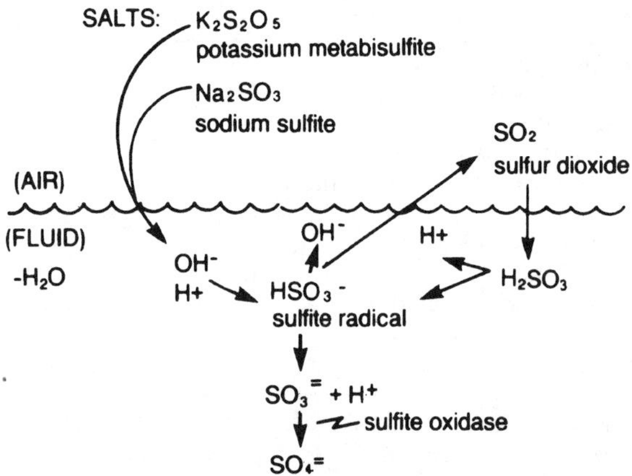

FIG. 71–1. Sulfite chemistry. Reprinted from *J Allergy Clin Immunol* 1984;74:469–472, with permission of C.V. Mosby Company.

Mechanism of Toxicity

The mechanism of hypersensitivity to sulfites has not been fully explained, and it is likely that there are several mechanisms of toxicity. Some investigators have suggested an IgE-mediated reaction, and in some cases an immunologic reaction may be involved. As mentioned above, there also appears to be a connection to sulfite oxidase deficiency in a small number of sensitive individuals. In addition, a cholinergic reflex mechanism has been suggested, in view of the observation, that many of the clinical manifestations reported with sulfite hypersensitivity are similar to those attributed to stimulation of the parasympathetic system. Stimulation of airway irritant receptors by inhaled sulfur dioxide has also been suggested as the mechanism for the immediate bronchospasm noted in some individuals. Inhalation of 1 to ppm of SO_2 causes bronchospasm in all subjects with asthma. However, only 4% to 10% of these cases are sensitive to oral sulfites, suggesting the existence of other factors that might explain this finding (16).

TABLE 71–4. *Toxic effects of sulfites noted in sensitive individuals*

Minor
Abdominal pain
Conjunctivitis
Diarrhea
Dizziness
Dysphagia
Flushing
Nausea
Pruritus
Rhinitis
Swelling of the tongue
Tachycardia
Tachypnea
Tingling
Urticaria
Weakness
Major
Anaphylaxis
Bronchospasm
Loss of consciousness
Seizures
Death

TABLE 71–5. *Treatment for sulfite reactions*

Prophylaxis
Cromolyn sodium
Nebulized atropine
Asthma (as needed)
Epinephrine
Aminophylline
Antihistamines

Diagnosis

A history of an allergic reaction, anaphylaxis, or bronchoconstriction occurring during ingestion of food (particularly salads) or beverages in a restaurant provides a strong clue to the diagnosis of sulfite sensitivity.

Laboratory Confirmation

Cutaneous tests for immediate hypersensitivity to common foods may be negative in most sulfite-sensitive individuals. Confirmation of sensitivity to sulfites may be obtained through provocative challenges delivered by ingestion or inhalation of sulfites.

Treatment

There is no specific treatment for sulfite sensitivity reactions. Treatment is determined on the basis of the presenting symptoms (Table 71–5). Patients should be cautioned to avoid the use of foods and drugs containing sulfites.

Treatment of symptoms consists of the usual measures for asthma or anaphylaxis, including administration of epinephrine, aminophylline, and antihistamines, together with other appropriate support. Reactions to sulfites have been blocked with nebulized cromolyn sodium (Intal) and nebulized atropine. A new drug, ketotifen (not yet available in the United States), has been shown to block metabisulfite-induced asthma.

MONOSODIUM GLUTAMATE

Monosodium glutamate (MSG) is a widely used food additive; it is also on the FDA listing of substances that are generally recognized as safe (18). MSG was discovered in the early 1900s when a chemist analyzed a seaweed commonly used as seasoning in Japanese cooking (19,20). MSG now appears on the market as a flavor enhancer and is found in seasoned salts, soy sauce, bouillons, meat bases, and certain cooked or frozen foods (21). It has also been suggested as the cause of the "Chinese restaurant syndrome," which is a benign, self-limiting process that has an excellent prognosis for immediate and rapid recovery (18,22). Chinese restaurant syndrome is a misnomer because symptoms similar to those produced by MSG have been reported after ingestion of substances that contained MSG but were not Chinese foods nor were eaten in Chinese restaurants (23).

Monosodium glutamate is the sodium salt of the amino acid, glutamic acid. It is commercially synthesized by taking protein, typically derived from wheat or soy, through an acid wash to unravel the amino acids. The neutralizing agent sodium hydroxide is then added to form the sodium salt of each amino acid, called hydrolyzed vegetable protein. Typically, MSG constitutes 10% to 30% of the mixture.

To restore lost flavor in nonfresh food, MSG is now added to a large percentage of canned, frozen, and prepared foods found in supermarket aisles. Chinese-restaurant food is a source of only a small fraction of the 85 million pounds of MSG that Americans now consume annually. Research on the MSG–headache link is currently important because there has been an enormous increase in both the variety and total consumption of foods containing MSG in the past decade.

There are several reasons for the expanded presence of MSG in food in the last 15 years. MSG use has proliferated beyond Chinese restaurants to most canned soups, sauces, dried food, frozen dinners, potato chips, canned meats, most diet foods, cured and lunch meat, and broths (Table 71–6) (24). MSG use also has increased because Americans consume more high MSG convenience foods such as fast and prepared foods and less fresh and homemade foods which almost never contain MSG.

Currently, the FDA permits the following terms on a food label to refer to MSG in food: *hydrolyzed vegetable protein*, *hydrolyzed plant protein*, *natural flavoring*, *flavoring*, and *seasoning*. The result of these labeling loopholes is that most MSG currently consumed cannot be identified in looking for the term *monosodium glutamate* or *MSG* on labels. Casual inspection of supermarket food labels reveals that more products use the terms *natural flavoring* or *hydrolyzed vegetable protein* than the term *monosodium glutamate*.

TABLE 71–6. *Monosodium glutamate and foods*

Canned soups
Sauces
Dried foods
Frozen dinners
Potato chips
Canned meats
Diet foods
Cured lunch meat
Broths

Mechanism of Toxicity

Glutamate is a nonessential amino acid with a function as an amino carrier between L-ketoglutarate and glutamine (25). L-Glutamic acid is present in large amounts in the central nervous system and has been suggested as a neurotransmitter. Glutamate is unique among amino acids by virtue of its direct utilization as an energy source by cerebral tissue (19).

Glutamate appears to have minimal peripheral effects but has excitatory effects at central sites that affect cardiovascular control (22). Glutamate also has numerous interactions with the tricarboxylic acid cycle and is an important precursor of glutathione and insulin as well as a critical source of urinary ammonium (26). Glutamate is also a known precursor for synthesis of acetylcholine, and extracellular sodium ions enhance acetylcholine synthesis in ganglia (23).

Pyroglutamate, which is formed from MSG when it is boiled, is similar to MSG but more readily crosses the blood–brain barrier (19). Although both MSG and pyroglutamate have been shown to cause Chinese restaurant syndrome, pyroglutamate provokes symptoms at lower concentrations than MSG, probably because of its greater permeation of the central nervous system (18).

Currently, it is thought that MSG produces a transient acetylcholinosis, which has signs and symptoms identical to those induced by acetylcholine (27). This appears to account for the multiple symptoms affected by MSG toxicity. There may be a familial tendency toward development of this sensitivity (28).

Toxicity

Symptoms related to MSG ingestion occur in a small percentage of the general public that is extremely sensitive to it (26). Affected individuals experience symptoms within 15 to 45 minutes of ingestion (29). Effects may last for up to several hours, and spontaneous resolution has been noted (13). Sometimes symptoms may not be noted for some hours after ingestion and may last for up to 2 days (23,30).

As mentioned, signs and symptoms of toxicity appear to be similar to those induced by acetylcholine (26) and may include dizziness, facial flushing, heartburn, palpitations, burning in the chest, chest tightness, tightness of the scalp, frontal or temporal headache, nausea, abdominal pain, paresthesia and numbness over the back of the neck, thirst, and lightheadedness (Table

TABLE 71–7. *Signs and symptoms of MSG reaction*

Adults
- Skin
  - Flushing
  - Scalp tightness
- Neurologic
  - Dizziness
  - Headache
  - Paresthesia
  - Lightheadedness
- Gastrointestinal
  - Heartburn
  - Burning in the chest
  - Nausea
  - Abdominal pain
  - Thirst
  - Chest tightness
- Miscellaneous
  - Palpitations

Children
- Shivering
- Shuddering
- Irritability
- Crying
- Abdominal pain
- Delirium

71–7) (31). Other symptoms described in adults have been a feeling of pressure behind the eyes and diaphoresis (28). In children, shivering and shuddering, irritability, crying, abdominal pain, and delirium have been described (21,27).

Reaction most commonly occurs after eating food on an empty stomach (32). This often occurs when clear soup or broth is eaten as a first course because MSG is frequently added to clear soups and broths in considerable quantities to obtain a pleasantly strong meat flavor (30). The rapid absorption of MSG under such circumstances may result in high serum concentrations that may overwhelm the blood–brain barrier, and trigger synthesis of acetylcholine.

Diagnosis

A thorough history and physical examination should be performed on all patients with signs and symptoms of MSG intoxication to rule out life-threatening disorders. Laboratory tests such as on serum electrolytes, complete blood cell count, serum glutamate concentrations, or roentgenography provide no additional information. There is no correlation between blood glutamate concentrations and the appearance of symptoms (25).

Treatment

Normally, MSG intoxication is benign and requires no treatment other than supportive care (27). In rare instances, patients may have cardiac symptoms that require electrocardiographic monitoring. In those instances, a 12-lead electrocardiogram should be obtained. Dysrhythmia, if noted, should be treated with standard antidysrhythmic therapy. Occasionally, bronchoconstriction may be noted and should be treated with the standard regimen, including β-specific nebulizers and intravenous xanthine derivatives.

REFERENCES

1. Mathison D, Stevenson D, Simon R: Precipitating factors in asthma. *Chest* 1985;87(Suppl.):50s–54s.
2. Metcalfe D: Diseases of food hypersensitivity. *N Engl J Med* 1989; 321:255–257.
3. Sampson H, Mendelson L, Rosen J: Fatal and near-fatal anaphylactic reactions to food in children and adolescents. *N Engl J Med* 1992; 327:380–384.
4. Kessler D: The federal regulation of food labeling. *N Engl J Med* 1989;321:717–725.
5. Swan G: Management of monosodium glutamate toxicity. *J Asthma* 1982;19:105–110.
6. Bush R, Taylor S, Busse W: A critical evaluation of clinical trials in reactions to sulfites. *J Allergy Clin Immunol* 1986;78:191–202.
7. Simon R: Sulfite sensitivity. *Ann Allergy* 1986;56:281–292.
8. Stevenson D, Simon R: Sulfites and asthma. *J Allergy Clin Immunol* 1984;74:469–472.
9. Baker G, Collett P, Allen D: Bronchospasm induced by metabisulfite-containing foods and drugs. *Med J Aust* 1981;2:614–616.
10. Schwartz H, Sher T: Bisulfite sensitivity manifesting as allergy to local dental anesthesia. *J Allergy Clin Immunol* 1985;75:525–527.
11. Dalton-Bunnow M: Review of sulfite sensitivity. *Am J Hosp Pharmacol* 1985;42:2220–2226.
12. Smilinske S: Review of parenteral sulfite reactions. *J Toxicol Clin Toxicol* 1992;30:597–606.
13. Wolf S, Nicklas R: Sulfite sensitivity in a seven-year-old child. *Ann Allergy* 1985;54:420–423.
14. Koepke J, Christopher K, Chai H, et al: Dose dependent bronchospasm from sulfites in isoetharine. *JAMA* 1984;251:2982–2983.
15. Jamieson D, Guill M, Wray B, et al: Metabisulfite sensitivity: case report and literature review. *Ann Allergy* 1985;54:115–121.
16. Anibarro B, Caballero T, Garcia-Ara C, et al: Asthma with sulfite intolerance in children: a blocking study with cyanocobalamin. *J Allergy Clin Immunol* 1992;90:103–109.
17. Napke E, Stevens D: Excipients and additives: hidden hazards in drug products and in product substitution. *Can Med Assoc J* 1984;131: 1449–1452.
18. Cochran J, Cochran A: Monosodium glutamania: the Chinese restaurant syndrome revisited. *JAMA* 1984;52:899.
19. Reif-Lehrer L: A questionnaire study of the prevalence of Chinese restaurant syndrome. *Fed Proc* 1977;36:1617–1623.
20. Settipane G: Adverse reactions to sulfites in drugs and foods. *J Am Acad Dermatol* 1984;10:1077–1080.
21. Schaumburg H, Byck R, Gerstl R, et al: Monosodium L-glutamate: its pharmacology and role in the Chinese restaurant syndrome. *Science* 1969;163:826–828.
22. Kerr G, Wu-Lee M, El-Lozy M, et al: Prevalence of "Chinese restaurant syndrome." *Research* 1979;75:29–33.
23. Ghadimi H, Kumar S, Abaci F: Studies on monosodium glutamate ingestion. *Biochem Med* 1971;5:447–456.
24. Oliver A, Rich A, Reade P, et al: Monosodium glutamate-related orofacial granulomatosis. *Oral Surg Oral Med Oral Pathol* 1991;71: 560–564.
25. Kenney R, Tidball C: Human susceptibility to oral monosodium L-glutamate. *Am J Clin Nutr* 1972;25:140–146.
26. Zautcke J, Schwartz J, Meuller E: Chinese restaurant syndrome: a review. *Ann Emerg Med* 1986;15:1210–1213.

27. Asnes R: Chinese restaurant syndrome in an infant. *Clin Pediatr* 1980;19:705–706.
28. Rubini, M: The many-faceted mystique of monosodium glutamate. *Am J Clin Nutr* 1972;24:169–171.
29. Scopp A: MSG and hydrolyzed vegetable protein induced headache: review and case studies. *Headache* 1991;31:107–110.
30. Wilkin J: Does monosodium glutamate cause flushing (or merely "glutamania")? *J Am Acad Dermatol* 1986;15:225–230.
31. Yang W, Purchase E: Adverse reactions to sulfites. *Can Med Assoc J* 1985;133:865–880.
32. Merritt J, Williams P: Vasospasm contributes to monosodium glutamate-induced headache. *Headache* 1990;30:575–580.

ADDITIONAL SELECTED REFERENCES

Bush R, Tasylor S, Holden K, et al: Prevalence of sensitivity to sulfiting agents in asthmatic patients. *Am J Med* 1986;81:816–820.

Ghadimi H, Kumar S: Current status of monosodium glutamate. *Am J Clin Nutr* 1972;25:643–646.

Sauber W: What is Chinese restaurant syndrome? *Lancet* 1980;1: 722–723.

Sher T, Schwartz H: Bisulfite sensitivity manifesting as an allergic reaction to aerosol therapy. *Ann Allergy* 1985;54:224–226.

Twarog F, Leung D: Anaphylaxis to a component of isoetharine (sodium bisulfite). *JAMA* 1982;248:2030–2031.

CHAPTER 72

Botulism

Botulism is an infrequent but devastating disease because the botulism toxin is one of the most dangerous toxins known (1). The disease should be considered a true medical emergency. The causative organism, *Clostridium botulinum*, is an anaerobic, spore-forming, Gram-positive, rod-shaped bacteria that is widely distributed in nature and is found mainly in the soil. These organisms elaborate the toxin, and a given strain of the organism produces only one toxin type (2).

The term *botulism* is derived from the Latin word *botulus*, meaning "sausage," because blood sausage was known for centuries to be associated with the symptom complex now recognized as botulism (3). Clinically, botulism can be classified into three major types on the basis of the cause of the disease and the age of the patient (1). These types are food-borne botulism, infant botulism, and wound botulism (4). Various strains of *C. botulinum* produce eight toxins in all (A, B, C_1, C_2, D, E, F, and G), differentiated by antigenic specificity and typically present in particular settings (5). For example, toxins A and B often come from inadequately processed vegetables or meat, and toxin E is associated with ingestion of fish and marine mammal products. All toxins are globular proteins approximately 150,000 daltons in molecular weight, and all act by the same mechanism. Most illness is caused by types A and B (5). There is a distinct geographic distribution of these toxins in the United States (1). Type A is evident primarily west of the Mississippi River, and type B is frequently seen in the eastern states (5). Type E is found predominantly in the Great Lakes region and in Alaska (7).

Clostridium botulinum produces a potent neurotoxin that causes progressive muscle paralysis. *C. botulinum* spores can survive a temperature of 100°C for several hours and moist heat at 120°C for 30 minutes (8). The toxin, however, is destroyed by boiling for 10 minutes. The spores germinate only under anaerobic and neutral or weakly acidic conditions if these are present for several days. Thus, the ingestion of formed toxin, not simply of spores, is required in the food-borne or adult form of botulism. In infant botulism, the toxin is produced by incubation of the spores within the gastrointestinal tract. Botulism, therefore, can occur after ingestion of preformed toxin or after ingestion of *C. botulinum* spores that germinate, proliferate, and then generate toxin in the gastrointestinal tract (5).

MECHANISM OF TOXICITY

Botulism toxin binds at the presynaptic clefts of cholinergic nerve terminals, blocking the release of acetylcholine at the neuromuscular junctions and peripheral autonomic synapses (3). This results in the clinical manifestation of autonomic dysfunction and generalized paralysis. The toxin binds to all ganglionic and postganglionic parasympathetic synapses as well as neuromuscular junctions (2). In the parasympathetic nervous system, both preganglionic and postganglionic fibers are involved early, which results in severe autonomic dysfunction (9).

On ingestion, botulism toxin is first transported across the intestinal wall into the serum. It then binds to a receptor on the surface of the presynaptic nerve membrane (8). The toxin or some part of it then crosses into the presynaptic terminal and combines with another internal receptor, which causes interference with acetylcholine release. This is an irreversible step leading to impairment of neurotransmitter release and resultant neuromuscular blockade. Although the presynaptic nerve can still propagate an impulse, there is no subsequent release of acetylcholine. Botulinum toxin that is absorbed into the bloodstream acts only on the peripheral nervous system; it does not cross the blood–brain barrier.

The effects of botulism toxin in some ways resemble those of curare except that the former acts presynaptically and its effects are only occasionally reversed by cholinesterase inhibitors (3).

WOUND BOTULISM

Wound botulism is a rare clinical entity and results from an infection of a wound by *C. botulinum* with subsequent in vivo production and systemic absorption of the toxin (3,10). Wound botulism clinically resembles food-borne disease but has a longer incubation period of approximately 10 days and has no gastrointestinal symptoms. Wound botulism has been associated with compound fractures, severe trauma, lacerations, puncture wounds, and hematoma (3). Such toxin-containing wounds may or may not look grossly infected. The process can occur in soil-contaminated traumatic wounds, as well as in surgical wounds; it is also associated with parenteral and intranasal cocaine abuse when *C. botulinum* infects needle sites and paranasal sinuses, respectively.

Wound botulism is diagnosed by positive would cultures in about two thirds of cases and by serum toxin detection in the other third. Wound botulism calls for treatment with antitoxin, debridement, and appropriate antibiotics.

FOOD-BORNE BOTULISM

Botulism is unknown after eating fresh food. Fermentation, pickling, canning, smoking, and similar processes that require anaerobic conditions enable *Clostridium botulinum* to produce its toxin. Inadequate processing of nonacidic foods and home canning procedures are responsible in a great majority of cases; because spore germination is inhibited at low pH, acidic foods are less frequently contaminated.

Typical food-borne botulism is caused by the ingestion of botulinum toxin elaborated by *Clostridium botulinum*. Toxin types are distinguished immunologically by using specific neutralizing antisera; types A, B, and E are the most common causes of human botulism (5,6).

Signs and Symptoms

Symptoms of botulism usually occur 12 to 36 hours after ingestion of contaminated food, although the incubation period can be as short as 4 hours or as long as 8 days (Table 72–1). Fever is usually not seen unless there is an infection from another source. Poisoning may cause anything from mild illness to death, which can occur within 24 hours of symptom onset.

TABLE 72–1. *Signs and symptoms of food-borne botulism*

Gastrointestinal
Nausea
Vomiting
Abdominal cramps
Abdominal distension
Constipation
Neurologic
Eye
Blurred vision
Diplopia
Photophobia
Ptosis
Mydriasis
Dizziness
Dysarthria
Respiratory
Respiratory failure
Laryngeal obstruction

Gastrointestinal

Early symptoms of botulism include nausea, vomiting, abdominal cramps, and abdominal distension. These effects are due to the toxin's local action on the gastrointestinal tract. Constipation is common; diarrhea is rarely found.

Neurologic

Systemic neurologic symptoms of botulism usually occur within 72 hours of gastrointestinal symptoms but may be delayed as long as 8 days. Early neurologic signs indicate a more severe infection and a worse prognosis (11). Presenting neurologic symptoms are bulbar paralysis and a descending motor paralysis (1). Various eye disorders may be early features and include blurred vision, diplopia, photophobia, ptosis, and mydriasis (2). The highest cranial nerves are usually affected first, so that diplopia may be the first presenting symptom (11). Dizziness and dysarthria may occur; and as the lower cranial nerves become involved, the patient may complain of dysphagia and a dry mouth. The motor nerves are then involved, and peripheral muscle weakness progresses. When the muscles of respiration are affected, fatal dyspnea may result. There is no sensory involvement, and the patient may remain mentally clear; myotactic reflexes also remain intact (2).

Cause of Death

The most serious effects of botulism are pulmonary infection or respiratory failure secondary to muscle dysfunction and bulbar paralysis. Although the most common cause of death is paralysis of the muscles of respiration, occasionally, patients may succumb to sudden laryngeal obstruction or unexpected cardiac arrest (1).

Diagnosis

The initial diagnosis of botulism is clinical and based on the history and physical examination. A correct diagnosis is difficult to make, and many times botulism is misdiagnosed in its early stages. Because most cases originate from tainted food, a careful history of ingestion of home-canned or home-prepared food should be sought. Definite diagnosis can be made by demonstration of toxin in serum or stool by the mouse inoculation test (3).

The differential diagnosis includes the Guillain–Barrè syndrome, acute poliomyelitis, myasthenia gravis, the Lambert–Eaton syndrome, tick paralysis, and chemical poisoning by atropine or organophosphorus compounds.

Laboratory Analysis

Botulism toxin may be detected in serum provided that blood is collected soon after the onset of clinical symptoms. Serum (10 mL) should be obtained before treatment, but treatment should not be delayed while awaiting laboratory confirmation because this may require more than 24 hours. The diagnosis is confirmed by observing the effects of injection of the patient's serum into mice by isolation of botulinum toxin from food residues.

Electromyography may help in the diagnosis by showing an increase in the abnormally small-amplitude muscle action potentials after repetitive nerve stimulation (staircase effect) (11). This is in contrast to findings in myasthenia gravis, in which repetitive nerve stimulation results in a decrease of the muscle action potentials (9).

Routine studies including a complete blood cell count, serum electrolytes, calcium and magnesium concentrations, blood urea nitrogen, hepatic enzymes, lumbar puncture, and a chest roentgenogram are usually normal but may be altered by secondary dehydration or pneumonitis.

Treatment

General Measures

Treatment is supportive, and early intervention is indicated. Effective treatment comprises three stages: respiratory care, removal of the nonabsorbed enterotoxin, and possible antitoxin therapy (2).

Respiratory Care

Respiratory impairment may present the most serious, life-threatening consequence of botulism poisoning. Respiratory muscle weakness often progresses rapidly and its severity is easily underestimated. Respiratory arrest still occurs commonly before mechanical support has been started.

Frequent careful clinical assessment and regular measurements of vital capacity are essential. These may be supplemented by maximal inspiratory and expiratory pressure estimations if these are practical (12). A rapid decrease in vital capacity, a vital capacity of only a third of the predicted value, or a value of approximately one liter should all suggest the need for ventilatory support. Ventilatory support may also be needed because of failure to clear secretions and because of the risk of aspiration even if the vital capacity is only mildly abnormal.

Aspiration pneumonia is common, and it is important that the method of ventilatory support should protect the airway. Modern methods of ventilatory assistance that are valuable for domiciliary use, such as negative pressure and nasal intermittent positive pressure ventilation, are not suitable. Positive pressure ventilation via an endotracheal tube is required (12).

A tracheostomy is usually needed, except in mild cases, because recovery of muscle function is usually slow. Ventilatory support is often needed for several weeks.

Gentamicin and other aminoglycosides should be avoided if possible in a patient with botulism because there have been reports of potentiation of the neuromuscular blockade with such agents.

Antitoxin

The use of antitoxin to botulism toxin is still open to debate. It appears that antitoxin has relatively little effect on toxin types A and B but appreciable effect on type E. It does not reverse any neurologic damage that may have already occurred but may slow or halt the progression of the disease by binding to circulating toxin. Both a bivalent and a trivalent equine-derived antitoxin are available. The bivalent antitoxin contains 10,000 international units of antibody to types A and B, and the trivalent antitoxin contains antibody to types A, B, and E. Both are currently available from the Centers for Disease Control. Dosage is one vial every 4 to 5 hours and may be repeated for 4 to 5 doses.

The decision to administer antitoxin must be based on the risk of its side reactions compared with its potential benefit. The percentage of side reactions from all types of botulism antitoxin is significant. Acute reactions include urticaria, skin rash, and anaphylaxis. The necessary medications and equipment should be readily available for the treatment of any serious side effects (10).

In instances in which the toxin type is unknown, the trivalent preparation is preferred. Before administering the antitoxin, inquiries should be made to determine whether there is a history of allergy, asthma, or hay fever. A skin test should be performed for horse serum sensitivity, and desensitization should be performed in the sensitive individual.

Botulinum toxin appears to be irreversibly bound to the nerve terminals and antitoxin is of no value once this binding has taken place. Recovery of function therefore depends on the formation of new motor endplates from the sprouting nerve terminals. Equine antitoxin, if given within the first 24 hours of symptom onset, can shorten the course and lower the chance of mortality from toxin A food-borne disease.

Human botulinogenic hyperimmune serum is under development but is not yet clinically available.

Guanidine

Because guanidine enhances release of acetylcholine from nerve terminals, its use has been suggested for treatment of botulism. Guanidine appears to be beneficial in patients with Eaton–Lambert syndrome, but clinical data have so far been inconclusive as to its effectiveness for botulism.

INFANT BOTULISM

Infant botulism was first described in 1976 and is now known to present with a diverse spectrum of clinical symptoms (9). It is not a new disease but rather a newly recognized manifestation of an old disorder (7,13). It is well established that *C. botulinum* is not a normal inhabitant of the infant gut (14). Extensive effort is being made to understand the factors that predispose some infants to colonization. Environmental and dietary factors have been evaluated because not only must the infant ingest spores, but the gut must be receptive (15).

Mechanism of Toxicity

No definitive food source can be implicated in most cases of infant botulism (16,17). In this disorder, the intestinal growth of the spores of *Clostridium botulinum* gives rise to subsequent systemic absorption of the toxin (18). The spores germinate in the gastrointestinal tract and produce botulism toxin in vivo (19). The altered intestinal flora and lack of clostridium-inhibiting bile-acids found in older individuals allow the bacteria to multiply in an infant's gastrointestinal tract (14). This mechanism is opposed to food-borne botulism, which results from the ingestion of preformed toxin. Most cases of infant botulism have been caused by either type A or B toxin, although recently a case caused by type F was reported (18).

The age of onset of infant botulism ranges from 2 to 8 months, with peak incidence being at 2 to 4 months of age. Only infants less than 1 year of age appear to have multiplication of spores in the gastrointestinal tract (7). The disease is endemic in California, Utah, and the southeastern areas of Pennsylvania (15). Honey is the only food source that correlates strongly with infant botulism, and therefore honey should be avoided during this period of life because evidence suggests that a small percentage of all honey is contaminated by botulism spores, which cannot be destroyed (20). The organism may survive passage through the infant stomach because of its alkaline pH and its relative lack of protease activity (5).

Signs and Symptoms

The severity of illness in patients with infant botulism varies. The typical clinical syndrome is characterized by variable constipation with subsequent progressive weakness, hypotonia, cranial nerve dysfunction, and hyporeflexia (Table 72–2) (9).

Gastrointestinal

Constipation is usually the first symptom, with the frequency of stool passage being less than 48 hours. Constipation may precede neuromuscular symptoms by as much as 3 weeks (21).

Neurologic

Cranial nerve dysfunction usually includes diminished gag reflex and poor sucking ability. These abnormalities then result in poor feeding. Other manifestations of motor cranial nerve dysfunction may include facial muscle weakness, ptosis, extraocular palsies, and sluggish pupillary light response (16). Cranial nerves VII, IX, X, and XI are almost always involved, and nerves III, IV, and VI are less frequently affected. The infant may appear to be alert despite profound weakness (20); this is characteristic of infant botulism. When the descending paralysis has affected bulbar musculature and has become generalized, loss of head control is prominent (9).

Weakness occurs in all symptomatic cases, and once present, usually progresses rapidly over 1 to 3 days. Subtle signs of weakness are a decrease in spontaneous movements and diminished response to noxious stimuli (21). The child will become more listless, more lethargic, and will sleep more than usual. The child's cry may begin to sound weak and feeble.

Muscular contractions that require frequent neuromuscular transmission such as sucking, swallowing, and head control are affected early. These functions are often the last to return during the recovery stage, and these chil-

TABLE 72–2. *Signs and symptoms of infant botulism*

Gastrointestinal
Constipation
Neurologic
Diminished gag reflex
Poor sucking ability
Facial muscle weakness
Ptosis
Extraocular palsy
Loss of head control
Hyporeflexia
Hypotonia
Weakness

TABLE 72–3. *Diseases to rule out in the differential diagnosis of infant botulism*

Diphtheria
Electrolyte imbalance
Guillain–Barrè syndrome
Metal encephalopathy
Meningitis
Metabolic encephalopathy
Myasthenia gravis
Reye's syndrome
Sepsis
Tick paralysis

dren often require prolonged tube feeding until sucking strength returns.

Diagnosis

Infant botulism is often initially misdiagnosed because its presentation can mimic other disease processes. Because infants are unable to describe their symptoms, the onset of illness can only be detected by careful observation (19). The differential diagnosis of infant botulism includes Guillain–Barrè syndrome, meningitis/encephalitis, dehydration/electrolyte derangement, Reye's syndrome, poliomyelitis, hypothyroidism, sepsis, myasthenia gravis, tick paralysis, diphtheria, cerebrovascular accident, and toxic exposures including organophosphate, heavy metals, and carbon monoxide (Table 72–3) (20).

Laboratory

Electromyographic abnormalities are the only relatively specific finding in infant botulism short of isolating the spores. Brief, small-amplitude, overly abundant action potentials are noted (10). The evoked muscle action potential is reduced because of impaired acetylcholine release (22). Supratetanic stimulation has been reported to result in the "staircase phenomenon" in almost all patients. This phenomenon is characterized by augmented muscle action potential with supratetanic stimulation and is not seen in muscle uninhibited by the botulinum toxin. In addition, as with the adult form of botulism, an incremental response to rapid, repetitive nerve stimulation is frequently noted. Routine laboratory studies including a complete blood cell count, serum electrolytes, and other tests will be normal unless secondarily affected by pneumonia or fluid and electrolyte shifts (16).

Confirmation of the diagnosis of infant botulism requires isolation of the organism or demonstration of specific toxin in stool samples. In contrast to the foodborne type, only rarely is the serum positive for organisms or toxin (22). The association of constipation with infant botulism frequently delays the procurement of stool for culture and toxin assay. Enemas are often used in an attempt to obtain stool for diagnosis; success is limited. Positive results of culture and toxin assays for botulism have been obtained by using enema effluent from colonic irrigation (22).

Evaluation of suspected patients includes complete blood count, metabolic and hepatic profiles, blood, urine, and spinal fluid cultures and analysis. These values are normal in infant botulism.

Physicians should maintain a high index of suspicion in all infants presenting with hypotonia with or without cranial nerve dysfunction. A second electromyogram should be considered if the initial examination results are negative and clinical suspicion remains high.

Cause of Death

Death from infant botulism has been caused by pulmonary complications (9) including aspiration pneumonia, which results from the diminished gag reflex combined with weakness and incoordination of the muscles of deglutition (20). Respiratory arrest secondary to manipulation for a lumbar puncture and ventilatory failure caused by paralysis of the muscles of respiration may also occur. There is suggestive evidence that infant botulism is the cause in some cases of sudden infant death syndrome (16).

Treatment

Supportive Care

Current management of infant botulism consists of supportive respiratory and nutritional care, which should be meticulous. The airway must be carefully maintained with either frequent positioning and suctioning or by intubation. All infants will be dehydrated on admission and will require intravenous fluids. Most cases will require nutritional supplementation. Patients should not be fed by mouth until they are able to gag and swallow. Mean time from hospitalization to resumption of oral feeding is about 50 days (22). Delayed gastric emptying and intestinal motility must be monitored and aspiration prevented. Nasogastric or nasojejunal feedings are usually successful with careful monitoring of residuals, but if doubt exists, total parenteral nutrition should be considered. Monitoring for apnea and bradycardia is essential in all patients (9).

Cathartics

It has been argued that laxatives, cathartics, and enemas may decrease the concentration of intestinal organisms or toxin. Because these sick infants are generally in a precarious metabolic condition and because fluid or electrolyte disturbances may result from injudicious or repeated purgation, use of cathartics is not advocated (10).

Antibiotics

Because penicillin has anticlostridial action it has been advocated for infant botulism (19). There appears to be no protective effect noted after administration either orally or parenterally, however. Some investigators have suggested that lysis of the organisms by penicillin may make more toxin available for absorption (13).

As with the adult form of botulism, aminoglycoside administration appears to worsen the muscle paralysis. In high doses, aminoglycosides have been demonstrated to produce nondepolarizing neuromuscular block. These drugs have been shown to contribute to the neuromuscular impairment, and because many of these infants are admitted for possible sepsis, antibiotics other than aminoglycosides should be given when there is a possibility of botulism.

Antitoxin

The efficacy of antitoxin is even less clear in infant botulism than in adult botulism because antitoxin neutralizes only circulating toxin and not that bound to nerves. Circulating toxin has only rarely been found in patients with infant botulism, so that the benefit of antitoxin is minimal (18). Antitoxin would not have any effect on the toxin-producing organisms in the gut; and because it is a horse serum product, it has substantial side effects, including serum sickness and anaphylaxis, and the potential for lifelong hypersensitivity to horse serum.

Recovery

Once symptoms of infant botulism reach a nadir, the patient's condition usually persists unchanged for 2 to 3 weeks before slow recovery of strength occurs (19). Toxin may be found in stool weeks to months after the patient has recovered (18). Recovery from botulism implies establishment of new anatomic pathways at the synapse because toxin binding is apparently irreversible (10).

The loss of function and a return of function appear to follow a relatively predictable course similar to that seen with nondepolarizing muscle relaxants such as curare. Movement of the fingers provides an early sign of returning muscle strength and is closely followed by incomplete eye opening.

Because the basic pathologic problem in infant botulism is self-limited, ideally all children should recover with a minimum of complications.

BOTULINUM TOXIN AS THERAPY

Ophthalmologists and neurologists have used local injections of botulinum toxin therapeutically in some patients with strabismus or focal movement disorders such as blepharospasm, hemifacial spasm, cervical dystonia, and spasmodic dysphonia. Minute amounts of botulinum toxin are injected into overactive muscles to produce transient local paralysis without systemic effects. Botulinum toxin therapy has yielded encouraging early results, and therapeutic trials continue to provide data for further assessment of efficacy.

REFERENCES

1. Sanders A, Seifert S, Kobernick M: Botulism. *J Fam Pract* 1983;16 987–1000.
2. Cherington M: Botulism: ten-year experience. *Arch Neurol* 1974;30: 432–437.
3. Hikes D, Manoli A: Wound botulism. *J Trauma* 1981;21:68–71.
4. Fullerton P, Gogna N, Stoddart R: Wound botulism. *Med J Aust* 1980;1:662–663.
5. Woodruff B, Griffin P, McCroskey L, et al: Clinical and laboratory comparison of botulism from toxin types A,B, and E in the United States, 1975–1988. *J Infect Dis* 1992;166:1281–1286.
6. Arnon S, Midura T, Damus K, et al: Honey and other environmental risk factors for infant botulism. *J Pediatr* 1979;94:331–336.
7. Aureli P, Fenicia L, Pasolini B, et al: Two cases of type E infant botulism caused by neurotoxigenic *Clostridium butyricum* in Italy. *J Infect Dis* 1986;154:207–211.
8. Shneerson J: Botulism: a potentially common problem. *Thorax* 1989; 44:901–902.
9. Arnon S: Infant botulism. *Annu Rev Med* 1980;31:541–560.
10. Keller M, Miller V, Berkowitz C, et al: Wound botulism in pediatrics. *Am J Dis Child* 1982;136:320–322.
11. Merson M, Hughes J, Dowell V, et al: Current trends in botulism in the United States. *JAMA* 1974;229:1305–1308.
12. Morse D, Rickard L, Guzewich J, et al: Garlic-in-oil associated botulism: episode leads to product modification. *Am J Public Health* 1990;80:1372–1373.
13. Roland E, Ebelt V, Anderson J, et al: Infant botulism: a rare entity in Canada? *Can Med Assoc J* 1986;135:130–131.
14. Oken A, Barnes S, Rock P, et al: Upper airway obstruction and infant botulism. *Anesth Analg* 1992;75:136–138.
15. Schreiner M, Field E, Ruddy R: Infant botulism: a review of 12 years experience at the Children's Hospital of Philadelphia. *Pediatrics* 1991;87:159–165.
16. Brougnton R, Campbell J, Wilson H: Infant botulism. *South Med J* 1981;74:257–258.
17. Thompson J, Glasgow L, Warpinski J, et al: Infant botulism: clinical spectrum and epidemiology. *Pediatrics* 1980;66:936–942.
18. Hoffman R, Pincomb B, Skeels M, et al: Type F infant botulism. *Am J Dis Child* 1982;136:270–271.
19. McCurdy D, Krishnan C, Hauschild A: Infant botulism in Canada. *Can Med Assoc J* 1981;125:741–743.
20. Brown L: Infant botulism and the honey connection. *J Pediatr* 1979; 94:337–338.
21. Jagoda A, Renner G: Infant botulism: case report and clinical update. *Am J Emerg Med* 1990;8:318–320.
22. Schmidt R, Schmidt T: Infant botulism: a case series and review of the literature. *J Emerg Med* 1992;10:713–718.

CHAPTER 73

Fish

Fish and shellfish are an increasing part of the diet of Americans, yet it has only been recently recognized that these animals are important causative agents in a number of neurologic and gastroenterologic disorders (1). This chapter is limited to a discussion of ciguatera and scombroid poisoning, which are the most common disorders caused by fish or shellfish (2,3). Disease arises from ingestion of a toxin known as ichthyosarcotoxin (4,5).

CIGUATERA

Ciguatera is a serious and sometimes fatal disease caused by the ingestion of various tropical marine fishes (6). It has been seen in islands of the Pacific and Caribbean Oceans (2). The term *ciguatera* is a misnomer; it is derived from the Spanish word for a similar disease caused by a poisonous marine snail or mollusk known as "cigua" (7). This animal is now known not to be a source of ichthyosarcotoxin (4,8,9). Ciguatera fish poisoning is the most common illness associated with fish ingestion in the U.S.

Toxicity from ciguatera is not confined to a single fish species but may result from ingestion of more than 400 species of herbivorous and carnivorous fish (Table 73–1) (10). Migratory bottom-dwelling shore fish caught near reefs located between 35°N and 35°S latitudes are those that typically cause ciguatera (1,5). Barracuda, jack, red snapper, grouper, and sea bass are commonly implicated in ciguatera (11,12). Ciguatera toxins rarely contaminate large pelagic or ocean-going fish such as tuna, marlin, or dolphin. The entire fish or just the flesh or viscera may be toxic; the highest concentration is within the liver, intestines, and gonads (6).

Ciguatera is a significant cause of morbidity in areas in which consumption of reef fish is common, including the Caribbean, southern Florida, Hawaii, the South Pacific, and Australia (13). Although ciguatera affects persons residing in tropical and subtropical coastal regions of the world, importation of fish and fish products from these areas has made the problem of concern in many other locations where they may be sold (4,8).

TABLE 73–1. *Fish associated with ciguatera*

Amberjack
Barracuda
Coral trout
Eel
Emperor
Grouper
Kingfish
Paddletail
Parrot fish
Red snapper
Sea bass
Squirrel fish
Yankee whiting

The chemical structure and action mechanism of the ichthyosarcotoxins that causes ciguatera are not clearly defined (6). Ciguatoxin, maitotoxin, scaritoxin, and perhaps palytoxin and okadaic acid are believed to be responsible for ciguatera. It is likely that other toxins will be discovered that play some part in the syndrome. The compounds are relatively heat-stable; therefore, cooking of the fish does not provide protection from illness (2,9). They are also stable in gastric fluids. The toxins have been identified as a low-molecular-weight lipid that is transmitted from fish to fish through the food chain; they are thought to be produced by the dinoflagellate *Gambierdiscus toxicus* (14). Until recently, ciguatera was blamed almost exclusively on the dinoflagellate *Gambierdiscus toxicus* first isolated and identified from the Gambier Islands where virtually all of the reef fish are said to be toxic. Recent research suggests that other dinoflagellates may play significant roles in the etiology of ciguatera in addition to *G. toxicus*, which has proven the most toxic. The severity of poisoning is related to the size of the fish because large predator fish accumulate the toxin from eating smaller fish, which "graze" on the dinoflagellates. The responsible dinoflagellates are found commonly as epiphytes on macroalgae from various phyla including red, brown, and green algae (15). Ciguatera-associated dinoflagellates are believed to live on dead coral where they thrive in a medium rich in algae, fungi, yeast, and bacteria (13).

Toxicity

Toxicity appears to be dose-related, with the worst reactions occurring in individuals who have had prior cases of ciguatera (9, 11). There is no uniformly reliable taste, appearance, or odor that distinguishes between contaminated and clean catch before ingestion. Sometimes, animals, usually pets, are fed parts of a fish to determine whether it is contaminated; if symptoms of poisoning do not develop, the catch is considered fit for human consumption (11). The disease is usually short-lived in most cases, and many patients do not seek medical attention (16). Although death is unlikely, signs and symptoms of the disease may be severe and produce long-term disability (5).

Ciguatera fish poisoning is a distinctive clinical syndrome characterized by a constellation of gastrointestinal, cardiovascular, and neurologic symptoms. More than 175 manifestations of symptoms have been noted in ciguatera (Table 73–2) (15). Gastrointestinal symptoms usually occur early and are of short duration. Neurologic manifestations may occur later in the course of the disease and may persist for weeks to months. The gastrointestinal symptoms are usually limited to a few days, whereas the neurologic symptoms may persist for weeks, months, or even years in some cases. Cardiovascular signs and symptoms may also be seen, with fairly profound hypotension and bradycardia noted (4).

The usual presentation involves a gastrointestinal illness with diarrhea, abdominal pain, nausea, and vomiting, appearing within 6 hours of ingestion (17). This may be followed by neurologic symptoms that include paresthesia of the extremities and perioral region, a sensation of burning or pain of the skin on contact with cold water, asthenia, headache, myalgia, and pruritus (13).

TABLE 73–2. *Signs and symptoms of ciguatera*

Gastrointestinal
Abdominal pain
Diarrhea
Nausea
Vomiting
Neurologic
Ataxia
Paresthesia
Temperature reversal
Vertigo
Miscellaneous
Arthralgia
Bradycardia
Diaphoresis
Fever
Hypotension
Myalgia
Respiratory paralysis
Weakness
Death

Gastrointestinal

Symptoms usually begin 2 to 6 hours after ingestion. Gastroenteritis with nausea, vomiting, diarrhea, and abdominal pain may appear initially (7,18). These symptoms usually subside without therapy within a few hours (12). Fever, diaphoresis, and sometimes bradycardia may accompany the gastrointestinal complaints (6,8). Though dehydration by vomiting and diarrhea may prove serious, gastrointestinal symptoms usually last only 1 or 2 days. Vomiting is less common with second attacks (19).

Neurologic

Typically, the patient also complains of neurologic symptoms such as numbness and tingling, ataxia, and vertigo (11). The neurosensory involvement is typically acral, affecting the perioral region and the distal extremities. Tingling of the mouth, tongue, or throat may therefore occur. Neurologic symptoms are usually the most bothersome and lingering complaints (2,12). Paresthesia, described as uncomfortable tingling sensations, most often develops in the extremities, oral cavity, and pharynx. Dysesthesia may be so painful that taking a shower seems unpleasant. In severe cases, a common complaint is that of "temperature reversal," that is, cold objects causing a burning sensation on contact with the fingertips, toes, or tongue (20). This phenomenon usually develops 2 to 5 days after the ingestion. Although the neurologic symptoms usually last no longer than a few days, they may occasionally recur for weeks or even months (4).

Ataxia and paresis most commonly manifest in the legs and less frequently in the extraocular muscles. Dental pain is often described as if the teeth are loose. Psychiatric disorders are often reported which may manifest as listlessness, fatigue, depression, neurosis, hysteria, frank malingering, and insomnia (13).

Cardiovascular

Cardiovascular symptoms are also associated with ciguatera. It has been demonstrated that ciguatoxin has positive inotropic effects on atrial muscle. Cardiovascular symptoms often present and disappear within 2 to 5 days. Extrasystoles may result indirectly by noradrenergic stimulation of myocardium as a result of ciguatoxin effects on neural channels. Bradycardia and hypotension are characteristic (20).

Miscellaneous

Arthralgia, myalgia, and weakness are also commonly observed (11). In extremely severe cases, there may be respiratory paralysis and death (21,22). Although ciguatera fish poisoning is not considered a fatal condition, there have been isolated reports of death (6,8).

Mechanism of Action of Ciguatera Toxin

Ciguatoxin increases the permeability of neural membranes to sodium, resulting in membrane depolarization (18). Studies suggest that the toxin causes a nerve-conduction block after initial neural stimulation (22). This action may explain some of the neurologic manifestations noted. Ciguatera toxin demonstrates some anticholinesterase activity (1,18,23).

Although ciguatoxin is the predominant toxin in ciguatera fish poisoning, other compounds may account for the variability in the clinical manifestations (21). Scaritoxin and maitotoxin produce both peripheral and central effects as well as cholinergic and α-adrenergic actions. Low doses cause hyperventilation, bradycardia, atrioventricular conduction defects, tachycardia, and transient hypertension (24).

Differential Diagnosis

The differential diagnosis of acute ciguatera must rule out other marine poisonings, botulism, bacterial food poisoning, eosinophilic meningitis, organophosphate poisoning, and monosodium glutamate ingestion in sensitive individuals (Table 73–3) (3,11). Because many toxic marine ingestions share clinical manifestations and because laboratory assays for specific toxins may not be immediately available, an accurate and detailed history, physical examination, and brief laboratory evaluation must be relied on to make the diagnosis (5).

Laboratory Analysis

Diagnosis is based entirely on clinical presentation; results of routine laboratory studies are normal, and there is no confirmatory laboratory test for the disease (21). The only widely recognized hematologic or biochemical abnormalities attributable to ciguatera that can be determined from laboratory tests are those secondary to the fluid and electrolyte disturbances associated with diarrhea and dehydration (4). Results of electromyography are usually normal. In uncomplicated cases, electroencephalograms and results of lumbar puncture have also been normal (23).

TABLE 73–3. *Conditions to rule out in the differential diagnosis of ciguatera*

Other marine poisonings
Botulism
Bacterial food poisoning
Eosinophilic meningitis
Organophosphate poisoning
Monosodium glutamate sensitivity

Efforts to establish the chemical identity of the heat-stable toxin and to develop assays for toxin in fish samples for use in outbreaks of ciguatera have met with only limited success (1). Definitive identification requires the use of an animal bioassay, radioimmunoassay, or rapid enzyme immunoassay (13). Unfortunately, the availability of these tests is limited, particularly in those areas of the world where ciguatera fish poisoning is a significant clinical problem (7,23).

Less elegant methods of detection include feeding contaminated fish to laboratory or domestic animals and observing them for clinical outcome.

Treatment

Treatment of ciguatera is supportive and symptomatic and consists of administration of antiemetic and antidiarrheal agents (as needed), fluids, and atropine when indicated for hypotension and bradycardia (16). Atropine may have no effect on musculoskeletal or neurologic symptoms (2). Pruritus may be relieved partially by H_1astamine antagonists. Although calcium, corticosteroids, pralidoxime, and vitamin B complex have been suggested, they have not been demonstrated to be useful. Respiratory support is necessary for the rare case in which respiratory paralysis occurs. Mannitol therapy has been used successfully in several case reports as therapy for the neurologic symptoms (16). The mechanism is hypothesized to be reduction of neuronal axonal edema and/or scavenging of hydroxyl free radicals (25).

SCOMBROID POISONING

Scombroid fish poisoning is the only form of ichthyosarcotoxism in which toxin is formed by the action of bacteria on fish flesh. Worldwide, scombroid poisoning is the most common cause of toxicity resulting from the ingestion of fish (7). It is also the only form of fish poisoning that is completely preventable with proper refrigeration and fish handling procedures (26).

Fish Associated with Scombroid Poisoning

Scombroid fish poisoning refers to the clinical syndrome that results from the ingestion of spoiled fish, usually of the families *Scombridae* and *Scomberesocidae* (27). This includes tuna, mackerel, skipjack, and bonito (26). However, nonscombroid fish, such as mahi-mahi, bluefish, amberjack, herring, sardines, and anchovies, as well as cheese, have also been implicated as causes of scombrotoxism.

Mechanism of Toxicity

Histamine was first suggested as the causative toxin in the 1940s, on the basis of a number of observations. Fish that have caused scombroid poisoning consistently contain large quantities of histamine. Scombroid fish contains substantial amounts of free histidine that can be decarboxylated to form histamine by enteric bacteria present in spoiled fish. Furthermore, the symptoms of scombroid fish poisoning resemble those of histamine toxicity, and improvement in symptoms has been reported after treatment with antihistamines (28).

The flesh of fish causing scombroid poisoning contains a great deal of histidine. In the presence of certain bacteria and the proper conditions, this histidine is broken down or decarboxylated to histamine, which causes symptoms when ingested. This bacterial enzymatic reaction occurs maximally at approximately 20°C and is prevented if bacterial growth is inhibited by adequate refrigeration. Scombrotoxin is heat-stable and is not destroyed by domestic or commercial cooking (26).

Although the exact nature of scombrotoxin is not known, it is believed to be made up of several substances that are histamine-related (5). Saurine was once postulated as one of these substances, but current evidence indicates that the active substance is a histamine salt (2).

Histamine is formed in foods largely from the growth of bacteria possessing the enzyme histidine decarboxylase. Fish such as tuna contain high concentrations of the amino acid histidine, in their muscle tissues, which can serve as a substrate for bacterial histidine decarboxylase (28). This enzyme converts histidine to histamine, and the histamine accumulates in the fish tissue.

One reason for the lingering doubt concerning histamine is that it has been impossible to reproduce the illness in normal subjects by administering histamine orally in doses comparable to those ingested when spoiled fish is eaten.

Toxicity

Symptoms of scombroid poisoning may develop within minutes to hours of ingestion of tainted fish. The symptoms are the same as those of any histamine-mediated reaction and include urticaria, itching, dizziness, and abdominal cramps (Table 73–4). Flushing of the face, neck, and upper trunk is the most characteristic and consistent symptom of scombroid poisoning (26). Nausea, vomiting, diarrhea, burning of the mouth and throat, and in more severe cases hypotension, bronchospasm, and respiratory distress may occur (29).

TABLE 73–4. Signs and symptoms of scombroid poisoning

Dermal
Urticaria
Pruritus
Flushing
Face
Neck
Trunk
Gastrointestinal
Nausea
Vomiting
Diarrhea
Burning of the mouth
Abdominal cramps
Miscellaneous
Bronchospasm
Hypotension
Respiratory distress

Serious complications are rarely encountered in cases of histamine poisoning. However, on rare occasions, serious cardiac and respiratory complications do occur. These more serious symptoms seem to occur in individuals with preexisting cardiac and respiratory conditions (30).

The duration of symptoms is typically short with complete remission often occurring within a few hours even without treatment. Occasionally, if left untreated, symptoms will persist for 24 to 48 hours.

Laboratory Analysis

The diagnosis of scombroid poisoning is primarily clinical (26). Blood histamine and urinary histamine metabolite concentrations are elevated in patients with scombroid poisoning, but measurements of this kind are usually not necessary or easy to obtain (2).

Treatment

Left untreated, symptoms of scombroid poisoning subside within 12 hours (28). Although fatalities have been reported, they are extremely rare. To avoid hypotension, intravenous fluid therapy may be initiated (25). Most patients suffering from scombroid fish poisoning will respond quickly to the administration of antihistamines. H_1 antagonists such as diphenhydramine or chlorpheniramine are the usual choices for treatment (31). However, H_2 antagonists such as cimetidine may also be effective in treating this illness. In severe cases accompanied by bronchospasm, bronchodilators should be administered (2).

Table 73–5 compares the various signs and symptoms with selected food poisoning.

TABLE 73–5. *Differential diagnosis of various food toxins*

Condition	Hypertension	Hypokalemia	Numbness and/or paresthesias	Weakness or paralysis	Respiratory paralysis	Cranial nerve involvement	Cardiac dysrhythmia	Nausea, vomiting, diarrhea
Ciguatera fish poisoning	-	-	++	-	+	+	+[a]	+++
Paralytic fish poisoning	-	-	++	++	+	-	-	++
Neurotoxic shellfish poisoning	-	-	++	-	-	-	-	++
Botulism	-	-	-	++	+	++	-	++[b]
Gastroenteritis	-	+[a]	-	+	+[a]	-	+[a]	+++

- Absent or usually absent.
+ Occasionally present.
++ Usually present.
+++ Always or almost always present.
[a]Seen mostly in children.
[b]Food-borne botulism.

REFERENCES

1. Cassanova M, Sanchez R, Marco R: Ciguatera poisoning. *Arch Neurol* 1982;39:387.
2. Dembert M, Strosahl K, Bumbarner R: Disease from fish and shellfish ingestion. *Am Fam Physician* 1981;24:103–108.
3. Lawrence D, Enriquez M, Lumish R, et al: Ciguatera fish poisoning in Miami. *JAMA* 1980;244:254–258.
4. Bagnis R, Kuberski T, Laugier S: Clinical observations on 3009 cases of ciguatera (fish poisoning) in the South Pacific. *Am J Trop Med Hyg* 1979;28:1067–1073.
5. Halstead B: Current status of marine biotoxicology—an overview. *Clin Toxicol* 1981;18:1–24.
6. Chretien J, Fermaglich J, Garagusi V: Ciguatera poisoning: presentation as a neurologic disorder. *Arch Neurol* 1981;38:783.
7. Hughes J, Merson M: Fish and shellfish poisoning. *N Engl J Med* 1976;295:1117–1120.
8. Russell F: Ciguatera poisoning: a report of 35 cases. *Toxicon* 1975; 13:383–385.
9. Sims J: A theoretical discourse on the pharmacology of toxic marine ingestions. *Ann Emerg Med* 1987;16:1006–1015.
10. Morris P, Campbell D, Freeman J: Ciguatera fish poisoning: an outbreak associated with fish caught from North Carolina coastal waters. *South Med J* 1990;83:379–382.
11. Ho A, Fraser I, Todd E: Ciguatera poisoning: a report of three cases. *Ann Emerg Med* 1986;15:1225–1228.
12. Morris J, Lewin P, Hargrett N, et al: Clinical features of ciguatera fish poisoning. *Arch Intern Med* 1982;142:1090–1092.
13. Swift A, Swift T: Ciguatera. *J Toxicol Clin Toxicol* 1993;31: 1–29.
14. Morris J: Ciguatera fish poisoning: barracuda's revenge. *South Med J* 1990;83:371–372.
15. Lange W, Lipkin K, Yang G: Can ciguatera be a sexually transmitted disease? *J Toxicol Clin Toxicol* 1989;27:193–197.
16. Lange W, Snyder F, Fudala P: Travel and ciguatera fish poisoning. *Arch Intern Med* 1992;152:2049–2053.
17. Senecal P, Osterloh J: Normal fetal outcome after maternal ciguatera toxin exposure in the second trimester. *J Toxicol Clin Toxicol* 1991; 29:473–478.
18. Rayner M: Mode of action of ciguatoxin. *Fed Proc* 1972;31: 1139–1145.
19. Williams R, Palafox N: Treatment of pediatric ciguatera fish poisoning. *Am J Dis Child* 1990;144:747–748.
20. Stommel E, Parsonnet J, Jenkyn L: Polymyositis after ciguatera toxin exposure. *Arch Neurol* 1991;48:874–877.
21. Geller R, Benowitz N: Orthostatic hypotension in ciguatera fish poisoning. *Arch Intern Med* 1992;152:2131–2133.
22. Fasano A, Hokama Y, Russell R, et al: Diarrhea in ciguatera fish poisoning: preliminary evaluation of pathophysiological mechanisms. *Gastroenterology* 1991;100:471–476.
23. Li K: Ciguatera fish poison: a cholinesterase inhibitor. *Science* 1965; 147:1580–1581.
24. Senecal P, Osterloh J: Normal fetal outcome after maternal ciguatera toxin exposure in the second trimester. *J Toxicol Clin Toxicol* 1991;29:473–478.
25. Palafox N, Jain L, Pinano A, et al: Successful treatment of ciguatera fish poisoning with intravenous mannitol. *JAMA* 1988;259: 2740–2742.
26. Dickinson G: Scombroid fish poisoning syndrome. *Ann Emerg Med* 1982;11:487–489.
27. Christman B: Scombroid fish poisoning. *N Engl J Med* 1991;325: 515–517.
28. Morrow J, Margolies G, Rowland J, et al: Evidence that histamine is the causative toxin of scombroid-fish poisoning. *N Engl J Med* 1991; 324:716–720.
29. Taylor S, Stratton J, Nordlee J: Histamine poisoning (scombroid fish poisoning): an allergy-like intoxication. *J Toxicol Clin Toxicol* 1989;27:225–240.
30. van Gelderen C, Savelkol T, van Ginkel L, et al: The effects of histamine administered in fish samples to healthy volunteers. *J Toxicol Clin Toxicol* 1992;30:585–596.
31. Deng J, Tominack R, Chung H, et al: Hypertension as an unusual feature in an outbreak of tetradotoxin poisoning. *J Toxicol Clin Toxicol* 1992;30:585–596.

PART XIV

VENOMOUS CREATURES

CHAPTER 74

Snakes

Snake venom poisoning is a medical emergency requiring immediate attention and the exercise of considerable judgment. Of the approximately 45,000 cases of snakebite that occur each year in the United States, about 8,000 are inflicted by venomous snakes and about 6,800 of these receive medical attention (1). Pit vipers are responsible for about 98% of all bites and for considerable morbidity (2). As more people have taken to outdoor activities, there has been an increase in the occurrence and treatment of both venomous and nonvenomous snakebites. Many physicians treating patients may be unfamiliar with the recognition of venomous bites, and accordingly, may be anxious about treatment protocols, which are controversial even among snakebite authorities (3).

TABLE 74–1. *Selective poisonous species of snakes*

***Crotalidae* (Pit vipers)**
Rattlesnakes
Copperhead
Water moccasin
Elapidae
Cobra
Coral snake
Krait
Tiger snake
Hydrophidae
Sea snake
Viperidae
Russell viper
Puff adder
Colubridae
Boomslang
Mangrove

TYPES OF SNAKES

Snakes are cold-blooded, carnivorous vertebrates that possess no mandibular joint, thereby permitting them to swallow their prey whole. Their teeth are curved backward, allowing them to pull food into the throat without its being chewed (4).

A great variety of venomous snakes are in existence. All are in the class *Reptilia*, order *Squamata*, and suborder *Ophidia*. The poisonous species all fall into one of the following families: *Crotalidae*, the pit vipers, such as the rattlesnakes; *Elapidae*, the elapids, which include the cobras and coral snakes; *Hydrophidae*, the sea snakes; *Viperidae*, including the true vipers such as the Russell viper and puff adder; and *Colubridae*, containing the boomslang and mangrove snake (Table 74–1).

The elapids include the most poisonous snakes in the world. The cobras, kraits, coral snakes, and tiger snakes fall into this family. They do not, however, account for the most deaths in either animals or humans.

There are only four types of venomous species that are indigenous to the U.S. Of these, three of the poisonous snakes are of the family *Crotalidae*, which include rattlesnakes, copperheads, and cottonmouths (commonly referred to as water moccasins). The coral snake is the only other native poisonous snake (3). At least one species of poisonous snake has been identified in every state except Alaska, Maine, and Hawaii (5).

Most of the deaths in the U.S. are attributed to the eastern diamondback rattlesnake (*C. adamanteus*), western diamondback rattlesnake (*C. atrox*), various subspecies of *Crotalus viridis*, and the timber rattlesnake (*C. horridus*) (1).

POISONOUS SNAKES

Pit Vipers

The pit vipers (*Crotalidae*) consist of rattlesnakes, copperheads, and cottonmouths. These snakes are distinguishable by a foramen, or pit, located between each eye and nostril (Fig. 74–1). The pit is a heat-sensitive organ that enables the snake to locate warm-blooded prey during nocturnal foraging (6). The pit viper's head appears triangular as a result of the venom glands located in the temporal region. They have elliptic pupils and two sharp, canalized fangs that are long and movable and that retract posteriorly when the mouth is closed.

Distinguishing feature	Poisonous (Pit viper)	Non-Poisonous
Pit	Pit	No Pit
Fangs	Fangs	No Fangs
Pupil	Elliptical	Rounded
Head Shape	Triangular (arrowhead)	Oval
Caudal Plate	Single Row or Rattle	Double Row

FIG. 74–1. Identification of snakes.

TABLE 74–2. *Deadly U.S. crotalids*

Eastern diamondback	*Crotalus adamanteus*
Western diamondback	*Crotalus atrox*
Western rattlesnake	*Crotalus viridis*
Sidewinder	*Crotalus cerastes*
Mojave rattlesnake	*Crotalus scutulatas*
Copperhead	*Agkistrodon contortrix*
Cottonmouth	*Agkistrodon piscivorus*

Rattlesnakes

The rattlesnakes are divided into two genera: *Crotalus* and *Sistrurus*. The genus *Crotalus* contains the more dangerous rattlesnakes, as well as a greater number of species, and is distributed over a far greater range. The main distinction between *Crotalus* and *Sistrurus* is that the former has small scales on the crown of the head while the latter has large plates. They both possess rattles which are a loosely articulated, but interlocking series of horny rings at the end of the tail, which, when vibrated, produce a hissing sound. This acts as a warning device by producing the buzzing sound one hears when the snake is aroused.

Rattlesnakes account for approximately 65% of all venomous snakebites in the U.S. each year. Most fatal bites result from the eastern diamondback rattlesnake (*Crotalus adamanteus*) or the western diamondback rattlesnake (*Crotalus atrox*), which are found from California to Arkansas (Table 74–2). Other species including the western rattlesnake (*Crotalus viridis*), found in the Great Plains to the Pacific coast, and the sidewinders (*Crotalus cerastes*), which dwell in the deserts of Arizona, Nevada, and southern California account for numbers of bites, few of which are fatal (7). The Mojave rattlesnake (*Crotalus scutulatas*), found in southern California, Nevada, Arizona, and western Texas, possesses the most potent neurotoxic venom of all rattlers but is responsible for only few bites per year (5).

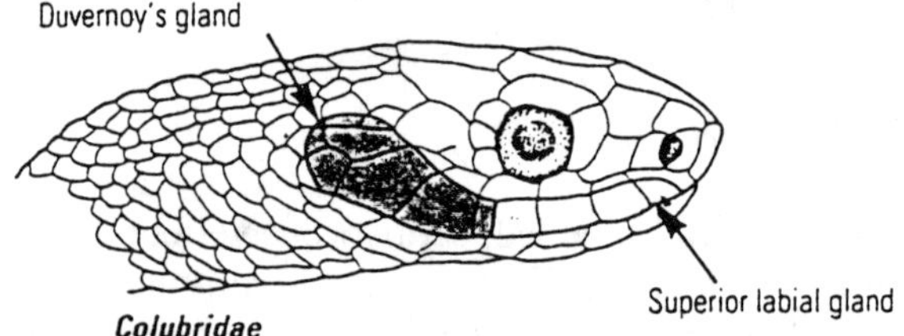

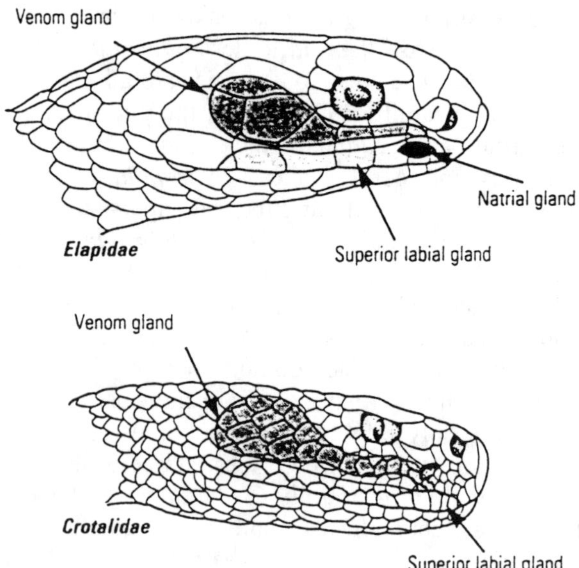

FIG. 74–2. Snake heads.

Moccasins

There are two species of moccasins: the cottonmouth (*Agkistrodon piscivorus*) and the copperhead (*Agkistrodon contortrix*). Both the cottonmouth and the copperhead are distinguished by their facial pits, elliptical pupils, the absence of rattles, and for the most part, the presence of a single row of scales on the underside of the tail. The copperheads and cottonmouth moccasin have large plates on the crown of their head and no rattles (Fig. 74–2). They do, however, vibrate their tails in the manner of a rattler.

Cottonmouth

The cottonmouth is an aquatic snake whose usual habitats includes swamps, lakes, streams, bayous, drainage ditches, and rice fields. Its distribution is the southeastern and southwestern sections of the U.S.

The cottonmouth passes through several distinct color phases, usually terminating in dark olive with darker crossbands. When disturbed, this snake will often open its mouth in a characteristically threatening manner. The inside of the mouth is white.

Copperhead

Copperheads have inverted "Y"s and hourglass configurations on their bodies. Their head varies in color from copper to various shades of brown. The average adult will vary in size from 24 to 36 inches. Its location is ubiquitous, being found on mountains, wooded hillsides, rock piles, rock quarries, and sawdust piles. It is not unusual for the copperhead to live within city limits and near suburban housing developments. When disturbed or stepped on, the copperhead can strike with lightning speed. The majority of bites by copperheads do not result in fatalities, but severe bites that are not treated may result in death.

SNAKE VENOM–GENERAL STATEMENT

The amount of venom that is injected is highly variable since it depends on many factors. Because snakes usually kill their prey before eating, the length of time since the snake has last eaten will affect the amount of venom the snake has available for injection into the poisoned victim. Therefore, snakes that have not eaten for some time will be capable of injecting larger amounts of venom into the victim. The amount of venom injected in the process of acquiring food is also believed to be related to the size of the prey. Venomous snakes are capable of regulating the amount of venom excreted from their fangs. If a snake is assuming a defensive stance, as in an encounter with a human, the amount of venom discharged is even more variable.

Snake venoms are complex mixtures, chiefly proteins, many having enzymatic activity. Although the enzymes contribute to the deleterious effects of the venom, the lethal property and some other toxic effects may be due to certain of the relatively small polypeptides (7). Crotalid venoms produce changes in capillary walls that can lead to the loss of fluid into tissues, particularly into the envenomated part, but sometimes into various organ systems, followed by the loss of electrolytes and proteins, and finally by the loss of red blood cells into the tissues. These phenomena are seen clinically as edema, ecchymosis, hypoproteinemia, and hemoconcentration (1).

The arbitrary grouping of snake venoms into categories such as "neurotoxins", "hemotoxins," and "cardiotoxins" is pharmacologically superficial and can lead to grave errors in clinical judgment. A so-called neurotoxin can produce marked cardiovascular changes or direct hematologic effects (7).

SIGNS AND SYMPTOMS OF CROTALID SNAKEBITE

General

The signs and symptoms of crotalid poisoning vary considerably, depending on the species of snake, the amount of venom injected, and other factors. It may be difficult to determine the severity of envenomation during the first several hours after a crotalid snake bite, and estimates of severity may need to be revised as poisoning progresses. A bite may appear minor at 1 hour but prove serious or even fatal at 3 hours. Not all crotalid snake bites result in envenomation; in approximately 20% of rattlesnake bites, the snake may not inject venom. Bites by rattlesnakes, cottonmouths, and copperheads usually cause immediate swelling, edema, and pain; but contrary to popular opinion, severe pain is not a constant finding (7). A preliminary physical examination should include inspection of the bite site to observe for fang marks, tooth marks, or both (4).

Symptoms and signs of pit-viper envenomation may include the presence of fang marks, swelling, pain, ecchymosis, weakness, various paresthesias, faintness, nausea, and vomiting, alterations in temperature, pulse, and blood pressure, fasciculations, urinary changes, early hemoconcentration followed by decreased hematocrit and platelet levels, petechiae, and shock (Table 74–3).

The most diagnostic sign of snakebite is rapid, progressive swelling. In most patients there is some swelling around the bite area within 5 to 10 minutes; and often, the swelling involves the entire finger, hand, toe, or food, depending on the species involved and the severity of the bite.

TABLE 74–3. *Signs and symptoms of pit viper envenomation*

Local findings	
	Fang marks
	Swelling
	Pain
	Ecchymosis
	Petechiae
Systemic findings	
	Weakness
	Paresthesia
	Faintness
	Nausea
	Vomiting
	Hemodynamic changes
	Fasciculations
	Hemoconcentration
	Shock

Puncture Wound

The number of puncture wounds may be one, two, or more depending on the number of fangs the snake has, the accuracy of the strike, and the number of strikes inflicted. Superficial lacerations produced by fangs usually do not result in envenomation because the discharge orifice of the fang lies somewhat above the tip.

Paresthesia

A common symptom following the bites by many rattlesnakes is paresthesia about the mouth, often the forehead and scalp, and sometimes of the fingers and toes. This is usually present following the bites of the Eastern diamondback rattlesnake (*Crotalus adamanteus*), the Pacific rattlesnakes (*C. viridis helleri* and *C. viridis oreganus*), most other *viridis* species, and some other species.

Ecchymosis

Ecchymosis is common in most cases of moderate or severe rattlesnake poisoning and usually appears around the bite within 3 to 6 hours. It is severe following bites by eastern and western diamondbacks, the prairie and Pacific rattlesnakes, and less severe following copperhead bites. The skin may appear tense and discolored; vesicles may form in the area of the bite within the first 8 hours, often becoming blood-filled (4).

Severe Envenomation

Severe envenomation may be accompanied by hypotension and shock, which generally occurs 30 minutes or more after the bite. Other frequent systemic manifestations are perioral paresthesias extending to the face and scalp along with tingling of the fingertips and toes after bites by eastern timber and western rattlesnakes. Skeletal muscle fasciculations occurring in the bitten area may occasionally become generalized secondary to the neurotoxic component of rattlesnakes such as the Eastern diamondback and Mojave rattlesnake (3).

In rare cases, a fang may penetrate a vein and the patient may lapse into shock, even before the swelling becomes obvious. In bites close to a vein, swelling may be minimal, even though the patient can be hypotensive and develop clotting deficits and hemorrhage.

Particularly following bites by the Mojave rattlesnake, respiratory distress may occur; and muscle fasciculations, spasms, and weakness are not uncommon. True paralysis may be seen in severe cases.

If the occurrence of edema and erythema have not manifested within 4 hours after a snakebite, it is generally safe to assume that the patient does not have pit viper envenomation (4).

Grading of Envenomation

Most of the suggested grading systems for crotalid bites are precarious, for they usually depend upon a few selected symptoms or signs and these are often stipulated for a specific time. It is more practical to grade envenomations as minimal, moderate, or severe, based on all clinical findings including laboratory data. One must then remember that the grading may need to be changed as the course of the poisoning or treatment progresses. Bites by

TABLE 74–4. *Grading of envenomation*

Grade	Types of symptoms
Minimal	Local swelling
	Erythema
	Ecchymosis
	No systemic manifestations
	Normal laboratory findings
Moderate	Above local findings
	Mild systemic manifestations
	Slight laboratory abnormalities
Severe	Marked swelling
	Marked erythema
	Marked ecchymosis
	Marked systemic manifestations
	Hypotension
	Tachycardia
	Respiratory compromise
	Neurologic changes
	Coagulopathy
	Abnormal prothrombin time (PT)
	Abnormal partial thromboplastin time (PTT)
	Abnormal platelet count
	Abnormal fibrinogen

the Mojave rattlesnake, for example, can give rise to minimal edema, local tissue changes, and pain, and therefore be graded as 1. The consequence can be the administration of insufficient antivenin resulting in a poor, or even fatal outcome. Diagnosis must therefore be established on the basis of all manifestations.

The grading of a poisoning in crotalid envenomations is often determined by the most severe symptom or sign. Minimal envenomation may present with swelling, erythema, and ecchymosis limited to the immediate area of the bite site (Table 74–4). There are either absent or insignificant systemic manifestations and laboratory findings are normal. A moderate bite might consist of the above positive findings, and in addition there may be systemic symptoms and signs that are present but not life-threatening. Laboratory parameters may be slightly altered but are not markedly abnormal. In severe envenomations, the swelling, erythema, and ecchymosis involve the whole extremity and is noted to be spreading rapidly. There are also marked systemic manifestations that may include hypotension, tachycardia, respiratory compromise, and neurologic changes. There is an abnormal coagulopathy profile including prothrombin time, partial thromboplastin time, platelet counts, and fibrinogen (1).

LABORATORY EXAMINATION FOR SNAKEBITE EXPOSURE

The following laboratory studies should be done: complete blood cell count; and determination of platelet, glucose, blood urea nitrogen, creatinine, and serum electrolyte concentrations (Table 74–5). Additional blood examinations should be obtained for transaminases, bilirubin, creatine phosphokinase, prothrombin time, partial thromboplastin time, thrombin time, and fibrinogen, and type and cross. A baseline urinalysis should be obtained. These tests can be repeated at appropriate intervals. An EKG should be obtained in all patients older than 40 years.

TABLE 74–5. *Laboratory studies in crotalid snakebite victims*

- Complete blood count
- Platelet count
- SMA-6 (Sequential Multiple Analysis—six different serum tests)
- Transaminases
- Bilirubin
- Creatine phosphokinase (CPK)
- Prothrombin time (PT)
- Partial thromboplastin time (PTT)
- Thrombin time
- Fibrinogen
- Type and crossmatch
- Urinalysis
- EKG (over 40 years)

TABLE 74–6. *Treatment of crotalid envenomation*

- **Pre-hospital**
  - History
    - Time of bite
    - Description of snake
    - Past medical history
      - ?Heart disease
      - ?Diabetes mellitus
      - ?Hypertension
      - ?Renal disease
      - ?Allergies
  - Treatment
    - Immobilization
    - Remove rings/constrictive items
    - Incision and suction (controversial)
    - Constriction band (controversial)
- **Hospital**
  - Treatment
    - Tetanus prophylaxis
    - Antibiotics
    - Antivenin skin testing
    - Antivenin

TREATMENT FOR CROTALID ENVENOMATION

After a crotalid snake bite, the bitten extremity and, preferably the bitten individual if practical, should be immediately immobilized to limit the spread of venom (Table 74–6). The bitten individual should be kept warm and transported to the nearest hospital as soon as possible; rings and/or other constrictive items should be removed (8). If the biting snake was killed, it should also be brought to the hospital for use in identification. Regardless of the bitten individual's clinical history, an intradermal sensitivity test should be performed before administration of the antivenin.

A detailed history of the envenomation along with the type of field therapy administered should be obtained. The history should include the time of the bite, a description of the snake, and whether it was killed and brought in for identification. The patient's past medical illnesses such as heart disease, diabetes mellitus, hypertension, and renal disease as well as allergies, asthma, exposure to horses, and previous administration of horse serum should be obtained.

There are few proven therapies for the prehospital treatment of pit viper envenomation. Suggested therapies have included immobilization of the bitten part, incision and suction, wound excision, cryotherapy, and the use of ligatures, including constriction bands and tourniquets. For many of these treatments, objective evidence of their efficacy is lacking, and some are believed to increase patient morbidity (9).

Immobilization

The affected part should be immobilized at the heart level and in a functional position. The patient should be kept warm, at rest, and should be given reassurance. Rings and constricting bands should be removed.

Incision and Suction

Incision and suction, if performed, should be done by a medical professional. If performed improperly, there is increased risk of wound infection and possible compromise and damage to neurovascular elements. An incision is made linearly through the skin, approximately 0.25 inch long and 0.125 inch deep over the fang puncture(s) (3). Suction, using Sawyer's "Extractor," applied directly over incisions or even over the fang punctures is of value during the first 30 to 60 minutes following the bite. The wound should be cleansed and covered with a sterile dressing.

Constriction Bands

Although constriction bands are discussed in nearly every article concerning the management of pit viper envenomation, there are a limited number of clinical or experimental studies on their use; the results of these studies have been mixed, with some reporting beneficial effects and others reporting ineffective or even detrimental outcomes.

Constriction bands have been recommended based on the belief that their use reduces systemic venom absorption without the marked increase in tissue damage seen with tourniquet use. At present, their clinical value is still unproven, and current medical opinion on their use is divided. Many authors discourage their use (9), yet many experts believe that an intermittently applied, lightly constricting tourniquet obstructing only lymphatic and superficial venous blood flow is very effective in delaying spread of venom and makes incision and suction more effective (3).

The potential risk of constriction band use is that local tissue damage may be increased, particularly if incorrectly applied, but this has not been tested experimentally.

Constriction Band vs. Tourniquet

Ideally, if constriction bands were useful in delaying systemic venom uptake without increasing local tissue damage, they could be used as a temporizing measure before arrival in the hospital, where a determination as to the need for additional treatment could be made. A constriction band is different from a tourniquet in that the band would be applied loosely enough so as to allow one finger to be inserted under the band. It should restrict only the superficial venous and lymphatic flow while arterial and deep venous flow would continue. In human beings, superficial venous and lymphatic flow is restricted at pressure of approximately 20 mm Hg. This distinguishes a constriction band from a tourniquet, which occludes all blood flow, both venous and arterial (9).

For patients subject to a delay of 30 minutes or longer before they are seen in a medical facility, a constriction band can be placed immediately proximal to the fang marks and suction applied over the punctures, using a Sawyer's First Aid Kit Extractor, which provides one atmosphere of negative pressure to the skin surface. This device appears to offer benefit if applied within the first 5 minutes following the bite (1).

Fasciotomy

Fasciotomy should be discouraged. It is usually unnecessary and reflects the use of insufficient antivenin during the first 12 hours of the poisoning. It may be necessary, however, when there is objective evidence via wick measurements of a constant, elevated intracompartment pressure above 40 mm Hg over an extended period of time and other evidence of severe vascular embarrassment. These, however, are very rare findings (7). Many authorities are now becoming more conservative with the use of a fasciotomy as initial treatment of envenomation.

Cryotherapy

The proponents of cryotherapy believe that cold in the form of ice packs or ice water applied to the site of the bite is useful in the reduction of pain, absorption of venom, and prevention of widespread scarring produced by other techniques. Most experts on snakebite do agree that there is no experimental evidence to support this method of therapy.

Electric Shock Treatment

Despite many attempts, investigators in the U.S. have been unable to demonstrate any beneficial effect from electric shock treatment, even when applied under ideal conditions. In 1990, the FDA banned the use of these devices and now there is required FDA approval before importing, manufacturing, advertising, or otherwise promoting a device delivering electric shock for the treatment of human beings or animals (10).

TABLE 74–7. *Usefulness of crotalid antivenin*

Rattlesnake (*Crotalus, Sistrurus*)
Copperhead
Cottonmouth
Fer-de-lance
Bothrops
Tropical rattler (*C. durissus*)
Cantil (*Agkistrodon bilineatus*)
Bushmaster (*Lachesis mutus*)

Miscellaneous

Tetanus prophylaxis should be instituted for any wound that broke the skin. Most authorities agree that antibiotics are indicated in most patients. A widely accepted approach is to administer a broad-spectrum antibiotic that provides appropriate Gram-negative coverage for the treatment of moderate to severe envenomations.

Antivenin

Crotalid antivenin contains venom-neutralizing globulins capable of neutralizing the toxic effects of venoms of crotalids native to North, Central, and South America, including rattlesnakes (*Crotalus*, *Sistrurus*), copperhead and cottonmouth moccasins, the fer-de-lance and other species of *Bothrops*, the tropical rattler (*C. durissus* and similar species), the Cantil (*A. bilineatus*), and bushmaster (*Lachesis mutus*) of Central and South America (Table 74–7) (11). The antivenin is not effective against the venoms of coral snakes and should not be used in the management of poisoning by these snakes.

Antivenin should not be routinely administered in every pit viper bite. It is unnecessary in most cases of copperhead bites, unless the envenomation is considered moderate to severe, or possibly when the victim is a small child. Water moccasin poisoning usually requires lesser doses of antivenin (7). Although antivenin appears to be effective in neutralizing the lethality of the venom, it is less effective in preventing local tissue damage (12).

ALLERGIC HISTORY AND SKIN TESTING

Before initiation of antivenin therapy, careful inquiry should be made concerning a history of allergy. In patients in whom antivenin is indicated, an intradermal sensitivity test should be performed before administration of the antivenin, regardless of the patient's clinical history. This is performed by the intracutaneous injection of 0.02 mL of saline-diluted serum at a site distant from the bite. The wheal site is observed for at least 10 minutes for the development of erythema, hives, pruritus, or other untoward effects. A syringe with epinephrine, 1:1,000, should be available to combat allergic reactions. In general, the shorter the interval between intradermal injection of the diluted antivenin and the beginning of a positive reaction, the greater the degree of sensitivity. If the individual does not have a history of allergy and the skin test is negative, the antivenin may be administered; however, a negative history of allergy and the absence of a reaction to a properly performed skin test do not preclude the possibility of an immediate sensitivity reaction. A negative skin test also does not indicate whether serum sickness will occur after administration of full doses of the antivenin (11).

Appropriate equipment for maintenance of an adequate airway and other supportive measures and agents (e.g., tourniquet, epinephrine, oxygen) for the treatment of anaphylaxis or other severe systemic reactions should be immediately and readily available whenever antivenin is administered.

Antivenin is administered to those patients who have demonstrated moderate to severe envenomation and have a negative skin test or conjunctival test (13). The demonstration of a negative skin or conjunctival test does not preclude the possibility of an anaphylactic reaction.

Immediate Sensitivity Reactions

If an immediate sensitivity reaction occurs, it usually occurs within 30 minutes after administration of the antivenin. Immediate sensitivity reactions may be most likely to occur in individuals with atopic sensitivity to horses. Signs and symptoms may develop within minutes after beginning, or during, administration of the antivenin

TABLE 74–8. Sensitivity reactions to antivenin

Immediate (within minutes)
Apprehension
Flushing
Itching
Urticaria
Edema
Face
Tongue
Throat
Dyspnea
Cyanosis
Nausea
Vomiting
Cardiovascular collapse
Delayed (5 to 24 days)
Malaise
Fever
Urticaria
Lymphadenopathy
Arthralgia
Nausea
Vomiting

and may include apprehension; flushing; itching; urticaria; edema of the face, tongue, and throat; cough; dyspnea; cyanosis; vomiting; and cardiovascular collapse (Table 74–8).

Treatment of Immediate Reaction

If a severe immediate sensitivity reaction occurs during administration of the antivenin, administration should be immediately discontinued, at least temporarily, and the patient given appropriate therapy as indicated. Immediate sensitivity reactions may usually be managed by temporarily interrupting administration of the antivenin or slowing its rate of administration and administering an antihistamine and/or epinephrine. If administration of the antivenin is temporarily interrupted and then reinitiated after control of the reaction, administration should be at a slower rate.

Delayed Sensitivity Reactions

Serum sickness, if it occurs, usually is evident 5–24 days after administration of the antivenin. The onset of serum sickness may be less than 5 days in some individuals, especially those who have received preparations containing equine serum in the past. Antivenin-induced serum sickness is generally dose-related. The usual manifestations of serum sickness are malaise, fever, urticaria, lymphadenopathy, edema, arthralgia, nausea, and vomiting. Neurologic manifestations such as meningism or peripheral neuritis occasionally occur. Peripheral neuritis usually involves the shoulder and arms. Pain and muscle weakness are frequently present, and permanent atrophy may develop. Although their efficacy is not clearly established, corticosteroids are commonly administered for the treatment of serum sickness reactions

Route of Antivenin Administration

Antivenin (*Crotalidae*) polyvalent is preferably administered by intravenous infusion. Antivenin must not be injected into a finger or toe.

For intravenous infusion, a 1:1 to 1:10 dilution of reconstituted antivenin in 0.9% sodium chloride or 5% dextrose injection is prepared. To avoid foaming, dilutions of the antivenin should be mixed by gentle swirling and should not be shaken.

The initial 5–10 mL of diluted antivenin should be infused over 3–5 minutes with careful observation of the patient; if no signs or symptoms of an immediate systemic reaction occur, the infusion is continued at the maximum safe rate of intravenous fluid administration. The rate of administration should be based on the severity of the signs and symptoms of envenomation and the patient's tolerance to the antivenin. Pregnancy is not a contraindication to administration of antivenin (3).

TABLE 74–9. *Antivenin dosage based on degree of envenomation*

Type of envenomation	Number of vials
No envenomation	None
Minimal envenomation	2–4
Moderate envenomation	5–9
Severe envenomation	10–15

Time of Antivenin Administration

The greatest danger from snakebite occurs within the first day or two after envenomation. The entire initial dose of antivenin should be administered as soon as possible and, to be most effective, within 4 hours after the bite. Antivenin is less effective when given after 8 hours and may be of questionable value when given after 12 hours; but in severe envenomations, it may be given even after 24 hours from the time of the bite. After 28 hours, antivenum is of questionable value although it may reverse coagulation deficits even after 30 hours.

Dosage

The following initial doses are recommended for children and adults: no envenomation, none; minimal envenomation, 20–40 mL (contents of 2–4 vials); moderate envenomation, 50–90 mL (contents of 5–9 vials); and severe envenomation, 100–150 mL or more (contents of 10–15 vials or more) (Table 74–9). Envenomation by large snakes may require relatively high doses, particularly in children or small adults. The dose of antivenin administered to children is not based on weight. The need for additional doses of antivenin is based on the clinical response to the initial dose and continuing assessment of the patient and severity of poisoning. If swelling continues to progress, systemic signs or symptoms of envenomation increase in severity, or new manifestations appear (e.g., hypotension, a decrease in hematocrit), an additional 10–50 mL (contents of 1–5 vials) should be administered.

Newer Fab Antivenin

An antivenin is now being investigated that consists of Fab fragments from sheep specific for crotalids. The production of these Fab fragments is generally by the same method as that for digitalis Fab fragments (1). When it is FDA-approved, as is expected, it should offer a quick, less toxic alternative than the available antivenin.

NON-PIT VIPERS

Coral Snakes

Coral snakes have permanent, immovable fangs and in order to inject its venom, the snake must bite and hang onto the area attacked. Because it must gain leverage to bite, it cannot bite a flat surface. Hence, few deaths are produced by coral snakes, even though it is one of the most poisonous snakes in the U.S. (15).

In the U.S. there are two genera of coral snakes—*Micruroides* (the Arizona coral snake, *Micruroides euryxanthus*) and *Micrurus* (two subspecies: the Eastern coral snake, *Micrurus fulvius fulvius*, and the Texas coral snake, *Micrurus fulvius tenere*) (Table 74–10). The *Micruroides* species is found in southern Arizona, with small population in western New Mexico. As a rule, they are very shy and elusive reptiles that uncommonly come into contact with humans (16). The Eastern coral snake is found from eastern North Carolina through the tip of Florida and in the coastal plain of the Gulf of Mexico to the Mississippi River. The Texas coral snake is found west of the Mississippi River in Louisiana, Arkansas, Texas, and northern Mexico. Coral snakes of the genus *Micrurus* also inhabit Mexico, Central America, and South America. They are small species with characteristic red and black bands separated by white or yellow bands. The tip of the nose is black. Some species may not be much larger than a pencil.

The Eastern coral snakes have completely black snouts and alternating continuous colored bands of red, yellow, and black, which encircle the body without interruption (16). The red and yellow bands are contiguous, and the red and black bands are wider than the interposed yellow bands. Rarely, coral snakes may be completely black, completely white, or partially pigmented. *M. f. fulvius* and *M. f. tenere* are very similar in appearance but can be differentiated by the amount and arrangement of black pigment found within the red bands, as well as by other characteristics. In contrast to crotalids, coral snakes have rounded pupils and lack facial pits. Adult *M. f. fulvius* usually vary from approximately 50 to 110 cm in length but may rarely be longer (1).

The coral snakes are nonaggressive and are usually not seen because they are undercover. Because they are shy, secretive, and nocturnal, they rarely bite humans. It is estimated that fewer than 20 coral snake bites occur annually in the U.S. Inquisitive small domestic animals or children may be bitten when traveling through underbrush.

The fangs of coral snakes are short, erect, and, unlike the hinged fangs of crotalids, fixed to the maxilla. The venom enters the fang at an opening in its base. The small size of the fangs makes it difficult for a coral snake bite to penetrate clothing. Most coral snake bites are inflicted on the upper extremities, particularly the hands and fingers, mainly because most bites occur as a result of handling the snakes. The biting mechanism of coral snakes differs from that of crotalid snakes. Crotalid snakes usually strike and withdraw rapidly; in contrast, coral snakes usually bite, hold on, and "chew," presumably so that a sufficient amount of venom can be introduced to immobilize its prey. The "chewing" action may result in more than one bite, and the victim may recall the snake "hanging on" for a "minute" or so.

TABLE 74–10. *Coral snakes found in the United States*

Micruroides
Arizona coral (*Micruroides euryxanthus*)
Micrurus
Eastern coral (*Micrurus fulvius fulvius*)
Texas coral (*Micrurus fulvius tenere*)

Coral Snake Venom

The most deleterious components of this venom appear to be various nonenzymatic, neurotoxic, low-molecular-weight polypeptides that cause a curare-like, postsynaptic, nondepolarizing blockade at the neuromuscular junction by binding competitively to the acetylcholine receptor. This blockade differs from that of curare in its delayed onset and extremely prolonged effect. Whereas many elapid venoms appear to contain a significant amount of acetylcholinesterase, this enzyme does not appear to play a major role in coral snake venom toxicity.

Unlike pit viper venoms, coral snake venom lacks significant proteolytic enzymatic functions, which explains the relative paucity or even total absence of local signs and symptoms following envenomation. There may be very mild swelling and pain or paresthesia at the bite site, but often the only local finding will be the presence of fang marks, which may be difficult to see.

Like crotalid snakebites, coral snake bites may not result in envenomation, and it has been estimated that envenomation may occur in less than 40–50% of coral snake bites. Although bitten individuals who exhibit one or more fang punctures seem most likely to have been envenomated, there is no reliable method to predict which bitten individuals may be envenomated by a coral snake bite. Even a dependable account that the biting snake did or did not "hang on" should not be used to predict the likelihood or severity of envenomation.

Diagnosis of Elapidae *Envenomation*

Elapidae envenomations differ markedly from pit vipers. There may be little or no pain or swelling immediately after the bite. Occasionally, there is a delay of 1 to 5 hours before the onset of these systemic symptoms

TABLE 74–11. *Diagnosis of* Elapidae *envenomation*

Local effects
Little/no early pain
Little/no early swelling
Scratch marks
Minimal tissue reaction
Slight erythema
Systemic effects
Anxiety
Diplopia
Drowsiness
Dysphagia
Dysphonia
Dyspnea
Euphoria
Headache
Lethargy
Motor paralysis
Respiratory depression
Salivation
Seizures
Tongue fasciculations
Weakness

from *Elapidae* envenomation (Table 74–11). They are characterized by ptosis, dysphagia, dysarthria, and intense salivation. Loss of deep tendon reflexes and respiratory depression occur later as a result of a potent neurotoxin.

Local effects of a coral snake bite may include scratch marks or fang puncture wounds (which may often be obscure); minimal to moderate edema or tissue reaction; erythema; and pain. If present, pain is usually minor and confined to the bite site but may radiate throughout a bitten extremity. Paresthesia and weakness of a bitten extremity may occur occasionally. In contrast to crotalid bites, in which moderate to severe envenomation usually can be predicted by rapid onset of local effects, severe and even fatal envenomation from a coral snake bite can be present without signs and/or symptoms of a substantial local tissue reaction. This fact, combined with the relative lack of local findings, may lead to a false sense of security on the part of the inexperienced treating physician. The earliest signs may be euphoria or drowsiness, followed by nausea and vomiting, excess salivation, bulbar paralysis, fasciculations, and later peripheral weakness progressing to paralysis.

Systemic signs and symptoms usually begin 1–7 hours after envenomation, although they may not occur for as long as 18 or more hours. It is well documented that there may be a total absence of local signs or symptoms of envenomation even in the face of a severe bite by the coral snake, and there may be significant delay in onset of any systemic findings. Once evident, systemic signs and symptoms may progress rapidly and precipitously. Paralysis has occurred within 2–3 hours after a bite and appears to be a bulbar-type paralysis, involving cranial motor nerves. Death from respiratory paralysis has occurred within 4 hours after a bite. Systemic signs and symptoms of envenomation may include euphoria; anxiety or apprehension; lethargy; drowsiness; headache; weakness; nausea; vomiting; bulbar signs such as fasciculations of the tongue, dysphagia, and paresis of the extraocular muscles; diplopia or blurring of vision; dysphonia; dyspnea; abnormal reflexes; seizures; motor weakness or paralysis, including complete respiratory paralysis, weak and irregular pulse, and occasional hypotension. Children appear to be prone to seizures following coral snake envenomations. The mechanism for this is unclear because snake neurotoxins do not appear to cross the blood–brain barrier to any significant degree, but the cause may be related to cerebral hypoxia secondary to respiratory failure (16). Cardiac failure has also been noted. Hemoglobinuria and cardiovascular shock have been observed in envenomed experimental animals. With vigorous supportive therapy and close observation, patients with complete respiratory paralysis have recovered, indicating that respiratory paralysis is reversible. Death is usually associated with respiratory and cardiac failure.

Laboratory

Although it is reasonable to obtain routine laboratory tests on admission, coral snake venom, unlike that of pit vipers, does not appear to cause any significant hematologic, electrolyte, or coagulation abnormalities in and of itself.

Management of Coral Snake Bite

Suspected coral snake envenomation should be considered a medical emergency requiring prompt evaluation and appropriate management. Clinicians responsible for the treatment of an envenomed patient should be familiar with the signs and symptoms of coral snake envenomation and current methods of first aid and general supportive therapy for venomous snakebites.

Field management of venomous snakebite is an area of much controversy, but it appears that most commonly recommended first aid measures used in pit viper envenomations are ineffective in coral snake bites. Coral snake venom is rapidly absorbed via the venous system as opposed to the lymphatic system, the major route of pit viper venom absorption. As a result, incision and suction and the use of constriction bands are not felt to be effective in retarding the spread of *Micrurus* venom.

As in all snake envenomations, keeping the patient calm and at rest while rapidly transporting him or her to a medical facility is of utmost importance. The bitten individual should be kept warm and transported to the nearest hospital as soon as possible; rings and/or other constrictive items should be removed. If the biting snake was killed, it should also be brought to the hospital for use in identification. Any individual who has been bitten by a coral snake and has any evidence of a break in the skin caused by the snake's teeth or fangs should be hospitalized for observation and/or treatment. The bite area should be cleansed with soap and water to remove any venom that may be present on the skin. The grading scales for severity of envenomation often used in pit viper bites should not be applied to coral snake envenomations because these scales are based primarily on local findings and early systemic systems. The bitten individual should be closely observed for at least 24 hours, including monitoring of respiratory rate every 30 minutes, vital signs, and neurologic status. Some clinicians suggest that it may be useful to monitor vital capacity as a means to detect incipient respiratory paralysis. Respiratory difficulties and/or paralysis can occur; therefore, facilities and personnel necessary for administration of oxygen, assisted or controlled respiration, and endotracheal intubation (or possibly tracheostomy) should be immediately and readily available, as well as an adequate supply of antivenin. Because hemoglobinuria has been observed in experimental animals envenomated by coral snakes, continuous bladder drainage with careful attention to urinary output and serum electrolyte balance is recommended in symptomatic individuals. Appropriate tetanus prophylaxis should be administered.

Coral snake envenomation may result in signs and symptoms involving the nervous system; thus, sedatives should be used with caution in bitten individuals. Because coral snake envenomation may also result in respiratory difficulties, including complete respiratory paralysis, the use of opiates that can depress respiration is contraindicated in bitten individuals.

Although acetylcholinesterase inhibitors might have a theoretical use in reversing neuromuscular blockade, no studies have been performed in humans to demonstrate their effectiveness in coral snake envenomations.

Antivenin

Hospital management of coral snake envenomation centers around the use of the specific antivenin manufactured by Wyeth–North American coral snake antivenin. It is important, before administering antivenin, to make every effort to identify the offending reptile positively as a coral snake because there are numerous mimics of this snake.

Antivenin to *Elapidae* is made from horse serum and has the same potential adverse effects as crotalid antivenin (4). For this reason, skin testing is advised. Before initiation of antivenin therapy, careful inquiry should be made concerning a history of allergic manifestation. In patients in whom antivenin is indicated, an intradermal sensitivity test should be performed before administration of the antivenin, regardless of the patient's clinical history. Appropriate equipment for maintenance of an adequate airway and other supportive measures and agents for the treatment of anaphylaxis or other severe systemic reactions should be immediately and readily available whenever antivenin is administered.

Indications for Antivenin

Once the snake has been identified, it is important to begin antivenin therapy as soon as possible if fang marks are present, even in the absence of any other signs or symptoms. Once systemic symptoms begin to occur, it may be difficult to reverse them or slow their progression, even with the use of antivenin.

After a negative skin test, the reconstituted antivenin should be diluted in normal saline solution or Ringer's lactate. There have been no human studies to determine the appropriate dosage of antivenin that should be used in coral snake envenomations (16). The usual recommended initial IV dose of the antivenin for children and adults is 30–50 mL (contents of 3–5 vials). Higher initial doses may be indicated in some individuals, depending on the nature and severity of the signs and symptoms of envenomation. Some clinicians suggest that 50–60 mL (contents of 5–6 vials) be given to bitten individuals if pain or neurologic signs or symptoms (e.g., paresthesia) are evident and that doses such as 80–100 mL (contents of 8–10 vials) be given if bulbar signs of paralysis are present. Envenomation by large snakes may require relatively high doses, particularly in children or small adults. The dose of antivenin administered to children is not based on weight. The need for additional doses of antivenin is based on the clinical response to the initial dose and continuing assessment of the patient and on severity of poisoning. If necessary, additional antivenin may be administered, usually in doses of 10–50 mL (contents of 1–5 vials). Venom yields determined under laboratory conditions suggest that some envenomed patients might require administration of a total dose of 100 mL or more (contents of 10 or more vials) of the antivenin to neutralize the venom injected by a biting snake.

It should be noted that the Wyeth antivenin is not effective in bites by the Arizona coral snake (*Micruroides*). However, the venom from this reptile is much less toxic than that of the *Micrurus* species and there has never been a reported fatality from the Arizona coral snake (1,16).

Sea Snakes

There are no sea snakes in North American coastal waters. However, sea snakes are quite common in tropical waters along the coasts of the Indian and Pacific Oceans. Human beings have far less contact with sea snakes than with terrestrial poisonous snakes. Persons encountering sea snakes are most often marine fishermen, and bites are considered an occupational hazard in the Indo-Pacific region (17).

Sea snakes are readily recognized by their flat tails and can be distinguished from sea eels by the presence of scales and the absence of gills and fins. All sea snakes are poisonous, possessing a pair of fangs connected by venom ducts and glands. Toxicity does not occur due to the lack of contact between these snakes and potential victims. Sea snakes will not be discussed further in this text.

NONPOISONOUS SNAKES

The *Colubridae* is a large family that consists primarily of nonpoisonous species, although, in reality, some poisonous varieties do occur. Although the vast majority of colubrids are considered harmless, about one third possess primitive rear "fangs" that are capable of penetrating human skin and delivering toxic saliva through chewing motions. In general, they produce no hazard to animals and only minimal danger to humans. The most dangerous snake in this family is the boomslang (*Dispholidus typus*), a non-American snake.

Garter snakes (*Thamnophis* sp) are members of the family *Colubridae*, which includes approximately 75% of all living species of snakes. Wandering garter snakes are ubiquitous and adaptable reptiles found in coastal areas and higher elevations in the U.S. and Mexico (14). They may be found in urban environments near abandoned lots or parks and are universally regarded as being nonpoisonous.

Harmless snakes, such as the garter snake, have round pupils, and do not possess fangs but contain small teeth that produce a typical bite pattern (14). In general, harmless snakebites are characterized by four rows of small scratches produced by the four rows of teeth in the snake's upper jaw, separated from two rows of small scratches produced by the two rows of teeth in the snake's lower jaw.

REFERENCES

1. Johnson C: Management of snakebite. *Am Fam Physician* 1991;44: 174–179.
2. Stolpe M, Norris R, Chisholm C, et al: Preliminary observations on the effects of hyperbaric oxygen therapy on Western Diamondback rattlesnake (*Crotalus arox*) venom poisoning in the rabbit model. *Ann Emerg Med* 1989;18:871–874.
3. Gold B, Barish R: Venomous snakebites. Current concepts in diagnosis, treatment, and management. *Emerg Clin North Am* 1992;10: 249–267.
4. White R, Weber R: Poisonous snakebite in central Texas. Possible indicators for antivenin treatment. *Ann Surg* 1991;213:466–472.
5. Curry S, Horning D, Brady P, et al: The legitimacy of rattlesnake bites in central Arizona. *Ann Emerg Med* 1989;18:658–663.
6. Chinonavanig L, Karnchanachetanee C, Pongsettakul P, et al: Diagnosis of snake venoms by a reverse latex agglutination test. *J Toxicol Clin Toxicol* 1991;29:493–503.
7. Russell F: Snake venom poisoning. *Vet Hum Toxicol* 1991;33: 584–586.
8. Jansen P, Perkin R, Van Stralen D: Mojave rattlesnake envenomation: prolonged neurotoxicity and rhabdomyolysis. *Ann Emerg Med* 1992; 21:322–325.
9. Burgess J, Dart R, Egen N, et al: Effects of constriction bands on rattlesnake venom absorption: a pharmacokinetic study. *Ann Emerg Med* 1992;21:1086–1093.
10. Dart R, Gustafson R: Failure of electric shock treatment for rattlesnake envenomation. *Ann Emerg Med* 1991;20:659–661.
11. Cardoso J, Fan H, Franca F, et al: Randomized comparative trial of three antivenoms in the treatment of envenomating by lance-headed vipers (*Bothrops jararaca*) in Sao Paulo, Brazil. *Quart J Med* 1993; 86:315–325.
12. Kelly J, Sadeghani K, Gottlieb S, et al: Reduction of rattlesnake-venom induced myonecrosis in mice by hyperbaric oxygen therapy. *J Emerg Med* 1991;9:1–7.
13. Troutman W, Wilson L: Topical ophthalmic exposure to rattlesnake venom. *Am J Emerg Med* 1989;7:307–308.
14. Gomez H, Davis M, Phillips S, et al: Human envenomation from a wandering garter snake. *Ann Emerg Med* 1994;23:1119–1122
15. Ismail M, Al-Bekairi A, El-Bedaiwy A, et al: The ocular effects of spitting cobras: I. the ringhals cobra (*Hemachatus haemachatus*) venom-induced corneal opacification syndrome. *J Toxicol Clin Toxicol* 1993;31:31–41.
16. Norris R, Dart R: Apparent coral snake evnenomation in a patient without visible fang marks. *Am J Emerg Med* 1989;7:402–405.
17. Coppola M, Hogan D: Venomous snakes of Southwest Asia. *Am J Emerg Med* 1992;10:230–236.

CHAPTER 75

Spiders

Arachnids belong to the phylum Arthropoda, the largest phylum in the animal kingdom. The arthropods contain the spiders, scorpions, insects, ticks, and caterpillars, among others. Some arthropods sting, others bite, while still others discharge a secretion that is toxic. Arthropods are invertebrates, with jointed bodies and legs. The animals of the Arachnida class possess appendages, which are bilaterally symmetric and capable of locomotion. The organism is covered by a cuticle and a strengthened exoskeleton (1).

Spiders are in the order Araneae, exist worldwide, and number approximately 30,000 species. Spiders are uniformly venomous, but most attack only other arthropods and are generally beneficial to humans. Of more than 2,000 genera of spiders known, only a few species have biting mechanisms strong and long enough and venom potent enough to be of significant danger to humans. Of these, 50 species have fangs that can penetrate human skin and are medically important to humans due to their ability to induce toxicity (2). The great majority of spiders either cannot effectively pierce human skin or never have the opportunity to do so. Or if they do, the venom at the most causes only trivial transient pain, a slight local reaction at the site where the venom is injected, or no reaction at all.

Spiders are ubiquitous in the continental U.S., but most spider bites either go unrecognized or require little medical attention. However, several spiders indigenous to the U.S., such as *Argiope*, *Chiracanthium*, *Loxosceles*, and *Phidippus* can cause a painful and necrotic wound (3).

All spiders feed on animal life. Their chelicerae, or "jaws" and venom are their means of capturing and subduing prey. The chelicerae are paired and composed of a relatively stationary base and a mobile fang. Fangs are hollow, with venom flowing into them from glands in the cephalothorax and exiting from a port at the tip. Spiders are only capable of seeing prey a few centimeters away. Consequently, prey is located by touch when landing on the web (1).

Generally speaking, spiders are either hunters or trappers. Trappers do so by way of spinning webs. Each species builds webs by its own characteristic invention to snare prey (4). Hunters, although they possess spinnerets and are capable of producing silk, do not spin such intricate webs. Instead they range and forage about or lie in wait for their prey. Once successful in locating a victim, the hunter grabs and devours the animal immediately.

The severity of the reaction to poisonous spider bites is dictated by many factors (4). The amount of venom injected may vary from almost none to a full dose, depending on the site of the bite, the length of time the fangs are in the tissues, and the quantity of venom in the gland sacs at the time of biting. Also, the reaction of individuals to the same amount of the same type of venom may vary widely, and the age and general state of the victim's health determine the severity of reaction.

Because the bite of the black widow spider or related species of the genus *Latrodectus* accounts for the majority of cases of arachnidism in the U.S., most physicians consider arachnidism synonymous with latrodectism. Though familiar with the rapid onset of cramping pains, diaphoresis, salivation, vomiting, and unconsciousness of latrodectism, many seem unaware of the gangro-cutaneous and other sequelae that may follow envenomation with the brown recluse spider (5).

Many members of the phylum Arthropoda secrete substances of a toxic nature to other animals and plants. Although all classes of Arthropoda presumably contain toxin-producing species, discussion will be limited to those insects and arachnids whose toxic secretions are of significant medical importance to humans.

BLACK WIDOW SPIDER BITE

Black widow spiders (*Latrodectus* sp) produce one of the most potent known venoms by volume (2). Although both male and female widow spiders are venomous, only the latter have fangs large and strong enough to penetrate the human skin. The black widow spider is easily recognized by the jet black body with the red hour-glass mark on the underside of the abdomen. The males are much smaller than the females and usually have yellow and red bands and spots over the back, as do the immature spiders. Immature females have red, brown, and cream markings on the dorsum of the abdomen and a cream hourglass marking (1).

Five species are found in the U.S., with at least one in every state except Alaska. The most common are *Latrodectus mactans* and *Latrodectus variolus*, which are located abundantly in southern and eastern states (2). These spiders are commonly known as the black widow, brown widow, or red-legged spider, depending on the species.

Female black widows are trappers. Black widows spin tangled webs of coarse silk in dark places, usually out-of-doors. Trash, rubble piles, and littered areas are usually most favored by the spider. Webs are placed in or close to the ground and in secluded, dimly lit areas that have access to flying insects. Other common preferred sites are abandoned rodent burrows, nests, barns, sheds, and garages. Prey is procured through entrapment, encirclement with silk, and consumption through venom liquefaction.

The female black widow is shy and nocturnal in habit. She does not leave her hidden web voluntarily and is completely out of her element away from the web. She is not aggressive and often may be subjected to extreme provocation without attempting to bite. However, the female black widow may rush out and bite when her web is disturbed or when she is accidentally trapped in clothing or shoes.

Venom

The venoms of *Latrodectus* sp are virtually identical and thought to act at the neuromuscular junction by binding to glycoproteins or gangliosides on the presynaptic membrane and opening cation channels. Large quantities of acetylcholine then are released from the presynaptic neuron while the reuptake of choline is inhibited simultaneously. The result is pain and cramping of large muscle groups (2).

Signs and Symptoms

Most bites occur on the extremities and generalized pain in the back or abdomen is the most frequent presenting complaint of patients seeking medical help. Pain at the bite site may only resemble that of a pinprick or may be painless (Table 75–1). Two tiny red marks are occasionally identifiable at the site of the bite. The middle of the site may be white, with surrounding erythema and a reddish-blue border (1).

Pain usually progresses from the bitten member up or down the arm or leg, finally localizing more or less in the abdomen and back. The abdominal muscles become rigid and board-like with severe cramps. In addition, nausea, depression, insomnia, tremors, speech defect, and a slight rise in body temperature may be noted. The symptoms may appear after a few hours or may be observed within a few minutes of the bite. Muscular spasms and cramps of the arms, legs, back, and abdomen may be quite painful at the height of the reaction. Limb pain and local adenopathy or lymph node pain are common. Local redness, swelling, urticaria, and piloerection usually follow. Bronchorrhea, vomiting, priapism, urinary retention, salivation, and diaphoresis may be pronounced for hours after envenomation. Other symptoms may include headache, ptosis and occasional eyelid edema, skin rash, conjunctivitis, salivation, inflammation at the site of the bite, and an increase in blood and cerebrospinal fluid pressures. Severe poisonings may lapse into coma, respiratory paralysis, and cardiovascular collapse (2).

TABLE 75–1. *Signs and symptoms of black widow spider bite*

Local
Pain (pinprick)
Two tiny red marks at site of bite
Systemic
Cholinergic
Salivation
Diaphoresis
Bronchorrhea
Generalized pain localizing to abdomen and back
Nausea
Vomiting
Nonspecific
Insomnia
Depression
Tremors
Hyperthermia
Piloerection
Headache
Urinary retention
Hypertension

Hypertension has been proposed to result from action of the venom on vasomotor centers in the brain stem and spinal medulla. It is also possible that acetylcholine liberated at cholinergic sympathetic ganglia may result in postganglionic release of norepinephrine-stimulating peripheral α-receptors, leading to vasoconstriction.

Diagnosis

Latrodectism has been confused with acute abdominal conditions, acute psychosis, acute renal failure, and meningitis. The astute examiner may prevent laparotomy by paying heed to the abrupt onset of abdominal rigidity without tenderness, and spontaneous restlessness instead of avoidance of movement.

Treatment

General Treatment

There are no first-aid measures of value for the widow spider bites. If the pain is intense, ice can be placed over the wound until the patient arrives at a medical facility. A variety of treatments have been tried for severe *Latrodectus* envenomations. Muscle relaxants, intravenous calcium gluconate, opioids, and *Latrodectus*-specific antivenin have been used with reported success (6).

Therapy is mainly supportive and should include stabilization of vital signs if necessary, and attention paid to secondary end-organ damage resulting from the release of acetylcholine and norepinephrine. Supplemental oxygen, intravenous access, and cardiac monitoring are indicated in the symptomatic young and old. As with any break in the skin, tetanus prophylaxis should be updated if required and antibiotic prophylaxis is not indicated for these bites.

Abdominal Pain

Although calcium salts have been recommended, there is limited scientific evidence supporting the use of calcium for *Latrodectus* envenomations. Data suggest that *Latrodectus* venom increases the permeability of the nerve terminal membrane to calcium and that high extracellular concentrations of calcium antagonize the releasing effects of black widow spider venom on neurotransmitters at nerve endings. Yet, most human experience with calcium gluconate is anecdotal, with symptoms often recurring within 20 minutes of infusion. In most cases, 10 mg of calcium gluconate administered intravenously or a relaxant such as methocarbamol, administered by slow intravenous push, will relieve the muscle cramps and pain. The calcium gluconate will often need to be repeated at 4-hour intervals for optimum effect. In the acute phase, diazepam may help with muscle cramps as well as for the less severe poisonings.

Antivenom

Antivenom is of equine origin and is recommended for patients who have hypertensive heart disease or respiratory distress, for pregnant patients who exhibit symptoms, and for those younger than 16 and older than 65 who show signs of latrodectism (1).

Patients with allergies to horse serum products and those who previously had received antivenin or horse serum products are at risk for immunoglobulin E-mediated immediate hypersensitivity reactions. As with all equine serum preparations, rapid administration of antivenin can induce histamine release and anaphylactoid signs and symptoms in most patients. Skin testing before administration may detect a highly allergic individual, but a negative skin test cannot rule out completely the occurrence of hypersensitivity reactions. The slow administration of antivenin, especially at the beginning of the infusion, usually is well tolerated.

One vial of antivenin can be added to 50 to 100 mL of 5% dextrose or normal saline solution and then infused over 20 to 30 minutes. The normal dose required is one to two vials, and prompt resolution is characteristic within 1 hour. Although pretreatment with histamine blockers may be beneficial in preventing histamine release, their efficacy in this situation is unproven. Patients receiving antivenin rarely require admission, and those who do predominantly are for observation following mild urticarial reactions that may be noted during antivenin infusion.

Patients with severe envenomations who are not candidates for antivenin should be treated with parenteral opioids or a combination of parenteral opioids and sedative-hypnotics such as diazepam or lorazepam. Many of these patients will need admission for observation and pain control, but symptoms usually resolve within 24 to 48 hours.

LOXOSCELES

The brown recluse spider belong to the order Araneae, family Loxoscelidae. There are 18 species in the genus *Loxosceles* found in and around North America, with 13 in the U.S. Six species in the U.S. are confirmed to cause necrotic arachnidism: *L. rufescens*, *L. laeta*, *L. reclusa*, *L. unicolor*, *L. arizonica*, and *L. devia*. Other species of *Loxosceles* have the same fiddle-backed marking on the carapace (7). *Rufescens* is bright to dull orange brown with yellow or orange legs. *Arizonica*, *unicolor*, *laeta*, and *devia* are all light brown to gray, lighter than *reclusa*, which may lull the patients and physician into a false sense of security (8). *Loxosceles reclusa* is the most common species in the U.S. and has been reported in at least 17 states. It is most prominent in the southern half of the Missouri-Ohio-Mississippi River basin and is also found in Tennessee, Kentucky, Georgia, Alabama, Indiana, Illinois, Iowa, Kansas, Oklahoma, Arkansas, Louisiana, and South Carolina (4). Common names include violin spider, Arizona brown spider, fiddle spider, brown recluse, and necrotizing spider (1).

Adult brown recluse spiders are from 7 to 13 mm in length and vary in color from yellow to dark brown. The violin-shaped dark marking on the cephalothorax immediately behind the eyes is the most conspicuous recognition characteristic (5). This band of darker color is broad behind the eyes, but narrows to a thin line near the middle of the back (Fig. 75–1). This mark distinguishes the brown recluse from other common brown spiders. The brown recluse is slightly smaller than the black widow and has an oval body with four long legs on each side of the thorax. Unlike black widow spiders, both sexes are of equal size and danger. Brown recluse spiders have six eyes present in three pairs. As most other spiders have eight eyes, this feature eliminates many spiders suspected of being a brown recluse.

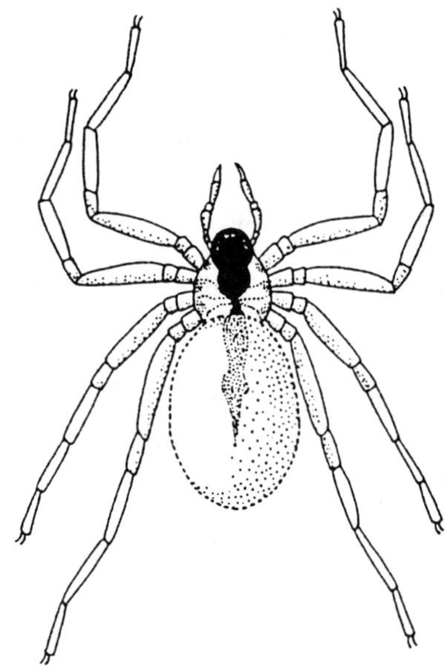

FIG. 75–1. *Loxosceles reclusa,* brown recluse spider. Note violin-shaped mark on the dorsum of the cephalothorax.

L. reclusa is usually nocturnal and lives in warm, dry areas, such as undisturbed cellars, crawl spaces, or abandoned buildings; woodpiles; fallen rocks; and similar sheltered areas. The largest populations may be found in indoor areas (4). Although timid and not aggressive toward humans, they will bite if molested or otherwise threatened. Human victims are often bitten while putting on clothing in which the spider is accidentally trapped and traumatized (5), when a sleeping individual rolls over onto a nocturnally active spider, or when one removes an article from a rarely disturbed storage area (4).

L. reclusa can live up to 6 months without food or water. It can tolerate temperature ranges from 8° to 43°C but prefers temperatures from 23° to 27°C (10).

Venom of *Loxosceles*

L. reclusa venom is very complex, being composed of at least eight different proteins (11). These include protease, alkaline phosphatase activity, lipase activity, sphingomyelinase D, and hyaluronidase activity (9). The exact venom components remain uncertain, but the same factors may be responsible for both local and systemic reactions. The hemolytic reaction is most likely the result of sphingomyelinase D present in the spider venom in a calcium-dependent reaction (12). In addition, sphingomyelin D has been shown to cause platelet aggregation resulting in the release of serotonin and thromboxane A_2, which could play a major role in causing the rapid coagulation and occlusion of small capillaries seen in *L. reclusa* envenomation.

Sphingomyelinase D acts directly on cell membranes. Sphingomyelinase D aggregates platelets, generates leukocyte chemoattractants, and liberates thromboxane B_2. This membrane damage along with the activity of brown recluse lipase results in a chain reaction of release of inflammatory mediators such as thromboxanes, leukotrienes, prostaglandins, and neutrophils. The cascade of injury is further reinforced by C-reactive protein and is complemented and compounded further by platelet aggregation and vascular thrombosis. Hemoglobinuria and resultant renal failure may result from the direct action of sphingomyelinase D on the sphingomyelin of the red cell membrane (1).

The initial injury is endothelial damage to the arterioles and venules, which become occluded with thrombi composed of leukocytes and platelets. Capillary stasis ensues followed by tissue infarction and mummification (13). Hemolysis of red blood cells occurs to some extent but is rarely clinically significant (9).

Signs and Symptoms

The clinical response to envenomation by *L. reclusa* ranges from a mild local reaction to severe systemic involvement and death (4).

Because the bite frequently occurs at night or the spider is crushed, *L. reclusa* is rarely positively identified as the cause of necrotic arachnidism, making the true incidence of *L. reclusa* envenomation difficult to determine accurately. The clinical manifestations may range from a mild erythema to a severe morbid stage without the typical cutaneous ulceration (9). In the majority of cases, envenomation of the brown recluse primarily produces a cutaneous reaction caused by the hemolytic and necrotizing venom to the spider (3).

Local Manifestations

The bite of the brown recluse spider typically presents the following picture. There may be mild transitory stinging at the time of the bite, but there is little associated early pain (Table 75–2). The patient may be completely unaware that he/she has been bitten and the spider is seldom seen. Only after 2 to 8 hours does pain, varying from mild to severe, begin. At the site of puncture, the first reaction of note is transient erythema, followed by a bleb or blister with an irregular area of ischemia. A zone of hemorrhage with induration, and a surrounding halo of erythema develops peripherally. The central ischemia may become stellate and the area, during the course of several days, turns dark in color and firm to touch (9). Within 7 days, the central area is depressed, sharply demarcated, dark and mummified. The area becomes indurated and between 7 and 14 days the eschar falls off, leaving an ulceration that will heal by secondary intention (4).

The two features of color and configuration help differentiate serious necrotic arachnidism from other ven-

TABLE 75–2. *Signs and symptoms of brown recluse spider envenomation*

Local symptoms
No early pain
Transient erythema
Bleb or blister
Zone of hemorrhage with induration
Central ischemia
Central area becomes sharply demarcated, dark and mummified
Systemic symptoms
Fever
Chills
Malaise
Nausea
Vomiting
Arthralgia
Myalgia
Generalized petechial rash
Severe systemic symptoms
Hemolytic anemia
Thrombocytopenia
Hemoglobinuria
Acute renal failure
Hemorrhage
Disseminated intravascular coagulation
Septicemia

omous bites that do not produce necrosis. The lesions of non-necrotic envenomations are mostly red and raised above the normal level of the skin, without any central depression (3).

Although the skin lesions are painful and disfiguring, death of envenomated patients is usually related to circulatory or renal failure. In nearly all fatal cases, hemolytic anemia, hemoglobinuria, and acute renal failure have been preterminal events (5).

In lesions destined to go on to significant necrosis, bullae and hemorrhage are usually evident by 24 hours, and a pale demarcated area is often present at 48 hours. The most extensive necrosis has long been recognized to occur in areas with increased subcutaneous fat. These areas—the thighs, abdomen, and buttocks—exhibit a more fragile, tenuous blood supply (1). In severe reactions, systemic symptoms begin around 36 hours and include morbilliform rash, urticaria, fever, nausea and vomiting, and occasional hemolysis or diffuse intravascular coagulation (14).

Systemic Manifestations

Systemic involvement is much less common than the local reaction (5). The systemic symptoms are directly proportional to the amount of envenomation but not to the severity of the skin lesions. Systemic symptoms usually present 24 to 72 hours after the bite occurs but before the typical ulceration has had time to develop and include fever, chills, malaise, weakness, nausea, vomiting, arthralgias, myalgias, generalized petechial rash, convulsions, disseminated intravascular coagulation, thrombocytopenia, and hemolytic anemia (15). The hemolysis can lead to hemoglobinemia, hemoglobinuria, renal failure, and death. The patient may think the cutaneous lesion is inconsequential and may neglect to mention it, or the physician may be so concerned about the systemic manifestations that he/she neglects to examine the skin. It is imperative, therefore, that any patient with hemolysis, thrombocytopenia, and hemoglobinuria be closely examined for any cutaneous manifestation of loxoscelism. Children are particularly susceptible, and the majority of reported fatal cases of loxoscelism have occurred in children less than 7 years of age (4). Death usually results from renal failure, hemorrhage into vital organs, or septicemia (16). Although in the absence of shock or other predisposing factors free hemoglobin is not toxic to the kidney, red blood cell stroma may initiate disseminated intravascular coagulation and acute renal failure (17).

Children with severe systemic reactions warrant hospitalization and close observation. If hemolysis occurs, then symptomatic support and packed red-cell transfusion are appropriate (14). Good hydration and monitoring of renal function are important to ensure that hemoglobinemia does not cause renal failure. Systemic steroids, although not of proven efficacy, may be administered in the acute phase (4 to 5 days) in an attempt to stop the destruction of red cells by the venom (4).

Diagnosis

The diagnosis of a brown recluse spider bite can be very difficult. If the patient does not bring the spider in for the examination, identification of the specific spider bite is difficult as well (4). The most important element in the diagnosis is the physician's knowledge of the disease and alertness in considering it. The diagnosis is usually based on clinical findings alone because the spider is rarely found and, if found, may not be recognized (9). Most patients are unable to say what bit them and do not come in for treatment until a necrotic lesion is already present (18).

There are five other species of spiders in the U.S. capable of producing necrotic lesions—*Chiracanthium*, *Argiope*, *Atrax*, *Lycosa*, and *Phidippus*—making the diagnosis of loxoscelism even more difficult (4). Routine laboratory tests are generally not helpful for diagnosis and prognosis of cutaneous arachnidism (3).

Laboratory

Laboratory findings in patients with systemic loxoscelism may include hematuria, hemoglobinuria, hemolytic anemia, leukocytosis, thrombocytopenia, hypofibrinogenemia, and increased fibrin split products

TABLE 75–3. *Laboratory abnormalities associated with brown recluse spider bite*

Hematuria
Hemoglobinuria
Hemolytic anemia
Leukocytosis
Thrombocytopenia
Hypofibrinogenemia
Increased fibrin split products

(Table 75–3) (4). These should be looked for by obtaining a complete blood count, urinalysis, platelet count, fibrinogen, clotting studies, and fibrin split products (19).

Treatment

The literature contains no controlled human studies evaluating treatment modalities for *L. reclusa* envenomation. However, there are numerous case reports advocating various treatment methods including steroids, local excision, polymorphonuclear leukocyte inhibitors, and most recently, hyperbaric oxygen therapy (20).

Conservative treatment for bites with cytotoxic reactions and necrosis remains the best course of treatment. The majority of cutaneous lesions can be managed simply with good wound care, elevation, ice packs, and immobilization. Heat should be avoided, because sphingomyelinase D activity increases as temperature rises. Cool compresses may help alleviate some of the inflammatory reaction (4). Tetanus prophylaxis should be administered, and an antianxiety–antipruritic agent may be helpful. Although bites can become secondarily infected, prophylactic antibiotics are controversial and probably not indicated; no clinical trials address this specific question (4). Steroids have not been proved effective, and antibiotics should be reserved for signs of infection (1). Adequate hydration to maintain a brisk urine output is essential.

Dapsone

A polymorphonuclear leukocyte inhibitor, dapsone, has been shown to decrease the amount of skin necrosis in animals (21). There are a few case reports of patients being treated with 50 to 200 mg/day showing marked decrease in pain, erythema, and induration (22). Although good results have been reported, adverse reactions to dapsone may include hepatitis, hemolysis, methemoglobinemia, and leukopenia. Adult patients who have a rapidly progressive severe bite may be started with low-dose therapy progressing from 50 to 500 mg/day, divided twice a day, for 2 weeks. Complete blood cell counts and methemoglobin levels should be monitored. When using dapsone, a dose-dependent hemolytic anemia may occur despite normal levels of glucose-6-phosphate dehydrogenase and, therefore, close monitoring of patients is imperative (22).

In combination with specific antivenom, dapsone may be helpful in severe cutaneous reactions to prevent extensive necrosis, even 48 hours after the bite (3).

Surgical Excision

Early wide surgical excision of the bite site has not proven to be effective in preventing the spread of necrosis (23). It is not possible to predict early in the course of envenomation which lesions will spontaneously regress. Surgery should probably be considered only for necrotic ulcers bigger than 1 to 2 cm in diameter. This should be performed after the borders of the lesion are well established, usually 1–2 weeks after the bite.

Antivenom

More recently, a specific antivenom to *L. reclusa* was developed and tested in vivo. When administered intradermally at the lesion site and within 24 hours of the bite, the specific antivenom was found to either block or markedly attenuate the cutaneous necrosis (3). This antivenom is not yet commercially available.

Systemic Loxoscelism

Systemic loxoscelism can be life-threatening and should be treated aggressively. Systemic steroids have a protective effect on red blood cell hemolysis and may also be beneficial in relieving other body complaints. The recommended dose of prednisone is 1 to 2 mg/kg/day for 2 to 4 days.

Clotting abnormalities and anemia should be treated as indicated with platelet transfusions and packed red blood cells (4).

TARANTULA

Tarantulas belong to the family Theraphosidae. The U.S. tarantula is related to and resembles its more deadly cousin *Atrax* sp, the funnel web of Australia. The large size and forbidding hairy appearance of the U.S. variety have given these spiders an undeserved reputation of dangerous aggression. Although wicked-looking and having a sinister reputation, most of the species of tarantula found in the United States, Mexico, Central America, and Trinidad have been described as harmless to humans, the bites having the feel and effect of pinpricks.

As members of suborder Orthognatha, they, like the funnel web, exhibit large vertically oriented fangs. The jaws of the tarantula work in a vertical plane rather than in a horizontal one as do those of the true spiders. To use the fangs in this plane, the tarantula must elevate the front of the body. When cornered by human beings or other animals, this position is taken and the fangs are used in a rake-like manner. Fortunately, the venom contained in sacs, held entirely within the base of the fangs, is little toxic to mammals. The strong jaws, however, can inflict slightly painful wounds. The U.S. tarantula is docile. Bites are rare and normally only elicit a low-grade histamine response at most. The wounds should be scrupulously cleansed and tetanus immunization updated.

Like tarantulas of the U.S., the funnel web spiders belong to the suborder Orthognatha. Unlike tarantulas of the U.S., they are irritable and possess venom that is deadly to humans. The toxic component, atraxotoxin, is a neurotoxin that acts directly on nerve membranes causing widespread release of neurotransmitters. Therefore, acetylcholine is released at motor endplates and acetylcholine, epinephrine, and norepinephrine through the autonomic nervous system.

REFERENCES

1. Allen C: Arachnid envenomations. *Emerg Med Clin North Am* 1992; 10:269–298.
2. Clark R, Wethern-Kestner S, Vance M, et al: Clinical presentation and treatment of black widow spider envenomation: a review of 163 cases. *Ann Emerg Med* 1992;21:782–787.
3. Alario A, Stahl R, Bancroft P: Cutaneous necrosis following a spider bite: a case report and review. *Pediatrics* 1987;79:618–621.
4. Gendron B: *Loxosceles reclusa* envenomation. *Am J Emerg Med* 1990;8:51–54.
5. Madrigal G, Erconani R, Wenzl J: Toxicity from a bite of the brown spider (*Loxosceles reclusus*). *Clin Pediatr* 1972;11:641–644.
6. Ennik F: Deaths from bites and stings of venomous animals. *West J Med* 1980;133:463–468.
7. Hobbs G, Harrell R: Brown recluse spider bites: a common cause of necrotic arachnidism. *Am J Emerg Med* 1989;7:309–312.
8. Hall R, Anderson P: Brown recluse spider bites: can they be prevented? *Missouri Med* 1981;78:243–244.
9. Arnold R: Brown recluse spider bites: five cases with a review of the literature. *JACEP* 1976;5:262–264.
10. Chu J, Rush C, O'Connor D: Hemolytic anemia following brown spider (*Loxosceles reclusa*) bite. *J Toxicol Clin Toxicol* 1978;12: 531–534.
11. Denny W, Dillaha C, Morgan P: Hemotoxic effect of *Loxosceles reclusus* venom: in vivo and in vitro studies. *J Lab Clin Med* 1964;64: 291–298.
12. Suarez G, Biggemann U, Schenone H: Effect of venom gland extracts of the south American brown spider, *Loxosceles laeta*, on in vitro protein synthesis. *Toxicon* 1983;21:553–557.
13. Magrina J, Masterson B: *Loxosceles reclusa* spider bite: a consideration in the differential diagnosis of chronic, nonmalignant ulcers of the vulva. *Am J Obstet Gynecol* 1981;140:341–343.
14. Eichner E: Spider bite hemolytic anemia: positive Coombs' test, erythrophagocytosis, and leukoerythroblastic smear. *Am J Clin Pathol* 1984;81:683–687.
15. Vorse H, Seccareccio P, Woodruff K, et al: Disseminated intravascular coagulopathy following fatal brown spider bite (necrotic arachnidism). *J Pediatr* 1972;80:1035–1038.
16. Murray L, Seger D: Hemolytic anemia following a presumptive brown recluse spider bite. *J Toxicol Clin Toxicol* 1994;32:457–460.
17. Hardman J, Beck M, Hardman P, et al: Incompatability associated with the bite of a brown recluse spider (*Loxosceles reclusa*). *Transfusion* 1983;23:233–236.
18. Rauber A: An unusual case of loxoscelism. *Vet Hum Toxicol* 1983; 25:43–46.
19. Russell F, Waldron W, Madoin M: Bites by the brown spiders *Loxosceles unicolor* and *Loxosceles arizonica* in California and Arizona. *Toxicon* 1969;7:109–117.
20. Butz W: Envenomation by the brown recluse spider and related species. A public health problem in the United States. *J Toxicol Clin Toxicol* 1971;4:515–524.
21. King L, Rees R: Dapsone treatment of a brown recluse bite. *JAMA* 1983;250:45.
22. Barrett S, Romine-Jenkins M, Fisher D: Dapsone or electric shock therapy of brown recluse spider envenomation? *Ann Emerg Med* 1994;24:21–25.
23. Auer A, Hershey F: Surgery for necrotic bites of the brown spider. *Arch Surg* 1974;108:612–618

CHAPTER 76

Scorpions

Scorpions are distributed throughout the tropics, arid deserts, and semi-arid grasslands, frequently concentrating in areas of human habitation to take advantage of shelter, water, and prey. They display the seasonal winter hibernation cycle of poikilotherms and the diurnal pattern of nocturnal predators. There are approximately 30 species of this genus confined to the New World. Of these, about seven are of considerable medical importance, and most of these species are found in Mexico (1).

The scorpion is very easily recognized because it so closely resembles a crab in appearance (Fig. 76–1). There is a long, segmented tail, which ends in a bulbous sac and conspicuous stinger. Black or yellowish in color, the scorpion can vary from 1.5 cm to 20 cm in length, depending on species and stage of development.

Scorpions are nocturnal creatures. During the day, they remain hidden under stones, bark, piles of lumber, etc., when outside. When indoors, they hide in closets, attics, shoes, stored newspaper, etc. They come out of seclusion at night to seek water and obtain insects, other arachnida, or small rodents upon which to feed.

In the United States, members of the genera *Hadrurus*, *Vejovis*, and *Uroctonus* are capable of inflicting a painful and often erythematous lesion; and only species of the genus *Centruroides* are sufficiently dangerous to warrant definitive medical care. The majority of scorpion species belong the the family *Vejovidae* (1) and most stings are, therefore, inflicted by members of this genus. The most deadly scorpion is *C. sculpturatus*, also known as *C. exilicauda*. Scorpions of the genus *Centruroides* are found throughout Arizona. Colonies are known to inhabit parts of Texas, New Mexico, Nevada, California, and northern Mexico (2).

The sting response is triggered by movement and situations in which scorpions become trapped in clothing or sleeping bags can result in multiple stings if movement persists. Most people are stung by scorpions when moving rocks, lumber, or other material where the creatures may be hiding. Stings may occur when a person puts on shoes or other clothing where a scorpion is concealed.

Venom

There are two very dissimilar types of scorpion venom. One has local effects but is comparatively harmless. The other contains a neurotoxin, which causes dramatic and sometimes fatal reactions. The venom of the lethal North American scorpion, *C. sculpturatus* is the most toxic. The venom of the other North American scorpion, *V. spinigerus*, appears to contain similar components but is less lethal and has a somewhat different mode of action.

Scorpion venoms are known to have an adverse effect on neuromuscular transmission. The venom simulates the symptoms of strychnine poisoning by acting chiefly on smooth and striated muscle, causing increased excitability and muscle contracture, trembling, and finally, paralysis.

Venoms of the *Centruroides* genus of Arizona and Mexico and *Leiurus quinquestriatus* are primarily neurotoxic. These venoms are composed of proteins and polypeptides. They affect sodium channels with resultant prolongation of action potentials as well as spontaneous depolarization of nerves of both the adrenergic and parasympathetic nervous systems. Stimulation of the adrenergic system results in a massive outpouring of catecholamines. Sympathetic overdrive manifestations may include tachycardia, hypertension, pulmonary edema, and seizures as well as perspiration, piloerection, and hyperglycemia. Components of a parasympathetic stimulation syndrome may also be present (manifested as the SLUG BAM acronym) (3).

Signs and Symptoms

The venom of nonlethal scorpions causes only local reactions such as sharp burning, swelling, and discoloration at the sting site, and rarely, anaphylaxis (Table 76–1).

The poisonous varieties, which possess very potent convulsant neurotoxic venoms, produce no local swelling or discoloration. The sharp pain first produced by the sting is quickly followed by paresthesia in the bite area,

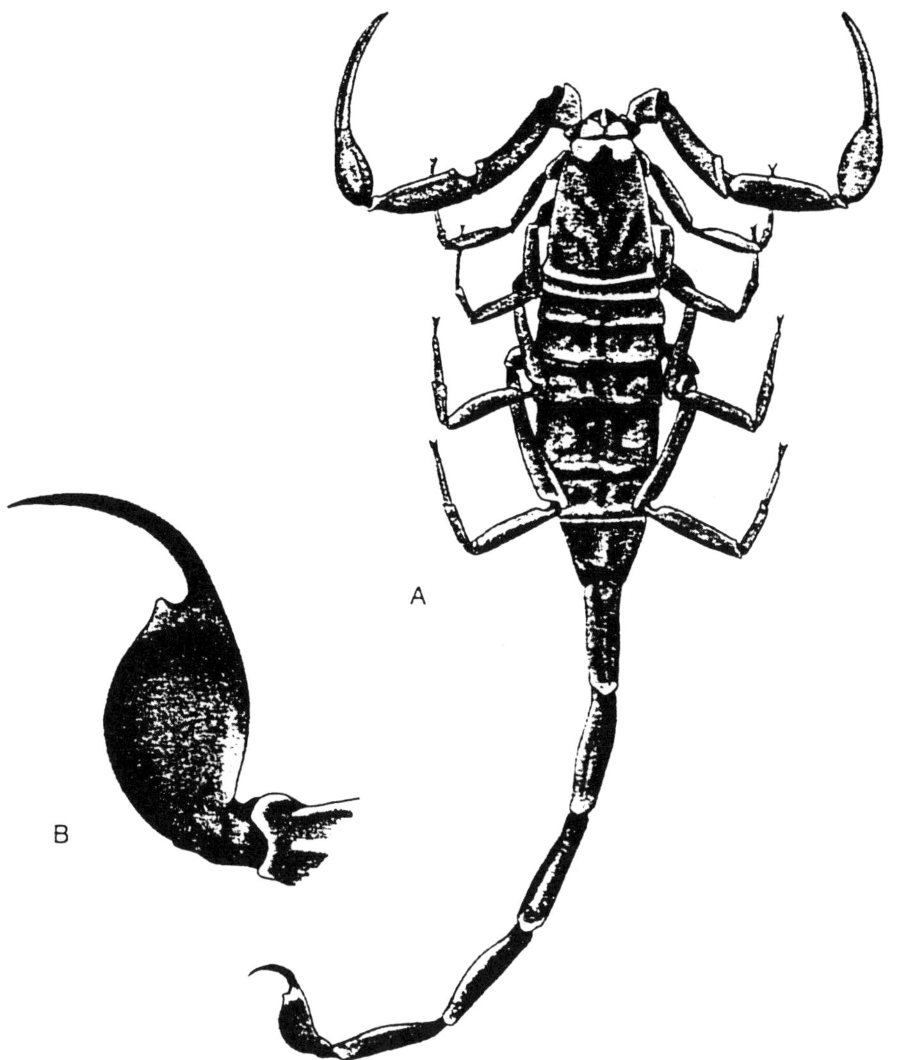

FIG. 76–1. A: Bark scorpion (*Centruroides sculpturatus*). **B**: Magnification of stinger (© Christopher Allen, DO, FACEP; illustration by Patti Smith.

which extends very rapidly. A period of hyperesthesia is followed by hypoesthesia and numbness or drowsiness.

If local symptoms are present, such as swelling, with or without discoloration and often extending along an extremity, the sting was doubtless from the less lethal species and will not usually progress to a systemic reaction unless there is anaphylaxis. On the other hand, complete lack of swelling at the site of the sting and/or evidence of hyperesthesia followed by hypoesthesia can be considered a danger signal, heralding a serious or even fatal reaction to the neurotoxin of a lethal species (4).

Initial neurologic disturbances reflect local tissue reaction and peripheral nerve effects. Immediate pain, erythema, and sensory alterations are common presenting complaints. Local muscle contractions may begin in close proximity to the sting site and follow the proximal advance of paresthesia and hyperesthesia. Sustained muscle spasm and paralysis reflect increased levels of acetylcholine or an anticholinesterase activity of the venom. Excessive peripheral neuromuscular activity may manifest as simple restlessness from apprehension or pain but may progress to uncontrollable spasm or opisthotonus.

Stings by the more toxic North American scorpions produce additional symptoms of skin flushing, parasympathetic activity, muscle fasciculations and twitching, hyperirritability and hyperactivity, hypertension, muscle weakness, and occasional paresthesia of the involved extremity (5).

Treatment

Local pain and paresthesias, both at the site and peripherally, are best treated with local compresses and

TABLE 76–1. *Signs and symptoms of scorpion envenomation*

Nonlethal
Local reaction
Burning
Swelling
Discoloration
Lethal
No local swelling
Paresthesia
Hyperesthesia
Muscle fasciculations
Hyperactivity
Hypertension
Muscle

oral analgesics. More severe symptoms may require airway support as well as intravenous antivenom (6).

Tachyarrhythmias may be treated with propranolol. Labetalol, or esmolol infusion, with additional α-adrenergic blocking effects, may be used when hypertension is a concern (4).

Other treatments for *C. sculpturatus* such as antihistamines, calcium, corticosteroids, and sympathomimetic drugs have been shown to have little value (7).

Antivenom

Since 1965, *Centruroides* scorpion antivenin has been made by lyophilizing micron-filtered hypersensitized goat serum. It is used within Arizona by special action of the Arizona State Board of Pharmacy (8).

The rapid and safe resolution of the severe symptoms of *Centruroides* scorpion envenomation following antivenin therapy has led some to recommend the use of antivenin in selected patients. Others, seeking to avoid any potential risk associated with the administration of a foreign protein, have recommended against its use. The fact that antivenin has not been subjected to Food and Drug Administration testing and production controls has also been cited as a cause for caution (9).

When making a decision about the use of antivenin, consideration must be given to the benefits of immediate symptom resolution, cost savings by management in and discharge from the ED, and the avoidance of sedation, paralysis, and intubation.

Antivenin is usually administered to severely poisoned patients such as the very young, the elderly, or those individuals with hypertension. Although a consideration of the risks and benefits may justify the administration of antivenin in severely envenomated children, there is less justification for the use of antivenin in less-affected children or adults (10).

Scorpion envenomations occurring outside the U.S. should be managed according to the venom toxicity of the offending species.

REFERENCES

1. Holmes H: Stings and bites. *Postgrad Med* 1990;88:75–78.
2. Bond G: Antivenin administration for *Centruroides* scorpion sting: risks and benefits. *Ann Emerg Med* 1992;21:788–791.
3. Gueron M, Ilia R, Sofer S: The cardiovascular system after scorpion envenomation. A review. *J Toxicol Clin Toxicol* 1992;30:245–258.
4. Reisman R: Stinging insect allergy. *Med Clin N Amer* 1992;76: 883–894.
5. Ennik F: Deaths from bites and stings of venomous animals. *West J Med* 1980;133:463–468.
6. Groshong T: Scorpion envenomation in eastern Saudi Arabia. *Ann Emerg Med* 1993;22:1431–1437.
7. Brown C, Shepherd S: Marine trauma, envenomations, and intoxications. *Emerg Med Clin N Amer* 1992;10:385–408.
8. Valentine M, Schuberth K, Kagey-Sobotka A, et al: The value of immunotherapy with venom in children with allergy to insect stings. *N Engl J Med* 1990;323:1601–1603.
9. Reisman R, Livingston A: Late-onset allergic reactions, including serum sickness, after insect stings. *J Allergy Clin Immunol* 1989;84: 331–337.
10. Lockey R: Immunotherapy for allergy to insect stings. *N Engl J Med* 1990;323:1632–1633.

CHAPTER 77

Bees

Many insects can cause systemic allergic reactions. Insect stings cause more deaths in the United States than bites from all other venomous animals. In the order *Hymenoptera*, these include the families *Apoidea* (bees), *Vespoidea* (wasps, yellow jackets, and hornets), and *Formicoidea* (ants). Of the ants, only those in the genus *Solenopsis* (fire ants) and the genus *Pogonomyrmex* (harvester ants) are known to cause IgE-mediated allergy in humans. Harvester ants are native to North America and are concentrated primarily in the southwestern US and Mexico (1).

Although a great deal of variation is found among the different species, the following characteristics are common to all members of this order: two pair of wings, three body segments (made up of a head, thorax, and abdomen), one pair of antennae, and, in the females, a tubular ovipositor that has been transformed into a stinging apparatus used for both offense and defense.

IMMUNOPATHOGENESIS

There are four basic mechanisms that can lead to mast-cell degranulation: (a) IgE-mediated hypersensitivity; (b) complement activation with synthesis of the anaphylatoxins c3 and c5a; (c) anaphylactoid substances that independently stimulate the mast cell; (d) inhibition of the arachidonic acid pathway. IgE-mediated allergic phenomena represent the classic hypersensitivity reaction, such as that seen in response to *Hymenoptera* stings (2).

The allergic reaction is a two-stage process. Sensitivity develops after the first sting when venom induces the production of venom-specific allergic (IgE) antibody, which then binds to tissue mast cells and circulating basophils. The second stage occurs when the patient is stung again. Re-exposure to the venom causes degranulation of mast cells and basophils with release of mediators, such as histamine, which cause the symptoms of anaphylaxis. This type of allergic reaction, therefore, requires four distinct stages as part of its evolution: (a) initial exposure to the allergen; (b) development of an IgE antibody in response to the allergen; (c) re-exposure to the same antigen; (e) antigen cross bridging on a pair of IgE antibodies affixed to a mast cell or a basophil (3).

Anaphylactic reactions from insect stings are mediated by IgE antibodies reacting with insect venoms. These antibodies can be detected by the immediate skin test reaction or in the serum by the radioallergosorbent test (RAST). No correlation exists between the degree of the allergic reaction and the levels of IgE antibody or the severity of the skin test reaction (4).

BEES

Bees may be "social" or "solitary." Solitary bees live alone, and each female bee prepares her own nest. Solitary bees survive for one season and include the carpenter bee, miner bees, mason bees, and cuckoo bees. Social bees maintain highly organized colonies, and include the bumblebee and honeybee. The honeybee is a fuzzy insect with alternating tan and black body stripes. It is usually seen pollinating clover and most often inflicts its sting when caught underfoot.

Stinging Mechanism

The stinging apparatus of the honeybee lies hidden inside a cavity at the posterior tip of the abdomen, from which it is extruded when the insect is ready to strike. When the stinger penetrates an insect, there is no more than the rapid thrust of the sting into a vulnerable area and its immediate withdrawal. When human skin is penetrated, the lancets become so firmly anchored by their barbs that withdrawal is impossible. In the struggle of the bee to free itself, or in the victim's attempt to brush it off, the whole stinging apparatus is usually avulsed. Damaged in this way, a bee soon dies. One should remember that the stinger, once imbedded, is neither absorbed nor does it disintegrate. Recent work has disclosed that yellow jackets also can leave stingers behind (5).

WASPS

Most wasps have slender bodies and four wings. The colors are quite assorted but most often are steel blue, black, yellow, or reddish. Typical wasps have a square head shield. Like the bees, wasps are also divided into the solitary and social varieties.

Solitary wasps are the most useful to humans because they destroy such a large number of harmful bugs, beetles, caterpillars, and flies. Examples of this group include the Mason, or Potter wasp, Mud daubers, and digger wasps. The social wasps include the yellow jackets and hornets.

Most of the social wasps inhabit the North temperate zone, and with cold weather arrival, the entire colony perishes except for an annual brood of queens which, after fertization, hibernate and start new colonies in the spring.

YELLOW JACKETS

These wasps, with black and yellow stripes, are approximately 17 mm in length. Their paper-covered nests are located hanging from bushes and trees, as well as in the ground.

Yellow jackets are very aggressive and are well known for their quick tempers and easy provocation. They tend to buzz around garbage cans, beverage containers, and various foods. They sometimes bite prior to stinging. The stinging female with her black face is easily distinguished from the nonstinging male which has a white or yellow face.

HORNETS

The most common variety of hornet, which is large and black with yellowish-white markings, builds large, round, pear-shaped nests, which generally hang from the stout limb of a tree at the edge of a forest. Unlike the wasp, which kills or paralyzes its prey, the hornet butchers it alive to facilitate transportation. Hornets usually do not attack unless the nest is threatened.

POLISTES

These wasps are usually reddish-brown, are elongated with a slender spindly-shaped abdomen. They differ from other wasps in that they seek the protection of houses and attics during the winter and become a nuisance when they emerge from hibernation in the spring. These insects are not aggresive. They sting only on strong provocation.

VENOM

An insect sting is an injection of venom by the female species through a modified ovipositor. The venom contains enzymes, which are the major allergens, as well as amines and peptides that encourage absorption of the venom. The most important allergens are (a) phospholipase A for the honeybee and (b) antigen 5, a protein of unknown function for vespids (yellow jackets, hornets, and wasps). Bee venom contains histamine and releases histamine in tissues by decarboxylation of histidine. Bee venom shares with wasp venom the presence of the spreading factor, hyaluronidase. As much as 10% of the hornet's venom consists of acetylcholine.

NORMAL REACTIONS TO BEE STINGS

For most persons, a sting is merely unpleasant and is followed by the development of a small hive and pruritus which may persist for several hours. When the sting is inserted, there is a sharp pinprick, followed by pain which lasts for several minutes. Within a few minutes, a small red area appears at the sting site and is gradually surrounded in turn by a whitish zone and a reddish flare. A wheal then forms and, as it subsides within a few hours, gives way to irritation, itching, and heat. All traces of the sting usually disappear within a few hours.

If the sting is located near the eyes, nose, or throat, the local reaction may cause more than the common amount of distress. Stings near the eyes are particularly hazardous since marked local reactions may result in atrophy of the iris, abscess of the lens, perforation of the globe, glaucoma, and changes in refraction.

LARGE LOCAL REACTIONS

About 10% of persons who are stung develop a large local reaction consisting of extensive and persistent swelling at the sting site. Occasionally, the reaction is severe enough to affect an entire extremity. These reactions are characterized by edema, pruritus, erythema, warmth, and pain; are limited to an area contiguous to the site of the sting; and usually peak within 24 to 48 hours. They persist for at least 48 to 72 hours and may last up to 5 days (1). Any degree of swelling, even if an entire limb is involved, is considered to be a local reaction, if it is continuous with the sting area, and no symptoms are apparent at areas distant to the sting site. Their pathogenesis involves IgE-mediated late-phase and cell-mediated hypersensitivity reactions (2).

SYSTEMIC REACTIONS AND ANAPHYLAXIS

Systemic allergic reactions to insect stings present in a variety of ways, ranging from those limited to the skin to reactions involving edema of the upper airway or bronchospasm; in the most severe episodes, there is cardiovascular collapse (1).

These reactions may first be indicated by dry hacking cough, sense of constriction in the throat or chest, swelling and itching about the eyes, massive urticaria, sneezing and wheezing, tachycardia, hypotension, pallor and a sense of impending disaster.

DELAYED SERUM-SICKNESS TYPE REACTION

Some patients have delayed reactions to stings. Some of these resemble serum sickness syndrome with symptoms including fever, lymphadenopathy, malaise, headache, urticaria, and polyarthritis. These symptoms may occur 10 to 14 days after the actual sting, and may occur after the first sting. Later, in such a patient, the response may become immediate and anaphylactic. The difference in the time onset of clinical manifestations rests on the fact that, at first, antibodies have to be formed but, thereafter, they are in production and become subject to the enhanced and accelerated phenomena.

DIAGNOSIS

The diagnosis of an insect sting reaction is usually obvious, and in contrast to insect bites, insect stings are always associated with pain. The allergic symptoms tend to occur within a short period, usually 10 to 15 minutes following the insect sting. When there is some delay in the onset of symptoms following the sting, this relationship may not be apparent. The identification of the insect responsible for the sting may be difficult.

Allergy Testing

Confirmation of stinging insect allergy is made by the detection of venom-specific IgE, carried out most easily by the simple immediate skin test. These tests are the most sensitive means of determining the presence of venom-specific IgE antibody. Five purified venoms are available for testing: honeybee, yellow jacket, yellow- and white-faced hornet, and wasp. Concentrations of venoms used for intracutaneous testing range from 0.001 to 1 μg/mL. Unequivocally positive or negative results are obtained in 95% of patients. Patients with relevant histories should be tested with appropriate dilutions of each of the available five single *Hymenoptera* venom preparations. Venom dilutions must be made with a special dilutent that contains human serum albumin (4).

Positive skin tests always must be interpreted in light of the clinical history. A positive skin test is not specific for anaphylactic allergy to venom because 85% of persons who have large local reactions also have positive skin tests (2).

Radioallergosorbent Test (RAST)

IgE antibodies reacting with venom also have been measured by the RAST. The RAST is not as sensitive as the skin test. Approximately 15–20% of the patients who have positive venom skin tests do not react in the RAST. Thus, the RAST should not be used as a routine diagnostic test. It may be of use when skin tests cannot be performed or when the reaction to skin tests in equivocal.

TREATMENT

Local

If the venom is deposited along with the stinger as with bee stings, it should be removed immediately, because contractions of the walls of the venom sac continue to inject additional venom long after the sting has been separated from the body of the insect.

The sting shafts are black with pieces of white tissue attached to them. The whole unit is about one-fourth the size of a match head. Squeezing or grasping with the fingertips will result in more venom being injected. The stinging apparatus should therefore be removed by scraping with a fingernail or knife blade. Once the residual parts have been removed, the sting site should be thoroughly cleansed with soap and water or an antiseptic solution.

Antihistamines can be given orally or parenterally, depending on the clinical findings. The need for other medications will depend on the clinical symptoms and may include the use of vasopressors, oxygen, and aerosol bronchodilators.

As a rule, acute reactions subside within a matter of minutes to hours, even without therapy. Rarely, the reaction may continue for long periods of time; if this occurs, steroids and restoration of plasma volume may be necessary.

Large Local Reactions

Large local reactions following insect stings, which are very common, are generally treated with the application of cold compresses and use of oral antihistamines and analgesics. If the swelling becomes extremely extensive and painful, steroid therapy is indicated with doses of prednisone, 20–40 mg daily, for several days.

Anaphylaxis

When confronted with a patient with a severe reaction, aqueous epinephrine 1:1,000 in a dose of 0.3–0.5 mL for adults (0.2–0.3 ml for children) should be given by deep subcutaneous injection, and the site massaged vigorously to hasten the rate of absorption. The patient should be closely observed because his response will determine whether or not the dose should be repeated.

Patients at risk for insect sting anaphylaxis are taught how to self-administer epinephrine and are advised to keep epinephrine and antihistamines available. Epinephrine is available in preloaded syringes and can be easily administered. Aerosols of epinephrine may be helpful in alleviating upper airway edema but usually are not absorbed in sufficient quantity to abort systemic reactions.

Oral or injectable antihistamines are usually administered to decrease the severity of hives or angioedema, but their use should not delay the administration of epinephrine for more serious reactions.

VENOM IMMUNOTHERAPY

The venoms used for immunotherapy are the same as those used for skin testing. Injection of purified insect venom, venom immunotherapy, is a highly effective prophylaxis for the prevention of subsequent sting reactions. Venom therapy stimulates production of serum venom-specific IgG, which is the immunologic corollary to clinical immunity (1).

Venom immunotherapy is indicated in individuals who have had a history of an acute allergic reaction following an insect sting and who have positive skin test reactions. The regimen begins with weekly injections of 0.01 μg and advances rapidly to 100 μg. The maintenance dose of 100 μg is given every 4 weeks for a year, after which the interval is lengthened to 6 to 8 weeks (5).

Immunotherapy is given once or twice a week for several months, then monthly or at longer intervals for at least 3 to 5 years. Such therapy causes a decrease in the serum level of venom-specific IgE and an increase in venom-specific IgG. These changes in antibody titers have been related to the efficacy of treatment.

Patients who have had venom anaphylaxis and who have positive venom skin tests are potential candidates for venom immunotherapy. Children who have had dermal symptoms as the only manifestation of the allergic reactions can be excluded and managed with symptomatic medication only.

All patients who have had the more severe symptoms of anaphylaxis, such as respiratory distress, hypotension, or upper airway edema, should receive venom immunotherapy regardless of age or the time interval since the sting reaction. Patients without systemic symptoms should not be given venom immunotherapy. Therefore, these patients should not have venom skin tests.

Almost all patients who have had large local reactions continue to have similar reactions following subsequent stings. These local reactions are not dependent on IgE antibody, which is present in more than half the individuals following large local reactions. The use of venom immunotherapy does not modify the large local reaction. In a small minority of patients anaphylaxis will develop with subsequent stings. For these reasons, patients with large local reactions are not considered candidates for venom immunotherapy, and these patients do not require venom skin tests.

Venom immunotherapy is 97% effective in reducing anaphylaxis from stings in adults with previous systemic reactions. Without therapy, almost 60% of such adults will have systemic reactions if stung again; some of these reactions may not respond even to properly administered epinephrine. More of the systemic reactions are potentially life-threatening in adults than in children (6).

REFERENCES

1. Reisman R, Livingston A: Late-onset allergic reactions, including serum sickness, after insect stings. *J Allergy Clin Immunol* 1989;84: 331–337.
2. Brown C, Shepherd S: Marine trauma, envenomations, and intoxications. *Emerg Med Clin N Amer* 1992;10:385–408.
3. Holmes H: Stings and bites. *Postgrad Med* 1990;88:75–78.
4. Graft D: Stinging insect allergy. *Postgrad Med* 1989;85:173–178.
5. Valentine M, Schuberth K, Kagey-Sobotka A, et al: The value of immunotherapy with venom in children with allergy to insect stings. *N Engl J Med* 1990;323:1601–1603.
6. Lockey R: Immunotherapy for allergy to insect stings. *N Engl J Med* 1990;323:1632–1633.

CHAPTER 78

Ants

Ants exist almost everywhere in the world, from the tropics to the Artic and Antartic. Their success as empire builders lies in their ceaseless industry, their high degree of organization and mutual cooperation, and their extreme specialization. Ants not only have queen, workers, and drones, as the bees do, but also have professional soldiers, that not only defend the nest but invade other colonies to carry off workers, which then become their slaves (1). Because the bites and stings of most ants are rarely more than a transient annoyance and only occasionally lead to allergic reactions, they will not be discussed here. Two types of ants will be discussed, the harvester ant and imported fire ant.

HARVESTER ANTS

These ants have a vicious sting and readily attack both humans and animals. They are colored black or red, have long legs, and are often 1 cm in length (Fig. 78–1). They live preferably in dry, warm, sandy places, where they excavate their nests to form low mounds bare of surrounding vegetation for a distance of several feet.

Harvester ants live on the seed cut from grasses and weeds, which they grind with their powerful mandibles and store within the nest. They have been known to kill small farm animals, which have blundered upon their nests, but severe reactions to multiple stings have rarely been reported in humans (3).

FIRE ANTS

These ants acquire their name from the fierce burning pain that is associated with their bites. The several species found indigenous to the United States are far less important than the imported tropical variety. In infested areas, fire ants account for 90% of all ant populations and stings from fire ants are more frequent than stings from other hymenoptera, becoming the most common cause of insect venom hypersensitivity (4).

In the early 1900s, fire ants were brought into the port city of Mobile, Alabama, on vegetation and produce from South America. Two species of fire ants were introduced; *Solenopsis richteri* and *Sonenopsis invicta*. The latter species has been much more aggressive and has spread rapidly throughout the southeastern U.S., displacing *S. richteri* and other ant species (1).

The genus *Solenopsis* is classified in the superfamily Formicoidea and family Formicidae.

Several other species of fire ants are found in the U.S., but most have been destroyed by the more aggressive, imported fire ants. These, and other less common species, have smaller colonies, are much less aggressive, and inflict less painful stings than *S. invicta* and *S. richteri*.

Life Cycle

Fire ants have four castes: female, male, major worker, and minor worker. The sexual forms are generally larger measuring 5–7 mm. The major workers measure 5–6 mm, and the minor workers 2–4 mm in length (5). Male and female ants have wings, but the female ants lose their wings after mating (6).

The fire ant's life cycle begins with the swarming of the male ants in the spring. The queens fly through the ant cloud until clasped by a male ant, at which time impregnation takes place. Sufficient sperm is deposited for the queen to produce 5–6 million eggs during a 6-year life span. After impregnation, the new queen disengages, lands, sheds her wings, burrows, and begins laying eggs. Within 3 years, the fire ant mound contains up to 250,000 ants with the queen deep inside. Mounds have tunnels that may radiate up to 130 feet. The ant colony moves up and down within the mound through these tunnels in response to temperature. Food is brought into the mound by worker ants. Because the queen is unable to digest solid food, she is fed liquids from other ants.

Envenomation

In stinging, the ant attaches itself to the skin with powerful mandible, arches its body, and injects 0.04–0.11 μL of venom through a stinger located in the distal abdomen. Although the mandibles are used for grasping, the venom

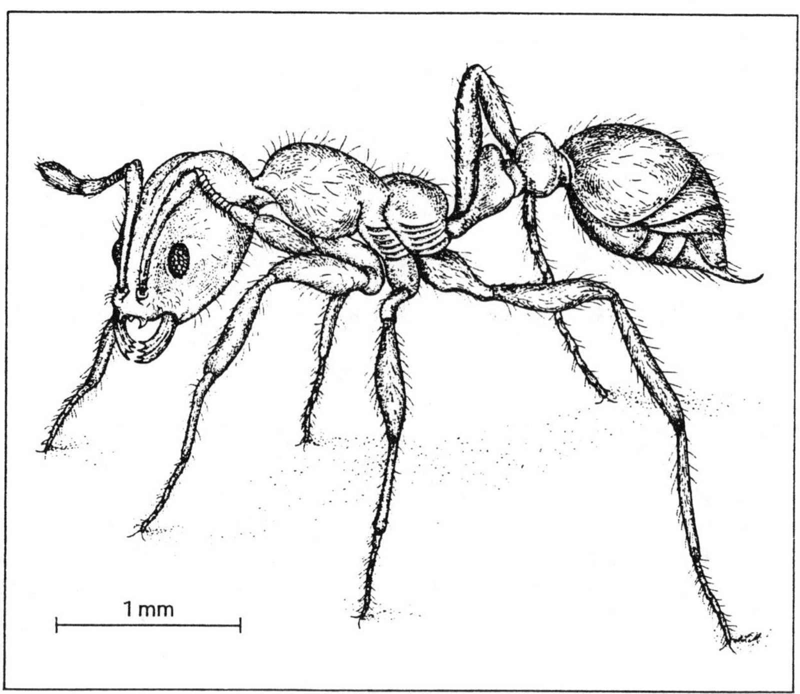

FIG. 78–1. The worker ant of the genus *Solenopsis* is 3 to 6 mm long. To sting, the ant attaches its mandible to the skin, arches its back at the peduncle, and injects venom through a stinger at the tip of its abdomen. If left undisturbed, the ant will rotate on its mandible and sting repeatedly. (From Lockey RF, *Hospital Practice*, March 15, 1990, p. 110, with permission of McGraw Hill, Inc.)

is introduced with a 0.5–1.0 mm stinger extruded from the abdomen.

Unlike bees and wasps, fire ants sting slowly, injecting their venom within seconds to minutes. Fire ant stings are, therefore, usually not immediately painful. If undisturbed, the ant will rotate its body about its mandibles to sting repeatedly. The venom induces an immediate, severe burning sensation at the site of the sting, followed by intense itching that may last for hours or days.

VENOM

Unlike other hymenoptera venoms which are primarily aqueous solutions containing a large percentage of protein, fire ant venom has an extremely low protein content. These proteins, including a phospholipase and a hyaluronidase, account for only 0.1% of fire ant venom by weight but are responsible for the IgE-mediated allergic response. The remaining portion of the fire ant venom are predominantly toxic alkaloids which are disubstituted piperidines. Venom alkaloids have no role in IgE-mediated responses but have cytotoxic, hemolytic, bactericidal, and insecticidal properties and activate the complement pathway. Venom alkaloids have some neurotoxic effects with reports of neuropathies, unconsciousness, seizures, and other neurologic manifestations. They also cause histamine release and tissue necrosis at the site of injection. These alkaloids are responsible for the pain and the typical findings that are characteristic of the local dermal reaction to fire ant stings (4). This aqueous fraction has been found to contain the allergenic activity of fire ant venom.

SIGNS AND SYMPTOMS

The venom induces an immediate, severe burning sensation at the site of the sting, followed by intense itching that may last for hours or days.

Reaction to imported fire ant stings can be divided into three categories: local, large local, and systemic (Table 78–1).

LOCAL REACTION

Almost all persons stung by imported fire ants have a wheal-and-flare reaction at the site of the sting. The wheal-and-flare reaction usually resolves within 30 minutes to an hour and evolves into a fully developed sterile pustule at the sting site within 24 hours. The epidermis covering the pustule sloughs off over a period of 48 to 72 hours. Healing takes place as the bottom of the lesion is covered with new epidermis. No treatment has been shown to prevent or resolve pustules (5).

TABLE 78–1. *Signs and symptoms of imported fire ant envenomation*

Local reaction
Wheat and flare reaction
Sterile pustule
Pruritis
Local necrosis
Large local reaction
Second phase of pruritis
Induration
May involve entire extremity
Systemic reaction
Pruritis
Hypotension
Respiratory distress
Angioedema
Urticaria
Gastrointestinal distress
Stridor
Syncope

Being sterile, the pustule usually heals spontaneously. The intense pruritus, however, prompts many patients to scratch off the pustule's thin epidermal covering, creating a direct route for secondary infection, which can cause considerable morbidity; sepsis and death have been reported. Local sepsis and, in some patients, particularly those with diabetes or impaired circulation, local necrosis, which may require surgical debridement and skin grafting, or occasionally, partial or complete amputation of a limb have been noted.

The intense inflammatory reaction and pustule that develop at the imported fire ant sting site probably result from the potent cytotoxins and hemolytics found in the alkaloid fraction of the venom. The toxins cause localized necrosis of the dermis and underlying connective tissue to create the characteristic sterile pustule that appears within 24 hours after almost all stings.

LARGE LOCAL REACTION

Large local reactions begin like normal local reactions but evolve into a second phase of pruritic erythema and induration that begins within 1 to 2 hours, becomes more prominent within 6 hours, and continues to expand for 24 hours. These painful reactions may eventually involve an entire extremity before they begin to subside, usually within 48 hours. Typical pustules that develop at the sting site are similar to those that occur in subjects without large local reactions except that eosinophils are more prominent in the infiltrate of pustular lesions from large local reactions (1). In extreme cases, the edema may cause compression of nerves or blood vessels. In some cases, the degree of induration present with late reactions suggests cellulitis. It is possible that a large local reaction is a form of dermal hypersensivity mediated by nonimmunologic mechanisms (7).

SYSTEMIC REACTION

Fatal anaphylactic reactions to the imported fire ant sting are less frequent nationally than those to other hymenoptera, but the true incidence remains unknown. In many parts of the South, however, the imported fire ant is the leading cause of insect-induced anaphylactic death. The prevalence of systemic allergic reactions is, in all likelihood, grossly underreported, because many persons who have systemic reactions do not realize the potential danger and, therefore, do not seek medical attention (2).

Systemic reactions involve signs and symptoms remote from the sting site. Manifestations include pruritis, hypotension, respiratory difficulty, upper airway edema, angioedema, urticaria, gastrointestinal distress, stridor, and syncope (5). Anaphylactic death is more common among adults than children, particularly in the elderly and those with coronary artery disease (4).

Diagnosis of Imported Fire Ant Sensitivity

Imported fire ant whole body extract (WBE) is the only commercial reagent available for diagnosis of and immunotherapy for persons who are hypersensitive to the insect. A commercial venom extract is available for experimental purposes only and has not been approved by the Food and Drug Administration for use in humans (8).

Imported fire ant WBE and venom are both valid for skin test and radioallergosorbent test (RAST) diagnosis of fire ant hypersensitivity. Venom RAST diagnosis is more sensitive but not more specific than WBE RAST. Both extracts can produce false-positive skin tests and RASTs in nonallergic subjects. WBE from hymenoptera other than the imported fire ant is not effective for diagnosis and therapy, unlike venom extract, probably because bee and vespid body enzymes biodegrade the venom proteins. This phenomenon does not appear to occur with imported fire ant WBE, which when properly prepared, contains most clinically important allergens.

TREATMENT

There is no treatment that will alter the evolution of local toxicity and the necrotic pustule. Topical steroids, systemic steroids, systemic antihistamines, sympathomimetics, local abrasion, treatment with povidone-iodine solution, and aspiration of pustules does not alter the pustule's clinical or pathologic course.

The management of choice for the pustular lesion caused by the imported fire ant is repeated cleansing of the site with soap and water, covering the lesion to prevent excoriation, and immediate treatment of secondary infection. Topical anesthetics or oral antihistamines may be used for pruritis. The airway must be established and maintained by using endotracheal intubation or cricothyrotomy if necessary. Intravenous fluids should be given to replenish depleted intravascular volume in the treatment of anaphylactic shock.

Late-phase imported fire ant sting reactions may respond to treatment with steroids and combinations of H1 and H2 receptor blocking agents (9).

Nonallergic local reactions do not usually require medical treatment, but the application of cold compresses may help to relieve the swelling and discomfort. The risk of secondary infection can be reduced by cleansing sting sites with soap and water and applying local antiseptics. The pustules can be covered with bandages to avoid excoriation.

Patients who suffer massive numbers of stings or who have severe complications may require supportive treatment in the hospital.

Large Local Reactions

Large local reactions may be treated with oral corticosteroids, oral H1 antagonists, and analgesics, which may help to relieve the discomfort associated with the reaction.

Meat tenderizer containing the proteolytic enzyme papain does not appear to be of any therapeutic value in the acute treatment of reactions to imported fire ant stings. There is no convincing evidence that epinephrine prevents or modifies the course of large local reactions. Elevation of the extremity plus treatment with glucocorticoids and antihistamines may prevent the need for decompressive surgery or amputation in such cases where compression of nerves are a concern (10).

Systemic Reactions

Treatment of anaphylactic reactions to the imported fire ant is the same as the treatment for other Hymenoptera previously discussed.

IMMUNOTHERAPY

Although fire ant venom is not commercially available, it has been collected and compared with the fire ant whole body extracts, commonly used for the diagnosis and treatment of allergic individuals. Although the test results indicate that venom is a better diagnostic antigen, fire ant whole body extracts can be prepared that contain sufficient allergen and are reliable for skin test diagnosis and therapy. Individuals at potential risk are tested with the whole body extract and are given immunotherapy with the same material (6). Studies have confirmed that imported fire ant whole body extracts contain clinically relevant allergens that are apparently effective for diagnosis and treatment of fire ant allergy. However, variability of skin test reactivity and treatment failures have been reported (7).

Although immunotherapy with venom preparations has been found to be highly effective and safe for prevention of future systemic reactions to Hymenoptera stings, at present, there are no reported trials of imported fire ant immunotherapy with standardized pure venom (11).

Because it is impossible for sensitized persons who live in infested areas to avoid fire ants, thousands of patients now receive immunotherapy with WBE. Treatment consists of weekly subcutaneous injections of the extract, with the dose increasing until an empirically determined maintenance dose, usually 0.5 mL of a 1:10 dilution of commercially available whole body extract is reached. This maintenance dose is then given approximately once a month. Uncontrolled observations suggest that this technique has a high level of efficacy but some failures of treatment have been reported (11).

Systemic reactions can occur during the administration of immunotherapy. It should, therefore, be performed only by clinicians experienced in the technique or under the guidance of an allergist–immunologist, and only when adequate means of treating systemic reactions are available. Patients should be informed of the risk and observed closely for 30 minutes after each injection (2).

REFERENCES

1. Stafford C, Hoffman D, Rhoades R: Allergy to imported fire ants. *South Med J* 1989;82:1520–1527.
2. Reisman R, Livingston A: Late-onset allergic reactions, including serum sickness, after insect stings. *J Allergy Clin Immunol* 1989;84: 331–337.
3. Freeman T, Hylander R, Ortiz A, et al: Imported fire ant immunotherapy: effectiveness of whole body extracts. *J Allergy Clin Immunol* 1992;90:210–215.
4. Hardwick W, Royall J, Petitt B, et al: Near fatal fire ant envenomation of a newborn. *Pediatrics* 1992;90:622–624.
5. Holmes H: Stings and bites. *Postgrad Med* 1990;88:75–78.
6. Reisman R: Stinging insect allergy. *Med Clin N Amer* 1992;76: 883–894.
7. Graft D: Stinging insect allergy. *Postgrad Med* 1989;85:173–178.
8. Stafford C, Hutto L, Rhoades R, et al: Imported fire ant as a health hazard. *South Med J* 1989;82:1515–1519.
9. Valentine M, Schuberth K, Kagey-Sobotka A, et al: The value of immunotherapy with venom in children with allergy to insect stings. *N Engl J Med* 1990;323:1601–1603.
10. Brown C, Shepherd S: Marine trauma, envenomations, and intoxications. *Emerg Med Clin N Amer* 1992;10:385–408.
11. Lockey R: Immunotherapy for allergy to insect stings. *N Engl J Med* 1990;323:1632–1633.

PART XV

ENVIRONMENTAL AGENTS

CHAPTER 79

Pesticides

Poisonings with various kinds of pesticides account for about 10% of all deaths caused by solid and liquid substances—a small but significant percentage of acute human poisonings. Since the mid-1940s more than 15,000 compounds, representing more than 35,000 different formulations, have been used as pesticides. The term *pesticide* is a general term that classifies these substances on the basis of their actions rather than chemically; the term encompasses insecticides, rodenticides, fungicides, herbicides, and fumigants. Because pesticides are manufactured for the purpose of destroying organisms that are considered undesirable for one reason or another, it is not surprising that all pesticides are capable of producing harm to humans (1).

Most pesticides are not pure compounds but complex mixtures containing various isomers, byproducts, and reactants. Either the active pesticidal ingredient or the solvent may cause toxicity. For example, liquid pesticides are formulated in petroleum distillates, such as kerosene, which may also have serious toxic potential apart from that associated with the pesticidal solute. Aspiration of the hydrocarbon may, therefore, be an additional hazard of the product.

Pesticide poisonings occur most often during the spring and summer months, when pesticides are used most frequently. Individuals who handle the concentrated pesticide, such as agricultural workers, formulators, loaders, and appliers, are at greatest risk.

RODENTICIDES

Many of the noninsecticide pesticides are extremely toxic and have limited usefulness because of their toxicity. The rodenticides comprise a group of pesticides that are toxic and have rather wide application but are restricted by government regulations.

A rodenticide is any commercially available product designed expressly to kill mice, rats, squirrels, gophers, and other small rodents. Rodenticides contain various toxins ranging in potency from the highly toxic phosphorus, monofluoroacetate, p-nitrophenolurea, strychnine, thallium, arsenic, and zinc phosphide compounds to the less toxic hydroxycoumarins and indanediones (Table 79–1) . There has yet to be an effective rodenticide developed that is nontoxic to humans.

TABLE 79–1. *Rodenticides*

Phosphorus
Monofluoroacetate
p-Nitrophenolurea
Strychnine
Thallium
Arsenic
Zinc phosphide
Hydroxycoumarins
Indanediones

PHOSPHORUS

Actions

Elemental phosphorus occurs in three forms: red, yellow or white, and black (2). Red and black phosphorus are nonvolatile, insoluble, and nonabsorbable and, therefore, nontoxic. Yellow phosphorus, however, is a toxic compound that causes severe local and systemic reactions (3). (White phosphorus, when exposed to light, turns yellow; hence, the names are synonymous (4). Yellow phosphorus is luminescent and highly flammable and spontaneously combusts in air. It is a general protoplasmic poison, causing damage to multiple organ systems including the gastrointestinal tract and cardiovascular, hepatic, and renal systems (4). Toxicity is increased when phosphorus is in the form of fine particles or emulsions or is dissolved in organic solvents such as alcohol, fats, and oils (5).

At one time, yellow phosphorus was used in match tips, fireworks, and unlicensed medical remedies. Numerous fatalities resulted from ingestion of these compounds (6). Matches that can be struck on any rough surface now contain either red phosphorus or phosphorus sesquisulfide together with potassium chlorate and glue.

Because of the increasing resistance of rodents to warfarin-containing substances (discussed later), yellow

TABLE 79–2. *Selected phosphorus-containing rodenticides by trade name*

Blue Death Rat Killer
Patterson's Zinc Phosphide Rodent Bait
Stearn's Electric Brand Paste
Common Sense Rat Preparation
J-O Electric Paste
Rat-Nip
Senco Paste

phosphorus has come back on the market as a rodenticide paste to be spread on crackers or bread. It may be present in concentrations of up to 5% (Table 79–2) (6).

Toxicity

Dermal Absorption

Phosphorus can be absorbed by all routes, including dermally and by inhalation (4). Skin contact produces painful second- and third-degree chemical and thermal burns. Phosphorus absorbed through the skin may produce a sudden and marked reversal of the ratio of serum calcium to phosphorus.

Gastrointestinal Absorption

Classically, phosphorus poisoning is divided into three phases (Table 79–3), although this description may not apply to many patients who ingest pesticide pastes (7). The initial symptoms may be painful second- and third-degree burns that develop a few minutes to hours after exposure. A gastroenteritis may follow, resulting from local irritation and causing nausea, vomiting, diarrhea, phosphorescent vomitus, and intense abdominal pain (5). Often, a garlic odor can be detected from the vomitus. In this phase, acute cardiovascular collapse may result from direct action of phosphorus on the myocardium (4,7). Many patients who ingest phosphorus paste may be asymptomatic when first seen in the emergency department, with the garlic odor and mucosal burns occurring in only a small percentage of cases (3).

The next phase is a lull or symptom-free period that may last for several weeks; during this time the patient appears to recover. The final phase represents systemic intoxication from the action of the absorbed phosphorus and involves the gastrointestinal tract, liver, heart, kidneys, and central nervous system (CNS). Death is usually attributed to irreversible shock, hepatic or renal failure, CNS or myocardial damage, or massive hematemesis.

TABLE 79–3. *Phases of acute phosphorus poisoning*

Phase 1
Painful burns
Gastroenteritis
Phosphorescent vomitus
Abdominal pain
Garlic odor of vomitus
Cardiovascular collapse
Phase 2
Symptom-free period
Phase 3
Gastrointestinal intoxication
Hepatic intoxication
Renal failure
CNS intoxication

Treatment

There is no antidote for acute yellow phosphorus poisoning (7). Treatment is directed toward removing the toxin as soon as possible after ingestion, preventing its absorption from the gastrointestinal tract, and providing intensive supportive care to maintain vital signs. Both the patient and clinician should be protected from further contact with the phosphorus to avoid burns of the skin and eyes. Cutaneous burns should be washed with copious amounts of water. If the phosphorus was ingested, gastric lavage with large quantities of potassium permanganate (1:5000) has been recommended to oxidize the phosphorus into the relatively harmless oxide. Although some investigators recommend administration of copper sulfate solution, this is contraindicated (5). Activated charcoal can adsorb phosphorus and, thus, should be administered (8).

FLUOROACETATE DERIVATIVES

Actions

Monofluoroacetate (Compound 1080, SMFA) is a white, odorless, tasteless crystalline compound that looks like flour or baking soda; it is usually mixed with a black dye. Fluoroacetamide (Compound 1081) is a related fluoroacetic derivative that has actions similar to those of fluoroacetate but has a somewhat slower onset of symptoms. Both compounds are highly effective poisons for all kinds of rodents but must be used with great caution because of their toxicity to other animals and humans. Because of their extreme toxicity, they are sold only to licensed pest-control operators (9).

Fluoroacetate occurs naturally as a constituent of a South African plant and is toxic when ingested, inhaled as dust, or absorbed through open wounds (it is not absorbed through the intact skin) (9,10). Its action is related not to its fluoride content but to the fact that it is converted to fluorocitrate in the body, which then interferes with the Krebs cycle by acting as a potent competitive inhibitor for the enzyme aconitase in the tricarboxylic acid cycle that normally converts citrate to isocitrate. The effects are especially noted in the heart and CNS (3).

Toxicity

Toxic symptoms are delayed for 2 to 3 hours after ingestion of fluoroacetate or absorption through broken skin because of the conversion of fluoroacetate to fluorocitrate. When symptoms begin they are usually severe (Table 79–4) (3,10).

General response to poisoning includes nausea and vomiting. Central nervous system effects include agitation, a depressed level of consciousness, apprehension, seizures, and coma. The cardiovascular effects may include ventricular ectopy, bigeminy, supraventricular or ventricular tachycardia and ventricular fibrillation and may lead to death (3).

Treatment

Treatment of fluoroacetate poisoning is mainly nonspecific and supportive. Contaminated clothing should be removed and the skin washed with soap and water. Seizures can be controlled with diazepam. There is evidence that an extrinsic supply of acetate ions, such as from glycerol monoacetate, has antidotal effects by competitively blocking the conversion of fluoroacetate to fluorocitrate in the tricarboxylic acid cycle. Although no clinical trials have confirmed the efficacy of this treatment, it is still advocated for acute ingestion. Glycerol monoacetate (0.24 g/kg), sodium acetate (0.12 g/kg), and ethyl alcohol are recommended (3). Another dosage regimen for glycerol monoacetate is to administer 0.5 mL/kg intramuscularly every 30 minutes for several hours and followed by a reduced dose for at least 12 hours. Monoacetin may also be administered in the same dosage. These compounds should be administered parenterally as soon as a definite diagnosis is made. Treatment can be expected to produce local edema, sedation, and vasodilation (3).

TABLE 79–4. *Symptoms of fluoroacetate poisoning*

General
Nausea
Vomiting
Central nervous system
Agitation
Lethargy
Apprehension
Seizures
Coma
Cardiovascular
Supraventricular tachycardia
Ventricular ectopy
Bigeminy
Ventricular tachycardia
Ventricular fibrillation

P-NITROPHENOLUREA

Actions

p-Nitrophenolurea, also known as Vacor, is a toxic, single-dose, quick-kill rodenticide. Vacor was introduced in 1975 and initially marketed as safe for humans (11). The manufacturer has withdrawn the product from the market because it has caused a significant number of deaths since it was introduced.

p-Nitrophenolurea is chemically related to alloxan and streptozocin, both of which are potent pancreatic beta-cell toxins and have been used for a number of years to induce diabetes in experimental animals and to treat islet cell carcinoma (12). All these substances, including Vacor, appear to act by interfering with nicotinamide metabolism in pancreatic beta cells, liver cells, and brain in rodents and humans, causing acute diabetes mellitus and autonomic dysfunction (12). Ingestion of as little as a single 30-g packet of the yellow-green powder has caused death (13).

Toxicity

Symptoms may be delayed in onset from 4 to 48 hours, which is the time necessary for enzyme interference to occur (Table 79–5) (11). Early symptoms may include nausea and vomiting, abdominal pain, and confusion. Later, the patient may complain of or exhibit chest pain, glycosuria, hyperglycemia, ketosis, seizures, and autonomic dysfunction (3,9).

The autonomic dysfunction may involve both sympathetic and parasympathetic nerves and may be manifested by postural hypotension (which is an early feature), hypothermia, dysphagia, dystonia, impaired pupillary responses, impotence, bowel and bladder dysfunction, and motor and sensory neuropathy (Table 79–6) (14). This neuropathy frequently develops within the first day after ingestion and produces the greatest degree of long-

TABLE 79–5. *Symptoms of p-nitrophenolurea poisoning*

Nausea
Vomiting
Abdominal pain
Confusion
Glycosuria
Hyperglycemia or hypoglycemia
Ketosis
Seizures
Autonomic dysfunction
Diabetic ketoacidosis

TABLE 79–6. *Autonomic dysfunctions associated with p-nitrophenolurea poisoning*

Postural hypotension
Hypothermia
Dysphagia
Dystonia
Impotence
Bowel and bladder dysfunction
Motor and sensory neuropathy

term disability in most patients (9,14). The neuropathic symptoms often progress over several days, and the greatest impairment usually occurs distally. A period of hypoglycemia may develop before hyperglycemia because of a sudden release of insulin stored in damaged pancreatic tissue. Late sequelae include cardiovascular collapse, respiratory failure, coma, and death. Death has been due to ketoacidosis, gastrointestinal perforation, cardiac dysrhythmias, and pneumonia (12).

Long-term sequelae in the form of glucose intolerance and neurologic dysfunction have been frequent among the survivors of acute intoxication. Some individuals have permanent insulin-dependent diabetes and long-term problems associated with autonomic dysfunction (13).

Treatment

Attempts at inducing emesis and catharsis may be ineffective because of the ileal and esophageal hypomotility produced by p-nitrophenolurea poisoning (13). These measures are still recommended, however, if the ingestion is recent enough. There are no supporting data to suggest that ion trapping and forced diuresis are of benefit, nor is there evidence that dialysis or hemoperfusion is efficacious in treating p-nitrophenolurea ingestion (14). The diabetes mellitus produced by Vacor may be difficult to manage in many cases. Regular eating may be difficult for some individuals because of gastrointestinal hypomotility and, in some cases, because of severe anorexia.

Specific treatment consists of administering niacinamide (nicotinamide), which interferes with the toxin's ability to reduce intracellular synthesis of nicotinamide adenine dinucleotide. When administered within a few hours of ingestion, niacinamide can prevent the development of pancreatic destruction and disturbances in autonomic function. N-methylniacinamide, niacin (nicotinic acid), and L-tryptophan, which are all precursors of nicotinamide adenine dinucleotide, have no effect on preventing depression of liver nucleotide concentration or on the development of diabetes mellitus. In addition, niacin should not be substituted for nicotinamide because the vasodilatory effects of niacin may add to the problems of blood pressure control (5,14). Niacinamide (500 mg) should be injected intravenously and followed by 100 to 200 mg intravenously every 4 hours for 2 to 3 days. If signs of toxicity develop, the frequency of injection should be increased to every 2 hours at a dosage not to exceed 3 g/day in adults or 1.5 g/day in children. Diabetic ketoacidosis should be managed with insulin (3).

Dihydroergotamine therapy, if instituted early in the course of an intoxication, has been shown to benefit some patients with severe postural hypotension (13,15).

THALLIUM

Actions

Thallium, an odorless and tasteless heavy metal, is a systemic poisoning with multisystem toxicities. It is among the most lethal poisons and produces one of the highest incidences of long-term sequelae, mainly neurologic. Thallium was discovered in the mid-1800s by a scientist searching for another element, tellurium. Thallium was used until the early 1900s to treat diseases such as syphilis, ringworm, and dysentery and until the 1950s in some countries as a depilatory paste. In industry, thallium may be encountered as a byproduct of the production or use of various metals and alloys, jewelry and optical lenses (16), thermometers, electronic equipment, and various pigments. Because of its high toxicity, its use as a rodenticide is now restricted to government agencies and it is available only by special permit (17).

In the United States, acute thallium poisoning has most often been caused by ingestion of thallium-containing insecticides or rodenticides. The latter are often prepared as wafers that are attractive to children as well as to rodents (Table 79–7) (18). Since the introduction of thallium sulfate (which is 60–80% thallium metal) as an effective odorless and tasteless rodenticide, suicidal and homicidal thallium poisonings have increased considerably (19). Poisoning from industrial exposure is expected to increase as well because glass and pharmaceutical firms have begun using thallium in manufacturing processes.

Thallium is especially toxic in its bivalent state as sulfate, acetate, and carbonate salts. The sulfide and iodide compounds are poorly soluble and, therefore, much less toxic (20). Thallium sulfate and other soluble salts are absorbed rapidly and completely through the intact skin and mucous membranes of the mouth and gastrointestinal tract (18).

TABLE 79–7. *Selected thallium-containing rodenticides by trade name*

Senco Corn Mix
Martin's Rat Stop
GTA Rat Bait
Gizmo Mouse Killer
Zelio Paste

Mechanism of Action

The effects of thallium are thought to be due to its interference with the metabolism of compounds containing sulfhydryl groups, especially those of the mitochondrial respiratory chain. Protein synthesis (particularly incorporation of cysteine) is inhibited, which may account for the symptom of alopecia (through prevention of keratinization; see next) (18).

In addition, cell membranes cannot distinguish between potassium and thallium ions because thallium behaves much like potassium in the body. Thallous ion has an affinity for sodium-potassium adenosine triphosphatase that is 10 times greater than that of potassium. Thallium is therefore preferentially transported into cells. Because it is similar to potassium, it substitutes for potassium in many physiologic reactions and depolarizes membranes in nerve and heart, antagonizes the effect of calcium on the heart, and corrects the cardiac effects of hypokalemia (18,19). Unlike lead and arsenic, thallium is soluble at physiological pH and, therefore, does not form complexes in bone (17).

Toxicity

Symptoms of thallium poisoning are mainly referable to the central nervous system and the gastrointestinal tract (Table 79–8) (18). The gastrointestinal symptoms may follow absorption of thallium by any route after a latent period of 12 to 24 hours. Symptoms may include abdominal pain, anorexia, nausea, diarrhea, and hemorrhagic gastroenteritis. Death may be secondary to respiratory paralysis or circulatory disturbances (16).

TABLE 79–8. *Signs and symptoms of thallium poisoning*

Gastrointestinal
Abdominal pain
Anorexia
Nausea
Diarrhea
Gastroenteritis
Gingival discoloration
Neurologic
Tremor
Paresthesia
Bilateral polyneuropathy
Irritability
Delirium
Coma
Pseudobulbar paralysis
Seizures
Somnolence
Facial palsy
Ocular
Ptosis
Strabismus
Mydriasis
Amblyopia
Optic atrophy
Autonomic
Fever
Tachycardia
Orthostatic hypotension
Urinary retention
Constipation
Dysrhythmias
Miscellaneous
Alopecia
Interference with nail growth
Lines in the gingiva
Liver necrosis
Renal tubular damage
Psychosis

General

In severe cases of thallium poisoning, delirium, seizures, coma, and death may occur but usually not earlier than 8 to 10 days after ingestion. More often the acute gastroenteritis subsides and the patient has an asymptomatic period of 3 to 4 days (20). This is gradually replaced by signs and symptoms referable to one or several systems. Intermittent intestinal colic, nausea and vomiting, diarrhea, stomatitis, excessive salivation, and gingival discoloration comparable to that of lead line may be noted. The gingival discoloration appears in some cases within 2 to 4 days of exposure and represents precipitated thallium in the gums at the base of the teeth (21).

Neurologic

Neuromuscular symptoms, such as tremors, paresthesias, and frank polyneuritis, have been described as bilateral painful legs and increase gradually until the patient may hardly be able to bear weight. The paresthesias usually begin as painful symptoms suggesting involvement of the smaller peripheral nerves that conduct sensory rather than motor impulses. Motor neuropathy follows with weakness; stretch reflexes are preserved until relatively late (21).

Mental changes are also frequent and may include poor concentration, irritability, somnolence, and occasional frank delirium; these may ultimately progress to coma. In serious or fatal cases of thallium poisoning, pseudobulbar paralysis due to peripheral neuritis of the cranial nerves is observed. In addition, paralysis of the ocular muscles, ptosis, strabismus, mydriasis, facial palsies, amblyopia, paralysis of the recurrent nerve, and optic atrophy accompanied by loss of vision have been noted (19,20).

Alopecia

Alopecia, which is usually due to a metabolic disturbance in the hair follicle, may occur simultaneously with severe polyneuritis approximately 14 days after exposure to thallium. It usually involves the entire scalp except for a small strip in the frontal area. Axillary, pubic, and facial hair may also be spared. Typically, a black pigmentation appears in the root of the hair and extends over its entire width. This is said to be specific for thallium and may be seen with the aid of a microscope. By the third week there is usually complete alopecia. If the patient recovers, normal growth usually ensues (18).

Aldrich–Mees Lines

Nail growth is impaired for a certain period, resulting in the appearance by the third or fourth week of typical semilunar white lines across the nails that parallel the growth of the nail and move toward the free edge. This is similar to Aldrich–Mees lines seen in arsenic poisoning (20).

Miscellaneous

Toxic psychosis and seizures that may proceed to status epilepticus, central necrosis of the liver, and damage to the renal tubular epithelium may also occur in thallium poisoning. Autonomic disturbances such as fever, tachycardia, labile blood pressure, orthostatic hypotension, urinary retention, constipation, xerostomia, and cardiac dysrhythmias also frequently occur.

Laboratory Analysis

Laboratory clues in diagnosis of thallium poisoning include slightly lowered serum potassium and a mild hypochloremic metabolic alkalosis due to the effects of thallium on the renal tubule (18). Examination of hair by chemical means is not useful because, unlike other metals, thallium is not incorporated into the hair matrix. Thallium concentrations in urine can be determined, and because thallium is not a normal constituent of the body any concentration may be considered significant (22).

Treatment

There is no known substance that can neutralize thallium that has been absorbed and fixed in the tissues, especially nervous system tissue. No treatment has been shown unequivocally to hasten excretion or to prevent death or permanent systemic damage (22). Thallium poisoning appears to be refractory to most antidotal agents, including chelating agents such as dimercaprol, calcium EDTA, and penicillamine. All antidotes proposed only neutralize the thallium in the intestinal tract and the percentage that, after reabsorption, is excreted into the colon. Both diphenylthiocarbazone (Dithizon) and diethyldithiocarbamate (Dithiocarb) have been suggested as antidotes because of their ability to form readily excreted complexes with thallium, but there has been limited experience with their use in humans. Recently, it has been shown that diethylthiocarbamate causes CNS toxicity by redistributing thallium to the CNS; it should, therefore, not be used until more information is available about its efficacy (18).

Gastric lavage with 1% sodium iodine should be performed as soon as possible after the diagnosis is made because it may be useful in converting the soluble thallium sulfate into insoluble thallium iodide. Oral administration of prussian blue (potassium ferric ferrocyanide) takes advantage of the high concentration of thallium in gastric secretions and in bile. Prussian blue is not absorbed from the gastrointestinal tract, and at the alkaline pH in small bowel, thallium is substituted for potassium in the crystal lattice of the complex and is excreted in the feces. Prussian blue should be administered as a colloidal solution at 250 mg/kg/day combined with 15% mannitol or 70% sorbitol (16).

Prevention and correction of fluid and electrolyte disturbances are important considerations, particularly if diarrhea is severe. If tachydysrhythmias occur, use of lidocaine or propranolol may be indicated. Shock may require the parenteral administration of fluids or vasopressors (18).

Peritoneal dialysis, hemoperfusion, and hemodialysis have, so far, not been shown to reduce significantly the total body load of thallium, although it is clear that hemoperfusion is more effective than dialysis in removing thallium from the blood compartment (16,23).

ANTICOAGULANT COMPOUNDS

Sweet clover disease was first described in 1924 as a hemorrhagic disorder of cattle following ingestion of spoiled clover silage. By 1939, bishydroxycoumarin was isolated from silage and identified as the toxic agent. Subsequently, warfarin (acetonylbenzylhydroxycoumarin)

TABLE 79–9. *Anticoagulant compounds used in rodenticides*

Hydroxycoumarins
Warfarin
Coumachlor
Long-acting hydroxycoumarins ("superwarfarins")
Warfarin-type
Brodifacoum
Bromadialone
Difenacoum
Indanedione-type
Chlorophacinone
Diphacinone
Pindone
Valone

has been shown to be about 50 times more lethal to rodents and so, warfarin has been used as a rodenticide as a 0.5% powdered concentrate (Table 79–9) (24). Common rats have appeared to show resistance to the regular warfarin rodenticides because of a reduction in the efficiency of vitamin K metabolism; this is a heritable factor. Because of this several "superwarfarin " compounds have been developed in the last decade to combat warfarin-resistant rat populations in the United States, Europe, and the United Kingdom (25). These derivatives of 4-hydroxycoumarin (brodifacoum, Talon; difenacoum, chlorophacinone, and bromodialone) possess 100 times the activity and at least 3 times the duration of action of the parent compound (Table 79–9) (26–28). All these compounds are available in supermarkets, drugstores, and hardware stores (Table 79–10) (30).

The indanedione anticoagulants contain many compounds that also have a longer duration of action than warfarin and are also referred to as superwarfarin compounds. These, too, induce profound changes in coagulation parameters (31), including chlorophacinone, diphacinone, pindone, and valone (Table 79–9). More caution is indicated with indanediones that are available in higher concentration baits than with 4-hydroxycoumarin compounds (32,33).

Anticoagulants have caused human intoxication in connection with therapeutic overdosage, homicide attempts, suicide attempts, and accidental substitution (3,29).

Pharmacokinetics

The superwarfarins exhibit two characteristics related to the increased rodenticidal activity and prolonged human toxic effects. First, these compounds bind irreversibly to epoxide reductase with 100-fold greater affinity than warfarin (34). Second, their pharmacologic half-life of 37 hours is at least 3 times that of warfarin (35). The longer duration of action for 2 to 5 days of these derivatives results from increased binding to lipophilic sites in the liver and, perhaps, in adipose tissue with prolonged release from these storage sites. The pharmacokinetics of brodifacoum in humans are unknown and the pharmacokinetics of the other superwarfarins have not been studied (25).

TABLE 79–10. *Hydroxycoumarin rodenticides by trade name*

Agicide rat and mouse bait
Black Flag rat and mouse killer
Black Jack mouse and rat killer
D-con
Hot Shot rat killer
Kelley's red mix
Parsons rat killer
Rat-kill
Ro-do
Speckman's Deth-rat
Vam-o
Voo-doo 42
Zord rodenticide

Mechanism of Action

The vitamin K-dependent blood proteins are synthesized in the liver in a precursor form. All the anticoagulant rodenticides act by interfering with the synthesis of vitamin K of which is essential for normal blood coagulation because it is a cofactor for the postribosomal synthesis of clotting factors II, VII, IX, and X (36); suppression of the hepatic formation of prothrombin and of factors VII, IX, and X produces clotting defects (Fig. 79–1). In addition, anticoagulant rodenticides cause direct capillary damage.

Warfarin and related compounds interfere with clotting factor synthesis by blocking the vitamin K-dependent gamma-carboxylation of glutamic acid residues in precursors of clotting factors II, VII, IX, and X (27). The warfarin receptor is thought to be associated with the enzyme vitamin K epoxide reductase. This enzyme is responsible for the continuous regeneration of vitamin K in the physiologically important vitamin K-epoxide cycle. During this cycle, vitamin K1 is converted to a biologically inactive metabolite called vitamin K1-2,3-epoxide. This epoxide is reduced back to the vitamin by a microsomal epoxide reductase. Because the coumarin anticoagulants inhibit the epoxide reductase step, they are referred to as indirect antagonists of vitamin K (36).

Warfarin is hydroxylated to inactive compounds by the mixed-function oxidase enzymes in the hepatic microsomes. These compounds are then excreted in the urine.

The superwarfarins are 100 times more potent than warfarin (25) because they have a greater affinity for vitamin K1 epoxide reductase, interrupt the vitamin K1-epoxide cycle at more than one site, and have considerably more

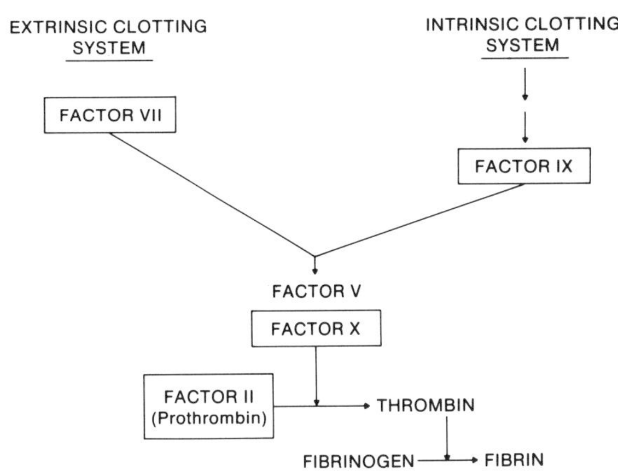

FIG. 79–1. Sites of warfarin action on the blood clotting system. Factors II, VII, IX, and X are inhibited.

anticoagulant ability than warfarin (27,37). The result is greater prolongation of clotting and prothrombin times. For example, brodifacoum and difenacoum have the same mechanism of action as warfarin but are far more powerful anticoagulants because of this increased duration of anticoagulation effect (38). The half-life of some long-acting anticoagulants may be as much as 10 times the average plasma half-life of warfarin (42 hours). In addition, they also have a larger apparent volume of distribution—approximately 6 times that of warfarin (0.17 L/kg) (39). Finally, there is a more sustained concentration of the long-acting preparations in the liver (40).

Because of the extreme differences in toxic potency and duration of action, it is of the utmost importance to differentiate long-acting compounds from that of warfarin (41).

Drug Interactions

There are many instances of drug interactions with warfarin and warfarin-like compounds. Mechanisms include interactions that increase plasma warfarin levels, alteration of the pharmacodynamics of warfarin without changing its plasma level, or by other mechanisms (Table 79–11).

Toxicity

Early after an overdose of a coumarin anticoagulant there are no discernible toxic signs and symptoms. Multiple doses of warfarin are usually required to cause alterations in anticoagulant activity; this does not appear to be true for the long-acting preparations. Bleeding may be the first manifestation of toxicity; if it is internal it may not be easily diagnosed. Later symptoms may consist of an upper gastrointestinal bleed, melena, epistaxis, cerebrovascular accident, easy bruising, and hematuria. Anemia, shock, and death may also occur.

Although the anticoagulant effect of warfarin can be expected to disappear within a few days, reports concerning human exposures to brodifacoum have been associated with clinical bleeding for more than 6 months. Slow systemic clearance and a large volume of distribution may explain brodifacoum's prolonged effect, whereas its potency may be due to hepatic accumulation, as evidenced by a high liver-to-serum ratio (42). The high lipid solubility and enterohepatic circulation of the long-acting anticoagulants are responsible for the prolonged duration of anticoagulant effects (43).

Diagnosis

Factitious purpura as a manifestation of warfarin ingestion is not an uncommon problem. Typically, it is seen in an emotionally disturbed patient with a history of mental illness. Acquired deficiency of the vitamin K-dependent blood coagulation proteins in an adult without vitamin K deficiency and without therapy with oral anticoagulants is

TABLE 79–11. *Drugs that alter prothrombin time by interacting with warfarin, according to type of interaction*

Pharmacokinetic (drugs that change warfarin levels)	Pharmacodynamic (drugs that do not change warfarin levels)	Mechanism unknown (drugs whose effect on warfarin levels is unknown)
Prolongs prothrombin time	**Prolongs prothrombin time**	**Prolongs prothrombin time**
Stereoselective inhibition of clearance of *S* isomer	Inhibits cyclic interconversion of vitamin K	Evidence for interaction convincing
Phenylbutazone	2nd- and 3rd-generation cephalosporine	Erythromycin
Metronidazole	Other mechanisms	Anabolic steroids
Sulfinpyrazone	Clofibrate	Evidence for interaction less convincing
Trimetoprim-sulfamethoxazole	Inhibits blood coagulation	Ketoconazole
Disulfiram	heparin	Flucomazole
Stereoselective inhibition of clearance of *R* isomer	Increases metabolism of coagulation factors	Isoniazid
Clinelidine[a]	Thyroxine	Piroxicam
Omeprazole[a]		Tamixifen
Nonstereoselective inhibitions of clearance of *R* and *S* isomers		Qunidine
Amiodarone		Vitamin B (megadose)
		Phenytoin
Reduces prothrombin time	**Inhibits platelet function**	**Reduces prothrombin time**
Reduces absorption	Aspirin	Penicillins
Cholestyramine	Other nonsteroidal antiinflammatory drugs	Griscofulvin[b]
Increases metabolic clearance	Ticlopidine	
Barbiturates	Moxalactam	
Rifampin	Carbenicillin and high doses of other penicillins	
Griscofulvin		
Carbamazepine		

[a]Causes minimal prolongation of the prothrombin time.
[b]Has been proposed to cause increased metabolic clearance.

due to accidental or factitious ingestion of vitamin K antagonists. Superwarfarin ingestion should be suspected in anyone who presents with an acquired bleeding disorder, prolongation of prothrombin time and partial prothrombin time, and a decrease in the levels of vitamin-K-dependent factors with no cause for vitamin K deficiency and no evidence of warfarin in the blood. The laboratory parameters that need to be monitored after superwarfarin ingestion are the same as those after warfarin ingestion. The prothrombin time becomes prolonged 24 to 36 hours after an overdose.

Laboratory Analysis

The principal diagnostic test for warfarin intoxication is a markedly reduced prothrombin time (44). Prolonged clotting and bleeding times may also be diagnostic indicators. With ingestion of the long-acting preparations, prothrombin activity should be monitored for a much greater period of time than is normally required for warfarin poisoning.

The superwarfarin agents are not detected in the serum warfarin assay. In addition, current toxicology screens of serum or urine do not identify superwarfarins. The analysis of vitamin K metabolites in serum is a sensitive method for detecting the presence of vitamin K antagonists. From these studies, one can make a presumptive diagnosis of anticoagulant poisoning allowing rational vitamin K therapy. Therefore, an elevated vitamin K epoxide–vitamin K ratio with undetectable warfarin levels strongly suggests an exogenous anticoagulant.

Treatment

Because deliberate ingestions usually involve large amounts, gastric emptying and activated charcoal are recommended in all such cases. Furthermore, vigilant follow-up and determination of prothrombin time is indicated over the next few days after ingestion. From a management perspective, all the anticoagulant rodenticides may be handled in the same way. Vitamin K specifically antagonizes the deficiencies associated with these anticoagulants, so that pharmacologic doses of vitamin K1 will provide the additional substrate necessary to resume the vitamin K1-epoxide cycle and continue the carboxylation process, thereby reversing the hypoprothrombinemia.

At present, there is no standard regimen for the administration of vitamin K1 as an antidote to coumarin anticoagulant poisoning. In the initial phases of poisoning, phytonadione (emulsified vitamin K1) is the preferred antidote rather than menadione or vitamin K3 (45). This is because the liver must metabolize vitamin K3 to vitamin K1, and this organ may be inhibited. The dose of vitamin K1 is 15 to 25 mg administered parenterally to an adult and 5 to 10 mg administered to a child. If the drug is administered intravenously, the dose should not exceed 1 mg/min (46). In a warfarin overdose, the duration of action of vitamin K may be shorter than normal and repeated administration may be necessary to restore clotting factor synthesis. Note that neither animal nor human data have been able to produce convincing recommendations for optimal vitamin K1 dosing (47). Theoretically, this dose should represent the total daily requirement which may vary greatly from individual to individual. High doses, up to 125 mg/day, have been used safely, titrated to the patient's coagulation status (38). Because the long-acting preparations can be detected in the urine for prolonged periods of time, oral vitamin K therapy can be used and may be necessary for at least 2 to 3 weeks (27); it may be required for as long as 1 year in some cases. Fresh frozen plasma may also be used as adjunctive treatment as necessary for serious bleeding episodes (48).

Adverse Effects

Phytonadione (vitamin K1) has been associated with anaphylactic deaths when given intravenously. Although this has usually been thought to occur only if the agent was infused rapidly, there have been reports of anaphylaxis occurring despite slow infusion of dilute phytonadione solutions. It is, therefore, recommended that this form of vitamin K be used intravenously only in acute emergencies where other routes are not feasible and the potential benefits outweigh the risks. Intramuscular and subcutaneous injections of phytonadione have not been associated with anaphylaxis; however, the former would be contraindicated in the face of a severe coagulopathy, and the latter, if not contraindicated, might result in slow absorption and delayed therapeutic effect.

Warfarin is hydroxylated to inactive compounds by the mixed-function oxidase system of the liver and then renally excreted. Phenobarbital can stimulate the activity of the microsomal oxidase system and has been used in some cases of superwarfarin poisoning to attempt to hasten degradation and excretion of the poison. Because of the lack of proven advantage of phenobarbital and the potential complications associated with sedating an anticoagulated patient, this therapy is unwarranted given the proven efficacy of vitamin K1 (49).

REFERENCES

1. Mortensen M: Management of acute childhood poisonings caused by selected insecticides and herbicides. *Pediatr Clin North Am* 1986;33: 421–445.
2. Maron B, Krupp J, Tune B: Strychnine poisoning successfully treated with diazepam. *J Pediatr* 1978;78:697–699.
3. Dipalma J: Human toxicity from rat poisons. *Am Fam Physician* 1981;24:186–189.
4. Simon F, Pickering L: Acute yellow phosphorus poisoning. *JAMA* 1976;235:1343–1344.
5. McCarron M, Gaddis G, Trotter A: Acute yellow phosphorus poisoning from pesticide pastes. *Clin Toxicol* 1981;18:693–711.

6. Marin G, Montoya C, Sierra J, et al: Evaluation of corticosteroid and exchange transfusion treatment of acute yellow phosphorus intoxication. *N Engl J Med* 1976;284:125–128.
7. Talley R, Linhart J, Trevino A, et al: Acute elemental phosphorus poisoning in man: cardiovascular toxicity. *Am Heart J* 1972;84:139–140.
8. Holt L, Holz P: The black bottle: a consideration of the role of charcoal in the treatment of poisoning in children. *J Pediatr* 1963;63: 306–314.
9. Peters K, Tong T, Katz K, et al: Diabetes mellitus and orthostatic hypotension resulting from ingestion of Vacor rat poison: endocrine and autonomic function studies. *West J Med* 1981;134:65–81.
10. Peters R, Spencer H, Bidstrup P: Subacute fluoroacetate poisoning. *J Occup Med* 1981;23:112–113.
11. Fretthold D, Sunshine F, Udinsky J, et al: Postmortem findings for a Vacor poisoning case. *Clin Toxicol* 1980;16:175–180.
12. Gallanosa A, Spyker D, Curnow R: Diabetes mellitus associated with autonomic and peripheral neuropathy after Vacor rodenticide poisoning: a review. *Clin Toxicol* 1981;18:441–449.
13. Benowitz N, Byrd R, Schamberlan M, et al: Dihydroergotamine treatment for orthostatic hypotension from Vacor rodenticide. *Ann Intern Med* 1980;92:387–388.
14. LeWitt P: The neurotoxicity of the rat poison Vacor. *N Engl J Med* 1980;302:73–77.
15. Jennings G, Ester M, Holmes R: Treatment of orthostatic hypotension with dihydroergotamine. *Br Med J* 1979;2:307.
16. Lehmann P, Favari L: Parameters for the adsorption of thallium ions by activated charcoal and prussian blue. *Clin Toxicol* 1984;22: 331–339.
17. Desenclos J, WIlder M, Coppenger G, et al: Thallium poisoning: an outbreak in Florida, 1988. *South Med J* 1992;85:1203–1206.
18. Davis L, Standefer J, Kornfeld M, et al: Acute thallium poisoning: toxicological and morphological studies of the nervous system. *Ann Neurol* 1980;10:38–44.
19. Moses H: Thallium poisoning. *Johns Hopkins Med J* 1978;142: 27–31.
20. Moeschlin S: Thallium poisoning. *Clin Toxicol* 1980;17:133–146.
21. Dumitru D, Kalantari A: Thallium poisoning. *Muscle Nerve* 1990;13:433–437.
22. Yokoyama K, Araki S, Abe H: Distribution of nerve conduction velocities in acute thallium poisoning. *Muscle Nerve* 1990;13: 117–120.
23. Kennedy P, Cavanagh J: Spinal changes in the neuropathy of thallium poisoning. *J Neurol Sci* 1976;29:295–301.
24. Hirsh J: Oral anticoagulant drugs. *N Engl J Med* 1991;324: 1865–1875.
25. Kruse J, Carlson R: Fatal rodenticide poisoning with brodifacoum. *Ann Emerg Med* 1992;21:331–336.
26. Jones E, Growe G, Naiman S: Prolonged anticoagulation in rat poisoning. *JAMA* 1984;252:3005–3007.
27. Barlow A, Gay A, Park B: Difenacoum (Neosorexa) poisoning. *Br Med J* 1982;285:541.
28. Bachmann K, Sullivan T: Dispositional and pharmacodynamic characteristics of brodifacoum in warfarin sensitive rats. *Pharmacology* 1983;27:281–288.
29. Fristedt B, Sterner N: Warfarin intoxication from percutaneous absorption. *Arch Environ Health* 1965;2:205–208.
30. Ross G, Zacharski L, Robert D, et al: An acquired hemorrhagic disorder from long-acting rodenticide ingestion. *Arch Intern Med* 1992; 152:410–412.
31. Park B, Scott A, Wilson A, et al: Plasma disposition of vitamin K1 in relation to anticoagulant poisoning. *Br J Clin Pharmacol* 1984;18: 655–662.
32. Lipton R, Klass E: Human ingestion of a "superwarfarin" rodenticide resulting in a prolonged anticoagulant effect. *JAMA* 1934;252: 3004–3005.
33. Mroczek W, Martin M: Warfarin-induced necrosis of skin. *Ann Intern Med* 1975;82:381–385.
34. Wells P, Holbrook A, Crowther N, et al: Interactions of warfarin with drugs and food. *Ann Intern Med* 1994;121:676–683.
35. Katona B, Wason S: Superwarfarin poisoning. *J Emerg Med* 1989;7:627–631.
36. Bell R: Metabolism of vitamin K and prothrombin synthesis: anticoagulants and the vitamin K-epoxide cycle. *Fed Proc* 1978;37: 2599–2604.
37. Watts R, Castleberry R, Sadowski J: Accidental poisoning with a superwarfarin compound (brodifacoum) in a child. *Pediatrics* 1990; 86:883–887.
38. Hoffman R, Smilkstein M, Goldfrank L: Evaluation of coagulation factor abnormalities in long-acting anticoagulant overdose. *J Toxicol Clin Toxicol* 1988;26:233–248.
39. Shearer M, Barkhan P: Vitamin K1 and therapy of massive warfarin overdose. *Lancet* 1979;1:266–267.
40. Murdoch D: Prolonged anticoagulation in chlorphacinone poisoning. *Lancet* 1983;1:355–356.
41. Chow E, Haley L, Vickars L, et al: A case of bromadiolone (superwarfarin) ingestion. *Can Med Assoc J* 1992;147:60–62.
42. Gurwitz J, Avorn J, Ross-Degnan D, et al: Aging and the anticoagulant response to warfarin therapy. *Ann Intern Med* 1992;116:901–904.
43. Hadler M, Shadbolt R: Novel 4-hydroxycoumarin anticoagulants active against resistant rats. *Nature (London)* 1975;253:275–277.
44. Lacy J, Goodin R: Warfarin-induced necrosis of skin. *Ann Intern Med* 1975;82:381–382.
45. Bjornsson T, Blaschke T: Vitamin K1 disposition and therapy of warfarin overdose. *Lancet* 1978;2:846–847.
46. Smolinske S, Scherger D, Kearns P, et al: Superwarfarin poisoning in children: a prospective study. *Pediatrics* 1989;84:490–494.
47. Weitzel J, Sadowski J, Furie B, et al: Surreptitious ingestion of a long-acting vitamin K antagonist/rodenticide, brodifacoum: clinical and metabolic studies of three cases. *Blood* 1990;76:2555–2559.
48. Chong L, Chau W, Ho C: A case of "superwarfarin" poisoning. *Scand J Haemotol* 1986;36:314–315.
49. Burucoa C, Mura P, Robert R, et al: Chorophacinone intoxication: A biological and toxicological study. *J Toxicol Clin Toxicol* 1989;27: 79–89.

ADDITIONAL SELECTED REFERENCES

Smith B: Strychnine poisoning. *J Emerg Med* 1990;8:321–325.

Gordon A, Richards D: Strychnine intoxication. *JACEP* 1979;8: 520–522.

Lambert J, Byrick R, Hammeke M: Management of acute strychnine poisoning. *Can Med Assoc J* 1981;124:1268–1270.

Teitelbaum D, Ott J: Acute strychnine intoxication. *Clin Toxicol* 1979;3:267–273.

Blain P, Nightingale S, Stoddart J: Strychnine poisoning: abnormal eye movements. *J Toxicol Clin Toxicol* 1982;19:215–217.

Edmunds M, Sheehan T, Van't Hoff W: Strychnine poisoning: clinical and toxicological observations on a nonfatal case. *Clin Toxicol* 1986; 24:245–255.

Sparagli G, Mannaioni P: Pharmacokinetic observations on a case of massive strychnine poisoning. *Clin Toxicol* 1973;6:533–540.

Herishanu Y, Landau H: Diazepam in the treatment of strychnine poisoning. *Br J Anaesth* 1972;44:747–748.

Baran R: Nail damage caused by weed killers and insecticides. *Arch Dermatol* 1974;110:467.

Sofola O, Odusote K: Sympathetic cardiovascular effects of experimental strychnine poisoning in dogs. *J Pharmacol Exp Ther* 1976;196:
29–34.

Dittrich K, Boyer M, Wanke L: A case of fatal strychnine poisoning. *J Emerg Med* 1984;1:327–330.

Boyd R, Brennan P, Deng J, et al: Strychnine poisuning. *Am J Med* 1983;74:507–512.

Oliver J, Smith H, Watson A: Poisoning by strychnine. *Med Sci Law* 1979;19:134–137.

Breckenridge A, Cholerton S, Hart J, et al: A study of the relationship between the pharmacokinetics and the pharmacodynamics of the 4-hydroxycoumarin anticoagulants warfarin, difenacoum and brodifacoum in the rabbit. *Br J Pharmacol* 1985;84:81–91.

Stowe C, Metz A, Arendt C, et al: Apparent brodifacoum poisoning in a dog. *J Am Vet Med Assoc* 1983;182:817–818.

CHAPTER 80

Insecticides

Pesticides represent a large group of chemicals that, in general, are described in terms of the organism they are intended to kill. Insecticides are pesticides used in the control of insects that may be either vectors of disease or destroyers of agricultural products. Insecticides include nicotine, organochlorines, pyrethrins, the acetylcholinesterase inhibitors, the organophosphates, and carbamates (1,2). This chapter is devoted to a discussion of the organochlorines which, for the most part, have been banned, and to a discussion of the pyrethrins, which are generally considered a safe group of insecticides (3). The acetylcholinesterase inhibitors are discussed in Chapter 81. Nicotine and strychnine are discussed in Chapters 83 and 84, respectively.

TABLE 80–1. *Chlorinated hydrocarbon insecticides*

Chlorinated ethane derivatives
Chlorophenothane (DDT)
Chlorinated cyclodienes
Chlordane
Dieldrin
Aldrin
Chlordecone (Kepone)
Endrin
Isobenzan
Heptachlor
Trichlor
Isodrin
Hexachlorcyclohexanes
Lindane (Kwell)

CHLORINATED HYDROCARBONS (ORGANOCHLORINES)

The chlorinated hydrocarbons were used extensively as insecticides from the mid-1940s until the 1960s and are now used only on a limited basis (4); many have been banned or severely restricted. Those still available are methoxychlor, kethane, and lindane.

Organochlorine insecticides comprise chlorinated ethane derivatives, of which chlorophenothane (DDT) is the best known; chlorinated cyclodienes, including chlordane, aldrin, dieldrin, heptachlor, and endrin; and other hydrocarbons, including such hexachlorcyclohexanes as lindane, toxaphene, and mirex (Table 80–1) (4).

Actions

Organochlorines are lipid-soluble, low-molecular weight compounds with a wide range of toxicities. Their principal action is generalized stimulation of the central nervous system by altering the transport of sodium and potassium ions across axonal membranes. Slowing of the repolarization of nerve cell membranes then results in the propagation of multiple action potentials for each stimulus (5).

All the chlorinated hydrocarbons have low water solubility; and because they are lipophilic, they generally distribute in parallel with the tissue concentration of total lipid (6). They are not well absorbed through the skin. They are degraded slowly in the environment and have been shown to accumulate in fish and animals, making them an environmental hazard (7). The widespread use of the organochlorine pesticides and other polyhalogenated hydrocarbons during the last 25 years has led to their ubiquitous presence in the environment.

Types of Organochlorine Insecticides/Chlorinated Ethane Derivatives (DDT)

DDT (trichloro-bis-p-chlorophenylethane), the prototype of the chlorinated hydrocarbons and of the chlorinated ethanes, was discovered during World War II and used with great success for controlling insect vectors of diseases such as typhus, malaria, and bubonic plague (8). The compound is credited with making as important contribution to human health as antibiotics (9). Extensive agricultural use of DDT did not begin until the late 1940s, when the compound became available for civilian use and was found to be effective for the control of a wide range of insects of agricultural importance. DDT has a wide margin of safety when used properly; and despite its previous widespread use, there is no documented, unequivocal report of a fatal human poisoning (9). Nevertheless, because of the accumulation of DDT in the animal kingdom and the environment, in 1972, DDT was banned in the United States for all but essential public health use and for a few minor uses in protecting crops for which there are no effective alternatives (10). A major reason for the Environmental Protection Agency ban of DDT was that it caused cancer in animals. DDT has been reported to induce liver tumors, lymphomas, and lung tumors in mice and liver tumors in some experiments with rats.

DDT is metabolized very slowly in human beings, so that DDT metabolites are detectable in the fat and sera of people long after exposures end. DDE (bis-p-chlorophenyldichloroethylene) is the principal metabolite stored in fat. Since 1951, there has been no progressive increase in human fat concentrations of DDT or DDE (8).

DDT acts primarily on the central nervous system, cerebellum, and higher motor cortex. DDT does not penetrate the skin well, and the dry powders and aqueous solutions are also poorly absorbed from the gastrointestinal and respiratory tracts (11).

Chlorinated Cyclodienes

Most chlorinated cyclodiene insecticides have been banned in the United States except for a few restricted and specialized uses. They are still used in some countries, however, and products containing them may still be found in American homes.

Seizures induced by the cyclodiene insecticides may be preceded by subjective complaints but frequently they occur with no prodromal signs and symptoms. Prodromal signs that have been reported include headache, visual disturbances, dizziness, diaphoresis, insomnia, nausea, vomiting, and malaise (7). An important difference between DDT and the chlorinated cyclodienes is that the latter are readily absorbed by intact skin (12).

Chlordane

Commercial chlordane contains chlordane, heptachlor, and trichlor (13,14). The results of human studies indicate that chlordane is even more dangerous than DDT. Chlordane was once widely used as an insecticide but currently is limited to professional underground application for termite control (15). Chlordane and heptachlor were banned from public use in 1976 (16). Human chlordane poisonings were never common, but even though the agent is no longer available to amateur gardeners, accidental poisoning still occurs (12).

Like most halogenated hydrocarbon insecticides, chlordane is slowly metabolized and is excreted primarily in the feces (17,18). Because of its storage in body fat, chlordane has a high degree of persistence and a high potential for cumulative neurotoxicity. Chlordane is absorbed dermally and by inhalation and is less toxic than heptachlor, to which it is chemically closely related (15).

Dieldrin, Endrin, and Isodrin

Dieldrin is the epoxide of aldrin that is also used as an insecticide. The corresponding stereo-isomers are endrin and isodrin. Endrin and isodrin are 2 to 3 times more poisonous than dieldrin and aldrin. Aldrin and dieldrin were banned in the United States as agricultural insecticides in 1974 (17). Especially when dissolved in oil, dieldrin is readily absorbed through the skin, respiratory mucosa, and the gastrointestinal tract. Dermal exposure results in systemic poisoning without skin irritation or local sensitization except secondary to the solvent or vehicle (17).

Hexachlorcyclohexanes

Although there are four common isomers of benzene hexachloride, the one most often used as an insecticide is γ-benzene hexachloride (lindane), which is commercially available as Kwell. γ-Benzene hexachloride is more properly called *hexachlorocyclohexane* because all the carbon double bonds in the benzene ring are saturated; benzene hexachloride is still used as a generic name for this compound, however (19). Lindane was formerly widely used as a crop insecticide in home and garden sprays and in products to control ectoparasites on livestock and pets. Although few human fatalities have occurred, many nonfatal poisonings have been reported (18).

Lindane is absorbed by all routes including the intact skin. It is more acutely toxic than DDT, although symptoms of poisoning are similar for both compounds. Some individuals appear to be more susceptible to poisoning by lindane than by DDT and violent tonic–clonic seizures have occurred in severe cases of acute poisoning. In addition, seizures and coma have been reported in children after prolonged topical use of lindane (12).

Kwell contains 1% lindane in a cream or lotion, which is intended principally for the treatment of scabies, and in a shampoo, which is intended for human and animal use in the treatment of head and pubic lice. When the toxicity of lindane is considered in the emergency department, it is important to distinguish between the topical form and the commercial-grade insecticide (18).

Lindane is partially metabolized in the liver to pentachlorophenol and other chlorinated phenols. Acute toxicity is very well recognized as stimulation of the central nervous system and convulsions, particularly in children. Chronic exposure induces liver enzyme activity and liver damage including tumor formation (19).

TABLE 80–2. *Features of poisoning with chlorinated hydrocarbon insecticides*

Paresthesia
Malaise
Headache
Nausea
Abdominal pain
Hyperexcitability
Muscle fasciculations
Seizures

Toxicity

The toxicity of the chlorinated hydrocarbons as a group varies widely. When absorbed systemically in significant quantities, any member of this group can produce paresthesias of the tongue, lips, and face; general malaise; headache; loss of appetite; nausea; vomiting; and abdominal pain (Table 80–2) (14). Neurologic manifestations include hyperexcitability, muscle fasciculations, and gross tremor, which may follow in rapid succession if the dose is sufficiently large. Seizures occur only with severe intoxication (12). The chlorinated cyclodienes stimulate the central nervous system (CNS) to a greater extent than DDT and tend to produce seizures before other less serious signs of illness appear (15). In addition, the chlorinated hydrocarbons sensitize the myocardium to epinephrine and may produce refractory ventricular dysrhythmias.

Treatment

Treatment for organochlorine poisoning consists of supportive therapy and decontamination. Therapy is directed toward efforts to remove the poison and to control the CNS effects including tremors and convulsions. Sympathomimetics such as epinephrine should be avoided because they may sensitize the myocardium and cause resultant refractory dysrhythmias. Diazepam or phenobarbital may be used to control seizures (18).

PYRETHRINS

Pyrethrum has been known and used as an insecticide for many years. *Pyrethrins* is a collective term that indicates naturally occurring insecticidal agents obtained from the flowers of the chrysanthemum plant (Chrysanthemum [Pyrethrum] cinerariaefolium) (Table 80–3) They can be prepared by drying and grinding the flowers to a powder (20). The powder may contain 1% to 3% of the active material. The pyrethrins are contained in most household insecticide sprays and powders. Pyrethrum is an insecticide found in more than 2,000 commercially available sprays and powders (21,22).

TABLE 80–3. *Pyrethrins and pyrethroids*

Allethrin
Barthrin
Bioallethrin
Bioresmethrin
Cyclethrin
Cypermethrin
Decamethrin
Dellamethrin
Dimethrin
Fenopropathrin
Fenvalerate
Flucythrinate
Fluvalinate
Jasmolin
Permethrin
Phenolthrin
Resmethrin
Tetramethrin
Transallethrin

Crude pyrethrum contains six active components formed by the combination of pyrethric acid and chrysanthemic acid with the three alcohols pyrethrolone, cinerolone, and jasmolone. The three esters of chrysanthemic acid are pyrethrin I, cinerin I, and jasmolin I, and are known collectively as the pyrethrins I fraction. The pyrethric acid esters are called pyrethrins II, cinerin II, and jasmolin II and comprise the pyrethrins II fraction.

Pyrethrin I is the most active for killing insects and pyrethrin II for rapid "knock-down" (21). These agents are toxic to houseflies, fleas, chiggers, mosquitoes, and the various body lice (23). The pyrethrins are not miticidal and are, therefore, not effective for the treatment of scabies. Pyrethrins have low toxicity to humans and are rapidly metabolized and leave virtually no residuum in the atmosphere. The pyrethrins are less toxic to mammals than all the other major classes of insecticide (21,24).

Synthetic Pyrethrins

Synthetic pyrethrins, called *pyrethroids*, are generally more effective at killing insects than the pyrethrins (Table 80–4). There are two classes of pyrethroids based on the chemical composition and clinical signs produced in poisoned animals (25). Type I pyrethroids (permethrin and resmethrin) lack an α-cyano group; poisoning by these compounds is characterized by ataxia, hyperexcitability, seizures, and tremors. Type II pyrethroids contain the α-cyano group (fenvalerate, dellamethrin, and cypermethrin). Poisoning by these compounds may involve inhibition of γ-aminobutyric acid activity resulting in incoordination, seizures, excessive salivation, and coarse whole-body tremors (20).

The first synthetic pyrethroids was allethrin, which had about the same insecticidal activity as the natural pyrethrins. It was not long before other pyrethroids

TABLE 80–4. *Signs and symptoms of pyrethrin overdose*

Ingestion
Nausea
Vomiting
Diarrhea
Abdominal cramps
Numbness
Tremors
Allergic reaction
Inhalation
Rhinitis
Sneezing
Mucosal edema
Cough
Shortness of breath
Bronchoconstriction
Chest pain

were developed that had greater insecticidal activity than the natural components. The first of these was bioresmethrin, to be followed by tetramethrin and d-phenothrin. These early or first generation pyrethroids were also unstable to light, thus, limiting their use in agriculture and animal husbandry.

The more common pyrethrin formulations are extracted in a suitable solvent or vehicle for use as household, garden, pet, or livestock spray (26). The vehicle may be an "inert" propellant but commonly has a hydrocarbon base for spray applications intended for a more persistent result. Without the use of such vehicles, pyrethrins are rather short-acting. There are also preparations containing mixtures of hydrocarbons with organochlorines, carbamates, and organophosphates. Many times, the pyrethrins have a synergist such as piperonylbutoxide added to the compound. Piperonylbutoxide is a synthetic piperic acid derivative that has little or no insecticidal activity but that potentiates the pyrethrins by inhibiting the hydrolytic enzymes responsible for their metabolism. Piperonylbutoxide increases insecticidal activity by 2 to 10 times (26).

Absorption

Neither the natural nor the synthetic pyrethrins are believed to be significantly absorbed through the intact skin. Despite this low order of primary toxicity, skin and inhalation contact in sensitive individuals may result in severe cutaneous and pulmonary sequelae.

Contact dermatitis, usually limited to mild parethesias, has resulted in severe erythema and vesiculations and is the most common adverse effect of pyrethrin exposure (27).

Metabolism

The relatively low toxicity in mammals is due to rapid metabolic breakdown by ester cleavage and oxidation. Pyrethrins I and II are quickly detoxified by hydrolysis of the relatively stable ester linkage to chrysanthemumic acid and alcohol. The mixed-function oxidase system of mammalian liver microsomes is responsible for such enzymatic oxidations. By substrate competition, insecticidal synergists, like piperonyl butoxide, are capable of inhibiting this system of liver enzymes (27). The implication is that the synergist might limit the enzymatic detoxification of some pyrethrins and ultimately enhance their toxicity.

Laboratory

No common laboratory tests are available to the emergency physician that have diagnostic or prognostic value. Plasma levels, even where available, are not clinically useful.

Toxicity

The belief that pyrethrins are nontoxic to humans appears to be well founded. Workers have handled the pure pyrethrins and doses have been taken orally without ill effect (21). Neither the natural nor the synthetic pyrethrins is significantly absorbed through intact skin (26). The main effect in sensitive individuals is an allergic reaction sometimes consisting of bronchoconstriction. Dermatitis secondary to the pyrethrins usually occurring after chronic exposure has also been noted (25). Paresthesias have been reported with the chronic use of one of the pyrethrins (22). More severe systemic reactions have not been reported (22,28). Asthma, vasomotor rhinitis, and anaphylaxis have also been reported.

Ingestion

Massive oral exposure may precipitate a neurologic syndrome ranging from numbness, excitability, tremors, and incoordination to paralysis and/or seizures (Table 80–4). It has been reported that death after massive oral doses may be due to respiratory failure. Oral and inhalation exposure has caused nausea, abdominal cramping, vomiting, and diarrhea (20).

Inhalation

The clinical manifestation of inhalation exposure to pyrethrins can be local or systemic in nature (27). Localized reactions confined to the upper respiratory tract include rhinitis, sneezing, scratchy throat, oral mucosal edema, and even laryngeal mucosal edema. Localized reactions of the lower respiratory tract are depicted by cough, shortness of breath, wheezing, and chest pain (29). A well-documented asthma-like reaction occurs with acute exposures in sensitized patients. Approximately 50% of persons sensitive to ragweed exhibit cross-reactivity to pyrethrum (20).

Treatment

Treatment of pyrethrin exposure is usually not necessary unless it is directed toward the allergic response. Decontamination is usually all that is necessary. Antihistamines may relieve allergic signs and symptoms. If the patient is manifesting bronchoconstriction, a bronchodilator should be administered. Kerosene and naphtha, which are common solvents in pyrethrin sprays, are generally more hazardous than the pyrethrins, and treatment may have to be directed toward effects of exposure to these compounds (28).

Pulmonary and allergic sequelae are treated symptomatically with airway maintenance, oxygen, and ventilatory assistance as dictated by patient status. Circulatory support may require intravenous fluids and, rarely, pressor agents. Pharmacologic treatment of bronchospasm and anaphylaxis uses the standard drugs and management protocols.

REFERENCES

1. De Palma A, Kwalick D, Zukerberg N: Pesticide poisoning in children. *JAMA* 1970;211:1979–1981.
2. Kline S, Bayer M: Insecticide poisoning. *Top Emerg Med* 1979;1: 73–83.
3. Hayes W: Epidemiology and general management of poisoning by pesticides. *Pediatr Clin North Am* 1970;17:629–644.
4. Sato A, Nakajima T: A structure-activity relationship of some chlorinated hydrocarbons. *Arch Environ Health* 1979;34:69–75.
5. Sanborn G, Selhorst J, Calabrese V, et al: Pseudotumor cerebri and insecticide intoxication. *Neurology* 1979;29:1222–1227.
6. Olson D, Sax L, Gunderson P, et al: Pesticide poisoning surveillance through regional poison control centers. *Am J Pub Health* 1991;81: 750–753.
7. Guzelian P, Vranian G, Boylan J, et al: Liver structure and function in patients poisoned with chlordecone. *Gastroenterology* 1980;78: 206–213.
8. Kreiss K, Zack M, Kimbrough R, et al: Cross-sectional study of a community with exceptional exposure to DDT. *JAMA* 1981;245: 1926–1930.
9. Wilson D, Locker D, Ritzen C, et al: DDT concentrations in human milk. *Am J Dis Child* 1973;125:814–817.
10. Rugman F, Cosstick R: Aplastic anaemia associated with organochlorine pesticide: case reports and review of evidence. *J Clin Pathol* 1990;43:98–101.
11. Austin H, Keil J, Cole P: A prospective follow-up study of cancer mortality in relation to serum DDT. *Am J Public Health* 1989;79: 43–46.
12. Rasmussen J: The problem of lindane. *J Am Acad Dermatol* 1981;5: 507–516.
13. Kutz F, Strassman S, Sperling J, et al: A fatal chlordane poisoning. *J Toxicol Clin Toxicol* 1983;20:167–174.
14. Olanoff L, Bristow W, Colcolough J, et al: Acute chlordane intoxication. *J Toxicol Clin Toxicol* 1983;20:291–306.
15. Aldrich F, Holmes J: Acute chlordane intoxication in a child: case report with toxicological data. *Arch Environ Health* 1969;19: 129–132.
16. Wang H, MacMahon B: Mortality of workers employed in the manufacture of chlordane and heptachlor. *J Occup Med* 1979;21:745–748.
17. Curley A, Garrettson L: Acute chlordane poisoning: clinical and chemical studies. *Arch Environ Health* 1969;18:211–215.
18. Morgan S, Stockdale E, Roberts R, et al: Anemia associated with exposure to lindane. *Arch Environ Health* 1980;35:307–310.
19. Kassner J, Maher T, Hull K, et al: Cholestyramine as an adsorbent in acute lindane poisoning: a murine model. *Ann Emerg Med* 1993;22: 1392–1397.
20. Paton D, Walker J: Pyrethrin poisoning from commercial-strength flea and tick spray. *Am J Emerg Med* 1988;6:232–235.
21. Casida J, Gammon D, Glickman A, et al: Mechanism of selective action of pyrethroid insecticides. *Annu Rev Pharmacol Toxicol* 1983; 23:413–438.
22. Knox J, Tucker S, Flannigan S: Paresthesia from cutaneous exposure to a synthetic pyrethroid insecticide. *Arch Dermatol* 1984;120: 744–746.
23. Smith D, Walsh J: Treatment of pubic lice infestation: a comparison of two agents. *Cutis* 1980;26:618–619.
24. Elliott M, Farnham A, Janes N, et al: Potent pyrethroid insecticides from modified cyclopropane acids. *Nature (London)* 1973;244: 456–457.
25. Martin J, Hester K: Dermatitis caused by insecticidal pyrethrum flowers. *Br J Dermatol Syph* 1941;53:127–142.
26. Taplin D, Meinking T: Pyrethrins and pyrethroids in dermatology. *Arch Dermatol* 1990;126:213–221.
27. Paton D, Walker J: Pyrethrin poisoning from commercial strength flea and tick spray. *Am J Emerg Med* 1988;232–235.
28. Carlson J, Villaveces J: Hypersensitivity pneumonitis due to pyrethrum. *JAMA* 1977;237:1718–1719.
29. Wax P, Hoffman R: Fatality associated with inhalation of a pyrethrin shampoo. *J Toxicol Clin Toxicol* 1994;32:457–460.

ADDITIONAL SELECTED REFERENCES

Arterberry J, Bonifaci R, Nash E, et al: Potentiation of phosphorus insecticides by phenothiazine derivatives: possible hazard, with report of a fatal case. *JAMA* 1962;182;110–112.

Benowitz N, Lake T, Keller K, et al: Prolonged absorption with development of tolerance to toxic effects after cutaneous exposure to nicotine. *Clin Pharmacol Ther* 1987;42:119–120.

Curley A, Kimbrough R: Chlorinated hydrocarbon insecticides in plasma and milk of pregnant and lactating women. *Arch Environ Health* 1969;18:156–164.

Hayes W, Curley A: Storage and excretion of dieldrin and related compounds: effect of occupational exposure. *Arch Environ Health* 1968; 16:155–162.

Hruban Z, Schulman S, Warner N, et al: Hypoglycemia resulting from Insecticide poisoning: report of a case. *JAMA* 1963;184:590–594.

Maibach H, Feldmann R, Milby T, et al: Regional variation in percutaneous penetration in man. *Arch Environ Health* 1911;23:208–211.

Thomas C, Aust S: Free radicals and environmental toxins. *Ann Emerg Med* 1986;15:1075–1083.

Warren M, Conrad J, Bocian J, et al: Clothing-borne epidemic. *JAMA* 1963;184:94–96.

Wolfe H, Durham W, Walker K, et al: Health hazards of discarded pesticide containers. *Arch Environ Health* 1961;3:531–537.

Young R, Jung F, Ayer H: Phorate intoxication at an insecticide-formulating plant. *An Ind Hyg Assoc J* 1979;40:1013–1016.

Byard J: Mechanisms of acute human poisoning by pesticides. *Clin Toxicol* 1979;14:187–193.

Zavon M: Poisoning from pesticides: Diagnosis and treatment. *Pediatrics* 1974;54:332–336.

Gehlbach S, Williams W, Perry L, et al: Nicotine absorption by workers harvesting green tobacco. *Lancet* 1975;1:478–480.

Manoguerra A, Freeman D: Acute poisoning from the ingestion of Nicotiana glauca. *J Toxicol Clin Toxicol* 1983; 19:861–864.

Gehlbach S, Williams W, Perry L, et al: Green tobacco sickness. *JAMA* 1974;229:1880–1883.

Mensch A: Nicotine overdose after a single piece of nicotine gum. *Chest* 1984;86:801–802.

Connolly G, Winn D, Hecht S, et al: The reemergence of smokeless tobacco. *N Engl J Med* 1986;314: 1020–1027.

Belanger G, Poulson T: Smokeless tobacco: a potential health hazard for children. *Pediatr Dent* 1983;5: 266–269.

Horan J, Linberg S, Hackett G: Nicotine poisoning and rapid smoking. *J Consult Clin Psychol* 1977;45: 344–347.

Battersby E, Cable J: Nicotine poisoning. *N Z Med J* 1964;63:367–369.

Garcia-Estrada H, Fischman C: An unusual case of nicotine poisoning. *Clin Toxicol* 1977;10:391–393. Rosenberg J, Benowitz N, Jacob P, et al: Disposition kinetics and effects of intravenous nicotine. *Clin Pharmacol Ther* 1980;28:517–522.

Kozlowski L, Appel C, Frecker R, et al: Nicotine, a prescribable drug available without a prescription. *Lancet* 1982;1:334.

McNabb M, Ebert R, McCusker K: Plasma nicotine levels produced by chewing nicotine gum. *JAMA* 1982; 248:865–868.

Malizia G, Andreucci G, Alfani F, et al: Acute intoxication with nicotine alkaloids and cannabinoids in children from ingestion of cigarettes. *Hum Toxicol* 1983;2:315–316.

Saxena K, Scheman A: Suicide plan by nicotine poisoning: A review of nicotine toxicity. *Vet Hum Toxicol* 1985; 27:495–497.

Atland P, Rattner B: Effects of nicotine and carbon monoxide on tissue and systemic changes in rats. *Environ Res* 1979;19:202–212.

Tonnesen P, Norregaard J, Sinonsen K, et al: A double-blind trial of a 16-hour transdermal nicotine patch in smoking cessation. *N Engl J Med* 1991;325:311–315.

Lavoie F, Harris T: Fatal nicotine ingestion. *J Emerg Med* 1991;9: 133–136.

Benowitz N: Cigarette smoking and nicotine addiction. *Med Clin N Amer* 1992;76:415–437.

Hipke M: Green tobacco sickness. *South Med J* 1993;86:989–992.

CHAPTER 81

AChE Inhibitors

The acetylcholinesterase (AChE) inhibitor insecticides comprise two distinctly different chemical groups that have the same basic mechanism of action but different toxicities. These two groups are the *organophosphates* and the *carbamates* (1). The organophosphate insecticides are most often involved in serious human poisoning (2–4). Formulations range from less than 1% to more than 95% of pure material. To date, several thousand organophosphate compounds have been synthesized, and more than 100 different products are currently marketed (5). Usually, organophosphates sold for household use are more dilute formulations (about 1% to 2%) compared to those sold for agricultural use (40% to 50%) (6). Access to these types of insecticides is difficult to control because of their overwhelming availability. They are found in flea collars, ant traps, fly paper, and various sprays for domestic and garden use; and they are used commercially to a great extent (7,8).

HISTORY

The organophosphates were produced during World War II when the Germans were unable to use nicotine as a pesticide and sought new compounds that could act as both insecticides and lethal gases (1). Scientists developed refinements of the alkyl esters of phosphoric acid, which were the prototypical organic phosphates that proved to be more effective as insecticides than nicotine and also very effective nerve gas. The most toxic of the organophosphates have been stockpiled as nerve gas for possible use in chemical warfare. Sarin and soman are two examples of these gases (9,10).

CLINICAL USES OF ACETYLCHOLINESTERASE INHIBITORS

The carbamates have been used in the treatment of myasthenia gravis and glaucoma (Table 81–1) (7). Carbamate use has decreased for these conditions because of the narrow margin of safety between therapeutic and toxic doses (5). The carbamates have also been used in the treatment of tachydysrhythmias and anticholinergic overdose (11).

TABLE 81–1. *Clinical uses of acetylcholinesterase inhibitors*

Myasthenia gravis
Glaucoma
Supraventricular tachydysrhythmias
Treatment of anticholinergic poisoning

ACETYLCHOLINESTERASE INHIBITORS AS INSECTICIDES

Like the chlorinated hydrocarbons, the acetylcholinesterase inhibitors have increased the yield of agricultural produce and have helped control insect vectors of malaria and other diseases (12). But, unlike the chlorinated hydrocarbons, the acetylcholinesterase inhibitors are rapidly hydrolyzed and, thus, residues of these materials on food have not been a problem (2). In addition, they do not accumulate in the environment or in the animal body. Because of these essential properties, they have replaced DDT (trichloro-bis-p-chlorophenylethane) and other chlorinated hydrocarbons. They do, however, have acute toxic effects and have caused numerous fatalities in humans and animals (13,14).

ABSORPTION

The organophosphate insecticides are absorbed by all routes, including the skin, gastrointestinal tract, conjunctiva, and respiratory tract. Clothing-borne epidemics have also been reported (15). Absorption in most instances of occupational poisoning has been through the skin and respiratory tract (16). The oral route is seen in those individuals who purposefully ingest the compound (17,18).

The carbamates are not appreciably absorbed through the intact skin and typically do not cause toxicity by this route (19,20).

TYPES OF CHOLINESTERASE

There are two general types of cholinesterase in the human body (2). Most cholinesterase in the nervous tissue and erythrocytes is acetylcholinesterase, which is the "true" enzyme that has an almost specific affinity for the naturally occurring substrate acetylcholine (21). The nonspecific enzyme pseudocholinesterase is made in the liver and found in serum and has the ability to hydrolyze a wide range of naturally occurring and synthetic esters in addition to acetylcholine (12,22). Although both may be affected by the acetylcholinesterase inhibitors and both can be measured by laboratory methods, only acetylcholinesterase is specific for organophosphate poisoning (1).

MECHANISM OF NEUROTRANSMISSION

The acetylcholinesterase inhibitors are powerful inhibitors of carboxylic esterase enzymes, including acetylcholinesterase and pseudocholinesterase (23,24). Acetylcholine is the neurotransmitter at the postganglionic parasympathetic nerve endings, preganglionic nerves to parasympathetic and sympathetic ganglia, somatic motor nerve endings to striated muscle, and certain synapses in the central nervous system (Figure 81–1) (14,25). Normally, acetylcholine is released at the nerve ending, crosses to the neuroreceptor site, and effects an action potential (20). It is then released from the site and is hydrolyzed by the enzyme acetylcholinesterase (4). The breakdown of acetylcholine occurs when it binds to an anionic site on acetylcholinesterase. The acetyl moiety next combines with an ester site on the enzyme and remains as the rest of acetylcholine cleaves off to form choline. Finally, the acetyl portion is rapidly hydrolyzed from the enzyme to form acetic acid and reactivated enzyme (9,26).

Effect of Organophosphates on Neurotransmission

The organophosphates are similar in chemical structure to the cholinesterase molecule. These compounds interfere with the normal process of neurotransmission by inhibiting acetylcholinesterase as a result of firm binding of phosphate radicals from the organophosphate to the active (anionic) site of the enzyme (24). A phosphorylated enzyme complex is then formed that has a much greater affinity for the enzyme than acetylcholine and results in an overabundance of acetylcholine at the neuroreceptor (17,27). The overabundance initially stimulates and then paralyzes transmission in cholinergic synapses and nerve endings, sparing adrenergic synapses, and results in profound sustained stimulation of the autonomic nervous system, skeletal muscle, and central nervous system (14,28). Without pharmacological intervention, the covalent binding of the phosphate radical to the active site of the cholinesterase transforms it to an inactive protein (24).

The Effect of "Aging"

The last reaction that modifies the enzyme-inhibitor complex in such a way that the organophosphate compound and enzyme cannot be separated and the enzyme cannot be reactivated by oximes is called "aging," and involves the formation of a monophosphoric acid residue that is bound to the enzyme protein. Before aging has occurred, administration of nucleophilic oximes, such as pralidoxime chloride, can reactivate the phosphorylated AChE but such treatment is ineffective after aging.

Effect of Carbamates on Neurotransmission

The carbamates are also cholinesterase inhibitors similar in usage to the organophosphates, however, they do

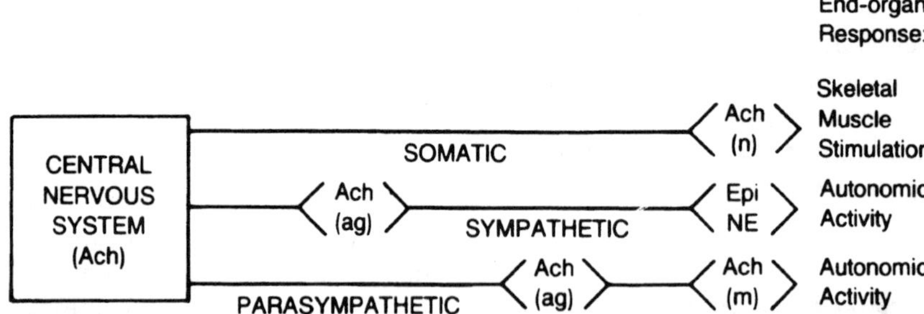

FIG. 81–1. Mechanism of transmission. Acetylcholine (Ach) in the central and peripheral nervous systems. Ach is the neurotransmitter at three peripheral sites: neuromuscular junction (n) and autonomic ganglia (ag) where nicotinic activity predominates; postganglionic parasympathetic receptors (m) where muscarinic activity predominates. In the CNS, nicotinic and muscarinic receptors are present. Norepinephrine (NE) acts at postganglionic sympathetic receptors, and epinephrine (Epi) is released from the adrenal medulla. Adapted from *Principles of Toxicology* 1984:129-152 by TA Gossel and JD Bricker, with permission of Raven Press. © 1984 Raven Press.

not contain a phosphate group and, therefore, have more reversible binding because the carbamate group can be cleaved off, although usually more slowly than the acetyl group of acetylcholine (20). Carbamates cause carbamolation of the ester site of the enzyme and, thus, prevent the enzyme acetylcholinesterase from de-esterifying acetylcholine. This complex is unstable, and spontaneous reactivation of cholinesterase occurs fairly rapidly (30). These compounds generally have a shorter duration of action and lower toxicity than the organophosphates. In addition, they do not cross the blood–brain barrier well, so that central cholinergic effects are absent or minimal. For most carbamates, a wider range exists between toxic and lethal doses than for the organophosphates (27).

Carbamates are often referred to as *reversible cholinesterase inhibitors.* This designation is not strictly correct because it implies that the carbamate is dissociated from the enzyme intact when in fact these compounds are covalently bound to the active site of the enzyme and are hydrolyzed in the same manner as acetylcholine (1).

CHARACTERISTICS OF ACETYLCHOLINESTERASE INHIBITORS

Organophosphates

The organophosphates that are of greatest toxicity are primarily used as agricultural insecticides to increase crop yield and decrease vectors of disease (Table 81–2). They include tetraethylpyrophosphate (TEPP), which is a direct-acting, water-soluble insecticide. TEPP was the first organophosphate insecticide; it was developed in the early 1800s but was considered too toxic for use.

Parathion, a chemical ester of thiophosphoric acid, is commercially available as a 25% emulsion or water-wettable powder or dust and is another very toxic agricultural insecticide (31–33). It is a yellow to dark-brown liquid of low vapor pressure that, because of its high toxicity, is not used in the home. It is one of the most commonly used agents in the United States and is responsible for a significant proportion of insecticide-related deaths. As little as one drop of concentrated material can be extremely dangerous (31). Most occupational accidents involving parathion are ascribed to dermal exposure (9). Although parathion is toxic, it is an indirect-acting compound that is converted by the liver to a more physiologically active and toxic form, paraoxon (5).

Phorate, mevinphos, demeton, disulfoton, and guthion are other very toxic agricultural insecticides. Generally stored as powders or emulsions, they are diluted by the user as needed.

TABLE 81–2. *Organophosphate pesticides in decreasing order of toxicity*

Highly toxic
Tetraethylpyrophosphate (TEPP, Bladan, Kilmite 40, Tetron, Kilmite, Vapatone)
Phorate (Thimet)
Disulfoton (Di-Syston)
Paraoxon (Mintacol)
Parathion (Thiophos, Etiolon, Alleron, Niagara Phoskil Dust)
Methylparathion (Dalt, Penncap-M)
Demeton (Systox)
Mevinphos (Phosdrin)
Sulfotepp (Bladafum, Dithione)
Methamidophos (Monitor)
Bomyl (Swat)
Guthion (Guthion)
Moderately toxic
Leptophos (Phosvel, Abar)
Diazinon (Diazide, Gardentox, Spectracide)
Ethion (Nialate)
Fenthion (Baytex, Entex, Sponon, Lysoff)
Coumaphos Acephate (Orthene)
Chlorpyrofos (Lorsban, Dursban)
Dimethoate (Cygon, Daphene, Defend)
Phostex Crufomate Merphos (Folex)
Trichlorfon (Dipterex, Dylox, Neguvon, Tugon)
Dichlorfenthion (Mobilawnr, Bromexr, Nemacider)
Fonofos (Dyfonate)
Dicrotophos (Bidrin)
Nalad (Dibrom)
Monocrotophos (Azodrin)
Phosphamidon (Dimercron)
Methidaton (Supacide)
Mildly toxic
Dichlorvos (DDVP, Vapona, No-Pest Strip)
Temephos (Abate, Abathion)
Chlorthion Malathion (Cythion, Karbofos, Malamar)
Ronnel (Korlan, Trolene, Viozene)

(Trade names).

From *JAMA* (1971;216:2131), © 1971, American Medical Association; and *Recognition and management of pesticide poisonings*, 3rd ed., by DP Morgan, U.S. Environmental Protection Agency, 1982.

Organophosphates of intermediate toxicity include coumaphos, crufomate, and trichlorfon. They are considered safe for use on domestic animals (7).

Organophosphates of low toxicity are available for use in the home and garden and include malathion, which is one of the most widely used organophosphates (34). Malathion is also one of the least toxic organophosphate insecticides, 100 to 1000 times less toxic than parathion (32,33). Like parathion, malathion is oxidized by the liver to malaoxon, which has stronger cholinesterase-inhibiting activity. Another less toxic organophosphate is dichlorvos, which is marketed as Vapona or DDVP and is incorporated into a plastic strip that slowly releases the vapor. DDVP is one of the few insecticides that have been tested directly on humans; it can be placed in the home and appears to be harmless when used as instructed.

Nerve Gas

The nerve agents are organophosphate compounds of a type first synthesized in 1850s, but their development as warfare agents did not occur until the 1930s. The first of the military nerve agents, known as tabun, or GA, was synthesized in 1936. Two years later, a second nerve agent was synthesized, now known as sarin, or GB. The four nerve agents are tabun, sarin, soman, and VX. Although commonly referred to as "nerve gas," these four agents actually exist under temperate conditions as clear, colorless liquids with high boiling points. They become aerosolized when dispersed by spraying or by an explosive blast from a shell or bomb.

Properties of Nerve Gases

Nerve agent vapors are four to six times denser than air. As a result, they tend to remain close to the ground and pose a risk, particularly to people occupying low areas and below-ground shelters. They are soluble in water as well as organic solvents and fat. After contact with water, they are hydrolyzed to products that are much less toxic than the parent compounds. Hydrolysis occurs slowly at neutral or acid pH but rapidly in the presence of alkali. As a result, alkaline solutions are effective decontaminates.

The "G-agents" are only moderately volatile; but due to their great toxicity, the vapors pose a significant inhalation hazard. Because of their tendency to evaporate, G-agents disperse within several hours and are described as nonpersistent. VX is much less volatile than the G-agents, but at ambient temperatures greater than 100°F, it also poses inhalation risks. It is a persistent agent that can remain where delivered for weeks or longer.

Although all four nerve agents are significantly hazardous by all routes and are percutaneous hazards, VX is least volatile and most efficiently absorbed through the skin.

Mechanism of Action

Like other organophosphate compounds, these agents act by binding to a serine residue at the active site of the cholinesterase molecule, thus, forming a phosphorylated protein that is inactive and incapable of breaking down acetylcholine (35). The resulting accumulation of toxic levels of acetylcholine at the synapse initially stimulates and then paralyzes cholinergic synaptic transmission.

The rate of aging varies greatly among the nerve agents. The half-time of aging is within minutes after soman exposure, about 5 hours after sarin exposure, and more than 40 hours after exposure to tabun and VX.

There is also evidence that nerve agents affect non-cholinergic mechanisms in the central nervous system (CNS). Antagonistic effects on GABA-ergic systems may explain convulsive activity after organophosphate poisoning.

Toxicity

Onset is more delayed after skin exposure to liquid nerve agents. A small droplet may cause no effects for as long as 18 hours. Clinical effects may occur 2 to 3 hours after thorough decontamination. Initial local effects of liquid, which are seldom noticed, include muscular fasciculations and sweating at the contamination site. A larger droplet also may cause gastrointestinal effects and complaints of malaise and weakness. Death after nerve agent exposure is due to respiratory failure resulting from depression of the respiratory center, paralysis of respiratory muscles, and obstruction caused by bronchospasm and bronchial secretions.

Metabolism of Organophosphates

The metabolism of parathion is typical of the organophosphates. There are two major routes of parathion metabolism: (a) hydrolysis to diethylphosphorothioate and paranitrol, and (b) oxidation of the sulfur moiety to give paraoxon. Paraoxon is then hydrolyzed to diethylphosphate and paranitrophenol (32).

Direct and Indirect Inhibitors

Some organophosphates are direct inhibitors of acetylcholinesterase, so that it is possible for them to produce local symptoms when absorbed from the eye, skin, or respiratory tract. Other compounds have only an extremely weak anticholinesterase action until they are transformed by the hepatic microsomal enzyme system to more toxic compounds. Serious illness caused by skin exposure to indirect inhibitors is, therefore, frequently delayed for several hours until the drug is metabolized (36). In massive poisoning, however, this lag may be absent.

Examples of direct inhibitors are TEPP and mevinphos, whereas parathion and malathion are examples of indirect-acting compounds (37). In addition, parathion and other compounds can be photo-oxidized outside the body to the more toxic metabolite, which then may enter the body and cause immediate symptoms (38).

Carbamates

Carbamate insecticides range from the highly toxic aldecarb, carbofuran, and tirpate, to the intermediately toxic aminocarb, bendiocarb, Bux, mimetan, and methomyl, to the minimally toxic fenethcarb and carbaryl (Table 81–3) (19). The carbamates are characterized by both a brevity

TABLE 81–3. *Carbamate insecticides*

Highly toxic
Aldecarb (Temik)
Carbofuran (Furadan)
Tirpate
Dimetilan (Snip Fly Bands)
Moderately toxic
Aminocarb (Matacil)
Bendiocarb (Ficam)
Befencarb (Bux)
Mimetan
Methomyl (Lannate, Nudrin)
Promecarb (Carbamult)
Methiocarb (Mesurol, Draza)
Propoxur (Unden)
Primicarb (Aphox, Rapid)
Minimally toxic
Fenethcarb
Ambenonium
Benzpyrinium
Carbaryl (Sevin)
Demecarium

(Trade names).

of action and a wide separation between the dose causing visible symptoms and the dose causing death.

Carbamates without insecticide activity have been used in medicine for many years (Table 81–4) (39). These include physostigmine for anticholinergic poisoning; pyridostigmine for myasthenia gravis; and neostigmine and edrophonium for paraoxysmal atrial tachycardia. These agents have been replaced by other more effective drugs (20).

TOXICITY

The general population is most likely to be exposed to organophosphates during domestic, garden, or medicinal use, or during accidental contamination arising from production, storage, transport, use, or disposal.

Clinical Features

Clinical manifestations of intoxication with the acetylcholinesterase inhibitors may be grouped according to whether the effects are muscarinic (from an overstimulation of the parasympathetic nervous system), nicotinic (from ganglionic and myoneural junction stimulation), or due to the action on the central nervous system (14). At low doses of organophosphates, muscarinic symptoms may predominate. In more severe intoxication, nicotinic and CNS symptoms may predominate. Acronyms have been devised for some of the signs and symptoms secondary to anticholinesterase inhibitor poisoning (Table 81–5 and Table 81–6).

TABLE 81–4. *Noninsecticide carbamates*

Edrophonium (Tensilon)
Neostigmine (Prostigmin)
Physostigmine (Antilirium)
Pyridostigmine (Mestinon)

TABLE 81–5. *Muscarinic effects of organophosphate and carbamate insecticide poisoning (Acronym: SLUG BAM)*

S	Salivation, secretions, sweating
L	Lacrimation
U	Urination
G	Gastrointestinal upset
B	Bradycardia, bronchoconstriction, bowel movement
A	Abdominal cramps, anorexia

Most organophosphate insecticides have a characteristic garlic odor, and patients who have ingested or absorbed these compounds usually retain such an odor on the breath, vomitus, or feces for several days (12). Organophosphates may be placed in another vehicle such as a hydrocarbon, in which case the hydrocarbon odor may be the primary odor (40).

Gastrointestinal effects are usually the first symptoms to appear after ingestion of these agents (Table 81–7). Sweating and muscle fasciculations may be noted early after dermal exposure and respiratory effects are first noted after inhalation (2). Clinical evidence of intoxication generally becomes apparent within a matter of minutes to an hour after the exposure (20), with the exact time depending on the severity and route of exposure. In mild intoxication, early complaints may be fatigue, headache, mild vertigo, weakness, loss of concentration, and blurred vision (11). Severe intoxication may result in muscular paralysis leading to sudden respiratory arrest (41); symptoms leading to death may occur within 5 minutes. The symptoms of organophosphate poisoning may be delayed especially if exposure is through skin application of an indirect acting agent (36). Compared with the organophosphates, the carbamates have a shorter duration of action and generally a lower toxicity; and although symptoms and signs of poisoning are similar, there is a more rapid decline of effects.

Muscarinic Effects

The muscarinic effects are usually the first to appear and may occur within minutes after exposure. Symptoms include headache, anorexia, nausea, sweating, blurred vision, epigastric and substernal tightness, and heartburn. More severe muscarinic symptoms may include abdominal cramps, vomiting, dyspnea, diarrhea,

TABLE 81–6. *Nicotinic effects of organophosphate insecticide poisoning (acronym: MTWtHF [days of the week])*

M	Mydriasis, muscle twitching, muscle cramps
T	Tachycardia
W	Weakness
tH	Hypertension, hyperglycemia
F	Fasciculations

TABLE 81–7. *Clinical features of organophosphate intoxication*

Muscarinic		Nicotinic	Central nervous system
Mild	Moderate to severe		
Anorexia Nausea Chest tightness Diaphoresis	Abdominal cramps Diarrhea Salivation Lacrimation Urination Defecation Wheezing Miosis Increased secretions Diaphoresis	Muscle twitching Fasciculations Cramps Weakness Mydriasis Tachycardia Hypertension Coma	apprehension Restlessness Giddiness Headache Tremors Ataxia Seizures

salivation, lacrimation, profuse sweating, pallor, wheezing, micturition, defecation, increased bronchial secretion, bradycardia, cardiac dysrhythmias, pulmonary edema, and miosis (20).

Miosis is one of the most characteristic signs and is seen in the early stages of almost all cases of moderately severe poisoning (14,42). Although miosis is often present, however, it is not a constant feature later in the exposure, and occasionally mydriasis may occur. Miosis develops as a consequence of marked parasympathetic stimulation of the iris, whereas mydriasis may be seen as a nicotinic effect of the organophosphates. Unilateral miosis by direct contact with a contaminated finger has also been noted (39).

Nicotinic Effects

The nicotinic effects of anticholinesterase inhibitor poisoning (Table 81–6) usually appear after muscarinic effects have reached moderate severity. These nicotinic effects may reflect a moderate to severe acute intoxication and may include muscle twitching and fasciculations (17). These symptoms are often first noted in the eyelids but in serious poisoning are more prominent in larger muscles (43). Muscle cramps and generalized and profound weakness may also be noted (44). These result from a depolarizing blockade of the neuromuscular junction. In addition, mydriasis, tachycardia, and hypertension may occur (45). Transient hyperglycemia and glycosuria are not uncommon findings in severe organophosphate poisoning and may simulate diabetic ketoacidosis (12,37,46). These nicotinic effects, as discussed earlier, have been attributed to stimulation of cholinergic preganglionic fibers to sympathetic ganglia and to the adrenal medulla as well as to a central increase in sympathetic vasoconstrictor tone.

Central Nervous System Effects

Organophosphates

In the CNS, acetylcholine receptors are distributed widely. With regard to organophosphate insecticide effects, the most important central nervous system locations are the respiratory and cardiovascular centers in the medulla (46). Central nervous system effects after organophosphate exposure are nonspecific and include anxiety, apprehension, restlessness, dizziness, giddiness, headache, tremors, ataxia, slurred speech, seizures, and coma (44).

Carbamates

Because the carbamates do not penetrate the central nervous system well, symptoms and signs are primarily muscarinic and nicotinic (30). If CNS symptoms do occur after carbamate poisoning, the possibility of a mixed intoxication or another cause should be strongly considered (1,39).

Causes of Death

Death from poisoning with acetylcholinesterase inhibitors usually results from respiratory failure caused by a combination of factors, including an overstimulation of all three receptor types (Table 81–8) (47). Bronchospasm, direct depression of the respiratory center with bradycardia and atrioventricular blocks, increased bronchial secretions, and decreased respiratory muscle strength all contribute (17). As mentioned, respiratory muscle paralysis results from nicotinic activity and excessive pulmonary secretions, bronchoconstriction, and pulmonary edema are consequences of muscarinic

TABLE 81–8. *Causes of death in acetylcholinesterase inhibitor exposure*

Muscarinic activity
Excessive pulmonary secretions
Bronchoconstriction
Pulmonary edema
Nicotinic activity
Respiratory muscle paralysis
Central nervous system activity
Respiratory center depression

activity (20,23), and respiratory center depression appears to be a centrally mediated event (19).

Intermediate Syndrome

The *intermediate syndrome* was first proposed as a distinct clinical entity in 1987. This syndrome occurs 24 to 96 hours after poisoning, after the patient has apparently survived the cholinergic phase of the overdose (5,48). Symptoms noted during this phase have been attributed to involvement of respiratory muscles as well as of muscles in the proximal limbs and of neck flexors. Paralytic symptoms have lasted as many as 18 days (49). Because of the respiratory muscle involvement, apnea may ensue. This syndrome is not responsive to atropine or pralidoxime and the patient may require ventilatory support (4).

Only certain organophosphates have been associated with the intermediate syndrome. These organophosphates are diazinon, bidrin, malathion, demethoate, methamidophos, monocrotophos, and parathion (Table 81–9) (50).

The clinical and EMG features of this syndrome do not correspond to any of the major human disorders of neuromuscular transmission. The clinical distribution of the involved muscles is reminiscent of myasthenia gravis, whereas depression of deep tendon reflexes is typical of the Eaton–Lambert Syndrome (51).

Many questions concerning the intermediate syndrome still have not been answered. Some of these questions involve the degree of environmental and genetic factors that influence the onset of this syndrome (52). It also appears that some organophosphates may have a higher affinity for nicotinic cholinesterases or distribute selectively to muscle producing a neuromuscular dysfunction that is longer lasting than at muscarinic sites (51). At present, we know very little about the type of damage at the motor end-plate or about risk factors associated with intermediate syndrome. It has been suggested that intermediate syndrome may be a manifestation of insufficient oxime therapy (53).

Delayed Neurotoxicity from Organophosphates

In addition to the intermediate syndrome, delayed neurotoxic effects of the organophosphates have also been reported 2 to 3 weeks after acute exposure and typically consist of a distal motor polyneuropathy (54). The cranial nerves and respiratory muscles are spared (4).

The mechanism of toxicity in delayed neurotoxicity is distinct from that in the acute phase. Effects are not responsive to either atropine or pralidoxime. The incidence of delayed toxicity after organophosphate poisoning is low (4).

The phosphorylation of a nervous system target protein called *neuropathy target esterase*, which has also been called *neurotoxic esterase* (54), has been considered to be a marker in animals of the subsequent development of a delayed neuropathy. A more accessible form of a similar human enzyme is found in peripheral blood leukocytes and platelets (55). At present, the monitoring of the peripheral form of the enzyme is being considered as a potential predictive test in humans for the development of a delayed neuropathy (56).

LABORATORY DETERMINATIONS

A diagnosis of intoxication is primarily based on a history of exposure to an organophosphate 6 hours or less before onset of illness and clinical evidence of diffuse parasympathetic stimulation. Laboratory verification is based on depression of plasma and red blood cell cholinesterase to activities substantially lower than those before exposure (Table 81–10) (2,57). To detect a decrease in activity, prior knowledge of a baseline activity measurement, which is unlikely, is required (58). Although having pre-exposure measurements of cholinesterase levels in individuals is preferred due to the narrower intra-individual variation, they are usually not available in cases with nonoccupational exposure to pesticides (59). In the absence of such pre-exposure measurements, sequential post-exposure measurements can be used to estimate the pre-exposure cholinesterase levels in the patients. In fact, the velocity of decline in cholinesterase activity is a more critical determinant than the absolute amount of the decline in predicting whether symptoms will manifest (58).

In actual practice, it is not feasible for laboratory determinations to aid in the diagnosis, but blood should be drawn in a heparinized tube before treatment is instituted, and the red blood cells and plasma should be separated by centrifugation and then frozen if they must be kept for

TABLE 81–9. *Organophosphates associated with the intermediate syndrome*

Bidrin
Demethoate
Diazinon
Malathion
Methamidophos
Monocrotophos
Parathion

TABLE 81–10. *Laboratory determinations in poisoning with acetylcholinesterase inhibitors*

Red blood cell cholinesterase
Serum cholinesterase
Alkylphosphate metabolites
Electrocardiogram
Chest roentgenogram
Serum electrolytes

analysis. The laboratory may, therefore, aid in confirmation because treatment must often be initiated before laboratory results are available (58).

Severe decreases in acetylcholinesterase activity are necessary before symptoms are seen. In acute poisoning, manifestations generally occur after more than 50% of red blood cell cholinesterase is inhibited; in mild poisoning, serum acetylcholinesterase activity is 20% to 50% of normal; in moderately severe poisoning, it is 10% to 20% of normal; in severe poisoning, it is less than 10% of normal (Table 81–11) (12).

There are clinically significant differences between the two cholinesterases. Depression of red blood cell (true) cholinesterase is considered a specific response to the organophosphates, whereas pseudocholinesterase activity may vary in a number of different diseases or toxic states, such as infectious hepatitis, chronic gastritis, chronic pneumonia, and carcinoma of the stomach and kidney, and in the malnourished elderly (Table 81–12) (58). In actuality, inhibition of pseudocholinesterase does not contribute to the cholinergic poisoning syndrome. Although the inactivation of plasma cholinesterase does not result in any significant deleterious effects, monitoring of plasma cholinesterase can be used to assess exposure to organophosphates with certain limitations (60).

If the red blood cell acetylcholinesterase has been completely and irreversibly inhibited by the organophosphates, recovery will take place at the same rate as new red blood cell regeneration (about 1% per day), whereas the enzyme in the plasma regenerates at a more rapid rate (approximately 25% in the first 7 to 10 days) (2,7). In severe poisoning, return to normal activity requires about 4 weeks for serum cholinesterase and about 5 weeks for erythrocyte cholinesterase (14).

In addition to cholinesterase activity, diagnosis of some of the organophosphates can be confirmed by detecting the poison or one of the alkyl phosphate metabolites, such as paranitrophenol, in blood or urine. These methods are typically used for monitoring purposes in the industrial setting, but it is unlikely that these tests would be available in an emergency setting (19).

An electrocardiogram should be obtained to examine for evidence of heart blocks and a chest roentgenogram, for evidence of atelectasis, aspiration, and pulmonary edema. Other laboratory findings that may be compatible with organophosphate poisoning but not diagnostic include hyperglycemia, hemoconcentration, leukocytosis, hypokalemia, acetonuria, and glycosuria (5). Hyperamylasemia and proteinuria have also been noted.

TABLE 81–11. *Serum acetylcholinesterase and symptomatology*

Percentage of normal	Symptoms
>50	No symptoms
20–50	Mild
10–20	Moderate
<10	Severe

TABLE 81–12. *Disease states that affect serum cholinesterase activity*

Acute infections
Anemia (some)
Carcinoma of stomach
Chronic gastritis
Chronic debilitating conditions
Chronic pneumonia
Malnutrition
Myocardial infarction
Parenchymal liver disease

TREATMENT

Exposure to the organophosphates and carbamates should be considered a medical emergency, and any patient with a diagnosis of insecticide poisoning should be hospitalized and kept under observation for at least 24 hours. Fatalities are usually the result of late recognition or inappropriate or insufficient therapy (5).

Treatment should consist of cardiopulmonary resuscitation, if necessary, and removal of the individual from further exposure (Table 81–13). Clothing, including boots and shoes, should be disposed of in plastic bags; and the skin should be decontaminated with generous amounts of soap or detergent and water. If possible, it is best that the patient be taken to a separate area for showering and instructed to wash the hair thoroughly and to clean the fingernails and the umbilicus (61). Oxygen should be administered and, if the compound was orally ingested, attempts should be made to retrieve the material with gastric lavage and subsequent administration of activated charcoal. A cathartic may not be necessary, especially if the patient already has diarrhea. Careful attention must be paid to the removal of secretions and maintenance of a patent airway. If pulmonary edema occurs it should be treated vigorously.

TABLE 81–13. *Treatment of poisoning with acetylcholinesterase inhibitors*

Cardiopulmonary resuscitation (if necessary)
Decontamination
Cardiac monitoring
Oxygen
Suction
Atropine
Adult: 2 to 4 mg or more as needed
Child: 0.015 to 0.05 mg/kg
Pralidoxime
Adult: 1 g over 15 to 20 minutes (repeat as needed)
Child: 25 to 50 mg/kg

If the patient is decontaminated outside the hospital facility, transportation to the hospital should be undertaken soon after decontamination is completed. Emergency department personnel should be notified in advance regarding the nature of the exposure so that proper arrangements can be made to avoid further contamination. The patient should be on a cardiac monitor because of the possibility of myocardial depression, heart block, or dysrhythmias. To avoid the possibility of respiratory arrest shortly after an overdose of organophosphates, patients should not be discharged from the hospital prematurely. If discharged, they should be informed to return if breathing difficulties appear (5).

Contraindicated Drugs

Drugs contraindicated in the treatment of acetylcholinesterase inhibitor intoxication include morphine and succinylcholine, as well as the methylxanthines, phenothiazines, barbiturates, and loop diuretics (Table 81–14).

Antidotal Therapy

The pharmacologic management of organophosphates relies on the administration of atropine, which ameliorates the muscarinic and CNS manifestations, and of pralidoxime, which ameliorates the nicotinic and CNS manifestations (2,17). Atropine should not be administered until cyanosis has been overcome because it may produce ventricular fibrillation in the presence of hypoxia (14).

Atropine acts by binding competitively to the same site as acetylcholine but without depolarizing the postsynaptic membrane (17). Nevertheless, it merely blocks certain actions of the acetylcholine already accumulated and does not reverse the fundamental biochemical lesion. The combination of both atropine and pralidoxime for organophosphate poisoning is more effective than either drug alone.

Poisoning with carbamate insecticides often does not require extensive treatment, and small doses of atropine may be all that is necessary (62). Pralidoxime is not necessary for carbamate poisoning, but if a patient presents with an unknown acetylcholinesterase inhibitor exposure, both atropine and pralidoxime should be administered because failure to administer pralidoxime can be lethal in an organophosphate poisoning (24).

Patients who require treatment with these antidotes should be observed closely and continuously for no less than 24 hours. Serious and sometimes fatal relapses can occur as a result of continuous absorption of the poison when decontamination is incomplete or if the effects of the antidotes dissipate.

TABLE 81–14. *Drugs contraindicated in the treatment of acetylcholinesterase inhibitor poisoning*

Barbiturates
Loop diuretics
Methylxanthines
Morphine
Phenothiazines
Succinylcholine

Atropine

Atropine blocks acetylcholine at the muscarinic receptors located primarily in smooth muscle and brain. Atropine is ineffective at nicotinic receptors located in striated (skeletal) muscle and sympathetic and parasympathetic ganglia. The significance of this receptor specificity is that atropine treatment fails to reverse muscle weakness and paralysis caused by acetylcholine accumulation at nicotine receptors. For this reason, even after atropine therapy, carbamate-poisoned patients may require ventilator support until AChE inhibition spontaneously reverses, and diaphragmatic and other respiratory muscle functions return.

Sufficient doses of atropine should be administered until muscarinic symptoms are relieved and signs of mild atropinization appear (63). Physicians unfamiliar with treating organophosphate poisoning tend to underdose with atropine; most fatalities occur as the result of underdosing. The dose of atropine may appear to be large, but the patient poisoned by cholinesterase inhibitors is able to tolerate it; failure to use the highest tolerable dose is far more serious than the effects of overdosage (64).

Because there is a possibility that hypoxic patients with pulmonary edema may develop ventricular tachycardia following atropinization, the hypoxia should be corrected with artificial ventilation if necessary before the administration of atropine (38).

Dosage

Atropine sulfate should be administered to an adult at a dose of 2 to 4 mg intravenously and should be repeated and/or increased until signs of atropinization appear. The pediatric dose of atropine is 0.015 to 0.05 mg/kg. Adequate atropinization is manifested by drying of secretions, dryness of the skin and mouth, mydriasis, flushing of the skin, and tachycardia. An important diagnostic clue is the failure of 1 to 2 mg of atropine to cause an anticholinergic effect. A mild degree of atropinization may need to be maintained for at least 48 hours; this should be titrated to the patient's physical signs. Although the average patient may need 40 mg of atropine per 24 hours, doses of more than 1 g per day have sometimes been required. Cases have been reported in which patients received up to 30 g of atropine over a 5-week period (65).

An atropine drip has been used by some physicians when patients require massive amounts of atropine for reversal of symptoms. A concentration of 1 mg/mL (100 1-mL vials) of atropine has been infused without dilution and titrated to effect (65).

Unlike agricultural organophosphate, insecticide patients who often require massive doses of atropine daily for a period of several days to weeks, the total dose required by nerve agent casualties over the first several hours usually is less than 20 mg.

Ipratropium has been effectively administered intratracheally, although there has been little experience with this regimen.

Pralidoxime

Pralidoxime (Protopam, 2-PAM), an oxime, was one of the few drugs ever developed based on the theory of how to correct a biochemical lesion (66). At least three soluble salts of pralidoxime are in use in different countries. Pralidoxime chloride, pralidoxime methane sulphonate, and obidoxime (Toxogonin) are identical in their action (67). In the United States, pralidoxime chloride is available and is probably safer than a number of other oximes studied. Unlike pralidoxime, obidoxime is able to cross the blood–brain barrier and to reactivate brain cholinesterases; however, this may not confer additional benefits over peripheral cholinesterase reactivators. Early work with obidoxime suggests that it has more side effects than pralidoxime.

Oximes are quaternary nitrogen-containing compounds that are thought to be unable to cross the blood–brain barrier and effect changes in the central nervous system (68). There is recent evidence, however, that this theory may not be correct (14,27,66,69,70). The most striking support for the central action of the oximes comes from clinical observations of prompt recovery from coma and seizures after the administration of pralidoxime not attributable to improvement in other parameters (14). Additionally, 2-PAM appears to reverse the CNS effects of organophosphate poisoning as evidenced by changes in EEG activity and reversal of coma without associated changes in other physiologic measurements (71).

Pralidoxime is specifically adapted to reactivate acetylcholinesterase by removal of the phosphate group bound covalently to the ester site. In patients with acetylcholinesterase inhibitor poisoning, removal of the phosphate group completely restores normal activity of the enzyme and can produce clinical improvement within minutes (1,17). It should be noted that oximes have been shown to benefit aldicarb intoxication (71).

Dosage

Pralidoxime is administered intravenously in a dose of 1 to 2 g in 100 mL of 5% dextrose in water over a 15-minute period (72,73). Recovery of consciousness and disappearance of toxic manifestations can occur within 10 to 40 minutes. The half-life of pralidoxime is 1 to 2 hours; and when manifestations recur in adult patients with severe poisoning, pralidoxime should be infused at a rate up to 500 mg/hour (12,14). Treatment of severe poisoning with pralidoxime may require higher doses or continuous infusions. Although there have not been any controlled studies to show the efficacy of continuous infusions (73), it has been suggested that the rate of 500 mg/hour be administered to a daily dose not to exceed 12 g in an adult. The initial pediatric dose of pralidoxime is 25 to 50 mg/kg (2). Plasma concentrations of 4 μ/mL are normally seen at the time of reversal of anticholinesterase effects of organophosphates (1).

Continuous Infusion

The continuous infusion of 2-PAM may offer several potential benefits in the treatment of organophosphate poisoning. First, the administration of a 2-PAM loading dose followed by a continuous infusion would permit rapid attainment of potentially effective serum concentrations that would be far below those previously associated with adverse effects (71). Accordingly, this form of therapy may reduce the occurrence of adverse effects previously associated with the intermittent, rapid intravenous infusion of larger doses of 2-PAM (65).

Second, continuous infusion of 2-PAM would be expected to produce sustained therapeutic serum concentrations that may more efficiently prevent the binding of the organophosphates to cholinesterases, thereby resulting in their sustained activation and continuous reactivation.

2-PAM therapy may be instituted with a 25 mg/kg intravenous dose given over 15 to 30 minutes, followed by a continuous infusion of 10 to 20 mg/kg/hour. Therapy with 2-PAM should be continued for at least 18 hours or longer, depending on the patient's clinical status and the properties of the suspected toxin. One would expect a continuous infusion rate of 10 to 20 mg/kg/hr to provide adequate serum concentrations of >4.0 mg/L for the management of organophosphate poisoning (71).

Timing of Treatment

Treatment with pralidoxime is more effective if it is started early because the alkyl phosphate of the organophosphate gradually undergoes a secondary irreversible reaction with the enzyme; this is known as aging. Inhibited acetylcholinesterase is not reactivated if it is already aged. This process of reversal is a time-dependent, nonenzymatic cleavage of the phosphate bond of the enzyme complex (27) and is due to the loss of an alkyl or alkoxyl group (28). Pralidoxime may, therefore, not be of benefit if given 36 to 48 hours after exposure to the insecticide (73).

Oximes are only moderately effective when given alone; and because they act in a manner different from that of atropine, the two drugs do not interfere with each other and can be administered at the same time. In addition, pralidoxime is most effective after a single exposure (74).

Side Effects

Side effects of therapeutic doses of pralidoxime have been minimal in normal subjects and practically nonexistent in individuals who have been poisoned. Complaints have included brief episodes of dizziness, blurred vision, diplopia, headache, nausea, and tachycardia (Table 81–15) (73). The material is rapidly excreted from the body, chiefly in the urine.

Pyridostigmine/Physostigmine Use in Nerve Gas

It is thought that those exposed to the risk of chemical warfare nerve agent attack may gain a measure of protection from organophosphates that "age" enzymes rapidly, by pretreatment with oral pyridostigmine, a carbamate compound that binds reversibly to cholinesterases and protects the enzyme from immediate exposure to organophosphates, which form a more stable bond. Also, pyridostigmine-treated red cells are still susceptible to reactivation by oximes (68).

The protective action of carbamates against organophosphate anticholinesterase poisoning probably depends on the ability of the carbamate to inhibit acetylcholinesterase forming a semi-stable carbamoylated enzyme that can spontaneously break down to liberate the enzyme. The fraction of the enzyme in the tissues that was carbamoylated would be protected against phosphorylation in subsequent poisoning by an organophosphate (75). The spontaneous decarbamoylation of the enzyme in parallel with the rapid removal would release sufficient acetylcholinesterase to maintain life. Studies on the effectiveness of pyridostigmine pretreatment in reversing the neuromuscular blockade produced by soman provide evidence that supports this hypothesis.

TABLE 81–15. *Side effects of pralidoxime*

Dizziness
Blurred vision
Diplopia
Headache
Nausea
Tachycardia

Carbamylation of 20% to 40% of the erythrocyte AChE is associated with antidotal enhancement. Carbamate pretreatment will not reduce the effects of the agents and, by themselves, carbamates provide no benefit. Pretreatment is not effective against Sarin and VX challenge and should not be considered a panacea for all nerve agents. It is of value for Soman intoxication when agent challenge is followed by atropine and an oxime. Pretreatment is ineffective unless standard therapy is administered after the exposure (76).

Because physostigmine is toxic at the amounts required, pyridostigmine is the drug of choice for pretreatment. The standard dosage is 30 mg orally every 8 hours for impending nerve agent attack. Because pyridostigmine does not cross the blood–brain barrier, it causes no central nervous system side effects or decrements in mental performance. For the same reason, however, it offers no protection against the CNS toxicity of nerve agents.

Carbamates must never be used after nerve agent exposure; in that setting, carbamate administration will worsen rather than protect from toxicity (75).

REFERENCES

1. Zweiner R, Ginsburg C: Organophosphate and carbamate poisoning in infants and children. *Pediatrics* 1988;81:121–126.
2. Milby T: Prevention and management of organophosphate poisoning. *JAMA* 1971;216:2131–2133.
3. Davies J, Davis J, Frazier D, et al: Disturbances of metabolism in organophosphate poisoning. *Ind Med Surg* 1967;36:58–62.
4. Davies J: Changing profile of pesticide poisoning. *N Engl J Med* 1987;316:807–808.
5. Tafuri J, Roberts J: Organophosphate poisoning. *Ann Emerg Med* 1987;16:193–202.
6. Byard J: Mechanisms of acute human poisoning by pesticides. *Clin Toxicol* 1979;14:187–193.
7. Selden B, Curry S: Prolonged succinylcholine induced paralysis in organophosphate insecticide poisoning. *Ann Emerg Med* 1987;16: 215–217.
8. DePalma A, Kwalick D, Zukerberg N: Pesticide poisoning in children. *JAMA* 1970;211:1979–1981.
9. Mortensen M: Management of acute childhood poisoning caused by selected insecticides and herbicides. *Pediatr Clin North Am* 1986;33: 421–444.
10. Done A: "Nerve gases" in the war against pests. *Emerg Med* 1973;5: 250–256.
11. Sofer S, Tal A, Shahak E: Carbamate and organophosphate poisoning in early childhood. *Pediatr Emerg Care* 1989;5:222–225.
12. Namba T, Hiraki K: PAM therapy for alkylphosphate poisoning. *JAMA* 1958;166:1834–1836.
13. Kopel F, Starobin S, Gribetz I, et al: Acute parathion poisoning. *J Pediatr* 1962;61:898–903.
14. Namba T, Nolte C, Jackrel J, et al: Poisoning due to organophosphate insecticides. *Am J Med* 1971;50:475–492.
15. Warren M, Conrad J, Bocian J, et al: Clothing-borne epidemic. *JAMA* 1963;184:94–96.
16. Goldman L, Beller M, Jackson R: Aldicarb food poisonings in California, 1985–1988: toxicity estimates for humans. *Arch Environ Health* 1990;45:141–147.
17. Namba T, Okazaki S, Taniguchi Y, et al: Inhibition by organophos-

phates and reactivation by oximes of tissue cholinesterase. *Naika Ryoiki* 1959;7:680–684.
18. Hayes W: Epidemiology and general management of poisoning by pesticides. *Pediatr Clin North Am* 1970;17:629–644.
19. Lyon J, Taylor H, Ackerman B: A case report of intravenous malathion injection with determination of serum halflife. *Clin Toxicol* 1987;25:243–249.
20. Garber M: Carbamate poisoning: the "other" insecticide. *Pediatrics* 1987;79:734–738.
21. Minton N, Murray V: A review of organophosphate poisoning. *Med Toxicol* 1988;3:350–375.
22. Arterberry J, Bonifaci R Nash E, et al: Potentiation of phosphorus insecticides by phenothiazine derivatives: possible hazard, with report of a fatal case. *JAMA* 1962;182:110–112.
23. Ahlgren D, Manz H, Harvey J: Myopathy of chronic organophosphate poisoning: a clinical entity? *South Med J* 1979;72:555–558.
24. Becker C, Sullivan J: Prompt recognition and vigorous therapy for organophosphate poisoning. *Emerg Med Rep* 1986;7:33–39.
25. Durham W, Hayes W; Organic phosphorus poisoning and its therapy. *Arch Environ Health* 1962;5:21–47.
26. Kline S, Bayer M: Insecticide poisoning. *Top Emerg Med* 1979;1: 73–83.
27. Lotti M, Becker C: Treatment of acute organophosphate poisoning: evidence of a direct effect on the central nervous system by 2-PAM (pyridine-2-aldoxime methylchloride). *J Toxicol Clin Toxicol* 1982; 19:121–127.
28. Fleisher J, Harris L: Dealkylation as a mechanism for aging of cholinesterase after poisoning with pinacolylmethylphosphonofluoridate. *Biochem Pharmacol* 1965;14:641–645.
29. Morgan DP: Recognition and management of pesticide poisonings, 3rd ed. US environmental Protection Agency. *JAMA* 1971;216: 2131.
30. Goldman L, Smith D, Neutra R, et al: Pesticide food poisoning from contaminiated watermelons in California, 1985. *Arch Environ Health* 1990;45:229–235.
31. Fredriksson T: Percutaneous absorption of parathion and paraoxon: decontamination of human skin from parathion. *Arch Environ Health* 1961;3:67–70.
32. Fredriksson T: Studies on the percutaneous absorption of parathion and paraoxon: rate of absorption of parathion. *Acta Derm Venereol (Stockh)* 1961;41:353–362.
33. Healy J: Ascending paralysis following malathion intoxication: a case report. *Med J Aust* 1959;1:765–767.
34. Goh K, Yew F, Ong K, et al: Acute organophosphate food poisoning caused by contaminated greef leafy vegetables. *Arch Environ Health* 1990;45:180–284.
35. Mortensen M: Pharmacological and toxicological considerations in the treatment of carbamate intoxications. *Am J Emerg Med* 1990;8: 83–84
36. Zavon M: Treatment of organophosphorus and chlorinated hydrocarbon insecticide intoxications. *Mod Treat* 1971;8:503–510.
37. Zadik Z, Blachar Y, Barak Y, et al: Organophosphate poisoning presenting as diabetic ketoacidosis. *J Toxicol Clin Toxicol* 1983;20: 381–385.
38. Weizman Z, Sofer S: Acute pancreatitis in children with anticholinesterase insecticide intoxication. *Pediatrics* 1992;90:204–206.
39. Miller D: Neurotoxicity of the pesticidal carbamates. *Neurobehav Toxicol Teratol* 1982;4:779–787.
40. Tabershaw I, Cooper W: Sequelae of acute organic phosphate poisoning. *J Occup Med* 1966;8:5–20.
41. Brown H: Electroencephalographic changes and disturbance of brain function following human organophosphate exposure. *Northwest Med* 1971;70:845–846.
42. Sim V: Anticholinesterase poisoning. *Clin Pharmacol* 1974;9:146–148.
43. Fisher J: Guillain-Barre syndrome following organophosphate poisoning. *JAMA* 1979;238:1950–1952.
44. Tsao T, Juang Y, Lan R, et al: Respiratory failure of acute organophosphate and carbamate poisoning. *Chest* 1990;98:631–636.
45. Dixon E: Dilatation of the pupils in parathion poisoning. *JAMA* 1957; 163:444–445.
46. Ramu A, Drexler H: Hyperglycemia in acute malathion intoxication in rats. *Isr J Med Sci* 1973;9:635–639.
47. Kass R, Kochar G, Lippman M: Adult respiratory distress syndrome from organophosphate poisoning. *Am J Emerg Med* 1991;9:32–33.
48. Senanayake N, Karalliedde L: Neurotoxic effects of organophosphate insecticides: an intermediate syndrome. *N Engl J Med* 1987;316: 761–763.
49. Bleecker J, Willems J, Neucker K, et al: Prolonged toxicity with intermediate syndrome after combined parathion and methyl parathion poisoning. *J Toxicol Clin Toxicol* 1992;30:333–345.
50. Haddad L: Organophosphate poisoning—intermediate syndrome? *J Toxicol Clin Toxicol* 1992;30:331–332.
51. De Bleecker J: Intermediate syndrome: prolonged cholinesterase inhibition. *J Toxicol Clin Toxicol* 1993;31:197–199.
52. Bleecker J, Neucker K, Willems: The intermediate syndrome in organophosphate poisoning: presentation of a case and review of the literature. *J Toxicol Clin Toxicol* 1992;30:321–329.
53. Benson B, Tolo D, McIntire M: Is the intermediate syndrome in organophosphate poisoning the result of insufficient oxime therapy? *J Toxicol Clin Toxicol* 1992;30:347–349.
54. Gadoth N, Fisher A: Late onset of neuromuscular block in organophosphate poisoning. *Ann Intern Med* 1978;88:654–655.
55. Besser R, Guttman L, Dillman U, et al: End-plate dysfunction in acute organophosphate intoxication. *Neurology* 1989;39:561–567.
56. Abou-Donia M, Lapadula D: Mechanisms of organophosphorus ester-induced delayed neurotoxicity: type I and Type II. *Annu Rev Pharmacol Toxicol* 1990;30:405–440.
57. Fournier F, Sonnier M, Dally S: Detection and assay of organophosphate pesticides in human blood by gas chromatography. *Clin Toxicol* 1978;12:457–462.
58. Coye M, Barnett P, Midtling J, et al: Clinical confirmation of organophosphate poisoning by serial cholinesterase analyses. *Arch Intern Med* 1987;147:438–442.
59. Sanz P, Rodriguez-Vicente M, Diaz D, et al: Red blood cell and total blood acetylcholinesterase and plasm pseudocholinesterase in humans: observed variances. *J Toxicol Clin Toxicol* 1991;29:81–90.
60. Rosenstock L, Keifer M, Daniell W, et al: Chronic central nervous system effects of acute organophosphate pesticide intoxication. *Lancet* 1991;338:223–227.
61. Markowitz S: Poisoning of an urban family due to misapplication of household organophosphate and carbamate pesticides. *J Toxicol Clin Toxicol* 1992;30:295–303.
62. Green M, Reid F, Kaminskis A: Correlation of 2PAM plasma levels after organophosphate intoxication. *Res Commun Chem Pathol Pharmacol* 1985;49:255–266.
63. Kort W, Kiestra S, Sangster B: The use of atropine and oximes in organophosphate intoxications: a modified approach. *J Toxicol Clin Toxicol* 1988;26:199–208.
64. Richards A: Malathion poisoning successfully treated with large doses of atropine. *Can Med Assoc J* 1964;91:82–92.
65. LeBlanc F, Benson B, Gilg A: A severe organophosphate poisoning requiring the use of an atropine drip. *Clin Toxicol* 1986;24:69–76.
66. Holland P, Parkes D: Plasma concentrations of the oxime pralidoxime mesylate (P2S) after repeated oral and intramuscular administration. *Br J Ind Med* 1976;33:43–46.
67. Bentur Y, Nutenko I, Tsipiniuk A, et al: Pharmacokinetics of obidoxime in organophosphate poisoning associated with renal failure. *J Toxicol Clin Toxicol* 1993;31:315–322.
68. Kurtz P: Pralidoxime in the treatment of carbamate intoxication. *Am J Emerg Med* 1990;8:68–70.
69. Rosenberg P: In vivo reactivation by PAM of brain cholinesterase inhibited by paraoxon. *Biochem Pharmacol* 1960;3:212–215.
70. Firemark H, Barlow C, Roth L: The penetration of 2PAM-C14 into brain and the effect of cholinesterase inhibitors on its transport. *J Pharmacol Exp Ther* 1964;145:252–265.
71. Farrar H, Wells T, Kearns G: Clinical and laboratory observations. Use of continuous infusion of pralidoxime for treatment of organophosphate poisoning in children. *J Pediatr* 1990;116:658–661.
72. Calesnick B, Christensen J, Richter M: Human toxicity of various oximes. *Arch Environ Health* 1967;15:599–608.
73. Thompson D, Thompson G, Greenwood R, et al: Therapeutic dosing of pralidoxime chloride. *Drug Intell Clin Pharmacol* 1987;21: 590–593.
74. Kurtz P: Pralidoxime in the treatment of carbamate intoxication. *Am J Emerg Med* 1990;8:68–70.
75. Deyi X, Linxiu W, Shuqiu P: The inhibition and protection of cholinesterase by physostigmine and pyridostigmine against soman poisoning in vivo. *Fund Appl Toxicol* 1981;1:217–221.

76. Dirnhuber P, French M, Green D, et al: The protection of primates against soman poisoning by pretreatment with pyridostigmine. *J Pharm Pharmacol* 1979;31:295–299.

ADDITIONAL SELECTED REFERENCES

Cavagna G, Locati G, Vigliani E: Clinical effects of exposure to DDVP (Vapona) insecticide in hospital wards. *Arch Environ Health* 1969;19: 112–123.

Dressel T, Goodale R, Ameson M, et al: Pancreatitis as a complication of anticholinesterase insecticide intoxication. *Ann Surg* 1978;189: 199–204.

Fredriksson T, Farrior W, Witter R: Studies on the percutaneous absorption of parathion and paraoxon: hydrolysis and metabolism within the skin. *Acra Derm Venereol (Stockh)* 1961;41:335–341.

Gaines T: Acute toxicity of pesticides. *Toxicol Appl Pharmacol* 1969;14: 515–534.

Gall D: The use of therapeutic mixtures in the treatment of cholinesterase inhibition. *Fund Appl Toxicol* 1981;1:214–216.

Goldin A, Rubinstein A, Bradlow B, et al: Malathion poisoning with special reference to the effect of cholinesterase inhibition on erythrocyte survival. *N Engl J Med* 1964;271:1289–1292.

Hruban Z, Schulman S, Warner N, et al: Hypoglycemia resulting from insecticide poisoning: Report of a case. *JAMA* 1963;184:590–594.

Levin H, Rodnitzky R: Behavioral effects of organophosphate pesticides in man. *Clin Toxicol* 1976;9:391–405.

Maibach H, Feldmann R, Milby T, et al: Regional variation in percutaneous penetration in man. *Arch Environ Health* 1971;23:208–211.

Maselli R, Jacobsen J, Spire J: Edrophonium: an aid in the diagnosis of acute organophosphate poisoning. *Ann Neurol* 1986;19:508–510.

Meller D, Fraser I, Kryger M: Hyperglycemia in anticholinesterase poisoning. *Can Med Assoc J* 1981;124:745–748.

Muller F, Hundt H: Chronic organophosphate poisoning. *S Afr Med J* 1980;57:344–345.

Namba T: Malathion poisoning. *Arch Environ Health* 1970;21:533–541.

Page L, Verhulst H: The oximes and organophosphate poisoning. *Am J Dis Child* 1962;103:185–190.

Pullicino P, Aquillina J: Opsoclonus in organophosphate poisoning. *Arch Neurol* 1989;46:704–705.

Sanborn G, Selhorst J, Calabrese V, et al: Pseudotumor cerebrii and insecticide intoxication. *Neurology* 1979;29:1222–1227.

Shemesh I, Bourvin A, Gold D, et al: Chlorpyrifos poisoning treated with ipratropium and dantrolene: a case report. *J Toxicol Clin Toxicol* 1988;26:495–498.

Sidell F, Borak J: Chemical warfare agents: II. Nerve agents. *Ann Emerg Med* 1992;21:865–871.

Sidell F: Soman and sarin: Clinical manifestations and treatment of accidental poisoning by organophosphates. *Clin Toxicol* 1974;7:1–17.

Victor S: Bell's palsy following organophosphate poisoning. *JAMA* 1978;239:1847–1848.

Wolfe, H, Durham W, Walker K, et al: Health hazards of discarded pesticide containers. *Arch Environ Health* 1961;3:531–537.

Young R, Jung F, Ayer H: Phorate intoxication at an insecticide-formulating plant. *Am Ind Hyg Assoc J* 1979;40:1013–1016.

Zavon M: Poisoning from pesticides: diagnosis and treatment. *Pediatrics* 1974;54:332–336.

CHAPTER 82

Herbicides

Herbicides are classified by their selectivity, mode of distribution, mode of action, time of application, and/or chemical structure. They tend to be more toxic to plants than to other life forms, but depending on the amount of chemical absorbed, toxic effects may be induced in any life form (1).

Herbicides have the lowest toxicity of the three major pesticide groups, yet the dangers posed by herbicidal chemicals to organisms and the environment are considerable. Most herbicidal poisonings are due to accidental spillage or intentional ingestion. These exposures can be equated to the herbicides' increased popularity and ready availability and the general lack of knowledge about the safe handling and use of these products. Many of these chemicals were used during wartime and are now marketed for civilian use by farmers and homeowners for killing weeds and controlling brush. From 900 C.E. until just before World War II, primarily inorganic compounds were used for the chemical control of weeds. However, these compounds were not very selective and tended to persist in the environment. Due to this persistence, damage to future crops was difficult to avoid.

Inorganic compounds still used today as herbicides include sodium arsenite, calcium cyanamide, cupric sulfate, mercurous chloride, potassium chlorate, and sodium chlorate. Of these, the arsenites and chlorates are still used frequently. The most powerful of the herbicides are paraquat and diquat, phenoxyacetic acid derivatives and the dinitrophenols. They are the subject of discussion in this chapter.

PARAQUAT

Paraquat (dimethylbipyridilium chloride, methylviologen) is a quaternary ammonium herbicide and the most important in a group of bipyridilium compounds used as herbicides (Table 82–1) (2). Other bipyridilium agents include diquat, difenzoquat, morfamquat, and chlormequat. These compounds are some of the most toxic poisons known to humans. Although the lung was once thought to be the target organ for the toxic effects of paraquat, it is now known that paraquat is a multi-system poison capable of causing toxicity to the kidneys, liver, brain, heart, and muscles (3).

TABLE 82–1. *Bipyridilium herbicides*

Chlormequat
Diquat
Difenzoquat
Morfamquat
Paraquat

Paraquat was first described in the latter part of the 19th century. It had been used as a redox indicator and was known as *methylviologen* until the 1950s when it began to be marketed as an herbicide. It is now a widely used, rapidly acting contact herbicide that is inactivated by soil, particularly clay. The inactivation is due to the tenacious binding of the compound to the soil (4).

Paraquat appears to react within plant cells in conjunction with sunlight to generate superoxide radicals, which in turn destroy plant cellular membranes and desiccate the leaves. If sprayed plants are harvested before exposure to sunlight, desiccation does not occur and unaltered paraquat remains on the plant (5).

Paraquat is used to control weeds and deep brush (6). It has been used in many countries, including Vietnam, as a defoliant. Not long ago, a government-sponsored aerial spraying program to destroy marijuana fields in Mexico was carried out. Mexican farmers, however, knowing that the action of paraquat depends on sunlight, began harvesting marijuana rapidly after spraying and wrapped the leaves in dark cloths for export to the United States. As a result, there was great concern for a time that marijuana contaminated with paraquat would cause poisoning in marijuana smokers. However, this has not been shown to occur (6,7).

Paraquat has produced many fatalities through indiscriminate usage and suicides, because ingestion of as little as 10 to 20 mL of a 20% solution of the concentrate can cause death. Although ingestion of large amounts of paraquat may be fatal within hours, death is usually delayed several weeks due to the insidious development of severe interstitial pulmonary fibrosis and subsequent fatal hypoxia.

ABSORPTION OF PARAQUAT

Paraquat is highly toxic to humans. Lethal poisoning can occur by absorption through the skin, inhalation, and ingestion. Paraquat is poorly absorbed from the gastrointestinal tract, with less than 5% of the ingested dose typically being absorbed. Although the absorption of paraquat by this route may be incomplete, it is nonetheless rapid, and symptoms of intoxication may be detected as early as 1 hour after ingestion. Because paraquat has an extremely low vapor pressure, the hazard of poisoning from inhalation is small. Only small amounts of paraquat can be absorbed through unbroken skin, but broken skin can readily absorb the herbicide causing severe or even fatal poisoning. This, however, is not a common mode of entry (3).

Most serious poisonings have involved liquid concentrates and most fatalities have occurred after ingestion of such preparations containing more than 25% paraquat. At this concentration, one or two mouthfuls may be fatal (5).

MECHANISM OF TOXICITY

Systemic toxicity in humans is thought to be mediated by the production of a superoxide anion, which through an intermediary, reacts with lipids to form hydroperoxides that interfere with pulmonary surfactant function (8,9). The result is cell damage producing inflammation, edema, and ultimately fibrosis. The formation of this toxic superoxide radical is more rapid under high oxygen tension, which is the proposed mechanism for the preferential site of paraquat toxicity in lung tissue (10).

Bipyridyl toxicity is due to the compound's ability to accept an electron and become reduced to a bipyridyl free radical. For paraquat, this occurs within the type I alveolar cells catalyzed by NADPH cytochrome P-450 reductase, while diquat toxicity occurs in the liver from flavoprotein, in the lens by glutathione reductase, or photochemically. The herbicidal activity of paraquat is dependent on active photosynthesis, during which it competes with nicotinamide-adenine dinucleotide phosphate (NADP) for electrons furnished by a transfer system in the chloroplast. Toxicity is as a result of reduction by NADPH–cytochrome P-450 reductase (NADPH is the reduced form of NADP) (3). The addition of a single electron to paraquat produces methylviologen, a free-radical resonating structure with a blue color (11). Methylviologen can react with molecular oxygen to regenerate paraquat ion and to yield such toxic and reactive products as hydrogen peroxide, superoxide anion, and peroxide anion (Fig. 82–1) (10). Superoxide ions are also responsible for other membrane lesions and secondary necrosis of the upper digestive tract, the liver, the renal tubules, and the adrenal glands. The survival time in fatally poisoned patients is highly variable, with death occurring anywhere from a few hours to 1 month after ingestion (3).

Paraquat also causes toxicity because the production of superoxide radicals initiates an arachidonic acid cascade that stimulates prostaglandin synthesis, leading to increased fluid flow into the intracellular space with subsequent pulmonary edema (2).

TOXICITY

Clinical Features

The major adverse effects of paraquat are corrosion of the gastrointestinal tract, pulmonary fibrosis, renal tubular necrosis, and hepatic necrosis (Table 82–2). Other lesions produced by paraquat include irritative dermatitis, nail damage, eye injury, and severe epistaxis (7,9,12–14). Although caustic agents may result in mouth ulcers and many toxins produce hepatic or renal failure, the constellation of signs and symptoms of painful oral ulceration with subsequent hepatic and renal failure should alert the physician to the possibility of paraquat poisoning. Symptoms of paraquat ingestion depend largely on the amount consumed. Subacute paraquat toxicity produces a unique two-stage sequential poisoning. Patients can die within the first 1 to 3 days of gastrointestinal ulceration and perforation. Patients surviving the first 7 days or *destructive phase* may appear to partially recover. Those who survive this phase but die later, gradually and inexorably develop pulmonary fibrosis and respiratory failure. Dur-

TABLE 82–2. *Clinical features of paraquat poisoning*

Local
Eye irritation
Mucous membrane irritation
Skin irritation
Gastrointestinal
Burning sensation
Ulceration
Esophageal perforation
Vomiting
Abdominal pain
Dysphagia
Respiratory
Tachypnea
Dyspnea
Cough
Cyanosis
Pulmonary edema
Pulmonary fibrosis
Renal
Tubular necrosis
Hepatic
Liver function test abnormalities
Jaundice
Cardiac
Conduction disturbances
Myocarditis

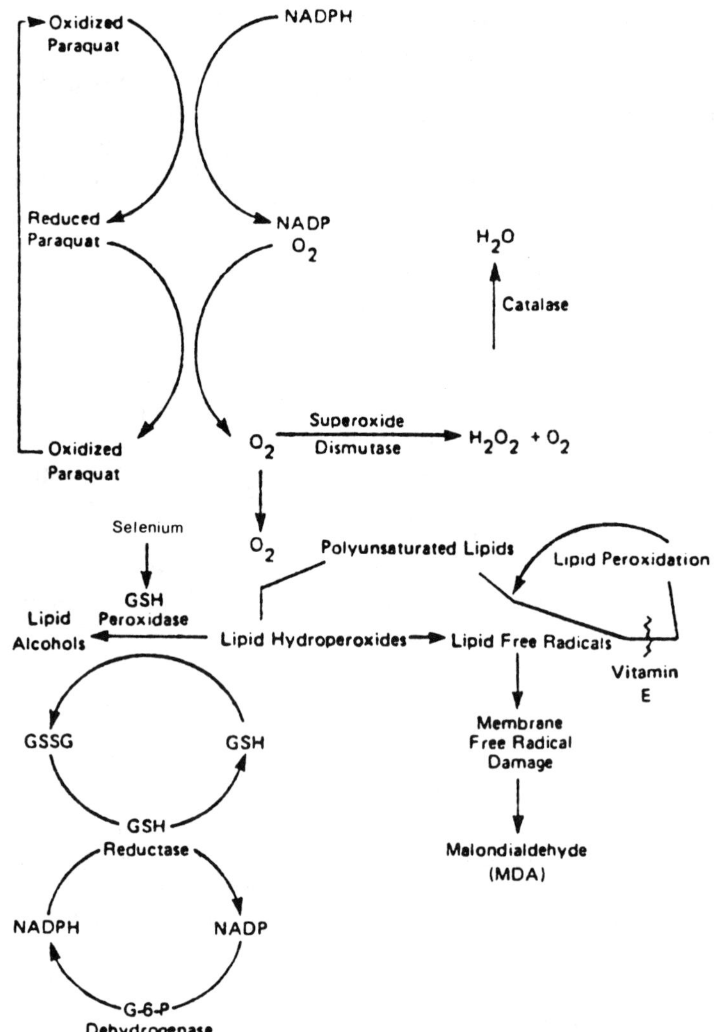

FIG. 82–1. Proposed mechanism of paraquat toxicity.

ing the next 3 to 14 days, called the *proliferative phase*, progressive pulmonary fibrosis and respiratory distress occur, producing dyspnea. Death occurs 10 to 21 days after initial exposure (15). The lung suffers from the disintegration of the alveolar epithelium producing moderate to marked alveolar and interstitial fibrosis. This disintegration produces bronchioles and alveoli that are seen as dilated areas of bullous emphysema.

Local Effects

The bipyridilium compounds may cause local skin lesions as a result of their corrosive nature. Dermal toxicity may also result from the effects of the wetting agent used for the paraquat (16). Paraquat may cause irritation of the eyes and mucous membranes and partial-thickness burns of the skin have been noted.

Gastrointestinal Effects

Initial gastrointestinal manifestations of paraquat poisoning include an immediate burning and ulceration of the mouth, tongue, throat, and esophagus (6). This is followed by vomiting, abdominal pain, dysphagia, and diarrhea. Esophageal perforation may occur. The initial phase of symptomatology may be followed by a latent period lasting up to 2 weeks, during which the patient appears to improve (17).

Respiratory Effects

Although paraquat causes multisystem damage, the highest tissue concentration is found in the lungs because there is active accumulation of paraquat in type II pneumocytes (2); consequently, there is more lung damage noted. Lung concentrations of paraquat may be 50 times higher than plasma concentrations. As just discussed, formation of the toxic superoxide radical causes membrane destruction and initiates an arachidonic acid cascade that stimulates prostaglandin synthesis, thereby, leading to toxicity (18).

Either the early or the delayed appearance of respiratory distress or failure is characteristic of paraquat poisoning. Selective binding and persistence of paraquat in lung tissue is considered the cause of pulmonary fibrosis, which is generally the lethal complication and can occur at any time between 5 and 30 days after ingestion (19). Massive doses of paraquat, however, may cause a fatal pulmonary edema and hemorrhage within 24 hours. The patient may develop dyspnea, tachypnea, and a nonproductive cough. As more damage develops, cyanosis is noted. Once symptoms are evident, the fibrosis progresses until death occurs secondary to the proliferative alveolitis; the alveolar walls become thickened and the patient dies from asphyxiation (16). The lethal amount of paraquat is relatively small and death may result from progressive hypoxemia even with aggressive respiratory treatment. The pathologic changes noted in the lung are identical to those from oxygen toxicity (20).

Lung damage was initially thought to imply a fatal outcome. However, there are reports of survivors who have developed varying degrees of lung damage, ranging from transient pleural effusions and resolving pulmonary infiltrates to persistent radiological change (17).

Renal Effects

Renal deterioration often begins 24 to 96 hours after paraquat ingestion. In most severe intoxication, renal tubular necrosis develops. The renal disorder may be observed before the development of pulmonary fibrosis. Microscopically, tubular damage is noted in the kidneys.

Hepatic Effects

Hepatic insufficiency has been reported to occur within 24 to 48 hours of ingestion and may manifest as abnormalities in liver function tests. Jaundice may also be noted. The hepatic disorders may also be observed before the development of pulmonary fibrosis.

Cardiac Effects

Cardiac involvement may consist of conduction disturbances, epicardial hemorrhage, and myocarditis. Respiratory difficulties may then ensue.

LABORATORY DETERMINANTS

For patients with paraquat poisoning, serial chest roentgenograms should be obtained and arterial blood gases measured to determine the onset of pneumonitis. Renal output should be carefully monitored for signs of renal involvement (4). Liver function studies are necessary to monitor hepatic involvement. Measurements of serum paraquat concentration may be useful for prognostic purposes, but the diagnosis must be made quickly, before concentrations can be determined, to increase the likelihood of effective intervention. A qualitative colorimetric urine test is also available; this makes use of sodium dithionite and sodium hydroxide. Two mL of 1% sodium dithionite in 1N sodium hydroxide is added to 10 mL of urine. If the solution turns blue, the urine is positive for bipyridilium compounds.

TREATMENT

Paraquat toxicity develops rapidly; thus, it is essential to institute therapy immediately, before confirmation of plasma paraquat concentrations is obtained. Treatment of paraquat intoxication is directed toward the removal of the material from the gastrointestinal tract and the prevention of further absorption by administering specific adsorbents. Initial treatment, therefore, consists of ipecac syrup or lavage, despite the corrosive nature of the compound.

Detoxification of Paraquat

Paraquat undergoes complete detoxification on contact with clay or earth, so that Fuller's earth (300 g of a 30% solution) or bentonite (200 to 500 mL of a 30% aqueous suspension) is an effective absorbent; the addition of 20% mannitol or 70% sorbitol may accelerate the passage of contents through the gastrointestinal tract (18,19). This therapy is most effective if given within 4 hours after ingestion of the herbicide. If neither of these adsorbents is available, then activated charcoal should be used. Many clinicians prefer activated charcoal because it is more readily available and can be administered more rapidly. There is no strong evidence that multiple-dose activated charcoal is effective, however (21).

Oxygen Therapy

It has been shown that lung damage from paraquat is enhanced by any concentration of oxygen. It is important, therefore, to give the patient hypoxic mixtures that protect the lung against the damage from hyperoxygenation (15,22,23). Early intubation and ventilation with positive-pressure breathing has been suggested as a method of administering low inspired oxygen tensions while facilitating adequate arterial oxygen pressure.

Methods to Enhance Excretion

When first introduced, charcoal hemoperfusion was thought to be a major advance in the management of paraquat poisoning. Subsequent clinical experience has not always been associated with success, however (11,24,25). Hemoperfusion may be of value in paraquat poisoning only if it is instituted before toxic concentrations accumulate in the lung (21,25). Paraquat has a large volume of distribution and, in most cases, toxic concentrations are reached in the lungs before hemoperfusion can be started (24,26). Furthermore, forced diuresis, dialysis, and hemoperfusion appear to offer minimal success because only a small fraction of the compound is removed (19,27). Dialysis is only useful if renal failure ensues (26).

The poor total body clearance by extracorporeal techniques and the rise in plasma paraquat concentrations for several hours after completion of hemoperfusion, is explained by the extensive tissue distribution of paraquat and its slow redistribution during the hemoperfusion process.

Hemodialysis or hemoperfusion, which has greater clearance values than hemodialysis or combinations of the two, usually follow gastrointestinal decontamination. The goal of these procedures is to remove paraquat from the bloodstream and prevent its uptake by the pneumocytes.

In human poisonings, hemoperfusion is frequently stalled until concentrations of paraquat in plasma are low and in target organs are high. The amount of paraquat that can be removed from the body by hemoperfusion at this time is small compared with the dose, despite efficient extraction of paraquat by the charcoal cartridges and high clearances and decreased plasma concentrations during the procedure (26).

Indications for Hemoperfusion

Hemoperfusion is considered for patients whose initial plasma concentrations are lower than 3 mg/L, those in whom the probability of survival lies between 20% and 70%, and those who present within a few hours of ingestion (4). Even in these groups, it is not proven that hemoperfusion, single or repeated, is useful. The likelihood of hemoperfusion being efficacious is probably greatest if it is begun within 10 to 12 hours after ingestion.

Other Therapies

Some investigators have tried to prevent the pulmonary complications of paraquat intoxication by using immunosuppressants and by attempting to prevent the formation of superoxide radicals (20). Superoxide dismutase, which is an enzyme that destroys superoxide radicals, has not been met with great success. Corticosteroids, fibrinolytic agents, and vitamin E (an antioxidant thought to be helpful as an oxygen scavenger) have all been tried but have not produced any beneficial results.

DIQUAT

Diquat (ethylene bipyridilium), an analog of paraquat, is considered much less toxic (27,28). It also is used as an herbicide and often is combined with paraquat. Diquat dibromide is sold under the Ortho label as a 35.3% solution of the product in water. Although poisoning by diquat is not as common, the signs and symptoms resemble those of paraquat but are milder (27).

Toxicity of Diquat

Diquat also forms a bipyridyl radical which disrupts cell membranes, but its clinical effects are different from those of paraquat. Unlike paraquat, diquat does not appear to produce pulmonary fibrosis. Diquat causes distension of the gastrointestinal tract by gastroenteric congestion and induces hyperexcitability and convulsions. Lung consolidation has only been reported after repeated doses. Because it is eliminated by the kidneys, it may cause renal damage leading to renal failure. A pre-renal component may add to this problem because of "third spacing" resulting in a decreased intravascular volume. Few fatalities have been associated with diquat intoxication (1).

Symptoms of systemic toxicity following acute ingestion include ulcerations of the gastric mucosa, vomiting, diarrhea, decreased gastrointestinal peristalsis, renal failure with oliguria or anuria, coma, and profound cardiovascular collapse (Table 82–3) (29).

CHLOROPHENOXY ACID HERBICIDES

The chlorophenoxy acid herbicides include such compounds as 2,4-dichlorophenoxyacetic acid (2,4-D) and 2,4,5-trichlorophenoxypropionic acid (2,4,5-T). These compounds are formulated as metal alkylamine salts or esters to produce material of low volatility. These compounds are among the most widely used for weed control and have been used for more than 40 years in the United States (30). Many millions of pounds of these herbicides are used domestically on an annual basis by railroads, utility firms, paper manufacturers, and farmers to clear land of wild growth (31).

Neither 2,4-D nor 2,4,5-T is absorbed appreciably through the intact skin, although 2,4,5-T appears to be

TABLE 82–3. *Signs and symptoms of diquat poisoning*

Gastrointestinal ulceration
Nausea
Vomiting
Diarrhea
Renal failure
Coma
Cardiovascular collapse

more irritating on the skin and mucous membranes than 2,4-D. There does not appear to be any consistent pattern of toxic symptoms except in scattered cases where a protracted peripheral neuropathy has been noted (1).

Mechanism of Action

The chlorophenoxy acid herbicides exert their toxic plant action by acting as growth hormones, altering a plant's metabolism to stimulate growth. During this process, the treated plants may develop high levels of nitrates or cyanide from rapid growth prior to wilting.

In humans, chlorophenoxy acids depress synthesis of ribonuclease, uncouple oxidative phosphorylation, demyelinate peripheral nerves, and elevate circulating levels of hepatic peroxisomes, such as CPK, LDH, AST (SGOT), and ALT (SGPT).

Clinical Manifestations and Treatment of Intoxication

Phenoxyacetic acid poisoning is surprisingly rare considering its widespread domestic use. Fatal self-poisoning is also rare, but there have been occasional reports of intoxication after overdose (32).

Signs and symptoms of overdose may include fatigue, nausea, vomiting, anorexia, diarrhea, muscle fasciculations, ataxia, and peripheral neuropathy (Table 82–4). Phenoxyacetic acid poisoning may also uncouple oxidative phosphorylation and produce pyrexia, hyperventilation, and hypoxemia. Hypersensitivity reactions involving respiratory complaints and dermatitis have also been reported (31). At higher doses when death is delayed, muscular and neural involvement results in stiffness of the extremities, ataxia, diminished coordination, muscle fibrillation, paralysis, and eventually, coma. Death is due to peripheral vascular collapse. Treatment is supportive and symptomatic.

Phenoxyacetic Acids and Dioxins

Although a thorough discussion of dioxins is beyond the scope of this book, recent reports concerning Agent Orange are worth mentioning. During the last few years, there has been great concern regarding the dioxins that have appeared as contaminants of 2,4,5–T (30). If the reaction temperature during synthesis of 2,4,5-T is allowed to rise too high, dioxin is produced (33); this does not occur with 2,4-D. Agent Orange, the defoliant used during the Vietnam war, is an equal mixture of 2,4-D and 2,4,5-T contaminated with 2,3,7,8-tetrachlorodibenzo-p-dioxin. The long-term effects of this dioxin contaminant have given rise to a great deal of controversy. A number of lawsuits have been based on alleged adverse health effects from exposures to Agent Orange, including sterility, birth defects, disfiguring skin diseases, malignancies, and other illnesses (33).

TABLE 82–4. *Signs and symptoms of phenoxyacetic acid poisoning*

Gastrointestinal
Nausea
Vomiting
Diarrhea
Anorexia
Neurologic
Muscular fasciculations
Ataxia
Peripheral neuropathy

DINITROPHENOLS

The dinitrophenols include 2,4 dinitrophenol, dinitrocresol, binapacryl, and dinoseb. They are rapidly absorbed through the skin, digestive tract, and lung. Plasma levels reach their highest concentration within a few hours. Dinitrophenols are metabolized to primary amines and their glucuronic acid conjugates.

Mechanism of Action

Dinitrophenols destroy cell membranes and uncouple oxidative phosphorylation by interfering with the normal coupling of carbohydrate oxidation to phosphorylation. This results in increased oxidative metabolism and oxygen consumption, ultimately depleting carbohydrate and fat stores. Metabolic activation and subsequent toxicity are increased by heat. Upon death, this uncoupling of oxidative phosphorylation causes rapid rigor mortis.

Toxicity

Acute

Acute poisoning in humans produce nausea, gastric upset, restlessness, a sensation of heat, flushed skin, sweating, rapid respiration, tachycardia, fever, cyanosis, and finally, collapse and coma (Table 82–5). Death is due to hyperthermia and respiratory or circulatory failure. Death or recovery occurs within 24 to 48 hours of exposure. The signs and symptoms reflect an elevated metabolic rate.

Chronic

Chronic exposure to dinitrophenols produces fatigue, restlessness, anxiety, excessive sweating, unusual thirst, and loss of weight. A yellow color to the conjunctiva

TABLE 82–5. *Signs and symptoms of dinitrophenol poisoning*

Acute
Nausea
Gastrointestinal upset
Tachypnea
Tachycardia
Hyperthermia
Cyanosis
Cardiovascular collapse
Coma
Chronic
Fatigue
Restlessness
Anxiety
Diaphoresis
Weight loss

and cataract formation have been demonstrated on chronic exposures to some dinitrophenols.

Treatment

If dermal exposure to one of the dinitrophenol herbicides occurs, the contaminated skin and hair should be bathed and shampooed promptly with soap and water. Further treatment consists of ice baths to reduce the elevated body temperatures and oxygen administration to assure vital tissue oxygenation. The clinical effects of dinitrophenol poisoning are enhanced when environmental temperatures are high.

PENTACHLOROPHENOL

Pentachlorophenol and its salts are used as insecticides, fungicides, herbicides, algacides, and disinfectants. Some 90% of pentachlorophenol is used for wood preservation and the treated product is commonly referred to as "penta-treated." Because pentachlorophenol is dissolved in oil and driven into the wood under pressure, the reference is often made to "pressure-treated wood."

Mechanism of Action

Pentachlorophenol is rapidly absorbed through the skin, digestive tract, and lung and is transported in the blood bound to albumin.

At low concentrations, pentachlorophenol uncouples oxidative phosphorylation in the mitochondria and inhibits mitochondrial and myosin adenosine triphosphatase (ATPase) at higher concentrations. It also inhibits cellular kinases, dehydrogenases, and reductases.

TABLE 82–6. *Signs and symptoms of pentachlorophenol poisoning*

Mild
Muscular weakness
Anorexia
Lethargy
Moderate
Tachypnea
Hyperpyrexia
Hyperglycemia
Glycosuria
Diaphoresis
Dehydration
Severe
Cardiovascular collapse
Respiratory failure
Hyperthermia

Toxicity

Pentachlorophenol is irritating to mucous membranes, the respiratory tract, and the skin. In mild intoxications, muscular weakness, anorexia, and lethargy occur (Table 82–6). Moderate intoxications cause accelerated respiration, hyperpyrexia, hyperglycemia, glycosuria, sweating, and dehydration. Lethal intoxication results in cardiac and muscular collapse, followed by death with the rapid onset of rigor mortis. Death is due to cardiac failure, respiratory failure or hyperthermia. Treatment is supportive (1).

REFERENCES

1. Smith E, Oehme F: A review of selected herbicides and their toxicities. *Vet Hum Toxicol* 1991;33:596–608.
2. Barabas K, Szabo L, Matkovics B: The search for an ideal antidote treatment in Gramoxone intoxication. *Gen Pharmacol* 1987;18: 129–132.
3. Thomas C, Aust S: Free radicals and environmental toxins. *Ann Emerg Med* 1986;15:1075–1083.
4. Pond S, Rivory L, Hampson E, et al: Kinetics of toxic doses of paraquat and the effects of hemoperfusion in the dog. *J Toxicol Clin Toxicol* 1993;31:229–246.
5. Smith L: Paraquat toxicity. *Philos Trans R Soc London Ser B* 1985; 311:647–657.
6. Smith R: Spraying of herbicides on Mexican marijuana backfires on U.S. *Science* 1978;199:861–864.
7. Landrigan P, Powell K, James L, et al: Paraquat and marijuana: epidemiologic risk assessment. *Am J Public Health* 1983;1784–788.
8. Bus J, Aust S, Gibson J: Superoxide and singlet oxygen-catalyzed lipid peroxidation as a possible mechanism for paraquat toxicity. *Biochem Biophys Res Commun* 1974;58:749.
9. Conradi S, Olanoff L, Dawson W: Fatality due to paraquat intoxication: confirmation by postmortem tissue analysis. *Am J Clin Pathol* 1983;80:771–776.
10. Bismuth C, Gardiner R, Dally S, et al: Prognosis and treatment of paraquat poisoning: a review of 28 cases. *J Toxicol Clin Toxicol* 1982;19:461–474.
11. Vale J, Crome P, Volans G, et al: The treatment of paraquat poisoning using oral sorbents and charcoal hemoperfusion. *Acta Pharmacol Toxicol* 1977;41(suppl):109–117.
12. Swan A: Exposure of spray operators to paraquat. *Chest* 1974; 65(suppl):65–67.

13. Baran R: Nail damage caused by weed killers and insecticides. *Arch Dermatol* 1974;110:467.
14. Wohlfahrt D: Fatal paraquat poisonings after skin absorption. *Med J Aust* 1982;1:512–513.
15. Fisher H, Clements J, Wright R: Enhancement of oxygen toxicity by the herbicide paraquat. *Am Rev Respir Dis* 1973;107:246–252.
16. Copland G, Kolin A, Shulman H: Fatal pulmonary in traalveolar fibrosis after paraquat ingestion. *N Engl J Med* 1974;291:290–292.
17. Hudson M, Patel S, Ewen S, et al: Paraquat induced pulmonary fibrosis in three survivors. *Thorax* 1991;46:201–204.
18. Meredith T, Vale J: Treatment of paraquat poisoning in man: methods to prevent absorption. *Hum Toxicol* 1987;6:49–55.
19. Hoffman S, Jederkin R, Korzets Z, et al: Successful management of severe paraquat poisoning. *Chest* 1983;84:107–109.
20. Franzen D, Baer F, Heitz W, et al: Failure of radiotherapy to resolve fatal lung damage due to paraquat poisoning. *Chest* 1991;1: 1164–1165.
21. Van de Vyver F, Guiliano R, Paulus C, et al: Hemoperfusion-hemodialysis ineffective for paraquat removal in life-threatening poisoning. *Clin Toxicol* 1985;23:117–131.
22. Brashear R, Sharma H, Deatley R: Prolonged survival breathing oxygen at ambient pressure. *Am Rev Respir Dis* 1973;108:701–704.
23. Rhodes M, Zavala D, Brown D: Hypoxic protection in paraquat poisoning. *Lab Invest* 1976;35:496–500.
24. Gelfand M, Winchester J, Knepshield J, et al: Treatment of severe drug overdosage with charcoal hemoperfusion. *Trans Am Soc Artif Intern Organs* 1977;23:599–604.
25. Mascie-Taylor J, Thompson J, Davison A: Hemoperfusion ineffective for paraquat removal in life-threatening poisoning. *Lancet* 1983;1:1376–1377.
26. Hampson E, Pond S: Failure of haemoperfusion and haemodialysis to prevent death in paraquat poisoning. A retrospective review of 42 patients. *Med Toxicol* 1988;3:64–71.
27. Williams P, Jarvie D, Whitehead A: Diquat intoxication: treatment by charcoal hemoperfusion and description of a new method of diquat measurement in plasma. *Clin Toxicol* 1986;24:11–20.
28. McCarthy L, Speth C: Diquat intoxication. *Ann Emerg Med* 1983; 12:394–396.
29. Manoguerra A: Full thickness skin burns secondary to an unusual exposure to diquat dibromide. *J Toxicol Clin Toxicol* 1990;28: 107–110.
30. Berwick P: 2,4-Dichlorophenoxyacetic acid poisoning in man. *JAMA* 1970;214:1114–1117.
31. O'Reilly J: Prolonged coma and delayed peripheral neuropathy after ingestion of phenoxyacetic acid weed killers. *Postgrad Med J* 1984; 60:76–77.
32. Cushman J, Street J: Allergic hypersensitivity to the herbicide 2,4-D in Balb/c mice. *J Toxicol Environ Health* 1982;10:729–741.
33. Tedschi L: Dioxin. *Am J Forensic Med Pathol* 1980;1:145–148.

ADDITIONAL SELECTED REFERENCES

Pommery J, Mathieu M, Mathieu D, et al: Atrazine in plasma and tissue following atrazine-aminotriazole-ethylene glycol-formaldehyde poisoning. *J Toxicol Clin Toxicol* 1993;31:323–331.

Siefkin A: Combined paraquat and acetaminophen toxicity. *J Toxicol Clin Toxicol* 1982;19:483–491.

Tungsanga K, Israsena S, Chusilp S, et al: Paraquat poisoning: Evidence of systemic toxicity after dermal exposure. *Postgrad Med J* 1983;59:338–339.

CHAPTER 83

Nicotine

Nicotine (methylpyridylpyrrolidine) is one of the most toxic and rapidly acting poisons. It was once widely used as a horticultural insecticide in vapor or spray form. Although it occurs naturally in tobacco products, it is also available as a colorless, volatile, and strongly alkaline liquid. Nicotine is a water-soluble liquid alkaloid. Initially, the solution is clear but turns a brown color on contact with air, closely resembling whiskey in appearance (1).

Tobacco leaves contain 2% to 5% of the alkaloid *Nicotiana tabacum* (2). The leaves are prepared as smoking and chewing tobacco and as snuff; tobacco has also been used in enemas and poultices (3–5). The use of smokeless tobacco, which is usually inserted between the cheek and gum, is becoming an increasingly widespread practice (6); the nicotine from the tobacco is quickly absorbed through the oral mucosa into the bloodstream (7).

Although it is one of the most widely abused drugs of modern times, serious or fatal overdoses of this agent are rare. Potentially ingestible forms of nicotine include nicotine alkaloid solution, nicotine sulfate pesticide solution, a concentrated Hare and Hound Repellant dust, cigarettes, cigars, pipe and chewing tobacco, and nicotine gum.

ABSORPTION

Nicotine is readily absorbed through the intact skin, respiratory tract, and mucous membranes (including the rectal mucosa). It is also incompletely absorbed through the gastrointestinal tract; absorption by this route is slow so that metabolic activity may be able to keep pace with absorption (5). Some cases of nicotine poisoning after dermal absorption have been due to careless handling of the compound when it was employed as an insecticide (8). Poisonings have also occurred from tobacco enemas used in the treatment of intestinal parasitic infestation, in skin contact with tobacco infusions or poultices, and from inhalation of insect sprays (9). A number of fatal poisonings have occurred in the last few years from "salads" prepared with wild flora that included wild tobacco.

Inhalation

Absorption of nicotine is facilitated by a huge alveolar surface area, thin alveolar epithelial and endothelial layers, and an extensible capillary bed. As a result of these anatomic factors, nicotine moves rapidly from the alveolar spaces into the systemic circulation.

Musous Membrane Absorption

The pH of tobacco smoke is important in determining the absorption of nicotine from different sites within the body. The pH of smoke from flue-cured tobaccos found in most cigarettes is acidic. At this pH, most of the nicotine is ionized and does not rapidly cross membranes. As a consequence, there is little buccal absorption of nicotine from cigarette smoke, even when it is held in the mouth. The absorption of nicotine from gum or smokeless tobacco is gradual, with blood levels peaking at the end of the chewing or snuff-taking period. Nicotine gum is buffered to an alkaline pH to facilitate absorption of nicotine through the mucous membranes of the mouth (10).

Oral

Orally ingested nicotine is less toxic than may be expected because the centrally mediated vomiting induced by the alkaloid usually causes emptying of the stomach before a fatal dose is absorbed and because there is a significant first-pass effect through the liver (3).

DOSAGE OF NICOTINE IN TOBACCO AND NICOTINE GUM

One tobacco cigarette contains approximately 20 to 30 mg of nicotine (11), although the usual dose absorbed from cigarette smoking is 1 to 2 mg. Cigars contain approximately 15 to 40 mg of nicotine. Cigarette butts contain approximately 25% of the original nicotine content. Clove cigarettes contain larger amounts of nicotine and poisonings have been reported from their use (12).

Nicotine gum (Nicorette), a relatively recent source of nicotine in the United States, has been used in Europe for more than 20 years (6,13). The gum is composed of a gum base and a natural extract of the tobacco plant bound to an ion-exchange resin, which provides a controlled release (14). One piece of gum contains 2 or 4 mg of nicotine. Because Nicorette is in gum form, some patients may not realize that it is a medication (5,7). Nevertheless, if used inappropriately, it is more dangerous than one ingested cigarette and produces blood nicotine concentrations equivalent to smoking half a cigarette per hour. In 30 minutes of chewing, 90% of the nicotine from the gum is released (15). If the gum is accidentally swallowed, the nicotine is poorly absorbed and the absorbed portion undergoes significant first-pass metabolism in the liver (13).

TOXICITY

Toxic effects from nicotine ingestion (Table 83–1) are usually rapid and, in severe cases, death may occur within a few minutes; ingestion of small amounts of nicotine may lead to rapid or gradual onset of symptoms. Nicotine acts on autonomic ganglia and postsynaptic neurons by first stimulating and then by depressing ganglia and nerve endings (16). The mechanism of stimulation is a direct acetylcholine-like action on the ganglia that is followed quickly by a prolonged ganglionic blockade due to persistent depolarization (3,6). A similar action occurs at the neuromuscular junction causing total paralysis of skeletal muscles and subsequent respiratory failure (11). This peripheral skeletal muscle paralysis does not affect all muscle groups simultaneously or equally (14). Respiratory failure from neuromuscular paralysis, which is one cause of death in nicotine overdose, usually occurs before central respiratory failure (9). The central nervous system is affected initially by stimulation of the medullary centers and later by depression (16). Nicotine also has a direct excitatory effect on smooth muscle leading to vasoconstriction and increased intestinal motility (15).

Usually, there is a spontaneous emesis as a result of stimulation of the chemoreceptor trigger zone; this may be accompanied by profuse salivation (16). There is simultaneous stimulation of both cholinergic and adrenergic postganglionic autonomic neurons, causing symptoms such as weakness, pallor from peripheral vasoconstriction, headache, dizziness, diaphoresis, prostration, and vomiting (12). In addition, there may be profuse diaphoresis, abdominal pain, diarrhea, hyperpyrexia, and mydriasis. In small doses, nicotine may produce miosis (12).

The cardiovascular responses are generally due to initial stimulation of sympathetic ganglia as a result of the release of norepinephrine. Tachycardia and hypertension may be observed. Hypotension may be followed by cardiovascular collapse and death.

TABLE 83–1. *Features of nicotine poisoning*

Gastrointestinal
Diarrhea
Emesis
Nausea
Salivation
Neurologic
Agitation
Coma
Confusion
Dizziness
Headache
Hyperpyrexia
Mydriasis
Seizures
Weakness
Neuromuscular
Decreased deep tendon reflexes
Depolarization blockade
Fasciculations
Hypotonia
Weakness
Dermal
Diaphoresis
Pallor
Cardiovascular
Asystole
Atrial fibrillation
Bradycardia
Cardiovascular collapse
Hypertension/hypotension
Sinus tachycardia
Respiratory
Tachypnea
Respiratory failure
Cholinergic
Bronchorrhea
Diaphoresis
Lacrimation
Salivation

Serious nicotine ingestions frequently result in rapid progression to hypotension and death. The most common mechanisms of death are respiratory arrest produced by peripheral neuromuscular blockade and cardiovascular collapse.

Nicotine does not cause any irreversible changes, and complete recovery can be expected in the patient who has had cardiovascular and respiratory support. Some of the nicotine dose is metabolized, whereas the remainder is eliminated in the urine (14).

Green Tobacco Sickness

The constellation of nausea, vomiting, headache, and weakness associated with handling green tobacco is called *green tobacco sickness*, a widespread illness known among tobacco field workers since the turn of the century (2,4). Although it has not been associated with mortality or long-term sequelae, it is responsible for significant discomfort (12).

Green tobacco sickness occurs almost exclusively in tobacco workers who crop tobacco leaves from plants in the field. In this process, the leaves are cracked, emitting a gummy substance that coats the workers' hands and skin. It has been hypothesized that the nicotine contained in the sap is absorbed cutaneously and causes green tobacco sickness (4,16).

Diagnosis and Laboratory Determinations

The diagnosis of nicotine poisoning is usually suggested primarily by the clinical history. Plasma nicotine concentrations are not clinically useful. The ingestion of more than 1 cigarette, 3 cigarette butts, 1 cigar butt, or any amount of nicotine gum should be considered potentially serious (14,17).

Nicotine is a commonly reported finding whenever urine toxicologic screens are performed. Nicotine or conitine, its metabolite, are found in the urine of all smokers and a large percentage of nonsmokers as a result of exposure to passive smoke. Toxicologic testing of neonates' first urine has been reported to be positive when the mother smokes and even in instances of maternal exposure to passive smoke (tertiary smoking).

Treatment

Prompt treatment for acute nicotine intoxication is essential. If skin contact has occurred, the contaminated clothing should be removed and the skin thoroughly washed with soap and water. Cutaneous nicotine poisoning may be prolonged as a result of continued absorption despite skin decontamination. Physicians should anticipate this possibility and be prepared to give intensive care for at least 12 to 24 hours (1).

Emesis is usually a spontaneous event if a significant amount of nicotine is absorbed so that emesis induction may not be necessary. If emesis has not occurred, the stomach should be emptied and activated charcoal and a cathartic should be administered. Hypotension may be treated with intravenous fluids and by placing the patient in Trendelenburg's position. If there is no response to these methods, pharmacologic treatment may be necessary (16).

Pharmacologic treatment may consist of atropine for parasympathetic excess and an α-blocking agent for increased sympathetic activity. Sympathomimetics may be required for symptomatic hypotension that cannot be corrected (1).

Nicotine itself produces no tissue damage and overdoses are potentially completely reversible with appropriate supportive care.

ADDICTION

With prolonged or repetitive exposure to nicotine, neuroadaption occurs. This results in an increased number of nicotine receptors in the brain. A consequence of neuroadaption is the emergence of nicotine withdrawal symptoms when nicotine use is abruptly stopped. Withdrawal symptoms include restlessness, irritability, anxiety, drowsiness, impatience, confusion, and impaired concentration. Most symptoms of the withdrawal syndrome reach maximal intensity 24 to 48 hours after cessation and gradually diminish in intensity over a period of 2 weeks. Other symptoms, such as a desire to smoke, particularly in stressful situations, persist for months or even years after cessation (18).

TREATMENT OF ADDICTION

The pharmacodynamics of gum and the transdermal system is somewhat different. The gum causes a gradual increase and decrease in nicotine levels in the body throughout the day. The user must repeatedly chew the gum to obtain nicotine over time, and nicotine levels fall overnight as the person sleeps. As with cigarette smoking, there is a daily cycle of neuroadaptation and abstinence with use of the chewing gum, but the amplitude of the cycles is blunted. Gum use has certain advantages and disadvantages.

Advantages include providing the smoker with a behavior that can be used when there is an urge to smoke, which offers a person some active control over nicotine-related mood changes. With intermittent use, allowing time for resensitization, the pharmacologic effects of nicotine persist in a stable manner from day to day. Disadvantages include the considerable effort needed to chew enough pieces of gum to obtain a reasonable level of nicotine in the body. Side effects include jaw fatigue, unpleasant taste, gastrointestinal upset, the risk of becoming dependent on nicotine gum and not being able to discontinue its use (18).

Clonidine has been reported to reduce tobacco withdrawal symptoms, including the intensity of craving for tobacco, presumably by acting on the α_2-adrenergic receptors of the central nervous system.

REFERENCES

1. Lavoie F, Harris T: Fatal nicotine ingestion. *J Emerg Med* 1991;9: 133–136.
2. Gehlbach S, Williams W, Perry L, et al: Nicotine absorption by workers harvesting green tobacco. *Lancet* 1975;1:478–480.
3. Manoguerra A, Freeman D: Acute poisoning from the ingestion of Nicotiana glauca. *J Toxicol Clin Toxicol* 1983;19:861–864.
4. Gehlbach S, Williams W, Perry L, et al: Green tobacco sickness. *JAMA* 1974;229:1880–1883.

5. Mensch A: Nicotine overdose after a single piece of nicotine gum. *Chest* 1984;86:801–802.
6. Connolly G, Winn D, Hecht S, et al: The re-emergence of smokeless tobacco. *N Engl J Med* 1986;314:1020–1027.
7. Belanger G, Poulson T: Smokeless tobacco: a potential health hazard for children. *Pediatr Dent* 1983;5:266–269.
8. Horan J, Linberg S, Hackett G: Nicotine poisoning and rapid smoking. *J Consult Clin Psychol* 1977;45:344–347.
9. Battersby E, Cable J: Nicotine poisoning. *N Z Med J* 1964;63: 367–369.
10. Tonnesen P, Norregaard J, Sinonsen K, et al: A double-blind trial of a 16-hour transdermal nicotine patch in smoking cessation. *N Engl J Med* 1991;325:311–315.
11. Garcia-Estrada H, Fischman C: An unusual case of nicotine poisoning. *Clin Toxicol* 1977;10:391–393.
12. Rosenberg J, Benowitz N, Jacob P, et al: Disposition kinetics and effects of intravenous nicotine. *Clin Pharmacol Ther* 1980;28:517–522.
13. Kozlowski L, Appel C, Frecker R, et al: Nicotine, a prescribable drug available without a prescription. *Lancet* 1982;1:334.
14. McNabb M, Ebert R, McCusker K: Plasma nicotine levels produced by chewing nicotine gum. *JAMA* 1982;248:865–868.
15. Malizia G, Andreucci G, Alfani F, et al: Acute intoxication with nicotine alkaloids and cannabinoids in children from ingestion of cigarettes. *Hum Toxicol* 1983;2:315–316.
16. Saxena K, Scheman A: Suicide plan by nicotine poisoning: a review of nicotine toxicity. *Vet Hum Toxicol* 1985;27:495–497.
17. Atland P, Rattner B: Effects of nicotine and carbon monoxide on tissue and systemic changes in rats. *Environ Res* 1979;19:202–212.
18. Benowitz N: Cigarette smoking and nicotine addiction. *Med Clin N Amer* 1992;76:415–437.

CHAPTER 84

Strychnine

ACTIONS

Strychnine is a white crystalline bitter-tasting alkaloid. Although initially isolated from the St. Ignatius bean, it is commercially produced from the seeds of the plant *Strychnos nux-vomicus*, a tree native to India (1,2). It is found in equal concentrations with the related alkaloid, *brucine*, a less potent compound. Brucine poisoning is not a major toxicologic problem, although this alkaloid may act as a local anesthetic. Strychnine was at one time a notorious agent in suicidal and homicidal poisonings and was included in various over-the-counter tonics, stimulants, veterinary preparations, cathartics, and laxatives (3). It can still be found in a number of preparations (4). The original commercial use of strychnine as an animal poison is its only legitimate use today.

Most preparations sold for household use contain 0.25% to 0.35% strychnine, although more concentrated forms are available. Cases of strychnine poisoning are now rare and are usually limited to accidental poisoning from strychnine-containing rodenticides (Table 84–1) or from substances of abuse that are cut with this alkaloid (5).

PHARMACOKINETICS

Strychnine is readily absorbed from the gastrointestinal tract and mucous membranes of the nose and mouth; symptoms of intoxication appear as early as 10 to 30 minutes after ingestion (6). Poisoning secondary to insufflation of strychnine mistaken for cocaine has been reported (1). Although strychnine acts only on the central nervous system, it does not preferentially bind to that tissue. Strychnine is largely detoxified in the liver and only a small amount is excreted unchanged in the urine (7). Strychnine has a half-life of approximately 10 hours and is eliminated by first-order kinetics. Spontaneous vomiting following oral exposure is unusual in strychnine poisoning (8).

TABLE 84–1. *Selected strychnine-containing rodenticides by trade name*

Kilmice
Gopher Death
Mologen Mouse Lure
Rat-Seed
Hot Springs Buttons
Elroy Mouse Bait
Mo-Go
Mice Doom Pellets
Mouse Seeds
Pied Piper Kwik Kill
Sanaseed
Sweeney's Poison Wheat
Gopher Go
Mouse Nots

MECHANISM OF ACTION

Strychnine is the prototype of chemicals that selectively block inhibitory neurons in the central nervous system, resulting in hyperexcitability. Strychnine competes with the neurotransmitter glycine for receptors in the spinal cord, brain stem, and higher centers. Because glycine mediates polysynaptic inhibition, strychnine blockade causes disinhibition with a resultant increase in motor neuron impulses reaching the muscles.

Tetanus toxin causes similar disinhibition but prevents release of glycine (Fig. 84–1) (6,9). Neuronal systems lacking specific synaptic inhibitory fibers are not excited by strychnine; thus, the cardiovascular and gastrointestinal systems are not directly affected (2,10,11).

TOXICITY

The clinical syndrome of strychnine poisoning is characteristic but not pathognomonic. Onset of symptoms usually begins within 15 to 30 minutes following ingestion and as soon as 5 minutes after inhalation. The first signs of strychnine poisoning may be myoclonus and a slight twitching of the limbs that is followed by sudden convulsions involving all muscles (Table 84–2). The initial event can also be a generalized seizure without any prodrome. These seizures may be painful because the patient may be awake and aware of the surroundings. Convulsive activity may occur spontaneously or may be excited by minor sensory input such as auditory or tactile

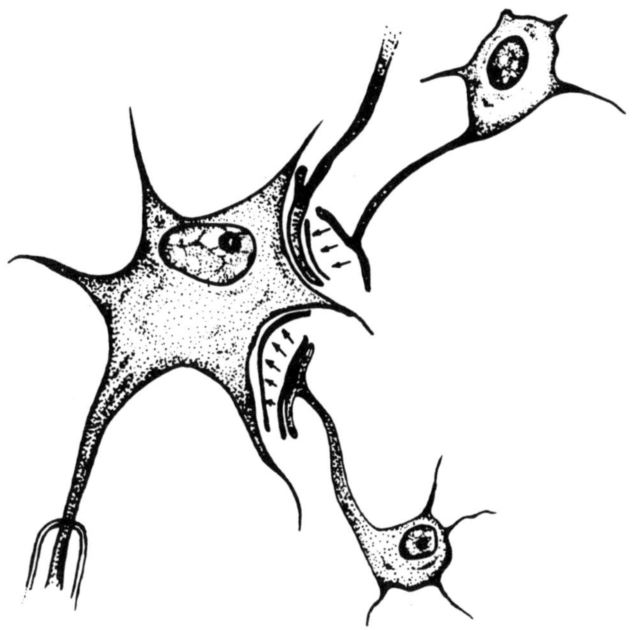

FIG. 84–1. Blockade of glycine uptake at the motor neuron by strychnine. Reprinted from *American Journal of Medicine* 1983;743:507–512; with permission of Technical Publishing Company. © 1983.

stimuli (11). The body arches backward in hyperextension (opisthotonos) with the arms and legs extended and the feet turned inward (12). The patient may exhibit trismus and facial contortions producing a characteristic fixed grinning expression (*risus sardonicus*) (1). Contraction of the muscles of the diaphragm together with spasm of the thoracic and abdominal muscles may arrest respiration (11). The convulsions may recur repeatedly; each lasts from 30 seconds to 2 minutes and is followed by a 10- to 15-minute interval during which the sensorium may be clear (13). The seizures may be followed by a period of depression. Patients seldom survive more than 5 untreated seizures, although some have survived 10 episodes (4). The muscle activity seen is usually distinguishable from seizures due to a cerebral cortical focus because the victim is usually conscious and may remain so in between convulsions. Death may be from respiratory failure, medullary paralysis, or asphyxia during the convulsive activity. Depending on the length of the seizure, cyanosis may develop. If death does not result from seizures or associated conditions, recovery may be complete (6,11).

TABLE 84–2. *Signs and symptoms of strychnine poisoning*

Hyperthermia
Myoclonus
Opisthotonos
Rhabdomyolysis
Risus sardonicus
Seizures
Trismus

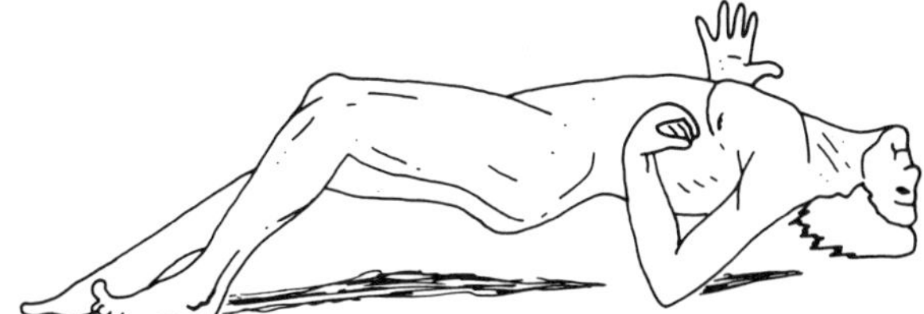

FIG. 84–2. Opisthotonos from a toxic overdose of strychnine. The body's weight in this example is supported by the head and feet.

Other problems associated with strychnine intoxication stem from the profound muscle spasms (2). Profound lactic acidosis secondary to the violent motor activity during seizures may occur (12). Once convulsions have been controlled, the lactic acidosis generally resolves without specific treatment because of the rapid metabolism of lactate. Rhabdomyolysis and hyperthermia from the extreme muscular activity during convulsions can lead to myoglobinuria and acute renal failure.

LABORATORY ANALYSIS

Strychnine can be detected by various laboratory methods (2), especially colorimetry and ultraviolet spectrophotometry. Rapid spot tests relying on color changes exist but lack specificity. The most specific method is gas chromatography with flame ionization. Serum strychnine concentrations can be measured but they correlate poorly with symptoms. Thin-layer chromatography (TLC) gives reliable qualitative information, whereas high-performance liquid chromatography provides quantitative data.

For most purposes, it is adequate to confirm strychnine poisoning with a qualitative test such as TLC. The urine and gastric aspirate are the most useful specimens for confirming the diagnosis. Strychnine resists postmortem putrefaction and tissue levels as low as 0.01 ppm are detectable. The quantitative tests are useful for research and forensic purposes.

TREATMENT

Appropriate management of strychnine poisoning requires prompt recognition and should be considered in all seizure patients. Treatment is directed toward establishing an airway to prevent asphyxia, controlling seizure activity to prevent trauma from involuntary movements, and decreasing any further absorption of the compound while treating the patient supportively (5). Adequate oxygenation and ventilation are of paramount importance, because most fatalities are secondary to respiratory compromise. This is best accomplished by early endotracheal intubation in the patient who manifests convulsions. Prophylactic intubation should be strongly considered in significant acute ingestions.

Aggressive control of convulsions is another key to successful management. The preferred method of controlling strychnine-induced seizure activity is the use of intravenous diazepam with or without a short-acting barbiturate (11,13,14). Diazepam is the drug of choice because it appears to act as a γ-aminobutyric acid agonist (4,9,14). The barbiturates provide the same agonist activity as benzodiazepines and should have the same efficacy (9,15). Neither the benzodiazepines nor the barbiturates antagonize the glycine receptor inhibition, so that even in large doses these drugs may not be completely effective (4).

If standard anticonvulsants do not control seizure activity, the patient should be pharmacologically paralyzed with pancuronium (1) to prevent the continued production of lactic acid and resultant metabolic acidosis and rhabdomyolysis, both of which are determining factors for long-term outcome (12). Pancuronium is advocated because it is a nondepolarizing neuromuscular blocking agent (7). Termination of muscle activity allows reversal of the lactic acidosis, hyperthermia, and rhabdomyolysis. Sodium bicarbonate is usually not necessary for the treatment of seizure-induced lactic acidosis in mild to moderate cases. Gastric lavage may then be performed and followed by administration of activated charcoal. An emetic should not be administered because the onset of convulsions is rapid and vomiting may actually elicit muscle spasms or at least complicate their management. Gastric lavage should always follow protection of the airway because pharyngeal stimulation may result in uncontrolled convulsions. Gastric emptying techniques are not advocated in the seizing patient because of the increased sensory stimulation. If respiratory depression occurs, respiration should be assisted or mechanically controlled (12).

Because the limiting factor in strychnine excretion through the kidney is its metabolism by microsomal liver enzymes, forced diuresis is usually of no appreciable benefit in drug removal (1,12). This is contrary to some reports that advocate diuresis for increasing excretion (3). In addition, acidification of the urine may predispose a patient with rhabdomyolysis to acute tubular necrosis and renal failure because the excretion of myoglobin is decreased in an acid urine. Intravenous fluid sufficient to maintain a brisk urine output is indicated pending assessment of myoglobinuria. In addition, peritoneal dialysis and hemodialysis appear to be of little benefit because of strychnine's rapid clearance from the blood (4,11).

REFERENCES

1. Gordon A, Richards D: Strychnine intoxication. *JACEP* 1979;8:520–522.
2. Lambert J, Byrick R, Hammeke M: Management of acute strychnine poisoning. *Can Med Assoc J* 1981;124:1268–1270.
3. Teitelbaum D, Ott J: Acute strychnine intoxication. *Clin Toxicol* 1979;3:267–273.
4. Blain P, Nightingale S, Stoddart J: Strychnine poisoning: abnormal eye movements. *J Toxicol Clin Toxicol* 1982;19:215–217.
5. Dipalma J: Human toxicity from rat poisons. *Am Fam Physician* 1981;24:186–189.
6. Edmunds M, Sheehan T, Van't Hoff W: Strychnine poisoning: clinical and toxicological observations on a nonfatal case. *Clin Toxicol* 1986;24:245–255.
7. Sparagli G, Mannaioni P: Pharmacokinetic observations on a case of massive strychnine poisoning. *Clin Toxicol* 1973;6:533–540.
8. Smith B: Strychnine poisoning. *J Emerg Med* 1990;8:321–325.
9. Baran R: Nail damage caused by weed killers and insecticides. *Arch Dermatol* 1974;110:467.
10. Sofola O, Odusote K: Sympathetic cardiovascular effects of experimental strychnine poisoning in dogs. *J Pharmacol Exp Ther* 1976;196:29–34.
11. Dittrich K, Boyer M, Wanke L: A case of fatal strychnine poisoning. *J Emerg Med* 1984;1:327–330.
12. Boyd R, Brennan P, Deng J, et al: Strychnine poisoning. *Am J Med* 1983;74:507–512.
13. Herishanu Y, Landau H: Diazepam in the treatment of strychnine poisoning. *Br J Anaesth* 1972;44:747–748.
14. Maron B, Krupp J, Tune B: Strychnine poisoning successfully treated with diazepam. *J Pediatr* 1978;78:697–699.
15. Oliver J, Smith H, Watson A: Poisoning by strychnine. *Med Sci Law* 1979;19:134–137.

CHAPTER 85

Hydrocarbons

Hydrocarbons are some of the most commonly used substances in industrialized society, and products containing hydrocarbons account for approximately 5% of all poisonings in children younger than 5 years of age (1,2). The ubiquity of these agents in the household and the fact that many, particularly furniture polishes, are pleasantly scented and colored, make them especially dangerous to young children, who often drink liquid hydrocarbons when left within reach by careless adults (3).

Hydrocarbons are organic compounds that consist only of carbon and hydrogen molecules (4). Hydrocarbon products are not pure substances but mixtures of saturated, unsaturated, ring, and straight-chain molecules (5). The liquid forms comprise molecules containing 5 to 15 carbon atoms that are arranged in aliphatic (straight-chain), alicyclic, and aromatic (benzene-based) structures with varying amounts of sulfur, nitrogen, and oxygen impurities (6,7).

Confusion has existed for many years as to the toxicity of hydrocarbons, partly because the hydrocarbon products are not a single class of compounds but may contain other more toxic compounds as well. For instance, fuels such as gasoline, petroleum naphtha, and kerosene, are among the most commonly ingested petroleum distillates; they carry a low systemic toxicity but are dangerous when their fumes are inhaled. Solvents and thinners, on the other hand, are more dangerous systemically because of their high content of benzene, toluene, xylene, and halogenated hydrocarbons. The toxicity of the various hydrocarbons must, therefore, be discussed in terms of the individual agents they contain (Table 85–1) (8).

TYPES OF HYDROCARBONS

Petroleum Distillates

Petroleum distillates (Table 85–2) are prepared by the fractionation of crude petroleum oil. All petroleum distillates are hydrocarbons but not all hydrocarbons are petroleum distillates (4). The petroleum distillates almost exclusively consist of the aliphatic hydrocarbons; in order of decreasing volatility, the major fractions are petroleum ether, gasoline, mineral spirits, kerosene, fuel oil, lubricating oils, paraffin wax, and asphalt or tar (8).

Mineral Seal Oil

Seal oil, which was originally obtained from seals and used primarily as fuel for lamps, is now gathered chiefly from petroleum; hence, it is termed *mineral seal oil* to distinguish it from the animal seal oil. It is almost exclusively used as a furniture polish (3). Mineral seal oil is not absorbed from the gastrointestinal tract; the only problem associated with ingestion is the potential for aspiration pneumonitis (5).

TABLE 85–1. *Hydrocarbons and their uses*

Product	Synonym	Use(s)
Benzene	Benzol	Paint thinner
Gasoline	Petroleum spirits	Fuel, paint thinner, glue thinner, high-performance fuel
Petroleum naphtha	Ligroin	Lighter fluid, high-performance fuel
VMP naphtha	Varnish naphtha	Paint thinner, varnish thinner
Turpentine	Pine oil	Paint thinner, shoe polish
Petroleum spirits	Mineral spirits, stodard solvent, white spirits	Paint solvent, dry cleaning agent, degreasing agent
Kerosene	Coal oil	Fuel, solvent, lighter fluid
Mineral seal oil	Signal oil, red furniture polish	Furniture polish
Fuel oil	Heating oil	Fuel
Petrolatum	Petroleum jelly	Laxative, ointment
Benzine	Petroleum ether	Dry cleaning agent, paint thinner, rubber solvent

Adapted, with permission, from “Hydrocarbon ingestion and poisoning” by E. Zieser in *Comprehensive Therapy* 1979;5:36. ©1979 Laux Publishing Company, Ayer, MA.

TABLE 85–2. *Petroleum distillates*

Asphalt
Fuel oil
Kerosene
Lubricating oils
Mineral seal oil
Naphtha
Paraffin wax
Petroleum ether (benzine)

Naphtha and Petroleum Ether

Naphthas are mixtures of aliphatics and aromatics that are obtained in the distillation of coal tar or petroleum (8). Petroleum naphthas include petroleum ether (more commonly known as benzine) and other compounds such as pentane and hexane. After ingestion, the major risk is that of aspiration pneumonitis.

Gasoline

Gasoline is the most commonly ingested distillate and consists of a mixture of aliphatic and acyclic hydrocarbons (mostly pentane and octane) but may also contain olefins, diolefins, cycloparaffins, and aromatic hydrocarbons in varying concentrations (9,10). Additives may be present, such as tetraethyl lead and cresyl phosphates but these do not pose a toxic hazard in acute ingestions (11,12). Gasoline is probably not absorbed well from the gastrointestinal tract but not enough data have been accumulated for this to be determined with any degree of certainty (13). After ingestion, the major risk is that of aspiration pneumonitis (14).

Kerosene

Kerosene or coal oil consists primarily of aliphatics and aromatics that may vary widely in composition (15). It is used as a paint thinner, degreaser and cleaner, and fuel oil in lamps and stoves. It continues to be a popular vehicle for many insecticides and fungicides (16). On prolonged or extensive contact with the skin, kerosene and its cogeners can produce epidermal necrolysis. After ingestion, the major risk is that of aspiration pneumonitis (9).

Other Distillates

Turpentine

Turpentine (oil of turpentine, spirits of turpentine), an oleoresin distillate, is a mixture of various pine species, camphenes, and other complex terpenes of low volatility. It is commonly used in mixing oil-based paints and in removing paint stains. Turpentine is readily absorbed from the gastrointestinal tract, skin, and respiratory tract. In addition to the risk associated with aspiration, turpentine acts both as a local irritant and a central nervous system (CNS) depressant (17).

Pine Oil Derivatives

Pine oil products are currently used in many households as cleaners and disinfectants. Accidental ingestion frequently occurs perhaps because of these products' pleasant aroma. In addition, because isopropyl alcohol is often a major constituent, a patient may ingest pine oil cleaner as an alternative to ethanol. Whereas the inert ingredients differ slightly among the various pine oil products, they consist of isopropyl alcohol, soaps, and trace chemicals such as ammonium hydroxide and benzoic acid in an aqueous solution. In assessing the toxicity of pine oil cleaner, the potential toxicity of the inert ingredients must be considered.

Pine Oil

The major toxic component of pine oil cleaner appears to be the pine oil itself. Pine oil is an essential or volatile oil related to turpentine. It is a colorless to pale yellow liquid with a pinaceous odor obtained from pitch-soaked pine wood by steam distillation or solvent extraction. Wood turpentine oil is produced similarly, the two oils being separated by fractional distillation or fractionation. Pine oil is the less volatile fraction (18).

Pharmacokinetics

Information regarding the pharmacokinetics of pine oil is limited. Several case reports indicate that pine oil is readily absorbed from the gastrointestinal tract, the rectum, and when used as an abortifacient, the uterus and vagina. After systemic absorption, it is metabolized and excreted in the urine.

Toxicity

Pine oil, when diluted in the form of pine oil cleaner, appears to produce much less severe pulmonary toxicity than petroleum distillates. Pulmonary toxicity is the most serious potential complication of any hydrocarbon ingestion. For pine oil cleaner, two distinct pathogenic mechanisms may be responsible: aspiration, either during ingestion or associated with emesis, and gastrointestinal absorption of pine oil with subsequent deposition in lung tissue. Pine oil odor on the breath appears to be a major diagnostic clue to intoxication.

Treatment

The treatment of pine oil cleaner ingestion depends on the level of unconsciousness of the individual, the time delay from exposure, and the volume ingested. Both pathogenic mechanisms responsible for the production of pneumonitis should also be considered (18).

When asymptomatic patients present early in the course of intoxication after ingestion of large volumes of pine oil cleaner (estimated to be 5 mL pure pine oil or approximately 1 oz Pine-Sol,) or when patients present with CNS depression, current treatment recommendations are gastric decontamination by gastric lavage followed by administration of activated charcoal and a cathartic. Patients presenting after ingestion of smaller volumes or those presenting hours after exposure may be treated by administration of activated charcoal and a cathartic followed by appropriate observation.

Coal Tar Derivatives

Coal tar derivatives, which include benzene, toluene, and xylene, are derived initially from the distillation of coal in the coking process and consist mainly of aromatic compounds. These compounds carry a greater risk of systemic toxicity than petroleum distillates.

The hydrocarbons most commonly ingested include petroleum solvents, dry cleaning fluids, spot removers, kerosene, lighter fluids, gasoline, and mineral seal oil (Table 85–2). The hydrocarbon derivatives are listed in Table 85–3 .

ROUTES OF ABSORPTION

Hydrocarbons can be absorbed orally, through the skin, or by inhalation (Table 85–4). Each of these modes of absorption is associated with different sites of toxicity (12). Ingestion is, by far, the most common route and may lead to chemical pneumonitis, CNS depression, and gastrointestinal irritation (17). Direct skin contact may lead to dermatitis or contact burns. The inhalation of a hydrocarbon as a drug of abuse may lead to CNS dysfunction; cardiac, renal, and liver toxicity; and lead poisoning (see Chapter 62) (20,21).

TABLE 85–3. *Other hydrocarbon distillates*

Coal tar
Benzene
Toluene
Xylene
Oleoresin
Turpentine

TABLE 85–4. *Routes of absorption of hydrocarbons with major associated medical problems*

Ingestion
Chemical pneumonitis
CNS depression
Gastrointestinal irritation
Dermal contact
Dermatitis
Contact burns
Inhalation (see Chapter 53)
CNS alteration
Cardiac dysfunction
Renal dysfunction
Lead toxicity
Liver dysfunction

PHYSICAL PROPERTIES OF HYDROCARBONS

The physical characteristics of the hydrocarbons can be described in terms of their viscosity, volatility, surface tension, and flammability. Viscosity is the most important property because it relates directly to the risk of pulmonary aspiration (2,5).

Viscosity is the property describing the ability of a substance to flow and the friction produced during flow (4). *Surface tension* is the force acting to maintain the integrity of a surface (22). The viscosity determines the likelihood of hydrocarbon entry into the lungs and the rate and extent of penetration into deep lung structures (20). A substance with low viscosity has less resistance to flow; consequently, even a small volume may be spread along the mucous membranes of the oral cavity and into the airway (23,24). Low viscosity and surface tension, therefore, increase the aspiration hazard (12).

The units of viscosity, *Saybolt seconds universal* (SSU), measure the time in seconds required for a sample liquid to flow through a calibrated orifice; the lower the viscosity, the less time required (6). Substances with viscosities less than 45 to 60 SSU represent the greatest aspiration hazard; those with viscosities greater than 100 to 250 SSU have a minimal risk (20).

Volatility is the ability of a liquid to evaporate rapidly and become a gas. The volatile hydrocarbons enter the central nervous system and other target organs most readily when absorbed by inhalation, ingestion, or rarely, prolonged or extensive dermal contact (4). Also, the most volatile hydrocarbons are the most flammable.

For toxicologic purposes, the hydrocarbons can be divided into four categories on the basis of these properties (Table 85–5) (4).

Low Viscosity, Low Volatility

The first group comprises substances with low viscosity and insignificant volatility, making pulmonary complications the sole toxic complication. Mineral seal oil is

TABLE 85–5. *Properties of hydrocarbons and associated toxicity*

Properties	Example	Systemic	Pulmonary
Low viscosity, low volatility	Mineral seal oil	0	++++
Intermediate viscosity, intermediate volatility	Gasoline, kerosene	+	+++
High volatility	Benzene, toluene, (xylene, chlorinated hydrocarbons)	+++	+
High viscosity, low volatility	Asphalt, tar, lubricating oils, mineral oil, fuel oil	0	0

the most commonly ingested product in this group. Systemic absorption of this compound is virtually nil (12).

Intermediate Viscosity, Intermediate Volatility

The second group is low to intermediate in viscosity and intermediate in volatility. These agents cause aspiration pneumonitis and include gasoline, kerosene, and other similar mixed hydrocarbons (11).

High Volatility

The third group contains the highly volatile substances whose viscosity is not important to their toxicity. These agents are mainly the aromatic agents and are responsible for central nervous system and systemic poisoning. Examples are the aromatic hydrocarbons toluene, xylene, benzene, and some chlorinated hydrocarbons.

High Viscosity, Low Volatility

The fourth group of hydrocarbons poses no hazard to either the pulmonary system or the CNS because they are of low volatility and high viscosity. This group contains asphalt or tar, lubricating oils, mineral oil, and fuel oil (23).

CLINICAL FEATURES OF INTOXICATION

Respiratory

Controversy has existed through the years as to whether the pulmonary insult from hydrocarbons is a result of systemic absorption or a direct effect of ingestion (14). Evidence has now conclusively shown that the hydrocarbons are aspirated directly into the lungs during ingestion or subsequent emesis and that they do not cause lung damage after absorption through the gastrointestinal tract (20).

Most patients brought to medical attention after hydrocarbon ingestion do not experience any pulmonary symptoms (1). Only 10% to 25% of patients develop clinical or roentgenographic evidence of pulmonary involvement (1). If aspiration does occur, chemical destruction of surfactant may develop resulting in severe ventilation and perfusion inequalities caused by alveolar and small airway closure. This leads to marked hypoxemia. Damage to the epithelial lining and pulmonary capillaries results in pathological findings such as interstitial inflammation, hyperemia, vascular thrombosis, hyaline membranes, and atelectasis (25).

The accidental aspiration of liquids from the mouth occurs in just a few seconds, and usually the volume of liquid aspirated is self-limiting in a conscious individual. As soon as the liquid enters the lungs, normal physiologic reflexes such as a momentary reflex cessation of breathing and the more active expulsive mechanism of coughing oppose further entry of the liquid. Symptoms occuring after ingestion of the hydrocarbon are due to hydrocarbon's rapid dispersion over the pharyngeal and glottic surfaces, with the more volatile components becoming gases on contact with the warm mucous membranes (Table 85–6) (26).

Initially, there may be a burning sensation in the mouth and throat that is followed by gagging, choking, coughing, and grunting respirations. These symptoms should be considered presumptive evidence of aspiration (20). An initial cyanosis, which is often noted within minutes of aspiration, may be due to the replacement of alveolar gas by the vaporized hydrocarbon (27).

Fever may occur 30 minutes to several hours after aspiration and bears no relation to the severity of the illness. It is part of the body's inflammatory response to a foreign substance rather than an indication of infection. Although infection may occur, its symptoms usually develop after the first 48 to 72 hours, with no particular

TABLE 85–6. *Respiratory symptoms of hydrocarbon ingestion*

Burning sensation in the mouth
Gagging
Choking
Cough
Grunting respirations
Cyanosis
Fever
Acute epiglottiditis (rare)

organism predominating (3). Acute epiglottiditis has also been reported with the presentation of severe sore throat, dysphagia, and progressive respiratory distress (28).

When signs and symptoms of aspiration are present, they usually progress during the first 24 hours and then subside over the next 1 to 4 days. Should death occur, it is attributable to pulmonary insufficiency and not CNS involvement.

Central Nervous System

In hydrocarbon poisoning, CNS symptoms are rare (7). When they do occur, they may include lightheadedness, lethargy, dizziness, headache, nausea, weakness, and fatigue that can progress to confusion, excitement, visual disturbances, seizures, and coma (Table 85–7).

Early theories regarding hydrocarbon poisoning tended to hold that CNS depression was a frequent and often serious complication of ingestion and that this was due to absorption into the systemic circulation (2). It has been shown that, although systemic absorption does occur, patients must ingest large doses (more than 4 to 5 mL/kg) for CNS toxicity to occur (20). The more likely mechanism for CNS dysfunction is hypoxia secondary to the pulmonary aspiration with subsequent respiratory damage. In other words, when CNS symptoms occur, they are secondary to hypoxia from the aspiration rather than from any direct CNS toxicity from the hydrocarbon (23). Although the aliphatic hydrocarbons typically produce CNS alterations secondary to hypoxia, the more volatile aromatic hydrocarbons such as benzene, toluene, and xylene are associated with a greater risk of systemic and CNS toxicity (2). Hypoxia need not be present for CNS symptoms to appear with these aromatic compounds.

Gastrointestinal

Gastrointestinal effects of hydrocarbon poisoning, such as nausea, vomiting, abdominal pain, and diarrhea, are usually mild and are due to direct mucosal irritation (4).

TABLE 85–7. *Central nervous system symptoms of hydrocarbon ingestion*

Lightheadedness
Lethargy
Dizziness
Confusion
Excitement
Headache
Visual disturbances
Seizures
Coma

Cutaneous

Hydrocarbons in direct contact with the skin can cause dermatitis and burns. Dermatitis may manifest as comedones, acne, folliculitis, or photosensitivity (4). Contact burns occur because of the fat-solvency properties of some of the hydrocarbons (9,30). Burns that have been described with prolonged contact consist of erythema, with blister formation noted within 24 hours (31). The burn is usually partial and healing occurs in approximately 21 days, leaving behind a pink-stained area representing the dyestuffs in the hydrocarbon (30).

In addition to local toxicity, certain hydrocarbons are readily absorbed through the skin and may cause toxic symptoms (32). Finally, the potential fire hazard posed by the hydrocarbons should always be considered; great care should be taken to avoid accidental ignition of hydrocarbons on the skin or clothing (30).

Systemic

Systemic toxicity has been associated with some of the hydrocarbons or additives to hydrocarbon products (Table 85–8); symptoms are related to the chemical composition and volatility of the ingested substance. For example, the aromatics have a greater degree of systemic toxicity than the aliphatics. Ingestions of these substances should be treated differently from ingestions of fuels and furniture polishes because of the greater risk of systemic toxicity. The risk of aspiration for these compounds is relatively minor (2).

Intravascular hemolysis may accompany hydrocarbon ingestion more frequently than previously thought and may result in significant hemoglobin loss. Patients with severe aspiration pneumonitis appear to be especially at risk (32).

TABLE 85–8. *Hydrocarbons and additives to hydrocarbon products that cause systemic toxicity (acronym: CHAMP)*

C	Camphor
H	Halogenated hydrocarbons
	Tetrachloroethane
	Trichloroethane
	Carbon tetrachloride
	Freons
A	Aromatic hydrocarbons
	Benzene
	Toluene
	Xylene
	Aniline dyes
M	Metals
	Mercury
	Lead
	Arsenic
P	Pesticides (see chapters 79–81)

TABLE 85–9. *Symptoms of benzene intoxication*

Aplastic anemia
Hepatic failure
Renal failure
Cardiac dysrhythmias
Respiratory depression
CNS depression

Benzene

Benzene, also known as *benzol*, is an aromatic hydrocarbon obtained by fractional distillation of light tar oil tar; it contains traces of carbon disulfide, phenol, toluene, xylene, and other substances (12).

Benzene is widely regarded as the most dangerous hydrocarbon used in industry today (6). It is rapidly absorbed upon ingestion, inhalation, or skin contamination, and has a particular affinity for nerve tissue. Symptoms of intoxication may include marked excitatory effects with subsequent depression and respiratory failure. Chronic poisoning is much more common than acute poisoning and may result in hematologic abnormalities such as leukopenia, aplastic anemia, and acute myeloblastic leukemia (Table 85–9) (12). Because of its toxic potential, benzene has been banned as an ingredient in products intended for use in the home (14).

Toluene and Xylene

Toluene, which is a product of the distillation of coal tar, is used in industry in the manufacturing of paint, rubber, and plastic cements (31). It has been described as causing a type I distal renal tubular acidosis and consequently carries a risk of causing systemic toxicity (6). A potentially serious and sometimes life-threatening reaction to repeated toluene abuse is hypokalemic muscle paralysis secondary to renal tubular acidosis (33). Characteristic symptoms of toluene intoxication include hallucinations, combativeness, blurred vision, ataxia, slurred speech, and stupor (Table 85–10) (34).

TABLE 85–10. *Symptoms of toluene and xylene intoxication*

CNS depression
Renal tubular acidosis
Cardiac dysrhythmias
Anion gap metabolic acidosis
Hypokalemia
Neuritis
Psychiatric disturbances
Bone marrow depression
Abdominal pain
Brain atrophy

Toluene is metabolized by benzyl alcohol to benzoic acid and is excreted largely as hippuric acid. This may contribute to an anion gap metabolic acidosis in addition to the hyperchloremic metabolic acidosis secondary to the renal tubular acidosis. Xylene toxicity is similar to that of toluene.

Substances Added to Hydrocarbon Products

In addition to systemically toxic hydrocarbons, there are certain additives to hydrocarbon products for which the hydrocarbon acts only as the solvent. The toxicity of the additive is of concern in such materials (4).

Camphor

Camphor can cause CNS stimulation and seizures (Table 85–11).

Metals

Metals attach to sulfhydryl groups in enzymes and cause multi-system organ failure (see Section X).

Aniline Dyes

Aniline dyes, which are manufactured from nitrobenzene, are sometimes added to hydrocarbons. Both aniline dyes and nitrobenzene can cause methemoglobinemia, hemolytic anemia, and CNS depression.

Halogenated Hydrocarbons

The halogenated hydrocarbons, such as carbon tetrachloride and trichloroethane, are in widespread use in both industry and the home and have potential multi-system toxicity (Table 85–12) (35,36). These hydrocarbons are excellent solvents for oils, waxes, and fats and are used as dry cleaning agents and surface degreasing compounds. In addition, they serve as vehicles for paints, varnishes, and other coatings. The most widely available halogenated hydrocarbon in household products is trichloroethane, which has replaced carbon tetrachloride in domestic solvents and cleaners.

TABLE 85–11. *Symptoms of camphor intoxication*

CNS stimulation
Seizures
Circulatory collapse
Enteritis

TABLE 85–12. *Symptoms of intoxication with halogenated hydrocarbons*

Cardiac dysrhythmias
Hepatitis
Nephritis
Gastroenteritis
CNS depression

LABORATORY DETERMINATIONS

Chest Roentgenography

Chest roentgenography is the single most important laboratory procedure in diagnosing hydrocarbon intoxication (Table 85–13); abnormalities usually appear within 12 hours after exposure (2,4,37). The roentgenogram can be obtained in the acute phase and may be positive even within 30 minutes after an aspiration (38).

Any pattern of infiltrate may be seen. Initially, the roentgenogram may disclose fine, punctate, mottled densities in the perihilar areas that extend into the midlung (26). Later, a patchy bibasilar infiltrate or atelectasis may be noted (12). The roentgenographic abnormalities are most often bilateral, reach their maximum at 72 hours, and usually clear within a few additional days without residual abnormality (39). Most patients with moderately severe to severe parenchymal disease show complete resolution of roentgenographic signs without complication. Clinical symptoms usually correlate poorly with roentgenographic findings because the film may often be positive in the absence of respiratory symptoms (12). In addition, resolution of the roentgenographic changes tends to lag behind clinical improvement (38).

In addition to the signs of chemical irritation, hemorrhagic bronchopneumonia and pulmonary edema may be noted in the most severe cases (26). Pleural effusion, pneumothorax, subcutaneous emphysema, pneumopericardium, pneumomediastinum, pneumatoceles, and cysts may form days after the aspiration of a hydrocarbon (26,28).

TABLE 85–13. *Laboratory studies in hydrocarbon intoxication*

Chest roentgenography
Bibasilar infiltrate
Atelectasis
Hemorrhagic bronchopneumonia
Pulmonary edema
Pleural effusion
Pneumothorax
Pneumomediastinum
Pneumatoceles
Arterial blood gases
Complete blood cell count
Serum electrolytes (for toluene or xylene poisoning)
Serum and urine metal concentrations
Methemoglobin concentration (for aniline or nitrobenzene poisoning)

Pneumatoceles are thought to result from overdistension and rupture of alveoli secondary to the intense inflammatory reaction in the bronchi (40). They form after consolidation has cleared; this may be within days or weeks of aspiration (41). Most pneumatoceles contain fluid that is easily demonstrated on frontal and lateral views of the upright chest. They may appear as unexpected findings on chest roentgenograms without evidence of pneumothorax or empyema (26,40).

Arterial Blood Gases

Arterial blood gases may be measured to ascertain the extent of hypoxemia. Values may reflect subtle abnormalities that may not be noted on the physical examination or radiographic studies (38).

Complete Blood Cell Count

Although an acute leukocytosis is often noted early after an ingestion as a result of the irritant effect of the hydrocarbon, a persistent increase in the white blood cell count after 48 hours is suggestive of bacterial superinfection. The degree of leukocytosis does not correlate well with severity of pneumonitis nor does a normal white blood cell count exclude a pneumonitis (39).

Miscellaneous

Serum electrolytes should be measured when chronic toluene ingestion or inhalation has occurred. Nitrobenzene and aniline cause a methemoglobinemia, so that methemoglobin concentrations should be measured. Serum and 24-hour urine concentrations of metals should be measured if these substances were ingested; values serve as a guide to chelation therapy.

With gas chromatography, quantitative hydrocarbon determinations from blood, urine, or expired air are possible (11). Such tests may help in the identification of the ingested substance but usually offer little help in clinical management and are, therefore, only necessary for forensic or medicolegal purposes (4,12,42).

TREATMENT

There are three important points concerning hydrocarbon ingestion that must be kept in mind for treatment planning. First, the average volume that a child can swallow in one mouthful is less than 1 teaspoon (2.5 to 5 mL); for an adult, the average volume is 3 teaspoons (37). Second, it is rare for a patient to ingest more than 2 tablespoons of a substance (1,4,15,44,45). Third, in general, the patient who is asymptomatic at the time of initial evaluation remains asymptomatic regardless of the findings on the initial chest roentgenogram.

Supportive Care

Supportive care is the mainstay of treatment of hydrocarbon exposure (Table 85–14). If the airway is obstructed it should be cleared and suctioned. Supplemental oxygen is indicated in all hypoxemic patients. In severe intoxications, constant positive airway pressure in spontaneously breathing patients and positive end-expiratory pressure in ventilated patients prevent airway closure, thus, improving the ventilation–perfusion ratios (1). Because this therapy has been associated with pneumothorax, however, it should be used with caution because these patients have lesions predisposing to pneumatoceles and pneumothorax (46).

Decontamination

Decontamination may be necessary if there was any spillage of the material on the skin or clothes; this is done to prevent skin irritation and burns as well as to decrease cutaneous absorption. Exposed skin should be cleansed with water and soap.

Prevention of Absorption

The most important principle in the treatment of a patient with a hydrocarbon pneumonitis is prevention of further hydrocarbon aspiration. Because large volumes of hydrocarbons in the gastrointestinal tract can generally be tolerated without severe systemic changes, vomiting should not be induced nor should gastric lavage be attempted unless it is absolutely necessary (20). There are differing reports as to the efficacy of activated charcoal, and although there is no contraindication to its use, it is probably not necessary or wise to administer an agent that may cause emesis (14).

TABLE 85–14. *Treatment of hydrocarbon exposure*

Supportive care
Oxygen
Decontamination
Bronchodilators (theophylline)
Contraindicated measures
Activated charcoal
Emesis or lavage (in general)
Prophylactic antibiotics
Corticosteroids
Oils

Administration of Oils

In the past, the use of vegetable and mineral oils was suggested for hydrocarbon ingestion because they were thought to act as miscible agents to minimize the risk of absorption. Not only is this therapy ineffective but it may increase the risk of lipoid pneumonitis, which is a nonfatal, low-grade, localized tissue reaction different and much less severe than a hydrocarbon pneumonitis (12).

Gastrointestinal Emptying Procedures

For most hydrocarbon ingestions, emesis or lavage does not improve the outcome and neither is indicated for ingestions of the volatile hydrocarbons. In contrast, the systemic toxicity associated with aromatic hydrocarbons, additives to hydrocarbon products, and halogenated hydrocarbons requires that these substances be removed by gastrointestinal emptying procedures (22).

Indications

Emesis appears to be superior to lavage in decreasing the aspiration hazard (2,12,44,47), although this is still an area of controversy. Emesis is indicated after the ingestion of benzene, toluene, halogenated hydrocarbons, camphor, heavy metals, pesticides, or any other systemically toxic ingredient (12) or if the dose of petroleum distillate ingested was greater than 4 to 5 mL/kg.

Contraindications

Emesis is not recommended if the patient has had a significant unprovoked emesis, is seizing, or lacks a gag reflex (12). In addition, the ingestion of mineral seal oil, kerosene, petroleum naphtha, fuel oil, mineral, and lubricating oils, and mineral spirits in any quantity need not be retrieved (2,8). Emesis is also contraindicated if the patient has ingested a high-viscosity, high surface tension liquid such as grease, petroleum jelly, paraffin wax, tar, glues, or asphalt.

Use of Bronchodilators

Bronchodilators may be necessary if bronchoconstriction is present (39). This condition occurs because of the direct irritant effect of hydrocarbons on the bronchioles. Bronchodilators, such as theophylline, may be beneficial in symptomatic patients (4). Epinephrine and other sympathomimetics should be avoided if the patient has ingested a material that can sensitize the myocardium to catecholamines and cause ventricular fibrillation (32).

Use of Antibiotics

Fever that follows hydrocarbon aspiration is the result of tissue damage rather than infection (39). Although the temptation is great to use antibiotics, they should not be used prophylactically because this may remove organisms that will be resistant to the antibiotic at a later time (48). The onset of fever after the first 48 hours may indicate secondary infection; treatment is then guided by appropriate bacterial cultures and Gram stain (20,39).

Use of Corticosteroids

Corticosteroids in theory may be of benefit in the prevention of pulmonary reaction and subsequent edema, fibrosis, and hemorrhage, but controlled clinical studies have not demonstrated a therapeutic or prophylactic role (49). In addition, corticosteroids have been shown to abolish the mononuclear response to pneumonitis and to decrease the protection against infection; they should, therefore, not be used (1,16,26).

Recommendations for Admission

If the patient is asymptomatic with a normal chest roentgenogram, no hospitalization is necessary if symptoms do not occur within a 6-hour period of observation (1). The same applies to the asymptomatic patient with an abnormal chest roentgenogram; a repeat roentgenography is optional. The symptomatic patient, even with a normal chest roentgenogram, should be admitted if symptoms persist or worsen (1). The asymptomatic individual who has ingested dangerous hydrocarbon additives should also be admitted (22).

REFERENCES

1. Anas N, Namasonthi V, Ginsburg C: Criteria for hospitalizing children who have ingested products containing hydrocarbons. *JAMA* 1981;246:840–843
2. Zieserl E: Hydrocarbon ingestion and poisoning. *Compr Ther* 1979;5: 35–42.
3. Shirkey H: Treatment of petroleum distillate ingestion. *Mod Treat* 1971;8:580–592.
4. Wasserman G: Hydrocarbon poisoning. *Crit Care Q* 1982;4:33–41.
5. Moriarty R: Petroleum distillate poisonings. *Drug Ther* 1979;9: 47–51.
6. Geehr E: Management of hydrocarbon ingestions. *Top Emerg Med* 1979;1:97–110.
7. Wolfsdorf J: Kerosene intoxication: an experimental approach to the etiology of the CNS manifestations in primates. *J Pediatr* 1976;88: 1037–1040.
8. Bratton L, Huddow J: Ingestion of charcoal lighter fluid. *J Pediatr* 1975;87:633–636.
9. Ainsworth R: Petro-vapor poisoning. *Br Med J* 1950;1:1547–1548.
10. Gurwitz D, Kattan M, Levison H, et al: Pulmonary function abnormalities in asymptomatic children after hydrocarbon pneumonitis. *Pediatrics* 1978;62:789–794.
11. Matsumoto T, Koga M, Sata T, et al: The changes of gasoline compounds in blood in a case of gasoline intoxication. *J Toxicol Clin Toxicol* 1992;30:653–662.
12. Goldfrank K, Kirstein R, Bresnitz E: Gasoline and other hydrocarbons. *Hosp Physician* 1979;15:32–38.
13. Hansen K, Sharp F: Gasoline sniffing, lead poisoning, and myoclonus. *JAMA* 1978;240:1375–1376.
14. Arena J: Emergency treatment of hydrocarbon product ingestion. *JAMA* 1973;226:213–217.
15. Cachia E, Fenech F: Kerosene poisoning in children. *Arch Dis Child* 1964;39:502–505.
16. Brown J, Burke B, Dajani A: Experimental kerosene pneumonia: Evaluation of some therapeutic regimens. *J Pediatr* 1974;84: 396–401.
17. Harris W: Toxic effects of aerosol propellants on the heart. *Arch Intern Med* 1973;131:162–166.
18. Brook M, McCarron M, Mueller J: Pine oil cleaner ingestion. *Ann Emerg Med* 1989;18:391–395.
19. Bass M: Sudden sniffing death. *JAMA* 1970;212:2075–2079.
20. Boeckx R, Postl B, Coodin F: Gasoline sniffing and tetraethyl lead poisoning in children. *Pediatrics* 1977; 60:140–145.
21. Hayden J, Comstock B: The clinical toxicology of solvent abuse. *Clin Toxicol* 1976;9:169–184.
22. Machado B, Cross K, Snodgrass W: Accidental hydrocarbon ingestion cases telephoned to a regional poison center. *Ann Emerg Med* 1988;17:804–807.
23. Gerarde H: Toxicological studies on hydrocarbons. *Toxicol Appl Pharmacol* 1959;1:462–474.
24. Panson R, Winek C: Aspiration toxicity of ketones. *Clin Toxicol* 1980;17:271–317.
25. Glaser H, Massengale D: Glue sniffing in children. *JAMA* 1962;181: 300–303.
26. Campbell J: Pneumatocele formation following hydrocarbon ingestion. *Am Rev Respir Dis* 1970;101:414–417.
27. Cohen S: The volatile solvents. *Public Health Rev* 1973;2:185–213.
28. Grufferman S, Walker F: Supraglottitis following gasoline ingestion. *Ann Emerg Med* 1982;11:368–370.
29. Coulehan J, Hirsch W, Brillman J, et al: Gasoline sniffing and lead toxicity in Navajo adolescents. *Pediatrics* 1983;71:113–117.
30. Hunter G: Chemical burns of the skin after contact with petrol. *Br J Plast Surg* 1968;21:338–341.
31. Binns H, Gursel E, Wilson N: Gasoline contact burns. *JACEP* 1978; 7:404–405.
32. Yaqoob M, Bell G, Percy D, et al: Primary glomerulonephritis and hydrocarbon exposure: a case-control study and literature review. *Quart J Med* 1992;83:409–418.
33. Algren J, Rodgers G: Intravascular hemolysis associated with hydrocarbon poisoning. *Pediatr Emerg Care* 1992;8:34–35.
34. Welch L, Kirshner H, Heath A, et al: Chronic neuropsychological and neurological impairment following acute exposure to a solvent mixture of toluene and methyl ethylketone (MEK). *J Toxicol Clin Toxicol* 1991;29:435–445.
35. Flowers N, Haran L: Nonanoxic aerosol arrhythmias. *JAMA* 1972; 219:33–37.
36. Flowers N, Haran L: The electrical sequelae of aerosol inhalation. Am Heart J 1972;83:644–651.
37. Daeschner C, Blattner R, Collins V: Hydrocarbon pneumonitis. *Pediatr Clin North Am* 1957;4:243–249.
38. Dice W, Ward G, Kelley J, et al: Pulmonary toxicity following gastrointestinal ingestion of kerosene. *Ann Emerg Med* 1982;11: 138–142.
39. Karlson K: Hydrocarbon poisoning in children. *South Med J* 1982;75:839–840.
40. Bergeson P, Hales S, Lustgarten M, et al: Pneumatoceles following hydrocarbon ingestion. *Am J Dis Child* 1975;129:49–54.
41. Scott P: Hydrocarbon ingestion: an unusual cause of multiple pulmonary pseudotumors. *South Med J* 1989;82:1032–1033.
42. Dollery C, Dows D, Draffan G, et al: Blood concentration in man of fluorinated hydrocarbons after inhalation of pressurized aerosols. *Lancet* 1970;2:1164–1166.
43. Jones D, Work C: Volume of a swallow. *Am J Dis Child* 1961; 102:427–429.
44. Press E, Done A: Solvent sniffing. *Pediatrics* 1967;39:451–461.

45. Press E: Cooperative kerosene poisoning study: evaluation of gastric lavage and other factors in the treatment of accidental ingestion of petroleum distillate products. *Pediatrics* 1962;29:648–662.
46. Gerarde H: Toxicological studies on hydrocarbons. *Arch Environ Health* 1963;6:325–341.
47. Ng R, Darawish H, Stewart D: Emergency treatment of petroleum distillate and turpentine ingestion. *Can Med Assoc J* 1974;111: 537–538.
48. Scalzo A, Weber T, Jaeger R, et al: Extracorporeal membrane oxygenation for hydrocarbon aspiration. *Am J Dis Child* 1990;144: 867–871.
49. Marks M, Chicoine L, Legere G, et al: Adrenocorticosteroid treatment of hydrocarbon pneumonia in children: a cooperative study. *J Pediatr* 1972;81:366–369.

ADDITIONAL SELECTED REFERENCES

Baldachin B, Melmed R: Clinical and therapeutic aspects of kerosene poisoning. *Br Med J* 1964;2:28–30.

Eade N, Taussig L, Marks M: Hydrocarbon pneumonitis. *Pediatrics* 1974;54:351–356.

Kirk L, Martin K: Sudden death from toluene abuse. *Ann Emerg Med* 1984;13:68–69.

Law W, Nelson E: Gasoline sniffing by an adult: report of a case with the unusual complication of lead encephalopathy. *JAMA* 1968;204: 1002–1004.

Massengale O, Glaser H, LeLievre R, et al: Physical and psychologic factors in glue sniffing. *N Engl J Med* 1963;269:1340–1344.

Polkis A, Burkett C: Gasoline sniffing: a review. *Clin Toxicol* 1977; 11:35–41.

Reinhardt C, Azar A, Maxfield M, et al: Cardiac arrhythmias and aerosol "sniffing." *Arch Environ Health* 1971;22:265–279.

Robinson R: Tetraethyl lead poisoning from gasoline sniffing. *JAMA* 1978;240:1373–1374.

Seshia S, Rajani K, Boeckx R, et al: The neurological manifestations of chronic inhalation of leaded gasoline. *Dev Med Child Neurol* 1978;2: 323–324.

Sperling F: In vivo and in vitro toxicology of turpentine. *Clin Toxicol* 1969;2:21–35.

Streicher H, Gabow P, Moss A, et al: Syndromes of toluene sniffing in adults. *Ann Intern Med* 1981;94:758–762.

Talker S, Anderson R, McCartney R, et al: Renal tubular acidosis associated with toluene "sniffing." *N Engl J Med* 1974;290:765–768.

Taylor G, Harris W: Cardiac toxicity of aerosol propellents. *JAMA* 1970;214:81–85.

Taylor G, Harris W: Glue sniffing causes heart block in mice. *Science* 1970;170:866–868.

Valpey R, Sumi S, Corass M, et al: Acute and chronic progressive encephalopathy due to gasoline sniffing. *Neurology* 1978;28: 507–510.

Young R, Grzyb S, Crismon L: Recurrent cerebellar dysfunction as related to chronic gasoline sniffing in an adolescent girl. *Clin Pediatr* 1977;16:706–708.

Brook M, McCarron M, Mueller J: Pine oil cleaner ingestion. *Ann Emerg Med* 1989;18:391–395.

APPENDIX A

Therapeutic Blood Concentrations of Selected Drugs

Drug	Therapeutic range
Analgesics	
Acetaminophen	10.0–20.0 μg/mL
Ibuprofen	10.0–50.0 μg/mL
Indomethacin	0.5–3.0 μg/mL
Pentazocine	0.14–0.6 μg/mL
Propoxyphene	50–200 ng/mL
Salicylate	10.0–25.0 mg/dL
Antibiotics	
Amikacin	15–25 μg/mL (peak)
	10–15 μg/mL (trough)
Chloramphenicol	15–25 μg/mL (peak)
	10–15 μg/mL (trough)
Gentamicin	<12.0 μg/mL (peak)
	<2.0 μg/mL (trough)
Kanamycin	20–25 μg/mL (peak)
	4–6 μg/mL (trough)
Tobramycin	<12.0 μg/mL (peak)
	<2.0 μg/mL (trough)
Anticonvulsants	
Carbamazepine	4.0–8.0 μg/mL
Ethosuximide	40–100 μg/mL
Phenobarbital	15.0–40.0 μg/mL
Phenytoin	10.0–20.0 μg/mL
Primidone	5.0–12.0 μg/mL
Valproic acid	50–100 μg/mL
Antihistamines	
Brompheniramine	12.0–17.0 ng/mL
Chlorpheniramine	10.0–40.0 ng/mL
Chlorphentermine	150.0–350.0 ng/mL
Cimetidine	0.2–2.5 μg/mL
Diphenhydramine	100–1000 ng/mL
Hydroxyzine	50.0–200.0 ng/mL
Methapyrilene	5.0–100.0 ng/mL
Antipsychotics	
Chlorpromazine	30.0–35.0 ng/mL
Haloperidol	5.0–20.0 ng/mL
Lithium	0.5–1.5 mEq/L
Mesoridazine	150–1000 ng/mL
Perphenazine	0.5 μg/dL
Prochlorperazine	100.0–500.0 ng/mL
Promazine	100.0–500.0 ng/mL
Promethazine	100.0–500.0 ng/mL
Thioridazine	100–150 μg/dL
Thiothixene	1.0 μg/dL
Trifluoperazine	80 μg/dL
β-**Adrenergic blocking agents**	
Atenolol	1.3 μg/mL
Propranolol	40.0–80.0 ng/mL

Drug	Therapeutic range
Benzodiazepines	
Alprazolam	8.0–37.0 ng/mL
Chlordiazepoxide	500–1000 ng/mL
Clonazepam	10.0–70.0 ng/mL
Clorazepate	300.0–1000.0 ng/mL
Diazepam	100.0–700.0 ng/mL
Flurazepam	10.0–140.0 ng/mL
Lorazepam	5.0–30.0 ng/mL
Oxazepam	200.0–500.0 ng/mL
Bronchodilators	
Dyphylline	5.0–15.0 µg/mL
Oxtriphylline	10.0–20.0 µg/mL
Theophylline	10.0–20.0 µg/mL
Cardiac drugs	
N-Acetylprocainamide	5.0–10.0 µg/mL
Amiodarone	0.5–3.0 µg/mL
Digitoxin	10.0–25.0 ng/mL
Digoxin	0.8–2.1 ng/mL
Diltiazem	100–200 ng/mL
Disopyramide	2.0–5.0 µg/mL
Flecainide	200–800 ng/mL
Lidocaine	1.2–5.0 µg/mL
Mexiletine	0.7–2.0 µg/mL
Procainamide	4.0–8.0 µg/mL
Quinidine	2.0–5.0 µg/mL
Tocainide	4.0–10.0 µg/mL
Verapamil	50.0–400.0 ng/mL
Central nervous system stimulants	
Amphetamine	20–100 ng/mL
Caffeine	5.0–14.0 µg/mL
Diethylpropion	100.0–300.0 ng/mL
Methamphetamine	10.0–50.0 ng/mL
Pheniramine	20.0–200.0 ng/mL
Phenmetrazine	50.0–250.0 ng/mL
Metals	
Arsenic	0.0–20.0 ng/mL
Cadmium	0.01–0.02 µg/dL
Copper	10.0–150.0 µg/dL
Iron	50–150 µg/dL
Lead	0.0–25.0 µg/mL
Mercury	0.5 µg/mL
Miscellaneous	
Carbamezapine	3–13 µg/mL
Cyanide	0.05 µg/mL
Isoniazid	1.0–7.0 µg/mL
Metronidazole	3.0–15.0 µg/mL
Narcotics	
Codeine	10–120 ng/mL
Hydrocodone	10.0–40.0 ng/mL
Hydromorphone	10.0–30.0 ng/mL
Meperidine	50–500 ng/mL
Morphine	40.0–150.0 ng/mL
Oxycodone	50.0–100.0 ng/mL
Propoxyphene	100.0–400.0 ng/mL

Drug	Therapeutic range
Sedative-hypnotics	
Amobarbital	2.0–10.0 μg/mL
Butabarbital	7.0–15.0 μg/mL
Butalbital	2.0–5.0 μg/mL
Chloral hydrate	2.0–10.0 μg/mL
Ethchlorvynol	1.0–6.0 μg/mL
Glutethimide	5.0–15.0 μg/mL
Hexobarbital	2.0–5.0 μg/mL
Mephobarbital	5.0–15.0 μg/mL
Meprobamate	8.0–24.0 μg/mL
Methaqualone	1.0–8.0 μg/mL
Metharbital	10.0–30.0 μg/mL
Methyprylon	4.0–10.0 μg/mL
Pentobarbital	0.5–3.0 μg/mL
Phenobarbital	15.0–40.0 μg/mL
Secobarbital	0.5–5.0 μg/mL
Thiopental	1.0–5.0 μg/mL
Tricyclic antidepressants	
Amitriptyline	100–250 ng/mL
Amoxapine	50–400 ng/mL
Desipramine	150–300 ng/mL
Doxepin	100–200 ng/mL
Imipramine	150–300 ng/mL
Maprotiline	150–400 ng/mL
Nortriptyline	50–150 ng/mL
Protriptyline	70–250 ng/mL
Trazodone	300–1600 ng/mL

APPENDIX B

Volumes of Distribution of Selected Drugs

Drug	Volume of distribution (liters per kilogram)
Acebutolol	1.2
Acetaminophen	0.75–1.0
Acetylsalicylic acid	0.1–0.3
Acyclovir	0.71
Alprazolam	12.0
Alprenolol	3.0
Amantadine	6.0
Aminoglycosides	0.2–0.5
Amiodarone	66.0
Amitriptyline	15
Amobarbital	2.4
Amphetamines	0.6
Amphotericin B	4.0
Atenolol	0.56
Atropine	2.4
Benzodiazepines	3.0–10.0
Bromide	>40
Bromocriptine	3.5
Caffeine	0.75
Carbamazepine	1.4
Captopril	0.70
Chloral hydrate	0.75–0.90
Chloramphenicol	0.9
Chlordiazepoxide	0.3
Chlorpromazine	10.0–35.0
Chlorpropamide	0.47
Cimetidine	1.0–2.0
Clonazepam	5.0–10.0
Clonidine	2.0
Clorazepate	1.0
Cocaine	2.0
Codeine	3
Dapsone	1.5
Desipramine	35.0
Diazepam	1.0–2.0
Digitoxin	0.54
Digoxin	7.0–10.0
Diltiazem	5.0
Diphenhydramine	3.0–4.0
Diphenoxylate	4.6
Disopyramide	0.6
Doxepin	20.0
Ethambutol	0.8
Ethanol	0.6
Ethchlorvynol	3.0–4.0
Ethosuximide	0.9
Fenoprofen	0.08–0.1

Drug	Volume of distribution (liters per kilogram)
Fentanyl	4.0
5-Fluorouracil	0.38
Flurazepam	22.0
Furosemide	0.2
Glutethimide	20–25
Halazepam	1.0
Haloperidol	18
Heparin	0.06
Ibuprofen	0.14
Indomethacin	0.3–0.9
Isoniazid	0.6
Ketamine	3.0
Labetalol	11.0
Lidocaine	1.5
Lithium	0.7–2.0
Lorazepam	1.3
Melphalan	0.63
Meperidine	4.5
Methadone	6.0–10.0
Methicillin	0.6
Methyldopa	0.29
Metoprolol	4.0–5.0
Metronidazole	1.1
Minoxidil	2.7
Morphine	3.0
Nadolol	2.0–3.0
Naloxone	3.0
Naproxen	0.09
Narcotics	3.0–5.0
Nicotine	2.6
Nifedipine	1.2
Nitrazepam	2.0
Nitroglycerin	3.3
Nortriptyline	18.0
Oxazepam	1.0–5.0
Oxyphenbutazone	0.14
Oxyprenolol	1.5
Pentazocine	5.0
Pentobarbital	1.0–2.0
Perphenazine	18.0–30.0
Phenobarbital	0.60–0.75
Phenothiazines	20.0–30.0
Phenylbutazone	0.02
Phenytoin	0.75
Pindolol	2.0
Practolol	1.6
Prazepam	4.5
Prazosin	0.6–1.0
Prednisone	1.0
Primidone	0.60
Procainamide	1.9
Propranolol	4.0
Protriptyline	22.0
Pyridostigmine	1.1
Quinidine	3.0
Rifampin	0.93

Drug	Volume of distribution (liters per kilogram)
Salicylate	0.1–0.3
Secobarbital	1.5
Sotalol	0.7
Temazepam	15
Tetracycline	3.0
Theophylline	0.46
Thiopental	2.3
Timolol	1.5
Tocainide	3.0
Tolmetin	0.04
Triazolam	1.5–2.5
Valproic acid	0.13
Verapamil	4.0–6.0
Warfarin	0.1

APPENDIX C

Street Names of Abused Drugs

Amphetamines

- Bam
- Beans
- Bennies
- Black and whites
- Black beauties
- Black birds
- Black cadillacs
- Black dex
- Black mollies
- Blacks
- Bombido
- Bombita
- Box cars
- Brown and clears
- Bumblebees
- Cartwheels
- Chalk
- Chicken powder
- Coast-to-coast
- Co-pilots
- Crank
- Crink
- Cris
- Criss-cross
- Cristina
- Crossroads
- Cross-tops
- Crystal
- Dex
- Dexies
- Dice
- Diet pills
- Double-cross
- Eye-openers
- Fives
- Footballs
- Green and clears
- Hearts
- Jelly babies
- Jelly beans
- Jolly beans
- L. A.
- LA turnabouts
- Lid poppers
- Lightning
- Little bomb
- Meth
- Minnibennies
- Nuggets
- Peaches
- Pep pills
- Pink hearts
- Powder
- Reducing pills
- Rhythm
- Roses
- Snow pellets
- Snow seals
- Speed
- Splash
- Spliven
- Sweets
- Thrusters
- Wake-ups
- Water

Barbiturates

- Block busters
- Blue
- Blue and reds
- Blue angels
- Blue birds
- Blue bullets
- Blue clouds
- Blue devils
- Blue dolls
- Blue heavens
- Bombita
- Christmas trees
- Double-trouble
- Downers
- Downs
- F-40
- F-66
- GBS
- Golf balls
- Goofballs
- Goofers
- Green dragons
- Lay back
- M and M's
- Marshmallow reds
- Mexican reds
- Mexican yellows
- Nebbies
- Nemmies
- Nimbies
- Nimby
- Nols
- Oral pob
- Peanuts
- Phennies
- Pink ladies
- Pinks

Purple rocks
Rainbows
Red
Red birds
Red devils
Red dolls
Red lilies
Reds
Reds and blues
Seccy
Seggy
Sleepers
Sleeping pills
Stopped
Stumblers
T-birds
Tooies
Tooties
Yellow bullets
Yellow dolls
Yellow jackets
Yellows

Chloral hydrate

Chlorals
Coral
Green frog
Jellies
Jelly beans
Joy juice
Knock-out drops
Mickey Finn
Peter

Cocaine

Base
Baseball
Basuco
Bazooka
Bernice
Bernies
Big bloke
Big C
Big flake
Big rush
Blotter
Blow
C
Candy
Carrie
Cholly
Coke
Corine
Corrine
Crack
Crystal
Dama blanca
Dama blance
Dream
Dust
Flake
Free base
Gift of the Sun God
Gin
Girl
Gold dust
Gravel
Green gold
Happy dust
Happy trails
Hard stuff
Heaven dust
Heaven leaf
Her
Hit
Jam
Joy powder
Lady
Leaf
Line
Noise candy
Nose
Nose candy
Pasta
Pimp
Rock
Roxanne
Schmack
She
Snort
Snowbirds
Snowcones
Snow flake
Snow seals
Star dust
Star-spangled powder
Supercoke
Toot
White girl
White lady
Whites

Combinations

Black dust = phencyclidine, heroin, embalming fluid
Blue velvet = paregoric + antihistamine
Boat = phencyclidine, heroin, embalming fluid
C and H = cocaine + heroin
C and M = cocaine + morphine
Dynamite = marijuana + heroin
Fours and dor's = codeine + glutethimide
Four-way = LSD + STP + methedrine + cocaine
F-66 = amobarbital + secobarbital
H and C = heroin + cocaine
Killer weed = phencyclidine + marijuana
Loads = codeine + glutethimide
Love trip = mescaline + MDMA
MDA = LSD + cocaine + heroin
OJ = marijuana + opium
Pineapple = heroin + methylphenidate
Pink wedges = LSD + STP + strychnine + cocaine
R and R = Seconal + wine
Snowball = cocaine + heroin
Speedball = cocaine + heroin
T's and blues = pentazocine + tripelenamine
Turps = terpin hydrate with codeine
Whiz bang = cocaine + heroin

Ethchlorvynol

Jelly beans
Mr. Green Jeans
Pickles

Fentanyl-like drugs

China white
Super heroin

Hashish and tetrahydrocannabinol

Black Russian
Crystal tea
Fingers

Gram
Keif
Kif
Kristal tea
Krystal tea
Quarter moon
Soles
Tac
THC

Heroin

Big H
Big Harry
Bindle
Blanco
Bombido
Boy
Brown
Brown sugar
Buju
Bundle
Butu
Caballo
Caca
Carga
China white
Chinese red
Chiva
Crap
Deuce
Dirt
Dogie
Doojee
Doper
Dujie
Dynamite
Flea powder
Foolish powder
H
Hairy
Half bundle
Half load
Hard candy
Hard stuff
Harry
Harry Jones
Henry
Hessle
Horse
Joy powder
Lady Jane
Little bomb
Mexican brown
Mexican mud
Nickel bag
Nickel deck
Nitroglycerin tabs
Noise
Pack
Pee
Persian brown
Powder
Quill
Salt
Scag
Scat
Shil
Shit
Skag
Skid
Smeck
Spoon
Stuff
Tecata
Thing
TNT
White stuff

Lysergic acid diethylamide (LSD)

Acid
Animal
Barrels
Battery acid
Beast
Big D
Black acid
Blotter acid
Blotter cube
Blue acid
Blue barrels
Blue cheers
Blue heaven
Blue microdot
Blue mist
Brown dots
California sunshine
Chief
Chocolate chips
Coffee
Contact lens
Crackers
Cube
Cupcakes
D
Domes
Double dome
Electric Kool Aid
Flats
Four-way
Ghost
Grape parfait
Green single domes
Hawaiian sunshine
The Hawk
Haze
Heavenly blue
Lime acid
LSD
Lucy in the Sky with Diamonds
Mellow yellow
Microdot
One-way
Orange barrels
Orange cupcakes
Orange mushrooms
Orance sunshine
Owskey's acid
Owsley
Paper acid
Pearly gate
Pink wedge
Pink witches
Purple barrels
Purple dragon
Purple flats
Purple haze

Purple hearts
Purple microdot
Purple wedge
Red dragon
Royal blue
Sandoz
Smears
Squirrels
Star
Sugar
Sugar lump
Sunshine
Ticket
Trips
Twenty-five
Vodka acid
Wafer
Wedding bells
Wedge
White lightning
Window glass
Window pane
Window pane acid
Yellow
Yellow dimples
Yellow kimples
Zen

Marijuana

Acapulco gold
Ace
Ashes
Baby
Bad seed
Bhang
Black mote
Block
Bobo' bush
Bomber
Boo
Brick
Broccoli
Bush
Butter
Butter flower
Can
Cannabis
Carmabis
Chiba-driba
Chicago green
Colorado cocktail
Columbian
Columbus black
Dagga
Dope
Doper
Dry high
Fine stuff
Fingers
Flower
Fu
Fuel
Gage
Ganja
Giggle smoke
Gold
Goof butt
Grash
Grass
Green
Griefo
Griffo
Guage
Hash
Hashish
Hashish oil
Hay
Hemp
Herb
Hot sticks
Indian Bay
Indian hat
Indian hemp
J
Jane
Jay
Jay joint
Jive
Jive stick
Joint
Joy smoke
Joy stick
Khat
Kick-stick
Killer weed
Kilo
Lid
Locoweed
Love weed
Mary
Mary Jane
Mexican Brown
MJ
Mohasky
Mojo
Mooters
Mootos
Mor-a-grifa
Mota
M.U.
Muggies
Muggles
Mutah
Panama gold
Panama red
Pat
Pod
Pot
Rainy-day woman
Reefer
Roach
Rope
Sativa
Seeds
Seeds and stems
Seeds and twigs
Smoke
Spilm
Spliff
Stack
Stick
Straw
Supergrass
Sweet Lucy
T

Tea
Texas stick
Thai stick
Twistum
Viper's weed
Weed
Yellow submarine
Ying gee

MDA, MDMA, DMT, and STP

Adam
AMT
Businessman's special
Businessman's trip
DET
DMT
DOB
DOM
Eve
Love drug
Love trip
Orange cupcakes
Serenity
Serenity, Tranquility, and Peace
Speed for lovers
Sweet tart
Syndicate acid

Methaqualone

AS
Citrexal
Disco biscuits
Love drug
Luding out
Luds
Paris 400
Q
Quads
Quas
714's
Soapers
Sopors

MPPP

New heroin
Synthetic demerol
Synthetic heroin

Nitrites

Ames
Amies
Amyes
Amys
Aymes
Boppers
Heart-on
Pearls
Poppers
Snappers

Opium

Big 0
Hop
Hophead
Joy plant
O
OJ
OP
Pin yen
Skee
Tar
Toys
When-shee
Yellow she baby
Yellow shee
Yen Shee Suey
Zero

Peyote and mescaline

Beans
Big chief
Button
Cactus
Cactus head
Hikori
Hukuli
Hyatari
Love trip
Mesc
Mescal
Mescal beans
Mescal button
Mese
P
Pink wedge
Seni
Tops
White light

Phencyclidine and ketamine

Angel dust
Angel hair
Angel mist
Crystal
Crystal joint
DOA
Dust
Dusted parsley
Elephant tranquilizer
Goon
Green
HCP
Hog
Horse tranquilizer
K
Kay jay
Killer weed
Kristal
Kristal joint
Love boat
Lovely
PCP
Pits
Purple
Rocket fuel
Sernyl
Special-la-coke
Super acid
Super C
Tic
Wack
White horizon

Psilocybin

God's flesh
Mexican mushroom
Mushroom
Simple simon

Subject Index

Index entries (page numbers) set in italics refer to figures and/or tables.